Handbook of Affective Disorders

Handbook of Affective Disorders

Edited by

Eugene S. Paykel MD FRCP FRCPsych
Professor of Psychiatry, University of Cambridge, Addenbrooke's Hospital,
Cambridge, UK

SECOND EDITION

THE GUILFORD PRESS
NEW YORK   LONDON

© Longman Group Limited 1982
© Longman Group Limited 1992

Published by The Guilford Press
A Division of Guilford Publications, Inc.
72 Spring Street, New York, NY 10012

This edition of *Handbook of Affective Disorders: Second Edition* is
published by arrangement with Churchill Livingstone,
London.

First edition 1982
Second edition 1992

All rights reserved

No part of this book may be reproduced, stored in a
retrieval system, or transmitted, in any form or by any
means, electronic, mechanical, photocopying, microfilm-
ing, recording, or otherwise, without written permission
from the publisher.

Printed in the United States of America

This book is printed on acid-free paper

Last digit is print number: 9 8 7 6 5 4 3 2 1

Library of Congress Cataloging-in-Publication Data

Handbook of affective disorders / edited by Eugene S. Paykel.
  —2nd ed.
      p. cm.
   Originally published: Edinburgh : New York : Churchill
Livingstone, 1992.
   Includes bibliographical references and index.
   ISBN 0-89862-674-9
   1. Affective disorders—Handbooks, manuals, etc.
I. Paykel, Eugene S.
   [DNLM: 1. Affective Disorders.   WM 171 H235]
RC537.H337 1992b
616.85'27—dc20
DNLM/DLC
for Library of Congress   92-1553
                                                   CIP

Preface to the Second Edition

Affective disorders are those disorders in psychiatry where mood disturbance is the central feature: in particular, the term is used for the states of depression and mania. Including the milder forms of clinical depression, affective disorders are probably the most common psychiatric disorders. Their recognition and treatment form a large part of the activities of most psychiatrists, and extend widely into the work of other doctors, psychologists, social workers and those in related helping professions. They have also been the focus of much research, accelerating in pace since the 1950s.

The first edition of the *Handbook of Affective Disorders* was published ten years ago. Since then, there has been steady advance with major developments in many diverse areas, including epidemiology, neurochemistry, neuroendocrinology, the recognition and treatment of seasonal affective disorders, cognitive therapy, psychotherapies, new drug treatments and the advent of molecular genetics.

The new edition has largely been rewritten. Reflecting the developments and the changes of emphasis now appropriate, the majority of chapters have new authors. The book is somewhat larger and has nine more chapters, but expansion has deliberately been limited and some chapters have been combined. Topics on which new separate chapters have been added include historical aspects, neuropsychology and imaging, studies of sleep, early environment, transcultural aspects, seasonal affective disorders, depression in medical settings, maintenance treatment (increasingly important as recurrence becomes a greater therapeutic problem than acute treatment), prediction of treatment response, use of anticonvulsants and interpersonal psychotherapy. The chapter on neurochemistry has been expanded to survey developments from which, after a period of uncertainty, a more consistent picture is starting to emerge.

The volume aims to provide a comprehensive handbook drawing together knowledge across a wide range of approaches and aspects of the field. The chapters have been contributed by experts chosen because they can speak with authority on their topics, and each has been asked to review present knowledge. The authors are international, derived particularly from Great Britain, the United States, Europe and Australasia. An explicit aim has been to encompass the varying approaches which should be incorporated in an eclectic orientation to psychiatry, ranging across the psychological, biological and social.

Depression has been given the greatest prominence, in view of its frequency. The continuities between milder and more severe forms seem more impressive than the differences, and both are covered. Mania receives somewhat less space since it is less common. Anxiety disorders, which previously were sometimes regarded as a facet of affective disorders, are now firmly separated in their own right, and in this volume are discussed mainly in relation to depression.

The book is divided into five parts. The first deals with descriptive aspects, including symptoms and their assessment, classification, history of the disorders, diagnosis and prognosis. The second part covers causative aspects, varying from biological and psychodynamic, together with epidemiology and underlying features such as personality. The third part deals with medication and physical treatments and the fourth with psychotherapeutic, cognitive and social approaches to treatment. Part Five deals with selected special aspects, including seasonal affective disorders, depression in relation to childbirth, childhood and adolescence, old age, bereavement, suicidal behaviour and depression in the special situations of general practice and medical settings.

It is hoped that the volume will be useful to students, postgraduate trainees, clinicians and research workers in psychiatry and related medical, scientific, nursing, psychological, social work and mental health disciplines.

Cambridge, 1992   E.S.P.

Acknowledgement

The Editor acknowledges with gratitude the assistance of Mrs Judy Goddard, who undertook a considerable share of the detailed editing, and whose flair and eye for detail made a substantial contribution to the work.

Contributors

Mohammed T. Abou-Saleh MB PhD ChB MPhil MRCPsych
Senior Lecturer in Psychiatry, University Department of Psychiatry, Royal Liverpool Hospital, Liverpool, UK

Nancy C. Andreasen MD PhD
Professor of Psychiatry, University of Iowa College of Medicine, Iowa City, Iowa, USA

Per Bech MD
Professor of Psychiatry, Frederiksburg General Hospital, Hillerød, Denmark

Aaron T. Beck MD DMS(Hon)
Professor of Psychiatry, University of Pennsylvania, Philadelphia, Pennsylvania, USA

Jules R. Bemporad MD
Director of Education, The New York Hospital–Cornell Medical Center, Westchester Division; Professor of Clinical Psychiatry, Cornell University Medical College, New York, USA

German E. Berrios MA(Oxon) MA FRCPsych FBPsS
Consultant and University Lecturer in Psychiatry, University of Cambridge; Director of Medical Studies and Fellow, Robinson College, Cambridge, UK

Paul Bridges MD PhD FRCPsych DPM
Consultant Psychiatrist and Senior Lecturer, Guy's Hospital and Geoffrey Knight National Unit for Affective Disorders, Brook Hospital, London, UK

Graham D. Burrows AO MD ChB BSc DPM FRANZCP FRCPsych
Professor and Director, Department of Psychiatry, University of Melbourne, Austin Hospital, Melbourne, Victoria, Australia

Dennis S. Charney MD
Professor of Psychiatry, Yale University School of Medicine, New Haven; Chief, Psychiatry Service, West Haven Veterans Administration Medical Center, West Haven, Connecticut, USA

Stuart Checkley BA BM BCh MRCP MRCPsych FRCPsych
Consultant Psychiatrist, Maudsley Hospital; Senior Lecturer, Metabolic Unit and Dean, Institute of Psychiatry, London, UK

John F. Clarkin PhD
Professor of Clinical Psychology in Psychiatry, Cornell University Medical College; Director of Psychology, The New York Hospital–Cornell Medical Center, Westchester Division, New York, USA

Zafra Cooper PhD
Senior Research Associate, Department of Psychiatry, University of Cambridge, Cambridge, UK

William Coryell MD
Professor of Psychiatry, University of Iowa College of Medicine, Iowa City, Iowa, USA

John L. Cox BM BCh DM(Oxon) MA DPM FRCPsych FRCP(Edin)
Professor and Head of Department of Psychiatry, School of Postgraduate Medicine and Biological Sciences, University of Keele; Consultant Psychiatrist, North Staffordshire Health Authority, Stoke-on-Trent, UK

Jonathan R. T. Davidson MD MB BS FRCPsych
Associate Professor of Psychiatry and Director, Anxiety Disorders Program, Department of Psychiatry, Duke University Medical Center, Durham, North Carolina, USA

Pedro L. Delgado MD
Department of Psychiatry, Yale University School of Medicine, New Haven, Connecticut, USA

Giovanni A. Fava MD
Associate Professor of Psychosomatic Medicine,
University of Bologna, Bologna, Italy

Max Fink MD
Professor of Psychiatry, State University of New York
at Stony Brook; Editor, *Convulsive Therapy*, New York,
USA

Paul Freeling OBE MB BS FRCGP
Professor of General Practice and Primary Care,
St George's Hospital Medical School, London, UK

Elliot S. Gershon MD
Chief, Clinical Neurogenetics Branch, Department of
Health and Human Sciences, National Institute of
Health, Bethesda, Maryland, USA

Ira D. Glick MD
Professor of Psychiatry, Cornell University Medical
College, New York, USA

Guy M. Goodwin DPhil MRCP MRCPsych
Clinical Scientist and Consultant Psychiatrist, MRC
Brain Metabolism Unit, Royal Edinburgh Hospital,
Edinburgh, UK

Ian M. Goodyer MD FRCPsych DCH
University Lecturer and Head, Section of
Developmental Psychiatry, Department of Psychiatry,
University of Cambridge, Addenbrooke's Hospital,
Cambridge, UK

William M. Grove PhD
Professor, Department of Psychology, University of
Minnesota, Minneapolis, Minnesota, USA

David A. F. Haaga PhD
Assistant Professor, Department of Psychology, The
American University, Washington DC, USA

Gretchen Haas PhD
Associate Professor of Psychiatry, University of
Pittsburgh School of Medicine, Western Psychiatric
Institute and Clinic, Pittsburgh, Pennsylvania, USA

Keith Hawton DM FRCPsych
Consultant Psychiatrist and Clinical Lecturer,
University Department of Psychiatry, University of
Oxford, Oxford, UK

George R. Heninger MD
Associate Chairman for Research; Director, Abraham
Ribicoff Research Facilities; Professor, Department of
Psychiatry, Yale University, New Haven, Connecticut,
USA

Robert M.A. Hirschfeld MD
Professor and Chairman, Department of Psychiatry
and Behavioral Sciences, University of Texas Medical
Branch, Galveston, Texas, USA

Florian Holsboer MD PhD
Professor of Psychiatry and Director, Max-Planck
Institute of Psychiatry, Munich, Germany

Neil Hunt MA MB BS MRCPsych
Clinical Research Fellow and Honorary Lecturer,
Department of Psychological Medicine, St
Bartholomew's Hospital Medical College, University of
London, London, UK

Eileen M. Joyce MA PhD MRCP MRCPsych
Senior Lecturer and Honorary Consultant, Academic
Department of Psychiatry, Charing Cross and
Westminster Medical School, London, UK

Peter R. Joyce BSc MB ChB PhD FRANZCP
Professor of Psychological Medicine, Christchurch
School of Medicine, Christchurch, New Zealand

Fiona K. Judd MD BS DPM FRANZCP
Associate Professor (Clinical), Department of
Psychiatry, University of Melbourne, Austin Hospital,
Heidelberg, Victoria, Australia

Gerald L. Klerman MD
Professor of Psychiatry and Associate Chairman for
Research, Cornell University Medical College, Payne
Whitney Clinic, New York, USA

David J. Kupfer MD
Professor and Chairman, Department of Psychiatry,
University of Pittsburgh School of Medicine, Western
Psychiatric Institute and Clinic, Pittsburgh,
Pennsylvania, USA

Julian Leff BSc MD FRCPsych MRCP
Professor of Social and Cultural Psychiatry; Director
MRC Social and Community Psychiatry Unit,
Institute of Psychiatry, London, UK

Joan L. Luby MD
Instructor in Psychiatry, Washington University School
of Medicine, Washington DC, USA

Alastair Macdonald MD MRCPsych
Senior Lecturer in Psychogeriatrics, United Medical
and Dental Schools (Guy's Campus), London, UK

William T. McKinney MD
Professor of Psychiatry, University of Wisconsin-
Madison Medical School, Madison, Wisconsin, USA

Myer Mendelson MD
Professor of Clinical Psychiatry, University of
Pennsylvania School of Medicine; Senior Attending
Psychiatrist, The Institute of the Pennsylvania
Hospital, Philadelphia, Pennsylvania, USA

Warwick Middleton MB BS FRANZCP
Deputy Director of Psychiatry, Royal Brisbane
Hospital; Senior Lecturer, University of Queensland,
Brisbane, Queensland, Australia

Elaine Murphy MD FRCPsych
Professor of Psychogeriatrics, United Medical and
Dental Schools, Guy's Hospital, London, UK

John I. Nurnberger Jr MD PhD
Professor of Psychiatry and Medical Neurobiology;
Director, Institute of Psychiatric Research, Indiana
University Medical Center, Indianapolis, Indiana, USA

Dan A. Oren MD
Senior Clinical Investigator, Unit of Outpatient
Studies, Clinical Psychobiology Branch,
National Institute of Mental Health, Bethesda,
Maryland, USA

Gordon Parker MD PhD FRANZCP
Professor and Head of School of Psychiatry, University
of New South Wales, Sydney, New South Wales,
Australia

Eugene S. Paykel MD FRCP FRCPsych
Professor of Psychiatry, University of Cambridge,
Addenbrooke's Hospital, Cambridge, UK

Carlo Perris MD
Professor of Psychiatry and Chairman, Department of
Psychiatry and WHO Collaborating Centre for
Research and Training in Mental Health, Umea
University, Umea, Sweden

Robert M. Post MD
Chief, Biological Psychiatry Branch, National Institute
of Mental Health, Bethesda, Maryland, USA

Lawrence H. Price
Department of Veterans Affairs Medical Center, West
Haven, Connecticut, USA

Robert F. Prien PhD
Director, Clinical Psychopharmacology Division of
Clinical Research, National Institute of Mental Health,
Rockville, Maryland, USA

Beverley Raphael MD FRANZCP FRCPsych FAASS
Professor and Head, Department of Psychiatry,

University of Queensland; Director of Psychiatric
Services, Royal Brisbane Hospital; Director, National
Centre for HIV Social Research, Royal Brisbane
Hospital, Brisbane, Queensland, Australia

Charles F. Reynolds III MD
Professor, Department of Psychiatry and Neurology,
University of Pittsburgh, Pittsburgh, Pennsylvania,
USA

Trevor W. Robbins BA MA PhD (Cantab)
University Lecturer, Department of Experimental
Psychology, University of Cambridge, Cambridge,
UK

Norman E. Rosenthal MD
Chief, Unit on Environmental Psychiatry, Clinical
Psychobiology Branch, National Institute of Mental
Health, Bethesda, Maryland, USA

Barbara J. Sahakian BA PhD (Cantab) Dip Clin Psych
University Lecturer and Tutor in Research,
Department of Experimental Psychology, University of
Cambridge, Cambridge, UK

Janine Scott MB BS MRCPsych
Consultation and Senior Lecturer, University
Department of Psychiatry, Royal Victoria Infirmary,
Newcastle Upon Tyne, UK

M. Tracie Shea PhD
Assistant Professor, Department of Psychiatry and
Human Behaviour, Brown University Medical School,
Providence, Rhode Island, USA

Trevor Silverstone DM FRCP FRCPsych
Professor of Clinical Psychopharmacology and Head,
Department of Psychological Medicine, St
Bartholomew's Hospital Medical College, University of
London, London, UK

Angela Lantz Smith MD BA
Resident in Psychiatry, St Luke's–Roosevelt Medical
Center, New York, USA

André Tylee MB BS MRCGP
Senior Lecturer, Division of General Practice and
Primary Care, St George's Hospital Medical School,
University of London, London, UK

Myrna M. Weissman MD
Professor of Epidemiology in Psychiatry and Chief,
Division of Clinical–Genetic Epidemiology, College of
Physicians and Surgeons of Columbia University, New
York, USA

George Winokur BA MD
Professor of Psychiatry, University of Iowa College of
Medicine, Iowa City, Iowa, USA

Irvin D. Yalom MD
Professor, Department of Psychiatry and Behavioral
Sciences, Stanford University School of Medicine,
Stanford, California, USA

Contents

PART 1

Descriptive aspects

1. Symptoms and assessment of depression

Per Bech

SYMPTOMS

Depressed mood and depressive states

In a medical sense depressed mood is a systemic symptom in the same way as fatigue and sleep disturbance. Since systemic phenomena can be produced both by organic disorders and by primary mental disorders they are often very difficult to classify. Thus, depressed mood and fatigue can be important indicators of cancer severity if ascribable to cancer itself, but they have another significance if due to severe depressive states associated with self-destructive behaviour.

Depressed mood, fatigue and sleep disturbance are also essential elements of minor forms of depressive states which Beard (1880) a century ago referred to as neurasthenia. When contrasted to manic states the cardinal triad of depression includes elements of emotional symptoms, motor retardation and negative beliefs (lowered self-esteem). Analogous to manic states the severity of depression can be graded into minor, major and psychotic syndromes. Bonhoeffer (1912) was among the first to exclude major depressive states from Beard's neurasthenia.

Minor states of depression

Mild states of depression are far more common than the more severe degrees. Around 10% of all patients seeking medical advice by their family doctor suffer from mild to moderate degrees of depression. However, doctors often fail to recognize this condition because there is no clear-cut categorized diagnosis of minor depression. Thus, these states are often concealed by a variety of somatic complaints or considered as anxiety or obsessive states. Furthermore, patients do not necessarily complain of feeling depressed: their presenting complaints may rather be vegetative symptoms of which some are systemic (fatigue and sleep distur-

bance) and some are localized (pains in the back, chest pain, nausea or abdominal discomfort or shortness of breath).

It is, therefore, understandable that many doctors feel more at ease in making a somatic rather than a psychiatric diagnosis in this situation. However, it is no help for the patients to be told that all the medical investigations have been negative. The symptoms of depression are as real to the patient as if he or she were suffering from a physical illness.

If a mental disorder is considered next, the minor depressive state is often misdiagnosed as anxiety neurosis, partly because anxiety is an essential component of depression and partly because many physicians find anxiety to be a socially more acceptable condition than depression, justifying the use of benzodiazepines instead of the more toxic antidepressants.

There is little doubt that by far the most frequent association of anxiety with other mental disorders is with depressive states. However, anxiety states occur as a separate syndrome from neurasthenia and depression although not with the same frequency as suggested by Freud (1959a), e.g. as stress disorders or panic disorders. The symptoms of anxiety states are mainly those of excessive stimulation of the sympathetic nervous system (autonomic hyperactivity). The inner tension often results in sleep disturbance which, in contrast to minor depression, is a problem of initial insomnia, i.e. the patient has difficulties in falling asleep, but having eventually fallen asleep he or she has no difficulties in maintaining sleep. In minor depression there is usually no initial insomnia but middle or late insomnia. Recent sleep EEG (electroencephalogram) studies have confirmed that anxiety states have prolonged REM (rapid eye movement) latency while minor depression has shortened REM latency (Kupfer & Thase 1989).

The minor depressive states can be distinguished clinically from anxiety states if the physician recalls the essential triad of depression: the mood of depression, decreased motor activity and negative beliefs (lowered self-esteem). In minor states this triad manifests itself by symptoms such as lack of interest, fatigue, work impairment, introversion and indecision. Recent studies in primary health care have shown that social impairment is related much more to depression than to anxiety states (Angst 1990). Finally, among the vegetative symptoms decreased appetite is more related to depression than to anxiety.

It is clear, as stated by Goldberg (1990), that the detection of a disorder is most important when it can be shown that an available intervention will favourably influence the further course. The more severe the depression, the more easily it can be shown that detection will shorten its course.

Studies carried out in primary health care have shown that in the majority of cases depression is a recurrent disorder (Angst 1990). Only in a minority of cases does depression take a chronic course or remain a single episode.

Recurrent minor depression as well as chronic minor depression have often been referred to as neurotic depression. Hence, neurosis covers both the minor degree of symptoms and the chronicity of symptoms. The minor depressive syndromes can, in contrast to the major degrees, become chronic without becoming more severe. Many of these chronic cases have often been through elaborate psychological tests in the search for neurotic personality processes. These cases may persist until they are correctly diagnosed and then suitably treated.

While the treatment of minor depression with antidepressants is a relatively simple matter today, the diagnosis is sometimes extremely difficult. Minor depression is, however, a clinical syndrome that can be detected by an interview directed towards the symptoms of depressed mood, anxiety, sleep disturbance (middle or late insomnia), fatigue and social impairment as evidenced by introversion, indecision and general work impairment.

Major depressive states

The triad of depression (mood of depression, retardation and negative beliefs) is much more clear-cut in these states than in the minor states. However, the intermixture of anxiety and depression is still very common. On the other hand, while autonomic hyperactivity is the main feature of anxiety in minor depression, other anxiety components do operate in major depression.

Thus, in elderly depressed patients with major depression it is the motor elements of anxiety (restlessness or agitation) that are predominant (agitated depression). In general, however, major depression has psychic elements of anxiety as an essential part (e.g. Hamilton 1989), including feelings of insecurity, worrying and apprehension which can produce periods of overpowering dread or panic (fears of insanity).

In major depression the mood of depression includes hopelessness and helplessness, which also can be considered as elements of negative cognitions of the future, such as feelings of apprehension. Hence, the quality of depressed mood is not simply a state of sadness. The prevailing element of negative beliefs (Beck 1967) is a sense of loss which is part of the lower self-esteem retrospectively experienced. Guilt is an experience of punishment for past misdeeds (prior to the current episode of depression). The most discriminant symptom when comparing anxiety states and major depressive states is guilt feelings (Breslau & Davis 1985).

Among the observable symptoms of major depression is the symptom of retardation which includes emotional (contact), intellectual (concentration difficulties) and motor and verbal activities. The interplay between emotional retardation and negative self-esteem is seen when the depressed woman is concerned directly about her lack of contact with her children and interprets this situation by saying that she has failed as a mother.

The concentration disturbance is often subjectively more pronounced than the objective evidence. In his book on a personal crisis Sutherland (1976), then working as Professor of Experimental Psychology, describes how he suffered from a major depressive state. He had severe difficulties in reading even a newspaper or watching television: 'I could concentrate on nothing except my own pain. . . . I spent the day longing for night to come.'

On examination, the severely depressed patient is rather immobile and the facial expression is often retarded. Conversation is marked by inertia: the depressed patient often does not speak spontaneously. The interplay between emotional and verbal retardation is often observed as an inertia in conversation increasing proportionally to the depth of the questions about the patient's personal problems which the physician is asking.

In the stage of major depression tiredness and pains are often very pronouncedly experienced by the patient as feelings of heaviness in arms and legs. In another description of a self-experienced depression Professor Gray (1983) says: 'Consider a person with acute 'flu' symptoms. If the symptoms continue day after day, week after week...that person, I predict, would come...near a severe depressive break down.' And Gray continues:

> Now consider a patient undergoing deep depression. In the early stage he begins to feel physically ill, and as the days pass his mental self-grooming decreases. At the start his optimism prevails... When tomorrow arrives, however, and he feels slightly worse, he learns that his optimism of the previous day was unjustified. This gradual unlearning of optimism continues... the patient has learned (correctly) that the future holds nothing but terrible suffering.

The preoccupation with bodily symptoms can lead to the conviction on the part of the patient that he or she is suffering from a severe physical illness. Thus, Sutherland (1976) was convinced that he suffered from a lung tumour although negative findings of physical investigations could reassure him for a brief while that his belief was unjustified. Preoccupations with bodily symptoms are often misdiagnosed as obsessions. On the other hand, true obsessive—compulsive behaviour is seen in major depression.

In contrast to the minor states of depression the major states less commonly become chronic. However, the daily experience that the future holds nothing but terrible suffering linked to the negative cognitions of guilt feelings and punishment increases the patient's wish to die. Thoughts of ending his or her life are common in major depression.

Patients living with responsible relatives and having a good treatment compliance can be treated at home for their major depression if it is not complicated by severe suicidal thoughts or by psychotic symptoms.

Psychotic depression

A small percentage of patients with major depression develop psychotic states in which the symptoms of guilt or hypochondria become delusional, i.e. the patient cannot even for a brief while understand that his or her view is unjustified. The hypochondriacal delusions often have a nihilistic quality, e.g. the ideas of being rotten inside, the bowels being blocked and withering away.

Depressive stupor is often connected with psychotic depression, but strictly speaking it indicates in itself no more than extreme motor retardation.

Loss of appetite and weight loss can be seen in the different stages of depression. However, in psychotic or nihilistic depression a total refusal of food can be observed and, in consequence, severe weight loss.

Depressed patients with suicidal behaviour, with stupor, or with severe agitation should all be treated in hospital.

Diagnostic types of depression

Endogenous and reactive depression are concepts that refer to aetiological theories. Thus, endogenous depression refers to a hereditary disorder characterized either by a bipolar course of episodes (i.e. depressive and manic episodes are alternating) or by recurrent depressive episodes (unipolar depression). Reactive depression refers to a depressive episode provoked by a single major life event or by enduring psychosocial circumstances.

The classical works on endogenous depression are the studies by Kraepelin (1902, 1921) while the classical studies on reactive depression are those of Wimmer (1916) and Freud (1959b). It is of great interest that the clinical descriptions of depression by Kraepelin, Wimmer and Freud are rather similar despite the differences between their aetiological theories (Bech 1990).

The term psychotic depression has been used by some authors synonymously with endogenous depression (e.g. Carney et al 1965, Roth et al 1983). Others such as Kraepelin (1921) and Hamilton (1960) use the term psychosis to cover degrees of severity and this is also the approach of the present author. As stated by Hamilton (1960) 'a schizophrenic patient who has delusions is not necessarily worse than one who has not, but a depressive patient who has is much worse.'

ASSESSMENT SCALES FOR DEPRESSION

Validity and reliability

Assessment scales or rating scales are methods for the assignment of numerals to clinical data (severity data or diagnostic data) according to rules of measurement. The theory behind the use of rating scales in depression is a model of measurement relevant to the fact that, on the one hand, no symptom is sufficient (pathognomonic) and, on the other hand, a limited number of symptoms is sufficient, if representative for the dimension under investigation. The psychometric concepts of content validity (the combination of symptoms into total scores) and of inter-observer reliability are important scientific aspects of rating scales in depressive disorders.

Content validity

Concerning scales measuring severity of depression the Thompson criteria (Thompson 1989) with some modification have been used:

1) mood of depression
2) anxiety
3) motor symptoms
4) cognitive symptoms (including both negative beliefs and indecision)
5) social impairment (including social functioning and social withdrawal)
6) vegetative symptoms.

Concerning scales for diagnosis, important aspects other than symptoms have been considered for the endogenous-reactive distinction:

1) psychosocial stressors
2) personality
3) onset, duration and persistence of clinical picture
4) previous episodes of depression
5) diurnal variation
6) reactivity of symptoms
7) biological symptoms (quality of depression, early awakening, weight loss)
8) psychological symptoms (anxiety, phobias, aggression).

Construct validity

There are two different psychometric methods of testing the evidence for adding up all items of a rating scale in order to derive an overall expression of the transmitted information (sufficient statistic). The most used but least conclusive method is principal component analysis (factor analysis). However, when a single dimension is expected (a 'common' or 'general' factor) there is no need to perform a complex factor analysis. Instead, a simple correlation analysis showing the coefficient between each item and the total score of the remaining items may be sufficient (item—total correlation, Bech & Rafaelsen 1980). The Cronbach coefficient alpha is an overall expression of the degree of positive correlations between items of a scale (Cronbach et al 1972).

The most conclusive method for testing whether the total score of a rating scale is a sufficient statistic is latent structure analysis. By this method the degree to which a scale is rankable is tested, i.e. whether a rank order of the items is consistent across age, sex and diagnosis. This hierarchical structure of items is, as stated by Feinstein (1987), the only guarantee for the transparency of the total score. By transparency Feinstein (1987) refers to the ability to see through a total score to determine what it contains. If all information in the individual items has been transmitted to the total score, the scale has optimal transparency. The most appropriate method of testing the hierarchical structure of a scale is Rasch analysis (Rasch 1960, Bech 1981). Another method is the Loevinger coefficient of hierarchical structure (Loevinger 1957). A Loevinger coefficient between 0.40 and 0.49 means a moderate tendency to hierarchical structure, while a coefficient of 0.50 or more means a clear structure (Mokken 1971). It should be emphasized that a high Cronbach coefficient alpha is not a sufficient condition for a high Loevinger coefficient (Wistedt et al 1990).

Concurrent validity

This covers the extent to which a scale correlates with a standard index, e.g. an internationally accepted rating scale. Scales that mutually correlate by a coefficient of 0.7 or more are considered to measure the same dimension (convergent validity). Correlation coefficients below 0.7 seem to indicate discriminant validity.

Inter-observer reliability

The process of rating by psychiatrists may give rise to rater bias which can be analysed by different methods, of which the intra-class coefficient (ICC) is an adequate extension of the overall agreement between different raters assessing the same patients (Bartko & Carpenter 1976). Another method is the Kendall concordance test (Siegel 1965), or less optimally, the Spearman correlation.

For self-rating scales the internal consistency of items has often been referred to as a reliability test, although more correctly it is a test of construct validity. The test-retest method is not relevant for measuring severity of depression as the scores will change in the period between the two tests due to the fluctuation of symptoms.

Self-rating scales for severity of depression

Table 1.1 shows the psychometric validity of first and

Table 1.1   Self rating scales for depression

Psychometric aspects	First generation scales			Second generation scales	
	Beck Depression Inventory (BDI-21) (Beck et al 1961)	Zung self-rating scale for depression (Zung 1965)	Carroll self-rating for depression (Carroll et al 1981)	Wakefield Inventory for depression (Snaith et al 1971)	Melancholia Sub-scale of Beck Inventory (BDI-12) (Bech et al 1975)
Content validity (% of item contribution)					
a. mood	10	15	8	25	8
b. anxiety	5	10	15	25	8
c. motor	0	5	15	8	0
d. cognitive	47	35	27	0	58
e. social	10	0	0	8	8
f. vegetative	29	35	35	33	16
Construct validity					
Factor analysis	3–7 factors	2 factors	–	–	–
Alpha coefficient	0.86 (0.76 - 0.95)	0.92	–	–	–
Loevinger coefficient	0.41	–	–	–	0.52
Concurrent validity —correlations with the Hamilton Depression Scale	0.73 (0.61–0.86)	0.56–0.79	0.80	0.87	0.79

second generation questionnaires specifically designed for measuring severity of psychiatric states.

The content validity shows in general that these scales cover few motor items but many cognitive items. The Beck Depression Inventory (BDI-21; Beck et al 1961) is still the most frequently used scale and covers most cognitive elements, in accordance with Beck's theory of negative cognitions in depression (Beck 1967). The second generation of scales derived from the BDI-21 are the Melancholia Subscale (BDI-12; Bech et al 1975) and the BDI-13, derived by item-total correlations (Beck & Beamesderfer 1974). The BDI-12 includes fewer vegetative symptoms and has been found to have a better discriminant validity than the BDI-21 in classifying responders to antidepressive therapy in patients with chronic pain disorders (Loldrup et al 1991).

The Wakefield Inventory (Snaith et al 1971) is a modification of the Zung scale (Zung 1965) and has been further modified by Snaith (1986) to reduce the

number of vegetative symptoms. The Carroll Depression Scale (Carroll et al 1981) is a self-rating version of the Hamilton Depression Scale (Hamilton 1960).

It is surprising how few studies have been devoted to the analysis of construct validity of the self-rating scales. Most research has been carried out on the Beck Depression Scale, and Steer et al (1986) and Beck et al (1988) have made useful overviews. In total, 13 studies have investigated the Beck scale with factor analysis and the range of factors isolated is three to seven. The relatively high alpha coefficient found in the various studies (Beck et al 1988) and shown in Table 1.1 is, however, no guarantee of a strong hierarchical structure (Green et al 1977). In the study of Loldrup et al (1991) a Loevinger coefficient of 0.41 was obtained for the BDI-21 (Table 1.1), which indicates a moderate hierarchical structure and accordingly a moderate transparency of the total score. So far, Rasch analysis of the self-rating scales for depression has not been performed.

Table 1.2 Observer rating scales for depression

Psychometric aspects	First generation scale	Second generation scales	
	Hamilton Depression Scale (Hamilton 1960, 1967)	Melancholia Scale (Bech & Rafaelsen 1980)	Montgomery-Åsberg Depression Scale (Montgomery & Åsberg 1979)
Content validity (% of item contribution)			
a. mood	18	18	30
b. anxiety	16	9	10
c. motor	12	18	0
d. cognitive	28	27	30
e. social	8	9	0
f. vegetative	28	18	30
Construct validity			
Factor analysis	general factor	general factor	general factor
Item—total correlation	acceptable	acceptable	acceptable
Latent structure analysis (Rasch)	more than one dimension	one dimension	more than one dimension
Concurrent validity (correlation with Hamilton)	–	0.97	0.82
Sensitivity to change during treatment			
Montgomery & Åsberg (1979)	less	–	most
Bech (1989)	most	–	less
Maier et al (1988)	least	most	less
Inter-observer reliability Intra-class coefficient	0.73	0.82	0.86

The correlation between the self-rating scales and the Hamilton scale (Table 1.1) is lowest for the Zung scale, but in general the coefficients are 0.7 or higher, indicating convergent validity. Strictly speaking, only the Carroll–Hamilton comparison investigated the correlation of the two scale administrations (self-ratings versus observer ratings) as the content of the Carroll and Hamilton scales is similar apart from observable elements such as motor symptoms and symptoms of insight.

The similarities and differences between self-rating scales and observer scales have been reviewed by Paykel and Norton (1986). Among the limitations in the applicability of self-rating scales were the following: a. correlations with observer scales are lower for observational items than for reported items and are lower for pretreatment measurement than post-treatment; b. furthermore, severely ill and psychotic depressives appear to underrate themselves whereas neurotic patients overrate themselves.

The trend in clinical research in depression seems to have followed the Paykel and Norton statement that self-rating scales have their main applicability in the minor forms of depression. The method appears to have been most useful in psychosomatic research when detecting minor psychiatric disorders. The General Health Questionnaire (Goldberg 1972) and the Symptom Checklist (SCL-90, Guy 1976) are often used for this purpose (Bridges & Goldberg 1989).

Observer rating scales for severity of depression

Table 1.2 shows the psychometric validity of first and second generation rating scales specifically designed for measuring severity of depressive states including sensitivity to rating changes in depression during treatment.

As expected the content validity shows that the Hamilton Depression Scale contains more motor items than the Carroll self-rating scale. The content validity of the Montgomery–Åsberg Scale is rather similar to the Zung self-rating scale for depression. The number of vegetative symptoms is lowest in the Melancholia Scale.

The construct validity of the Hamilton scale has been extensively evaluated whereas only a few studies applying factor analysis have been performed on the Montgomery–Åsberg Scale and the Melancholia Scale (Lecrubier et al 1983, Chambon et al 1990). The Montgomery–Åsberg Depression Scale was constructed on the basis of the Comprehensive Psychopathological Rating Scale (Åsberg et al 1978) by item — total correlations, and the 10 items with the highest coefficients were selected (Montgomery & Åsberg 1979). Other depression subscales have been derived from the Comprehensive Scale (Perris 1986). The Melancholia Scale was constructed on the basis of the Hamilton Depression Scale and the Cronholm–Ottosson Depression Scale (Ottosson 1960) and includes 11 items (Bech & Rafaelsen 1980).

The Hamilton Depression Scale is by far the most frequently used depression scale. As early as his first study Hamilton (1960) used principal component analysis and found that the first factor only had a weak correlation with the total score. However, in his second study (Hamilton 1967) he obtained a substantial correlation coefficient (0.92) between the first factor and the total score. These findings indicate that the total score gives reasonable information about the state of the patient, although in some populations it is not always sufficient. It should be recalled that the 1960 study included more severe depressives than the 1967 study. When reviewing all studies that have used factor analysis with his scale, Hamilton concluded (1987) that the first factor measured severity of depression and that the second factor separated anxiety from retarded depression.

The homogeneity of the Hamilton Scale in different populations using total–item correlations has been investigated by Paykel (1990). He found that the Hamilton symptoms were more homogeneous in patients treated for depression in general practice than in depressed inpatients or outpatients treated by psychiatrists.

Latent structure analysis of the Hamilton scale by use of Rasch models has shown that only a subgroup of items have a hierarchical structure (Bech et al 1981). This was the background on which the Melancholia Scale was constructed (Bech & Rafaelsen 1980). This scale has been shown to fulfill the Rasch model, in contrast to the Hamilton and Montgomery–Åsberg Scales (Maier & Philipp 1985, Allerup 1986, Maier et al 1988, Chambon et al 1990).

The capacity to see through a total score of a rating scale, its transparency, is therefore most pronounced for the Melancholia Scale. Its total score is a sufficient statistic. The transparency of the Hamilton Scale is most pronounced for score values below 25 (Bech et al 1975). It is of great interest that Paykel et al (1988) found that a Hamilton score of 12 or less indicated a depression where placebo is as effective as tricyclic antidepressants. A total score of 13–15 or of 16–24 indicated that tricyclics were superior to placebo. In this way the terminology of the total scores has been standardized in a form of predictive validity. The detection of a disorder is most important when it can be shown that an available intervention will favourably influence the course of the patient's disorder. A Hamilton score of 13 seems to be the cut-off score for the treatment of depression with tricyclics, according to the work by Paykel et al (1988). Furthermore, the differentiation of dysthymia and major depression appears due to intensity of symptoms (Berrios & Bulbena-Villarasa 1990) and not to specific symptom profiles.

Sensitivity to measurement of change in depressed patients during treatment was the basis for construction of the Cronholm–Ottosson Depression Scale (Ottosson 1960). The Montgomery–Åsberg Scale was introduced as a scale that was better than the Hamilton Scale in differentiating responders from non-responders to antidepressant treatment (Montgomery & Åsberg 1979). However, Maier et al (1988) have found the Melancholia Scale more sensitive than the Montgomery–Åsberg or Hamilton Scales.

The Hamilton Depression Scale has been used in many different versions in respect of both number of items and item definitions. The most frequently used version is the one included in the Early Clinical Drug Evaluation Program (ECDEU) battery of scales (Guy 1976). This version was not fully accepted by Hamilton (1987). In collaboration with Hamilton a revised version of his scale was derived in which the 17 items were published together with the six extra Melancholia Scale items (Bech et al 1986).

The Clinical Interview for Depression is a rating scale developed by Paykel (1986) in which the Hamilton Scale is included. This scale contains items relevant for making the distinction between endogenous and reactive depression as well as items covering panic attacks, phobic anxiety and obsessive symptoms. A principal component analysis 'Paykel 1986' showed that two factors clearly correspond to depression and to anxiety. The depression factor included the group of symptoms of the Hamilton Scale that fulfilled the Rasch model of unidimensionality of severity of depression (Bech et al 1981).

In general, the observer scales for depression have a better construct validity than self-rating scales and their applicability covers the whole range of depressive states. Moreover, they can be completed with minimal patient cooperation (bedside scales). Their inter-observer reliability is high (Table 1.2). The function of measurement in primary clinical research is in connection with Popper's dialectic of conjecture and refutation in order to test the null hypothesis, which postulates no difference between the treatments under investigation (Popper 1976). The best psychometric scale puts the null hypothesis at greatest risk.

The Hamilton scale has a very high degree of international use which is an important aspect of a scale in relation to secondary research, i.e. in drawing conclusions across studies (meta-analysis). The exclusive reliance on one rating scale only might, however, restrict construct validity. By use of more than one scale it is possible to evaluate not only to what extent the scales agree but also to what extent they do not seem to measure the same dimension (i.e. discriminant validity). The Clinical Interview for Depression (Paykel 1986) is a good example of an extension to more than one scale which does not extend the interview markedly. The Hamilton Depression Scale/ Melancholia Scale (Bech et al 1986) is another example, as is the attempt to extract the Hamilton scale from the Comprehensive Psychopathological Rating Scale (Nilson & Axelsson 1989).

Diagnostic observer rating scales for depression

Table 1.3 shows the psychometric validity of the first and second generation of rating scales designed for diagnosis of depression.

The content should be quite different from that of severity, but in the first Newcastle Scale (Carney et al 1965) 30% of the items are severity symptoms while 20% of the second Newcastle Scale (Gurney 1971, Roth et al 1983) include severity symptoms. This might explain the correlation between severity scales and diagnostic scales (endogenous depression) found in some studies (Bech 1981).

Course of symptoms during the depressive episode under investigation (onset, duration, persistence, diurnal variation and reactivity) takes 50% of the item content in the 1971 Newcastle Scale but 0% in the 1965 version. Thus, the two Newcastle Scales focus on different aspects of clinical depression. The Diagnostic Melancholia Scale (Bech et al 1988) is derived from the Newcastle scales, from which the severity symptoms have been excluded as have previous episodes and the onset of current episode.

The construct validity of the two Newcastle Scales has been examined by use of factor analysis and by discriminant function analysis. By these multivariate methods the various items of the scales have been given positive and negative diagnostic weights. In this way the information contained in the scales has been transmitted to one single diagnostic dimension with endogenous depression at one end and reactive depression at the other.

The score distribution of the Newcastle Scales has been used as a validation criterion (Carney et al 1965, Carney 1986). A genuine boundary between endogenous and reactive depression should, according to this hypothesis, manifest itself by a 'point of rarity' around the middle of the Newcastle dimension. In fact, a bimodal distribution of the 1965 Newcastle scores was found by Carney et al (1965) with the point of rarity of scores around +6. A score of +6 or more indicates endogenous depression and a score of +5 or less indicates reactive depression. There has, however, been an extensive debate in the literature about the distribution of the Newcastle scores which has been summarized by Carney (1986). The most impressive argument against using score distribution on a single dimension was that stressed by Eysenck (1970), who argued that the scores on each of the diagnostic dimensions (endogenous and reactive) should be considered separately.

The Diagnostic Melancholia Scale is scored in accordance with the suggestions of Eysenck (1970), i.e. with subscores for endogenous and subscores for reactive depression. Five items are endogenous items (the three biological symptoms, diurnal variation and the day-to-day persistence of symptoms) and five other items are

Table 1.3 Observer rating scales for diagnosis of depression

Psychometric aspects	First generation scales		Second generation scale
	Newcastle Scale (1965) (Carney et al 1965, Roth et al 1983)	Newcastle Scale (1971) (Gurney 1971, Roth et al 1983)	Diagnostic Melancholia Scale (Bech et al 1988)
Content validity (% of item contribution)			
a. psychosocial stressors	10	10	10
b. personality	10	0	10
c. onset, duration, persistence of current episode	0	30	20
d. previous episodes	10	0	0
e. diurnal variation of symptoms	0	10	10
f. reactivity of symptoms	0	10	10
g. biological symptoms (quality, early awakening, weight loss)	20	10	30
h. psychological symptoms (anxiety, phobias, aggression)	20	10	10
i. severity symptoms (psychotic, motor, guilt)	30	20	0
Construct validity			
Factor analysis	two factors	two factors	–
Latent structure analysis (Rasch)	–	–	two dimensions
Score distribution	bimodal and unimodal	bimodal and unimodal	unimodal
Number of dimensions	one	one	two
Inter-observer reliability			
Intra-class coefficients	0.44–0.81	0.34–0.71	0.51–0.62

reactive items (psychosocial stressors, personality deviation, reactivity of symptoms, somatic anxiety (stress item) and duration of symptoms). It has been found that both groups of symptoms fulfil the Rasch model (sufficient statistic), but no simple mathematical relationship between the two subscores was obtained. It was also found that around 32% of major depressive patients score high on both subscores, indicating mixed endogenous—reactive depression.

A more comprehensive depression scale for the diagnosis of depression than the Newcastle Scales and the Diagnostic Melancholia Scale is the WHO Schedule for Standardized Assessment of Depressive Disorders (WHO-SADD; Sartorius et al 1983, Jablensky et al 1986). This is a very interesting scale that produces three profiles for the description of a depressed patient: a demographic profile, a symptomatological profile, and a past history profile. However, the formulation of the diagnosis is a clinical judgment as there is no inbuilt diagnostic score or algorithm. Attempts have been made to extract the Newcastle Scales and the Diagnostic Melancholia Scale from WHO-SADD (Bech et al 1984). The Clinical Interview for Depression (Paykel 1986) also includes items from which the 1965 Newcastle Scale and the Diagnostic Melancholia Scale can be extracted.

REFERENCES

Allerup P 1986 Rasch model analysis of a rating scale. Danish Institute for Educational Research. Copenhagen

Angst J 1990 Depression and anxiety: a review of studies in the community and in primary health care. In: Sartorius N, Goldberg D, de Girolamo G, Costa e Silva J A, Lecrubier Y, Wittchen H-U (eds) Psychological disorders in general medical settings. Hogrefe & Huber, Toronto, p 60–68

Åsberg M, Perris C, Schalling D, Sedvall G (eds) 1978 The CPRS – development and applications of a psychiatric rating scale. Acta Psychiatrica Scandinavica (suppl) 271

Bartko J J, Carpenter W T 1976 On the methods and theory of reliability. Journal of Nervous and Mental Diseases 163: 307–317

Beard G M 1880 A practical treatise on nervous exhaustion (neurasthenia). Treat EB, New York

Bech P 1981 Rating scales for affective disorders: Their validity and consistency. Acta Psychiatrica Scandinavica 64 (suppl 295): 1–101

Bech P, Rafaelsen O J 1980 The use of rating scales exemplified by a comparison of the Hamilton and the Bech—Rafaelsen melancholia scales. Acta Psychiatrica Scandinavica 62 (suppl 255): 128–131

Bech P, Gram L F, Dein E, Jacobsen O, Vitger J, Bolwig T G 1975 Quantitative rating of depressive states. Acta Psychiatrica Scandinavica 51: 161–170

Bech P, Allerup P, Gram L F, Reisby N, Rosenberg R, Jacobsen O, Nagy A 1981 The Hamilton Depression Scale. Evaluation of objectivity using logistic models. Acta Psychiatrica Scandinavica 63: 290–299

Bech P, Gjerris A, Andersen J, Rafaelsen O J 1984 World Health Organization Schedule for Standardized Assessment of Depressive Disorders (WHO/SADD). Item combinations and inter-observer reliability. Psychopathology 17: 244–252

Bech P, Kastrup M, Rafaelsen O J 1986 Mini-compendium of rating scales for states of anxiety, depression, mania, schizophrenia with corresponding DSM-III syndromes. Acta Psychiatrica Scandinavica 73 (suppl 326): 1–37

Bech P, Allerup P, Gram L F, Kragh-Sørensen P, Rafaelsen O J, Reisby N, Vestergaard P 1988 The Diagnostic Melancholia Scale (DMS): Dimensions of endogenous and reactive depression with relationship to the Newcastle scales. Journal of Affective Disorders 14: 161–170

Beck A T 1967 Depression: clinical, experimental, and theoretical aspects. University of Pennsylvania Press, Philadelphia

Beck A T, Beamesderfer A 1974 Assessment of depression: the Depression Inventory. In: Pichot P (ed) Psychological measurement in psychopharmacology. Karger, Basel, p 151–169

Beck A T, Ward C H, Mendelson M, Mock J, Erbaugh J 1961 An inventory for measuring depression. Archives of General Psychiatry 4: 561–571

Beck A T, Steer R A, Garrison R 1988 Psychometric properties of the Beck Depression Inventory: twenty-five years of evaluation. Clinical Psychology Review 8: 77–100

Berrios G E, Bulbena-Villarasa A 1990 The Hamilton Depression Scale and the numerical description of the symptoms of depression. In: Bech P, Coppen A (eds) The Hamilton Scales. Springer, Berlin, p 80–92

Bonhoeffer K 1912 Zur Differentialdiagnose der Neurasthenie und endogenen Depression. Berliner Klinische Wochenschrift 49: 1–4

Breslau N, Davis GC 1985 Refining DSM-III criteria in major depression. An assessment of the descriptive validity of criterion symptoms. Journal of Affective Disorders 9: 199–206

Bridges K, Goldberg D 1989 Self-administered scales of neurotic symptoms. In: Thompson C (ed) The instruments of psychiatric research. John Wiley, Chichester, p 157–176

Carney M W P 1986 The Newcastle Scale. In: Sartorius N, Ban T A (eds) Assessment of depression. Springer, Berlin, p 201–212

Carney M W P, Roth M, Garside R F 1965 The diagnosis of depressive syndromes and prediction of ECT response. British Journal of Psychiatry 121: 35–40

Carroll B J, Feinberg M, Smouse P E, Rawson S G, Greden J F 1981 The Carroll Rating Scale for depression. Development, reliability and validation. British Journal of Psychiatry 138: 194–200

Chambon O, Cialdella P, Kiss L, Poncet F 1990 Study of the unidimensionality of the Bech–Rafaelsen Melancholia Scale using Rasch analysis in a French sample of major depressive disorders. Pharmacopsychiatry 23: 243–245

Cronbach L J, Gleser G C, Nanda H, Rajaratnem N 1972 The generalizability of behavioral measurements. John Wiley, New York

Eysenck H J 1970 The classification of depressive illness. British Journal of Psychiatry 117: 241–250

Feinstein A R 1987 Clinimetrics. Yale University Press, New Haven

Freud S 1959a The justification for detaching from neurasthenia a particular syndrome: the anxiety neurosis (first published in Neurologisches Zentralblatt 1895). Collected papers, vol 4. Basic Books, New York, p 76–106

Freud S 1959b Mourning and melancholia (first published in 1917) Collected papers, vol 4. Basic Books, New York, p 152–170

Goldberg D 1972 The detection of psychiatric illness by questionnaires. Oxford University Press, Oxford

Goldberg D 1990 Reasons for misdiagnosis. In: Sartorius N, Goldberg D, de Girolamo G, Costa e Silva J A, Lecrubier Y, Wittchen H-U (eds) Psychological disorders in general medical settings. Hogrefe & Huber, Toronto, p 139–145

Gray E G 1983 Severe depression: a patient's thoughts. British Journal of Psychiatry 143: 319–322

Green S B, Lissitz R W, Mulaiek S A 1977 Limitations of coefficient alpha as an index of test unidimensionality. Educational and Psychological Measurement 37: 827–838

Gurney C 1971 Diagnostic scales for affective disorders. Proceedings of the Fifth World Conference of Psychiatry, Mexico City, p 330

Guy W (ed) 1976 Early clinical drug evaluation (ECDEU) assessment manual for psychopharmacology. Publication No. 76–338. National Institute of Mental Health, Rockville

Hamilton M 1960 A rating scale for depression. Journal of Neurology, Neurosurgery and Psychiatry 23: 56–62

Hamilton M 1967 Development of a rating scale for primary depressive illness. British Journal of Social and Clinical Psychology 6: 278–296

Hamilton M 1987 Assessment of psychopathology. In: Hindmarch I, Stonier P D (eds) Human psychopharmacology. Measures and methods. John Wiley, Chichester, p 1–18

Hamilton M 1989 Frequency of symptoms in melancholia (depressive illness). British Journal of Psychiatry 154: 201–206

Jablensky A, Sartorius N, Gulbinat W, Ernberg G 1986 The WHO instruments for the assessment of depressive disorders. In: Sartorius N, Ban T A (eds) Assessment of depression. Springer, Berlin, p 61–81

Kraepelin E 1902 Clinical psychiatry (translated by R Defendorf) MacMillan, London

Kraepelin E 1921 Manic-depressive insanity and paranoia. E & S Livingstone, Edinburgh

Kupfer D J, Thase M E 1989 Laboratory studies and validity of psychiatric diagnosis: has there been progress? In: Robins L N, Barret J E (eds) The validity of psychiatric diagnosis. Raven Press, New York, p 177–202

Lecrubier Y, Steru L, Lancrenon S, Lavoisy J 1983 Les déprimes ambulatoires en pratique de ville: une enquête épidemiologique. Actualités Psychiatriques 2A: 19–26

Loevinger J 1957 Objective tests as instruments of psychological theory. Psychological Reports 3: 635–694

Loldrup D, Hansen H J, Langemark M, Olesen J, Bech P 1991 (in press). The validity of the Melancholia Scale (MES) in predicting outcome of antidepressants in chronic idiopathic pain disorders. European Psychiatry

Maier W, Philipp M 1985 Comparative analysis of observer depression scales. Acta Psychiatrica Scandinavica 72: 239–245

Maier W, Philipp M, Heuser I, Schlegel S, Buller R, Wetzel H 1988 Improving depression severity assessment. Reliability, internal validity and sensitivity to change of three observer depression scales. Journal of Psychiatric Research 22: 3–12

Mokken R J 1971 A theory and procedure of scale analysis. Mouton, Paris

Montgomery S A Åsberg M 1979 A new depression scale designed to be sensitive to change. British Journal of Psychiatry 134: 382–389

Nilsson A, Axelsson R 1989 Psychopathology during logterm lithium treatment of patients with major affective disorders. Acta Psychiatrica Scandinavica 80: 375–388

Ottosson J-O 1960 Experimental studies of the therapeutic action of electro-convulsive therapy in endogenous depression. Acta Psychiatrica et Neurologica Scandinavica 35 (suppl 145): 69–97

Paykel E S 1986 The Clinical Interview for Depression. In: Sartorius N, Ban T A (eds) Assessment of depression. Springer, Berlin, p 304–315

Paykel E S 1990 Use of the Hamilton Depression Scale in general practice. In: Bech P, Coppen A (eds) The Hamilton Scales. Springer, Berlin, p 40–47

Paykel E S, Norton K R W 1986 Self-report and clinical interview in the assessment of depression. In: Sartorius N, Ban T A (eds) Assessment of depression. Springer, Berlin, p 356–366

Paykel E S, Hollyman J A, Freeling P, Sedgwick P 1988 Predictors of therapeutic benefit from amitriptyline in mild depression: a general practice placebo controlled trial. Journal of Affective Disorders 14: 83–95

Perris C 1986 Rating of depression with a subscale of the CPRS. In: Sartorius N, Ban T A (eds) Assessment for depression. Springer, Berlin, p 90–107

Popper K 1976 The unended quest. Fontane, London

Rasch G 1960 Probalistic models for some intelligence and attainment tests. Danish Institute for Educational Research, Copenhagen (Reprinted 1980 University of Chicago Press, Chicago)

Roth M, Gurney C, Mountjoy C Q 1983 The Newcastle rating scales. Acta Psychiatrica Scandinavica 68 (suppl 310): 42–54

Sartorius N, Davidian H, Ernberg G, Fenton F R, Fuji I, Gastpar M, Gulbinat W, Jablensky A, Kielholz P, Lehmann H E, Naraghi N, Shimizu M, Shinguku N, Takahashi R 1983 Depressive disorders in different cultures. World Health Organization, Geneva

Siegel S 1956 Nonparametric statistics. McGraw-Hill, New York

Snaith R P 1986 The development of four self-assessment depression scales. In: Sartorius N, Ban T A (eds) Assessment of depression. Springer, Berlin, p 153–158

Snaith R P, Ahmed S N, Mehta S, Hamilton M 1971 Assessment of the severity of depressive illness: the Wakefield self-assessment depression inventory. Psychological Medicine 1: 143–149

Steer R A, Beck A T, Garrison R 1986 Applications of the Beck Depression Inventory. In: Sartorius N, Ban T A (eds) Assessment of depression. Springer, Berlin, p 123–142

Sutherland S 1976 Breakdown. A personal crisis and a medical dilemma. Weidenfeld & Nicholson, London

Thompson C 1989 Theory of rating scales. In: Thompson C (ed) The instruments of psychiatric research. John Wiley, Chichester, 1–17

Wimmer A 1916 Psykogene sindssygeformer in Sct Hans Mental Hospital 1816–1916. Jubilee Publication Gad, Copenhagen, 85–216

Wistedt B, Rasmussen A, Pedersen L, Mulm U, Träskman-Bendz L, Wakelin J, Bech P 1990 The development of an observer scale for measuring social dysfunction and aggression. Pharmacopsychiatry (in press)

Zung W W K 1965 A self-rating depression scale. Archives of General Psychiatry 12: 63–70

2. Symptoms and assessment of mania

Trevor Silverstone   Neil Hunt

Descriptions of the manic syndrome can be found in the classical writings of Hippocrates and Arateus. However, it was not until the end of the last century that Kraepelin (1921) delineated manic depressive illness as a clinical entity, stressing the close relationship between the syndromes of depression and mania. Leonhard further dissected manic depression into unipolar and bipolar types on the basis of genetic susceptibility (Leonhard et al 1962). This dichotomy has since been confirmed by a number of clinical and genetic studies, reviewed in chapter 5 (e.g. Angst et al 1973, Perris 1966).

SYMPTOMS

Diagnosis

There is general uniformity among the various diagnostic systems as to which symptoms constitute the manic syndrome. Most recent research in bipolar disorder has used either the Research Diagnostic Criteria (RDC) of Spitzer, Endicott & Robins (1978) or the criteria in the *Diagnostic and Statistical Manual*, 3rd edn (revised) (DSM-IIIR; Table 2.1) (American Psychiatric Association 1987). The forthcoming tenth edition of the *International Classification of Diseases*, devised by the World Health Organization, uses a descriptive approach rather than the checklist method of the other two.

The main diagnostic difficulties arise between mania, hypomania and schizoaffective disorder (see below).

The description of the symptoms of mania given by Kraepelin (1921) can hardly be bettered, and many of the illustrations given below are from his text. Most of the others come from interviews we recently conducted on a series of 68 patients fulfilling RDC criteria for bipolar disorder.

Table 2.1 Diagnostic criteria for manic episode (DSM-IIIR; American Psychiatric Association 1987)

A. A distinct period of abnormally and persistently elevated, expansive or irritable mood.

B. During the period of mood disturbance, at least three of the following symptoms have persisted (four if the mood is only irritable) and have been present to a significant degree:
   1) inflated self-esteem or grandiosity
   2) decreased need for sleep, e.g. feels rested after only 3 hours of sleep
   3) more talkative than usual or pressure to keep talking
   4) flight of ideas or subjective experience that thoughts are racing
   5) distractibility, i.e. attention is too easily drawn to unimportant or irrelevant external stimuli
   6) increase in goal directed activity (either socially, at work or school, or sexually) or psychomotor agitation.
   7) excessive involvement in pleasurable activities which have a high potential for painful consequences.

C. Mood disturbance sufficiently severe to cause marked impairment in occupational functioning or in usual social activities or relationships with others, or to necessitate hospitalization to prevent harm to self or others.

D. At no time during the disturbance have there been delusions or hallucinations for as long as 2 weeks in the absence of prominent mood symptoms.

E. Not superimposed on schizophrenia, schizophreniform disorder, delusional disorder or other psychotic disorder.

F. It cannot be established that an organic factor initiated and maintained the disturbance.

Mood changes

The fundamental symptom required to make the diagnosis of mania is a change in the mood of the subject. This is either an elevation of mood out of keeping with the subject's circumstances or increased irritability. Self reports are often expressed in terms such as 'an intense sense of wellbeing', 'too good to be true' (Lerner 1980), 'cheerful in a beautiful world'. The change of mood may be described in religious terms such as 'having become one with God'. Elation may also be inferred from the 'tendency to joke and to make facetious remarks', or patients may be seen to indulge in behaviours generally associated with a heightened mood such as laughing, singing and dancing. The similarity to states of cheerful drunkenness probably reflects the disinhibition found in both states as much as any change in mood. Astrup et al (1959) described the mood state in excited schizophrenia as an ecstasy state unlike the typical manic elation.

The subjective improvement in mood, though generally recognized, may not be regarded as pathological by the patient, so that patients are often presented for treatment by their relatives rather than themselves. Angst et al (1973) reported that admission was less common in later episodes of manic depression and this may reflect the increasing insight into the serious import of the mood change. A few patients regard this enhancement of mood as worth seeking rather than avoiding and so are reluctant to take measures to prevent recurrence.

One of the main lines of evidence used by Kraepelin to support his view that mania and depression were closely related was the occurrence of mixed affective states. Many patients experience some depression during a manic episode; in one series nearly half were considered 'dysphoric manics' (Post et al 1989). Dysphoria is more frequent in severe mania, when there may be rapid changes between laughter and tears. In such cases despite obvious overactivity and pressure of speech depressive ideas are expressed. At times the depressive ideas may be in direct contradiction to the apparent mood of the patient. Patients with mixed symptoms have been noted to have a poorer outcome in terms of length of episode (Keller et al 1986). It has also been suggested that they have a less good response to lithium (Secunda et al 1987).

Inflated self regard (grandiosity)

The presence of grandiosity may be apparent either from the ideas expressed or through overt behaviour. Patients may exaggerate their own achievements or importance within believable limits, claiming that they do important jobs and know famous people. They lose their sense of modesty and boast of their successes, both real and imagined. They sometimes describe

feeling a change within themselves 'a great power inside me'. These changes in self regard can become delusional and are the most common form of delusion found in mania. However grandiose delusions are not specific to mania, occurring also in schizophrenic psychoses.

Sometimes the ideas of power and status are clearly delusional. Patients may describe themselves in grandiose ways such as 'the son of Zeus', 'Mrs King David'. In other cases the delusions are difficult to pin down in the patient's playfulness and rush of ideas. Patients occasionally act on their delusions; they may demand to be called by a title or even go to the palace to claim their rightful place on the throne. However distractibility often prevents such plans from being carried out.

Increased energy and activity

Patients may report that they have solved difficult, even insuperable problems and tackled numerous challenging tasks. However it is often apparent from the report of relatives that many projects have been started but few completed. Though there is an increase in energy, the coherence of activity is lost so that it becomes futile; examples are washing and rewashing the curtains and covering the house with wet drapes. The night-time activities in particular can become extremely disruptive for the family; Winokur et al (1969) reported this to be a common reason for presentation. Patients may start to run rather than walk, be unable to sit or stand still, and spend their time running purposelessly up and down the ward. They can report feeling incredibly strong and fit and that they feel little fatigue. Indeed, staff often tire before the patient. While death from exhaustion was reported in severe mania in the early part of the century, careful analysis of these cases suggests there may have been more obvious physical causes, such as infections (Derby 1933).

Increased talkativeness (pressure of speech)

Increased talkativeness is another facet of the pressure of activity. Patients often talk with little or no prompting and the pressure of speech may lead to them continuing to talk even when left alone. Speech is not only profuse but also loud, with patients bellowing and even screaming. Some sing at the top of their voices, others use foreign languages or phrases. There is an abundance of words as well as ideas so that common phrases, slang, puns and rhymes pepper the speech.

Interruption can be difficult and may provoke irritation. Ideas pass abruptly from one topic to another but the origin and flow of the ideas is usually apparent. These changes in speech can also be reflected in writing, both in quantity and style.

Flight of ideas

Flight of ideas is the characteristic thought disorder found in mania. There is digression from one idea to others similar or frequently associated with it, without regard to the goal of the original train of thought. Sudden changes in topic may also occur when the patient is distracted by his environment. Even when flight of ideas is severe it is generally distinguishable from the thought disorder of schizophrenia which appears more disorganized and 'ideationally fluid' (Solovay et al 1987). The thought disorder of mania was found to be extravagantly combinatory, with humour and flippancy. Formal schizophrenic-type thought disorder is uncommon in manic episodes (Jampala et al 1989).

The example below is from a patient who was telephoned at home; the goals of his speech are continually lost as he is distracted either by connected ideas or what is happening in his flat.

> It's 9:45 for the telephone therapy, telephone therapy's the best in the world. People are cleaning up the house, working very hard, there's Flash on the floor, the dog doesn't like Flash. There's a flash in my eye as I'm looking at the trees, there's not much oxygen from the trees. There's water on the floor, *agua*. Run the water, don't block the sink.

Astrup et al (1959) found that flight of ideas was the commonest type of disturbed thinking in manic depressives but was extremely rare in schizophrenics. Racing thoughts are generally considered to be the subjective experience of flight of ideas; this has also been described in depressive states by Kraepelin and more recently by Braden & Ho (1981). Manic patients may describe their thoughts as 'teeming', and feel their head to be 'full of thoughts'. In mania, although the thoughts are racing they are generally progressive, in contrast to the picture in depression where the same thoughts are often going round and round.

Decreased need for sleep

A reduced need for sleep was experienced by all of our patients during a manic swing. It appears to be a qualitatively different experience from sleep loss in depression, which is rarely welcomed by the subject. Small amounts of sleep are experienced as refreshing and patients may not sleep for several days in a row. One of our patients described this as 'becoming a 24-hour person'. The universality of this symptom and its presence in the early or prodromal period make it a useful early-warning sign to patients and their families. It has also been found that sleep deprivation can precipitate mania in susceptible subjects and this has been suggested as the precipitating mechanism in puerperal mania (Wehr et al 1987). Symptomatic treatment of sleep loss in the early stages may be a useful treatment strategy.

Decreased attention

Decreased attention span both to internal and external cues may underlie the thought disorder found in mania. It is not thought that there is any serious disorder of perceptive processes but that the patient digresses with uncommon ease to any fresh stimulus. This distractibility, along with increased energy, explains much of the change which is observed in speech and activity.

Loss of inhibitions

A lack of normal critical sense is another hallmark of mania. Kraepelin illustrated his passage on mania with a picture of a man with both a pipe and a cigar in his mouth! Clothing may be inappropriately garish and bright; patients may wear vivid make-up and bedeck themselves with jewellery and other unusual forms of decoration. In the more severe states, patients become unkempt and dishevelled as they find no time for self-care.

Patients are frequently overfamiliar, talking to complete strangers to whom they may make inappropriate sexual and personal comments. They may demand preferential treatment because they are so busy and important and are easily irritated when their unreasonable demands are not met. Some spend lots of money, or give away their earnings in an extravagant gesture. The spending power now available with credit cards can rapidly lead to financial difficulties. Patients have been known to fly abroad or frequent places of ill-repute that they would normally avoid. It is not uncommon for manic patients to make public spectacles of themselves. Winokur et al (1969) found hypersexuality in 65% of his sample but noted that promiscuity was not common and that sexual activity was generally appropriately directed. Unwanted pregnancy can occur in a setting of hypersexuality due to lack of contraceptive caution.

Aggression is a common feature of mania and is generally related to being thwarted or restrained but can at times be gratuitous. Patients can be quick to take offence and may react with outbursts of rage, violence and destructiveness.

Psychotic symptoms

In our series, 47 of the 68 patients, when manic, were either deluded (29) or hallucinating (6) or both (12) (we excluded patients diagnosed as schizoaffective). A similar proportion (48%) of patients were deluded in the series of Winokur et al (1969). Leff et al (1976) found that 57% of the UK- and Danish-born samples they studied were psychotic, but this occurred more commonly in immigrants (94%). Manic patients are more likely to show psychotic features than those admitted with depression (Black & Nasrallah 1989).

Most commonly, the delusions in mania are grandiose, but paranoid delusions may also occur. Astrup et al (1959) reported that delusions of persecution were less common in manic depressives (half of whom were unipolar) than in schizophrenics, but did occur in 13%. Paranoid delusions may be an early symptom of mania and this should be considered in the differential diagnosis of patients presenting with paranoid ideas. Astrup found that manic-depressive patients with paranoid delusions had a poorer prognosis. Winokur reported that 35% of patients with a mixture of depression and elation had depressive delusions.

In mania the delusions tend not to be as fixed and persistent as in schizophrenia. It is often difficult to be sure of the fixed false nature of an idea when the patient presents it in a jocular, swaggering manner.

Auditory hallucinations were the most common type of hallucination in Astrup's series occurring in 40%. The incidence in manic-depression was again lower than in schizophrenia. Winokur reported a rate of 21% and noted that these occurred in the most severely manic group. Auditory hallucinations often reflect the prevailing delusions and may be grandiose. One of our patients heard a voice across the courtyard saying 'you've got class'. Another described a chorus in the sky singing hymns. Visual changes may occur, these range from the experience of the world as having 'an increased brightness' to complex visual imagery; 'a volcanic island surrounded by a turquoise sea'. Clear visual hallucinations are unusual and organic states should be considered when they occur.

Frequency of symptoms

Winokur et al (1969) reported on the frequency of symptoms in 61 patients who were consecutively admitted to hospital for mania. They found that all of the patients were overactive, and that 90% or more were sleeping less and overtalkative. In our own study, based on a structured interview of 68 patients, we found that nearly half (32/68) had experienced all seven of the criteria in RDC. As Winokur points out, while there are advantages to selecting consecutive patients, there is a bias towards those with frequent relapses of sufficient severity to warrant admission. Table 2.2 shows the frequency of the individual symptoms in the two studies.

Table 2.2   Frequency of symptoms present in mania (percentage)

	Winokur et al	Hunt & Silverstone
Elevated or irritable mood	98/85	100
Increased energy and activity	100	100
Decreased attention	100	90
Increased talkativeness	99	100
Flight of ideas or racing thoughts	93	81
Decreased need for sleep	90	100
Inflated self regard (may be delusional)	86	74
Loss of inhibitions	75 (sexual only)	100

Such studies suggest that the individual symptoms of mania are intimately related to each other. This has been confirmed in a cluster analysis of psychiatric syndromes, in which the manic cluster and paranoid schizophrenia were the most robust (Everitt et al 1971). Not only is the clinical picture relatively consistent across patients, but recurrent episodes are often similar both in phenomenology and course.

Personality

The difference from usual self (Hudgens et al 1967) coming on over a short period of time is one of the hallmarks of mania. In general, however the personalities of subjects between episodes appear much more normal than is the case in schizophrenia. Astrup et al (1959) noted that, in contrast to schizophrenia, a change of personality was not a prodromal symptom of manic depression. A proportion of bipolar patients experience subsyndromal mood swings (cyclothymia) both before the onset of their first major affective episode and between episodes. Fichtner et al (1989) found marked cyclothymia in 70% of 27 bipolars between episodes but also found a similar proportion in schizophrenics.

The presence of 'negative symptoms' such as affective flattening, loss of volition and decreased sociability, which are often found among patients with schizophrenia, are not common among euthymic bipolars (Montague et al 1989).

Onset

Sclare & Creed (1990) reported that the three most common initial symptoms were increased activity, reduced sleep and elated mood. The time between onset and admission was found to vary from 2 days to more than 4 months. Though the prodromal period is hard to define it is often clear that mania can have a rapid onset, especially when it follows a switch from depression. Molnar et al (1988) reported a mean of 20 days between onset and peak severity of mania. Post et al (1981) reported that those with a rapid onset tended to have a poorer prognosis.

Pattern of illness

Approximately 50% of the patients in our series presented with mania as their first episode while the remainder had experienced a previous episode of major depression. Similar figures have been obtained in other studies – 61% in the study by Winokur et al (1969). Winokur also reported that 50% of the manic episodes (including recurrences) that he observed were immediately preceded by depression. Though the majority of patients experience both manic and depressive episodes, some are only afflicted by mania. An out-patient study of bipolar patients found that 16% had never been treated for depression (Nurnberger et al 1979). Evidence from clinical and family studies suggests that unipolar mania should not be considered a separate entity from bipolar disorder (Pfohl et al 1982).

A third of patients end their episode of mania with a switch into depression. This is more common in those patients with a prior history of depression and a family history of affective disorder (Lucas· et al 1989). Following recovery from an episode of mania the next episode is as likely to be depression as mania (Petterson 1977).

Dunner & Fieve (1974) coined the term 'rapid cyclers' for those patients who experienced more than four affective episodes in a year, not necessarily separated by a symptom-free interval. They found 13% of their bipolar outpatients were rapid cyclers. In our series only three patients (4%) fulfilled the criteria for rapid cycling. The most commonly reported associated factors in rapid cycling are use of antidepressants (Wehr & Goodwin 1987) and hypothyroidism, both clinical and biochemical (Bauer et al 1990). Apart from cycle length there are no other particular clinical features which distinguish it from other forms of bipolar disorder.

Time course

Kraepelin (1921) described episodes of mania lasting a few days but stated that the majority lasted several months. He also recognized that, despite an episode lasting a long time, 'one could still hope with great probability for complete restoration of health'. Bratfos & Haug (1968) reporting on a population admitted in the 1950s stated that 8/9 episodes of mania lasted less than 7 months. More recently Keller (1988) reported that 64% recovered within 8 weeks, and 83% within a year. This was faster than patients with pure depressive or mixed/cycling episodes. Interest in chronic mania has waned over the century (Hare 1981). In our own study there were no patients who persistently filled the criteria for mania for more than 5 consecutive months. It may be that chronic manics are now classified as rapid cyclers, having more than four episodes per year, or that they exhibit persistent symptoms but not the entire syndrome. Alternatively, those patients with chronic and therefore severe mania may be included among the schizoaffective group.

SYMPTOMATOLOGY IN RELATED CONDITIONS

Schizomania

Definitions of mania generally exclude those patients with schizophrenic symptoms, such as third-person auditory hallucinations and passivity experiences. Data from the clinical course and family history has been used to determine whether schizomania should be considered as nosologically closer to bipolar disorder or schizophrenia (Kendell 1985). Kraepelin's view that the main differentiation should be made on the longitudinal course of the illness has clinical relevance. There is evidence to suggest that schizomania runs a course of relapse and remission which is either similar to bipolar disorder (Maj 1985, Pope et al 1980) or at least better prognostically than schizophrenia (Levinson & Levitt 1987). Taylor & Abrams (1973) described 52 patients with an admission diagnosis other than mania, mainly schizophrenia. However they all fulfilled research criteria for mania but in addition experienced auditory hallucinations, had first-rank symptoms of Schneider or displayed catatonia. These patients were similar to bipolars in gender distribution, age of onset, family history and treatment response. The authors concluded that first-rank symptoms of schizophrenia are not diagnostically decisive when manic symptoms are present. As in classical mania the phenomenology appears to be stable between episodes (Brockington et al 1980).

Family studies suggest that schizomanics with a mainly affective course have similar family histories to other affective disorder patients (both bipolar and unipolar) (Gershon et al 1982). These lines of evidence suggest that schizomania may be a severe from of mania, though schizoaffective patients are clearly a heterogenous group, both in their illness and the way they have been defined (Maj 1989). The Research Diagnostic Criteria distinguish between schizoaffective patients who are mainly affective and those who are mainly schizophrenic. The latter group have persistent schizophrenic symptoms between their mood swings.

Hypomania

Hypomania is the mild variant of mania and is generally defined by the severity of incapacity, though some use the term for non-psychotic mania. Symptoms are the same as in mania but of lesser severity. Inflated self esteem and elevation of mood are common, but patients may not have a change in sleep pattern. They may claim an increased facility for work but this is often dogged by distractability and irritability.

While there are no specific features of hypomania, there is some evidence of the stability of this diagnosis over time. Recurrent episodes of hypomania and depression without any episodes of mania has been termed bipolar II illness (Coryell et al 1989).

Cyclothymia

Cyclothymia denotes the recurrent experience of some of the symptoms of mania and depression where the episodes do not meet the criteria for the full syndromes of mania or depression. Cyclothymia is classified in RDC as a personality disorder but in DSM-IIIR as an affective disorder. This latter categorization particularly reflects the research of Akiskal, who has linked cyclothymia to bipolar affective disorder (Akiskal et al 1983). There are no specific symptoms of cyclothymia that are not features of the major affective disorders. The term hyperthymia is sometimes used to describe those patients who persistently exhibit elevation of mood but not the full manic or hypomanic syndromes.

MANIA IN PARTICULAR PATIENT GROUPS

Postnatal women

Manic symptoms are common among women who develop a psychiatric illness severe enough to warrant admission soon after childbirth. Meltzer & Kumar (1985) found that 33% of puerperal admissions with an onset within 2 weeks of childbirth could be diagnosed as manic. Brockington et al (1981) reported that 30% of puerperal psychoses could be classified as manic and a further 13% schizomanic.

Confusion can be an additional symptom in puerperal mania (Brockington et al 1981). Kadrmas et al (1979) found that while Schneiderian symptoms were more common in puerperal mania than mania at other times, the prognosis was better. However Platz & Kendell (1988) found the prognosis for puerperal mania to be no better. Bipolars who have children are clearly at considerable risk of relapse in the puerperium, but relapse is by no means inevitable (Winokur 1988). Many women who experience manic or depressive episodes outside the postpartum period have had their first affective episode in the puerperium. This was the case for 45% of the parous women in our series.

The mentally handicapped

Mania can occur in mental handicap, but there are difficulties in making the diagnosis. Periodic changes in behaviour, with increased vocalization, activity and aggression, raise the possibility of bipolar disorder. A review of the literature found that mentally handicapped patients could be identified as being manic using the symptomatology of DSM-III (Sovner & Hurley 1983). The presence of a family history of affective disorder is common and treatment with lithium can be beneficial (Rivinus & Harmatz 1979). A seasonal pattern of relapse may give a clue to the diagnosis (Arumainayagam & Kumar 1990).

Children

That bipolar disorder can occur in adolescence is clear, but the status of mania in younger children is less so (British Medical Journal 1979). There are reports of manic symptoms in children as a distinct change in behaviour rather than a persistent hyperactivity (Varanka et al 1988) and a literature review of psychotic prepubertal children using the DSM-III criteria suggested that about 20% could be considered manic (Weller et al 1986). Whether this leads to adult bipolar disorder is uncertain. It is unusual to find a history of onset occurring before the age of 15 among adult bipolar patients (Joyce 1984, Angst et al 1973).

The elderly

Shulman & Post (1980) studied the case notes of 67 elderly patients with mania. While they did not compare the symptomatology with that in a younger group they found that these patients did fulfil the criteria of Feighner et al (1972) for mania, suggesting a similar clinical picture. Two other case note studies found the classical symptoms of mania to be present in the elderly (Glasser & Rabins 1984, Yassa et al 1988).

Organic factors are more common in the elderly and genetic factors less prominent. In the series of Shulman & Post (1980) a quarter had evidence of cerebral organic impairment. Similar findings were reported by Stone (1989), who found a short-term memory loss to be the most common clinical sign of organic impairment; a small proportion went on to develop dementia within 3 years.

ASSESSMENT

A full assessment of mania, once the diagnosis is made, should take into account the precipitants and risks associated with the condition as well as the severity.

Precipitants

Medication

Rapid cessation of treatment with prophylactic lithium

can precipitate relapse within 2–3 weeks after discontinuation (Mander & London 1988).

Whether antidepressants are responsible for switches from depression into mania is still disputed, as it has been difficult to separate out the natural occurrence of mania following depression from the effects of antidepressant treatment (Wehr et al 1987). Antidepressant treatment, particularly with monoamine reuptake inhibitors, has also been implicated in the genesis of rapid cycling. In a study of 51 rapid-cycling patients, 73% had been taking antidepressants at the time of onset of rapid cycling, and in 50% the cycling stopped or slowed when these drugs were withdrawn (Wehr et al 1988).

Life events

Retrospective case note studies have suggested that life events play a role in precipitating a manic episode, particularly the first attack (Ambelas 1979, Leff et al 1976). In a study where the effects of a hurricane on bipolar patients were examined, the relapsers were noted to have been less stable clinically prior to the hurricane (Aronson & Shukla 1987). However a recent study (Sclare & Creed 1990) using a sophisticated life-event instrument did not find an increased rate of events occurring prior to relapse compared to the 6 months after recovery.

Illicit drug use

Use of drugs such as amphetamines can either mimic mania or precipitate it in bipolar patients (Silverstone & Cookson 1982). Anabolic steroids in the large doses used by athletes and body-builders can also result in mood changes, and occasionally produce frank mania in people who have not experienced mania outside this situation (Pope & Katz 1988).

Physical disorders

Assessment of a manic patient is not complete without consideration of the numerous physical disorders that can lead to a full manic syndrome (Krauthammer & Klerman 1978). Mania occurring after physical disorders has been termed 'secondary mania'. The phenomenology of secondary mania may include confusion, but this is not invariable. The presence of organic factors is common in the elderly (Stone 1989). Robinson et al (1988) found that when mania occurred after brain injury, involvement of the right hemisphere was the most common site.

Season

Kraepelin noted that some of his patients showed a seasonal pattern to their illness, many becoming depressed in the autumn and winter and improving in the summer. Admission rates for mania in a number of countries show a seasonal variation with a peak in spring or summer. It is not known whether it is day length, amount of sunshine or another climatic variable which is important in determining such seasonal variation (Silverstone & Romans-Clarkson 1989).

Risk

Manic episodes can lead to serious social and financial consequences with loss of employment, divorce and debt (Carlson et al 1974). The best guide to the likelihood of such events occurring during a particular manic episode is what happened in previous episodes. Admission should be considered if the costs of previous episodes have been high. Information should always be sought from relatives and close friends as that from the patient may be unreliable, particularly when insight is lacking.

Though aggression is common, serious crimes of violence are not. Petterson (1977) noted that there was no evidence of an increased criminality among bipolars when compared to the general population in Sweden. However, in a study of patients admitted to hospital by court order, manics constituted one third of all those suffering from affective disorder (Gibbens & Robertson 1983).

Tsuang (1978) in his follow up of the Iowa 500 found that suicide accounted for 11% of the deaths in the manic group, at least five times that of the controls. In another study Black et al (1978) found the main suicide risk to be in those bipolars with an index admission for depression. It is likely that suicide usually occurs during periods of depression. Suicidal thoughts do occur in mania when there are also depressive features; Winokur et al (1969) report a figure of 7% for this. Serious injury occasionally occurs due to misapprehension of risks or as a result of grandiose ideas. One of our patients lost an arm and part of a leg when he thought he was fast enough to outrun a train.

Rating scales

Monitoring change in the severity of the manic disturbance can be useful both clinically and for research on therapeutic interventions. The Brief Psychiatric Rating Scale (Overall & Gorham 1962) is a general psychopathology scale which rates some of the symptoms that occur in mania, such as excitement, hostility and grandiosity. Although this scale is useful in many types of study on inpatients, more specific scales have been devised for assessment of mania. Unlike the depression rating scales, which focus on subjective experience, manic scales concentrate on rating behaviour. All the scales discussed below have shown good validity and reliability; indeed reliability is generally better in manic than in depressive rating scales.

Beigel et al (1971) designed a scale for use by the nursing staff, consisting of 26 items, though only 11 of them were found to correlate well with global measures. Petterson et al (1973) published a seven-item interview scale for use by physicians. Bech & Rafaelsen (Bech et al 1979) and Young et al (1978) constructed 11-item clinician rated scales based on the earlier work. These two scales include items on mood, activity, speech, aggression, sleep, sexual interest and insight; the Young scale also has an item on appearance. Severity of each symptom is scored on a 0–4 scale, except that in the Young scale the four items on irritability, delusions, aggression and pressure of speech are rated up to 8.

For most purposes the Bech & Rafaelson or the Young Scales are adequate, though for more detailed assessment of symptomatology there is the larger 28-item scale devised by Blackburn et al (1977). This scale includes specific items on hallucinations, persecutory ideas and religiosity as well as rating depression and emotional lability. Physician-rated scales generally relate to a short period of observation; there can be advantages in nurse-rated scales which take into account behaviour throughout the day. The mania rating scale of Beigel et al (1971) has been adapted by Brierley et al (1988), who produced a nine-item behaviour rating scale to be completed by the nursing staff which is related to the entire period of observation. Behaviours rated include overactivity, overtalkativeness and disinhibition as well as mood items on irritability and elation. This scale was found to have good reliability and validity when compared to the Young scale.

REFERENCES

Akiskal H S, Hirschfeld R M, Yerevanian B I 1983 The relationship of personality to affective disorders. Archives of General Psychiatry 40: 801–810

Ambelas A 1979 Psychologically stressful events in the precipitation of manic episodes. British Journal of Psychiatry 135: 15–21.

American Psychiatric Association 1987 Diagnostic and statistical manual of mental disorders (3rd edn.—revised) American Psychiatric Association, Washington, DC

Angst J, Baastrup P, Grof P, Hippius H, Poldinger W, Weis P 1973 The course of monopolar depression and bipolar psychoses. Psychiatrica Neurologica et Neurochirugica 76: 489–500

Aronson T A, Shukla S 1987 Life events and relapse in bipolar disorder: the impact of a catastrophic event. Acta Psychiatrica Scandinavica 75: 571–576

Arumainayagam M, Kumar A 1990 Manic-depressive psychosis in a mentally handicapped person. British Journal of Psychiatry 156: 886–889

Astrup C, Fossum A, Holmboe R 1959 A follow-up study of 270 patients with acute affective psychoses. Acta Psychiatrica et Neurologica Scandinavica 34 (suppl 135)

Bauer M S, Whybrow P C, Winokur A 1990 Rapid cycling bipolar affective disorder. Archives of General Psychiatry 47: 427–432

Bech P, Bolwig T G, Kramp P, Rafaelson O J 1979 The Bech—Rafaelsen mania scale and the Hamilton depression scale. Acta Psychiatrica Scandinavica 59: 420–430

Beigel A, Murphy D L, Bunney W 1971 The manic-state rating scale. Archives of General Psychiatry 25: 256–262

Black D W, Nasrallah A 1989 Hallucinations and delusions in 1715 patients with unipolar and bipolar affective disorders. Psychopathology 22: 28–34

Black D W, Winokur G, Nasrallah A 1987 Suicide in subtypes of major affective disorder. Archives of General Psychiatry 44: 878–880

Blackburn I M, Loudon J B, Ashworth C 1977 A new scale for measuring mania. Psychological Medicine 7: 453–458

Braden W, Ho C K 1981 Racing thoughts in psychiatric inpatients. Archives of General Psychiatry 38: 71–75

Bratfos O, Haug J O 1968 The course of manic-depressive psychosis. Acta Psychiatrica Scandinavica 44: 89–112

Brierley C E, Szabadi E, Rix K J, Bradshaw C 1988 The Manchester nurse rating scales for the daily simultaneous assessment of depressive and manic ward behaviours. Journal of Affective Disorders 15: 45–54

British Medical Journal 1979 Manic states in affective disorders of childhood and adolescence (editorial). British Medical Journal 1: 214–215

Brockington I F, Wainwright S, Kendall R E 1980 Manic patients with schizophrenic or paranoid symptoms. Psychological Medicine 10: 73–83

Brockington I, Cernik K, Schofield E et al 1981 Puerperal psychosis. Archives of General Psychiatry 38: 829–833

Carlson G A, Kotin J, Davenport Y B, Adland M 1974 Follow up of 53 bipolar manic-depressive patients. British Journal of Psychiatry 124: 134–139

Coryell W, Keller M, Endicott J, Andreasen N, Clayton P, Hirschfeld R 1989 Bipolar II Illness: course and outcome over a five-year period. Psychological Medicine 19: 129–141

Derby I M 1933 Manic-depressive 'exhaustion' deaths. Psychiatry Quarterly 7: 436–449

Dunner D L, Fieve R R 1974 Clinical factors in lithium carbonate prophylaxis failure. Archives of General Psychiatry 30: 229–233

Everitt B S, Gourlay A J, Kendell R E 1971 An attempt at validation of traditional psychiatric syndromes by cluster analysis. British Journal of Psychiatry 119: 399–412

Feighner J, Robins E, Guze S, Woodruff R A, Winokur G, Munoz R 1972 Diagnostic criteria for use in psychiatric research. Archives of General Psychiatry 31: 665–672

Fichtner C G, Grossman L S, Harrow M, Goldberg J F, Klein D N 1989 Cyclothymic mood swings in the course of affective disorders and schizophrenia. American Journal of Psychiatry 146: 1149–1154

Gershon E S, Hamovit J, Guroff J J et al 1982 A family study of schizoaffective, bipolar I, bipolar II, unipolar and normal control probands. Archives of General Psychiatry 39: 1157–1167

Glasser M, Rabins P 1984 Mania in the elderly. Age and Ageing 13: 210–213

Gibbens T C, Robertson G 1983 A survey of the criminal careers of hospital order patients. British Journal of Psychiatry 143: 362–369

Hare E 1981 The two manias: a study of the evolution of the modern concept of mania. British Journal of Psychiatry 138: 89–99

Hudgens R W, Morrison J R, Barcha R G 1967 Life events and onset of primary affective disorders. Archives of General Psychiatry 16: 134–145

Jampala V C, Taylor M A, Abrams R 1989 The diagnostic implications of formal thought disorder in mania and schizophrenia: a reassessment. American Journal of Psychiatry 146: 459–463

Joyce P R 1984 Age of onset in bipolar affective disorder and misdiagnosis as schizophrenia. Psychological Medicine 14: 145–149

Kadrmas A, Winokur G, Crowe R 1979 Postpartum mania. British Journal of Psychiatry 135: 551–554

Keller M B 1988 The course of manic depressive illness. Journal of Clinical Psychiatry 49 (suppl 11): 4–7

Keller M B, Lavori P W, Coryell W et al 1986 Differential outcome of pure manic, mixed/cycling and pure depressive episodes in patients with bipolar illness. Journal of the American Medical Association 255: 3138–3142

Kendell R E 1985 The diagnosis of mania. Journal of Affective Disorders 8: 207–213

Kraepelin E 1921 Manic-depressive insanity and paranoia (trans. Barclay R M). E & S Livingstone, Edinburgh

Krauthammer C, Klerman G 1978 Secondary mania. Archives of General Psychiatry 35: 1333–1339

Leff J P, Fischer M, Bertelsen A 1976 A cross-national epidemiological study of mania. British Journal of Psychiatry 129: 428–442

Leonhard Von K, Korff I, Schulz H 1962 Die Temperamente in den Familien der monopolaren und bipolaren phäsischen Psychosen. Psychiatrica et Neurologica 143: 416–434

Lerner Y 1980 The subjective experience of mania. In: Belmaker R H, van Praag H M (eds) Mania: an evolving concept. MTP Press, Lancaster

Levinson D F, Levitt M E 1987 Schizoaffective mania reconsidered. American Journal of Psychiatry 144: 415–425

Lucas C P, Rigby J C, Lucas S B 1989 The occurrence of depression following mania. British Journal of Psychiatry 154: 705–708

Maj M 1985 Clinical course and outcome of schizoaffective disorders. Acta Psychiatrica Scandinavica 72: 542–550

Maj M 1989 A family study of two subgroups of schizoaffective patients. British Journal of Psychiatry 154: 640–643

Mander A J, Loudon J B 1988 Rapid recurrence of mania following abrupt discontinuation of lithium. Lancet 2 July: 15–17

Meltzer E S, Kumar R 1985 Puerperal mental illness, clinical features and classification: a study of 142 mother and baby admissions. British Journal of Psychiatry 147: 647–654

Molnar G, Feeney M G, Fava G A 1988 Duration and symptoms of bipolar prodromes. American Journal of Psychiatry 145: 1576–1578

Montague L R, Tantam D, Newby D, Thomas P, Ring N 1989 The incidence of negative symptoms in early schizophrenia, mania and other psychoses. Acta Psychiatrica Scandinavica 79: 613–618

Nurnberger J, Roose S P, Dunner D L, Fieve R R 1979 Unipolar mania: a distinct clinical entity? American Journal of Psychiatry 136: 1420–1423

Overall J E, Gorham D R 1962 The brief psychiatric rating scale. Psychological Reports 10: 799–812

Perris C 1966 A study of bipolar (manic-depressive) and unipolar recurrent depressive psychoses. Acta Psychiatrica Scandinavica (suppl 194)

Petterson U 1977 Manic-depressive illness: a clinical, social and genetic study. Acta Psychiatrica Scandinavica (suppl 269)

Petterson U, Fyro B, Sedval G 1973 A new scale for the longitudinal rating of manic states. Acta Psychiatrica Scandinavica 49: 248–256

Pfohl B, Vasquez N, Nasrallah H 1982 Unipolar vs bipolar mania: a review of 247 patients. British Journal of Psychiatry 141: 453–458

Platz C, Kendell R E 1988 A matched-control follow-up and family study of 'puerperal psychoses'. British Journal of Psychiatry 153: 90–94

Pope H G, Katz D L 1988 Affective and psychotic symptoms associated with anabolic steroid use. American Journal of Psychiatry 145: 487–490

Pope H G, Lipinski J F, Cohen B M, Axelrod D T 1980 'Schizoaffective disorder': an invalid diagnosis? American Journal of Psychiatry 137: 921–927

Post R M, Ballenger J C, Rey A C, Bunney W E 1981 Slow and rapid onset of manic episodes: implications for underlying biology. Psychiatry Research 4: 229–237

Post R M, Rubinow D R, Uhde T W et al 1989 Dysphoric mania. Archives of General Psychiatry 46: 353–358

Robinson R G, Boston J D, Starkstein S E, Price T R 1988 Comparison of mania and depression after brain injury: causal factors. American Journal of Psychiatry 145: 172–178

Rivinus T M, Harmatz J S 1979 Diagnosis and lithium treatment of affective disorder in the retarded: five case studies. American Journal of Psychiatry 136: 551–554

Sclare P, Creed F 1990 Life events and the onset of mania. British Journal of Psychiatry 156: 508–514

Secunda S K, Swann A, Katz M M, Koslow S H, Croughan J, Chang S 1987 Diagnosis and treatment of mixed mania. American Journal of Psychiatry 144: 96–98

Shulman K, Post F 1980 Bipolar affective disorder in old age. British Journal of Psychiatry 136: 26–32

Silverstone T, Cookson J 1982 The biology of mania. In: Granville-Grossman K (ed) Recent advances in clinical psychiatry 4. Churchill Livingstone, Edinburgh

Silverstone T, Romans-Clarkson S 1989 Bipolar affective disorder: causes and prevention of relapse. British Journal of Psychiatry 154: 321–335

Solovay M R, Shenton M E, Holzman P S 1987 Comparative studies of thought disorders. Archives of General Psychiatry 44: 13–20

Sovner R, Hurley A D 1983 Do the mentally retarded suffer from affective illness? Archives of General Psychiatry 40: 61–67

Spitzer R, Endicott J, Robins E 1978 Research Diagnostic Criteria: rationale and reliability. Archives of General Psychiatry 35: 773–782

Stone K 1989 Mania in the elderly. British Journal of Psychiatry 155: 220–224

Taylor M A, Abrams R 1973 The phenomenology of mania. Archives of General Psychiatry 29: 520–522

Tsuang M T 1978 Suicide in schizophrenics, manics, depressives and surgical controls. Archives of General Psychiatry 35: 153–155

Varanka T M, Weller R A, Weller E B, Fristad M A 1988 Lithium treatment of manic episodes with psychotic features in prepubertal children. American Journal of Psychiatry 145: 1557–1559

Wehr T A, Goodwin F K 1987 Can antidepressants cause mania and worsen the course of affective illness? American Journal of Psychiatry 144: 1403–1411

Wehr T A, Sack D A Rosenthal N E 1987 Sleep reduction as a final common pathway in the genesis of mania. American Journal of Psychiatry 144: 201–204

Wehr T A, Sack D A, Rosenthal N E, Cowdry R W 1988 Rapid cycling affective disorder: contributing factors and treatment responses in 51 patients. American Journal of Psychiatry 145: 179–184

Weller R A, Weller E B, Tucker S G, Frista d M A 1986 Mania in prepubertal children: has it been underdiagnosed? Journal of Affective Disorders 11: 151–154

Winokur G 1988 Postpartum mania. British Journal of Psychiatry 153: 843–844

Winokur G, Clayton P, Reich T 1969 Manic depressive illness. C V Mosby, St Louis

Yassa R, Nair V, Nastase C, Camille Y, Belzile L 1988 Prevalence of bipolar disorder in a psychogeriatric population. Journal of Affective Disorders 14: 197–201

Young R C, Biggs J T, Ziegler V E, Meyer D A 1978 A rating scale for mania: reliability, validity and sensitivity. British Journal of Psychiatry 133: 429–435

3. Concepts, diagnosis and classification

William M. Grove   Nancy C. Andreasen

The concept of affective disorder is historically very old (see Chapter 4). Our modern system of classification comes chiefly from Kahlbaum and Kraepelin. Kahlbaum coined the terms 'dysthymia' (a chronic form of melancholia) and 'cyclothymia' (a disorder characterized by a fluctuating mood; Kahlbaum 1863). Kraepelin (1921) worked out a comprehensive system for classifying psychoses which drew on concepts developed by his predecessors. In the Kraepelinian synthesis, all disorders were seen as discrete. 'Melancholia' was retained to refer only to episodes in the elderly. Depressive disorders occurring in younger patients were named 'manic-depressive illness'. Manic-depressive illness was distinguished from the other psychotic disorder which occurs in younger patients, dementia praecox, on the basis of course, age and type of onset, heredity, presumed aetiology and clinical symptoms.

Kraepelin recognized that many depressed patients were prone to cycle into mania and therefore unified mania and depression into 'manic-depressive illness'. This illness tended to be relatively severe, episodic, recurrent, having a good prognosis and a full *restitutio ad integrum* between episodes. Since then, other complementary or competing systems have been developed, often in an attempt to account for mild, chronic or diagnostically confusing depressive syndromes.

DELINEATING AFFECTIVE DISORDERS

The concept of affective disorder has involved some longstanding controversies, including whether depression is a disease which strikes people or an understandable response to an unhappy situation; the relationship between states of elation and depression; the number and nature of kinds of depression. These issues have not been fully resolved and they represent major issues confronting the affective disorders nosologist. They may be summarized as two basic questions: 1) What are the limits of the affective disorders? 2) What methods for subtyping affective disorder, especially depression, are most useful?

Finding limits to affective disorders involves deciding on boundaries with normality on the one hand and with other disorders on the other hand.

The boundaries between depression and normality

There is currently controversy about when a normal fluctuation in mood becomes depression. Some investigators define depression quite broadly and view it as a constellation of characteristic symptoms seen on interview or self-report. When these symptoms are present, even if they have been triggered by recent life events or have been relatively brief in duration, depression is considered to be present. This point of view is often used to argue that there is a high prevalence of 'undiagnosed depression' in the general population. Other investigators argue that such symptoms may constitute demoralization, simple unhappiness or bereavement (Frank 1973, Wing et al 1978, Clayton et al 1972). They attempt to exclude relatively mild, brief or situational disorders from the fold. Usually those who conceptualize depression narrowly are interested in delineating a disorder with a characteristic prognosis, course or aetiology. If they are researchers, they often wish to isolate homogeneous groups which may have some common (usually biological) basis.

Diagnostic criteria, structured interviews and computerized diagnostic systems represent efforts to demarcate depressions different from and more severe than demoralization, simple unhappiness or grief. Various examples of such approaches include the Present State Examination and its computerized system

CATEGO (Wing et al 1974), the criteria of Feighner et al (1972), the Research Diagnostic Criteria (RDC) (Spitzer et al 1978), DSM-IIIR (American Psychiatric Association 1987) and ICD-10 (World Health Organization 1990a). These systems attempt to narrow the concept of depression by requiring a specified number of depressive symptoms, usually four to six, which have been present for a specified time period, usually 2–4 weeks. Even when such approaches are used, some investigators worry that the definition is still too overinclusive to have either clinical utility in predicting treatment response or research utility in isolating homogeneous groups. In such cases, workers often turn to even narrower conceptualizations of depression and require that the disorder be endogenous, recurrent or incapacitating.

The distinction between mania and normality is usually much less difficult, as attested by the diagnostic reliability for mania being consistently higher than that for depression (Grove 1987). When one begins to speak of hypomania or cyclothymia, however, similar problems of demarcation arise. The solutions are usually the same as in the case of depression: the use of criteria and structured interviews. A psychometric approach has been taken by Depue (Depue et al 1981) with initially very favourable results.

The boundary between affective disorders and schizophrenia

This boundary is especially unclear. Many patients present with a clinical picture which combines affective and more typical schizophrenic symptoms (e.g. Schneiderian first-rank symptoms). The concept of schizoaffective disorder was first introduced by Kasanin (1933), who defined it as an acute psychosis with a mixture of schizophrenic and affective symptoms which was likely to have a relatively good prognosis.

Formerly, schizoaffective disorder was considered a type of schizophrenia. The relation of schizoaffective illnesses to the schizophrenias and to affective disorders was reviewed several times in the 1970s (Ollerenshaw 1973, Welner et al 1974, Procci 1976, Pope & Lipinski 1978), and it was often concluded that schizoaffective disorders ought to be moved entirely to within the affective illnesses. Although such reviews were useful, they tended to blur potentially distinct concepts like acute schizophrenia, good prognosis schizophrenia or episodic schizophrenia. Brockington & Leff (1979) reported that the concordance between extant research definitions of schizoaffective disorder was extremely poor, suggesting that data from different studies could only be pooled with great caution.

Several problems arise in the definition of schizoaffective disorder. First, investigators do not agree on whether it should be defined cross-sectionally or longitudinally. Cross-sectional definitions emphasize the simultaneous coexistence of both affective and schizophrenic symptoms. Longitudinal approaches emphasize both a mixture of symptoms and a characteristic course, typically one with acute onset and relatively complete remission. Each of these approaches has additional problems in definition. The cross-sectional approach must determine how long the symptoms must coexist and what to do with cases in which one type of symptom remits while the others persist for a relatively long period. For example, should a patient who continues to have bizarre delusions and hallucinations for 4 months after recovery from affective symptoms be considered to be schizophrenic, schizoaffective or to have some other diagnosis? Problems with the longitudinal approach involve those of getting a reliable history of mode of onset, quality of previous remissions and premorbid functioning level. The longitudinal approach is represented by DSM-IIIR (based solely on the relative durations of schizophrenic-like and affective syndromes, ignoring remissions and mode of onset), while the RDC and ICD-10 are primarily cross-sectional.

During the past decade the nosology of schizoaffective disorder, while still quite problematic, has been somewhat clarified by family and longitudinal studies. It seems useful to distinguish, following Van Eerdewegh et al (1987) and DSM-IIIR, between schizo-bipolar and schizo-unipolar disorders. This amounts to asking whether a given patient has ever had a clear-cut manic syndrome. On the whole, schizo-bipolar patients seem to have illnesses more similar to affective disorder than to schizophrenia (Clayton 1982). However, some patients even within the schizo-bipolar class can be found who have a more schizophrenia-like course. Patients with phenomenologically 'mainly schizophrenic' schizo-bipolar disorder have been found to have a worse outcome than those with ordinary bipolar illness (Levinson & Levitt 1987).

With regard to course and family history, schizo-unipolar patients appear to be a heterogeneous group lying on average between affective disorders and schizophrenia (Clayton 1982). They are probably more like schizophrenics in family history (Endicott et al 1986, Angst et al 1979), but have risks of schizophrenia in their relatives only about half of the magnitude of the relatives of those schizophrenics themselves.

There is still uncertainty about how to classify patients with unusual, mood-incongruent psychotic features who do not appear to have a chronic course. DSM-IIIR and ICD-10 classify them with the major affective disorders (*vide infra*), while the RDC places them under schizoaffective disorders.

The boundary between affective and anxiety disorders

This is another definitional issue as murky as schizo-affective disorder. The principal problems are those of phenomenological, diagnostic and aetiological (chiefly familial or genetic) overlaps between major depression, panic disorder and perhaps also generalized anxiety disorder. One particularly vexing problem is so-called 'comorbidity', i.e. patients garner two or more (often several) diagnoses, sometimes for what seem clinically to be facets of the same disorder. These problems are discussed in chapter 6.

BASIC CONTROVERSIES CONCERNING SYSTEMS OF CLASSIFICATION

The classification of affective disorders has served as the battleground for a number of key issues which also apply to psychiatric nosology in general. These include the following questions: Should the classification be categorical or dimensional? Should it be unitary, dichotomous, or multiple? What are the proper methods for determining the validity of a classification system?

Unitary versus multiple approaches

Aubrey Lewis (1938) was among the first to raise this issue in a convincing and troubling way. He suggested that the varying states of depression may form a continuum by stating that the various classifications 'are nothing more than attempts to distinguish between acute and chronic, mild and severe: and where two categories only are presented, the one—manic depressive — gives the characteristics of acute severe depression, the other of chronic mild depression.' Lewis's point of view implies that depression should be considered a unitary condition and should not be further subtyped. Kendell (1968, 1976, Kendell & Gourlay 1970) has been the most eloquent advocate of this position in more recent times; in the section below

on endogenous depression we discuss his ideas and data.

Advocates of subtyping depression have been many. Most of the popular subtypes are dichotomous: endogenous versus reactive, psychotic versus neurotic, primary versus secondary, bipolar versus unipolar and so on. Most of these dichotomous systems grow out of clinical experience and represent attempts to define subtypes which will predict outcome or response to treatment. In addition, attempts to develop classifications on a quantitative basis have also yielded several systems. These tend to be more complex than the clinical systems. For example, Paykel (1971), Overall et al (1966) and Andreasen & Grove (1982) have developed systems composed of three or four subtypes by using mathematical approaches such as factor analysis or cluster analysis. Such classifications will be discussed in more detail later in this chapter.

Even if Kendell's hypothesis that depression is a continuum is correct, it may nonetheless be useful to identify pseudosubtypes, for the same reason that it is useful to speak of some people as 'tall'. Employing category words need not imply reifying them. Investigators interested in identifying correlates of depression (e.g. genetic or neurochemical variation, treatment response) need to divide the broad category of depressive illness for study. Consequently, the search for meaningful subtypes is likely to continue.

Categorical versus dimensional approaches

The categorical versus dimensional controversy is related to the above controversy, but is distinct. It has been discussed and reviewed by Eysenck (1970) and Kendell (1976).

The typological approach conceptualizes psychiatric illnesses as discrete entities, sometimes mutually exclusive. For example, a patient cannot have both affective disorder and schizophrenia, nor can he fall somewhere between the two. The key questions are then: What are the proper classes? and How can we best assign class labels to illness episodes? This approach allies psychiatry to the so-called 'medical model' and assumes that specific diseases can be identified, with the ultimate goal of identifying aetiologies.

While not incompatible with either the medical model or a search for aetiology, the dimensional approach is more often used by investigators who work from a psychometric or empiric approach to classification. In its pure form, the dimensional approach stresses the use of a number of different descriptive dimensions or factors in characterizing patients. For example, a patient who presents with depressive symptoms might be evaluated on such dimensions as severity of symptoms, types of symptoms and underlying personality factors. If the dimensional approach were applied very broadly, then such factors as family history, life events and social supports might also be used to describe a given patient. The relationship between these factors or dimensions may be studied statistically through factor analysis, which may be used to reduce a large number of variables to a smaller, more workable set. Nevertheless, the major problem with dimensional approaches is their complexity. Because many dimensions are usually involved, this approach is difficult to apply clinically or even to use in research.

The validation of diagnostic groups

The ultimate test of any diagnostic system is its construct validity. Construct validity refers to the extent to which diagnostic category membership has consistent and meaningful relationships to measures of other constructs, as theory (e.g. aetiological theory) states it ought to. In construct validation, the underlying theory and measures of key theoretical constructs are tested at the same time.

Perhaps because construct validation requires a well-articulated theory, which we currently lack for psychopathology, most attempts to validate classification systems in psychiatry have emphasized aspects of predictive validity. Predictive validity assesses the degree to which various 'predictors', e.g. treatment outcome or family history, are differently associated with various subtypes of affective disorder. The validity of such subtypes, such as the bipolar — unipolar or endogenous — reactive distinction, has been explored through examining whether such groups respond to a specific treatment, such as electroconvulsive therapy or lithium. In addition, outcome and course variables are often explored, looking at such variables as frequency of recurrence and extent of remission. Investigators who explore these validity factors recognize, of course, that they are not foolproof: responses to specific therapies, for example, do not necessarily separate diseases. Many infectious diseases respond to penicillin and disorders as diverse as multiple sclerosis and psoriasis respond to corticosteroids.

Identifying a specific aetiology is the ultimate proof of any nosological category. In the case of affective disorders, as in most of psychiatry, questions abound but answers are few. Familial and genetic aspects have been examined, with conflicting findings about linkage. Other investigators have identified factors which may be associated with endogenous or severe depression, such as neuroendocrine or neurotransmitter abnormalities, but such findings have not been consistently replicated in different centres. We seem to be far from an aetiological classification of the affective disorders.

CLINICAL CLASSIFICATIONS OF AFFECTIVE DISORDER

Since no classification scheme has established ascendancy, several competing systems are currently in use. These may be divided into two groups: those used in clinical practice and those used in research. While this distinction is somewhat arbitrary and some research classifications are often used clinically, nevertheless these two approaches to classification tend to reflect different needs and therefore to arrive at different solutions to the various nosological issues described above. Clinical systems require adequate coverage. A place must be found for every patient who is seen. Consequently, the classes in clinical systems tend to be relatively broad and inclusive. On the other hand, researchers need to identify homogeneous groups and can usually afford to have large numbers of unclassified patients. During the past several decades, however, clinical and research systems have become more similar, due to the development of diagnostic criteria for the clinical systems.

Two major systems of classification are currently used clinically, the International Classification of Diseases (World Health Organization 1978) (ICD) and the third Diagnostic and Statistical Manual of the American Psychiatric Association, revised (1987) (DSM-IIIR). Both are currently under revision. ICD-10 (World Health Organization 1990a) is sufficiently crystalized that the final version (to be published in 1991 or 1992) should not differ much from the one summarized here. On the other hand, the deliberations of the DSM-IV mood disorders work group are not so far advanced, so we can only alert the reader to options being considered for DSM-IV (personal communication, Rush 1990).

ICD-10

Because it must be used by psychiatrists from all over the world, who represent a variety of conceptual backgrounds, and also because it must serve the needs

Table 3.1   Classification of affective disorders in ICD-10

F25 Schizoaffective disorders	Current episode mixed
Manic type	Currently in remission
Depressive type	**F32 Depressive episode**
Mixed type	Mild
F30 Manic episode	Without somatic symptoms
Hypomania	With somatic symptoms
Mania	Moderate
Without psychotic symptoms	Without somatic symptoms
With psychotic symptoms	With somatic symptoms
Mood-congruent versus incongruent psychotic symptoms	Severe
	Without psychotic symptoms
F31 Bipolar affective disorder	With psychotic symptoms
Current episode hypomanic	**F33 Recurrent depressive disorder**
Current episode manic	Current episode mild
Without psychotic symptoms	Current episode moderate
With psychotic symptoms	Current episode severe
Mood-congruent vs. incongruent psychotic symptoms	Without psychotic symptoms
	With psychotic symptoms
Current episode depressed	**F34 Persistent affective disorders**
Mild or moderate	Cyclothymia
Without somatic symptoms	Dysthymia
With somatic symptoms	
Severe	
Without psychotic symptoms	
With psychotic symptoms	

of patients in a variety of economic and social situations, ICD-10 provides an inclusive classification system. It resembles the RDC and DSM-IIIR in many ways, most notably in that it gives explicit diagnostic criteria. An additional system of research criteria is being developed in which the definitions are slightly more restrictive (World Health Organization 1990b).

In ICD-10, five categories (excluding schizoaffective disorder) are used to define the major forms of affective disorder. These form a four-level hierarchical tree requiring four digits for complete coding that subspecify the kind of affective disorder (see Table 3.1). The organizing principles of the hierarchy are that the most important variable is episode polarity (current and lifetime presence of mania versus depression versus both), then severity (mild/moderate versus severe), then, for severe depression, presence versus absence of psychotic symptoms and, for mild or moderate depression, presence of the somatic syndrome (endogenous or melancholic symptoms). In addition, optionally

psychotic symptoms can be specified as mood-congruent or -incongruent.

The concept of mania embodied in ICD-10 is quite similar to that in DSM-IIIR. By contrast, the ICD-10 and DSM-IIIR definitions of a depressive episode are more discrepant. ICD, in its draft research criteria, requires 'two of the following' (for mild or moderate) or all three of the following (for severe): 1) 'depressed mood . . . for most of the day and almost every day, largely uninfluenced by circumstances, . . . for at least two weeks'; 2) 'marked loss of interest or pleasure . . .'; 3) 'decreased energy and increased fatiguability' (italics added). At either threshold, this is stronger than the DSM, which requires only 'depressed mood most of the day nearly every day' or 'markedly diminished interest or pleasure'. ICD further requires two (for mild) or three (for moderate or severe) of the following: 4) loss of confidence and self-esteem; 5) 'unreasonable feelings of self-reproach or excessive and inappropriate guilt'; 6) suicidal thoughts, suicidal behaviour or recurrent thoughts of death; 7) trouble making decisions or concentrating; 8) agitation or retardation; 9) sleep disturbance; 10) *change* in appetite (italics added). (Quotations are used when the ICD definition of a symptom differs notably from DSM-IIIR.) The requirement of only two symptoms from 4)–10) will probably make mild depression in ICD-10 milder than DSM-IIIR major depression, although the requirement of at least two of 1)–3) might have a countervailing effect.

ICD-10 differentiates patients with and without what it calls 'somatic symptoms' or 'somatic syndrome'. The latter is used to qualify mild or moderate depressive episodes. It is relatively close to the RDC diagnostic subtype of endogenous depression. It consists of the presence of at least four of the following: 1) loss of interest or loss of pleasure; 2) lack of responsivity of the depressed mood to events or activities; 3) early morning awakening; 4) mood worse in mornings; 5) marked retardation or agitation; 6) marked loss of appetite; 7) loss of 5% or more of body weight in the past month; 8) marked loss of libido. As one can see, the concept of 'somatic syndrome' includes only cross-sectional symptoms, and ignores premorbid personality, response to treatments, and so on. In this it is like the RDC and DSM-III, but unlike the Newcastle group's concept of endogenous depression and unlike DSM-IIIR.

While the above gives a broad outline of the hierarchical scheme and the chief criteria, upon scanning Table 3.1 the reader will see that ICD-10 is actually not so simple as portrayed. In addition to polarity, severity and somatic syndrome, ICD-10 also classifies patients according to whether their illnesses are recurrent and by their duration of illness (episodic versus persistent affective disorders, i.e. cyclothymia, dysthymia).

The ICD category of schizoaffective disorder is for patients who, within the same episode of illness and simultaneously or within a few days of each other, in addition to a full affective syndrome of mania, depression or both, show definite schizophrenic symptoms. There is no requirement that the psychotic symptoms persist in the event of a remission of the affective symptoms, which makes this classification similar to the RDC and unlike DSM-IIIR.

DSM-IIIR and DSM-IV

The classification of affective disorders in DSM-IIIR is summarized in Table 3.2. Almost all affective disorders are grouped under a single heading.

Under DSM-IIIR as under ICD-10, an affective syndrome of depression or mania is diagnosed and then, depending on the lifetime history, the patient's illness is classified. In DSM-IIIR, there is no minimum duration required for a manic illness, but an option under consideration for DSM-IV is to return to the DSM-III requirement of 1 week's duration (any duration if hospitalized) or 3 days for hypomania (both durations being compatible with ICD-10).

Table 3.2   Classification of affective disorders in DSM-IIIR

Mood disorders

Bipolar disorders
  With mania
    Course: Manic, depressed, or mixed
    Features: With psychotic features
          Mood-congruent or -incongruent or without psychotic features
  Cyclothymia
  Not otherwise specified (e.g. hypomania, bipolar II)

Depressive disorders
  Major depression
    Course: Single episode or recurrent
    Features: With psychotic features
          Mood-congruent or -incongruent or without psychotic features
    Features: Melancholic type or not
    Features: With or without seasonal pattern
  Dysthymia
    Features: Early or late onset

Psychotic disorders not elsewhere classified

Schizo-affective disorder
  Course: Bipolar or depressive type

Adjustment disorders

With depressed or anxious mood or mixed emotional features

With depressed mood

Illnesses meeting criteria for depression, mania or hypomania are then subdivided into 'bipolar disorder' and 'major depression', which are distinguished by whether a manic episode has ever occurred. Because evidence suggests that the great majority of manics eventually experience depression, a separate category for unipolar mania was not included as it was in ICD-10. Rather, manic patients who have never displayed depressive symptoms are classified under 'bipolar disorder, currently manic'. Bipolar disorder is subdivided into three groups: currently manic, currently depressed, and mixed (for those patients who cycle within a single episode). An option being considered by the DSM-IV work group is to move bipolar II patients (i.e. those with full depressive episode(s), hypomania(s) but without full-blown mania) from the residual category 'bipolar disorder, not otherwise specified' into a more specific niche such as 'Bipolar disorder with hypomania'. This would emphasize the link between bipolar II and bipolar I illnesses as suggested by considerable data. Alternatively, the bipolar II patient could appear as a coded subtype of depressive episode, e.g. 'depressive episode with hypomania'.

There has been an upswing of interest in the group of bipolar patients who have many episodes close together (e.g. four or more episodes in one year). They are commonly called 'rapid cyclers' although they may have short 'well' intervals between switches. They comprise 13% or more of bipolar patients (Dunner & Fieve 1974). They present extraordinary treatment challenges and so clinicians have been keen to study them. Rapid cycling bipolars have a much rockier course (Roy-Byrne et al 1985) and they are decidedly less likely to respond to lithium (Dunner & Fieve 1974), as compared to non-rapid cycling bipolar patients. There seems to be an association between thyroid abnormalities and rapid cycling (Cowdry et al 1983), which may not be a result of lithium treatment. The great majority of rapid cyclers are women (Dunner & Fieve 1974). In view of the profound clinical significance of rapid cycling, it is not surprising that a proposal has been made that DSM-IV recognize either a modifying term or a coded designation for this condition.

The term 'major depression' is used for most unipolar depressions. Major depression is further subclassified at the fourth digit as a single episode or recurrent. It is further subclassified at the fifth digit on the basis of the presence of 'melancholia', psychotic features and seasonal pattern. In DSM-IIIR the term 'melancholia' corresponds to the British concept of 'endogenous' depression and ICD-10 'somatic' depression. Because there were objections to the term 'endogenous', based on arguments that not all such depressions 'come from within' or are unprecipitated, the term 'melancholic' was used. In DSM-III, the 'melancholic' subtype diagnosis was based on symptoms only, while in DSM-IIIR it explicitly considers personality features and previous good recovery from a depressive episode. The DSM-IV work group is debating whether to return to a purely symptomatic basis for 'melancholia', perhaps empha-

sizing symptoms such as psychomotor retardation, anhedonia, unreactive mood, distinct quality of mood and mood worse in mornings. This would be partly similar to ICD-10 and partly different, since ICD also considers vegetative symptoms important.

There has been controversy over the years about whether a form of depression with atypical features constitutes a distinct nosological entity. It was long ago proposed that presence of 'atypical' depressive symptoms was a predictor of good response to monoamine oxidase inhibitors (West & Dally 1959). However, studies following up this claim have used varied definitions of 'atypical depression'. Paykel et al (1983) noted three possible meanings of the term: anxious depression, reversed functional shift (i.e. weight gain, hypersomnia; now often referred to as reversed vegetative symptoms), and simply non-endogenous depression. Liebowitz and colleagues (1984) published data indicating that good monoamine oxidase inhibitor treatment outcome could be predicted by presence of at least two of the following symptoms: 1) overeating, increased appetite, or weight gain; 2) oversleeping; 3) leaden paralysis (the feeling that one's extremities are so extraordinarily heavy that one practically cannot move them); and 4) exquisite sensitivity to interpersonal rejection. A proposal to introduce in DSM-IV an 'atypical or reverse vegetative symptom depression' subtype of depressive episode based on these criteria is under review by the mood disorders work group.

DSM-IIIR requires the diagnostician to note whether psychotic features, such as delusions or hallucinations, are present and whether these are mood-congruent or mood-incongruent. The DSM-III decision to include under mood disorders depression with mood incongruent delusions and hallucinations was reached after considerable debate; it has been affirmed in DSM-IIIR and will probably remain unchanged in DSM-IV. A number of patients formerly designated as having schizoaffective disorder are classified among the mood disorders under DSM-IIIR. There is a proposal for DSM-IV to separate severity and psychotic features. At present, these two episode characteristics compete for a coding digit, so that both cannot be ascribed to a given patient.

The 'seasonal pattern' qualifier is the result of accumulating evidence that some patients have an undulating course corresponding to the seasons, generally with depressions during winter and remissions during summer (corresponding to the duration of daylight in the area) (Rosenthal et al 1984). Multiple studies have suggested that, unlike non-seasonal depressions, seasonal depressions respond to therapy involving artificial sunlight falling on the face (e.g. Wehr et al 1986, Yerevanian et al 1986).

Consideration is being given to adding a qualifier to depressive episodes if they begin during the post-partum period (say, 2 months after delivery). It is not known whether this qualifier will actually be included nor how it would be implemented in coding digits.

DSM-IIIR places mild affective conditions together with severe ones which they otherwise phenomenologically resemble. This leads to classifying cyclothymic disorder and dysthymic disorder as affective disorders rather than as personality disorders. Both refer to relatively persistent disorders and are defined as lasting at least two years. Cyclothymic disorder refers to cases in which the mood swings between mild depression and mild hypomania, while dysthymic disorder refers to chronic, mild depressive syndromes. ICD-10 also has a dysthymia category. In DSM-IV it is anticipated that the dysthymia category will remain, but the diagnostic criteria may be modified based on an ongoing field trial. Since many patients meet criteria for dysthymia, but also suffer episodes of major depression, another option for DSM-IV is to develop modifying terms for the course of illness in major depression (e.g. major depression with or without antecedent dysthymia and good or poor interepisode recovery). Other mild depressive syndromes which are not severe enough to meet criteria for major depression or chronic enough to meet criteria for dysthymic disorder, may appear under adjustment disorder with depressed, anxious or mixed mood.

Developing a system with good reliability was one of the major goals of the DSM effort. Consequently, the authors attempted to keep overlap between categories to a minimum. Each category is defined with explicit diagnostic criteria. Although efforts were made to draw on recent research in classification, not all research was accepted. For example, the classification does not use the common distinction between primary and secondary depression. Because the classification system was written to meet the needs of both clinicians and researchers, some researchers may find the definition of major depression to be too broad or overinclusive and may choose other methods (e.g. ICD-10) for defining narrower or more homogeneous groups.

SYSTEMS OF CLASSIFICATION USED IN RESEARCH

To distinguish between classification systems used for research and for clinical purposes is to some extent arbitrary. Many of the classification systems discussed in this section have been developed by investigators who believe that their primary utility is clinical; i.e. they believe that these categories enjoy significant predictive validity because they define groups which are homogeneous in terms of response to treatment or outcome. Nevertheless, many of the classification systems developed through research have had strikingly little impact on clinical systems such as ICD or DSM.

The bipolar–unipolar distinction

The subdivision of affective disorders into bipolar and unipolar types is perhaps the most widely accepted throughout the world. Although many investigators who have explored and supported the bipolar–unipolar distinction are adherents of a Kraepelinian approach to diagnosis, this distinction runs counter to the Kraepelinian synthesis. That is, rather than grouping all severe forms of affective disorder under a single heading, manic-depressive illness, it separates them on the basis of the occurrence of mania into at least two groups which are considered to represent distinct and different illnesses.

Originally proposed by Leonhard (1979), this distinction has received considerable support through the work of Perris (1966, 1968, 1969, 1971), Winokur et al (1969) and many other investigators. The reader is referred to chapter 5 for a full review of the evidence for the validity of the unipolar–bipolar distinction.

One problem with the bipolar–unipolar distinction is whether the bipolar group should be further subdivided. Dunner et al (1976a,b) have developed some evidence for dividing bipolar subjects into two groups, bipolar I and bipolar II and this distinction has often been made in the American literature. Bipolar II patients differ from bipolar I patients in that they suffer either from hypomania or mild mania and have not required hospitalization for the elated phase of bipolar illness. Bipolar I patients, on the other hand, have been hospitalized for mania. Bipolar II patients tend in some regards to resemble bipolar I patients in terms of their family history and response to treatment (Dunner et al 1976a,b). However, it would be premature to include bipolar II illnesses with bipolar I; Endicott et al (1985) and Coryell et al (1984) have provided evidence from the American NIMH Collaborative Studies of the Psychobiology of Depression–Clinical that bipolar II 'breeds true' in families, so that it may turn out to be a separate entity or group of entities.

The subtyping of unipolar disorders is also at present

an open question. One can subtype by family history, by biological 'marker' characteristics (e.g. sleep architecture abnormalities, neuroendocrine dysfunction) or by symptoms and course. By far the most attention has gone to the latter sort of subtyping (e.g. the psychotic–neurotic distinction).

Yet another issue in the bipolar–unipolar dichotomy is the relationship of relatively mild disorders, particularly cyclothymia. Akiskal et al (1978a) reported on a series of cyclothymic patients in terms of family history, longitudinal course and pharmacological response profile. They found the cyclothymic group to resemble bipolar I patients in having a strong, positive family history for affective illness, to have many more affective episodes during a two to three year follow-up period than a 'pseudocyclothymic' group, and to be more likely to develop hypomania in response to tricyclic therapy. 35% of the cyclothymic group developed either clear-cut depression or clear-cut hypomania or mania during the 2–3-year follow-up period. These findings seem to argue for the possibility of considering cyclothymic personality to be within the biological family of affective disorders, perhaps as a bipolar II variant.

Splitting bipolar and unipolar disorders has usually been motivated by a desire to identify pure nosologic classes for study. For example, the bipolar II distinction was originally developed in order to remove a group of patients from the unipolar class so as to keep unipolar depressions more 'pure'. That is, when it was recognized that depressed patients who had experienced hypomania usually came from families with a high prevalence of bipolarity, it was reasoned that such patients might in fact represent a mild form of bipolar disorder. If the research strategy involves studying unipolar depression, then such an approach seems quite reasonable. On the other hand, if one is emphasizing bipolar disorder, then bipolar II patients may represent a questionable group. Although not all these subtypes of affective disorder may represent true nosologic classes, the most appropriate approach at present seems to be to identify as many subtypes as possible, to study them separately and to use data gathered in this way eventually to make a decision concerning which really represent true nosological classes.

The primary–secondary distinction

Originated by Munro (1966), the primary–secondary distinction has been emphasized primarily by the St Louis group in the United States. Woodruff et al (1967)

proposed that the broad category of depressive disorders be broken down into two mutually exclusive groups on the basis of natural history. Primary depression was defined as a depressive syndrome occurring in a patient with no prior history of any other psychiatric illness. All other depressions were secondary, for example those in persons with histories of alcoholism, panic disorder or hysteria. Woodruff and his associates (Woodruff et al 1967, Guze et al 1971) anticipated that the course and prognosis of secondary depression would resemble that of the antecedent disorder and that it might require a different type of treatment from primary depression. Because of the variability and potential influence of the various antecedent diagnoses on course and treatment, secondary depression was thought to be a less homogeneous disorder than primary depression.

Although the distinction seems clear, several problems have emerged. Originally it was presented as subtyping of unipolar depressions only. Winokur (1972a) first divides affective disorders into bipolar and unipolar; only unipolar disorders are further subdivided, into primary and secondary depression. Data of Andreasen et al (1988) suggest that Winokur's scheme is correct and that the primary–secondary distinction makes little difference within the bipolar group.

A second issue concerns what qualifies as an antecedent diagnosis. The original descriptions defined secondary affective disorder as occurring after either medical or psychiatric disorder. With time, however, most investigators have chosen to eliminate medical illnesses from the definition because so many patients could be diagnosed as having secondary depressions. The nature of antecedent psychiatric diagnoses also presents problems. The early discussions of secondary depression emphasized antecedent disorders such as alcoholism, hysteria or antisocial personality. Other investigators have studied depressions secondary to drug addiction and schizophrenia (Weissman et al 1977) or disorders characterized by high levels of anxiety such as panic disorder, phobic disorder and obsessive-compulsive disorder (Andreasen & Winokur 1979a). There is some question whether secondary affective disorders should be defined as secondary to all disorders which may occur in the nomenclature, including, e.g., nicotine dependence and sleepwalking. Investigators who use diagnostic schemes such as the Research Diagnostic Criteria (Spitzer et al 1978) have limited antecedent diagnoses to those defined by their research criteria.

While many investigators believe that the primary–

secondary distinction is of great importance, their confidence may rest on shaky grounds. One consistent finding is that secondary depression has an earlier age of onset than primary depression (Clayton 1983). However, this might simply be due to comparing patients with two disorders (secondary) rather than one (primary), i.e. a selection bias. Weissman et al (1977), Andreasen & Winokur (1979a) and Grove et al (1987a) found only minimal differences in cross-sectional phenomenology. That primary and secondary depressions have similar depressive symptom phenomenology is also supported by studies comparing primary depression to depression secondary to panic disorder (Dubé et al 1986, Grunhaus et al 1986). Sleep studies have produced conflicting results (Akiskal et al 1982, Dubé et al 1986, Grunhaus et al 1986, Thase et al 1984). The first three studies showed more sleep architecture abnormalities in primary depression but the latter investigation, which alone controlled for severity and age, did not.

Weissman et al (1977) and Andreasen & Winokur (1979) found no differences in treatments received or apparent treatment response, while Zorumski et al (1986) reported a universal response to ECT in primary depression compared to 58% response among secondary patients. These ECT findings await replication.

Familial illness data are equivocal. Two studies have indicated that patients with secondary depression have a higher familial rate of alcoholism and drug abuse (Andreasen & Winokur 1979a, Grove et al 1987b), mostly due to the high frequency of these disorders as primary diagnoses in secondary depressed probands. In the former study, there was an increased rate of major depression in relatives of secondary probands; in the latter, a marginally increased rate of secondary depression only. In another study, no differences in overall rate for any type of affective illness or depression were found, but primary patients tended to have a higher familial prevalence of bipolar illness (Akiskal et al 1978a).

The data suggest, then, that the distinction between primary and secondary depression may not be as useful as was originally alleged. It has slowly been dropping out of use.

The endogenous–reactive distinction

The endogenous–reactive distinction enjoys wide but controversial support. Among all the methods currently available for subclassifying depressive syndromes, this dichotomous classification has been the most thoroughly studied by researchers and the most widely used by clinicians.

Nevertheless, the distinction has problems in definition and delineation. The endogenous–reactive distinction is often used as if synonymous with the psychotic–neurotic distinction. In fact, the dichotomy is sometimes referred to as the endogenous–neurotic distinction. To further add to the confusion, as these four terms have become widely used as the names for subtypes of depression almost all have lost their original meaning.

The original concept of 'endogenous' depression was that, as the name indicates, the depression 'arose from within' in contrast to an 'exogenous' or 'reactive' depression which was caused from without. Endogenous depressions, examined in a large series of factor analytic studies, have consistently been found to have a set of characteristic symptoms, including terminal sleep disturbance, psychomotor retardation, distinct quality of mood, weight loss, difficulty in concentrating, severely depressed mood and inability to respond to affectively pleasant changes in the situation or environment (Carney et al 1966, Kiloh & Garside 1963, Kiloh et al 1972, McConaghy et al 1967, Mendels & Cochrane 1968, Rosenthal & Klerman 1966). The rather consistent appearance of these symptoms in different studies of endogenous depression has led some investigators to conclude that endogenous depression might best be defined phenomenologically. Deciding whether or not a particular depression has been precipitated by some outside factor can be quite difficult. On the one hand, most patients can identify some unhappy life situation or event which could be essentially causal and pure endogenous depressions, in the sense of having absolutely no identifiable precipitating factors, are quite rare. On the other hand, some patients clearly develop and sustain a severe endogenous-like incapacitating depression in the face of some painful life event. In fact, most studies which have examined the relationship between endogenous-like depressive syndromes and life events has found life stresses to occur almost as often in endogenous as in non-endogenous depressions (e.g. Leff et al 1970, Thomson & Hendrie 1972, Brown et al 1979, Benjaminsen 1981, Hirschfeld 1981, Matussek & Neuner 1981, Grove et al, 1987c).

In view of these facts, it is now common to define endogenous depression phenomenologically. This approach was taken in the Research Diagnostic Criteria (Spitzer et al 1978). The identifying symptoms are those which have previously been identified in the

factor analytic studies, such as terminal sleep disturbance, diurnal variation, distinct quality of mood and
non-reactivity of mood in the face of pleasurable events.
The American DSM definition is close to the British
concept of endogenous depression in that it includes
more than symptoms (e.g. premorbid personality,
previous response to somatic therapies) in the
definition.

Most studies exploring this dichotomy compare
endogenous to neurotic depression. The term
'neurotic' also carries multiple meanings with it, such
as a disorder arising from internal psychological
conflict, a disorder characterized primarily by anxiety, a
disorder which is likely to be chronic and mild or a
disorder which is to be treated with psychotherapy
rather than medication. Indeed, the term 'neurotic'
carries connotations quite different from 'reactive', the
old opposite of 'endogenous'. Factor analysts apparently preferred the term 'neurotic' because of the items
which load at the other extreme on a bipolar endogenous–neurotic factor: responsivity of mood, self-pity,
variability of illness, immaturity, hysterical features,
inadequacy, initial insomnia, irritability, hypochondria,
obsessionality, sudden onset and precipitating factors.

The validity of this distinction has been a matter of
continuous and vigorous debate, proceeding on two
levels, clinical and statistical. Some of the older studies
evaluating the validity of this concept are summarized
in Table 3.3. The clinical and neurochemical or
neuroendocrine findings in support of the concept of
endogenous depression appear relatively strong. The
endogenous syndrome has sometimes been found to be
a useful predictor of response to somatic treatment,
whether it be tricyclics or ECT. Older follow-up studies
indicated that endogenous depression generally had a
better long term outcome. Further, considerable
evidence, though not wholly consistent, suggests that
endogenous depression is statistically associated with
abnormal neuroendocrine response (e.g. cortisol non-
suppression after dexamethasone).

However, recent studies cloud this picture. For
example, in the Collaborative Studies of the
Psychobiology of Depression, clinical presence of an
endogenous syndrome was associated with *worse*
outcome in the index episode and more morbidity in 5-
year follow-up (Grove et al 1987c). Similarly, negative
responses to ECT or doctor's-choice treatment have
been reported by others (Abou-Saleh & Coppen 1983,
Copeland 1983, Zimmerman et al 1985a).
Additionally, family studies do not support the reasonable expectation that endogenous depression would be
more familial than non-endogenous depression
(Andreasen et al 1986).

Table 3.3 Validation of the endogenous–neurotic distinction

Response to treatment

Endogenous depression predicts good response to antidepres-
sants
(Raskin & Crook 1976, Rao & Coppen 1979, Paykel 1972b,
Bielski & Friedel 1976)

Endogenous depression mostly predicts good response to
ECT
(Carney et al 1966, Carney & Sheffield 1972, Abou-Saleh &
Coppen 1983)

Prognosis and outcome

Endogenous depression mostly predicts good short- and long-
term outcome
(Paykel et al 1974, Carney & Sheffield 1972, Kay et al 1969,
Copeland 1983, Grove et al 1987c)

Neurochemical and neuroendocrine studies

Endogenous depression usually predicts breakaway from
dexamethasone suppression
(Carroll et al 1976, Carroll et al 1981, APA Task Force on
Laboratory Tests in Psychiatry 1987, Davidson et al 1984,
Zimmerman et al 1985c).

Endogenous depression shows different response to methylamphetamine challenge
(Checkley 1979)

Decreased brain dopamine consumption in retarded or 'vital'
depression
(van Praag & Korf 1971)

Statistical studies of endogenous depression have
become more positive, albeit guardedly so, as methods
have advanced. In early work, the graphing of discriminant analysis scores yielded a bimodal distribution,
suggesting that endogenous and neurotic depression
represented two distinct illnesses (Carney et al 1966,
Carney & Sheffield 1972, Garside et al 1971). On the
other hand, investigators working primarily in London
obtained clearly unimodal distributions (Kendell 1968,
Kendell & Gourlay 1970, Ni Bhrolchain 1979, Ni
Bhrolchain et al 1979). Possible reasons for this
discrepancy have been reviewed in several articles
(Kendell 1976, Eysenck 1970). As Fleiss (1972) has
indicated, such distributions cannot be interpreted
simply by eye since a unimodal distribution could
reflect two independent populations with some degree
of overlap in the middle. The existence of a syndrome
with symptoms like those the Newcastle group attribute
to endogenous depression has been confirmed by a
plethora of cluster analytic and taxometric studies

(Pilowsky et al 1969, Fleiss 1972, Paykel 1971, 1972a, 1972b, Raskin & Crook 1976, Byrne 1978a, Andreasen et al 1980, Matussek et al 1981, Andreasen & Grove 1982, Parnowski 1986, Young et al 1986, Grove et al 1987c).

The major problem with the endogenous–neurotic distinction is with its neurotic half. Investigators now recognize that this group is heterogeneous. Akiskal et al (1978b) reviewed the nosological status of neurotic depression and presented data from a short-term follow-up on such patients, concluding that the concept was no longer meaningful. The somewhat related concept of atypical depression was reviewed by Paykel et al (1983) and was found to include concepts of anxious depression, depression with reversed functional shift and simply non-endogenous depression. Winokur (1985) proposed positive diagnostic criteria for neurotic depression, but we know of no follow-up validating studies. For the time being, the logical approach to this morass is, in our view, to keep the baby but to throw out the bath-water. Endogenous depression, perhaps renamed to 'vegetative' (Young et al 1986) or 'nuclear' (Grove et al 1987c) depression to shed the connotations of an unprecipitated illness, appears to be a useful concept for research purposes. Such depressions should be distinguished from other types of depression and the latter group explored in more detail for meaningful subtypes.

On the other hand, it remains to be seen whether the chief correlates of endogenous depression, namely full recovery and good response to somatic therapies, are empirically robust enough to recommend the concept for routine clinical use. DSM-IIIR puts previous response to somatic therapy on the list of criteria for melancholia, perhaps in an effort to restore this part of endogenous depression's predictive power.

Pure depression versus depression spectrum disease versus non-familial depression

This method for subtyping depressive disorders was first proposed by George Winokur and his associates. It exemplifies the use of a familial methodology in developing a nosological system. In an early study, Winokur et al (1971) subdivided a group of depressed patients on the basis of age at onset. They noted that the early-onset group tended to contain more females than the later-onset group, and that the male relatives of the early-onset group tended to have a higher prevalence of alcoholism and antisocial personality while the female relatives tended to have more depression. This led them

to propose that alcoholism, antisocial personality and depression might compose a spectrum of related disorders that tended to be familially and perhaps genetically related and that tended to express itself as alcoholism or antisocial personality in males and depression in females. This familial pattern has been explored in several additional investigations by Winokur and others and his earlier findings confirmed (Winokur 1979).

As this system continued in use, however, problems arose. The early definition described pure depression as depression occurring in males over 40 with a family history of affective disorder and depression spectrum disease as depression occurring in females under 40 with a family history of antisocial personality, alcoholism and affective disorder; this did not provide for classification of late-onset females, men with a family history of alcoholism and the like. Nor could it classify the patient with no family psychiatric history. Consequently, another scheme was developed based simply on family history (Andreasen & Winokur 1979b). This system is hierarchical. First, affective disorders are divided into primary and secondary; secondary cases are not further divided. Primary cases are subsequently divided into unipolar and bipolar; bipolars are considered homogeneous. Finally, primary unipolar cases are subdivided into three groups: 1) non-familial depression (patients with no family history of any major psychiatric illness as defined by the Research Diagnostic Criteria); 2) pure depression (patients who have a family history of depressive disorder only); and 3) depression spectrum disease (those patients with a family history of alcoholism, antisocial personality, hysteria or drug abuse, either alone or in combination with depression).

The validity of this system has been explored chiefly in relation to the dexamethasone suppression test; results from investigators working at (or trained at) Iowa consistently indicate that depression spectrum patients are normal suppressors while pure depressive disease patients show higher rates of early escape from dexamethasone-induced cortisol suppression (Schlesser et al 1979, 1980, Coryell et al 1982, Zimmerman et al 1985b). In addition, the insulin tolerance test glucose response has also been reported to differentiate the groups, with depression spectrum patients having normal tests and pure and sporadic depressives showing abnormalities (Lewis et al 1983). Attempts to validate the Winokur classification by investigators at other centres have been less uniformly successful. Amsterdam et al (1982) and Rudorfer et al (1982) could not replicate dexamethasone test differences between the familial subtypes, but Targum et al (1982) did so. Perris et al (1983b) did not find clinical differences, though most clinical studies indicate that depression spectrum disease is less severe and that non-familial (sporadic) depression tends to resemble pure depression (Andreasen & Winokur 1979b, Winokur 1979, Behar et al 1980, Zimmerman et al 1986; but see van Valkenburg et al 1983). Patients with sporadic and pure depression tended to have a better response to antidepressants, while patients with depression spectrum disease tended to respond to major tranquillizers. The sporadic and pure depressives tended to come from a higher socioeconomic class and to have less parental divorce than the depression spectrum disease patients. Depression spectrum patients had more aggressive and less socialized personalities as measured by questionnaire in one study (Perris et al 1983a) but rated presence of abnormal premorbid personality did not differentiate spectrum patients in another report (Behar et al 1981). Thus, this classification contains some validity, especially in relation to hypothalamic–pituitary–adrenal axis abnormalities, but appears not to replicate well in other centres and so remains controversial.

Taxonometric systems of classification

Factor analysis permits exploration of the relationships between *symptoms*, but does not directly provide new classifications of *persons* (or, more properly, their illness). Principal methods for developing such new classifications are heuristic ones such as cluster analysis and mathematical model-based methods such as latent class analysis. Collectively, these have been called taxonometric techniques.

The first use of taxonometrics in affective disorders was one of exploration, frequently using cluster analysis or the conceptually related method inverse factor analysis. Originally, much of this work was done on relatively unselected patient populations and very broad arrays of sign and symptom data, following the unabashedly inductivist approach advocated by Sneath & Sokal (1973). This approach was supported by arguments that clinical approaches had as yet failed to yield a clearly reliable, strikingly valid classification; that taxonometric approaches could process much more data than the human mind; that such systems would not be hamstrung by preconceptions and so could find new taxa.

However, this atheoretical approach lost much of its charm as investigators found that cluster analysis and kindred methods, applied in this fashion, had a host of conceptual and technical problems. First, there are many methods of cluster analysis and many ways to measure interpatient similarity. Few have been studied with reference to their ability to give correct results when a correct classification is known in advance. It is discouraging that patients classified one way by one method will often be classified quite differently by another (Byrne 1978b). There is the difficult problem of the appropriate number of clusters to interpret (Milligan & Cooper 1985). The fundamental problem is that all commonly used taxonometric methods will yield groups, whether they are real or fictive. Therefore, multiple independent validity checks must be invented and applied in order to know whether results are spurious (see chapter 4 of Jain & Dubes 1988, Meehl & Golden 1982).

A number of studies using taxonometric methods have been conducted, reviewed by Blashfield & Morey (1979) and Grove (1984); most were cited above in connection with endogenous depression. The studies vary widely in the quality of the data which they have entered and the appropriateness of methods used to generate clusters. Only a few investigators have insisted on repeated replications of clusters or the use of independent validators such as response to treatment (e.g. Paykel 1972a,b Overall et al 1966, Raskin & Crook 1976, Andreasen et al 1980, Andreasen & Grove 1982, Grove et al 1987c). These studies have yielded a varying number of subtypes ranging from two (Pilowsky et al 1969, Grove et al 1987c) to four (Paykel 1971, Raskin & Crook 1976, Andreasen & Grove 1982). Paykel's four categories included psychotic depressives, anxious depressives, hostile depressives and young depressives with personality disorder. Raskin's four classes included agitated depressions, neurotic depressions, endogenous depressions and young patients with personality disorder. Thus, the Paykel and Raskin classifications are strikingly similar. Andreasen & Grove, studying a heterogeneous population of patients with a depressive syndrome (with or without other features), found four groups: endogenous depressions, strictly defined psychotic depressions, moderately severe depressions and cycling or mixed bipolar depressions. Schizoaffective episodes mostly went into an unclassifiable residuum. Other cluster studies which have found two or three groups have also consistently isolated a class which corresponds to severe, psychotic or endogenous depression. Thus, as stated earlier, these studies give some mathematical validation to at least one traditional subtype.

Biologically derived classification systems

Investigators and clinicians agree that the ideal classification system would group together patients who share a common aetiology and who are likely to have a characteristic response to specific treatments and a characteristic outcome. Although such a classification system is still beyond our grasp, several lines of investigation have been pursued. These involve attempts to subdivide depressed patients either on the basis of low urinary MHPG excretion or on the basis of levels of 5-HIAA in the cerebrospinal fluid. These relationships have been reviewed by several investigators (Schildkraut et al 1978a,b, Asberg et al 1976, Goodwin et al 1978). The strong and obvious advantage of such classification systems is that they speak to the biology of depressions, hopefully linking phenomenology to some of its most important causes. Such classifications also have theoretical appeal, in that they may be linked to specific neurotransmitter hypotheses concerning the aetiology of affective disorders. Ultimately, the resolution of these controversies must await the availability of more definitive measures of brain activity, metabolism and structure.

REFERENCES

Abou-Saleh M T, Coppen A 1983 Classification of depression and response to antidepressive therapies. British Journal of Psychiatry 143: 601–603

Akiskal, H S, Djenderedjian A H, Bolinger J M et al 1978a The joint use of clinical and biological criteria for psychiatric diagnosis. II. Their application in identifying subaffective forms of bipolar illness. In: Akiskal H S, Webb W L (eds) Psychiatric diagnosis: exploration of biological predictors. Spectrum, New York, p 133–145

Akiskal H S, Bitar A H, Puzantian V R et al 1978b The nosological status of neurotic depression. Archives of General Psychiatry 35: 756–766

Akiskal H S, Lemmi H, Yerevanian B, King D, Belluomini 1982 The utility of the REM latency test in psychiatric diagnosis: a study of 81 depressed outpatients. Psychiatry Research 7: 101–110

American Psychiatric Association 1987 Diagnostic and statistical manual of mental disorders, 3rd edn—revised. American Psychiatric Association, Washington

Amsterdam J D, Winokur A, Caroff S N, Conn J 1982 The dexamethasome suppression test in outpatients with primary affective disorder and healthy control subjects. American Journal of Psychiatry 139: 287–291

Andreasen N C, Grove W M 1982 The classification of depression: traditional versus mathematical approaches. American Journal of Psychiatry 139: 45–52

Andreasen N C, Winokur G 1979a Secondary depression: familial, clinical and research perspectives. American Journal of Psychiatry 136: 62–66

Andreasen N C, Winokur G 1979b Newer experimental methods for classifying depression. Archives of General Psychiatry 36: 447–452

Andreasen N C, Grove W M, Maurer R 1980 Cluster analysis and the classification of depression. British Journal of Psychiatry 137: 256–265

Andreasen N C, Scheftner W, Reich T, Hirschfeld R M A, Endicott J, Keller M 1986 The validation of the concept of endogenous depression: a family study approach. Archives of General Psychiatry 43: 246–251

Andreasen N C, Grove W M, Coryell W H, Endicott J, Clayton P J 1988 Bipolar versus unipolar and primary versus secondary affective disorder: which diagnosis takes precedence? Journal of Affective Disorders 15: 69–80

Angst J, Felder W, Lohmeyer B 1979 Schizoaffective disorders: results of a genetic investigation, I. Journal of Affective Disorders 1: 139–153

APA Task Force on Laboratory Tests in Psychiatry 1987 The dexamethasone suppression test: An overview of its current status in psychiatry 144: 1253–1262

Asberg M, Thoren P, Traskman L et al 1976 'Serotonin depression'—a biochemical subgroup within the affective disorders? Science 191: 478–480

Behar D, Winokur G, van Valkenburg C, Lowry M 1980 Familial subtypes of depression: a clinical view. Journal of Clinical Psychiatry 41: 52–56

Behar D, Winokur G, van Valkenburg C, Lowry M, Lachenbruch P A 1981 Clinical overlap among familial subtypes of unipolar depression. Neuropsychobiology 7: 179–184

Benjaminsen S 1981 Primary non-endogenous depression and features attributed to reactive depression. Journal of Affective Disorders 3: 245–259

Bielski R J, Friedel R O 1976 Prediction of tricyclic antidepressant response. Archives of General Psychiatry 33: 1479–1489

Blashfield R K, Morey L C 1979 The classification of depression through cluster analysis. Comprehensive Psychiatry 20: 516–526

Brockington I F, Leff J P 1979 Schizoaffective psychosis: Definitions and incidence. Psychological Medicine 9: 91–99

Brown G W, Ni Bhrolchain M, Harris T O 1979 Psychotic and neurotic depression: Part 3. Aetiological and background factors. Journal of Affective Disorders 1: 195–211

Byrne D G 1978a Cluster analysis applied to self-reported depressive symptomatology. Acta Psychiatrica Scandinavica 57: 1–10

Byrne D G 1978b A note on cluster analysis and depression: disparities in results produced by the application of different clustering methods. Australian and New Zealand Journal of Psychiatry 12: 99–102

Carney M W P, Sheffield B F 1972 Depression and the Newcastle scales: their relationship to Hamilton's scale. British Journal of Psychiatry 121: 35–40

Carney M W P, Roth M, Garside R F 1966 The diagnosis of depressive syndromes and the prediction of ECT response. British Journal of Psychiatry 111: 659–674

Carroll B, Curtis C G, Mendels J 1976 Neuroendocrine regulation in depression. Archives of General Psychiatry 33: 1039–1044

Carroll B, Feinberg M, Greden J F et al 1981 A specific laboratory test for melancholia: standardization, validation, and clinical utility. Archives of General Psychiatry 38: 15–22

Checkley S A 1979 Corticosteroid and growth hormone response to methylamphetamine in depressive illness. Psychological Medicine 9: 107–155

Clayton P J 1982 Schizoaffective disorders. Journal of Nervous and Mental Disease 170: 646–650.

Clayton P J 1983 A further look at secondary depression. In Clayton P J, Barrett J E (eds) Treatment of depression: old controversies and new approaches. Raven Press: New York, p169–191

Clayton P J, Halikas J A, Maurice W L 1972 The depression of widowhood. British Journal of Psychiatry 120: 71–77

Copeland J R M 1983 Psychotic and neurotic depression: discriminant function analysis and five-year outcome. Psychological Medicine 13: 373–383

Coryell W, Gaffney G, Burkhardt P E 1982 The dexamethasone suppression test and familial subtypes of depression – a naturalistic replication. Biological Psychiatry 17: 33–42

Coryell W, Endicott J, Reich T, Andreasen N, Keller M 1984 A family study of bipolar II disorder. British Journal of Psychiatry 145: 49–54

Cowdry R, Wehr T, Zis A, Goodwin F 1983 Thyroid abnormalities associated with rapid cycling bipolar illness. Archives of General Psychiatry 40: 414–420

Davidson J, Lipper S, Zung W W K, Strickland R, Krishnan R, Mahorney S 1984 Validation of four definitions of melancholia by the dexamethasone suppression test. American Journal of Psychiatry 141: 1220–1223

Depue R A, Slater J, Wolfstetter-Kausch H, Klein D, Goplerud E, Farr D 1981 A behavioral paradigm for identifying persons at risk for bipolar depressive disorder: a conceptual framework and five validation studies. Journal of Abnormal Psychology 90: 381–437

Dubé S, Jones D A, Bell J, Davies A, Ross E, Sitaram N 1986 Interface of panic and depression: clinical and sleep EEG correlates. Psychiatry Research 19: 119–133

Dunner D, Fieve R 1974 Clinical factors in lithium carbonate prophylaxis failure. Archives of General Psychiatry 30: 229–233

Dunner D L, Gershon E S, Goodwin F K 1976a Heritable factors in the severity of affective illness. Biological Psychiatry 11: 31–42

Dunner D L, Stallone F, Fieve R R 1976b Lithium carbonate and affective disorders. Archives of General Psychiatry 33 117–120

Endicott J, Nee J, Andreasen N, Clayton P, Keller M, Coryell W 1985 Bipolar II: combine or keep separate? Journal of Affective Disorders 8: 17–28

Endicott J, Nee J, Coryell W et al 1986 Schizoaffective, psychotic, and nonpsychotic depression: differential familial association. Comprehensive Psychiatry 27: 1–13

Eysenck H J 1970 The classification of depressive illnesses. British Journal of Psychiatry 117: 241–250

Feighner J P, Robins E, Guze S B et al 1972 Diagnostic criteria for use in psychiatric research. Archives of General Psychiatry 26: 56–73

Fleiss J L 1972 Classification of the depressive disorders by numerical typology. Journal of Psychiatric Research 9: 141–153

Frank J D 1973 Persuasion and healing. Johns Hopkins University Press, Baltimore

Garside R F, Kay D W K, Wilson I C, Deaton I D, Roth M 1971 Depressive syndromes and the classification of patients. Psychological Medicine 1: 333–338

Goodwin F K, Muscettola G, Gold P W et al 1978 Biochemical and pharmacological differentiation of affective disorder: an overview. In: Akiskal H S, Webb W L (eds) Psychiatric diagnosis: exploration of biological predictors. Spectrum, New York, p 313–336

Grove W M 1984 The numerical taxonomy of endogenous depression. Unpublished doctoral dissertation, University of Minnesota

Grove W M 1987 The reliability of psychiatric diagnosis. In: Last C G, Hersen M (eds) Issues in diagnostic research. Plenum Press, New York

Grove W M, Andreasen N C, Clayton P J, Winokur G, Coryell W H 1987a Primary and secondary affective disorders: baseline characteristics of unipolar patients. Journal of Affective Disorder 13: 249–257

Grove W M, Andreasen N C, Winokur G, Clayton P J, Endicott J, Coryell W H 1987b Primary and secondary affective disorders: unipolar patients compared on familial aggregation. Comprehensive Psychiatry 28: 113–126

Grove W M, Andreasen N C, Young M et al 1987c Isolation and characterization of a nuclear depressive syndrome. Psychological Medicine 17: 471–484

Grunhaus L, Rabin D, Harel Y, Greden J F, Feinberg M, Hermann R 1986 Simultaneous panic and depressive disorders: clinical and sleep EEG correlates. Psychiatry Research 17: 251–259

Guze S B, Woodruff R A, Clayton P J 1971 'Secondary' affective disorder: A study of 95 cases. Psychological Medicine 1: 426–428

Hirschfeld R M A 1981 Situational depression: validity of the concept. British Journal of Psychiatry 39: 35–46

Jain A K, Dubes R C 1988 Algorithms for clustering data. Prentice Hall, Englewood Cliffs

Kahlbaum E 1863 Die Grüppierung des psychischen Krankheiten. Danzig, 1863. Cited in Jelliffe S E 1931 Some historical phases of the manic-depressive synthesis. Association for Research in Nervous and Mental Disease 11: 3–47

Kasanin J 1933 The acute schizoaffective psychoses. American Journal of Psychiatry 13: 97–126

Kay D W K, Garside R F, Roy J R et al 1969 'Endogenous' and 'neurotic' symptoms of depression: a 5- to 7-year follow-up of 104 cases. British Journal of Psychiatry 115: 389–399

Kendell R E 1968 The classification of depressive illnesses. Oxford University Press, Oxford

Kendell R E 1976 The classification of depressions: a review of contemporary confusion. British Journal of Psychiatry 129: 15–28

Kendell R E, Gourlay J 1970 The clinical distinction between psychotic and neurotic depressions. British Journal of Psychiatry 117: 257–266

Kiloh L G, Garside R F 1963 The independence of neurotic depression and endogenous depression. British Journal of Psychiatry 109: 451–463

Kiloh L G, Andrews G, Neilson M, Bianchi G N 1972 The relationship of the syndromes called endogenous and neurotic depression. British Journal of Psychiatry 121: 183–196

Kraepelin E 1921 Manic-depressive insanity and paranoia. E & S Livingstone, Edinburgh

Leff M J, Roatch J F, Bunney W E Jr 1970 Environmental factors preceding the onset of severe depressions. Psychiatry 33: 291–311

Leonhard K 1979 The classification of endogenous psychoses, 5th edn, Robins E (ed), Berman R (tr). Irvington, New York

Levinson D F, Levitt, M E M 1987 Schizoaffective mania reconsidered. American Journal of Psychiatry 144: 415–425

Lewis A J 1938 States of depression: their clinical and aetiological differentation. British Medical Journal 2: 4060ff

Lewis D A, Kathol R G, Sherman B M, Winokur G, Schlesser M A 1983 Differentiation of depressive subtypes by insulin insensitivity in the recovered phase. Archives of General Psychiatry 40: 167–170

Liebowitz M R, Quitkin F M, Stewart J W, McGrath P J, Harrison W, Rabkin J, Tricano E, Markowitz J S, Klein D F 1984 Phenelzine *v* imipramine in atypical depression. Archives of General Psychiatry 41: 669–677

McConaghy N, Joffe A D, Murphy B 1967 The independence of neurotic and endogenous depression. British Journal of Psychiatry 113: 479–484

Matussek P, Neuner R 1981 Loss events preceding endogenous and neurotic depressions. Acta Psychiatrica Scandinavica 64: 340–350

Matussek P, Soeldner M, Nagel D 1981 Identification of the endogenous depressive syndrome based on the symptoms and the characteristics of the course. British Journal of Psychiatry 138: 361–372

Meehl P E, Golden R R 1982 Taxometric methods. In Kendell P C, Butcher J N (eds) Handbook of research methods in clinical psychology. John Wiley, New York; p 127–181

Mendels J, Cochrane C 1968 The nosology of depression: the endogenous-reactive concept. American Journal of Psychiatry 124 (suppl): 1–11

Milligan G W, Cooper M C 1985 An examination of procedures for determining the number of clusters in a data set. Psychometrika 50: 159–179

Munro A 1966 Some familial and social factors in depressive illness. British Journal of Psychiatry 112: 429–441

Ni Bhrolchain M 1979 Psychotic and neurotic depression: 1. Some points of method. British Journal of Psychiatry 134: 87–93

Ni Bhrolchain M, Brown G W, Harris T O 1979 Psychotic and neurotic depression: 2. Clinical characteristics. British Journal of Psychiatry 134: 87–93

Ollerenshaw D P 1973 The classification of the functional psychoses. British Journal of Psychiatry 122: 517–530

Overall J E, Hollister L E, Johnson M et al 1966 Nosology of depression and differential response to drugs. Journal of the American Medical Association 195: 946–948

Parnowski T 1986 Psychopathological pattern of depression in affective disorders: A cluster analysis. Acta Psychiatrica Scandinavica 73: 139–146

Paykel E S 1971 Classification of depressed patients: a cluster analysis derived grouping. British Journal of Psychiatry 118: 275–288

Paykel E S 1972a Correlates of a depressive typology. Archives of General Psychiatry 27: 203–210

Paykel E S 1972b Depressive typologies and response to amitriptyline. British Journal of Psychiatry 120: 147–156

Paykel E S, Klerman G L, Prusoff B A 1974 Prognosis of depression and the endogenous-neurotic distinction. Psychological Medicine 4: 57–64

Paykel E S, Parker R R, Rowan P R, Rao B M, Taylor C N 1983 Nosology of atypical depression. Psychological Medicine 13: 131–139

Perris C 1966 A study of bipolar (manic-depressive) and unipolar recurrent depressive psychoses. Acta Psychiatrica Scandinavica (suppl) 194

Perris C 1968 Genetic transmission of depressive psychoses. Acta Pychiatrica Scandinavica (Suppl) 203

Perris C 1969 The separation of bipolar (manic-depressive) from unipolar recurrent depressive psychoses. Behavioral Neuropsychiatry 1: 17–25

Perris C 1971 Abnormality on paternal and maternal sides: observations in bipolar (manic-depressive) and unipolar depressive psychoses. British Journal of Psychiatry 119: 207–210

Perris H, Eisemann M, Ericsson U, von Knorring L, Perris C 1983a Personality characteristics of depressed patients classified according to family. Neuropsychobiology 9: 99–102

Perris H, Eisemann M, Ericsson U, von Knorring L, Perris C 1983b Attempts to validate a classification of unipolar depression based on family data. Neuropsychobiology 9: 103–107

Pilowsky I, Levine S, Boulton D M 1969 The classification of depression by numerical taxonomy. British Journal of Psychiatry 115: 937–945

Pope H G, Lipinski J F 1978 Diagnosis in schizophrenia and manic-depressive illness. Archives of General Psychiatry 35: 811–828.

Procci W R 1976 Schizo-affective psychosis: fact or fiction? Archives of General Psychiatry 33: 1167–1178

Rao V A R, Coppen A 1979 Classification of depression and response to amitriptyline therapy. Psychological Medicine 9: 321–325

Raskin A, Crook T H 1976 The endogenous–neurotic distinction as a predictor of response to antidepressant drugs. Psychological Medicine 6: 59–70

Rosenthal S H, Klerman G L 1966 Content and consistency in the endogenous depressive pattern. British Journal of Psychiatry 112: 471–481

Rosenthal N E, Sack D A, Gillin J C, Lewy A J, Goodwin F K, Davenport Y, Mueller P S, Newsome D A, Wehr T A 1984 Seasonal affective disorder: a description of the syndrome and preliminary findings with light therapy. Archives of General Psychiatry 41: 72–80

Roy-Byrne P, Post R, Uhde T, Porcu T, Davis D 1985 The

longitudinal course of recurrent affective illness. Acta Psychiatrica Scandinavia 71 (Suppl 117) 3–34

Rudorfer M V, Hwu H-G, Clayton P J 1982 Dexamethasone suppression test in primary depression: significance of family history and psychosis. Biological Psychiatry 17: 41–48

Schildkraut J J, Orsulak P J, Schatzberg A F et al 1978a Toward a biochemical classification of depressive disorders: I. Differences in urinary excretion of MHPG and other catecholamine metabolites in clinically defined subtypes of depression. Archives of General Psychiatry 35: 1427–1433

Schildkraut J J, Orsulak P J, LaBrie R A, et al 1978b Toward a biochemical classification of depressive disorders: II. Application of multivariate discriminant function analysis to data on urinary catecholamines and metabolites. Archives of General Psychiatry 35: 1436–1439

Schlesser M A, Winokur G, Sherman B M 1979 Genetic subtypes of unipolar primary depressive illness distinguished by hypothalamic—pituitary adrenal axis activity. Lancet 1: 739–741

Schlesser M A, Winokur G, Sherman B M 1980 Hypothalamic—pituitary—adrenal axis activity in depressive illness: its relationship to classification. Archives of General Psychiatry 37: 737–743

Sneath P H A, Sokal R R 1973 Numerical taxonomy. Freeman, San Francisco

Spitzer R L, Endicott J, Robins E 1978 Research diagnostic criteria: rationale and reliability. Archives of General Psychiatry 35: 773–782

Targum S D, Byrnes S M, Sullivan A C 1982 Subtypes of unipolar depression distinguished by the dexamethasone suppression test. Journal of Affective Disorders 4: 21–27

Thase M E, Kupfer D J, Spiker D G 1984 Electroencephalographic sleep in secondary depression: a revisit. Biological Psychiatry 19: 805–814

Thomson K C, Hendrie H C 1972 Environmental stress in primary depressive illness. Archives of General Psychiatry 26: 130–132

Van Eerdewegh M M, Van Eerdewegh P, Coryell W et al 1987 Schizoaffective disorders: bipolar–unipolar subtyping. Journal of Affective Disorders 12: 223–232

van Praag H M, Korf J 1971 Retarded depression and the dopamine metabolism. Psychopharmacologia 19: 199–203

van Valkenburg C, Akiskal H S, Puzantian V 1983 Depression spectrum disease or character spectrum disorder? Comprehensive Psychiatry 24: 589–595

Wehr T A, Jacobsen F M, Sack D A, Arendt J, Tamarkin L, Rosenthal N E 1986 Phototherapy of seasonal affective disorder: time of day and suppression of melatonin are not critical for antidepressant effects. Archives of General Psychiatry 43: 870–875

Weissman M M, Pottenger M, Kleber H et al 1977 Symptom patterns in primary and secondary depression. Archives of General Psychiatry 34: 854–862

Welner A, Croughan J L, Robins E 1974 The group of schizoaffective and related psychoses – critique, record, follow-up, and family studies: I. A persistent enigma. Archives of General Psychiatry 31: 628–631

West E D, Dally P J 1959 Effects of iproniazid in depressive syndromes. British Medical Journal 1: 1491–1494

Wing J K, Cooper J E, Sartorius N 1974 The measurement and classification of psychiatric symptoms. Oxford, Oxford University Press

Wing J K, Mann S A, Leff J P et al 1978 The concept of a 'case' in psychiatric population surveys. Psychological Medicine 8: 203–217

Winokur G 1972a Depression spectrum disease: description and family study. Comprehensive Psychiatry 13: 3–8

Winokur G 1972b Family history studies: VIII. Secondary depression is alive and well and. . . . Disease of the Nervous System 33: 94–99

Winokur G 1979 Unipolar depression: is it divisible into autonomous subtypes? Archives of General Psychiatry 36: 47–52

Winokur G 1985 The validity of neurotic-reactive depression: new data and reappraisal. Archives of General Psychiatry 42: 1116–1122

Winokur G, Clayton P J, Reich T 1969 Manic depressive illness. C V Mosby, St Louis

Winokur G, Cadoret R, Dorzab J, Baker M 1971 Depressive disease: a genetic study. Archives of General Psychiatry 24: 135–155

Woodruff R A, Murphy G E, Herjanic M 1967 The natural history of affective disorders: I. Symptoms of 72 patients at the time of index hospital admission. Journal of Psychiatric Research 5: 255–263

World Health Organization 1978 Mental disorders: glossary and guide to their classification in accordance with the ninth revision of the International Classification of Diseases. WHO, Geneva

World Health Organization 1990a ICD-10. 1990 draft of chapter V, Mental and behavioural disorder – clinical descriptions and diagnostic guidelines. WHO, Geneva

World Health Organization 1990b ICD-10 1990 Chapter 5. Mental and behavioural disorders. Diagnostic criteria for research. May 1990 Draft for Field Trials. WHO, Geneva.

Yerevanian B L, Anderson J L, Grota L J, Bray M 1986 Effects of bright incandescent light on seasonal and non-seasonal affective disorder. Psychiatry Research 18: 355–364

Young M A, Scheftner W, Klerman G L, Andreasen N C, Hirschfeld R M A 1986 The endogenous subtype of depression: a study of its internal construct validity. British Journal of Psychiatry 148: 257–267

Zimmerman M, Coryell W, Pfohl B 1985a The treatment validity of DSM-III melancholic subtyping. Psychiatry Research 16: 37–43.

Zimmerman M, Coryell W, Pfohl B 1985b Importance of diagnostic thresholds in familial classification. Archives of General Psychiatry 42: 300–304

Zimmerman M, Coryell W, Pfohl B, Stangl 1985c Four definitions of endogenous depression and the dexamethasone suppression test. Journal of Affective Disorders 8: 37–45

Zimmerman M, Coryell W, Pfohl B 1986 Validity of familial subtypes of primary unipolar depression. Archives of General Psychiatry 43: 1090–1096

Zorumski C F, Rutherford J L, Burke W J, Reich T 1986 ECT in primary and secondary depression. Journal of Clinical Psychiatry 47: 298–300

4. History of the affective disorders

German E. Berrios

INTRODUCTION

The group of conditions nowadays called 'affective disorders' has resulted from the convergence of certain *words* (e.g. 'affective' and its cognates), *concepts* (theoretical notions accounting for 'mood'-related experiences) and *behaviours* (observable changes in action and speech associated with whatever the neurobiology of these disorders happens to be). Each order of elements has had a different history and their evolution has been asynchronous. The three components were only put together during the early part of the twentieth century. Since there is no reason to expect that this convergence was 'written in the nature of things', its explanation belongs more to history than to science. If the convergence hypothesis is correct, then those who believe that the history of the conditions now called mania and melancholia starts with the Greeks must be mistaken, for their anachronistic approach, at best, only chronicles the history of the words.

One of the problems confronting the historian is that the phrase 'affective disorders' refers to a diffuse family of subjective and objective behavioural disturbances. In current English-speaking psychiatry, for example, it names the depressive and manic syndromes, combinations thereof and occasionally some of their accompanying anxiety symptoms (Zerssen 1988). 'Affective' (the operative word) has itself a long and noble history and is part of a panoply of terms which include emotion, passion, feeling, sentiment, mood, affective equivalent, dysthymia, cyclothymia, dysphoria, etc. Although these terms name overlapping subjective states, they have different semantic provenances. Basically, it is unclear whether they all refer to some fundamental unitary mental function or to combinations of functions (Berrios 1985a). Sentiment, emotion and passion have been customarily distinguished from mood, affect and feeling in terms of criteria such as duration, polarity, intensity, insight, saliency, association with an inner or outer object, bodily sensations and motivational force. They are defined as short-lived, more or less intense feeling states, which appear related to a recognizable object (Ribot 1897); emotion and passion (the latter of which is an intense version of the former) are assumed to be accompanied by bodily changes and hence to possess motivational properties (Leeper 1948).

Mood and affect, on the other hand, are defined as longer lasting and more or less *objectless* states capable of providing a background feeling tone to the individual (Ketal 1975, Owens & Maxmen 1979). Upon this baseline of mood, short-lived emotions or ideas of congruent (synthymic) or incongruent (catathymic) value can be superimposed (Bash 1955). The tone and consistency of experiences ordinarily called 'mood and affect' are probably controlled by neuroendocrine variables and subject to both genetic and environmental control. In clinical practice, patients suffering from an affective disorder are expected to 'describe' their feeling state, in spite of the fact that some aspects of their illness (e.g. psychotic symptoms) may prevent them from behaving as rational observers. This, in addition to the fact that they may be experiencing novel and strange sensations, make their so-called 'privileged' position doubtful. The fact that psychiatrists are successful in identifying mood states is reassuring, not least to the historian, and suggests that a well-structured descriptive system is in operation: for example, that doctor and patient share systems of signals of cultural and/or evolutionary origin (Krueger 1928, Mantegazza 1878, Gruber 1981, Darwin 1872). A complete history of the affective disorders should include an analysis of the words involved in the naming of feeling states (for this see Berrios 1985a).

The history of the affective disorders

Our current notions of depression and mania date from the second half of the nineteenth century and emerged from the transformation of the old notions of melancholia and mania. The ideological changes that made them possible included the development of faculty psychology and the new anatomoclinical model of disease, and the inclusion of subjective experiences into the symptomatology of mental disorders (Berrios 1987, 1988a, 1988b). The concept of mania was first narrowed down and the residuum redefined (under the influence of faculty pyschology) as a primary disorder of *affect and action*. The pre-nineteenth century notion of melancholia was equally refurbished; this was facilitated by Esquirol's concept of lypemania which emphasized the *affective* nature of the disorder (Esquirol 1820). Once the right conceptual conditions were available, the new clinical versions of mania and melancholia were combined into the new concept of alternating, periodic, circular or double form insanity (Foville 1882; Ritti 1876, Mordret 1883). This process culminated with Kraepelin's concept of 'manic-depressive insanity' which included most forms of affective disorder under the same umbrella (Kraepelin 1921).

The transformation of melancholia into depression

'Melancholia', wrote John Haslam (1809), 'the other form in which this disease (madness) is supposed to exist, is made by Dr Ferriar to consist in "intensity of idea". By intensity of idea I presume is meant, that the mind is more strongly fixed on, or more frequently recurs to, a certain set of ideas, than when it is in a healthy state...' (pp 32–33). Haslam's perception was correct. Up to the period of the Napoleonic Wars, melancholia was but a rag-bag of insanity states whose only common denominator was the presence of few (as opposed to many) delusions. In practice this means that cases of schizophrenia might have been so catalogued. Sadness and low affect (which were no doubt present in some cases) were *not* considered as definitory symptoms. Indeed, states of non-psychotic depression, of the type that nowadays would be classified as DSM-IIIR 'major depression' would not have been called 'melancholia' at all. During the eighteenth century these states were classified as 'vapours', 'spleen', or 'hypochondria', i.e. what Cullen called 'neuroses', and Sydenham and

Willis, the previous century, had called 'nervous disorders'.

The term 'depression'

To search for the origins of the term and the concept of 'depression' the historian does not need to go beyond the middle of the nineteenth century (Jackson 1986). As we have seen a number of conceptual changes had determined that 'melancholia' could no longer be: 1) a subtype of mania; 2) a primary disorder of intellect; or 3) irreversible. What emerged was a form of partial insanity defined as a primary disorder of emotions whose features (whether clinical or aetiological) reflected a general state of loss, inhibition, reduction and decline. Thus constituted, 'melancholia' was renamed 'depression', a term that had been popular in mid-nineteenth century cardiovascular medicine to refer to a reduction in function (Berrios 1988b). The word was first used metaphorically as 'mental depression'; soon after, the adjective 'mental' was dropped.

By 1860 it appears in medical dictionaries: 'applied to the lowness of spirits of persons suffering under disease' (Mayne 1860, p 264). The first edition of Régis's (1885) Manual (which was to go through many editions) defined depression thus: 'is the state opposed to excitation. It consists in a reduction in general activity ranging from minor failures in concentration to total paralysis...' (p 77). Physicians also preferred the word depression to melancholia or lypemania, perhaps because it evoked a 'physiological' explanation. For example Sir William Gull (1894) used it as early as 1868 in his article on 'hypochondriasis': 'its principal feature is mental depression, occurring without apparently adequate cause...' (p 287). By the end of the century 'depression' was defined as: 'a condition characterized by a sinking of the spirits, lack of courage or initiative, and a tendency to gloomy thoughts. The symptom occurs in weakened conditions of the nervous system, such as neurasthenia and is specially characteristic of melancholia' (Jastrow 1901, p 270). Savage (1898) in his very popular *Insanity and the Allied Neuroses* (studied by countless clinical students in the UK) defined melancholia as 'state of mental depression, in which the misery is unreasonable...' (p 151). Adolph Meyer (1901) continued campaigning in favour of the new word after the end of the century. Thus constituted, a legion of depressive symptoms and states (both subjective and objective) began to be recognized. These ranged from stupor or 'melancholia attonita' (Berrios 1981) to nihilistic delusions (Cotard 1882).

Kraepelin (1921) legitimized the term by using it in an adjectival manner and amongst the 'depressive states' he included melancholia simplex, stupor, melancholia gravis, fantastic melancholia and delirious melancholia.

British psychiatry took some time to catch up. The same group of disorders continued sailing under the name 'melancholia' as shown by the famous *Nomenclature of Diseases* drawn up by a Joint Committee appointed by the Royal College of Physicians of London (RCP 1906). Therein 'melancholia' was classified as a 'disease of the nervous system' (code 146) exhibiting acute, recurrent or chronic states. The Committee advised that 'the variety when known should be returned according to the following categories: agitated, stuporous, hypochondriacal, puerperal, climacteric, senile and from acute or chronic disease or from injury' (p 37).

There was some disagreement concerning the taxonomic position of the new melancholia. Because its symptoms were frequent in clinical practice, and often found accompanying other forms of insanity, the new melancholia was classified in a number of ways. Some saw it as: 1) a stage in the development of a unitary psychosis (e.g. Griesinger 1861); 2) a separate disease, either self-contained or part of a cycle including euphorias and/or stupor (e.g. Baillarger 1854); 3) a development of the subject's personality, i.e. an exaggeration of acquired vulnerabilities (e.g. Freud 1917); or 4) a manifestation of a tainted pedigree (e.g. Magnan and degeneration theory; Saury 1886). These hypotheses were not considered as exclusive and the manner of their combination engendered much debate. This is partly explained by the fact that the logic of justification and falsification which operated amongst nineteenth-century alienists was based on the marshalling of single cases and of counter-examples. Although the statistical notion of the 'law of error' (Gaussian distribution) (Hilts 1967) was already available, it had not yet penetrated the methodology of medicine. So case reports exhibiting minor deviations from the idealized type created difficulty and forced alienists to declare them as new forms.

In the eighth edition of his *Textbook*, Kraepelin (1921) cut the Gordian knot by creating an overinclusive notion which included all forms of depression and mania, even including the notion of 'involutional melancholia' (Berrios 1991). This omnibus concept was characterized by: 1) a periodic course; 2) a good prognosis; and 3) endogenicity (i.e. not related to precipitants); all three criteria demanded standards of clinical description and observation which at the time were difficult to achieve (Berrios 1991). They also led to surprising conclusions, for example, that some paranoias, neurasthenias or (even) changes in bowel habit (without other accompanying features) may be hidden forms of manic-depressive illness (Kraepelin 1921). These less recognizable Kraepelinian views are rarely mentioned nowadays, perhaps because of selective reading; only those amongst his clinical statements are quoted which are intelligible to current psychiatrists. In Kraepelin, the concept of affective disorder can be said to be at its most overinclusive; indeed, the history of the affective disorders after 1910 is no more than the analysis of the fragmentation of the Kraepelinian notion.

In the period between Esquirol and Kraepelin seven assumptions were made with regards to the affective disorders (Berrios 1985a, 1987, 1988a, 1988b). These conditions were: 1) to be a 'primary' pathology of affect (Bolton 1908); 2) to have a stable psychopathology (Foville 1882); 3) to have brain representation (Ritti 1876); 4) to be periodic in nature (Falret 1854, Baillarger 1854); 5) to be genetic in origin (Foville 1882); 6) to appear in individuals with recognizable personality predisposition (Ritti 1876); and 7) to be endogenous in nature (Kraepelin 1921, Chaslin 1912). These assumptions were made on the basis of clinical observation, logical reasoning and ideology, and not surprisingly, each has a different conceptual history.

The classification of the affective disorders

During the nineteenth century, the drive to classify the affective disorders had various origins (Berrios 1987). There was, first, the taxonomic impetus affecting the whole of medicine; second, the internal need to tidy up the nosology of psychiatry; third, the influence of faculty psychology and the ever looming presence of degeneration theory; and, late in the century, the need to identify homogenous clinical groups for neuropathological study, particularly in relation to the differential diagnosis between melancholia and dementia (Mairet 1883, Dumas 1894, Berrios 1985b).

From the vantage point of the twentieth century, the eighteenth-century concept of insanity is only superficially intelligible. Not sufficient emphasis has been placed on the fact that it was 'atemporal' in the sense that it constituted a state of mind *sub specie aeternitatis*; remissions being explained away as 'lucid intervals'. This meta-theoretical notion was concealed by the fact that during the eighteenth century medical practitioners made great use of life-events to explain the 'onset' of insanity thereby giving the impression that mental disorders could exist in a temporal context; this is a mirage. The concept of insanity as a medical 'disease' only achieved full meaning during the nineteenth century when time was truly incorporated as a dimension of disease. This longitudinal view becomes evident in Kahlbaum (Katzenstein 1963), Wernicke and Kraepelin (Berrios & Hauser 1988). Up to the time of Kahlbaum there had been much debate as to what 'subsisted' or 'endured' in a mental disease, i.e. the symptoms, oscillations in psychological energy or brain changes. Symptoms were the favourite choice to play this ontological role; this explains the proliferation of reported new 'diseases' (which were simply different symptom patterns). First with Kahlbaum, and then with Kraepelin (who followed him closely) this was to change as their ontological demands included that the symptom cluster persisted in time (i.e. the course of disease) and that it had some sort of identifiable brain representation. This drastically reduced the number of insanities. Even then, Kraepelin's nosology was unable to escape the curse of the 'intermediate' cases. Growing increasingly sceptical late in life, he was to relinquish his separatist view (Kraepelin 1920). The French followed a different path, for they could not escape degeneration theory, a wide view of the nature of disease which also provided a sharp taxonomic principle (Berrios & Beer 1991).

This proliferation of mental disorders is an interesting feature of nineteenth-century alienism. It resulted from the fact that in psychiatry the anatomoclinical model of disease was far more difficult to implement, and alienists ended up with many symptom descriptions (Berrios 1984). In fact, the nineteenth century had inherited a simple classification for the insanities: phrensy, mania, melancholia and dementia had been defined on theoretical grounds (e.g. Pinel 1809). The dismantling of the old theory of the insanities led to the simultaneous availability of various conceptual dichotomies which were instrumental in the analysis and classification of the affective disorders: 1) total versus partial insanity; 2) acquired versus inherited disorder; 3) acute versus chronic disease course; 4) anatomical versus functional basis; 5) reversible versus irreversible disorder; 6) exogenous versus endogenous origin; 7) relevant versus irrelevant personality-related factors; and 8) form versus content of symptoms.

NINETEENTH-CENTURY FRANCE

During the first half of the nineteenth century classificatory fashions originating in France had a commanding influence on the rest of Europe. Pinel was perhaps the last great man to use melancholia and mania in the old, classical sense. Esquirol, Georget, Billod, Baillarger, Falret, Marcé, Morel, Linas and Magnan implemented major changes in these categories. Their work, however, had not yet been completed when the Kraepelinian view took France by storm, splitting the ranks of her alienists (Ey 1954, Rouart 1936). Some, like Deny & Camus (1907), supported the notion of an overinclusive manic depressive illness; others stuck to the old views and the debate continued well into the 1930s.

Pinel

Pinel (1809) had defined melancholia as an insanity characterized by a circumscribed number of delusions (*délire exclusif*). His conception of melancholia was wide:

> Melancholia frequently remains stationary for many years without its central delusion changing in character, and without causing much physical or psychological change. It can be seen in patients with this condition detained at Bicêtre for twelve, fifteen, twenty, or even thirty years, that they are still victims of the delusions that originated their admission . . . some having a more mobile character, and after observing the agitated behaviour of some lunatics, develop a manic state . . . others, after many years undergo a sort of internal revolution, and their delusions change. One of these patients, already advanced in years, had believed for years that he had been imprisoned by his parents who wanted his fortune, more recently however, he began to fear that we wanted to poison him . . . (pp 167–168)

Pinel included under melancholia all forms of chronic psychosis, including schizophrenia.

Esquirol and lypemania

But this was soon to change. Under the influence of faculty psychology, and believing that melancholia was a primary disorder of emotions, Esquirol (1820) criticised the old usage: 'the word melancholia, consecrated in popular language to describe the habitual state of sadness affecting some individuals, should be left to poets and moralists whose loose expression is not subject to the strictures of medical terminology' (p 148). Prichard (1835) had a similar view and Rush (1812), after criticising Cullen's usage, advised against the use of the word 'melancholia', coining instead 'tristimania'. But of all these new terms, it was 'lypemania' that survived the longest. Esquirol (1820) defined it as 'a disease of the brain characterized by delusions which are chronic and fixed on specific topics, absence of fever, and *sadness which is often debilitating and overwhelming*. It must not be confused with mania which exhibits generalized delusions and excited emotions and intellect nor with monomania that exhibits specific delusions and expansive and gay emotions, nor with dementia characterized by incoherence and confusion of ideas resulting from weakening...' (pp 151–152). Esquirol even reported a clinical and epidemiological profile for the new disease: rates for lypemania were found to increase between May and August (p 159); the age group most affected were those between 25 and 45 (p 161); in 110 of 482 cases 'heredity' seemed to have played a role; common causes included domestic crisis, grief and disturbed relationships (p 166); about a third of his cohort died, often of tuberculosis.

The term lypemania had its critics. Delasiauve (1856) called it too *'élastique*... apart from being less imprecise was no different in terms of contents from the old word melancholia' (p 382). Delasiauve was here referring to the fact that Esquirol had kept *circumscribed delusions* (a vestige of the old intellectualistic notion) as a defining criterion. He was, of course, right as it is clear that paranoia and the delusional disorders were still included under lypemania (Sèrieux & Capgras 1909, p 293). Delasiauve suggested that the boundaries of lypemania be narrowed further to refer to: 'an exaggeration and persistence of feelings of *depression*' (p 384). The highest point in the history of lypemania was reached in the work of Billod (1856), who attempted a classification and refinement of its psychopathology. Billod accepted that lypemania had to be defined on the basis of sad delusions and affect and suggested a fourfold classification: lypemania with sad delusions and sadness; sad delusions and no sadness; sad delusions and mixed or alternating affective disorder (this included the bipolar states); and no sad delusions and sadness. This contrived symmetry allowed the recognition of various clinical subtypes. Some of these have since disappeared (e.g. ironic or religious lypemania) others (e.g. hypochondriacal, stuporous or irritable lypemania) are still sailing current seas only under a different name.

The term 'lypemania' did not catch on in Germany, Austria, Switzerland or Great Britain, where the word 'melancholia' was maintained. Prichard (1835) paid no attention to it. Griesinger (1861), who regularly quoted Esquirol, did not take any notice either. Feuchtersleben (1847) mentioned the term once, but did not acknowledge its origins. Bucknill & Tuke (1858) did mention the word lypemania, but continued using 'melancholia' on the excuse that Esquirol himself had stated that the two terms could be used interchangeably (p 147). Lypemania is an example of what historians call a 'bridge' category: it died away after catalysing the transition of melancholia from its old intellectualistic to its modern emotional definition.

NINETEENTH-CENTURY GERMANY

It has been customary to accept the view (Bolton 1908), started by Deny & Camus (1907), that during most of the nineteenth century the German contribution to the history of the affective disorders was negligible, and that it only became important after the work of Krafft-Ebing, Weygandt, Kraepelin and Dreyfus. This view is anachronistic in that it judges 'importance' with regards to current concepts. Under the influence of German Romanticism alienists such as Reil, Heinroth and Griesinger expressed views on the affective disorders which closely reflect the growing importance of affect and passion in the development of mental illness (Berrios 1985a). For example, Heinroth (1975) wrote:

> The origin of the false notions of patients suffering from melancholia... is being erroneously attributed to the intellect... here the intellect is not at fault... it is the disposition which is seized by some depressing passion, and then has to follow it, and since this passion becomes the dominating element, the intellect is forced by the disposition to retain certain ideas and concepts. It is not these ideas or concepts which determine the nature and the form of the disease. (p 190–191)

Writings by German alienists from this period also reflect an anti-cartesian approach, for example, by classifying the insanities in terms of the 'single principle of cerebral development, both physical and psychological' (Roubinovitch 1896).

Griesinger

The concepts of melancholia and mania are more difficult to elucidate in the work of Griesinger. In spite of his great influence and reputation, Griesinger had limited clinical psychiatric experience (Wahrig-Schmidt 1985) (he was in his middle twenties when he wrote the first edition of his book on mental pathology and therapeutics), and hence based his definitions on borrowed cases and theoretical views. With regards to his views on the affective disorders a number of sources can be identified: 1) Herbartian associationism, which allowed him to identify 'the elementary symptoms (units of analysis) of insanity'; 2) Broussais's notion of 'irritation' and general views on pathological changes in vital energy, leading to the claim that mental disorders result from an increase or a decrease in vitality; and 3) the 'unitarian' view, that there only was one form of insanity which changed in its symptomatic expression through time (Rennert 1968). Thus, although Griesinger's clinical description of melancholia has a 'modern' ring, it should not be forgotten that it belongs to a different conceptual world in which there were no independent psychiatric diseases but only successive symptom clusters reflecting the oscillations of a vital principle (Griesinger 1861).

Kahlbaum

The views of Kahlbaum (1863) on melancholia and mania are confusing because he included both syndromes under the term 'dysthymia' (which he attributed to Carl Friedrich Flemming). (On the history of this concept see also Bronisch 1990.) Flemming, one of the great leaders of German asylum psychiatry (Kolle 1963) published in 1859 an extraordinary book on *The Pathology and Therapy of the Psychoses* where a full chapter is dedicated to the syndromes resulting from the primary disorders of the emotions (pp 56–80) (Flemming 1859). Kahlbaum put forward an original classification, based on a longitudinal concept of disease (Katzenstein 1963). The third group in this classification were the 'vecordias' (defined as idiopathic disturbances of mental life, with onset after puberty, and which have more or less specific symptoms). They were subdivided, according to faculty psychology, into disturbance of intellect (paranoia), volition (diastrophia) and emotions (dysthymia). The latter included 'dysthymia melana' and 'elata' according to whether there was a predominance of sad affect (*Vorwalten trauriger Affecte*) or elated affect (*freudiger Affecte*) (p 134). With regard to melancholia, Kahlbaum said: 'In our view melancholia is not a disease but a syndrome (*ein Symptomenkomplex*)' (p 97).

Krafft-Ebing

In Krafft-Ebing (1879) the definition and classification of melancholia and mania is described in a 'modern' voice. As Bercherie (1980) has perceptively noticed, Krafft-Ebing's taxonomic principles are based on a series of dichotomies. First, the psychoses are divided into those with and without intellectual retardation; second, the latter into those with (organic) or without (functional) identifiable brain pathology; third, the functional psychoses are split into those developing in degenerates (i.e. those with family loading of mental illness: psychoneurosis) and in 'normals'; finally, the psychoneuroses are divided into melancholia, mania, acute and hallucinatory insanity. Melancholia, Krafft-Ebing defined as a 'painful inhibition of psychological functions' and mania an an exalted facilitation. This classification reigned supreme in Germany until the time of Kraepelin.

Kraepelin and the notion of 'involutional melancholia'

The synthetic views of Kraepelin have been reported and commented on sufficiently in the literature not to require further rehearsal (Jackson 1986, Rouart 1936, Ey 1954). However, there is still much confusion with regards to the history of the concept of involutional melancholia (Arnaud 1899, Dana 1904, Gaupp 1905, Berger 1907, Ducosté 1907, Phillips 1912a,b. Treadway 1913, Gibson 1918, Fishbein 1949, Ey 1954, Cordeiro 1973). Let us first quote a standard definition: 'The term customarily refers to agitated depressions occurring for the first time in life after the age 45–50, in contrast to manic-depressive illness which manifests itself at an early age' (Post 1965, p 103). The conventional story is that up to the seventh edition of his textbook Kraepelin considered involutional melancholia as a separate disease and that, when confronted by the evidence collected by Dreyfus (1907), he decided to include it in the eighth edition under the general heading of manic depressive insanity (Sérieux 1907, Post 1965, Kendell 1968, Jackson 1986). Indeed, this account was first presented by Kraepelin himself:

> The fact that states of depression are specially frequent at the more advanced ages, had already before this forced the supposition on me, that the processes of involution in the body are suited to engender mournful or anxious moodiness; it was one of the reasons which caused me to make a special clinical place for a portion of these forms under the name melancholia. After the purely clinical foundations of this view were shaken by the investigations of Dreyfus, our representation also now lets the causal significance of age appear in a light somewhat different from my former view (Kraepelin 1921, p 169).

The story is, however, more complex than that and it is unlikely that the findings of Dreyfus alone caused Kraepelin's change of heart. For example, Thalbitzer (1926) claimed that his own work had also been influential (p 41). In fact, in the eighth edition Kraepelin abandoned not only involutional melancholia but the entire group of 'senile psychoses'. More to the point, the reasons which in the first place led him to consider involutional melancholia as a separate disease had been many: depression became more frequent with age, in older age groups psychomotor agitation was more frequent than retardation, outcome worsened with age, and melancholia often became complicated by 'mental weakness', that is, cognitive impairment (Kraepelin 1921, p 190). In the eighth edition, Kraepelin twice felt obliged to justify his change of opinion. In the first explanation he mentioned Dreyfus; in the second he stated that further experience had taught him that 'the arguments in favour of the separation of melancholia were not sound' (p 191) for

> dementias could be explained by the appearance of senile or arteriosclerotic disease; that other cases after very long duration of illness, some of them displaying manic symptoms, had still recovered. The frequency of depressive attacks in advanced age we have come to recognize as an expression of a general law which governs the change of colouring of the attack in the course of life. Lastly, the substitution of anxious excitement for volitional inhibition has proved to be behaviour which we meet with in advancing age in those cases also which decades previously had fallen ill in the usual form . . . (p 191).

This account was confirmed many years later in his autobiography (Kraepelin 1983, p 74).

Dreyfus and his monograph

By quoting Dreyfus in the eighth edition, Kraepelin burdened the young man (who was only 26 when he started the research) with the responsibility of having been the cause of his change of heart. Dreyfus, a Swiss psychiatrist, was born in Basle in 1879 and died in Zürich in 1957. He trained in Würzburg, Giessen and Heidelberg. He came to work with Kraepelin in Munich in 1905. He then moved to Frankfurt where he was promoted in 1916 to a University lecturership. He remained in this city until 1934 when he had to escape to Switzerland.

To test the hypothesis that involutional melancholias had a bad prognosis (i.e. patients did not recover) Kraepelin asked Dreyfus (1907) to find out what had happened to all the cases he had diagnosed in 1892 as

'melancholia' whilst he was working at the Heidelberg Clinic. 'Melancholia' at the time was being used by Kraepelin as a shorthand for 'involutional melancholia'. The rest he called 'depressive states'. Dreyfus completed the follow-ups in 1906, so the longest was about 14 years. He included 85 cases, of which he described 44 in exquisite detail, sometimes even transcribing daily entries during the index episode. In more than half of the total sample Dreyfus managed personal follow-ups. A statistical analysis of Dreyfus's data (for details see Berrios 1991) shows that only 43 subjects improved, and that the only significant correlation of outcome was with age! ($r=0.30$; $p<0.01$). When the sample is divided by sex, the correlation disappears for the males; in the females it goes up to $r=0.39$ ($p<0.01$). The rate of spontaneous recovery seems to have been much higher in younger depressives (Kraepelin 1921, Brush 1897). So, Dreyfus's conclusion that the natural history of involutional melancholia was no different from that of depression affecting younger subjects does not seem to have been warranted by his own data, particularly because he did not include a control group. Indeed, he did not notice that in his female patients outcome was correlated with age.

The great synthesis suggested by Kraepelin in the eighth edition of his textbook created as many problems as it solved. The history of the affective disorders in Europe and other parts of the world since his work could be described as the attempts at solving the various clinical problems and contradictions that his views created (Soukhanoff & Gannouchkine 1903, Deny 1909, Rocha 1906, Lange 1928, Rouart 1936, Ey 1954). For example, these issues were discussed in a famous meeting of New York Neurological Society on 1 November 1904 with the participation of great men such as Dana, Starr, Collins, Meyer, Parsons and Diefendorf. Dana reported a personal series of 400 cases of melancholia and divided them into two groups. One included cases with onset during 'involution or change of life'; this form was chronic and incurable, and was characterized by 'hypochondriacal and obsessive ideas, dysthesia, somatic delusions, hallucinations, self-accusations and at times suicidal ideas and impulses (Dana 1904, p 1033). A second group included cases starting in early life with no 'definite picture' which, according to Dana, Kraepelin wanted to classify under the manic-depressive umbrella. Dana believed that this latter group could also show the clinical features of the 'involutional type' but that in spite of these it often had a good prognosis. Dana's was not the first large American series of melancholics to be reported. Brush, from the Sheppard Asylum in Baltimore, read a paper at a 1897 meeting of the British Medical Association describing 100 cases of acute melancholia and emphasizing the high incidence of physical disease (Brush 1897). The same year Weir Mitchell (1897) reported a series of 3000 cases of melancholia which he studied to test the hypothesis that cases were more 'apt to relapse in the spring or summer'. He found no evidence of seasonal changes. But European views remained predominant in the USA during this period. Smith Ely Jelliffe (1911) read a paper before the 66th Meeting of the American Medico-Psychological Association on 'Cyclothemia, the mild forms of manic depressive psychoses and the manic depressive constitution' and did not once quote an American colleague. On these mild forms, however, British psychiatrists had a great deal to say during the first 30 years of the twentieth century (see below).

NINETEENTH-CENTURY GREAT BRITAIN

Prichard

British psychiatric taxonomy took an important step forward in the work of James Cowles Prichard (1835). Although influenced by French views, Prichard showed rare originality in view of the fact that, once again, he may not have had a great deal of clinical psychiatric experience (Stocking 1978). Prichard classified melancholia as a subtype of 'moral insanity' (in fact, a disorder of the emotions): 'the faculty of reason is not manifestly impaired, but a constant feeling of gloom and sadness clouds all the prospects of life... this tendency to morbid sorrow and melancholy, as it does not destroy the understanding, is often subject to control when it first arises, and probably receives a peculiar character from the previous mental state of the individual....' (p 18). Mania, in turn, was defined by Prichard in much wider terms, as a form of 'raving madness' and on this he followed closely pre-nineteenth century views. There is little doubt that his striking clinical descriptions do include cases of acute psychotic mania but also organic deliria and some schizophrenias. Mania was for Prichard a harbinger of 'chronic and advanced states of madness' (p 79).

Bucknill & Tuke

When presenting their own classification, Bucknill & Tuke (1858) limited themselves to listing various psychiatric conditions. Melancholia and mania are described as separate entities but not classified as subtypes of 'emotional insanity' (except the subsyndrome that they called 'melancholia without delusions'; p 178). This listing without higher level grouping must be considered as a curious departure from contemporary fashion which, since the time of Pinel and certainly of Esquirol, had dictated a threefold grouping for all insanities. Bucknill & Tuke listed six forms of melancholia: simple (non-psychotic), complicated (psychotic), acute, chronic, remittent and intermittent. Mania, in turn, was considered as a general form of madness, as with Prichard.

Maudsley

Maudsley's (1895) views on mania and melancholia closely follow the British tradition. He called melancholia 'insanity with depression' and made it tantamount to Bucknill & Tuke's 'simple melancholia' (i.e. non-psychotic depression). He also described a second group called 'melancholia with delusions' which more or less corresponds to the current concept of psychotic depression: 'in this form of depression the sad feeling is accompanied by a fixed sad idea or by a set of fixed sad ideas which crystallize, so to speak, out of or about it... out of the melancholic gloom emerge dimly and shape themselves by degrees positive delusions of thought...' (p 188). In this category he included melancholia with stupor, acute delirious melancholia and hypochondrial melancholia, and discussed symptoms such as suicide, homicide and hallucinations. Maudsley's analysis of mania was symmetrical with that he afforded to melancholia. Mania was 'insanity with excitement' and included mania without delusion or simple mania where: 'there is an extraordinary excitement, *without* positive derangement, of feeling and thought: quickened thought flushed with elated and aggressive feeling...' (p 234) and 'recovery not taking place, what other issues has acute mania? The next most common event is that it becomes *chronic*, the excitement subsiding but the derangement continuing...' (p 262). Nodding in the general direction of the Continent, Maudsley concludes with regards to alternating recurrent insanity (*folie circulaire*): 'there is still one issue more of acute or rather subacute mania which it remains to take notice of – where it ends by being transformed, its seeming ending being but the beginning of an opposite-complexioned disorder. When the acute symptoms are past... the patient falls instead into an abject melancholy depression.' (p 276).

The 1906 *Nomenclature of Diseases*

This pre-Kraepelinian view of both melancholia and mania came to an end in Great Britain towards the turn of the century after the rapid acceptance of the Kraepelinian view (Bolton 1908). This acceptance was made official in the fourth edition of the *Nomenclature of Diseases* drawn up by the Joint Committee of the Royal College of Physicians of London (RCP 1906), whose psychiatric members were George Savage and Percy Smith. '*Mania*: acute, recurrent and chronic' (145.) appears as a separate disorder including seven subtypes (a to g): hysterical, puerperal, epileptic, alcoholic, senile, from other acute and chronic disease or from injury, and delirious. '*Melancholia*: acute, recurrent or chronic' (146.) also appears under a different heading with seven subtypes (a to g): agitated, stuporous, hypochondriacal, puerperal, climacteric, senile, and from other acute or chronic disease or from injury. Finally, '*Circular insanity, alternating insanity*' (147.) is included without subdivisions. This classification lasted until the great British debate of the 1920s.

Aetiological views

Little has been written on late nineteenth-century British *aetiological* views on the affective disorders. This section will limit itself to listing the most popular hypotheses. G M Robertson, then a senior assistant at the Morningside Asylum (later to become Professor of Psychiatry at Edinburgh), published in 1890 a provocative paper suggesting a 'modular' approach: 'what explanation is there of the existence of these symptoms of melancholia . . . in answering this question we must know that we are investigating a function of an organ which has become diseased; the function being the production of depressed or painful emotion . . .' (Robertson 1890, p 53). Influenced by Darwin and Romanes, Robertson went on to identify a number of symptoms of melancholia (e.g. catalepsy) which he considered as the expression of vestigial behaviours. 10 years later John Turner (1900) asked another important crucial question: 'very perplexing to the student of insanity is the question as to how states of exaltation or depression arise . . . To what changes in the nervous system do they correspond? . . . Are these changes localized in different parts of the nervous system in mania and melancholia?' (p 505). Turner decided against the modular view and adopted a Jacksonian stance (for an account of J H Jackson's views see Berrios 1985c):

'whilst both melancholia and mania are associated with a dissolution of the nervous system, in the former case the reduction takes place along sensory lines of the reflex nervous arc, and in the latter along motor lines' (p 506). But perhaps the most accomplished paper on 'the cerebral localization of melancholia' was written by Bernard Hollander (1901) who, after reviewing the literature concluded that: 'a certain relation exists between the central area of the parietal lobe, namely, the angular and supramarginal gyri, and melancholic states of mind' (p 485).

Great Britain and the Continent

It has been shown that until the turn of the century views on the affective disorders in France, Germany and Great Britain were more or less uniform. This is not very surprising as free communication existed (indeed more than nowadays) between alienists of these three nations. (As evidence for this, see international list of contributors in Tuke's Dictionary – Tuke 1892). Most European alienists shared the belief that mania and melancholia: 1) resulted from a primary pathology of the emotions; 2) could be combined in various ways; 3) resulted from cerebral disease; 4) were inherited; and 5) could recover. Kraepelin's synthesis, although resisted in France, served to reinforce this uniformity. This commonality of views lasted well into the 1920s when national differences began to appear. These originated from the selective attention that alienists in each country paid to different aspects of the affective disorders. The British continued worrying about clinical description, severity and classification, the French about inheritance and environmental triggers, and the Germans, influenced by Kretschmer's original thinking, debated a great deal the question of constitution and personality factors. As an illustration of the internal debates that led to national differences we shall explore the British debate on classification.

TWENTIETH-CENTURY GREAT BRITAIN

During the 1920s British views began to depart from those held in the Continent. This divergence resulted from uncertainties concerning the nosological position of certain forms of affective disorders which were called 'neurotic, reactive, exogenous, psychogenic or constitutional'. The view that these clinical forms might need to be included with the rest of manic depressive syndromes was based on a number of arguments: 1) clinical observation; 2) challenge to Kraepelin's dichotomous view; 3) the growth of the psychodynamic hypothesis that there might be a 'continuity' between all forms of depression; and 4) the influence of Meyerian psychiatry.

As we have seen, during most of the nineteenth century the classification of mania and melancholia (whatever their definition) had not been difficult. Symptom pattern, presence or absence of delusions, course, and whether or not the two were combined proved sufficient taxonomic criteria. As we have also seen, the cases requiring classification were collected from the most severe end of the affective disorders (i.e. hospitalized patients). Classifications were, therefore, not encumbered by the large number of minor and non-psychotic affective disorders which up to the First World War were mainly seen in private consulting rooms and which were called hypochondria, hysteria, neurasthenia, agoraphobia or psychasthenia. Indeed, clinical analysis of cases reported under all these rubrics (for example, 'cyclical neurasthenics') (Sollier 1893, Saukanoff 1909) shows that they were mostly non-psychotic manic-depressive states.

Apart from the social changes which led to differential patterns of care (e.g. the foundation of the Maudsley hospital with its emphasis on 'neurotic' outpatients), one of the most important factors in the rekindling of the classificatory debate in Great Britain was the dismembering of the clinical concept of neurasthenia. The complex reasons for this process are beyond the scope of this chapter, but suffice it to say that not all the cases set asunder by this fragmentation could be taken over by its successor, the disease called psychasthenia (Janet 1903). Many of those were to constitute the large group that Montassut (1938) analysed in his masterly monograph on the 'constitutional depressions'. In addition, psychodynamic ideas were beginning to have some impact (Newcombe & Lerner 1981), particularly in relation to mechanisms such as 'reactivity' and the question of the relationship between personality and depression. A good illustration of this influence is to be found in the British debate over the clinical place of the minor or 'neurotic' depressions.

Mapother

In 1926, Edward Mapother, then superintendent of the Maudsley Hospital (Petrie 1940), presented a controversial paper at the Nottingham Meeting of the British Medical Association (Mapother 1926). He stated that his problem was 'what *meaning* should be attached to

the term 'manic depressive psychosis'. He believed that 'the range of the term was a matter of convention; at present there is no agreement, and no one with the authority to impose it' (p 872). And in a Meyerian fashion he continued: 'All would probably agree that under the heading are included cases of functional mental disorder which show as their predominant features one of a contrasting pair of anomalous *types of reaction*: 1) The depressive reaction . . . ; and 2) the manic reaction'. He asked whether all cases with these symptoms should be included or only some, as some 'cases merge into those where constitutional symptoms of one kind or the other are pretty constantly present'. With surprising scepticism he added: 'it is unproven and improbable that any mental syndrome is due to a specific cause, and consequently there is no more likelihood of a constant course in mania or depression than in jaundice' (p 872). He challenged the distinction between neuroses and psychoses which had 'really grown out of practical differences particularly as regards certification and asylum treatment' and concluded that since a distinction could not be made, it was nonsense to try and differentiate between neurotic (anxiety neurosis) and psychotic depression.

E. Farquhar Buzzard, who was chairing, disagreed with the view that these two conditions could not really be distinguished, and so did Thomas A. Ross, from the Cassel Hospital, who stated that 'if Dr Mapother would carefully study mental states he would find that they would lead him to perceive fundamental differences between the psychoses and the psychoneuroses' (p 877); he then added that these doubts could originate from the fact that 'only a small section of the psychoneurotic group found its way to the Maudsley Hospital'! Then, it was the turn of a young Scottish psychiatrist working under Ross; his name was Robert Dick Gillespie (Henderson 1945). He rose to say that he was surprised about Mapother requiring that a 'meaning should be attached to the term manic depressive psychosis' and that

the failure (by Mapother) to mention clinical criteria he would have regarded as an accident, were it not for the remark later in the paper that details of mental state were utterly unreliable (p 878) . . . this tendency more or less unconscious to depreciate clinical differentiation gave the key to Dr Mapother's subsequent surprising classification of all psychoneurosis as a subdivision of the manic depressive psychosis . . . the truth was that the latter was essentially a clinical conception, and that an attempt to define something that had been differentiated on purely clinical grounds in terms of the academic psychology after McDougall was likely to fail'.

Then Gillespie flew his own colours:

> The task of psychopathology at present was not so much
> the discovery of a physical basis – that was not psycho-
> pathology, and smacked of the pseudo-physiologizing of
> the latter half of the nineteenth century... – but the
> unravelling of the meaning and origin of mental symptoms
> as such... it was to be regretted that Dr Mapother had
> made no mention of McCurdy's work on the manic
> depressive psychosis... his work did much to upset what
> might be called the 'psychiatrist's fallacy' – that thought
> always followed emotion. Emotion probably more often
> followed thought. (p 879)

These statements by Gillespie, of great importance to
the history of the affective disorders in Great Britain,
deserve further exploration.

Gillespie and the Cambridge connection

Robert Dick Gillespie (1897–1945) had trained under
D.K. Henderson in Glasgow and A. Mayer in
Baltimore; after a meteoric career he succeeded Sir
Maurice Craig at Guy's. In his relatively short life he
wrote with great originality on fatigue, sleep, hypochondria and depression. In 1926 there was a good reason
for Gillespie to mention McCurdy. In fact, these two
great men were to collaborate between 1927 and 1929
while Gillespie held the Pinsent-Darwin Research
Studentship in Mental Pathology at Cambridge.
McCurdy (1886–1947) was a Canadian psychologist
and psychiatrist (Banister & Zangwill 1949) who
trained first as a biologist at Toronto University and
then as a physician at Johns Hopkins. After doing
postgraduate work in neuropathology under Alzheimer
in Munich, he returned to New York as a psychiatric
assistant to August Hoch.

It is suggested in this chapter that the change in views
on the nature of the affective disorders shown by
Gillespie between the Nottingham debate and the
publication of his classical paper on the 'Clinical differentiation of types of depression' (1929) was due to
McCurdy's influence. In this latter paper Gillespie
reviewed the literature in detail, particularly the work of
Kraepelin, Lange, Cimbal and Kretschmer, searching
for depressive states that might be dependent on
personality or on environment. He also reported 25
cases which he classified into reactive (14),
autonomous (7) and involutional (3). He stated that
the three could be distinguished in terms of family
history, symptoms, personality and response to life
events. These criteria, in fact, he had borrowed from
McCurdy (1925). In view of this, Kendell's (1968)
comments that Gillespie provided no 'justification for

his assumption that classification on the basis of
reactivity was more useful or more valid than that based
on another criterion...' (p 5) is perhaps too harsh.
Gillespie's paper must be read in conjunction with
McCurdy's book, where both conceptual and therapeutic justifications (certainly not statistical, for at the
time such a form of demonstration was not part of the
scientific canons of medicine) are provided.

Buzzard and the 'milder forms'

In 1930, Sir E. Farquhar Buzzard (who had been
knighted since chairing the BMA Nottingham meeting
in 1926), returned to the issue of milder depressives
without cyclothymia: 'We frequently see depressed
patients who do not give this history of preceding
elation or depression. A source of anxiety may be ascertained and its importance as an aetiological factor has
to be measured. The sequence of events suggests that
anxiety precipitated or caused depression' (Buzzard
1930, p 881). Buzzard went on to identify the distinguishing features:

> Having referred to the difficulty of diagnosis in the milder
> forms – and the milder the form, the more difficult the
> diagnosis... let me emphasize those (clinical points)
> which I have come to regard as most helpful: 1) the type of
> depression...; 2) the loss of all natural and accustomed
> interests...; 3) the self-reproach...; 4) the preservation
> of sleep...; 5) the history of hypomanic phase...; 6) the
> coincident physical disturbances...; 7) the family history,
> particularly of suicide and alcoholism... (pp 882–883)

In the ensuing discussion H. Crichton-Miller
'regretted the title of the discussion... the term 'manic-
depressive psychosis' may be correct enough for use in
mental hospitals but it suggests too much. The term
'cyclothymia', on the other hand, covers the subject
under discussion: it includes the milder manifestations...' (p 883). He also emphasized how important
it was to know the subject's pre-morbid personality, and
criticized Kretschmer for his over-simplistic distinction between 'cycloids' and 'schizoids'. Crichton-Miller
was interested in the 'physiological aspects' of the
disease:

> In the first place periodicity appears to be a
> physiological rather than a psychological quality... in
> the second place there is great similarity between the
> euphoria of alcoholic intoxication and the exaltation of
> the cyclothymic... thirdly there is similarity between
> the depression associated with chronic intestinal
> absorption and the depressed phase of
> cyclothymia... fourthly the commonest example of
> cyclothymia occurs in some women in relation to the
> menstrual cycle (p 886).

He concluded 'the problem is not one for the psychologist, but for the biochemist'. (The term cyclothymia had been in use since the late nineteenth century; see: Soukanoff 1909, Jelliffe 1911, Deny 1908, Bagenoff 1911.)

Next, George Riddoch emphasized stress and the psychological aspects of the disease, and Henry Yellowlees felt that Kraepelin's taxonomy and psychology were out of date, and that the real clinical issue was to *differentiate the milder forms from neurasthenia*. He concluded that they were talking about a physical disease and that psychological treatments were not indicated. W.R. Reynell agreed, and Helen Boyle (the only lady doctor to intervene in the debate) put forward an eclectic view based on Golla's endocrinological work (thyroid disorders) and Stoddart's psychodynamic theory. E.B. Strauss, who had spent some time at Marburg working under Kretschmer (whose translator into English he was to become) defended the views of his teacher, and emphasized the notion of 'reactive depression' which he defined as: 'a condition precipitated by an intolerable situation in the patient's life. It is allied to true neurasthenia, prison psychosis, and the like. Whether the condition is entirely exogenous or whether a current conflict stirs up and allies itself to unconscious mechanisms, may be debated by psychoanalysts' (p 895).

The 'milder forms' in the Continent

A similar debate (although under a different terminological garb) took place in France and Germany. It concerned the diagnosis and aetiology of the 'milder forms' of affective disorders. As mentioned above, the Kraepelinian synthesis had been based on the description of asylum cases, and had left out a large group of disorders composed of protracted griefs, dysphorias, minor depressions, anxiety disorders and neurasthenias. Clinical decisions as to the nature of this group became important in the context of out-patient and private practice.

In comparison with his major contribution to the clinical and nosological aspects of the affective disorders, Kraepelin had been reticent on the role played by other modulatory factors, such as the 'personality'. On this the French were far more advanced (see the magnificent work by Binet 1892 and Ribot 1884). After 1890, psychodynamic models and treatments also became increasingly important: in this regard, France was, perhaps, the most permeable of the three nations (Hesnard 1971). The breaking up of the old group of 'neuroses' (e.g. neurasthenia and psychasthenia) (Berrios 1985d) set asunder a large number of clinical states which (as the British debate showed) after a period of indeterminacy began to be considered as the 'milder' forms of manic depressive illness. To many, this solution was not satisfactory and the Continental response is well expressed in the work of Courbon (1923), Rouart (1936), Benon (1937) and Montassut (1938). The British debate flared up in the 1930s, as a result of the work of Aubrey Lewis (1934, 1938): this has been well analysed by Kendell (1968) and is not discussed further.

REFERENCES

Arnaud S 1899 La senescenza precoce nei melancolici. Rivista di Patologia Nervosa e Mentale 4: 362–367

Bagenoff T 1911 La cyclothymie. In: Marie A (ed) Traité international de psychologie pathologique, vol 2. Alcan, Paris, p 709–722

Baillarger J F 1854 De la folie à double-forme. Annales Médico-Psychologiques 6: 367–391

Banister H, Zangwill O L 1949 John Thompson McCurdy (1886–1947). British Journal of Psychology 40: 1–4

Bash K W 1955 Lehrbuch der allgemeinen Psychopathologie. Georg Thieme, Stuttgart

Benon R 1937 La mélancolie. Marcel Vigné, Paris

Bercherie P 1980 Les fondements de la clinique. Editions du Seuil, Paris

Berger K 1907 Über die Psychosen des Klimakteriums. Monatschrift für Psychiatrie und Neurologie 22: 13–52

Berrios G E 1981 Stupor: a conceptual history. Psychological Medicine 11: 677–688

Berrios G E 1984 Descriptive psychopathology: conceptual and historical aspects. Psychological Medicine 14: 303–313

Berrios G E 1985a The psychopathology of affectivity. Psychological Medicine 15: 745–758

Berrios G E 1985b 'Depressive pseudodementia' or 'melancholic dementia': a 19th century view. Journal of Neurology, Neurosurgery and Psychiatry 48: 393–400

Berrios G E 1985c Positive and negative symptoms and Jackson: a conceptual history. Archives of General Psychiatry 42: 95–97

Berrios G E 1985d Obsessional disorders during the 19th century. In: Bynum W F, Porter R, Shepherd M (eds) The anatomy of madness, vol 1. Tavistock, London, p 166–187

Berrios G E 1987 Historical aspects of the psychoses: 19th century issues. British Medical Bulletin 43: 484–497

Berrios G E 1988a Melancholia and depression during the 19th century: a conceptual history. British Journal of Psychiatry 153: 298–304

Berrios G E 1988b Depressive and manic states during the 19th century. In: Georgotas A, Cancro R (eds) Depression and mania. Elsevier, New York, p 13–25

Berrios G E 1991 Affective disorders in old age: a conceptual history. International Journal of Geriatric Psychiatry 6: 337–346

Berrios G E, Beer D 1991 The concept of unitary psychosis: a conceptual history (submitted for publication)

Berrios G E, Hauser R 1988 The early development of Kraepelin's ideas on classification: a conceptual history. Psychological Medicine 18: 813–821

Billod E 1856 Des diverses formes de lypémanie. Annales Médico-Psychologiques 2: 308–338

Binet A 1892 Les altérations de la personnalité. Alcan, Paris

Bolton J S 1908 Maniacal-depressive insanity. Brain 31: 301–318

Bronisch T 1990 Dysthyme Störungen. Nervenarzt 61: 133–139

Brush E N 1897 An analysis of one hundred cases of acute melancholia. British Medical Journal 2: 777–779

Bucknill N J C, Tuke D H 1858 A manual of psychological medicine. John Churchill, London

Buzzard E F 1930 Discussion on the diagnosis and treatment of the milder forms of the manic-depressive psychosis. Proceedings of the Royal Society of Medicine 23: 881–895

Chaslin P 1912 Eléments de sémiologie et clinique mentales. Asselin et Houzeau, Paris

Cordeiro J C 1973 Etats délirants du troisième age. L'Encephale 62: 20–55

Cotard J 1882 Du délire des négations. Archives de Neurologie 4: 152–170; 282–296

Courbon P 1923 De la dualité étiologique de la manie et de la mélancolie. L'Encephale 18: 27–31

Dana C L 1904 A discussion on the classification of the melancholias. Medical Record 66: 1033–1035

Darwin C 1872 The expression of the emotions in man and animals. John Murray, London

Delasiauve L J F 1856 Du diagnostic différentiel de la lypémanie. Annales Médico-Psychologiques 3: 380–442

Deny G 1908 La cyclothymie. La Semaine Medicale 15: 169–171

Deny G 1909 Représentation schématique et nomenclature des différentes formes de la psychose maniaque-dépressive. L'Encéphale 4: 363–366

Deny G, Camus P 1907 La psychose maniaque-dépressive. Baillière, Paris

Dreyfus G L 1907 Die Melancholie. Ein Zustandsbild des manisch-depressiven Irreseins. Gustav Fischer, Jena

Ducosté M 1907 De L'involution présénile dans la folie maniaque-dépressive. Annales Médico-Psychologiques 65: 299–303

Dumas G 1894 Les états intellectuels dans la mélancolie. Alcan, Paris

Esquirol J E 1820 Mélancolie. In: Dictionnaire des sciences médicales par une Société de Medicins et de Chirurgiennes. Panckoucke, Paris

Ey H 1954 Les psychoses périodiques maniaco-depressives. Étude 25. In: Études Psychiatriques vol 3. Desclée de Brouwer, Paris, p 429–518

Falret J P 1854 Mémoire sur la folie circulaire. Bulletin de l'Académie de Médicine 19: 382–415

Fishbein I L 1949 Involutional melancholia and convulsive therapy. American Journal of Psychiatry 106: 128–135

Flemming C F 1859 Pathologie und Therapie der Psychoses. August Hirschwald, Berlin

Foville A 1882 Folie à double forme. Brain 5: 288–323

Freud S 1917 Trauer und Melancholie. Gesammelte Werke (1963), vol 10. Fischer, Frankfurt

Gaupp R 1905 Die Depressionszustände des höheren Lebensalters. Münchener Medizinische Wochenschrift 22: 1531–1537

Gibson E T 1918 A clinical summary of 106 cases of mental disorder of unknown etiology arising in the fifth and sixth decades. American Journal of Insanity 75: 221–249

Gillespie R D 1929 The clinical differentiation of types of depression. Guy's Hospital Reports 79: 306–344

Griesinger W 1861 Die Pathologie und Therapie der psychischen Krankheiten für Aerzte und Studierende. Adolphe Krabbe, Stuttgart

Gruber H E 1981 Darwin on Man. University of Chicago Press, Chicago

Gull W W 1894 A collection of the published writings of W W Gull (ed T Acland). (2 vols). New Sydenham Society, London

Haslam J 1809 Observations on madness and melancholia, 2nd edn. Callow, London

Heinroth J C 1975 Textbook of disturbances of mental life (2 vols, Tr J Schmorak). Johns Hopkins University Press, Baltimore.

Henderson D K 1945 Robert Dick Gillespie. American Journal of Psychiatry 102: 572–573

Hesnard A 1971 De Freud à Lacan. Les Editions ESF, Paris

Hilts V L 1967 Statist and statistician: three studies in the history of nineteenth century English statistical thought. PhD Dissertation, Harvard University

Hollander B 1901 The cerebral localization of melancholia. Journal of Mental Science 47: 458–485

Jackson S W 1986 Melancholia and depression. Yale University Press, New Haven

Janet P 1903 Les obsessions et la psychasthénie. Alcan, Paris

Jastrow J 1901 Depression. In: Baldwin J M (ed) Dictionary of philosophy and psychology, vol 1. McMillan, London, p 270

Jelliffe S E 1911 Cyclothemia. The mild forms of manic-depressive psychosis and the manic-depressive constitution. American Journal of Insanity 67: 661–675

Kahlbaum K 1863 Die Gruppirung der psychischen Krankheiten und die Eintheilung der Seelenstörungen. A W Kafemann, Danzig

Katzenstein R 1963 Karl Ludwig Kahlbaum und sein Beitrag zur Entwicklung der Psychiatrie. Juris, Zürich

Kendell R E 1968 The classification of depressive illness. Oxford University Press, Oxford

Ketal R 1975 Affect, mood, emotion and feeling: semantic considerations. American Journal of Psychiatry 132: 1215–1217

Kolle K 1963 Carl Friedrich Flemming. In: Kolle K (ed) Grosse Nervenärzte, vol 3. George Thieme, Stuttgart, p 61–68

Kraepelin E 1920 Die Erscheinungsformen des Irreseins. Zeitschrift für die gesamte Neurologie und Psychiatrie 62: 1–29

Kraepelin E 1921 Manic-depressive insanity. E & S Livingstone, Edinburgh

Kraepelin E 1983 Lebenserinnerungen. Springer, Berlin

Krafft-Ebing R 1879 Lehrbuch der Psychiatrie. Enke, Stuttgart

Krueger F 1928 Das Wessen der Gefühle. Archiv für die gesamte Psychologie 65: 91–128

Lange J 1928 Die endogenen un reaktiven Gemütserkrankungen. In: Bumke O (ed) Handbuch der Geisteskrankheiten, vol 2. Springer, Berlin

Leeper R W 1948 A motivational theory of emotion to replace emotion as a disorganized response. Psychological Review 55: 5–21

Lewis A 1934 Melancholia: a clinical survey of depressive states. Journal of Mental Science 80: 277–378

Lewis A 1938 States of depression. British Medical Journal 2: 875–878

McCurdy J T 1925 The psychology of emotion. Morbid and abnormal. Kegan Paul, Trench, Trubner, London

Mairet D 1883 De la démence mélancolique. Masson, Paris

Mantegazza P 1878 Fisionomia e mimica (English translation: Physiognomy and Expression, no date) Walter Scott, London

Mapother E 1926 Discussion on manic-depressive psychosis. British Medical Journal 2: 872–879

Maudsley H 1895 The pathology of mind. A study of its distempers, deformities and disorders. MacMillan, London

Mayne R G 1860 An expository lexicon of the terms, ancient and modern in medicine and general science. John Churchill, London

Meyer A 1901 Melancholia. In: Baldwin J M (ed) Dictionary of philosophy and psychology, vol 2, McMillan, London, p 61–62

Mitchell S W 1897 An analysis of 3000 cases of melancholia. Transactions of the Association of American Physicians 12: 480–487

Montassut M 1938 La dépression constitutionnelle. Masson, Paris

Mordret E 1883 De la folie à double forme. Baillière, Paris

Newcombe N, Lerner J C 1981 Britain between the wars: the historical context of Bowlby's theory of attachment. Psychiatry 44: 1–12

Owens H, Maxmen J S 1979 Mood and affect: a semantic confusion. American Journal of Psychiatry 136: 97–99

Petrie A A W 1940 Edward Mapother. Journal of Mental Science 106: 747–749

Phillips J G P 1912a Involutional conditions. In: Mott F W (ed) Early mental disease. The Lancet Extranumbers 2. Wakley & Son, London, p 90–92

Phillips J G P 1912b Psychoses associated with senility and arteriosclerosis. In: Mott F W (ed) Early mental disease. The Lancet Extranumbers 2. Wakley & Son, London, p 146–148

Pinel P 1809 Traité médico-philosophique sur l'aliènation mentale. J A Brosson, Paris

Post F 1965 The clinical psychiatry of late life. Pergamon Press, Oxford

Prichard J C 1835 A treatise on insanity and other disorders affecting the mind. Sherwood, Gilbert & Piper, London

RCP 1906 The nomenclature of diseases, 4th edn. HMSO, London

Régis E 1885 Manuel pratique de médicine mentale. Doin, Paris

Rennert H 1968 Wilhelm Griesinger und die Einheitpsychose. Wissenschaftliche Zeitschrift der Humboldt-Universität 17: 15–16

Ribot T 1884 Les maladies de la personalité. Alcan, Paris

Ribot T 1897 The psychology of emotions. Walter Scott, London

Ritti A 1876 Folie à double forme. In: Dechambre A (ed) Dictionnaire encyclopédique des sciences médicales. Masson, Paris

Robertson G M 1890 Melancholia, from the physiological and evolutionary points of view. Journal of Mental Science 36: 53–67

Rocha D da 1906 La psychose maniaque-dépressive. Annales Médico-Psychologiques 64: 250–262

Rouart J 1936 Psychose maniaque dépressive et folies discordantes. Doin, Paris

Roubinovitch J 1896 Des variétés cliniques de la folie en France et en Allemagne. Octave Doin, Paris

Rush B 1812 Medical inquiries and observations upon the diseases of the mind. Kimber & Richardson, Philadelphia

Saury H 1886 Étude clinique sur la folie héréditaire. Delahaye & Lecrosnier, Paris

Savage G H 1898 Insanity and allied neuroses. Cassell, London

Sérieux P 1907 Review of Dreyfus's book, L'Encephale 2: 456–458

Sérieux P & Capgras J 1909 Les folies raisonnantes. Le délire d'interprétation. Alcan, Paris

Sollier P 1893 Sur une forme circulaire de la neurasthénie. Revue de Médicine 13: 1009–1019

Soukhanoff S 1909 La cyclothymie et la psychasthénie. Annales Médico-Psychologiques 67: 27–38

Soukhanoff S & Gannouchkine P 1903 Étude sur la mélancolie. Annales Médico-Psychologiques 61: 213–238

Stocking Jr G W 1978 Introduction. In: Prichard J C Researches into the physical history of man (repr). University of Chicago Press, Chicago, p ix-cx

Thalbitzer S 1926 Emotions and insanity. Kegan Paul, Trench, Trubner, London

Treadway W L 1913 The presenile psychoses. Journal of Nervous and Mental Disease 40: 375–387

Tuke D H 1892 A Dictionary of psychological medicine. Churchill, London

Turner J 1900 A theory concerning the physical conditions of the nervous system which are necessary for the production of states of melancholia, mania, etc. Journal of Mental Science 46: 505–512

von Feuchtersleben E 1847 The principles of medical psychology. London, Sydenham Society

Wahrig-Schmidt B 1985 Der junge Wilhelm Griesinger. Gunter Narr, Tübingen

Zerssen D v 1988 Definition und Klassifikation affektiver Störungen aus historischer Sicht. In: Zerssen D von, Möller H J (eds) Affektive Störungen. Springer, Berlin, p 3–11

5. Bipolar–unipolar distinction

Carlo Perris

A distinction between bipolar (manic-depressive) and unipolar (either depressive or manic) recurrent affective disorders is firmly established in the most widely accepted international classification systems, e.g. in the ninth revision of the WHOs International Classification of Diseases (ICD–9; World Health Organization 1978), the forthcoming tenth revision (ICD–10), and in the *Diagnostic and Statistical Manual,* third edition revised (DSM-IIIR) of the American Psychiatric Association (1987). The manuals include both sketchy clinical descriptions and detailed diagnostic criteria for giving an appropriate diagnostic label. In both manuals the crucial distinctive feature is the occurrence of both *manic* and *depressive* episodes in the bipolar subgroup. The distinction between bipolar and unipolar affective disorders is, however, relatively recent. Previously, the label manic-depressive psychosis was used for both depressed and manic patients independently of whether they had also shown episodes of the opposite polarity.

HISTORICAL BACKGROUND

Kraepelin's effort to systematize knowledge about mental diseases available at the end of the last century occurred at a time when Sydenham's suggestion that 'all Diseases should be reduced to certain and definite Species' was still influential. We can easily recognize the fundamental elements upon which he based his classificatory work. These were: the severity of the disorder (psychotic); the identification of groups of symptom-complexes with the same evolutions and outcomes; and the assumption that heredity played a prominent role in the causation of these disorders.

Kraepelin (1913) not only recognized the importance of Falret's and Baillarger's earlier identification of circular manic-depressive states but also progressively refined and extended his view of 'manic-depressive

insanity' (MDI) in successive editions of his *Textbook of Psychiatry.* Thus, under the heading MDI he finally included 'on the one side, the whole domain of the so-called periodic or circular insanities, on the other hand, the simple mania, a greater part of the morbid states termed melancholia, and also a not inconsiderable number of cases of amentia'. Kraepelin's conception of MDI embraced in the end 'all cases of affective excess' including those at a personality level.

Kraepelin strongly believed in the hereditary aetiology of non-organic psychotic disorders. According to his own findings, a hereditary loading occurred in 80% of patients. In particular, he stated that psychiatric morbidity occurred in 36% of the parents of average patients, and in 40% of the parents of patients with more severe and frequent episodes. However, when considering the figures it should be kept in mind that case reports written around the turn of the century referring to hereditary loading do not necessarily imply that the same disorder occurred in the patient as among his/her first degree relatives. Kraepelin, in commenting upon hereditary factors in his MDI patients, stated that about one-third of their relatives had suffered from some mental disorder or alcoholism, most frequently from MDI. He excluded, however, the occurrence among relatives of MDI patients of epileptic and arteriosclerotic psychoses and of dementia praecox (Kraepelin 1913, p 1354).

Kraepelin's very wide conception of MDI gave rise to criticism in many quarters. Noticeable is the warning against the overextension of the term MDI issued by Adolf Meyer, who as early as 1905 had introduced Kraepelin's classification into the United States. In particular, Meyer stressed the fact that there were many 'depressions' that did not show the characteristics of MDI. In Germany, in his *Allgemeine Psychopathologie* Jaspers (1913) wrote:

Just as the rings made on the water by raindrops are first small and distinct and then grow larger and larger, swallow each other and then vanish, so from time to time in psychiatry there emerge diseases which constantly enlarge themselves until they perish with their own magnitude. Esquirol's monomania, the paranoia of the eighties and Meynert's amentia are all examples of this. Hebephrenia and catatonia, which were clearly defined, grew into dementia praecox which seemed to have no limits and *folie circulaire* into manic-depressive insanity which seemed equally ill-defined. (English translation 1963, p 568)

Later on, while British psychiatrists, challenged by the classical reports by Mapother (1926) and Lewis (1934, 1936), became involved in the debate as to whether 'endogenous' and 'exogenous' depression should be regarded as a unitary disorder varying in severity or as several discernible reaction types and disease entities, German psychiatrists, mainly scholars from the school of Wernicke, rejected the comprehensive definitions of MDI and dementia praecox suggested by Kraepelin and proposed a classification of endogenous psychoses comprised of several subgroups.

One of the most consistent proponents of a more detailed classification of endogenous psychoses was Leonhard who, in several articles and in successive editions of his *Aufteilung der endogenen Psychosen* (1957–1971; first published in English in 1979), proposed a division of the 'endogenous' psychoses into four main groups, and several subgroups as shown in Table 5.1.

In Leonhard's classification – as in that proposed earlier by Kleist (1953) – the course variable was used not only to separate 'endogenous affective disorders' from other 'endogenous' psychoses (e.g. the 'non-systemic' and 'systemic' schizophrenic disorders) but also to differentiate two large groups within the affective psychoses. This second differentiation referred to the occurrence of both depressive and manic phases in the same patient (bipolar form: i.e. true manic-depressive psychosis) or the occurrence of recurrent episodes of

psychotic depression or mania, without episodes of the opposite polarity (unipolar forms). Thus, the new classification element of 'polarity' of the phenomenological pattern became for Leonhard a decisive factor in the differentiation of affective disorders of an 'endogenous type'.

In his textbook, Leonhard (1957–1971) described in detail the clinical pictures of both the bipolar and unipolar forms of the illness, and reported abstracts of 83 case histories.

Both in Leonhard's original work and in a paper by one of his pupils (von Trostorff 1968) there is documentation of hereditary factors in both the unipolar and the bipolar forms of affective disorders, and that these are more pronounced in the bipolar form.

Leonhard and his associates also carried out a thorough investigation of temperamental characteristics in both bipolar and unipolar psychoses (Leonhard 1963, Leonhard et al 1962). These studies were extended to include members of their families, following a procedure previously adopted by Hoffman (1921). Leonhard concluded that bipolar manic-depressive patients were characterized by cyclothymic temperaments and unipolar depressives by 'subdepressive' temperaments, and also that similar personality characteristics could be found to some extent in the parents, siblings and children of the patients.

Unfortunately, Leonhard's work remained unnoticed for a long time outside Germany. Not until the middle of the 1960s did two comprehensive investigations of recurrent depressive psychosis appear, almost simultaneously but independently of each other, in which Leonhard's idea of polarity was taken into account – one by Angst (1966) in Switzerland and one by the author (Perris 1966, Perris & d'Elia 1964) in Sweden. The main results of these investigations appeared to be surprisingly consistent in most respects (Angst & Perris 1968) and supported Leonhard's hypothesis.

Table 5.1 Leonhard's classification of phasic psychoses and schizophrenia

Affective psychoses			Cycloid psychoses	Unsystematic schizophrenia	Systematic schizophrenia
Bipolar	**Monopolar**				
Manic-depressive	Depression	Mania	Anxiety—happiness psychosis	Affect laden paraphrenia	Paranoid forms
	a. agitated	a. unproductive	Agitated—retarded	Cataphasia (schizophasia)	Hebephrenic forms
	b. hypochondriacal	b. hypochondriacal	Confusion psychosis	Periodic catatonia	Catatonic forms
	c. with self-blaming	c. exalted	Hyperkinetic-hypokinetic motility psychosis		
	d. with reference etc	d. confabulatory etc			

Since that time a distinction between these two forms of affective disorder has been taken into account in almost all the psychiatric literature.

DEFINITION OF BIPOLAR AND UNIPOLAR AFFECTIVE DISORDERS

It is necessary at this juncture to comment upon the definitions of bipolar and unipolar affective disorders.

a. Bipolar affective disorder: In my original work (Perris & d'Elia 1964, Perris 1966) in order to achieve a satisfactory level of homogeneity a proband had to have suffered from both manic and depressive phases irrespective of whether hospital treatment had been received for both or only one. Information was based on hospital research, doctors' questionnaires and personal interviews with the patients and *at least* one first-degree relative. Short-term euphoria associated with treatment (mostly ECT) was not taken into account. As 'probably' bipolar I defined those patients who had experienced either manic or depressive phases according to a doctor's diagnosis and whose relatives reported that phases of different polarity had occurred but had not received medical attention.

b. Unipolar affective disorder: depression: For a proband to be defined as having a unipolar depressive *psychosis*, I required that the patient should have suffered from at least three episodes of illness separated from each other by intervals of complete symptomatic remission. Illnesses were required to show a global depressive pattern and impaired reality judgment severe enough to warrant hospital admission. I defined as '*probably*' unipolar patients who had experienced two separate depressive episodes consistent with the description given above, and who had reached the age of 60.

Patients who did not fulfil these criteria were defined as having 'unspecified affective disorders'.

c. Unipolar affective disorder: mania: In my original study a small number of patients were included who at the time of the study had suffered from one or more episodes of mania without having any history of depressive cycles. This distinction was derived from Leonhard's classification. However, I was unable to find more than 17 cases among the hospital records of 1539 patients which were scrutinized and many of these were still young enough to be at risk of depression. Hence I was unable to draw any conclusions from the study of this small group of patients. Results of later studies by other authors (Abrams & Taylor 1974, Abrams et al 1979, Nurnberger et al 1979, Pfohl et al 1982a, b) have consistently been against a distinction between unipolar mania and bipolar disorder.

In the American literature (Dunner et al 1970) bipolar patients have been divided into bipolar I and II. Bipolar I includes those who have suffered from clear-cut episodes of mania and depression, bipolar II those patients who have received medical attention for episodes of depression and have in their history short episodes of hypomania. Winokur and his associates also include among bipolars those patients who have suffered from depression and have a family history of certain bipolar psychosis in any first degree relative. Patients belonging to this subgroup have been labelled bipolar III by Depue & Monroe (1978).

Other studies have used less stringent definitions, particularly for unipolar depressive psychosis. With some exceptions (e.g. Bertelsen et al 1977, Smeraldi et al 1978) many investigations have not required any particular number of episodes in order to define a patient as 'unipolar', so that, patients of any age

Table 5.2 Course in bipolar patients in relation to type of first episode. Number of patients who changed polarity (i.e. became bipolar) in successive episodes

Number of patients		Episode						
		2nd	3rd	4th	5th	6th	7th	8th
First episode mania								
Male	20	11	5	1	3	—	—	—
Female	25	13	6	3	—	1	—	2
Total	45	24	11	4	3	1	—	2
First episode depression								
Male	36	24	10	2	—	—	—	—
Female	50	26	12	9	1	1	1	—
Total	86	50	22	11	1	1	1	—

suffering their first episode of depression have been regarded as unipolars.

Even the earlier occurrence of three separate episodes of psychotic depression does not completely eliminate the risk of misclassification. An analysis of my bipolar probands (Perris 1968), shown in Table 5.2, indicated that only 16% of patients changed polarity after three depressive episodes and only 4% after four episodes. Similar findings have been reported by Angst (1973) who, in a series of 400 bipolar patients from an international study, analysed the first 10 episodes. He calculated that the risk of misdiagnosing a patient as unipolar was about 13%. Since both sets of calculations refer to bipolar patients who exhibited episodes of mania the risk of misdiagnosing a bipolar patient as unipolar will be much smaller after three episodes of depression in unselected series.

More recently, Clayton (1981), on the basis of a survey of the literature, has estimated that between 5% and 18% of unipolar patients become bipolar. Akiskal et al (1978) found that 18% of patients defined as 'neurotic' depressives at the index episode had become bipolar during a 4-year follow-up. These results should be taken as a warning against giving the label 'unipolar' to patients at their first episode of depression.

FREQUENCY OF BIPOLAR DISORDERS

At the time of the first edition of this Handbook no clear-cut epidemiological information was available about the incidence and prevalence of bipolar manic-depressive psychosis in the general population. An indirect estimate, from older studies in which the proportion of patients who had suffered from both depression and mania was given, suggested that bipolar manic-depressive psychosis is a relatively rare disorder comprising between 10 and 40% of these series.

More recently, a few epidemiological studies have taken this distinction into account. In a population study carried out in New Haven in the USA, Weissman & Myers (1979) ascertained the lifetime prevalence of bipolar affective disorder to be 1.2%. Faravelli & Incerpi (1985) reported the 1-year prevalence of bipolar disorder in a representative population sample in Florence to be 1.7%, while that of 'atypical bipolar disorder' (according to DSM-III criteria) was 0.3%. On the other hand, Hällström (1984) found a point prevalence of major depressive episode of 6.9% in a Swedish urban female population, but no instances of bipolar disorder. Weissman et al (1988) in the NIMH Epidemiologic Catchment Area Study probability

sample of over 18 000 adults from five USA communities, found a cross-site lifetime prevalence for bipolar disorder of 1.2%, without sex difference.

At the present time no clear-cut information is available concerning the relative frequency of bipolar and unipolar affective disorders in different ethnic groups. In a WHO study of in- and outpatients with affective disorder in four cultures (Jablensky et al 1981) the rate of bipolar disorder ranged from 6.5% in Teheran to 28.3% in Basle.

Further information on epidemiological studies is given in chapter 8.

GENETIC STUDIES

Family studies

The genetics of affective disorder are dealt with more thoroughly in chapter 9 but aspects relevant to the bipolar-unipolar distinction will be reviewed here. The original results of the family studies by Angst and Perris are summarized in Table 5.3, in which only the findings concerning the risks of affective disorders in the parents and siblings of the probands are given. However, neither study found any increased risk of schizophrenia in the families of either group.

Table 5.3   Diagnostic differentiation of secondary cases (parents and siblings) in studies of Angst and Perris

	Bipolar or manic	Unipolar depressive	Other depressive and suicide cases
Bipolar probands			
Angst	3.7 + 1.5	11.2 + 2.5	3.1 + 1.4*
Perris	10.8 + 1.4	0.58 + 0.03	8.6 + 1.2
Unipolar probands			
Angst	0.29 + 0.03	9.1 + 1.6	2.3 + 0.8*
Perris	0.35 + 0.02	7.4 + 1.1	6.8 + 1.0

*only suicide

As shown in the table, the occurrence of bipolar disorder in relatives of unipolar probands was particularly low and almost the same in both studies, while that of unipolar disorder was significantly higher. Results concerning the relatives of bipolar probands were less consistent. The risk of unipolar disorder was almost negligible in the study of Perris, but in Angst's was even higher than that of bipolar illness. Among the secondary cases in my investigation, however, there was

Table 5.4 Morbidity risk (%) for affective disorders in first degree relatives of unipolar probands

Study	Bipolar	Unipolar	Unspecified and suicide	Total affective disorders
Gershon et al (1974)	2.1	11.5	—	13.6
Trzebiatowska (1977)	—	7.5	5.0	12.5
Smeraldi et al (1978)	0.6	8.0	4.3	12.9
Mendlewicz (1979)	2.4	27.2	—	29.6
Taylor et al (1980)	4.1	8.3	—	—
Jakimow-Venulet (1981)	0.5	15.3	—	15.8
Perris et al (1982)	0.8	17.4	—	18.2
Stancer et al (1987)	1.4	24.4	—	—

Table 5.5 Morbidity risk (%) for affective disorder in first degree relatives of bipolar probands

Study	Bipolar	Unipolar	Unspecified and suicide	Total affective disorders
Winokur et al (1967)	10.2	20.4	—	30.6
Helzer et al (1974)	4.6	10.6	—	15.2
Goetzl et al (1974)	2.8	13.7	—	16.5
Gershon (1974)	3.8	6.8	—	10.6
Mendlewicz & Rainer (1974)	17.7	22.4	—	—
Pettersson (1974)	4.6	2.7	5.7	13.0
James & Chapman (1975)	6.4	13.2	—	19.6
Trzebiatowska (1977)	10.0	—	6.0	16.0
Johnson & Lehman (1977)	15.5	19.8	—	—
Smeraldi et al (1978)	5.8	7.1	3.9	16.8
Mendlewicz (1979)	18.6	20.4	—	41.4
Taylor et al (1980)	4.8	4.2	—	—
Jakimow-Venulet (1981)	11.8	6.1	—	17.9
Stancer et al (1987)	4.4	18.7	—	24.6

a high number of suicides and of cases with a depressive disorder that did not fulfil the definition of psychotic unipolar depression. Cumulatively, the morbidity risk for any affective disorder in each subgroup proved to be quite similar in both studies (in bipolar families 21.0% and 20.0% respectively, in unipolar families 11.7% and 14.6%). Also in line with Leonhard's original assumption, the family loading in bipolar families was significantly higher than that in relatives of unipolar probands.

Since then many studies have been carried out. The main findings are shown in Tables 5.4 and 5.5.

The total risk of affective disorder in the unipolar family studies in Table 5.4 is 18.1%, consistent with the earlier findings as is the ratio of bipolar to unipolar disorder. Higher risks of unipolar disorders were found by Mendlewicz (1979) and by Stancer et al (1987), possibly due to broader definitions of 'unipolar depression' in the classification of their secondary cases.

In the studies of bipolar disorder (Table 5.5) the total risk for affective disorder is 20.2%, almost the same as in the two earlier studies. Again the studies by Mendlewicz stand out as showing high rates. In bipolar families the average risk of a bipolar disorder is 8.6% with considerable variation among the different studies. The average risk of unipolar disorder 'is 12.8%. It should be noted, however, that the significant difference in total family loading between bipolar and unipolar families found by Angst and Perris does not occur in the average figures from the studies reviewed in Table 5.4 and 5.5.

It is evident that bipolar disorder aggregates in the relatives of probands with a bipolar disorder compared with the relatives of unipolar probands. In contrast, the risk of unipolar disorder appears to be quite high in bipolar families, and higher than that originally found by Perris. This may be due to the secondary cases which were left unclassified because they did not fit the definition of either unipolar or bipolar disorder, but which might have represented unipolar disorders.

On the other hand, since Kraepelin it has been known that the first episode of MDI is most often one of depression. Shorter periods of observation in the relatives (siblings and children in particular) would underestimate the risk of mania. Also, differences in the risk periods taken into account to calculate the number of relatives at risk ('*Bezugssiffer*') greatly influence the values which are obtained.

One finding which appears to be consistent in the family studies discussed so far is the very low risk of bipolar disorder in unipolar families. One exception is the study by Taylor et al (1980), who found a morbidity risk of 4.1%. However, in the more recent NIMH and Yale studies (Weissman et al 1984) the rates of bipolar I disorder in relatives of probands with a severe major depression (which could be assumed to correspond with what has been called 'unipolar depression' in most studies) were 1.5% and 0.8% respectively. Also, Rice et al (1987) found the risks of bipolar illness in relatives of bipolar probands to range from 5.7% to 7.2% depending on whether only an interview or a family study approach had been adopted in the ascertainment of secondary cases. In contrast, the risk (per cent) of bipolar disorder in relatives of unipolar probands was found to be 1.1-1.7. Hence, if it is assumed that family aggregation indicates a hereditary component, the relative absence of bipolar disorder in the families of unipolars strongly supports the 'genetic' distinction between unipolar and bipolar disorder.

On the other hand, the occurrence of (less strictly defined) 'unipolar' cases in bipolar families might speak against a clear-cut genetic distinction between bipolar and unipolar illnesses. However, in families of healthy controls who had never suffered from any affective disorder, the risks of major and minor depression were found to be 5.9% and 2.5% respectively in the study by Weissman and her co-workers (Weissman et al 1984). Hence it might be that many so-called 'unipolar' cases in bipolar families represent depressions which are not necessarily genetically related to the bipolar disorder observed in the proband.

Both bipolar and unipolar disorder have been divided into subgroups according to different historical and clinical variables. As concerns the bipolars, the proposed division into bipolar I, II, and III has already been mentioned. Other subdivisions include age at onset or course characteristics (e.g. whether predominantly manic, predominantly depressive or almost equally comprising manic and depressive episodes, or whether mania is to be regarded as 'primary' or 'secondary'). Also, different subgroupings have been used in family studies of unipolar probands (e.g. mild/severe; primary/secondary; endogenous/non-endogenous; with or without melancholia; early or late onset; pure disease versus spectrum disease versus sporadic disease; psychotic/non-psychotic). However, since these studies do not bear directly on the distinction between unipolar and bipolar disorder rather than the heterogeneity of patients labelled as 'unipolar', they will not be reviewed here.

Twin studies

The results of twin studies (reviewed by Zerbin-Rüdin 1969, 1979, Bertelsen et al 1977, Kringlen 1985) also support a distinction between unipolar and bipolar disorder. Kringlen, in particular, emphasizes that the MZ/DZ ratio (4.9 for bipolar, 2.3 for unipolar disorder in the study by Bertelsen et al) clearly declines from bipolar disorder via psychotic major depression to nonpsychotic major depression and depressive adjustment disorder. In Kringlen's view this finding clearly indicates the significance of hereditary factors in bipolar affective disorders, whereas it is less conclusive concerning depressive disorders. In particular, Kringlen raises the question of whether the DSM-III diagnosis of major depression covers too broad a heterogeneous group to be useful in genetic studies. In a very recent twin study by McGuffin and co-workers (1990) the nature versus nurture issue in the causation of depression has been particularly addressed. As in previous studies, the authors found significantly higher monozygotic than dizygotic concordance. However, applying an additive model in which depression is considered as a threshold, they also found that both genetic factors and shared family environment make substantial and significant contributions to the familiality of depression. This conclusion is in keeping with results by our group (Perris et al 1987), which show that probands from families with at least one affected parent also experience the rearing attitudes of their parents as more dysfunctional (depriving) than patients without affected parents.

There are no studies in the literature of twins reared apart bearing on the issue of a distinction between unipolar and bipolar disorder. Price (1968) was able to identify 12 pairs reared apart. Eight of them were concordant in a broad sense. Not one of them was bipolar. Kringlen (1985) reports on one such pair in his own series; the proband had typical manic attacks while the co-twin was normal.

Studies of adoptees

Adoption studies are still few and their results are inconsistent. Mendlewicz & Rainer (1977) investigated morbidity among biological and adoptive parents of bipolar adoptees and compared their findings with those obtained from biological parents of bipolar non-adoptees, from biological and adoptive parents of normal adoptees and from biological parents of poliomyelitic patients. The major finding was that psychopathology in the biological parents was in excess of that found in the adoptive parents. In addition, the frequency of psychopathology in the biological parents of bipolar adoptees was similar to that of the parents of non-adopted bipolars. However, the difference in psychopathology between the biological and adoptive parents was statistically significant only if it included the total affective spectrum, i.e. bipolar and unipolar cases, schizoaffective psychosis and cyclothymia, rather than only bipolar cases. In a recent study of adoptees from Sweden (von Knorring 1983) comprising 115 adoptees with affective disorders (49% mostly depressive) and substance abuse (51%), and 115 matched controls, there was no significant correlation between specific diagnoses in biological parents and their adopted offspring. Neither bipolar adoptees nor bipolar parents (either biological or adoptive) were included in von Knorring's series.

Studies of association and linkage

Ever since Winokur and his associates (1969) presented some evidence of a possible linkage of bipolar disorder with different markers on the X-chromosome, a number of studies have been published. These are reviewed in chapter 9. Here, however, it should be pointed out that positive results which have been reported are obtained only if all affectively ill subjects in the pedigrees investigated are considered.

To sum up, the conclusions of the previous edition of this chapter seem to be still valid and may be summarized:

a. Genetic factors may be relevant in determining the form of the disorder.

b. MDI as described by Kraepelin probably comprises genetically heterogeneous subgroups.

c. There is evidence suggesting that unipolar depression as presently defined in most studies is genetically distinct from bipolar depression.

d. There is also evidence suggesting that a genetic influence is greater in the causation of bipolar than of unipolar disorder. A large proportion of non-bipolar depressed patients do not have any apparent heredity loading at all in their family.

e. The genetic transmission of bipolar and unipolar recurrent depression is still unclarified, nor do we know what is actually genetically transmitted.

f. Very likely a distinct genetic liability for depression and mania respectively must be taken into account, which together with other non-genetic factors contribute to the occurrence of the manifest disorders.

SOCIODEMOGRAPHIC VARIABLES

Sex distribution

It is generally accepted that affective disorders occur more frequently in women than in men and several explanations have been proposed to explain this difference. However, none of the single variables explored so far (e.g. methodological, endocrine, psychosocial and genetic factors) is enough to account for the increased rates of depression among women. Also, there is some suggestion (Klerman 1988) that the male/female differences have narrowed in recent decades. However, in the original studies by Angst and Perris the sex distribution was almost equal in bipolar disorder, although women clearly outnumbered men in unipolar depression. More recent results by Rice et al (1984) and by others are

Table 5.6   Mean scores and s.d. on the three factors in the different sub-groups

	Rejection		Emotional warmth		Overprotection	
Fathers						
1. Unipolar	33.7*	8.5	44.1*	10.4	28.9	5.7
2. Bipolar	34.1	10.1	46.3	15.4	29.4	6.0
3. Healthy controls	35.6	8.4	49.2	9.8	31.0	7.1
Mothers						
1. Unipolar	34.7*	9.8	44.2***	11.1	31.5	6.4
2. Bipolar	35.3	9.5	49.5	13.2	32.2	7.0
3. Healthy controls	36.1	9.0	52.2	8.7	34.8	7.8

* $p < 0.05$; *** $p < 0.001$ when compared with controls

consistent with the conclusion that there is no sex difference in bipolar illness.

Family environment

Both Angst (1966) and Perris (1966) found that the position in the sibship of bipolar and unipolar probands did not differ from the expected values in a random population, and there were no differences between the groups concerning seriously disturbed environments during childhood. In a more recent large series, Perris & Perris (1979) found that a disturbed childhood environment seemed to be shared by patients with bipolar, unipolar and other psychiatric disorders but were not specific to the kind of disorder. In particular, there were no significant differences in parental deprivation by separation or death. Significantly more bipolar than unipolar probands were 5 years or more older than their next sibling, but the relevance was unclear. In a later study (Perris et al 1986a) parental loss by death did not differentiate subjects with a bipolar or unipolar disorder from their healthy siblings.

In the 1966 series Perris found that the onset of a unipolar disorder occurred earlier where there was a

Table 5.7   Mean scores and s.d. on the three EMBU factors in depressives with (A) and without (B) affective disorders

EMBU factor	A		B		p	
	mean	s.d.	mean	s.d.		
Rejection						
Father	38.3	11.5	34.3	9.4	<0.05	
Mother	37.8	10.6	34.4	8.3	<0.10	<0.05
Both parents	74.2	20.6	65.3	18.6	<0.02	
Emotional warmth						
Father	44.3	11.0	46.5	10.6		
Mother	45.3	12.0	47.7	10.3		
Both parents	87.4	24.6	89.7	24.3		
Overprotection						
Father	30.5	7.7	30.1	7.0		
Mother	32.6	7.3	32.4	6.9		
Both parents	61.6	14.4	59.6	15.1		

disturbed childhood environment. More recently, Perris et al (1986b) found that unipolar patients, compared with healthy subjects, had experienced the rearing attitudes of both their parents as more rejecting and more lacking emotional warmth (see Table 5.6). This finding is in line with several others in the literature (Parker 1983, Alnaes & Torgersen 1990).

In the Swedish series bipolar patients did not show any difference when compared with healthy controls. However, in a replication study comprising Italian patients (Perris et al 1985) even the bipolar patients scored their parents as rejecting and lacking emotional warmth. When the experiences of dysfunctional parental rearing reported by the Swedish unipolar patients were analysed in relation to age at onset (Perris et al 1987) statistically significant differences between early and late onset patients were found. In particular, early onset patients reported a more dysfunctional rearing attitude in both their parents (see Table 5.7).

Joyce (1984(a)) did not find any difference in parental bonding in bipolars compared with healthy controls. On the other hand, Glassner & Haldipur (1985) suggest that a significant majority of bipolar subjects compared with matched controls have been treated as the special child of the family.

Clayton (1981) points out that several studies have found a positive association between bipolar disorder and high socioeconomic status. This finding might be related to the fact that bipolar patients are often described as already high achievers at a young age (Coryell et al 1989, Glassner & Haldipur 1985).

Age at onset

There is general agreement in the literature that the onset of bipolar disorder occurs on average at a younger age than that of unipolar recurrent depression. In fact, both in Angst's and Perris's investigations, the mean age of onset showed a peak in the age group 25–29 years in the bipolars and 40–44 years in the unipolars. Winokur et al (1969) reported a median age at onset of 24 years in their series of bipolar patients. In the follow-up study of bipolar patients by Carlson et al (1974) the average age of onset was 30 years. Joyce (1984(b)), in a series of 200 hospitalized bipolar patients, found that the most common age of onset was 15–19 years. Among 200 bipolars investigated by Clayton (1981) 20% were ill by 20 years, 49% by 30 years, and 89% by 50 years. Gammon et al (1983) underscore that bipolar disorder is moderately frequent in adolescent inpatients although it is often unrecognized. A significantly earlier

onset in bipolar patients compared with unipolars was also found in an international study of a large series of Italian and Swedish patients (Smeraldi et al 1987). Also, the presence of at least one affected parent was significantly related to an earlier onset independently of polarity.

More recently, Klerman (1988) has reviewed the evidence for an increase in depression among adolescents and young adults. Since it is not yet known to what extent such an increase is determined by an increase of unipolar depression occurring for the first time at a young age, it is possible that the bipolar/unipolar difference in age of onset will considerably narrow in the near future.

Current family environment

Concerning the current family environment, Perris (1966) found that the occurrence of divorce was significantly higher in bipolar than in unipolar probands. More recent studies (Mayo 1970, Brodie & Leff 1971, Carlson et al 1974, Hoover & Fitzgerald 1981, Coryell et al 1985, Lesser 1983) confirm the high frequency of divorce and of marital conflict among bipolar patients. Lesser, in particular, underscores that undiagnosed 'hypomania' is often the cause of marital disruption. It should be noted that marital maladjustment has also been reported in non-bipolar depressed patients (Weissman & Paykel 1974, Merikangas et al 1985a). Findings in Angst's and Perris's series concerning celibacy rate and fertility did not distinguish bipolar from unipolar patients, nor did they distinguish patients as a whole from the Swiss and Swedish general populations.

A number of authors (Gershon et al 1971, Dunner et al 1976, Merikangas & Spiker 1982, Negri et al 1981, Waters et al 1983) have reported on the possible occurrence of assortative mating in patients with an affective disorder. Assortative mating seems to occur more frequently in men than in women and in bipolars than unipolars. However, the results reported so far are not consistent and do not allow any definite conclusion.

Life events

The issue of life events and social stress in patients suffering from an affective disorder is dealt with more extensively in chapter 10. At this juncture it may suffice to point out that stressful events seem to be important in the occurrence of bipolar as well as unipolar affective disorders. The occurrence of stressful events prior to onset did not distinguish bipolar from unipolar patients either in Angst's or in Perris's series. Similar results have been obtained by Brodie & Leff (1971) and by Mayo (1970) and, more recently, by H. Perris (1984). Glassner & Haldipur (1983) reported a higher number of life events in late onset (>20 years) than in early-onset bipolars. Joffe et al (1989) did not find any difference in life events between bipolar and manic patients. On the other hand no relationship was found between life events and the onset of mania in a recent study by Sclare & Creed (1990).

PERSONALITY CHARACTERISTICS

As mentioned earlier, Leonhard suggested some differences in personality structure between bipolar and unipolar patients, and also among the relatives of patients belonging to the two groups. There is a great deal of information concerning personality characteristics and psychometric measures in bipolar and unipolar patients available in the literature (see chapter 12). However, most of the studies are biased by the fact that patients were investigated in a phase of illness and not a symptom-free period.

In a first study (Perris 1966) of comparable groups of bipolar and unipolar patients investigated during a symptom-free period, using the Marke — Nyman Temperament Scale (MNT) (Nyman & Marke 1962), bipolar patients were found to score lower on the stability scale whereas unipolar patients scored lower on the validity scale. These findings were verified later by Hirschfeld & Klerman (1979), who also found that measures of stability, validity and solidity distinguished unipolar but not bipolar patients from published norms. Metcalfe et al (1975) also found significantly lower validity scores in recovered unipolar patients compared with healthy controls. A significantly lower score on stability in bipolars as compared with controls was reported by Bech & Rafaelsen (1979).

In a subsequent study (Perris 1971) using the Maudsley Personality Inventory (Eysenck 1959) a significantly higher N-score was found in unipolar patients than bipolars. However, this difference was evident only at the time of discharge from hospital and disappeared when the patients were re-examined on follow-up. Results by Bech & Rafaelsen (1979) are consistent with these findings.

In another study Strandman (1978) and Perris & Strandman (1980) used the Cesarek and Marke Personality Schema (CMPS) (Cesarek & Marke 1968) and found that 'dominance', 'exhibition' and 'autonomy' were psychogenic needs associated with bipolar disorder whereas 'defence of status' and 'guilt feelings' were more marked in unipolar patients. They also found that the characteristics of unipolar depressives remained unchanged whether investigated in a depressive phase or in a phase of recovery. A difference in 'autonomy' between bipolar and unipolar patients has also been reported by Bech & Rafaelsen (1979).

A series of papers on the personality characteristics of bipolar and unipolar patients has been published by Donnelly & Murphy (1973a,b) and Donnelly et al (1975). Using the MMPI these authors found that the bipolar group had significantly higher scores than unipolar patients on the Ma scale and significantly lower scores on the Pt scale. They also documented a greater tendency to endorse socially desirable response sets in bipolar than in unipolar patients. Finally, in a study of Rorschach responses Donnelly et al (1975) found that the bipolar style of response was characterized by selective attention to the more objective aspects of the ink-blots, while the unipolar style was characterized by a more subjective approach. Primary response to colour was found only in bipolar patients. The feasibility of Rorschach studies in identifying personality markers of bipolar patients has been confirmed by Last et al (1984).

A series of articles on the personality characteristics of bipolar and unipolar patients has been published by Hirschfeld and his co-workers (Hirschfeld et al 1983a,b, 1986). Recovered non-bipolar female depressives compared with the normal population were found to be introverted, submissive and passive with increased interpersonal dependency but normal emotional strength. A comparison of recovered bipolar and unipolar patients failed to show any marked intergroup difference. On the other hand, both groups substantially differed from a never-ill group on measures of emotional strength.

The psychological functioning of bipolar patients in remission was investigated in 35 patients by MacVane et al (1978) and the results were compared with those obtained in 35 matched healthy controls. The study failed to show any significant differences on measures of positive mental health and of external orientation between patients and controls. Murray & Blackburn (1974) applied the Cattell 16 Personality Factor Scale to carefully defined bipolar and unipolar patients and reported significant differences in 'emotional stability', 'surgency', 'adventurousness' and 'extraversion', where the unipolar scored lower, and in 'anxiety', where the unipolar scored higher than the bipolar patients.

A very thorough study of the personality characteristics of unipolar patients has been carried out by von Zerssen (1977). In this study unipolar patients achieved higher scores than both bipolar patients and non-psychiatric controls on the scale representing the 'melancholic type' described by Tellenbach (1961), a result confirmed by Frey (1977). This personality pattern comprises features such as orderliness, conscientiousness, meticulousness, conventional thinking and dependency on close personal relationships, and closely corresponds to the characteristics found by Perris & Strandman (1980). More recently, von Zerssen & Pössl (1990) presented evidence for an association between the 'manic type' of personality and a predominantly manic course of an affective illness, and between the 'melancholic type' of personality and a unipolar depressive course. Matussek & Feil (1983) compared the personality characteristics of bipolar and unipolar patients with those of healthy controls by using a battery of five self-rating questionnaires. Unipolar patients were found to lack autonomy while bipolar patients had a hypomanic drive toward success and achievement and were anancastic and aggressive.

In a series of investigations from our department (Perris et al 1983, 1984, von Knorring et al 1984) recovered patients who had suffered from a bipolar or unipolar depressive episode were studied by means of a Swedish personality inventory (Karolinska Sjukhusets Personlighetsinventorium; KSP) aimed at measuring stable personality traits and their results were compared with those by a series of mentally healthy individuals. Bipolar patients scored slightly differently from unipolars in many variables but none of the differences was significant. On the other hand, the former patients scored differently from the healthy controls in almost all the personality variables covered by the KSP, with the exception of the variable 'social desirability', on which all groups scored alike. A factor analysis of the results yielded three principal factors: factor 1 covering variables reflecting anxiety proneness, psychasthenia, suspicion and guilt; factor 2 (bipolar) covering different aspects of aggression; and factor 3 comprising the variables 'impulsiveness' and 'monotony avoidance'. By applying a discriminant analysis 81.3% of the subjects could be correctly classified as former depressed patients or healthy volunteers. From those studies it was concluded that although intergroup differences may occur, the main characteristics of the personality of the depression-prone individual seem to be anxiety, psychasthenia (covering such traits as orderly, conscientious, bound to routine), suspicion and guilt. Such characteristics are shared by both bipolars and unipolars. Depression-prone individuals also show a higher level of inhibited aggression and a lower level of manifest aggression than healthy controls.

In more recent studies (e.g. Charney et al 1981) the relationship of personality disorder to depressive subtype has been investigated. Personality disorder was found to be significantly more common in unipolar non-melancholic depressed patients than in unipolar melancholic and bipolar depressed patients. On the other hand, the difference in the prevalence of personality disorder between unipolar melancholic and bipolar patients was not significant.

In summary, there is reasonable agreement in the literature that unipolar patients may be characterized by a particular personality make-up which distinguishes them from never-ill controls. On the other hand, the personality characteristics on self-report questionnaires of bipolar patients in a recovery phase show less pronounced and inconsistent differences from those of healthy controls. Investigations in which projective techniques have been used, suggest that personality markers can be identified in bipolar patients as well.

SYMPTOMATOLOGY, COURSE AND OUTCOME

Symptomatology

Investigations concerned with possible differences in symptomatology between bipolar and unipolar patients are still few and inconclusive. Moreover, those available are limited to a single episode and might be biased by the fact that the authors were aware of the final diagnosis of the patients. Leonhard (1957–1971) suggested the occurrence of a stereotyped symptom picture in repeated episodes of psychotic unipolar depression and of a more pronounced symptomatic variability in the repeated depressive episodes of bipolar patients. He documented this assumption with a series of case reports in his textbook. Unfortunately no later studies of this issue have been published. In Perris's 1966 series, there were a few unipolar patients who manifested a stereotyped delusional pattern in successive episodes even when the interval between the episodes had been of several years. However, the available hospital records were limited. Charney & Nelson (1981) and Helms & Smith (1983) have reported that between 92 and 95% of the patients with psychotic depression have had previous and/or subsequent episodes of a psychotic severity. Unfortunately no detailed analysis of delusional content or other psychotic characteristics in those patients have been reported by the authors. Stability of psychotic symptomatology across episodes has been reported also by Winokur et al (1985). In a cross-sectional study of 23 bipolar patients in a depressive episode and 32 depressed unipolars rated on a depression symptom scale there were no differences (Perris, 1966).

Beigel & Murphy (1971) reported that higher levels of physical activity, overt expression of anger and somatic complaints differentiated the depression of their unipolar patients from that of the bipolar patients, who tended to be less active and more socially withdrawn. Ayuso & Sáiz (1981) reported that unipolar patients scored significantly higher than bipolar patients on several items of the Hamilton scale (somatic and psychic anxiety, loss of weight, guilt, obsessive symptoms etc). Casper et al (1985) investigated the occurrence of somatic symptoms and found that only appetite loss differentiated unipolar from bipolar patients. In their review of behavioural characteristics of bipolar and unipolar patients, Depue & Monroe (1978) suggest that psychotic unipolar and bipolar I groups are associated with two different behavioural profiles. Unipolar depressives more frequently show increased psychomotor activity, insomnia, somatic complaints and hypochondriasis. Bipolar patients in a depressed phase, instead, appear to be characterized by psychomotor retardation, hypersomnia, fewer somatic complaints and perhaps less anxiety. Also, Gurpegui et al (1985) reported that unipolar patients show more frequent somatic symptoms (loss of weight, reduced appetite, autonomic disturbances, muscular tension and reduced sexual interest), whereas bipolar patients show more frequent hostile feelings. Taken together, those findings seem to suggest possible symptom differences between unipolars and bipolars. However, it is impossible to exclude the influence of confounding factors (e.g. age, severity and duration of the depressive episode). In studies from our department no differences in pain as a symptom between bipolar and unipolar depressives were found (von Knorring et al, 1983). Female patients, however, reported pain significantly more often than male patients, independently of polarity. Young et al (1990) did not find gender-related differences in endogenous symptoms, global severity of depression or impairment in functioning in a large series of non psychotic unipolar depressives.

In various studies (Andreasen & Akiskal 1983, O'Grady 1990) the occurrence of Schneiderian first-rank symptoms in patients with affective disorders has been reported. Such symptoms, according to Andreasen & Akiskal, are found especially in manics. Ries (1985) suggests that catatonia may be at least as common in bipolar disorder as it is in schizophrenia. To what extent results concerning the occurrence of first-rank symptoms and/or catatonia are due to a widened concept of 'affective disorder' that also encompasses patients who would previously have been labelled as schizoaffective is unclear. Other aspects of this broadening have been the inclusion of the variable 'mood incongruent delusions' among the DSM criteria of affective disorders and the extension of the label 'bipolar' to schizoaffective disorders. Winokur (1984), in an attempt to contribute a possible explanation for the confusing issues concerning psychotic unipolar or psychotic bipolar illnesses or schizoaffective disorder has suggested that a trait or propensity to psychosis is transmitted totally independently of the major affective illness.

Thus, summing up, it seems that no consistent symptomatological differences between unipolar and bipolar depressed patients have been found which would allow a correct diagnosis in the absence of information about disease course. The differences reported by the authors surveyed in this section are suggestive but not yet conclusive, since they might have been due to the influence of confounding factors which have not been completely controlled.

Course and outcome

Data in the literature agree that bipolar patients show a higher frequency of relapse over their lifetime than unipolars, and that this difference is not due to an earlier onset of the bipolar form. Results of recent studies (e.g. Fukuda et al 1983) are consistent with this assumption. Studies are reviewed in detail in chapter 7.

Older follow-up studies yielded inconsistent findings, mainly because no consistent distinction between bipolar and unipolar forms was made, and because no systematic methodology was adhered to. Leonhard reported in his *Textbook* the course of the illness in 117 bipolar patients. The number of phases per patient averaged 5, without significant differences between men and women. Predominant manic colouring occurred in 17.9%, predominant depressive in 25.6% and equally pronounced manic and depressive in 56.4% of the episodes. In my series (Perris 1968) with a follow-up ranging between 17 and 23 years, the average number of episodes per patients was 6.5 in bipolars and 4.3 in unipolars.

In a methodologically elegant study Angst and his co-workers (Angst & Weiss 1967, Grof et al 1973) have been able to show that the average duration of morbid episodes is shorter than previously believed. Bipolar patients are likely to suffer from episodes which do not last on average longer than 3 months, while the average duration of unipolar episodes is about 4 months. However, it should be kept in mind that pronounced differences in treatment imply that old and new long-term studies are hardly comparable. According to Angst and associates, the length of an affective episode remains relatively constant for each patient, apparently independently of the number of episodes that precede it. Frequency of episodes shows an increase during the first 10 years of the illness and thereafter reaches a ceiling value. Age at onset seems to play an important role in the sense that the older the patient is at the first onset of the illness, the more likely is an early relapse; this means that the intervals between episodes become shorter.

Carlson et al (1974), who studied the global outcome of 53 bipolar patients followed up for about 3 years on average, reported that only 57% had remained well since the initial hospitalization. 17% had exhibited partial remission only, 12% were chronically ill and 4% had committed suicide during the follow-up period. The findings of Carlson et al are quite similar to those obtained by Winokur et al (1969) and to those reported by Jääskeläinen (1976). Keller et al (1986) have reported a prospective follow-up study bearing on the issue of the persistent risk of chronicity in recurrent episodes of nonbipolar depressive disorder. In their series of 101 patients they found a 22% probability that the first episode would last at least 1 year. The findings taken together throw some doubt on the opinion currently held that affective disorders have a good prognosis. Kerry et al (1983), however, studied 27 patients with histories up to 65 years duration and more than 100 manic-depressive attacks and found that a complete recovery without any cognitive deterioration had occurred. On the other hand, Roukema et al (1984) suggested that when the manic patient deteriorated and reached the 'end-state of the illness' his symptoms were almost similar to those of schizophrenia. In her review Clayton (1981) points out that the question of chronicity in bipolar affective disorder is still unanswered. It seems, however, that between one-third and 45% of bipolar patients show a chronic course characterized by the presence of symptoms, social decline or both.

Mortality, suicide and suicide attempts

Early studies suggested an increased mortality in MDI but had not taken into account a distinction into bipolar and unipolar forms. Calculations made by Perris and d'Elia (in Perris 1966, p 172–183) indicated an increased mortality in bipolar but not in unipolar patients with a shortening of life expectancy by 26% in the bipolar and of only 4% in the unipolar patients. The increased mortality in bipolar patients, which is not due to any particular cause of death, was confirmed later by several other authors (Rorsman 1968, Pettersson 1974, Jääskeläinen 1976, Tsuang & Woolson 1977).

Perris and d'Elia (in Perris 1966, p 172–183) did not find any difference in rate of suicide between unipolars and bipolars. Other authors (Dunner et al 1976, Morrison 1982), however, have reported a higher rate in bipolars. More recently, Rihmer et al (1990) found 47 bipolars (46 bipolar II, and 1 bipolar I), and 53 unipolars among 100 consecutive suicide victims. Since the composition of the subgroups in this study was similar for age and sex the possible confounding effect of these variables can be excluded. It remains unclear, however, whether the over-representation of bipolar II reflects a true higher suicide-proneness in this group or is, at least in part, due to a higher frequency of bipolar II in the Hungarian population. In this context, it should be emphasized that bipolar II women also showed the highest rate of suicide attempts in a study by Goldring & Fieve (1984).

The occurrence of attempted suicide in 138 bipolars and 139 unipolars with a 20-year follow-up has been reported by d'Elia & Perris (1969). 26% of bipolar and 21% of unipolar patients attempted suicide one or more times during the follow-up. The occurrence of a suicide attempt was significantly higher in female than in male bipolars whereas no sex difference was found in the unipolar group. The frequency of suicide attempts after the sixth episode was still about 9% in the bipolar group ($n=74$), while there were no suicide attempts by unipolar patients after the 6th episode ($n=25$). Bipolar patients, especially females, showed a tendency to make suicide attempts earlier in the course of the depressive episode than unipolar patients.

Biological variables

The literature concerning the biochemistry of affective disorders in unipolar and bipolar disorders will not be reviewed in detail since there are authoritative reviews in other chapters in this Handbook. Unfortunately, none of the biochemical variables investigated so far has shown consistent differences between bipolars and unipolars and none of these variables can be safely assumed to represent a confirmed trait or marker of either disorder. Differences in blood enzymes (MAO, COMT, DBH), biogenic amine metabolites, plasma amino acids, TSH/TRH responses, melatonin suppression by light etc which have been reported seem more to reflect 'state' intergroup differences.

Peterson et al (1984) have reported that an abnormal uncoupler-accelerated efflux of 5-hydroxytryptamine from platelets significantly distinguishes bipolar patients from both unipolars and healthy controls. Such finding suggests an aberration in the mechanisms of serotonin storage and transport.

Several studies have focused on possible differences in dexamethasone suppression test (DTS) response in bipolar and unipolar patients (Gurpegui et al 1985, Joyce 1984c, Coryell & Schlesser 1983, Coryell et al 1985, Zisook et al 1985, Feinberg & Carroll 1984, Hayes & Ettigi 1983). However, the results of these studies have proved to be inconsistent.

A recent review of neurophysiological and neuroanatomical studies in affective disorders is reported elsewhere (Perris 1988). Only a few studies have taken into account a distinction between bipolar and unipolar disorder. In my 1966 series, no specific electroencephalographic (EEG) abnormalities were found which distinguished between the two types of disorder. Differences reported in other studies using dynamic EEG procedures have probably been due to the clinical characteristics of the morbid episode at the time of investigation rather than a trait difference. Several studies have been concerned with the issue of laterality of the abnormalities, but again the inconsistent results appear to be related to 'state' variables. Several studies have focused on the EEG characteristics of sleep (see chapter 19). One of the most consistent findings in those studies seems to be a shortened REM latency, which may be a psychobiological marker for primary depression (Kupfer 1976). Duncan et al (1979) have compared night sleep measures and REM sleep architecture in unipolar and bipolar depressed patients. Both groups showed significant differences in REM architecture when compared with healthy controls. Also, bipolar patients showed significantly greater fragmentation of REM periods than unipolar patients. Studies of evoked potentials, also carried out extensively in our department, have failed to show consistent differences between bipolars and unipolars.

A few investigations have been concerned with electrodermal activity (EDA) in subtypes of depression (Williams et al 1985, Iacono et al 1983). The EDA of the patients with affective disorder was found to be uniformly depressed across all tasks and conditions. However, no differences were found between unipolar and bipolar patients.

Several computerized tomographic studies (CT scans) of patients suffering from affective disorders have been reported and are described in chapter 18. These studies show ventricular enlargement in a small proportion of patients suffering from affective disorders, but not specifically so for either bipolars or unipolars. Possibly patients with enlarged ventricles have a poorer outcome and an increased mortality compared with patients without ventricular enlargement.

To my knowledge, no post-mortem studies bearing on the distinction between bipolar and unipolar affective disorder have been reported.

RESPONSE TO TREATMENT

In a catamnestic study Perris and d'Elia (in Perris 1966, p 153–165) found that unipolar patients required on average more ECT than bipolars for a depressive episode. Strömgren (1973) reported similar response rates in patients with unipolar and bipolar depression. Planned therapeutic trials directly comparing acute treatment response in bipolar and unipolar patients are still few in number. This may be due to the difficulty of collecting a series of depressed bipolar patients large enough to permit comparisons within a reasonable span of time. Also, the likely heterogeneity of patients subsumed under the heading 'unipolar' makes the results of such comparisons of uncertain interpretation.

Both groups of depressives appear to show the same responsiveness to antidepressants (Angst & Perris 1968) although Bunney et al (1970) reported a better response to tricyclics in unipolar than in bipolar depressed patients. On the other hand, only bipolar patients are likely to show a clear-cut syndrome-shift in connection with treatment. In particular, Goodwin et al (1970) found that a consistent hypomanic response in patients treated with L-dopa only occurred in bipolar depressives and suggested that this test could be used to differentiate between bipolars and unipolars.

The issue of the choice of drug for the prevention of recurrence in patients with unipolar or bipolar disorder is discussed in chapter 25. Prien (1988) reviewed this question and also reported on a consensus conference convened by the National Institutes of Health and NIMH in 1984. In unipolar disorder the tricyclics have a logistical advantage over lithium since most acute unipolar depressions are treated with an antidepressant so that continuation with the same drug avoids a switch of drug. Lithium should always be preferred when there is suspicion of a latent or undiagnosed bipolar disorder.

In a careful multidimensional study of long-term lithium therapy, Smigan (1984) found lithium to be effective in preventing relapses in about two-thirds of patients defined as bipolar or unipolar in a strict sense. Other authors (Maj et al 1985, Grof 1990) have presented evidence that a positive family history of bipolar illness is the best predictor of a positive response to long-term lithium treatment.

ACKNOWLEDGEMENT

Mrs Doris Cedergren skilfully contributed to the collection of references and to the preparation of the manuscript.

REFERENCES

Abrams R, Taylor M A 1974 Unipolar mania. Archives of General Psychiatry 30: 441–443

Abrams R, Taylor M A, Hayman M A, Krishna R 1979 Unipolar mania revisited. Journal of Affective Disorders 1: 59–68

Akiskal H S, Bitar A H, Puzantian V R et al 1978 The nosological status of neurotic depression. Archives of General Psychiatry 35: 756–766

Alnaes R, Torgersen S 1990 Parental representation in patients with major depression, anxiety disorder and mixed conditions. Acta Psychiatrica Scandinavica 81: 518–522

American Psychiatric Association 1987 Diagnostic and statistical manual of mental disorders, 3rd edn (revised). American Psychiatric Association, Washington

Andreasen N C, Akiskal H S 1983 The specificity of Bleulerian and Schneiderian symptoms: a critical reevaluation. Psychiatria Clinica of North America 6: 41–54

Angst J 1966 Zur Ätiologie und Nosologie endogener depressiver Psychosen. Monographien aus dem Gesamtgebiete der Neurologie und Psychiatrie. Springer, Berlin

Angst J 1973 Discussion. In: Angst J (ed) Classification and prediction of outcome of depression. Schattauer, Stuttgart, p 85–86

Angst J, Perris C 1968 Zur Nosologie endogener Depressionen. Vergleich der Ergebnisse zweier Untersuchungen. Archiv für Psychiatrie 210: 373–386

Angst J, Weis P 1967 Periodicity of depressive psychoses. Excerpta Medica International Congress Series 129: 703–710

Ayuso J L, Saiz J 1981 Las depresiones. Interamericana, Madrid

Bech P, Rafaelsen O J 1979 Personality and manic-melancholic illness. Read at the WPA Symposium on Psychopathology of depression, Helsinki, June

Beigel A, Murphy D L 1971 Unipolar and bipolar affective illness. Archives of General Psychiatry 24: 215–220

Bertelsen A, Harvald B, Hauge M 1977 A Danish twin study of manic-depressive disorders. British Journal of Psychiatry 130: 330–351

Brodie K H, Leff M J 1971 Bipolar depression. A comparative study of patient's characteristics. American Journal of Psychiatry 127: 1086–1090

Bunney W E Jr, Brodie H K H, Murphy D L 1970 Psychopharmacological differentiation between two subgroups of depressed patients. Proceedings of the 78th Annual Convention of the American Psychological Association 5: 829–830

Carlson G A, Kotin J, Davenport Y B, Adland M 1974 Follow-up of 53 bipolar manic depressive patients. British Journal of Psychiatry 124: 134–139

Casper R C, Redmond D E Jr, Katz M M, Schaffer C B, Davis J M, Koslow S H 1985 Somatic symptoms in primary affective disorder. Presence and relationship to the classification of depression. Archives of General Psychiatry 42: 1098–1104

Cesarek L, Marke S 1968 Mätningar av psykogena behov med frågeformulärsteknik. Skandinaviska Testförlaget, Stockholm

Charney D S, Nelson J C 1981 Delusional and nondelusional unipolar depression. Further evidence for distinct subtypes. American Journal of Psychiatry 138: 328–333

Charney D S, Nelson J C, Quinlan D M 1981 Personality traits and disorder in depression. American Journal of Psychiatry 138: 1601–1604

Clayton P J 1981 The epidemiology of bipolar affective disorder. Comprehensive Psychiatry 22: 31

Coryell W, Schlesser M A 1983 Dexamethasone suppression test response in major depression: Stability across hospitalizations. Psychiatry Research 8: 179–189

Coryell W, Smith R, Cook B, Moucharafieh S, Dunner F, House D 1985 Serial dexamethasone suppression test results during antidepressant therapy: Relationship to diagnosis and clinical change. Psychiatry Research 10: 165–174

Coryell W, Endicott J, Keller M et al 1989 Bipolar affective disorder and high achievement: A familial association. American Journal of Psychiatry 146: 983–988

d'Elia G, Perris C 1969 Selbstmordversuche im Laufe unipolarer und bipolarer Depressionen. Archiv für Psychiatrie und Nervenkrankheiten 212: 339–356

Depue R A, Monroe S M 1978 The unipolar–bipolar distinction in the depressive disorders. Psychological Bulletin 88: 1001–1030

Donnelly E F, Murphy D L 1973a Social desirability and bipolar affective disorder. Journal of Consultative and Clinical Psychology 41: 469

Donnelly E F, Murphy D L 1973b Primary affective disorder: delineation of a unipolar depressive subtype. Psychological Review 32: 744–746

Donnelly E F, Murphy D L, Scott W H 1975 Perception and cognition in patients with bipolar and unipolar depressive disorders. Archives of General Psychiatry 32: 1128–1131

Duncan W C Jr, Pettigrew K D, Gillin J C 1979 REM architecture changes in bipolar and unipolar depression. American Journal of Psychiatry 136: 1424

Dunner D L, Fleiss J L, Addonizio G, Fieve R R 1976 Assortative mating in primary affective disorders. Biological Psychiatry 11: 43–51

Dunner D L, Gershon E S, Goodwin F K 1970 Heritable factors in the severity of affective illness. Paper read at the Annual Meeting of the American Psychiatric Association, San Francisco, May

Eysenck H J 1959 Manual of the Maudsley Personality Inventory. London

Faravelli C, Incerpi G 1985 Epidemiology of affective disorders in Florence. Preliminary results. Acta Psychiatrica Scandinavica 72: 331–333

Feinberg M, Carroll B J 1984 Biological 'markers' for endogenous depression. Effect of age, severity of illness, weight loss, and polarity. Archives of General Psychiatry 41: 1080–1085

Frey R 1977 Die premorbide Persönlichkeit von monopolar und bipolar Depressiven. Archiv für Psychiatrie und Nervenkrankheiten 224: 161–173

Fukuda K, Etoh T, Iwadate T, Ishii A 1983 The course and prognosis of manic-depressive psychosis: a quantitative analysis of episodes and intervals. Tohoku Journal of Experimental Medicine 139: 299–307

Gammon G D, John K, Rothblum E D, Mullen K, Tischler G L, Weissman M M 1983 Use of a structured diagnostic interview to identify bipolar disorder in adolescent inpatients: frequency and manifestations of the disorder. American Journal of Psychiatry 140: 543–547

Gershon E S, Dunner D L, Sturt L, Goodwin F K 1971 Assortative mating in the affective disorders. Read at the Annual Meeting of the American Psychiatric Association. Washington, May

Glassner B, Haldipur C V 1983 Life events and early and late onset of bipolar disorder. American Journal of Psychiatry 140: 215–217

Glassner B, Haldipur C V 1985 A psychosocial study of early-onset bipolar disorder. Journal of Nervous and Mental Disease 173: 387–394

Goetzl U, Green R, Shybrow P, Jackson R 1974 X-linkage revisited. A further family study of manic-depressive illness. Archives of General Psychiatry 31: 665–672

Goldring N, Fieve R R 1984 Attempted suicide in manic-depressive disorder. American Journal of Psychotherapy 38: 373–383

Goodwin F K, Murphy D L, Brodie K H, Bunney W E 1970 L-Dopa, catecholamines and behaviour: a clinical and biochemical study in depressed patients. Biological Psychiatry 2: 341–366

Grof P, Angst J, Haines T 1973 The clinical course of depression: practical issues. In: Angst J (ed) Classification and prediction of outcome of depression. Schattauer, Stuttgart

Grof P 1990 Family study of lithium. Presented at the IGSAD meeting in Umeå, Sweden, 23–25 May

Gurpegui M, Casanova J, Cervera S 1985 Clinical and neuroendrocrine features of endogenous unipolar and bipolar depression. Acta Psychiatrica Scandinavica 72(suppl 320): 30–37

Hällström T 1984 Point prevalence of major depressive disorder in a Swedish urban female population. Acta Psychiatrica Scandinavica 69: 52–59

Hayes P E, Ettigi P 1983 Dexamethasone suppression test in diagnosis of depressive illness. Clinical Pharmacology 2: 538–545

Helms P M, Smith R E 1983 Recurrent psychotic depression. Journal of Affective Disorders 5: 51–54

Helzer J E, Winokur G 1974 A family interview study of male manic depressives. Archives of General Psychiatry 31: 73

Hirschfeld R M A, Klerman G L 1979 Personality attributes and affective disorders. American Journal of Psychiatry 136: 67–70

Hirschfeld R M A, Klerman G L, Clayton P J, Keller M B 1983a Personality and depression. Empirical findings. Archives of General Psychiatry 40: 993–998

Hirschfeld R M A, Klerman G L, Clayton P J, Keller M B, McDonald-Scott P, Larkin B H 1983b Assessing personality: Effects of the depressive state on trait measurement. American Journal of Psychiatry 140: 695–699

Hirschfeld R M A, Klerman G L, Keller M B, Andreasen N C, Clayton P J 1986 Personality of recovered patients with bipolar affective disorder. Journal of Affective Disorders 11: 81–89

Hoffman H 1921 Die Nachkommenschaft bei endogenen Psychosen. Monographien aus dem Gesamtgebiete der Neurologie und Psychiatrie. Springer, Berlin

Hoover C F, Fitzgerald R G 1981 Marital conflict of manic-depressive patients. Archives of General Psychiatry 38: 65–67

Iacono W G, Lykken D T, Peloquin L J, Lumry A E, Valentine R H, Tuason V B 1983 Electrodermal activity in euthymic unipolar and bipolar affective disorders. A possible marker for depression. Archives of General Psychiatry 40: 557–565

Jääskeläinen J P K 1976 The course and prognosis of unipolar and bipolar depression (in Finnish with English summary). Psychiatrie Fennica Monograph No 7

Jablensky A, Sartorius N, Gulbinat W, Ernberg G 1981 Characteristics of depressive patients contacting psychiatric services in four cultures. A report from the WHO Collaborative study on the assessment of depressive disorders. Acta Psychiatrica Scandinavica 63: 367–383

Jakimow-Venulet B 1981 Hereditary factors in the pathogenesis of affective illnesses. British Journal of Psychiatry 139: 450–456

James N M, Chapman C J 1975 A genetic study of bipolar affective disorder. British Journal of Psychiatry 126: 449–456

Jaspers K 1913 Allgemeine Psychopathologie. Springer, Berlin (English translation by Hoenig J, Hamilton M W. Manchester University Press, 1963)

Joffe R T, MacDonald C, Kutcher S P 1989 Life events and mania: a case-controlled study. Psychiatry Research 30: 213–216

Johnson G S F, Lehman M M 1977 Analysis of familial factors in bipolar affective disorders. American Journal of Psychiatry 34: 1074–1083

Joyce P R 1984a Parental bonding in unipolar affective disorder. Journal of Affective Disorders 7: 319–324

Joyce P R 1984b Age of onset in bipolar affective disorder and misdiagnosis as schizophrenia. Psychological Medicine 14: 145–149

Joyce P R 1984c The dexamethasone suppression test in acute mania. Journal of Affective Disorders 7: 281–286

Keller M B, Lavori P W, Rice J, Coryell W, Hirschfeld R M A 1986 The persistent risk of chronicity in recurrent episodes of nonbipolar major depressive disorder: A prospective follow-up. American Journal of Psychiatry 143: 24–28

Kerry R J, McDermott C M, Orme J E 1983 Affective disorders and cognitive performance. A clinical report. Journal of Affective Disorders 5: 349–352

Kleist K 1953 Die Gliederung der neuropsychischen Erkrankungen. Monatsschrift für Psychiatrie und Neurologie 125: 526–554

Klerman G L 1988 The current age of youthful melancholia. Evidence of increase in depression among adolescents and young adults. British Journal of Psychiatry 152: 4–14

Kraepelin E 1913 Psychiatrie. III Band. J A Barth, Leipzig

Kringlen E 1985 Depression research: a review with special emphasis etiology. Acta Psychiatrica Scandinavica (suppl 319) 71: 117–130

Kupfer D J 1976 REM latency: a psychobiological marker for primary depressive disease. Biological Psychiatry 77: 159–174

Last U, Belmaker R H, Rosenbaum M 1984 Rorschach markers in euthymic manic-depressive illness. Neuropsychobiology 12: 96–100

Leonhard K 1957–1971 Aufteilung der endogenen Psychosen 1st–4th edn. Akademie, Berlin

Leonhard K 1963 Die präpsychotische Temperamente bei den monopolaren und bipolaren phasischen Psychosen. Psychiatric Neurology 146: 105–115

Leonhard K, Korff I, Schulz H 1962 Die Temperamente in den Familien der monopolaren und bipolaren phasischen Psychosen. Psychiatric Neurology 143: 416–434

Lesser A L 1983 Hypomania and marital conflict. Canadian Journal of Psychiatry 28: 362–366

Lewis A 1934 Melancholia: a historical review, and a clinical survey of depressive states. Journal of Mental Science 80: 1–42, 277–378

Lewis A 1936 Melancholia: prognostic study and case material. Journal of Mental Science 82: 488–558

McGuffin P, Katz R, Rutherford J 1990 Nature, nurture and depression. A twin study. Psychological Medicine (in press)

MacVane J R, Lange J D, Brown W A, Zayat M 1978 Psychological functioning of bipolar manic-depressives in remission. Archives of General Psychiatry 35: 1351–1354

Maj M, Arena P, Lovero N, Pirozzi R, Komali D 1985 Factors associated with response to lithium prophylaxis in DSM III major depression and bipolar disorder. Pharmacopsychiatry 18: 309–313

Mapother E 1926 Manic-depressive psychosis. British Medical Journal 2: 872–879

Matussek P, Feil W B 1983 Personality attributes of depressive patients. Results of group comparisons. Archives of General Psychiatry 40: 783–789

Mayo J A 1970 Psychosocial profiles of patients on lithium treatment. International Pharmacopsychiatry 5: 190–202

Mendlewicz J 1979 Genetic forms of manic illness and the question of atypical mania. In: Shopsin B (ed) Manic illness. Raven Press, New York

Mendlewicz J, Rainer J D 1974 Morbidity risk and genetic transmission in manic depressive illness. American Journal of Human Genetics 26: 692–701

Mendlewicz J, Rainer J D 1977 Adoption study supporting genetic transmission in manic-depressive illness. Nature 268: 327–329

Merikangas K R, Spiker D G 1982 Assortative mating among in-patients with primary affective disorder. Psychological Medicine 12: 753–764

Merikangas K R, Prusoff B A, Kupfer D J, Frank E 1985a Marital adjustment in major depression. Journal of Affective Disorders 9: 5–11

Merikangas K R, Weissman M M, Pauls D L 1985b Genetic factors in the sex ratio of major depression. Psychological Medicine 15: 63–69

Metcalfe M, Johnson A L, Coppen A 1975 The Marke— Nyman Temperament Scale in depression. British Journal of Psychiatry 126: 41–48

Meyer A 1905 quoted by Mendelson M 1974 In: Psychoanalytic concepts of depression. Spectrum, New York, p 5–6

Morrison J R 1982 Suicide in psychiatric practice population. Journal of Clinical Psychiatry 43: 348–352

Murray L G, Blackburn I M 1974 Personality differences in patients with depressive illness and anxiety neurosis. Acta Psychiatrica Scandinavica 50: 183–191

Negri F, Melica A M, Zuliani R, Gasperini M, Macciardi F, Smeraldi E 1981 Genetic implications in assortative mating of affective disorders. British Journal of Psychiatry 138: 236–239

Nurnberger J, Roose S P, Dunner D L, Fieve R R 1979 Unipolar mania: a distinct clinical entity. American Journal of Psychiatry 136: 1420–1423

Nyman G E, Marke S 1962 Sjöbring's differentiella psykologi. Gleerup, Lund

O'Grady J C 1990 The prevalence and diagnostic significance of Schneiderian first-rank symptoms in a random sample of acute psychiatric in-patients. British Journal of Psychiatry 156: 496–500

Parkar G 1983 Parental overprotection. Grune & Stratton, New York

Perris C 1966 A study of bipolar and unipolar recurrent depressive psychoses. Acta Psychiatrica Scandinavica 42 (suppl 194)

Perris C 1968 The course of depressive psychoses. Acta Psychiatrica Scandinavica 44: 238–248

Perris C 1971 Personality patterns in patients with affective disorders. Acta Psychiatrica Scandinavica (suppl 221): 43–51

Perris H 1984 Life events and depression. Part 2. Results in diagnostic sub-groups, and in relation to the recurrence of depression. Journal of Affective Disorders 7: 25–36

Perris C 1988 Neurophysiological and neuroanatomical studies of depression and mania. In: Georgotas A, Cancro R (eds) Depression and mania. Elsevier, New York, p 213–243

Perris C, d'Elia G 1964 Pathoplastic significance of the premorbid situation in depressive psychoses. Acta Psychiatrica Scandinavica (suppl 180): 87–100

Perris C, Perris H 1979 Status within the family and early life experiences in patients with affective disorders and cycloid psychoses. Psychiatria Clinica 11: 155–162

Perris H, Strandman E 1980 Psychogenic needs in depresssion. Archiv für Psychiatrie und Nervenkrankheiten 227: 97–107

Perris C, Perris H, Ericsson U, von Knorring L 1982 The genetics of depression. A family study of unipolar and neurotic-reactive depressed patients. Archiv für Psychiatrie und Nervenkrankheiten 232: 137–155

Perris C, Eisemann M, Ericsson U, von Knorring L, Perris H 1983 Patterns of aggression in the personality structure of depressed patients. Archiv für Psychiatrie und Nervenkrankheiten 233: 89–102

Perris C, Eisemann M, von Knorring L, Perris H 1984 Personality traits in former depressed patients and in healthy subjects without past history of depression. Psychopathology 17: 178–186

Perris C, Maj M, Perris H, Eisemann M 1985 Perceived parental rearing behaviour in unipolar and bipolar depressed patients. Acta Psychiatrica Scandinavica 72: 172–175

Perris C, Holmgren S, von Knorring L, Perris H 1986a Parental loss by death in the early childhood of depressed patients and of their healthy siblings. British Journal of Psychiatry 148: 165–169

Perris C, Arrindell W A, Perris H, Eisemann H, van der Ende J, von Knorring L 1986b Perceived depriving parental rearing and depression. British Journal of Psychiatry 148: 170–175

Perris C, Perris H, Eisemann M 1987 Perceived parental rearing practices, parental affective disorders and age at onset in depressed patients. International Journal of Family Psychiatry 8: 183–199

Peterson L-L, Bartfai T, Ernster L 1984 Uncoupler-accelerated efflux of 5-hydroxytryptamine from platelets of healthy subjects and patients with unipolar and bipolar depression. Psychiatry Research 13: 141–150

Pettersson U 1974 Manisk depressiv sjukdom. Doctoral Thesis, Karolinska Institute, Stockholm

Pfohl B, Vasquez N, Nasrallah H 1982a The mathematical case against unipolar mania. Journal of Psychiatric Research 16: 259–265

Pfohl B, Vasquez N, Nasrallah H 1982b Unipolar vs bipolar mania: a review of 247 patients. British Journal of Psychiatry 141: 453–458

Price J 1968 The genetics of depressive behaviour. In: Coppen A J, Walk A (eds) Recent development in affective disorders. Headley Brothers, Ashford, p 37–54

Prien R F 1988 Maintenance treatment of depressive and manic states. In: Georgotas A, Cancro R (eds) Depression and mania. Elsevier, New York. pp 439–451

Rice J, Reich T, Andreasen N C et al 1984 Sex-related differences in depression. Familial evidence. Journal of Affective Disorders 7: 199–210

Rice J, Reich T, Andreasen N C et al 1987 The familial transmission of bipolar illness. Archives of General Psychiatry 44: 441–447

Ries R K 1985 DSM-III implications of the diagnoses of catatonia and bipolar disorder. American Journal of Psychiatry 142: 1471–1474

Rihmer Z, Barsi J, Arató M, Demeter E 1990 Suicide in subtypes of primary major depression. Journal of Affective Disorders 18: 221–225

Rorsman B 1968 Dödligheten bland psykiatriska patienter. Läkartidningen 65: 149–156

Roukema R, Fadem B, James B, Rayford F 1984 Bipolar disorder in a low socioeconomic population. Difficulties in diagnosis. Journal of Nervous and Mental Disorders 172: 76–79

Sclare P, Creed F 1990 Life events and the onset of mania. British Journal of Psychiatry 156: 508–514

Smeraldi E, Negri F, Melica A M 1978 A genetic study of affective disorders. Acta Psychiatrica Scandinavica 56: 382–398

Smeraldi E, Macciardi F, Holmgren S, Perris H, von Knorring L, Perris C 1987 Age at onset of affective disorders in Italian and Swedish patients. Acta Psychiatrica Scandinavica 75: 352–357

Smigan L 1984 Some clinical, biological and psychological aspects of long-term lithium therapy. Umeå University medical dissertations, New Series No 130

Stancer H C, Persad E, Wagener D K, Jorna T 1987 Evidence for homogeneity of major depression and bipolar affective disorder. Journal of Psychiatric Research 21: 37–53

Strandman E 1978 Psychogenic needs in patients with affective disorders. Acta Psychiatrica Scandinavica 58: 16–29

Strömgren L S 1973 Unilateral versus bilateral electroconvulsive therapy. Investigation into the therapeutic effect in endogenous depression. Acta Psychiatrica Scandinavica (suppl 240)

Taylor M A, Abrams R, Hayman M A 1980 The classification of affective disorders. A reassessment of the bipolar-unipolar dichotomy. A clinical, laboratory and family study. Journal of Affective Disorders 2: 95–109

Tellenbach H 1961 Melancholie. Springer, Berlin

Trzebiatowska-Trzeciak O 1977 Genetical analysis of unipolar and bipolar endogenous affective psychoses. British Journal of Psychiatry 131: 478–485

Tsuang M T, Woolson R F 1977 Mortality in patients with schizophrenia, mania, depression and surgical conditions. British Journal of Psychiatry 130: 162–166

von Knorring A L 1983 Adoption studies on psychiatric illness. Umeå University Medical Dissertations, New Series No 101

von Knorring L, Perris C, Eisemann M, Eriksson U, Perris H 1983 Pain as a symptom in depressive disorders. I. Relationship to diagnostic subgroup and depressive symptomatology. Pain 15: 19–26

von Knorring L, Perris C, Eisemann M, Perris H 1984 Discrimination of former depressed patients from healthy volunteers on the basis of stable personality traits assessed by means of KSP. European Archives of Psychiatry and Neurological Sciences 234: 202–205

von Trostorff S 1968 Uber di hereditäre Belastung bei den bipolaren und monopolaren phasischen Psychosen. Schweizer Archiv für Neurologie, Neurochirurgie und Psychiatrie 102: 235–243

von Zerssen D 1977 Premorbid personality and affective psychoses. In: Burrows (ed) Handbook of studies on depression. Excerpta Medica, Amsterdam, p 79–103 von Zerssen D, Pössl J 1990 The premorbid personality of patients with different subtypes of an affective illness. Journal of Affective Disorders 18: 39–50

Waters B, Marchenko I, Abrams N, Smiley D, Kalin D 1983 Assortative mating for major affective disorder. Journal of Affective Disorders 5: 9–17

Weissman M M, Myers J K 1979 Affective disorders in a US urban community. Archives of General Psychiatry 35: 1304–1311

Weissman M M, Paykel E S 1974 The depressed woman – a study of social relations. University of Chicago Press, Chicago

Weissman M M, Gershon E S, Kidd K K et al 1984 Psychiatric disorders in the relatives of probands with affective disorders. Archives of General Psychiatry 41: 13–21

Weissman M M, Leaf P J, Tischler G L 1988 Affective disorders in five United States communities. Psychological Medicine 18: 141–153

Williams K M, Iacono W G, Remich R A 1985 Electrodermal activity among subtypes of depression. Biological Psychiatry 20: 158–162

Winokur G 1984 Psychosis in bipolar and unipolar affective illness with special reference to schizo-affective disorder. British Journal of Psychiatry 145: 236–242

Winokur G, Clayton P, Reich T 1969 Manic depressive illness. C V Mosby, St Louis

Winokur G, Scharfetter C, Angst J 1985 Stability of psychotic symptomatology (delusions, hallucinations), affective syndromes, and schizophrenic symptoms (thought disorder, incongruent affect) over episodes in emitting psychoses. European Archives of Psychiatry and Neurological Sciences 234: 303–307

World Health Organisation 1978 Mental disorders: glossary and guide to their classification in accordance with the ninth revision of the International classification of Diseases. WHO, Geneva

Young M A, Sheftner W A, Fawcett J, Klerman G L 1990 Gender differences in the clinical features of unipolar major depressive disorders. Journal of Nervous and Mental Disease 178: 200–203

Zerbin-Rüdin E 1969 Zur Genetik depressiver Erkrankungen. In: Hippius, Selbach (eds) Das depressive Syndrom. Urban & Schwarzenberg, Munich, p 37–56

Zerbin-Rüdin E 1979 Genetics of affective psychoses. In: Schou M, Strömgren E (eds) Origin, prevention and treatment of affective disorders. Academic Press, New York

Zisook S, Janowsky D S, Overall J E, Risch S C 1985 The dexamethasone suppression test and unipolar/bipolar distinctions. Journal of Clinical Psychiatry 46: 461–465

6. Anxiety disorders and their relationship to depression

Fiona K. Judd   Graham D. Burrows

ANXIETY DISORDERS

Anxiety is generally experienced as unpleasant with a subjective feeling of foreboding. It accompanies any situation which threatens an individual's well-being. Such situations include conflict and other types of frustration, threat of physical harm, threat to self esteem and pressure to perform beyond one's capabilities. Anxiety is regarded as pathological when it is more frequent, more severe or more persistent than the individual is accustomed to or can tolerate. Manifestations of anxiety include both somatic and psychological symptoms.

Freud (1894) described the major features of anxiety neurosis. These included awareness of threat, irritability and poor concentration, and a constellation of possible somatic symptoms such as palpitations, difficulty breathing, tremor, sweating, giddiness, paraesthesiae and gastrointestinal disturbance.

The introduction of behaviour therapy (Wolpe 1958) led to the subcategorization of anxiety neurosis. Desensitization was demonstrated to be effective in the treatment of phobic anxiety but not of generalized anxiety (Marks et al 1968). Simple phobias showed a particularly favourable response to desensitization and exposure therapy (Watson et al 1971), more so than agoraphobia. The International Classification of Diseases (ICD-9; World Health Organization 1978) includes anxiety states, phobic state, obsessive compulsive disorder, acute stress reaction, all of which may be considered forms of pathological anxiety, as separate disorders.

Further changes in the classification of anxiety disorders were introduced in the American Psychiatric Association (APA) Diagnostic and Statistical Manual of Mental Disorders (DSM-III) in 1980 (American Psychiatric Association 1980). Panic disorder was delineated as a separate diagnostic category. The separation of panic from generalized anxiety followed the observation by Klein and colleagues (Klein & Fink 1962, Klein 1964) that imipramine reduced panic attacks but not generalized anxiety. Subsequently Klein (1981) suggested that panic leads to the development of agoraphobia. The latter concept has been

Table 6.1 Classification of anxiety disorders ICD-9 versus DSM-III/IIIR

ICD-9 (1978)	DSM-III (1980)	DSM-III-R (1987)
Anxiety states	Generalized anxiety disorder	Generalized anxiety disorder
	Panic disorder	Panic disorder (without agoraphobia)
Phobic state	Agoraphobia ± panic	Panic disorder with agoraphobia
	Social Phobia	Social phobia
	Simple Phobia	Simple phobia
		Agoraphobia without history of panic
Obsessive–compulsive disorder	Obsessive–compulsive disorder	Obsessive–compulsive disorder
Acute reaction to stress		
Adjustment reaction	Adjustment disorder	Adjustment disorder
	Post-traumatic stress disorder	Post-traumatic stress disorder

Table 6.2   Classification of anxiety disorders ICD-10 versus DSM-IIIR

ICD-10 (draft)			DSM-IIIR
Phobic disorders			
agoraphobia	–	without panic disorder	agoraphobia without history of panic disorder
	–	with panic disorder	panic disorder with agoraphobia
social phobia			social phobia
specific phobias			simple phobia
Other anxiety disorders			
panic disorder			panic disorder without agoraphobia
generalized anxiety disorder			generalized anxiety disorder
mixed anxiety and depressive disorder			—
Obsessive-compulsive disorder			obsessive-compulsive disorder
Reaction to severe stress and adjustment disorders			
acute stress reaction			—
post-traumatic stress disorder			post-traumatic stress disorder
adjustment disorder			adjustment disorder

incorporated in the recent revision of DSM-III, DSM-IIIR (American Psychiatric Association 1987) (Table 6.1).

Studies of the association between anxiety disorders and depression are rendered difficult by problems of classification. These include the classificatory system used and its underlying theoretical assumptions, and whether a hierarchical or comorbidity approach to diagnosis is adopted.

The classification of anxiety disorders adopted by the APA is still debated. This is highlighted by the differences between the DSM-IIIR (American Psychiatric Association 1987) and draft ICD-10 (World Health Organization 1988) classifications (Table 6.2). The controversy surrounds two categories: panic disorder, and mixed anxiety and depressive disorder. These areas of controversy reflect two important conceptual issues: delineation of the boundaries of the group of anxiety disorders and classification of the disorders within those boundaries.

Conceptually panic and phobic disorders are viewed differently in DSM-IIIR and ICD-10. The APA classification follows Klein's (1981) model and views agoraphobia as a secondary feature of panic disorder. A separate category of agoraphobia without history of panic disorder is available for those individuals who do not describe panic attacks. By contrast the ICD-10 regards panic attacks occurring in an established phobic situation as an expression of the phobia, which is given diagnostic preference. Panic disorder is reserved for

individuals with recurrent spontaneous panic attacks in the absence of phobic symptoms.

Mixed anxiety and depressive disorder (ICD-10) does not appear in DSM-IIIR, nor is there any category equivalent to it. This diagnosis is used when symptoms of anxiety and depression are both present, but only to a mild or moderate degree, and when neither is clearly predominant. If one set of symptoms predominates a simple diagnosis of anxiety or depression is made; if both syndromes are present and severe two diagnoses are given.

HIERARCHICAL OR COMORBIDITY APPROACHES

Considerable overlap in symptomatology exists between the various anxiety disorders and between anxiety and depressive disorders. In order to deal with this, many classificatory systems have contained explicit or implicit hierarchies of disorders, with associated exclusionary rules reflecting the assumptions of the hierarchy. For example, for some DSM-III disorders a diagnosis is excluded if its symptoms are 'due to' a co-existing disorder which occupies a higher position in the hierarchy. Any of the anxiety disorders may be excluded by major depression. Arbitrary exclusion systems such as this allow clinicians to make a single diagnosis but may obscure true relationships among disorders or syndromes.

An alternative to the hierarchical approach is to

define coexisting complications of a disorder. Thus symptoms which are concurrent with a more pervasive disorder, but which are not a typical feature of the pervasive disorder, are considered to be a coexisting complication and to warrant a separate diagnosis. This approach has been adopted by DSM-IIIR.

Adopting a comorbidity rather than hierarchical approach has widespread implications for understanding of the relationship between anxiety disorders and depression. For example, the study of Leckman and colleagues (1983a), demonstrating that a history of anxiety disorder was associated with increased prevalence of both anxiety and depression, suggests that anxiety is not an integral part of depression. If so, this has implications for not only familial aggregation but possibly also for aetiology and treatment.

ANXIETY DISORDERS AND DEPRESSION

Three major conceptual models for the relationship between anxiety and depression exist: unitary, dualist and anxious-depressive.

The unitary model

This proposes that anxiety and depression are variants of the same disorder and differ quantitatively. The suggestion is that anxiety and depression be regarded as two symptomatic stages of affective disorder with the ratio of anxiety and depressive symptoms varying over time, so that the diagnosis depends upon when in the course of illness the assessment is made (Gersh & Fowles 1979). It is supported by studies demonstrating change in diagnosis with time (Kendell 1974).

Further support for the unitary position comes from studies of patients with anxiety neurosis, which demonstrate a high prevalence of depressive symptoms (Fawcett & Kravitz 1983, Roth et al 1972) or a high rate of secondary depression (Clancy et al 1978, Dealy et al 1981). Studies reporting favourable treatment response of anxious patients to antidepressants (Kelly & Walter 1969a, Sargant & Dally 1962, Tyrer et al 1988) and of depressed patients to anxiolytics (Henry et al 1969, Hollister et al 1967, Overall et al 1966, Tiller et al 1989) further support the unitary view.

Advocates of the unitary model have suggested that anxiety may be an aetiological factor for depression. Depression may be preceded by prodromal periods of chronic anxiety (Hays 1964). A recent study of depressive disorders in childhood (Kovacs et al 1989) found 41% had anxiety disorders in conjunction with an index episode of depression, in most cases antedating and dovetailing into the depression. While this supports the unitary hypothesis, the frequent persistence of anxiety after the depression has remitted supports a dualist view. Schapira & colleagues (1972) found that long-standing anxiety states subsequently acquire depressive characteristics. Clancy et al (1978) found that the development of secondary depression in their anxious patients was usually delayed for several years after the onset of anxiety.

Depression and anxiety rating scales contain common factors of anxiety and depression (Mendels et al 1972, Johnstone et al 1980). A high correlation between anxiety and depression measured by rating scales has been replicated by several researchers (Costello & Comrey 1967, Crown & Crisp 1966, Cockett 1969).

The dualist view

The most well-known research advocating the position that anxiety and depression are distinct and separate entities comes from the Newcastle group.

Roth et al (1972), Gurney et al (1972) and Schapira et al (1972) have compared biographical, clinical and prognostic data of patients with anxiety states and depressive illness and demonstrated that these two disorders are separate, not simply clinical variants of an affective disturbance.

In a prospective study of 145 patients, Roth et al (1972) compared patients with anxiety states and depressive illness in respect of a wide range of clinical, early life and personality features. Overlap in respect of affective disturbance between the two groups was large. Severe episodic depressed mood was recorded in the majority of the anxious group, but severe persistent depression was significantly more common among the depressed group. Severe episodic tension was commonly found in depressed patients, but severe persistent tension was significantly more frequent amongst the anxious patients.

Patients with anxiety more often reported social anxiety and maladjustment than depressed patients. They described themselves as being poor mixers and more easily hurt by trivial remarks or criticisms. They also reported suffering more often from some degree of anxiety caused by the stress of everyday life. Within the anxious group, personality traits of dependence and immaturity were also recorded more often. Higher neuroticism scores and lower extroversion scores on the Maudsley Personality Inventory were found in those with anxiety states compared to depressive states (Kerr et al 1970).

The age of onset of illness among the anxiety states was lower than amongst patients with a depressive illness. The duration of illness was significantly shorter amongst the depressed group. A significantly higher number of patients with anxiety states reported more severe and more numerous stresses in association with the onset of illness.

A principal component analysis carried out on 58 items obtained from the study of the total patient group produced a bipolar component with anxiety symptoms at one pole and depressive symptoms at the other. Symptoms related to depression included early wakening, retardation, persistent depression, short duration of illness, depression worse in the morning and delusions. Symptoms associated with anxiety included temporal lobe features, panic attacks, agoraphobia, unreality feelings, dizzy attacks, hysterical symptoms, obsessional symptoms, attacks of unconsciousness, other phobias, reactivity of depression and marked tension. The emergence of this bimodal (anxiety versus depression) component confirmed the hypothesis of Roth et al that within the affective population studied there were two distinct syndromes corresponding to anxiety and depression. The anxiety features contained in this component are very similar to the diagnostic features of panic disorder (DSM-III).

Gurney et al (1972), in the same patient population, carried out a discriminant function analysis using a multiple regression programme in which the dependent variable was the initial clinical diagnosis (anxiety state/depressive illness). The sought to determine whether or not two patient groups corresponding to the clinical states of anxiety and depression could be confirmed by discriminant function analysis. 13 items were isolated as being of great value in discriminating between anxiety states and depressive illness. Features related to anxiety were the presence of neurotic traits in childhood, excessive dependence, physical stress associated with the onset of the illness, panic attacks, situational phobias (agoraphobia), derealization, anxiety symptoms and compulsive symptoms. Features associated with depression were a low neuroticism score, depressed mood, early waking, suicidal tendencies and retardation. Panic attacks accounted for about one-third of the predicted variance. The distribution of patients' scores based on the 13 items were clearly bimodal. There was a close correspondence between the two groups defined by discriminant function analysis and the originial clinical diagnosis of anxiety

state and depressive illness. There findings confirmed the hypothesis that patients with anxiety states and depressive illnesses fall into two distinct clinical groups.

Schapira et al (1972) followed up patients originally studied by Roth et al (1972), on average 3.8 years after the initial key assessment. Patients who had been admitted to hospital with anxiety states did significantly less well than those with depressive illness. All symptoms studied at follow-up were more frequent and more severe in the anxiety group of patients. The nature of the symptomatology present in the two groups at follow-up differed. Symptoms generally associated with anxiety differentiated between the two groups. Prominent among these symptoms were agoraphobia, depersonalization, derealization and perceptual distortions. Features associated with depression failed to discriminate between the groups. 24 patients in the original anxiety group had a further breakdown during the follow-up period, while 12 in the depressive group suffered from subsequent illness during follow-up. Only one of the anxiety patients suffered from a depressive illness during this time, and two of the depressed patients from an anxiety state, demonstrating that diagnostic crossover between the two groups was very unusual. The findings of this follow-up study suggested that a distinction between anxiety states and depressive illness was both valid and useful. It further confirmed the differentiation between syndromes made 3.8 years previously on the basis of the initial clinical observations.

Subsequently, evidence from a variety of sources has supported the dualist view.

Discriminant analysis studies

Prusoff & Klerman (1974) were able by discriminant function analysis of the 58-item Symptom Checklist (SCL) to separate 364 outpatients clinically diagnosed as depressed, from an equal number diagnosed as anxious. Depressed patients reported themselves as more severely impaired on most items and factors. The depression factor contributed most to the discrimination. When levels of depression were held constant, the anxious patients reported more somatization. Downing & Rickels (1974) separated a mixed anxiety-depression group into distinct subgroups by discriminant function analysis of items from a physician checklist and self-report symptom checklist. Patients were clinically diagnosed as having mixed anxiety-depression. Derogatis et al (1972) also used the 58-item SCL in a study of 641 anxious patients and 251 depressed neurotics. Factor analysis revealed five symptom constructs – somatization, obsessive-compulsive symptoms, interpersonal sensitivity, depression and anxiety. Differences observed tended to involve qualitative distinctions in individual affective components in the anxiety and depression dimensions.

Psychophysiological measures

Both similarities and differences between anxiety and depression are found on psychophysiological studies. Anxious patients show high levels of electrodermal activity and slow habituation of skin conductance responses to repeated auditory stimuli (Lader & Wing 1964). Agitated depressives are more aroused than retarded depressives and, like anxious patients, habituate more slowly than controls to auditory stimuli. Retarded depressives show almost no electrodermal activity (Lader & Wing 1969); lower forearm blood flow has been noted in non-agitated compared to agitated depressives (Kelly & Walter 1969b). Increased pulse rate is also found in agitated but not in retarded depressives (Lader & Wing 1969).

Treatment studies

When first introduced it was suggested that anxiety symptoms responded to benzodiazepines, while depressive symptoms responded to tricyclic antidepressants (TCA) or monoamine oxidase inhibitors (MAOI). More recently, studies have demonstrated that TCA and MAOI are effective for the treatment of panic disorder (Judd et al 1986) and TCA, especially clomipramine, are effective for the treatment of obsessive-compulsive disorder (Murphy et al 1989). For generalized anxiety, the position remains unclear. In a recent review, Liebowitz et al 1988 examined a variety of studies in which TCA were used for the treatment of anxiety. Their analysis of the literature revealed that, although several studies demonstrated that TCA were effective for patients with mixed anxiety-depression, only one study which required predominant anxiety to be present showed TCA to be more beneficial than benzodiazepines.

Rating scales

Most instruments developed to measure anxiety and depression reflect the overlap between these two disorders. For example the Hamilton Depression Rating Scale (HDRS) includes items on insomnia, agitation,

psychic and somatic anxiety. Thus, it is not surprising that the score on HDRS correlates highly with measures of anxiety. Two relatively simple physician-rating scales have been developed by Raskin and by Covi (Lipman et al 1981) to evaluate depression and anxiety respectively. In a large collaborative study of primarily depressed and primarily anxious patients, the Raskin and Covi scales reliably differentiated between diagnostic groups (Lipman 1982). Statistically significant differences were also found when the mean scores of the anxious and depressed groups were contrasted on the Hamilton Anxiety and Depression Scales. Further exploration of the differences in symptomatology between anxious and depressed patients identified the symptoms which were rated higher by anxious than by depressed patients. There were: fear of fainting, numbness or tingling, heart pounding or racing, difficulty breathing, panic attacks, phobic avoidance, hot and cold spells and lump in the throat. Interestingly, as with the Newcastle group's findings (Roth et al 1972, Gurney et al 1972), these symptoms correspond to DSM-III/DSM-IIIR categories of panic and agoraphobia. Symptoms rated highest by depressed patients included feelings of hoplessness, anhedonia, loss of interest, suicidal ideation, crying, disturbed sleep and feeling of worthlessness.

Family history

Roth et al (1972) found that neurotic illness and personality disorder were more common in first-degree relatives of anxious patients. In a family study of major depression, Leckman et al (1983b) found that first-degree relatives of probands with depression and an anxiety disorder had higher rates of both anxiety and depression than those of probands with depression only. Torgersen (1985), in a study of neurotic twin probands, has demonstrated that hereditary factors appear to be important in the development of anxiety neurosis, while childhood environmental factors seem important in the development of neurotic depression. The concordance for pure anxiety neurosis was almost four times as high in MZ as in DZ twins. No significant differences existed between MZ and DZ twins of neurotic depressive probands, with concordance rates being high in both twin groups.

The anxious–depressive position

This view proposes a mixture of the two syndromes, phenomenologically different from either primary anxiety or primary depression. Although controversial, considerable evidence exists which suggests a distinct 'anxious depression' syndrome may exist, separate from other depressive syndromes and differentiated according to phenomenology and treatment response. The controversy surrounding this view relies on determining the difference between anxious depression and major depression with a concomitant anxiety disorder, and delineating the place of concepts such as atypical depression, which some (West & Dally 1959) but not all (Liebowitz et al 1984a) define as including prominent anxiety. Studies using factor analysis (Overall et al 1966), cluster analysis (Paykel 1971) and discriminant function analysis (Torgersen 1985) have identified groups suffering from both anxiety and depression.

DEPRESSION IN PATIENTS WITH ANXIETY DISORDERS

Panic disorder and agoraphobia

Studies demonstrating separation between anxiety and depressive disorders have consistently identified anxiety items of which the prominent features are symptoms characteristic of panic attacks (Roth et al 1972, Gurney et al 1972, Lipman 1982). McNair & Fisher (1978) suggested that the bipolar principal components factor in the study of Roth et al (1972), which was interpreted as anxiety versus depression, might be more precisely named panic anxiety versus endogenous depression. Thus, although it is still considered by many to be a controversial diagnosis, a great deal of research focusing on the relationship between anxiety and depression has involved the study of patients with panic disorder.

Phenomenology

A variety of early studies has documented a high incidence of secondary depression in patients with panic attacks (Woodruff et al 1972, Dealy et al 1981, Clancy et al 1978).

More recent studies have specifically assessed the relationship between panic disorder and depression. Breier et al (1984) examined the historical report of the longitudinal course of symptoms in 60 patients with panic disorder or agoraphobia with panic attacks. Two-thirds of patients had a current or past history of major depression. Half of those with major depression had at least one major depressive episode prior to and temporally separate from the onset of panic attacks. Patients with a history of depression had more severe anxiety

symptoms and longer duration of panic disorder than those with no history of depression. Van Valkenberg et al (1984) compared clinical and family data in four groups of patients: panic disorder only, panic with secondary depression, depression only, depression and secondary panic attacks. Patients with panic disorder only were older at first onset of panic attacks than those with panic and secondary depression. No differences between the two groups with respect to treatment response, psychosocial outcome or family history of psychiatric diagnosis were found. By contrast, patients with depression and secondary panic attacks had a later age of onset of panic attacks than both other groups with panic, and also a trend towards more chronic depression, poor treatment response, poor psychosocial outcome and greater family history of depression. The findings of these two studies are consistent with the hypothesis that patients with depression secondary to panic represent a more severe variant of panic disorder.

Family history

Several studies have documented an increased prevalence of affective disorder in families of patients with agoraphobia (Klein 1964, Bowen & Kohut 1979, Munjack & Moss 1981), while others (Buglass et al 1977) have failed to do so. Studies of patients with anxiety neurosis (Noyes et al 1978) and with panic disorder (Crowe et al 1980) have not demonstrated an increased risk of depression in relatives of probands compared with control populations.

Two studies (Leckman et al 1983b, Weissman et al 1984) do suggest an association between depression and panic disorder. Leckman et al (1983b) found an increased risk of depression, panic and phobic disorders in adult relatives of depressed probands with panic disorder. In an extension of this study, Weissman et al (1984) examined the risk of psychiatric disorder in the children aged 6–17 years of probands with major depression and specific anxiety disorders. Findings paralleled those observed in adult first-degree relatives. Depression plus panic or agoraphobia in adult probands conferred an increased risk of major depression and anxiety disorders (separation anxiety) in young children. These two studies suggest a relationship between depression and panic disorder.

Treatment response

Tricyclic antidepressants (TCAs) and monoamine oxidase inhibitors (MAOIs) are effective in alleviating panic attacks (Judd et al 1986). The mode of action of antidepressants in panic disorder has been questioned. Marks et al (1983) suggested that anti-panic effect occurred only in those with at least moderately depressed mood, and that this improved concomitantly with reduction of phobic anxiety symptoms. A series of studies by Zitrin and colleagues (1978, 1980, 1983), in which patients with depression were excluded, demonstrated antipanic efficacy of imipramine.

Benzodiazepines were earlier thought to be of little benefit in panic disorder. However, a series of studies have demonstrated the efficacy of high-dose benzodiazepines for treatment of this disorder (Judd et al 1990).

Biological findings

The dexamethasone suppression test has been extensively used in the study of depression where a non-suppression rate of approximately 50% has been found in endogenous depression (Carroll et al 1981). DST results for patients with panic disorder and agoraphobia have consistently shown a low rate of non-suppression similar to that of normal controls, suggesting that the biological basis for panic attacks differs from that of depressive illness (Judd et al 1987). Platelet serotonin uptake is increased in panic disorder (Norman et al 1986) and decreased in depressive illness (Meltzer et al 1983, Tuomisto et al 1979). Infusion of sodium lactate reliably produces panic in patients with panic disorder (Liebowitz et al 1984b). A similar rate of panic is seen with lactate infusion in patients with major depression and secondary panic (McGrath et al 1985, Cowley et al 1986), but not depression only (McGrath et al 1985). Sleep EEG recordings clearly differentiate between patients with panic disorder and those with depression. Depressed patients have shorter REM latency, higher REM density and more total REM; panic disorder patients do not differ significantly from controls (Uhde et al 1984). Patients with simultaneous major depression and panic disorder have REM values somewhere between those of patients with either disorder alone (Grunhaus et al 1986).

Social phobia

Although there is a high degree of comorbidity between agoraphobia, social phobia and panic attacks, demographic and clinical data support a distinction between social phobia and agoraphobia (Marks 1970, Aimes et al 1983). While depressed patients often show social withdrawal and social phobic patients often describe dysphoric symptoms, studies specifically assessing the association of social phobia and depression are lacking.

Family studies of social phobia compared to normals, other anxiety disorders or depression have not been reported.

Treatment studies in social phobia have focused on response to the antidepressants and beta-blockers. Many treatment studies have included social phobic together with agoraphobic patients. These suggest MAOI efficacy for social phobics (Judd et al 1986). An open study of patients with DSM-III social phobia has confirmed this (Liebowitz et al 1986). Beta-blockers have been shown to benefit patients with social phobia (Gorman et al 1985). Tricyclic antidepressants have not been specifically evaluated for social phobia, nor have benzodiazepines.

Few biological studies of social phobia exist. Social phobics show a much lower rate of panic after sodium lactate infusion than do patients with panic attacks (Liebowitz et al 1985).

Obsessive–compulsive disorder (OCD)

Once thought to be rare, obsessive–compulsive disorder is now recognised as a major source of psychological distress, with a lifetime prevalence of 2–3% (Robins et al 1984).

Phenomenology

Although it has generally been classified with the anxiety disorders, it has been argued that OCD would be more appropriately classified with the affective disorders or in its own category (Insel et al 1985). Lifetime history of major depression is reported in up to 50% of patients with OCD (Welner et al 1976, Goodwin et al 1969), with a similar number reported to be depressed at the onset of the disorder (Rachman & Hodgson 1980). Obsessional symptoms are also common in depressive illness. Depression and OCD are differentiated by demographic features. Obsessive-compulsive disorder affects males and females equally and has an early age of onset, with 30% first experiencing symptoms before they are 15 years old.

Family history

Few family studies are available and no consistent results have been found. Insel et al (1983) reported an increased prevalence of affective disorders in first-degree relatives of patients with OCD, but Coryell (1981) found no relationship between OCD and family history of affective disorder.

Treatment

The antidepressant clomipramine has well-demonstrated efficacy in OCD (e.g. Marks et al 1980, Mavissakalian & Michelson 1983, Rappaport & Ismond 1982, Thoren et al 1980). Two of these studies (Rappaport & Ismond 1982, Thoren et al 1980) found no relationship between pretreatment levels of depression and response of obsessive-compulsive symptoms to clomipramine, while in the other two studies good treatment response was related to high pretreatment levels of depression. More recent studies have demonstrated the efficacy of fluvoxamine (Price et al 1987, Goodman et al 1989) and fluoxetine (Jenike et al 1989). Two of these studies specifically assessed pretreatment depression and found no relationship to improvement in obsessive-compulsive symptoms (Jenike et al 1989, Goodman et al 1989).

Biology

Some similarities in response to biological tests between patients with OCD and depression have been noted. The dexamethasone suppression test has shown variable results. Two studies (Insel et al 1982a, Cottraux et al 1984) found that one-third of patients were non-suppressors. By contrast Lieberman et al (1985) found a non-suppression rate no greater than for normal controls. It is of note that the patients in the study of Insel & colleagues (1982a) were currently depressed or had recently recovered from depression. Some patients with OCD who were not currently depressed have been shown to have decreased REM latency (Insel et al 1982b) and blunted growth-hormone response to clonidine (Siever et al 1983), both of which have also been observed in depressed patients.

A variety of research in addition to treatment studies suggests abnormalities of serotonergic function in patients with OCD. High pretreatment levels of CSF 5-hydroxyindoleacetic acid (5-HIAA) (Thoren et al 1980) and increased platelet 5-HT levels (Flament et al 1985) are associated with treatment response to clomipramine. Oral m-chlorophenylpiperazine (mCPP), a selective 5-HT receptor agonist, exacerbates compulsive symptoms (Zohar et al 1987). These abnormalities of serotonergic function together with the response to biological tests do suggest an overlap at the neurobiological level between OCD and depression.

Post-traumatic stress disorder

By definition, post-traumatic stress disorder (PTSD) occurs only in response to some unusual environmental precipitant. Systematic clinical and epidemiological data are lacking. A high prevalence of concurrent psychiatric diagnoses has been reported in patients with PTSD (Sierles et al 1983, Green et al 1985, Davidson et al 1985). Most commonly, these are depression, other anxiety disorders, alcohol and substance abuse.

One reported family study of PTSD found an increased rate of alcohol and drug abuse, anxiety and depression in first-degree relatives (Davidson et al 1985). The patterns of prevalence of psychiatric disorder in relatives suggested a closer genetic relationship between PTSD and generalized anxiety than between PTSD and depression. Tricyclic antidepressants and MAOI are both claimed to be of value in the treatment of PTSD. At present reports are mainly confined to uncontrolled case reports (Van der Kolk 1987).

Generalized anxiety disorder

Particular difficulty in studying the relationship of generalized anxiety disorder (GAD) and depression stems from the way in which GAD is conceptualized. The DSM-III category of GAD was that of a residual category, created for those patients with significant anxiety but not panic, phobias, obsessions or compulsions. DSM-IIIR defines a more specific syndrome. GAD as defined in ICD-10 is similar to this, but not as narrowly defined. The ICD-9 concept of anxiety state is much broader than either the DSM-III or DSM-IIIR GAD category.

These differences in definition, coupled with the controversy as to whether mixed anxiety and depression represents a separate category lead to difficulties in defining the relationship between GAD and depression.

REFERENCES

Aimes P, Gelder M, Shaw P 1983 Social phobia. A comparative clinical study. British Journal of Psychiatry 142: 174–179

American Psychiatric Association 1980 DSM-III: Diagnostic and Statistical Manual of Mental Disorders, 3rd edn. American Psychiatric Association, Washington

American Psychiatric Association 1987 Diagnostic and Statistical Manual of Mental Disorders, 3rd edn – revised. American Psychiatric Association, Washington

Bowen R C, Kohut J 1979 The relationship between agoraphobia and primary affective disorders. Canadian Journal of Psychiatry 24: 317–322

Breier A, Charney D S, Heninger G R 1984 Major depression in patients with agoraphobia and panic disorder. Archives of General Psychiatry 41: 1129–1135

Buglass D, Clark J, Henderson A S 1977 A study of agoraphobic housewives. Psychological Medicine 7: 73–86

Carroll B J, Feinberg M, Greden J F et al 1981 A specific laboratory test for the diagnosis of melancholia. Archives of General Psychiatry 38: 15–22

Clancy J, Noyes R, Hoenk P R, Slymen D J 1978 Secondary depression in anxiety neurosis. Journal of Nervous and Mental Diseases 166: 846–850

Cockett R 1969 A short diagnostic self-rating scale in the pre-adult remand setting. British Journal of Psychiatry 115: 1141–1150

Coryell W 1981 Obsessive-compulsive disorder and primary unipolar depression. Comparisons of background, family history, course and mortality. Journal of Nervous and Mental Disease 169: 220–224

Costello C G, Comrey A I 1967 Scales for measuring depression and anxiety. Journal of Psychology 66: 303–319.

Cottraux J A, Bouvard M, Claustrat B et al 1984 Abnormal dexamethasone suppression test in primary obsessive-compulsive patients. A confirmatory report. Psychiatry Research 13: 157–165

Cowley D S, Dager S R, Dunner D L 1986 Lactate-induced panic in primary affective disorder. American Journal of Psychiatry 143: 646–648

Crowe R R, Pauls D L, Slymen D J, Noyes R 1980 A family study of anxiety neurosis. Morbidity risk in families of patients with and without mitral valve prolapse. Archives of General Psychiatry 37: 77–79

Crown S, Crisp H H 1966 A short clinical diagnostic self-rating scale for psychoneurotic patients. British Journal of Psychiatry 112: 917–923

Davidson J, Swartz M, Storck M, Krishnan R R, Hammett E 1985 A diagnostic and family study of post-traumatic stress disorder. American Journal of Psychiatry 142: 90–93

Dealy R S, Ishiki D M, Avery D H, Wilson L G, Dunner D L 1981 Secondary depression in anxiety disorders. Comprehensive Psychiatry 22: 612–618

Derogatis L R, Lipman R S, Covi L, Richards K 1972 Factorial invariance of symptom dimensions in anxious and depressive neuroses. Archives of General Psychiatry 27: 659–665

Downing R W, Rickels K 1974 Mixed anxiety-depression. Fact or myth? Archives of General Psychiatry 30: 312–317

Fawcett J, Kravitz H M 1983 Anxiety syndromes and their relationship to depressive illness. Journal of Clinical Psychiatry 44: 8–11

Flament M F, Rapoport J L, Berg C J et al 1985 Clomipramine treatment of childhood obsessive-compulsive disorder: a double-blind controlled study. Archives of General Psychiatry 42: 977–983

Freud S 1894 The justification for detaching from neurasthenia a particular syndrome: the anxiety neurosis. In: Strachey J (trans) Collections: Standard edition of the complete works of Sigmund Freud, vol 3. Hogarth Press, London, p 90–117

Gersh F S, Fowles D C 1979 Neurotic depression. The concept of anxious depression. In: Depue R A (ed) The psychobiology of the depressive disorders: implications for the effects of stress. Academic Press, New York, 81–104

Goodman W K, Price L H, Rasmussen S A, Delgado P L, Heninger G R, Charney D S 1989 Efficacy of fluvoxamine in obsessive-compulsive disorder. A double-blind comparison with placebo. Archives of General Psychiatry 46: 36–44

Goodwin P, Guze S, Robins E 1969 Follow up studies in obsessional neurosis. Archives of General Psychiatry 20: 182–187

Gorman J, Liebowitz M, Fyer A, Compeas R, Klein D 1985 Treatment of social phobia with atenolol. Journal of Clinical Psychopharmacology 5: 298–301

Green B L, Lindy J D, Grace M C 1985 Post-traumatic stress disorder. Toward DSM-IV. Journal of Nervous and Mental Diseases 173: 406–411

Grunhaus L, Rabin D, Harel Y et al 1986 Simultaneous panic and depressive disorders: clinical and sleep EEG correlates. Psychiatry Research 17: 251–259

Gurney, Roth M, Garside R F, Kerr T A, Schapira K 1972 The relationship between anxiety states and depressive illnesses. Part 2. British Journal of Psychiatry 121: 162–166

Hays P 1964 Modes of onset of psychotic depression. British Medical Journal 2: 779–784

Henry B W, Markette J R, Emken R L, Overall J E 1969 Drug treatment of anxious depression in psychiatric outpatients. Diseases of the Nervous System 30: 675–679

Hollister L E, Overall J E, Shelton J, Pennington V, Kimbell I, Johnstone M 1967 Amitriptyline, perphenazine and amitriptyline-perphenazine combination in different depressive syndromes. Archives of General Psychiatry 17: 486–493

Insel T R, Kalin B H, Guttmacher L B et al 1982a The dexamethasone suppression test in patients with primary obsessive-compulsive disorder. Psychiatry Research 6: 153–160

Insel T R, Gillin J C, Moore A 1982b Sleep in obsessive-compulsive disorder. Archives of General Psychiatry 39: 1372–1377

Insel T R, Hoover C, Murphy D C 1983 Parents of patients with obsessive-compulsive disorder. Psychological Medicine 13: 807–811

Insel T R, Zahn T, Murphy D L et al 1985 Obsessive compulsive disorder: anxiety disorder? In: Tuma A H, Maser J D (eds) Anxiety and the anxiety disorders. Lawrence Erlbaum, Hillsdale, N J, p 577–596

Jenike M A, Buttolph L, Baer L, Ricciardi J, Holland A 1989 Open trial of fluoxetine in obsessive-compulsive disorder. American Journal of Psychiatry 146: 909–911

Johnstone E, Cunningham Owens D G, Frith C D et al 1980 Neurotic illness and its response to anxiolytic and antidepressant treatment. Psychological Medicine 10: 321–328

Judd F K, Norman T R, Burrows G D 1986 Pharmacological treatment of panic disorder. International Clinical Psychopharmacology 1: 3–16

Judd F K, Norman T R, Burrows G D, McIntyre I M 1987 The dexamethasone suppression test in panic disorder. Pharmacopsychiatry 20: 99–101

Judd F K, Norman T R, Burrows G D 1990 Pharmacotherapy of panic disorder. International Review of Psychiatry 2: 399–410

Kelly D H W, Walter C J S 1969a A clinical and physiological relationship between anxiety and depression. British Journal of Psychiatry 115: 401–406

Kelly D H W, Walter C J S 1969b The relationship between clinical diagnosis and anxiety assessed by forearm blood flow and other measurement. British Journal of Psychiatry 114: 611–626

Kendell R E 1974 The stability of psychiatric diagnoses. British Journal of Psychiatry 124: 352–356

Kerr T A, Schapira K, Roth M, Garside R F 1970 The relationship between the Maudsley Personality Inventory and the course of affective disorders. British Journal of Psychiatry 116: 11–19

Klein D F 1964 Delineation of two drug responsive anxiety syndromes. Psychopharmacologia 5: 397–408

Klein D F 1981 Anxiety reconceptualized. In: Klein D F, Rabkin J (eds) Anxiety: new research and changing concepts. Raven Press, New York, p 235–265

Klein D F, Fink M 1962 Psychiatric reaction patterns to imipramine. American Journal of Psychiatry 119: 432–438

Kovacs M, Gatsonis C, Pavlavskas S L, Richards C 1989 Depressive disorders in childhood. IV. A longitudinal study of co-morbidity with and risk for anxiety disorders. Archives of General Psychiatry 46: 776–782

Lader M H, Wing L P 1964 Habituation of the psychogalvanic reflex in patients with anxiety states and in normal subjects. Journal of Neurology, Neurosurgery and Psychiatry 27: 210–218

Lader M H, Wing L P 1969 Physiological measures in agitated and retarded depressed patients. Journal of Psychiatric Research 7: 89–100

Leckman J F, Merikangas K R, Pauls D L, Prusoff B A, Weissman M W 1983a Anxiety disorders and depression: contradictions between family study data and DSM III conventions. American Journal of Psychiatry 140: 880–882

Leckman J F, Weissman M M, Merikangas K R, Pauls D L, Prusoff B A 1983b Panic disorder and major depression: increased risk of depression, alcoholism, panic and phobic disorders in families of depressed probands with panic disorder. Archives of General Psychiatry 40: 1055–1059

Lieberman J A, Kane J M, Sarentakos S et al 1985 Dexamethasone suppression tests in patients with obsessive-compulsive disorder. American Journal of Psychiatry 142: 747–751

Liebowitz M R, Quitkin F M, Stewart J W et al 1984a Phenelzine v imipramine in atypical depression. A preliminary report. Archives of General Psychiatry 41: 669–677

Liebowitz M R, Fyer A J, Gorman J M et al 1984b Lactate provocation of panic attacks. Clinical and behavioral findings. Archives of General Psychiatry 41: 764–770

Leibowitz M, Fyer A, Gorman J et al 1985. Specificity of lactate infusions in social phobic vs panic disorders. American Journal of Psychiatry 142: 947–950

Liebowitz M, Fyer A, Gorman J, Campeas R, Levin A 1986 Phenelzine in social phobia. Journal of Clinical Psychopharmacology 6: 93–98

Liebowitz M R, Fyer A J, Gorman J M et al 1988 Tricyclic therapy of the DSM-III anxiety disorders. A review with implications for further research. Journal of Psychiatric Research 22: (suppl 1) 7–31

Lipman R S 1982 Differentiating anxiety and depression in anxiety disorders: use of rating scales. Psychopharmacology Bulletin 18: 69–77

Lipman R S, Covi L, Downing R W et al 1981 Pharmacotherapy of anxiety and depression: rationale and study design. Psychopharmacology Bulletin 17: 91–95

McGrath P J, Stewart J W, Harrison W, Quitkin F M, Rabkin J 1985 Lactate infusion in patients with depression and anxiety. Psychopharmacology Bulletin 21: 555–557

McNair D M, Fisher S. 1978 Separating anxiety from depression. In: Lipton M A , Dimascio M, Killam K F (eds) Psychopharmacology: a generation of progress. Raven Press, New York, p 1411–1418

Marks I M 1970 The classification of phobic disorders. British Journal of Psychiatry 116: 377–386

Marks I M, Gelder M G, Edwards G 1968 Hypnosis and desensitization for phobias: a controlled prospective trial. British Journal of Psychiatry 114: 1263–1274

Marks I M, Stern R S, Mawson D, Cobb J, McDonald R 1980 Clomipramine and exposure for obsessive-compulsive rituals. British Journal of Psychiatry 136: 1–25

Marks I M, Gray S, Cohen D et al 1983 Imipramine and brief therapist-aided exposure in agoraphobics having self-exposure homework. Archives of General Psychiatry 40: 153–162

Mavissakalian M, Michelson L 1983 Tricyclic antidepressants in obsessive-compulsive disorders. Anti-obsessional or antidepressant agents? Journal of Nervous and Mental Disease 171: 301–306

Meltzer H G, Arora R C, Tricou B J, Fang V S 1983 Serotonin uptake in blood platelets and dexamethasone suppression test in depressed patients. Psychiatry Research 8: 41–47

Mendels J, Weinstein N, Cochrane C 1972 The relationship between anxiety and depression. Archives of General Psychiatry 27: 649–653

Munjack D L, Moss H B 1981 Affective disorder and alcoholism in families of agoraphobics. Archives of General Psychiatry 38: 869–871

Murphy D L, Zohar J, Benkelfat C, Pato M T, Pigott T A, Insel T R 1989 Obsessive-compulsive disorder as a 5-HT subsystem-related behavioural disorder. British Journal of Psychiatry 155 (suppl 8): 15–24

Norman T R, Judd F K, Gregory M et al 1986 Platelet serotonin uptake in panic disorder. Journal of Affective Disorders 11: 69–72

Noyes R, Clancy J, Crowe R, Hoenk P R, Slymen D J 1978 The familial prevalence of anxiety neurosis. Archives of General Psychiatry 35: 1057–1060

Overall J E, Hollister L E, Johnson M, Pennington V 1966

Nosology of depression and differential response to drugs. Journal of the American Medical Association. 195: 946–948

Paykel E S 1971 Classification of depressed patients: a cluster analysis derived grouping. British Journal of Psychiatry 118: 275–288

Price L H, Goodman W K, Charney D S, Rasmussen S A, Heninger G R 1987 Treatment of severe obsessive-compulsive disorder with fluvoxamine. American Journal of Psychiatry 144: 1059–1061

Prusoff B, Klerman G L 1974 Differentiating depressed from anxious neurotic outpatients. Use of discriminant function analysis for separation of neurotic affective states. Archives of General Psychiatry 30: 302–309

Rachman S J, Hodgson R J 1980 Obsessions and compulsions. Prentice-Hall, Englewood Cliffs, NJ Rapoport J, Ismond D R 1982 Biological research in child psychiatry. Journal of the American Academy of Child Psychiatry 21: 543–548

Robins L N, Helzer J E, Weissman M M et al 1984 Lifetime prevalence of specific psychiatric disorders in three sites. Archives of General Psychiatry 41: 949–958

Roth M, Gurney C, Garside R F, Kerr T A 1972 The relationship between anxiety states and depressive illnesses – Part 1. British Journal of Psychiatry 121: 147–161

Sargant W, Dally P 1962 Treatment of anxiety states by antidepressant drugs. British Medical Journal 1: 6–9

Schapira K, Roth M, Kerr T A, Gurney C 1972 The prognosis of affective disorders: the differentiation of anxiety states and depressive illnesses. British Journal of Psychiatry 121: 175–181

Sierles F S, Chen J J, McFarland R E, Taylor M D 1983 Post-traumatic stress disorder and concurrent psychiatric illness: a preliminary report. American Journal of Psychiatry 140: 1177–1179

Siever L J, Insel T R, Jimerson D C et al 1983 Growth hormone response to clonidine in obsessive-compulsive patients. British Journal of Psychiatry 142: 184–187

Thoren P, Asberg M, Cronholm B, Jornested L, Traskman L 1980 Clomipramine treatment of obsessive-compulsive disorder. Archives of General Psychiatry 37: 1289–1294

Tiller J, Schweitzer I, Maguire K, Davies B 1989 Is diazepam an antidepressant? British Journal of Psychiatry 155: 483–489

Torgersen S 1985 Hereditary differentiation of anxiety and affective neuroses. British Journal of Psychiatry 146: 530–534

Tuomisto J, Tukiainen R, Ahlfors U G 1979 Decreased uptake of 5-hydroxytryptamine in blood platelets from patients with endogenous depression. Psychopharmacology 65: 141–147

Tyrer P, Murphy S, Kingdon D et al 1988 The Nottingham study of neurotic disorder: comparison of drug and psychological treatments. Lancet 2: 235–240

Uhde T W, Roy-Byrne P, Gillin C H et al 1984 The sleep of patients with panic disorder: preliminary findings. Psychiatry Research 12: 251–259

Van der Kolk B 1987 The drug treatment of post traumatic stress disorder. Journal of Affective Disorders 13: 203–213

Van Valkenburg C, Akiskal H S, Puzantian V, Rosenthal S, 1984 Clinical, family history and naturalistic outcome – comparisons with panic and major depressive disorders. Journal of Affective Disorders 6: 67–82

Watson J P, Gaind R, Marks I M 1971 Prolonged exposure: a rapid treatment for phobias. British Medical Journal 1: 13–15

Weissman M M, Leckman J F, Merikangas K R, Gammon G D, Prusoff B A 1984 Depression and anxiety disorders in patients and children. Results from the Yale Family Study. Archives of General Psychiatry 41: 845–852

Welner A, Reich T, Robins I, Fishman R, Van Doren T 1976 Obsessive-compulsive neurosis: record, family and follow-up studies. Comprehensive Psychiatry 17: 527–539

West E D, Dally P J 1959 Effect of iproniazid in depressive syndromes. British Medical Journal 1: 1491–1494

Wolpe J 1958 Psychotherapy by reciprocal inhibition. Stanford University Press, Stanford

Woodruff R A, Guze S B, Clayton P J 1972 Anxiety neurosis among psychiatric outpatients. Comprehensive Psychiatry 13: 165–170

World Health Organization 1978 International classification of diseases, 9th revision. WHO, Geneva

World Health Organization 1988 International classification of diseases, 10th edn – draft. WHO, Geneva

Zitrin C M, Klein D F, Woerner M G 1978 Behavior therapy, supportive psychotherapy, imipramine and phobias. Archives of General Psychiatry 35: 307–316

Zitrin C M, Klein D F, Woerner M G 1980 Treatment of agoraphobia with group exposure in vivo and imipramine. Archives of General Psychiatry 37: 63–72

Zitrin C M, Klein D F, Woerner M G, Ross D C 1983 Treatment of phobias. Comparison of imipramine hydrochloride and placebo. Archives of General Psychiatry 40: 125–138

Zohar J, Mueller E A, Insel T R, Zohar-Kadouch R C, Murphy D L 1987 Serotonergic responsivity in obsessive-compulsive disorder: comparison of patients and healthy controls. Archives of General Psychiatry 44: 946–951

7. Course and outcome

William Coryell   George Winokur

Natural history will vary within even the most discrete illnesses. This variability necessarily increases when disorders reflect mixed ætiologies and, as the affective disorders arise from causes which are presumptively mixed and notoriously obscure, their outcomes are especially diverse and difficult to predict. Nevertheless, the literature on course and outcome contains important consistencies and some predictions can be made with confidence.

Long-term follow-up studies are, by necessity, 'naturalistic'. The investigator does not assign or control treatment but allows the subject to seek treatment, or not, as he or she would under ordinary circumstances. Nor can treatment be 'controlled for' since the causal relationships between treatment and course are bi-directional (outcome also causes treatment) and cannot be disentangled. Generalizability is always a concern since patients in different samples may seek, or have access to, different treatment modalities. There is, however, no viable alternative. Research attempts to specify and control treatment in the long run quickly result in small and highly biased samples. The solution, of course, lies in replication across studies. The features and predictors of course which reappear despite sample differences are robust and should be clinically applied. Most assertions in the following review will therefore reflect findings reported by at least two independent investigators.

The reader should be aware of other biases affecting essentially all follow-up studies. Researchers typically draw their samples from university-based centres, and ill individuals who seek help elsewhere, or who fail to seek help altogether, are not characterized. The literature therefore probably describes the more impaired and complicated end of an illness spectrum.

Invariably, a significant proportion of subjects is lost to follow-up, through refusal, death or simple disappearance. The baseline features of these individuals are rarely described and they may differ in important ways from those who do complete follow-up. Moreover, follow-up studies are finite and are usually substantially less than lifelong. Figures which describe the likelihood of various outcomes (i.e. chronicity, relapse, recovery) must be viewed accordingly.

BIPOLAR AFFECTIVE DISORDER

Definition

Though the syndrome of mania was recognized in antiquity, its widespread use to subdivide affective disorder is a relatively recent development (Leonhard et al 1962, Winokur et al 1969, Perris 1966, Angst 1966). Most of the older follow-up studies failed to apply this division. Yet, due in large part to the advent of lithium treatment, this separation is now the most widely accepted of the various dichotomies proposed for affective disorder. Numerous other subdivisions exist but these generally apply to unipolar disorder rather than to bipolar disorder. The following is organized accordingly.

The diagnostic importance given mania has led to particular interest in its boundaries. Most operational definitions of mania have specified a minimum duration and number of symptoms (Feighner et al 1972, Spitzer et al 1978, American Psychiatric Association 1987). Patients not infrequently describe some of the required symptoms but lack the specified minimum number and/or duration. The label most often applied to this symptom cluster is hypomania and the corresponding disorder is usually termed 'bipolar II'. Only recent follow-up studies have separated bipolar I and bipolar II patients; earlier ones were silent on the issue.

Onset

Onset may be dated from the first symptoms, the first syndrome or the first treatment; the corresponding mean ages will vary accordingly. Regardless of the definition used, though, the mean age of onset for bipolar illness rarely exceeds 33 years (Baastrup et al 1970, d'Elia et al 1974, Loranger & Levine 1978, Petterson 1977, Carlson et al 1974, Clayton et al 1965, Dunner et al 1976a, Perris 1968, Winokur et al 1969, Woodruff et al 1971, Abrams & Taylor 1980, Bland & Orn 1982, Akiskal et al 1983, Coryell et al 1985a, Angst 1986, Endicott et al 1985, Blumenthal et al 1987). The incidence of onset falls rapidly in later years. For example, 88% of a series of 393 collected by Angst et al (1973) had an onset before 49 years of age. Sex apparently does not affect age of onset (Dunner et al 1976a, Perris 1968, Wertham 1928, Winokur 1975, Endicott et al 1985, Burke et al 1990).

Mean ages of onset described for bipolar illness are consistently lower than those given for unipolar illness. Several studies suggest that bipolar II illness too begins earlier than unipolar illness (Endicott et al 1985, Coryell et al 1985a, Blumenthal et al 1987, Angst 1986) but several do not (Ayuso-Gutierrez & Ramos-Brieda 1982, Kupfer et al 1988).

The proportion of bipolar patients who begin their illness with mania rather than depression varies widely across reported cohorts. Perris (1968) reported that 34% of 131 bipolar probands had a first episode featuring mania but, of the 150 bipolar patients described by Dunner et al (1976b), 79% had mania at the outset of illness. Other authors (Winokur et al 1969, Carlson et al 1974, Petterson 1977) have reported intermediate proportions and the balance of the literature indicates that mania occurs in over half of the initial attacks in bipolar patients.

Duration

On the natural duration of a manic attack, Kraepelin (1921) remarked '. . . the great majority extend over many months.' Other case series collected before the advent of effective somatic treatment (about 1945) bear him out (see Table 7.1). Wertham (1928) collected the largest series and, among 2000 cases, the most frequent duration was four months. These figures are longer than those generated by more contemporary studies by a factor of two or more (Table 7.1). One-half of the episodes described by Coryell et al (1989), for instance, lasted one month or less. Figure 7.1 illustrates this graphically; these episodes were observed prospectively among patients followed after recovery from an index mania or depression. While some differences are apparent across centres, at all centres the likelihood of recovery increased most rapidly in the initial 10 weeks following episode onset.

Table 7.1 Duration of manic episodes

Author	n (episodes)	Mean duration (months)
Patients followed before 1945		
Swift 1907	74	7
Wertham 1928	2 000	8
Lundquist 1945	95	13
Coryell (unpublished)	68	8
Patients followed after 1945		
Winokur et al 1969	91	1.8
Angst et al 1973	2 798	2.7
Coryell et al 1989	81	2.6

According to many reports, age and recurrence affect the length of manic episodes. They are not consistent as to the nature of these effects, however. MacDonald (1918), Wertham (1928) and Lundquist (1945) all found that older patients had longer first attacks. In Lundquist's patients, the duration of subsequent attacks was stable in younger patients but tended to shorten in late onset patients. Rennie (1942) found a similar consistency of episode duration in younger 'cyclothymia' patients but a lengthening with recurrence in older patients. Without dividing by age, Swift (1907) noted that first attacks averaged 7 months in length while the mean duration of second attacks was 11.5 months. Finally, Angst et al (1973) much later described a large series of episodes and concluded that episode length remains stable for given individuals regardless of episode number.

Manic episode durations seem unrelated to the quality or quantity of most symptoms. However, high levels of depressive symptoms apparently portend a poor short-term outcome (Himelhoch et al 1976, Secunda et al 1987, Cohen et al 1988). Likewise, Keller et al (1986a), in a more systematic follow-up, found that patients who entered the study with a mixture of manic and depressive syndromes or who had cycled within the index episode, took a substantially longer time to recover than did patients who began follow-up in a purely manic episode.

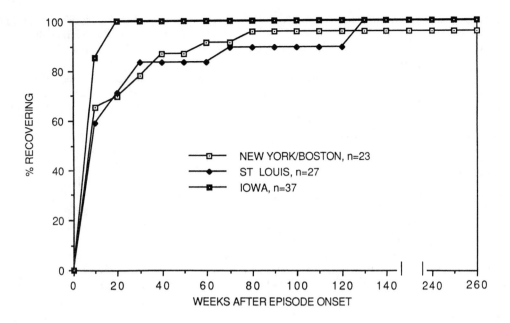

Fig. 7.1   Time to recovery from the first prospectively observed episode of mania during a 5-year follow-up (from the NIMH Collaborative Program on the Psychobiology of Depression – Clinical Studies)

Recovery

The recovery rate cited in a given study depends largely on the length of follow-up and the definition of recovery peculiar to that study. Poort (1945) and Bratfos & Haug (1968) reported relatively high rates of chronicity associated with index episodes (56% and 45% respectively). Both authors apparently included as chronic individuals incapacitated for much of the follow-up period by a high relapse frequency and significant numbers of these 'chronic' patients had had at least some asymptomatic periods. For instance, 22 of 58 unipolar and bipolar patients listed as chronic in the Bratfos study had been 'free from symptoms' at the time of discharge and none of the patients listed as chronic in the Poort study (1945) had failed to recover from their first attack. At the other extreme, Wertham (1928) reported that only 14 of 2000 hospitalized manics (0.7%) had symptoms persisting longer than 5 years. Since Wertham used centralized statistics limited to hospital admissions in a given area, this figure probably reflects the proportion of patients requiring chronic hospitalization.

Other studies have noted the importance of length of follow-up in rates of recovery. Winokur et al (1969) found that rates of full recovery increased markedly as follow-up lengths moved to 3 years. Morrison et al (1973), using routinely obtained follow-up material and charts from the Iowa 500 cohort, likewise found a strong relationship between the likelihood of recovery and follow-up lengths when these ranged to less than 5 years. Recovery rates noted when observation extends beyond 3 years appear more stable, however. Lundquist (1945) and Rennie (1942) performed relatively long follow-ups and concluded that, of manics, 8% and 11% respectively did not recover from their index episode. Four of the eight non-recovered manics in the Lundquist study developed schizophrenia so that the actual proportion with true chronic mania was 4%. Likewise, Stenstedt (1952) followed 49 manics over 2–20 year periods and found only two (4%) to have taken a chronic course. Most recently, the Collaborative Depression Study (Coryell et al 1989) found that only eight (5.1%) of 166 patients who began the follow-up in an episode of bipolar illness failed to recover. With the exclusion of those who were re-diagnosed at the end of follow-up as having schizophrenia or schizoaffective disorder, mainly of schizophrenic type (5.1%), only six (3.8%) of 158 failed to recover. The cumulative proportion recovering increased most rapidly in the first 6 months but changed very slowly after one year (Fig. 7.1).

In summary, then, it appears that manic episodes typically resolve within several months. Those which fail to remit, at least temporarily, within several years or those which evolve into schizophrenia are quite uncommon. Less uncommon are courses in which rapidly recurrent, severe episodes produce chronic social and vocational impairment (Welner et al 1977).

Long-term course

Proportions of patients having no further attacks following the index episode show wide variation across studies (Table 7.2). Kraepelin (1921) observed the majority of 459 manic patients for over 20 years and noted that 208 (45%) had only one attack. Only 30% of the sample had three or more attacks. In a later, lengthy follow-up of first admission manics, Lundquist (1945)

noted that 55% of those who remained diagnostically stable had only one attack. In most of the more recent follow-ups, however, the single episode course is the exception (Bratfos & Haug 1968, Angst et al 1973, Carlson et al 1974, Coryell et al 1989). Differences in follow-up length cannot reconcile these studies since the Kraepelin and Lundquist studies were among the longest. Also, Rennie (1942) and Poort (1945) relied chiefly on mailed questionnaires but reported some of the highest relapse rates while Stendstedt (1952), who carried out personal follow-up interviews of all probands, found considerably lower rates. Some of these disparities might be explained in other ways, however. In many earlier studies, episodes ended only with discharge; since the lengths of hospital stay were typically much greater in the first half of this century, a single episode by this definition may have subsumed several as defined by more contemporary criteria. Alternatively, contemporary treatment may bring about

Table 7.2 Percentage of single episode courses in unipolar and bipolar illness

Author	Follow-up (years)	Intake period ending	Unipolar n	Unipolar %	Bipolar n	Bipolar %
Kraepelin 1921	10–40	before 1920	440	60	459	45
Rennie 1942	25 (approx)	1916	142	18	66	8
Lewis 1936	7–8	1929	61	23	—	—
Lundquist 1945	10–30	1931	171	61	95	55
Poort 1945	10 (approx)	1932	75	33	51	23
Stendstedt 1952	2–20	1948	239	58	49	32
Winokur 1975	2–20	1944	—	—	30	33
Shobe & Brion 1971	18	1953	105	43	15	33
Kay et al 1969	5–7	1959	104	28	—	—
Bratfos & Haug 1968	1–12	1961	126	44	23	13
Angst et al 1973	1–12	1972	626	5	393	0.5
Carlson et al 1974	1–12	1970	—	—	53	4
Nystrom 1979	10	1971	83	19	—	—
Bland & Orn 1982	15 (approx)	1980	75	55	27	26
Smith & North 1988	11	1980	58	29	—	—
Lehman et al 1988	11 (approx)	1984	65	22	—	—
Lee & Murray 1988	18	1984	65	5	—	—
Kiloh et al 1988	15	1985	133	37	—	—
Coryell et al 1989a	5	1987	442	33	53	11

symptom-free periods which are less stable than those which occur more naturally with the simple passage of time.

The time to relapse has as much clinical importance as time to recovery, yet far fewer studies have examined the variables which might predict it. According to at least three (Kraepelin 1921, Angst et al 1973, Dunner et al 1979) the time to relapse decreases over the first two or three episodes. In the longer two of these studies, symptom-free episodes then stabilized in length. Lundquist (1945), however, noted that relapse was no more likely after a second episode than after a first. Others have found tentative evidence that episodes cluster over time (Winokur 1975, Saran 1969). Finally, it must be remembered that an apparent decrease in interval length may be in part artefactual since larger intervals are more likely than shorter ones to be missed near the end of a finite period of observation.

Age of onset has also been related to interval lengths but the results here are inconsistent as well. Swift (1907) and MacDonald (1918) both noted an association between an age of onset over 40 years and a relatively short first interval. Lundquist (1945), on the other hand, made his only age division at 30 years and noted that the older patients had a longer first interval. Finally, Dunner et al (1979) detected no relationship between age of onset and relapse interval.

A bipolar course which features frequent shifts between mania and euthymia or depression is now designated 'rapid cycling'. The concept has particular importance since rapid cycling is the most often cited predictor of a poor outcome to lithium therapy. Unfortunately, the four available studies relevant to this condition concur only that females show a marked predominance (Dunner et al 1977, Kukopoulos et al 1980, Wehr et al 1988, Nurnberger et al 1988), though none have clearly implicated menopause (Kukopoulos et al 1980, Wehr et al 1988) or hypothyroidism (Wehr et al 1988, Nurnberger et al 1988). Two studies provided follow-up data and both found a correspondence between rapid cycling and the use of tricyclic antidepressants (Wehr et al 1988, Kukopoulos et al 1980, Kukopoulos et al 1983).

The dominance of one pole over another may exhibit some stability from one episode to the next (Lundquist 1945, Perris 1968, Quitkin et al 1981) and this has led some authors to consider the existence of manic-prone and depression-prone forms of bipolar disorder (Angst 1978, Quitkin et al 1986). The apparent stability is only modest, however, and follow-up studies have yet to determine whether or not such predominance extends beyond two contiguous episodes.

The likelihood of an eventual diagnostic revision to schizophrenia is low. Rennie (1942), Bratfos & Haug (1968), Carlson et al (1974) and Faravelli & Poli (1982) all reported no evolution to schizophrenia among their manic probands. Other lengthy follow-up studies have reported schizophrenic outcomes in 8–9% of patients who began with a diagnosis of mania (Lundquist 1945, Tsuang et al 1981). Moreover, of 70 patients who began a recent 5-year follow-up with mania and either mood-congruent or mood-incongruent psychotic features, six (8.6%) had psychotic features present throughout the final 6 months (Coryell et al 1990c).

All of the above factors – episode lengths, symptom-free intervals, the likelihood of relapse, syndrome predominance and diagnostic evolution – interact with environmental and constitutional specifics to determine the overall impact of the illness. That 'global outcome' has been defined in numerous ways is understandable and consensus across studies is elusive. Table 7.3 illustrates some of the ways in which outcome categories in bipolar illness have been defined. While percentages in the best outcome categories tend to be substantial, so do percentages in the worst outcome categories. It is clear that the prognosis is not uniform; many patients experience little disability while many others experience a great deal.

Given the variance in outcome definitions across studies, the inclusion of other disorders for comparison within studies can provide important perspective to the data. The most commonly afforded comparison is to unipolar illness. Several have found no outcome differences between unipolar and bipolar disorders (Hastings 1958, Bland & Orn, 1982); several others have revealed modest trends favouring unipolar illness (Tsuang et al 1979, Grossman et al 1984, Coryell et al 1989) and still others have noted that, on average, bipolar patients have markedly poorer outcomes (Shobe & Brion 1971, Bratfos & Haug 1968, McGlashan 1984). Only Lundquist (1945) noted a strong trend favouring bipolar patients over unipolar patients. Thus, the literature yields a composite in which bipolar illness is at least somewhat more malignant in the long run than is unipolar illness.

In cross-section, bipolar disorder shares clinical features with schizophrenia and, in fact, the boundaries between these illnesses have varied markedly over time and settings (Baldessarini 1970). Outcome comparisons between these illnesses are, though surprisingly

Table 7.3   Long-term prognosis in bipolar illness

Study (*n*)	Length of follow-up (years)	Baseline	% with good outcomes	% with poor outcomes
Rennie 1942 (66)	25 (approx)	1913–1916	30 'recovered for 5 years or longer'	?
Lundquist 1945 (86)	10–30	1912–1921	78 'never had any further mental troubles' outside of attacks	15 did not 'socially' recover.
Tsuang et al 1979 (86)	40	1934–1944	43 'absence of psychiatric "symptoms" at time of follow-up'	25 'incapacitating' psychiatric symptoms at time of follow-up
Hastings 1958 (66)	6–12	1938–1944	41 'may have spent a short time in a state hospital; . . . soon paroled and never returned'	27 'had continuous trouble of the type for which he was hospitalized'
Shobe & Brion 1971 (15)	18	1949–1953	47 'not incapacited in any degree' during follow-up period	53 'unable to work or to function socially most of the time'
Bratfos & Haug 1968 (42)	1–12	1952–1961	?	45 'not free of symptoms for any length of time'
Carlson et al 1974 (53)	1–12	1960–1970	57 'well' since hospitalization	28 non-remitting with various levels of severity
Grossman et al 1984 (33)	1.5	~1982	33 'good according to index of overall functioning'	39 'poor' according to index of overall functioning
McGlashan 1984 (19)	15	1945–1975	11 'recovered'	32 'continuously incapacitated'

rare, consistent in their results. In three studies, measures indicated substantially better outcomes for patients with bipolar illness than for those with schizophrenia (Tsuang et al 1979, Bland & Orn 1982, Grossman et al 1984). In the fourth study (McGlashan 1984) outcome for 15 bipolar patients was only slightly better than that for schizophrenic patients but much worse than that for unipolar patients. These subjects were particularly chronic as they began the follow-up and their outcomes may be less typical than those described in other studies.

It appears, then, that outcome in bipolar illness is on average slightly worse than that for unipolar illness but substantially better than that for schizophrenia. The range of possible outcomes remains quite large, however, and there is little to guide the clinician in distinguishing good prognosis from poor prognosis bipolar patients. Several authors have noted an association between premorbid personality and outcome.

Both MacDonald (1918) and Kraepelin (1921) noted the poor prognostic implications of cyclothymic personality and Wertham (1928) mentioned that a 'manic constitution' was a possible predictor of chronic mania. More recently, the presence of rapid cycling (Dunner et al 1977, Kukopuolos et al 1980, Wehr et al 1988, Nurnberger et al 1988) and, in particular, mixed states (Himmelhoch et al 1976, Secunda et al 1987) have been associated with poor short-term treatment response. If these features are stable qualities of a given patient's illness, they might be expected to predict a poorer overall outcome in the long run. Evidence is emerging, however, that, in many cases, rapid cycling may be a transient phenomenon (Coryell et al in press).

According to some authors, an adolescent onset portends a poor outcome (Olsen 1961) as the evolution of psychosocial adjustment may be particularly sensitive to disruption at this period. Mania in adolescence is, in fact, more often misdiagnosed than is mania during adulthood (Coryell & Norten 1980, Ballenger et al 1982, Kendell 1985), possibly because psychotic features are more likely with an adolescent onset (Ballenger et al 1982, McGlashan 1988, Rosen et al 1983). Misdiagnosis may, in itself, have negative consequences as long as it persists. However, direct comparisons of adolescent onset and adult onset bipolar disorders have shown little overall difference in outcome (Carlson et al 1977, McGlashan, 1988).

Mortality and suicide

With rare exceptions (Martin et al 1985), follow-up studies have regularly found excess mortality among bipolar patients. This excess has been attributed both to natural and to unnatural causes but, again with few exceptions (Weeke & Vaeth 1986), excess mortality due to natural causes is confined to samples identified before 1950 (Tsuang et al 1980, Derby 1933). This excess natural mortality has been due largely to cardiovascular deaths and may reflect the exhaustion to which these patients were prone before the advent of effective treatment. Derby (1933), for instance, found a 22.5% death rate among 4341 patients, hospitalized with mania between 1912 and 1932. One-third of these cases were admitted with 'cardiac symptoms' and 40% appeared, clinically, to die of 'exhaustion'.

While more contemporary samples have shown little excess mortality from natural causes, the liability to suicide has remained high (Perris 1966, Petterson 1977, Morrison 1982, Weeke & Vaeth 1986, Black et al 1987). The literature is divided as to whether the likelihood of suicide among bipolar patients is as high as that among unipolar patients. According to some authors the risk for eventual suicide is lower for bipolar patients than for unipolar patients (Black et al 1987, McGlashan 1984). According to others it is higher (Morrison 1982, Dunner et al 1976a), while still others have found little or no difference in risk (Perris 1966, Scheftner et al in press, Tsuang 1978, Weeks & Vaeth 1986).

UNIPOLAR AFFECTIVE DISORDER

Since bipolar illness does not always begin with a manic episode, any large group labelled as unipolar is likely to contain at least some bipolar patients. The quantity and importance of this contamination and the diagnostic measures necessary to limit it are uncertain and many

follow-up studies of depression fail to mention the development of mania altogether. An incomplete list of those which have done so (Table 4), reveals high variability and a median value of approximately ten percent. Higher and lower rates of switching apparently do not simply reflect the length of follow-up. The differences between diagnostically stable and diagnostically unstable samples are obscure.

A diagnosis of unipolar disorder grows more secure with the recurrence of unipolar depressive episodes. Angst et al (1978), for instance, used both retrospective and prospective views to determine that 70% of bipolars were correctly diagnosed within three episodes. The proportion diagnosed correctly rose slowly thereafter and was 83% by six episodes. Dunner et al (1976b) used the initial hospitalization for unipolar depression as a starting point and determined that approximately 90% of those who eventually developed mania did so by their third subsequent episode.

Table 7.4 The likelihood of mania during the follow-up of previously unipolar patients

Study	Number followed	Length of follow-up (years)	Number (%) developing mania
Akiskal et al 1983	206	3	41 (19.9)
Strober & Carlson 1982	60	0.5–4	12 (20.0)
Dunner et al 1976	102	0.5–5	2 (2.0)
Coryell et al 1989	442	5	19 (4.3)
Rao & Nammalvar 1977	102	3–13	36 (37.5)
Nystrom 1979	83	10	4 (4.8)
Lehman et al 1988	63	11	0 (0)
Angst et al 1978	203	15	20 (9.8)
Lee & Murray 1988	65	18	10 (15.4)
Winokur & Wesner 1987	225	35	22 (9.7)

Do depressed patients who will eventually become manic exhibit distinguishing features? At least two of the three relevant studies (Strober & Carlson 1982, Akiskal et al 1983, Winokur & Wesner 1987) agree that the following features increase the risk of an eventual bipolar course—young age, psychomotor retardation, guilt, a high familial loading for affective disorder and a family history of mania.

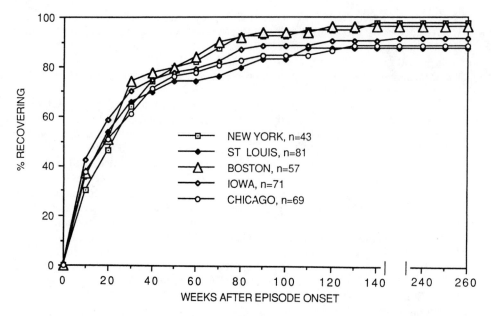

Fig. 7.2   Time to recovery from the first prospectively observed episode of major depression during a 5-year follow-up (from the NIMH Collaborative Program on the Psychobiology of Depression – Clinical Studies)

Onset

As might 'be expected from the greater heterogeneity of unipolar affective disorder, mean and median ages of onset are more variable across studies than they are for bipolar illness. In studies involving both conditions, onset is consistently later for unipolar disorder (Angst et al 1973, Perris 1968, Prien et al 1974, Woodruff et al 1971, Clancy et al 1974, Burke et al 1990). Onset may also be less abrupt; in at least two studies unipolars reported longer durations at hospitalization than did manic patients (Winokur 1985a, Winokur et al 1990).

Duration

Unipolar depressives tend to have episodes similar to or slightly longer in duration than those of bipolars reported in the same study (Angst et al 1973, Bratfos & Haug 1968, Lundquist 1945, Rennie 1942, Swift 1907, Coryell et al 1989). As shown in Figure 7.2, the likelihood of recovery increases most rapidly in the first 6 months after onset, somewhat less rapidly in the next 6 months and very slowly thereafter.

A later age of onset may be associated with longer duration (Angst et al 1973, Lundquist 1945,

MacDonald 1918). Some authors have reported that episode duration increases with recurrence, particularly with late onset individuals (Rennie 1942, Swift 1907, MacDonald 1918) but other authors have reported stable durations in recurrent attacks (Angst et al 1973, Lundquist 1945).

Recovery

Since the definition of recovery varies widely from study to study, within-study comparisons of recovery rates for different conditions are more meaningful than comparisons across studies. Among those which compared unipolar and bipolar groups in this way, recovery rates were higher for unipolar illness in some (Bratfos & Haug 1968; Shobe & Brion 1971, Morrison et al 1973), but higher for bipolar illness in others (Hastings 1958, Lundquist 1945, Rao & Nammalvar 1977). Still others found no difference (Coryell et al 1989) and conclusions are obviously limited.

As with bipolar illness, recovery rates cited for unipolar illness are affected by follow-up length (Winokur & Morrison 1973). Recent, high intensity follow-ups (Keller et al 1984, Coryell et al 1989) suggest that the relationship between recovery rate and follow-up length is most pronounced during the first

1–2 years following intake. Recoveries continue to accumulate beyond that point but do so much more slowly (Fig. 7.2).

The longer follow-up efforts consistently identify a small group of patients who fail to recover. Older patients (Watts 1956, Bratfos & Haug 1968, Winokur & Morrison 1973, Rao & Nammalvar 1977, Keller et al 1986b), those with psychotic features (Kay et al 1969, Lundquist 1945, Poort 1945) and those already chronically ill (Kay et al 1969, Keller et al 1984) are overrepresented in this group. However, even among those who are already chronically ill, there is a substantial likelihood of recovery. Among depressed outpatients already ill for 2 or more years, Akiskal et al (1981) found that 66% showed 'clinical response to thymoleptic treatment'. In another sample of 129 similarly chronic patients (mostly inpatients), 77.5% recovered during a 5-year follow-up (Coryell et al 1990c).

Long-term course

While multiple episode courses are more common among bipolar patients (Table 7.2), a large proportion of unipolar patients relapse as well among the predominantly hospitalized series included in most long-term follow-ups published so far. Factors which increase the risk for relapse among unipolar patients include a history of recurrence (Gonzales et al 1985, Keller et al 1983), young age (Gonzales et al 1985, Keller et al 1983, Giles et al 1989) and a diagnosis of secondary depression (Keller et al 1983, Rabkin et al 1986).

The fact that a given episode follows a recovery does not ensure against chronicity (Keller et al 1986b, Lehman et al 1988) and the likelihood of chronicity may persist unchanged even after three or four recurrences (Lehman et al 1988). As with bipolar illness, then, the long-term outcome can be very good or it can be very poor. Indeed, a substantial proportion remain highly symptomatic at the end of lengthy follow-up periods. In a 5–7-year follow-up by Key et al (1969), 14% of 104 depressed patients had Hamilton Rating Scale (Hamilton 1967) scores of 15 or more. Shobe & Brion (1971) and Lee & Murray (1988) each conducted 18-year follow-ups; in the first study 15% were 'unable to work or function most of the time' and, in the second, 19% had 'chronic residual symptoms or chronic severe stress and handicap'. Few replicable predictors of long-term outcome have emerged, unfortunately. Several diagnostic sub-types have proven helpful in predicting the near future and these will be discussed below.

A more surprising development is one of diagnostic change. Such outcomes are, in fact, quite rare among patients with primary unipolar depression (Murphy et al 1974, Faravelli & Poli 1982). The most fundamental change is to schizophrenia and most of the authors who have noted such revisions have cited low figures of zero (Faravelli & Poli 1982), 2% (Coryell et al 1980, Rennie 1942), 4% (Lewis 1936, Guze et al 1983) or 6% (Lundquist 1945, Tsuang et al 1981). Four studies have noted that such diagnostically unstable patients were significantly more likely to have psychotic features (Guze et al 1983, Rennie 1942) or 'characteristics' of schizophrenia (Coryell et al 1980, Poort 1945) when first given a diagnosis of depression.

Mortality

As with bipolar illness, almost all relevant studies of unipolar depressive disorder have shown evidence of excess mortality. While some have noted excess deaths attributed to cancer or cardiovascular disease (Murphy et al 1987, Murphy et al 1988) most have found that unnatural deaths accounted for all excess mortality in unipolar disorder (Black et al 1987, Martin et al 1985, Scheftner in press, Tsuang et al 1980, Rorsman et al 1982, Weeke & Vaeth 1986).

Psychological autopsies of completed suicides have consistently found depressive illness to be the most common preceding disorder (Robins et al 1959, Dorpat & Ripley 1960, Barraclough et al 1974, Chynoweth et al 1980). The proportion of deaths attributable to suicide among depressed patients is higher with shorter follow-up periods of observation since the risk for suicide in this population is highest during the first 1–2 years after hospitalization (Black et al 1987, Fawcett et al 1987). As this period lengthens, the proportion of deaths due to suicide stabilizes at approximately 15% (Guze & Robins 1970, Coryell 1981a, Coryell et al 1982b; Tsuang 1978).

Most attempts to identify clinical predictors of suicide within patient populations have followed suicide attempters or other diagnostically mixed groups. Within such heterogeneous samples, hopelessness may be the single most robust predictor of completed suicide (Beck et al 1985, 1990). Those studies which have focused on depressed populations have reached little consensus, however. Males were at higher risk for eventual suicide in two studies (Barraclough & Pallis 1975, Modestin & Kopp 1988) but not in two others (Black et al 1987, Fawcett et al 1987). Nor have diagnostic subtypes of depression proven to be useful predictors. Specifically, the presence of delusions was proposed as a risk factor in one study (Roose et al 1983) but appeared unimportant in two others (Coryell & Tsuang 1982, Black et al 1988). The single most replicable risk factor for suicide among patients with depression is a history of suicide attempts. Three studies have found strong relationships between a history of such behaviour at the beginning of follow-up and the risk for ultimate suicide (Fowler et al 1979, Modestin & Kopp 1988, Barraclough & Pallis 1975); a fourth (Fawcett et al 1987) found a strong supporting trend. Finally, laboratory evidence of hypothalamic – pituitary – adrenal axis hyperactivity may provide an additional index of suicide risk. In three of these studies, depressed patients who eventually committed suicide were significantly more likely to have shown abnormal cortisol escape from dexamethasone suppression (Coryell & Schlesser 1981, Carroll et al 1980, Norman et al 1990).

SUBDIVISION OF UNIPOLAR ILLNESS

Divisions based on phenomenology or presumed aetiology

Most of these divisions have been bipartite. Labels for one side of this dichotomy have been 'endogenous', 'vital', 'psychotic' and 'vegetative'. While these are not conceptually synonymous, they have often been used interchangeably. This applies as well to labels for the converse condition — 'neurotic', non-endogenous', 'non-psychotic' 'reactive' or 'situational'. However, when Klerman et al (1979) applied operational criteria for those conditions to a series of 90 patients with unipolar illness, the overlap between theoretically distinct groups was large. They noted that, as a possible result of such confusion, evidence validating various subdivisions of unipolar illness was scant compared to the evidence bearing on the bipolar–unipolar division.

As late as 1969, Kay et al remarked on the absence of long-term follow-up studies comparing course and outcome among 'endogenous' and 'neurotic' groups. Since then at least five such studies have appeared but the results have been far from consistent. Kay et al (1969) used factor analysis to identify 31 patients with endogenous depression and 39 with neurotic depression. Endogenous patients had a more favorable course over a 5–7-year follow-up period despite having significantly more re-admissions. Likewise Paykel et al

(1974), in a much shorter follow-up of 10 months, noted that endogenous depressives were more likely to experience full remission. Lee & Murray (1988), on the other hand, found a direct correspondence between endogenicity, as measured with a diagnostic index, and poor outcome during an 18-year follow-up. Copeland (1983) used a definition for 'psychotic' depression which resembled that described by the RDC (Spitzer et al 1978) and DSM-IIIR (American Pyschiatric Association 1987) for endogenous depression or melancholia. Patients with psychotic depression had higher relapse rates and more re-admissions but were as likely as patients with 'neurotic' depression to rate themselves as 'entirely well' or 'very well' at various times in the 5-year follow-up. Kiloh et al (1988) used their own definitions for endogenous and neurotic depression and found very little difference in outcome during another 18-year follow-up. Finally, the high intensity follow-up conducted by the National Institute of Mental Health Collaborative Depression Study found no relationship between the RDC endogenous/nonendogenous distinction and the likelihood of recovery from the index episode, of relapse, or of recovery from the first prospectively observed episode (Keller et al 1983, Keller et al 1984, Keller et al 1986b).

A reconciliation of these disparate findings is not possible. Among other important design differences, each study used its own definition of endogenous or psychotic depression. In particular, some studies gave considerable weight to long-standing personality problems and a stormy lifestyle in this distinction while others did not. Some authors have suggested that it is these enduring traits, rather than cross-sectional symptom quality, which most effectively identify patients with 'neurotic-reactive' depression (Winokur 1985b, Winokur et al 1987, Zimmerman et al 1987). In support of this, two studies have found significant relationships between high Maudsley Personality Inventory neuroticism scores and a prospectively determined liability to chronicity (Weissman et al 1978, Hirschfeld et al 1986).

Before the advent of tricyclic antidepressants, most investigators considered mood-congruent delusions to be simply another depressive symptom. The emergence of delusions as important predictors of poor tricyclic antidepressant response (Hordern et al 1963) led to the designation of delusional depression as a diagnostic subtype. Indeed, delusional depression may have some prognostic significance beyond acute treatment response. This significance, however, apparently varies with the passage of time and across patient samples. One study, for instance, found that more delusional patients than nondelusional patients had returned to their normal selves 6 months after intake (Coryell et al 1986a) while another found instead, modest differences favoring non-delusional depression at 6 months (Coryell et al 1987). Three studies have found more substantial differences favoring non-delusional depression in short-term follow-ups (Coryell et al 1982a, Murphy 1983, Robinson & Spiker 1985) but in other studies (Coryell & Tsuang 1982, Coryell et al 1987) the prognostic advantage attached to nonpsychotic depression dissipated over time.

The presence of psychotic features may allow several other predictions as well. First, delusions are likely to reappear in subsequent episodes (Baldwin 1988, Kettering et al 1987). Second, two studies (Coryell et al 1987, Coryell et al 1986a) concur that the degree of improvement at discharge among delusional patients is more strongly correlated with clinical status later in follow-up than it is among non-delusional patients.

Divisions based on chronology of psychiatric diagnoses

The distinction between primary and secondary unipolar depression first proposed by Woodruff et al (1967) depends on the relative chronology of affective and non-affective diagnoses. A first depression preceded by one of 13 non-affective psychiatric illnesses is termed 'secondary'. This approach avoids both unfounded assumptions regarding aetiology and the ambiguities arising from the multiple concepts of endogenous and neurotic depression. The concept also embodies a compelling analogy to the relationships between many medical syndromes and diseases. Hypertension, for instance, is a well-recognized syndrome which can be primary or which can occur as a complication of a number of discrete diseases.

A recent review (Coryell 1988a) found consensus that patients with secondary depression, in comparison to those with primary depression, exhibit a lower female to male ratio, develop their first episode of depression at a younger age, view the depressed state as less distinct from their usual selves, have a lower likelihood of psychotic features, more often express suicidal thoughts and behaviours and less often show an abnormal escape from dexamethasone suppression.

Most follow-up studies which have distinguished primary from secondary depression have been limited to observation periods of 6 months–2 years. They have

consistently associated secondary depression with a lower recovery rate (Akiskal et al 1978, Coryell et al 1985b,c, Keller et al 1984) and higher relapse rate (Keller et al 1983, Rabkin et al 1986).

Depressions may also arise secondary to medical illness. Other than the observation that these conditions often improve as the medical illness improves (Moffic & Paykel 1975, Light et al 1986) very little data is available to describe course beyond the acute treatment response. One group has followed patients who developed depression after cerebrovascular accidents (Robinson et al 1984, Robinson et al 1986). Depression in this sample appeared quite persistent but the data afforded no direct comparisons to patients with primary depression or to patients with depression secondary to functional illness or to other medical conditions. Winokur et al (1988) did provide such a comparison. They noted that patients with depression secondary to medical illness were more likely than those with depression secondary to psychiatric illness to show marked improvement on follow-up and to exhibit a single episode course.

Divisions based on family history

When early-onset and late-onset unipolar depressive cohorts are compared, the former group features female relatives with depression and male relatives with alcoholism and/or sociopathy. In a late-onset cohort, male and female relatives have equal rates of depression and there is very little alcoholism (Winokur et al 1971). Moreover, depressed patients with alcoholic relatives are more likely to be labelled 'reactive-neurotic' on clinical and historical bases (Perris et al 1982), to have a personality disorder (Pfohl et al 1984) or to have a 'character spectrum disorder' (Akiskal et al 1981). Such findings led Winokur and his colleagues to suggest a subdivision of primary unipolar depression based on patterns of familial psychopathology (Winokur et al 1978). Thus, depressive spectrum disease (DSD) applies to those patients with a family history of alcoholism or antisocial personality and pure depressive disease (PDD) designates patients with a family history only of depression. Sporadic depressive disease (SDD) requires an absence in the family history of alcoholism, antisocial personality or depression.

Only three studies have compared these subtypes by course and outcome (Van Valkenberg et al 1977, Smith & North 1988, Zimmerman et al 1988). In comparison to FPDD patients, patients with DSD were more likely to present with non-serious suicide attempts (Smith &

North 1988, Zimmerman et al 1986), precipitating events (Smith & North 1988, Zimmerman et al 1986) and a history of divorces or separations (Smith & North 1988, Zimmerman et al 1986, Van Valkenberg et al 1977). In one short-term follow-up (Zimmerman et al 1988) and in another much longer one (Smith & North 1988), DSD patients were much less likely to be symptom-free for extended periods. Thus, in historical and prognostic terms, DSD patients follow a course predicted by the traditional concepts of neurotic-reactive depression.

SCHIZOAFFECTIVE DISORDER

As with any other diagnostic dichotomy, the separation of affective disorder and schizophrenia leaves a diagnostically uncertain group. The term schizoaffective has become relatively popular in the past 15 years but many labels have been applied to this group. To add confusion, the term schizoaffective has itself been redefined numerous times. Despite these vagaries in terminology and the usual methodological differences existing across studies, follow-ups of schizoaffective disorder have generated highly consistent results.

When compared to schizophrenic patients, patients with schizoaffective conditions have consistently better outcomes (Tsuang et al 1976, Brockington et al 1980a, b, Pope et al 1980, Coryell et al 1982a, VanPraag & Nijo 1984, Coryell et al 1984, Grossman et al 1984, Coryell & Zimmerman 1987). When compared to typical affective disorder patients, however, patients with a schizoaffective (or equivalent) diagnosis have poorer outcomes at at least trend levels (Angst et al 1970, Tsuang et al 1976, Pope et al 1980, Angst 1980, Brockington et al 1980a, Himmelhoch et al 1981, Coryell et al 1982a, Brockington & Meltzer 1983, VanPraag & Nijo 1984, Grossman et al 1984, Maj 1985, Coryell & Zimmerman 1987, Winokur et al 1990, Coryell et al 1990a, b). Because these differences have, in many instances, been small and statistically insignificant, authors have sometimes concluded that no difference existed. This was more often the case when schizoaffective disorder was compared to mania; differences between these groups have been smaller than those between schizoaffective depression and more typical depression (Brockington et al 1980a,b, Maj 1985, Coryell et al 1990a, 1990c). Schizoaffective patients also have familial loadings for schizophrenia and affective disorder which are intermediate between schizophrenia and affective disorder proband groups (see Coryell 1988b for a review). Together with the

previously noted outcome patterns, these findings support a conceptual position of diagnostic uncertainty. Accordingly, the label schizoaffective disorder is equivalent to 'undiagnosed', the differential diagnoses are schizophrenia and affective disorder, and the passage of time will, in many cases, result in a more meaningful diagnosis.

Given a label of schizoaffective disorder, what historical or clinical features predict long term outcomes? Since outcome differences between mania and schizoaffective mania are smaller than those between depression and schizoaffective depression, a bipolar diagnosis should imply a relatively good prognosis for schizoaffective depression. Two studies have, in fact, shown this (Maj et al 1987, Coryell et al 1990a). Not surprisingly, a history of schizophrenia-like symptoms present for 2 or more years is also a powerful predictor of a poor outcome (Coryell et al 1990c, Coryell & Zimmerman 1988). Finally, a history of schizophrenia-like symptoms present, at some point, in the absence of an affective syndrome, comprises a particularly grave prognostic sign, both for schizoaffective depression (Brockington et al 1980a, Coryell et al 1990a, Maj et al 1987) and for schizoaffective mania (Coryell et al 1990b).

ANXIETY STATES

The operationalized subdivision of anxiety disorders into panic, phobic and obsessive-compulsive is a relatively recent development. Most of the older follow-up studies lumped these conditions under the generic label of 'anxiety states'. The literature reveals some consistency, nevertheless. Table 7.5 lists the older follow-up studies chosen by Greer (1969) as methodologically adequate and supplements them with seven more recent studies. With the exception of Schapira et al (1972) and Krieg et al (1987), these newer studies specifically described patients who would, for the most part, meet DSM-III criteria for panic disorder or agoraphobia with panic attacks.

Those studies which specified an outcome category of 'no symptoms' or 'no impairment' consistently showed that fewer than one in five patients had this outcome, regardless of follow-up length. More variable were the proportions of patients who were 'unimproved' or who, at follow-up, continued to have moderate to severe symptoms. However, many of these results cluster near the median value of one-third.

Only two studies included a group with depressive disorders for comparison (Schapira et al 1972, Coryell

Table 7.5 Long-term outcome in anxiety states

Author	Length of follow-up (years)	n	% good outcomes	% poor outcomes
Wheeler et al 1950	20	60	12 'well' no symptoms or disability in final 5 yrs	15 symptoms, with moderate to severe disability
Miles et al 1951	2–12	62	23 'markedly improved'	42 'essentially unchanged'
Eitinger 1955	10	29	41 'improved'	24 'no improvement' or deteriorated
Blair et al 1957	1–6	81	52 'much improved'	8 'not improved'
Greer & Cawley 1966	5	37	27 'recovered'	24 'no change', 'worse'
Schapira et al 1972	1–6	66	18 'well'	26 'ill', unimproved
Noyes & Clancy 1976	5	57	16 no symptoms or impairment in final 6 months	33 'moderate' to 'severe' impairment
Noyes et al 1980	4–9	112	12 no symptoms or impairment	31 'moderate' to 'severe' impairment'
Coryell et al 1983	1–10	100	17 no symptoms or impairment	32 'unimproved'
Krieg et al 1987	6–8	40	5 'no impairment'	68 'marked' to 'severe' impairment
Faravelli & Albanesi 1987	1	53	15 recovered without relapse	45 full DSM III syndrome persisted
Noyes et al in press	2–4	89	10 no symptoms at follow-up	34 'moderate' to 'severe' or 'extreme' symptoms

et al 1983). Both found that recovery rates for anxiety states were substantially lower than those for depressive disorders at all follow-up points. Both also found scant overlap between outcome predictors for anxiety disorders and those for depressive disorders.

Among the various clinical and historical features tested as long-range outcome predictors, overall symptom severity has emerged most consistently as an indicator of poor prognosis (Miles et al 1951, Kerr et al 1974, Faravelli & Albanosi 1987, Noyes et al in press). At least three studies have noted relationships between poor outcome and abnormal personality traits evident at baseline (Noyes & Clancy 1976, Noyes et al in press, Faravelli & Albanosi 1987). In the most detailed of these (Noyes et al in press), the presence of a DSM-III personality disorder strongly predicted both the number and intensity of anxiety symptoms as well as the extent of disability and social maladjustment at follow-up. Low socioeconomic status (Noyes et al 1980, Coryell et al 1983) and the duration of symptoms present at baseline evaluation (Noyes & Clancy 1976, Coryell et al 1983) have also predicted poorer outcomes.

Anxiety symptoms may complicate primary depression (Coryell et al 1988) and, conversely, depressive symptoms may complicate anxiety disorders (Clancy et al 1978). The prognostic significance of the latter development has been mentioned only infrequently, though it occurs often (Krieg et al 1987, Maier & Buller 1988, Noyes et al 1980). On the other hand, two studies have considered the prognostic consequences of panic attacks in the context of primary depression (Van Valkenberg et al 1984, Coryell et al 1988). In both, panic attacks were associated with a relatively poor outcome. There are, as yet, no reports analogously describing the prognostic significance of obsessions, compulsions or phobias as complications of primary depression.

Some, but not all, anxiety disorders carry increased risks for suicide. This has been appreciated only recently; 'anxiety neurosis' has appeared infrequently in psychological autopsy studies and an influential prospective study found only one suicidal outcome (Wheeler et al 1950). However, other studies have found substantially higher rates (Kerr et al 1969, Harris 1938) and one found a risk for suicide equal to that of a matched sample with primary depression (Coryell et al 1982b). Obsessive-compulsive disorder, on the other hand, apparently carries little risk for suicide (Coryell 1981b, Coryell 1984). Finally, the excess mortality seen among patients with panic disorder may not be limited to unnatural causes. An excess in deaths due to cardio-vascular disease has arisen among males in three samples (Coryell et al 1982b, Sims 1984, Coryell et al, 1986b). There are possible explanations but none enjoys consensus.

CONCLUSION

Numerous factors—the mercurial definition of terms, occult sample differences and variable treatment experiences — account for inconsistent conclusions across studies. Certain findings have nevertheless emerged with sufficient regularity to warrant clinical application.

Most bipolar patients experience onset in their second or third decade. They are very likely to recover from a given episode but are also very likely to relapse. Mixed or cycling presentations are associated with poor short-term outcomes. Longer-term outcomes may be very good or very poor; there are presently no reliable predictors of these alternatives. However, fewer than 10% develop an eventual schizophrenia-like course. Excess mortality for natural causes was significant in the first half of the century but appears rare now. Death from suicide remains a significant problem, however.

Onset for unipolar illness is more variable than that for bipolar illness but is regularly later, on average, than that for bipolar illness. Roughly 10% of depressed patients without such a history eventually develop mania, though the likelihood of this drops markedly with three or more unipolar episodes. While relapses are less frequent than those experienced by bipolar patients, they are quite likely, particularly in samples

from the past several decades. Most recoveries take place in the first 6 months of follow-up and the likeli-hood of recovery continues to rise thereafter but does so much more slowly beyond 2 years. Nevertheless, many patients who present with an already chronic condition go on to recover.

Factors associated with a poor short-term outcome in unipolar depression are a pre-existing non-affective disorder and the presence of psychotic features. The endogenous versus non-endogenous distinction has shown less consistency as an outcome predictor. Uni-polar patients may experience somewhat better long-term outcomes than bipolar patients. As with bipolar illness, however, there are no reliable long-term out-come predictors. Unnatural deaths account for excess mortality in unipolar illness and 15% eventually die by suicide.

Schizoaffective disorder, however defined, tends to follow a course intermediate between affective disorder and schizophrenia. A relatively good prognosis is associated with a bipolar diagnosis, an acute onset and the absence of a history in which schizophrenia-like symptoms existed without a concurrent affective syndrome.

Fewer than 20% of patients with anxiety states show full recovery on follow-up and this compares unfavourably to outcome in primary depression. Severity and the presence of abnormal personality traits predict poorer outcomes in anxiety states. Panic disorder, but probably not obsessive-compulsive disorder, carries a substantial risk for suicide.

The literature supports considerably more conclu-sions than it did when the first edition of this book appeared. Researchers are now sensitive to many of the factors which have confounded the interpretation of past efforts. It seems likely that the accumulation of knowledge on the course of the affective disorders will continue to accelerate.

REFERENCES

Abrams R, Taylor M A 1980 A comparison of unipolar and bipolar depressive illness. American Journal of Psychiatry 137: 1084–1087
Akiskal H S, Bitar A H, Puzantian V R, Rosenthal T L, Walker P W 1978 The nosological status of neurotic depression. Archives of General Psychiatry 35: 757–766
Akiskal H S, King D, Rosenthal T L, Robinson D, Scott-Strauss A 1981 Chronic depressions – part I. Clinical and familial characteristics in 137 probands. Journal of Affective Disorders 3: 297–315
Akiskal H S, Walker P, Puzantian V R, King D, Rosenthal

T L, Dranon M 1983 Bipolar outcome in the course of depressive illness. Journal of Affective Disorders 5: 115–128
American Psychiatric Association 1987 Diagnostic and statistical manual of mental disorders, 3rd edn. – revised. American Psychiatric Association, Washington, DC
Angst J 1966 Zur Aetiologie und Nosologie endogener depressiver Psychosen. Eine genetische, soziologische und klinische Studie. Monographien aus dem Gesamtgebiete der Neurologie und Psychiatrie, Heft 112. Springer Verlag, Berlin
Angst J 1978 The course of affective disorders II. Typology of

bipolar manic depressive illness. Archiv für Psychiatrie und Nervenkrankheit 226: 65–73

Angst J 1980 Course of unipolar depressive, bipolar manic depressive and schizoaffective disorders. Results of a prospective longitudinal study. Fortschritte der Neurologie-Psychiatrie 48: Abstract 3–30

Angst J 1986 The course of major depression, atypical bipolar disorder, and bipolar disorder. In: Hippius H et al (eds) New results in depression research. Springer Verlag, Berlin, p 26–35

Angst J, Weis P, Grof P, Baastrup P C, Schou M 1970 Lithium prophylaxis in recurrent affective disorder. British Journal of Psychiatry 116: 604–614

Angst J, Baastrup P, Grof P, Hippius H, Poldinger W, Weis P 1973 The course of monopolar depression and bipolar psychosis. Psychiatria, Neurologia and Neurochirurgin 76: 489–500

Angst J, Felder W, Frey R, Stassen H H 1978 The course of affective disorders I. Change of diagnosis of monopolar, unipolar, and bipolar illness. Archiv für Psychiatrie und Nervenkrankheit 226: 57–64

Ayuso-Gutierrez J L, Ramos-Brieda J A 1982 The course of manic depressive illness. Journal of Affective Disorders 4: 9–14

Baastrup P C, Poulsen J C, Schou M, Thomsen K, Amdisen A 1970 Prophylactic lithium: double blind discontinuation in manic depression recurrent depressive disorders. Lancet 2: 326–330

Baldessarini, R J 1970 Frequency of diagnosis of schizophrenia vs. affective disorders from 1944 to 1968. American Journal of Psychiatry 127: 759–763

Baldwin R 1988 Delusional and nondelusional depression in late life – evidence for distinct sub-types. British Journal of Psychiatry 152: 39–44

Ballenger J C, Reus V I, Post R M 1982 The 'atypical' clinical picture of adolescent mania. American Journal of Psychiatry 139: 602–606

Barraclough B M, Pallis D J 1975 Depression followed by suicide: a comparison of depressed suicides with living depressives. Psychological Medicine 5: 55–61

Barraclough B, Bunch J, Sainsbury P 1974 A hundred cases of suicide: clinical aspects. British Journal of Psychiatry 125: 355–73

Beck A T, Steer R A, Covacs M, Garrison B 1985 Hopelessness and eventual suicide: a ten year prospective study of patients hospitalized with suicidal ideation. American Journal of Psychiatry 142: 559–563

Beck A T, Brown G, Berchick R J, Stewart B L, Steer R A 1990 Relationship between hopelessness and ultimate suicide: a replication with psychiatric outpatients. American Journal of Psychiatry 147: 190–195

Black D, Winokur G, Hasrallah A 1987 Suicide in subtypes of major affective disorder. Archives of General Psychiatry 44: 878–880

Black D W, Winokur G, Nasrallah A 1987 Is death from natural causes still excessive in psychiatric patients? A follow-up of 1593 patients with major affective disorder. Journal of Nervous and Mental Disease 175: 674–680

Black D W, Winokur G, Nasrallah A 1988 Effect of psychosis on suicidal risk in 1593 patients with unipolar and bipolar affective disorders. American Journal of Psychiatry 145: 849–852

Blair R, Gilroy J M, Pilkington F 1957 Some observations on out-patient psychotherapy. British Medical Journal 1: 318–321

Bland R C, Orn H 1982 Course and outcome in affective disorders. Canadian Journal of Psychiatry 27: 573–578

Blumenthal R, Egeland J, Sharpe L, Nee J, Endicott J 1987 Age of onset in bipolar and unipolar illness with and without delusions or hallucinations. Comprehensive Psychiatry 28: 547–554

Bratfos O, Haug J O 1968 The course of manic depressive psychosis: a follow-up investigation of 215 patients. Acta Psychiatrica Scandinavica 44: 89–112

Brockington I F, Meltzer H Y 1983 The nosology of schizo-affective psychoses. Pscychiatric Developments 4: 317–338

Brockington I F, Kendell R E, Wainwright S 1980a Depressed patients with schizophrenic or paranoid symptoms. Psychological Medicine 10: 665–675

Brockington I F, Wainwright S, Kendell R E 1980b Manic patients with schizophrenic or paranoid symptoms. Psychological Medicine 10: 73–83

Burke K C, Burke J D, Regier D A, Rae D S 1990 Age of onset of selected mental disorders in five community populations. Archives of General Psychiatry 47: 511–518

Carlson G A, Cotin J, Davenport Y B, Adland M 1974 Follow-up of 53 bipolar manic depressive patients. British Journal of Psychiatry 125: 134–139

Carlson G A, Davenport Y B, Jamison K 1977 A comparison of outcome in adolescent and late onset bipolar manic depressive illness. American Journal of Pscyhiatry 134: 919–922

Carroll B J, Greden J F, Feinberg M 1980 Suicide, neuroendocrine dysfunction and CSF 5-HIAA concentrations in depression. In: Angrist (ed) Recent advances in neuropsychopharmacology – proceedings of 12th CINP Congress. Pergamon Press, Oxford, p 307–313

Chynoweth R, Tonge J, Armstrong J 1980 Suicide in Brisbane – a retrospective psychosocial study. Australian and New Zealand Journal of Psychiatry 14: 37–45

Clancy J, Tsuang M T, Norton B, Winokur G 1974 The Iowa 500: a comprehensive study of mania, depression and schizophrenia. Journal of the Iowa Medical Society 64: 394–398

Clancy J, Noyes R, Hoenk P R, Slymen D J 1978 Secondary depression in anxiety neurosis. Journal of Nervous and Mental Disease 166: 846–850

Clayton P J, Pitts F N, Winokur G 1965 Affective disorder IV. Mania. Comprehensive Psychiatry 6: 313–322

Cohen S, Kahn A, Robison J 1988 Significance of mixed features in acute mania. Comprehensive Psychiatry 29: 421–426

Copeland J R M 1983 Psychotic and neurotic depression: discriminate function analysis and 5-year outcome. Psychological Medicine 13: 373–383

Coryell W 1981a Diagnosis specific mortality: Primary unipolar depression and Briquet's syndrome (disorder). Archives of General Psychiatry 38: 939–942

Coryell W 1981b Obsessive-compulsive disorder and primary unipolar depression. Journal of Nervous and Mental Disease 169: 220–224

Coryell W 1984 Mortality after thirty to forty years: panic disorder compared with other psychiatric illnesses. In:

Grimspoon L (ed) Psychiatry update. American Psychiatric Association Annual Review, vol III

Coryell W 1988a Secondary depression. In: Michels R, Cavenar J, Cooper A, Guze S B, Judd L L, Klerman G, Solnit A (eds) Psychiatry. J B Lippincott, Philadelphia, p 1–9

Coryell W 1988b Nosology: Schizo-affective and schizophreniform disorders. In: Tsuang M T, Simpson J C (eds) Handbook of schizophrenia: nosology, epidemiology and genetics III. Elsevier, Amsterdam, p 27–39

Coryell W, Norten S G 1980 Mania during adolescence. Journal of Nervous and Mental Disease 168: 611–613

Coryell W, Schlesser M A 1981 Suicide and the dexamethasone suppression test in unipolar depression. American Journal of Psychiatry 138: 1120–1121

Coryell W, Tsuang M T 1982 Primary unipolar depression and the prognostic significance of delusions. Archives of General Psychiatry 39: 1181–1184

Coryell W, Zimmerman M 1987 Progress in the classification of functional psychoses. American Journal of Psychiatry 144: 1471–1474

Coryell W, Zimmerman M 1988 Diagnosis and outcome in schizo-affective depression: a replication. Journal of Affective Disorders 15: 21–27

Coryell W, Lowry M, Wasek P 1980 Diagnostic instability and depression. American Journal of Psychiatry 137: 48–51

Coryell W, Tsuang M T, McDaniel J 1982a Psychotic features in major depression: is mood congruence important. Journal of Affective Disorders 4: 227–236

Coryell W, Noyes R, Clancy J 1982b Excess mortality in panic disorder. Archives of General Psychiatry 39: 701–703

Coryell W, Noyes R, Clancy J 1983 Panic disorder and primary unipolar depression. Journal of Affective Disorders 5: 311–317

Coryell W, Lavori P, Endicott J, Keller M, VanEerdewegh M 1984 Outcome in schizo-affective, psychotic and nonpsychotic depression. Archives of General Psychiatry 41: 787–791

Coryell W, Endicott J, Andreasen N, Keller M 1985a A comparison of bipolar II and nonbipolar major depression among the relatives of affectively ill probands. American Journal of Psychiatry 142: 817–821

Coryell W, Zimmerman M, Pfohl B 1985b Short-term prognosis in primary and secondary major depression. Journal of Affective Disorders 9: 265–270

Coryell W, Pfohl b, Zimmerman M 1985c Outcome following electroconvulsive therapy: a comparison of primary and secondary depression. Convulsive Therapy 1: 10–14

Coryell W, Zimmerman M, Pfohl B 1986a Outcome at discharge and six months in major depression: the significance of psychotic features. Journal of Nervous and Mental Disease 174: 92–96

Coryell W, Noyes R, House J D 1986b Mortality among outpatients with anxiety disorders. American Journal of Psychiatry 143: 508–510

Coryell W, Endicott J, Keller M 1987 The importance of psychotic features to major depression: course and outcome during a two-year follow-up. Acta Psychiatrica Scandinavica 75: 78–85

Coryell W, Endicott J, Andreasen N et al 1988 Depression and panic attacks: the significance of overlap as reflected in follow-up and family study data. American Journal of Psychiatry 145: 293–300

Coryell W, Keller M, Endicott J, Andreasen N, Clayton P, Hirschfeld R 1989 Bipolar II Illness: course and outcome over a five-year period. Psychological Medicine 19: 128–141

Coryell W, Keller M, Lavori P, Endicott J 1990a Affective syndromes, psychotic features and prognosis I. Depression. Archives of General Psychiatry 47: 651–657

Coryell W, Keller M, Lavori P, Endicott J 1990b Affective syndromes, psychotic features and prognosis. II Mania. Archives of General Psychiatry 47: 658–664

Coryell W, Endicott J, Keller M 1990c Chronic affective disorder: outcome during a five-year follow-up. American Journal of Psychiatry 147: 1627–1633

Coryell W, Endicott J, Keller M (in press) Rapidly Cycling affective disorder: demographics, diagnosis, family history and course. Archives of General Psychiatry

d'Elia G, von Knorring L, Perris C 1974 Non-psychotic depressive disorders: a ten year follow-up. Acta Psychiatrica Scandinavica 225 (suppl): 173–186

Derby I M 1933 Manic depressive 'exhaustion' deaths. Psychiatric Quarterly 7: 435–449

Dorpat T L, Ripley H S 1960 A study of suicide in the Seattle area. Comprehensive Psychiatry 1: 349–359

Dunner D L, Gershon E S, Goodwin F K 1967a Heritable factors in the severity of affective illness. Biological Psychiatry 11: 31–42

Dunner D L, Fleiss J L, Fieve R R 1976b The course of development of mania in patients with recurrent depression. American Journal of Psychiatry 133(8): 905–908

Dunner D L, Russek F D, Russek B, Fieve R R 1977 Rapid cycling manic depressive patients. Comprehensive Psychiatry 18(6): 186–189

Dunner D L, Murphy D, Stallen F, Fieve R R 1979 Episode frequency prior to lithium treatment in bipolar manic-depressive patients. Comprehensive Psychiatry 20: 511–515

Eitinger L 1955 Studies in neurosis. Acta Psychiatrica et Neurologica Scandinavica (suppl 101) 1–47

Endicott J, Nee J, Andreasen N, Clayton P, Keller M, Coryell W 1985 Bipolar II: combine or keep separate? Journal of Affective Disorders 8: 17–28

Faravelli C, Albanesi G 1987 Agoraphobia with panic attacks: one-year prospective follow-up. Comprehensive Psychiatry 28: 481–487

Faravelli C, Poli E 1982 Stability of the diagnosis of primary affective disorder. Journal of Affective Disorders 4: 35–39

Fawcett J, Sheftner W, Clark D, Hedeker D, Gibbons R, Coryell W 1987 Clinical predictors of suicide in patients with major affective disorders: A controlled prospective study. American Journal of Psychiatry 144: 35–40

Feighner J P, Robins E, Guze S B, Woodruff R A, Winokur G, Munoz R 1972 Diagnostic criteria for use in psychiatric research. Archives of General Psychiatry 26: 57–63

Fowler R C, Tsuang M T, Kronfol Z 1979 Communication of suicidal intent and suicide in unipolar depression. Journal of Affective Disorders 1: 219–225

Giles D, Jarrett R, Biggs M, Guzick D, Rush A 1989 Clinical predictors of recurrence in depression. American Journal of Psychiatry 146: 764–767

Gonzales L R, Lewinsohn P M, Clark G N 1985 Longitudinal follow-up of unipolar depressives: An investigation of predictors of relapse. Journal of Consulting and Clinical Psychology 53: 461–469

Greer S 1969 The prognosis of anxiety states. In: Lader M H (ed) Studies of anxiety. Royal Medico-psychological Association, London, p 151–157

Greer H S, Cawley R H 1966 Some observations on the natural history of neurotic illness. Archdall Medical Monograph No 3. Australasian Medical Publishing Co, Sydney

Grossman L S, Harrow M, Fudala J L, Meltzer H Y 1984 The longitudinal course of schizoaffective disorders. Journal of Nervous and Mental Disease 172: 140–149

Guze S B, Robins E 1970 Suicide and primary affective disorders. British Journal of Psychiatry 117: 437–438

Guze S B, Cloninger R, Martin R L, Clayton P J 1983 A follow-up and family study of schizophrenia. Archives of General Psychiatry 40: 1273–1276

Hamilton M 1967 Development of a rating scale for primary depressive illness. British Journal of Social and Clinical Psychology 6: 278–296

Harris A 1938 The prognosis of anxiety states. British Medical Journal 2: 649–654

Hastings, D W 1958 Follow-up results in psychiatric illness. American Journal of Psychiatry 114: 1057–1066

Himmelhoch J M, Mulla D, Neil J F, Detre T P, Kupfer D J 1976 Incidence and significance of mixed affective states in a bipolar population. Archives of General Psychiatry 33: 1062–1066

Himmelhoch J M, Fuchs C Z, May S J, Symons B J, Neil K S 1981 When a schizoaffective diagnosis has meaning. Journal of Nervous and Mental Disease 169: 277–282

Hirschfeld R M A, Klerman G L, Andreasen N C, Clayton P J, Keller M B 1986 Psycho-social predictors of chronicity in depressed patients. British Journal of Psychiatry 148: 648–654

Hordern A, Holt N F, Burt C G, Gordon W F 1963 Amitriptyline in depressive states. British Journal of Psychiatry 109: 815–825

Kay D W K, Garside R F, Roy J R, Beamish P 1969 Endogenous symptoms in neurotic syndromes of depressions: a 5 to 7 year follow-up of 104 cases. British Journal of Psychiatry 115: 389–399

Keller M B, Lavori P W, Lewis C E, Klerman G L 1983 Predictors of relapse in major depressive disorder. Journal of the American Medical Association 250: 3299–3304

Keller M B, Klerman G L, Lavori P W, Coryell W, Endicott J, Taylor J 1984 Long-term outcome of episodes of major depression. Journal of the American Medical Association 252: 788–792

Keller M B, Lavori P W, Coryell W et al 1986a Differential outcome of pure manic, mixed/cycling, and pure depressive episodes in patients with bipolar illness. Journal of the American Medical Association 255: 3138–3142

Keller M B, Lavori W, Rice J, Coryell W, Hirschfeld R M A 1986b The persistent risk of chronicity in recurrent episodes of nonbipolar major depressive disorder: a prospective follow-up. American Journal of Psychiatry 143: 24–28

Kendell R 1985 The diagnosis of mania. Journal of Affective Disorders 8: 207–213

Kerr T A, Schapira K, Roth M 1969 The relationship between premature death and affective disorders. British Journal of Psychiatry 115: 1277–1282

Kerr T A, Roth M, Schapira K 1974 Prediction of outcome in anxiety states and depressive illnesses. British Journal of Psychiatry 124: 125–33

Kettering R, Harrow M, Grossman L, Meltzer H 1987 The prognostic relevance of delusions in depression: a follow-up study. American Journal of Psychiatry 144: 1154–1160

Kiloh L G, Andrews G, Neilson M 1988 The long-term outcome of depressive illness. British Journal of Psychiatry 153: 752–757

Klerman G L, Endicott J, Spitzer R, Hirschfeld R M A 1979 Neurotic depressions: a systematic analysis of multiple criteria and meanings. American Journal of Psychiatry 136: 57–61

Kraepelin E 1921 Manic-depressive insanity and paranoia. E & S Livingstone, Edinburgh

Krieg J C, Bronisch T, Wittchen H U, VonZerssen D 1987 Anxiety disorders: a long-term prospective and retrospective follow-up study of former inpatients suffering from an anxiety neurosis or phobia. Acta Psychiatrica Scandinavica 77: 36–47

Kukopulos A, Reginaldi D, Laddomada P, Floris G, Serra G, Tondo L 1980 Course of the manic depressive cycle and changes caused by treatments. Pharmakopsychiatrie Neuro-psychopharmakologie 13: 156–167

Kukopulos A, Caliari B, Tundo A et al 1983 Rapid cyclers, temperament and antidepressants. Comprehensive Psychiatry 24: 249–258

Kupfer D J, Carpenter L L, Frank E 1988 Is bipolar II a unique disorder? Comprehensive Psychiatry 29: 228–236

Lee A S, Murray R M 1988 The long-term outcome of Maudsley depressives. British Journal of Psychiatry 153: 741–751

Lehman H E, Fenton F R, Deutsch M, Feldman S, Engelsmann F 1988 An 11-year follow-up study of 110 depressed patients. Acta Psychiatrica Scandinavica 78: 57–65

Leonhard K, Korff I, Shulz H 1962 Die Temperamente in den Familien der monopolaren und bipolaren phasischen Psychosen. Psychiatrie Neurologie 143: 416–430

Lewis A 1936 Melancholia: prognostic study and case material. Journal of Mental Science 82: 488–558

Light R W, Merrill E J, Despars J, Gordon G H, Mutalipassi L R 1986 Doxepin treatment of depressed patients with chronic obstructive pulmonary disease. Archives of Internal Medicine 146: 1377–1380

Loranger A W, Levine P 1978 Age at onset of bipolar affective illness. Archives of General Psychiatry 35: 1345–1348

Lundquist G 1945 Prognosis and course in manic depressive psychoses. A follow-up study of 319 first admissions. Acta Psychiatrica et Neurologica 35(suppl 1): 1–96

MacDonald J B 1918 Prognosis in manic-depressive insanity. Journal of Nervous and Mental Disease 47: 20–30

McGlashan T H 1984 The Chestnut Lodge follow-up study. II. Long-term outcome of schizophrenia in the affective disorders. Archives of General Psychiatry 41: 586–601

McGlashan T 1988 Adolescent versus adult onset of mania. American Journal of Psychiatry 145: 221–223

Maier W, Buller R 1988 One-year follow-up of panic disorder. European Archives of Psychiatry and Neurological Science 238: 105–109

Maj M 1985 Clinical course and outcome of schizo-affective disorders. Acta Psychiatrica Scandinavica 72: 542–550

Maj M, Starace F, Kemali D 1987 Prediction of outcome by historical, clinical and biological variables in schizoaffective disorder, depressed type. Journal of Psychiatric Research 21: 289–295

Martin R L, Cloninger C R, Guze S B, Clayton P J 1985 Mortality in a follow-up of 500 psychiatric outpatients. Archives of General Psychiatry 42: 47–54

Miles H H W, Barrabee E L, Finesinger J E 1951 Evaluation of psychotherapy: with a follow-up study of 62 cases of anxiety neurosis. Psychosomatic Medicine 13: 83–105

Modestin J, Kopp W 1988 Study on suicide in depressed inpatients. Journal of Affective Disorders 15: 157–162

Moffic H S, Paykel E S 1975 Depression in medical inpatients. British Journal of Psychiatry 126: 346–353

Morrison J R 1982 Suicide in a psychiatric practice population. Journal of Clinical Psychiatry 43: 348–352

Morrison J, Winokur G, Crowe R, Clancy J 1973 The Iowa 500 – the first follow-up. Archives of General Psychiatry 29: 678–682

Murphy E 1983 The prognosis of depression in old age. British Journal of Psychiatry 142: 111–119

Murphy G E, Woodruff R A, Herjanic M, Fischer J R 1974 Validity of the diagnosis of first degree affective disorder. Archives of General Psychiatry 30: 751–756

Murphy J M, Monson R R, Olivier D C, Sobol A M, Leighton A H 1987 Affective disorders and mortality. Archives of General Psychiatry 44: 473–480

Murphy E, Smith R, Lindesay J, Slattery J 1988 Increased mortality rates in late life depression. British Journal Psychiatry 152: 347–353

Norman W H, Brown W A, Miller I W, Keitner G I, Overholser J C 1990 The dexamethasone suppression test and completed suicide. Acta Psychiatrica Scandinavica 81: 120–125

Noyes R, Clancy J 1976 Anxiety neurosis: a five year follow up. Journal of Nervous and Mental Disease 162: 200–205

Noyes R, Clancy J, Hoenk P R, Slymen D J 1980 The prognosis of anxiety neurosis. Archives of General Psychiatry 37: 173–178

Noyes R, Reich J, Christiansen J, Suelzer M, Pfohl B, Coryell W (in press) Outcome of panic disorder: Relationship to diagnostic subtypes and comorbidity. Archives of General Psychiatry

Nurnberger J, Guroff J J, Hamovit J, Berrettini W, Gerson E 1988 A family study of rapid cycling bipolar illness. Journal of Affective Disorders 15: 87–91

Nystrom S 1979 Depressions: Factors related to ten-year prognosis. Acta Psychiatrica Scandinavica 60: 225–238

Olsen T 1961 Follow-up study of manic depressive patients whose first attack occurred before the age of 19. Acta Psychiatrica Scandinavica 37(suppl 162): 45–52

Paykel E S, Klerman G L, Prusoff B A 1974 Prognosis of depression in the endogenous – neurotic distinction. Psychological Medicine 4: 57–64

Perris C 1966 A study of bipolar (manic depressive) and unipolar recurrent depressive psychoses. I. Genetic investigation. Acta Psychiatrica Scandinavica 194 (suppl): 15–44

Perris C 1968 The course of depressive psychoses. Acta Psychiatrica Scandinavica 44: 238–248

Perris H, Von Knorring L, Perris C 1982 Genetic vulnerability for depression and life events. Neuropsychobiology 8: 241–247

Petterson V 1977 Manic depressive illness. Acta Psychiatrica Scandinavica 269 (suppl).

Pfohl B, Stangl D, Zimmerman M 1984 The implications of DSM-III personality disorders for patients with major depression. Journal of Affective Disorders 7: 309–318

Poort R 1945 Catamnestic investigations on manic-depressive psychoses with special reference to the prognosis. Acta Psychiatrica et Neurologica 20: 59–74

Pope H G, Lipinski J F, Cohen B M, Axelrod D T 1980 'Schizoaffective disorder': an invalid diagnosis? A comparison of schizoaffective disorder, schizophrenia, and affective disorder. American Journal of Psychiatry 137: 921–927

Prien R F, Klett J, Caffey E M 1974 Lithium prophylaxis in recurrent affective illness. American Journal of Psychiatry 131(2): 198–203

Quitkin F M, Kane J, Rifkin A, Ramos-Lorenzi J R, Nayak D V 1981 Prophylactic lithium carbonate with and without imipramine for bipolar I patients. Archives of General Psychiatry 38: 902–907

Quitkin F M, Rabkin J G, Prien R F 1986 Bipolar disorder: are there manic-prone and depressive-prone forms? Journal of Clinical Psychopharmacology 6: 167–172

Rabkin J G, McGrath P, Stewart J W, Harrison W, Markowitz J S, Quitkin F 1986 Follow-up of patients who improved during placebo washout. Journal of Clinical Psychopharmacology 6: 274–278

Rao A V, Nammalvar N 1977 The course and outcome of depressive illness: a follow-up study of 122 cases in Madurai, India. British Journal of Psychiatry 130: 392–396

Rennie T A C 1942 Prognosis in manic-depressive psychosis. American Journal of Psychiatry 98: 801–814

Robins E, Murphy G E, Wilkinson R H, Gassner S, Kayes J 1959 Some clinical considerations in the prevention of suicide based on a study of 134 successful suicides. American Journal of Public Health 49(7): 888–899

Robinson R G, Spiker D G 1985 Delusional depression: a one year follow-up. Journal of Affective Disorders 9: 79–83

Robinson R G, Starr L B, Price T R 1984 A two year longitudinal study of mood disorders following stroke. British Journal of Psychiatry 144: 256–262

Robinson R G, Lipsey J R, Rao K, Price T R 1986 Two-year longitudinal study of post-stroke mood disorders: comparison of acute onset with delayed onset depression. American Journal of Psychiatry 143: 1238–1244

Roose S P, Glassman A H, Walsh B T, Woodreng S, Vital-Herne J 1983 Depression, delusions and suicide. American Journal of Psychiatry 140: 1159–1162

Rorsman B, Hangell O, Lanke J 1982 Mortality in the Lundby Study. Neuropsychobiology 8: 188–197

Rosen L N, Rosenthal M E, Dunner D L, Fieve R R 1983 Social outcome compared in psychotic and nonpsychotic bipolar I patients. Journal of Nervous and Mental Disease 171: 272–275

Saran B M 1969 Lithium. Lancet 1: 1208–1209 (letter)

Schapira K, Roth M, Kerr T A, Gurney C 1972 Prognosis of affective disorders: the differentiation of anxiety states from depressive illnesses. British Journal of Psychiatry 121: 175–181

Scheftner W A, Fogg L, Young M, Fawcett J (in press) Five-year mortality experience in affective disorders. Archives of General Psychiatry

Secunda S K, Swann A, Katz M M, Koslow S H, Croughan J, Chang S 1987 Diagnosis and treatment of mixed mania. American Journal of Psychiatry 144: 96–98

Shobe F O, Brion P 1971 Long-term prognosis in manic depressive illness. Achives of General Psychiatry 24: 334–337

Sims A 1984 Neurosis and mortality: investigating and association. Journal of Psychosomatic Research 28: 353–362

Smith E, North C 1988 Familial subtypes of depression: a longitudinal perspective. Journal of Affective Disorders 14: 145–154

Spitzer R L, Endicott J, Robins E 1978 Research diagnostic criteria: rationale and reliability. Archives of General Psychiatry 35: 773–782

Stenstedt A 1952 A study in manic depressive psychosis. Acta Psychiatrica et Neurologica (suppl 79), 3–85

Strober M, Carlson G 1982 Bipolar illness in adolescents with major depression. Archives of General Psychiatry 39: 549–555

Swift H M 1907 The prognosis of recurrent insanity of the manic depressive type. American Journal of Insanity 64: 311–326

Tsuang M T 1978 Suicide in schizophrenics, manics, depressives and surgical controls. Archives of General Psychiatry 35: 153–155

Tsuang M T, Dempsey G M, Rauscher F 1976 A study of 'atypical schizophrenia'. Archives of General Psychiatry 33: 1157–1160

Tsuang M T, Woolson R F, Fleming J A 1979 Long term outcome of major psychosis. I. Schizophrenia and affective disorders compared with psychiatrically symptom free surgical controls. Archives of General Psychiatry 36: 1295–1301

Tsuang M T, Woolson R F, Fleming J A 1980 Causes of death in schizophrenia and manic depression. British Journal of Psychiatry 136: 239–242

Tsuang M T, Woolson R, Winokur G, Crowe R 1981 Stability of psychiatric diagnosis: schizophrenia and affective disorder over a 30- to 40-year period. Archives of General Psychiatry 38: 535–539

VanPraag H M, Nijo L 1984 About the course of schizoaffective psychoses. Comprehensive Psychiatry 25: 9–22

Van Valkenburg C, Lowry M, Winokur G, Cadoret R 1977 Depression spectrum disease vs pure depressive disease. Journal of Nervous and Mental Disease 165(5): 341–347

Van Valkerburg C, Akiskal H S, Puzantian V, Rosenthal T 1984 Anxious depression: clinical, family history, and naturalistic outcome – comparisons with panic and major depressive disorders. Journal of Affective Disorders 6: 67–82

Watts, C A H 1956 The incidence and prognosis of endogenous depression. British Medical Journal 1: 1392–1397

Weeke A, Vaeth M 1986 Excess mortality of bipolar and unipolar manic-depressive patients. Journal of Affective Disorders 11: 227–234

Wehr T, Sack D, Rosenthal N, Cowdry R 1988 Rapid cycling affective disorder: contributing factors and treatment responses in fifty-one patients. American Journal of Psychiatry 145: 179–184

Weissman M M, Prusoff B A, Klerman G L 1978 Personality in the prediction of long term outcome of depression. American Journal of Psychiatry 135: 797–800

Welner A, Welner Z, Leonard M A 1977 Bipolar manic-depressive disorder: a reassessment of course and outcome. Comprehensive Psychiatry 18(4): 327–332

Wertham, F I 1928 A group of benign chronic psychoses: prolonged manic excitements. American Journal of Psychiatry 9: 17–78

Wheeler E O, White P D, Reed E W, Cohen M E 1950 Neurocirculatory asthenia (anxiety neurosis, effort syndrome, neuroasthenia): a 20 year follow-up study of 173 patients. Journal of the American Medical Association 142: 878–888

Winokur G 1975 The Iowa 500: heterogeneity and course in manic-depressive illness – bipolar. Comprehensive Psychiatry 16: 125–131

Winokur G 1985a Comparative studies of familial psychopathology in affective disorders. In: Sakai T, Tsuboi T (eds) Genetic aspects of human behaviour. Igaku-Shoin, Tokyo, p 87–96

Winokur G 1985b The validity of neurotic-reactive depression. Archives of General Psychiatry 42: 1116–1122

Winokur G, Morrison J 1973 The Iowa 500: follow-up of 225 depressives. British Journal of Psychiatry 123: 543–548

Winokur G, Wesner R 1987 From unipolar depression to bipolar illness: twenty-nine who changed. Acta Psychiatrica Scandinavica 76: 59–63

Winokur G, Clayton P J, Reich T 1969 Manic depressive illnesss. CV Mosby, St Louis

Winokur G, Cadoret R, Dorzab J, Baker M 1971 Depressive disease: a genetic study. Archives of General Psychiatry 24: 135–144

Winokur G, Behar D, Van Valkenburg C, Lowry M 1978 Is a familial definition of depression both feasible and valid? Journal of Nervous and Mental Disease 166: 764–768

Winokur G, Black D, Nasrallah A 1987 Neurotic depression: a diagnosis based on pre-existing characteristics. European Archives of Psychiatric and Neurological Sciences 236: 343–348

Winokur G, Black D, Nasrallah A 1988 Depressions secondary to other psychiatric disorders and medical illnesses. American Journal of Psychiatry 145: 233–237

Winokur G, Black D, Nasrallah A 1990 The schizoaffective continuum: non-psychotic, mood-congruent and mood-incongruent. In: Tsuang M T, Marneros A (eds)

Affective and schizoaffective disorders. Springer Verlag, Berlin

Woodruff R A, Murphy G E, Herjanic M 1967 The natural history of affective disorders I. Symptoms of 72 patients at the time of index hospital admission. Journal of Psychiatric Research 5: 255–263

Woodruff R A, Guze S B, Clayton P J 1971 Unipolar and bipolar primary affective disorder. British Journal of Psychiatry 119: 33–38

Zimmerman M, Coryell W, Pfohl B 1986 Validity of familial subtypes of primary unipolar depression. Archives of General Psychiatry 43: 1090–1096

Zimmerman M, Coryell W, Stangl D, Pfohl B 1987 Validity of an operational definition for neurotic unipolar major depression. Journal of Affective Disorders 12: 29–40

Zimmerman M, Coryell W, Pfohl B, Stangl D 1988 Prognostic validity of the familial subtypes of depression. European Archives of Psychiatry and Neurological Sciences 237: 166–170

PART 2

Causative aspects

8. Epidemiology

Angela L. Smith   Myrna M. Weissman

INTRODUCTION

In the previous edition of this Handbook we presented an exhaustive review of current understanding of the epidemiology of affective disorders (Boyd & Weissman 1982). We confined the discussion to available data primarily from population surveys and, in a few instances, to case register data published in the English language. We described the epidemiology in terms of depressive symptoms, non-bipolar and bipolar disorders, although this division did not fit any usual diagnostic scheme. We focused on community surveys because it was our contention that they yielded the most complete information on incidence and prevalence, since these data were unbiased by factors determining who sought treatment. We recognized that the division of the discussion into depressive symptoms, bipolar and non-bipolar disorders was unorthodox. Our review of the literature led us to conclude that there was a fair amount of international agreement that some people have depressive symptoms that were not of sufficient intensity to warrant a clinical diagnosis. There was also some agreement that bipolar disorder (defined by one or more episodes of mania) was a distinct diagnostic entity. However, people with clinical depression who were not bipolar constituted a heterogeneous group. There was considerable international disagreement about how to define or subdivide this latter group, who represented the majority of depressives. Therefore, we presented this group with depression as an aggregate under the title 'non-bipolar depression'.

We also noted that the study of the epidemiology of affective disorders or any psychiatric disorder was hindered by major differences in diagnostic classifications used over time, between countries and among investigators and clinicians within countries. The same terms had different meanings in different diagnostic schemes and different terms had similar meanings in different diagnostic schemes (Klerman 1980).

At the time of the preparation of that chapter, there were a number of epidemiological studies under way that were taking advantage of the improvements in diagnostic specification and reliability. Over the previous decade, it had been increasingly recognized that to obtain reliable data that could be used comparatively among studies, among countries and over time, the rules of case definition and a standardized procedure of examination had to be developed. Advances in systematic diagnosis and case assessment took place in the mid-1970s and were applied to epidemiological studies in the 1980s. This chapter will present the results of many of these studies, which for the first time provide us with independent cross-national comparisons among data obtained by similar methods. This review will focus on three major categories of affective disorder following DSM-III criteria: bipolar disorder, major depression and dysthymia. In addition, new epidemiological surveys not reported in the previous review using the Present State Examination (PSE) (Wing et al 1974) and ICD-9 criteria (World Health Organization 1978) will be described. We still think, as noted in the 1982 chapter and for the same reasons, that community survey data provide the most unbiased estimates of rates. In order to place these studies in perspective, the historical context will be reviewed. However, the reader interested in examining the epidemiological survey data on affective disorders prior to 1980 is referred to our 1982 edition of this chapter (Boyd & Weissman 1982) as well as to a review by Charney & Weissman (1988).

Historical trends in the USA

The history most pertinent to the present 'state of art'

psychiatric epidemiology may best be construed as encompassing three generations of increasingly sophisticated techniques aimed at establishing true prevalence of mental disorder in communities (Dohrenwend & Dohrenwend 1982, Weissman & Klerman 1978).

The first known United States study of this nature was conducted by Dr Edward Jarvis in Massachusetts in 1855. He sought to determine the prevalence of 'insanity' and 'idiocy' indirectly by examining the reports of key informants as well as hospital and other records. He then analysed the data according to sociodemographic factors such as sex, age, residence and economic status.

Subsequent studies in the United States were similarly characterized by the use of indirect methods of ascertainment and constitute the 'first generation' of epidemiological studies. In comparison with future research, these studies were characterized by their incomplete 'case' assessments, diagnosed unreliably at face value by clinicians. Nevertheless, such research contributed significantly to future epidemiological directions. For example, Faris & Dunham (1967) demonstrated the significance of social variables in their classic examination of mental hospital admission rates in Chicago during the 1930s.

During the Second World War, military psychiatrists and social scientists investigated phenomena such as combat fatigue and stress reactions. Studies were conducted with rigorous precision reflected in advanced sampling and survey techniques. In particular, they relied on direct interviews of community residents, a distinction of 'second-generation' studies; moreover, data from these interviews were exposed to statistical analysis.

Data derived from screening questionnaires on scales of impairment used in the World War II studies disclosed an apparent correlation between psychiatric symptomatology and the environmental stresses of combat. Thus, the identification of external 'stress' as an important precipitating factor of mental illness was established, akin to the previous decade's recognition of the role played by social factors in disease evolution. Subsequent studies in civilian settings proposed analogous 'stress' factors such as poverty, social class, rapid social change and urbanization.

The unanticipated finding that psychiatric reactions had also occurred among those men previously screened as mentally fit for selective service focused even more attention on precipitating stresses rather than predisposing vulnerabilities. In addition, the publicized prevalence of psychiatric disorder implied in the high rejection rates for selective service created heightened awareness of mental health problems and the need for information. This new public insight prompted federal support for epidemiological studies in the general population at the close of the war.

The consequent community surveys of the 1950s and 1960s adopted not only the methodology of direct interview developed during the military experience, but also the unifying concept of stress as the mediator of mental illness. The latter was consistent with defining mental health and mental illness along one continuum, an orientation based on the theories of Adolph Meyer. Thus, rejecting the Kraepelinian models (Kraepelin 1921) of discrete psychiatric disorders, these newer studies chose to measure overall impairment, independent of specific diagnosis, and to attribute aetiology to social factors. Representative community surveys included the Stirling County Study (Leighton et al 1963), the Baltimore Morbidity Survey (Pasaminick et al 1956) and the Midtown Manhattan Study (Srole et al 1962). Overall, these studies reported high rates of impairment (e.g. 81% in the Midtown Manhattan Study). Other studies, such as that of Hollingshead & Redlich (1958), established social class as a variable associated with treated mental illness, especially schizophrenia.

The development of methodology and attention to psychosocial variables engendered significant contribution to the understanding of psychiatric disorders and the use of mental health services; however, the intentional failure to establish rates for specific psychiatric disorders was severely to limit application of previous findings to the issues of public policy and to the research in psychopharmacology, genetics and neuropsychiatry that would emerge in the 1970s.

In response to this recognition, as well as to the research gaps identified by Jimmy Carter's Presidential Commission on Mental Health (PCMH) in 1977, a 'third generation' of epidemiological studies was to evolve in the 1980s. Its convergence with the allied fields of clinical psychiatry and basic research is readily observed in the development of reliable and systematic techniques of assessment by direct interview or family history. This refined methodology is actually the legacy of the psychopharmacological revolution, initiated almost three decades earlier.

The psychopharmacological revolution, begun in the 1950s, initiated a resurgence of interest in descriptive psychopathology as the basis for diagnostic assessment. The development of subsequent pharmacotherapies and their clinical trials was motivated by the desire to find the most appropriate medication for the individual patient. Furthermore, clinical trials required the selection of homogeneous groups of patients to test reliably the efficacy and safety of the drugs, to propose and verify aetiological hypotheses, to allow comparisons between studies and finally to foster communication with the practising clinician.

The US experience in standardized assessment

The Washington University Department of Psychiatry in St Louis strove to meet these needs in the 1970s and recommended use of operational criteria in establishing the diagnosis of a number of psychiatric illnesses (Feighner et al 1972). These diagnostic criteria were subsequently incorporated into the Research Diagnostic Criteria (RDC) published in 1978 by Spitzer and colleagues. As noted by the authors, 'the RDC were developed to enable research investigators to apply a consistent set of criteria for the description or selection of samples of subjects with functional psychiatric illness ... the affective disorders are subclassified into a number of nonmutually exclusive subcategories to permit testing of hypotheses relevant to affective illness.' DSM-III, published in 1980, was based on the above approach. DSM-IIIR was an interim modification, and in 1992 DSM-IV will be ready (American Psychiatric Association 1987).

For the affective disorders, diagnoses by the RDC and DSM-III differ slightly in their requirements for duration and accessory symptomatology. More importantly, the RDC additionally require presence of impairment indicated variably by help-seeking behaviour, use of medication or disruption of socio-occupational role functioning.

A logical extension of the operational criteria set forth by the RDC was the development of standardized instruments that could quantify the duration and intensity of the requisite symptom patterns experienced by the research subject. A structured interview, the Schedule for Affective Disorders and Schizophrenia (SADS) was designed to supplement the RDC (Spitzer et al 1978). Its purpose was to obtain information on a patient's functioning and symptoms. It elicited details on the current episode as well as historical information.

The application of the standardized instruments in epidemiological research proved feasible in a pilot study of 511 community residents by Weissman & Myers in 1975–1976 (Weissman & Myers 1978, Myers & Weissman 1980). This was the first study to demonstrate the feasibility of obtaining clinical psychiatric diagnosis using the new structured diagnostic methods in epidemiological surveys. The findings set the stage for the funding of a large epidemiological study, the Epidemiologic Catchment Area Study (ECA).

A limitation in broader application of the SADS for a multisite survey prompted by the PCMH of 1977 was that it required clinically-trained interviewers. In response, Robins, in association with several collaborators, developed the Diagnostic Interview Schedule (DIS) (Robins et al 1981). The DIS is a highly structured interview for use by lay interviewers in epidemiological surveys. It is designed to elicit the elements of diagnosis (symptom severity, frequency and distribution) and is capable of generating computer diagnosis in terms of DSM-III or RDC.

The UK experience

A parallel development in psychiatric diagnosis occurred in the UK. Wing and his collaborators developed the Present State Examination (PSE), which incorporated standard methods of defining, eliciting and recording symptoms in an interview. The PSE has been widely tested in large-scale international studies and has a reasonably high degree of reliability (Cooper et al 1972, World Health Organization 1978, Wing et al 1974, Orley & Wing 1979). The Present State Examination schedule contains 140 items, which can be rated either on the basis of subjective experiences described by the patient as having occurred during the previous 4 weeks or from observations made by the examiner during the interview. A computer programme (CATEGO) can be applied to the resulting symptom profile in order to achieve classifications of varying degrees of complexity related to ICD-9 (World Health Organization 1978).

Wing and colleagues (1978) pointed out that in outpatient psychiatric work, in liaison psychiatry and, above all, in community surveys, a serious problem arises as to where to establish the threshold for a diagnosis. They constructed an Index of Definition (ID), incorporated in a computer program, which was applied to symptom or syndrome profiles derived from the PSE. The ID, which is a scale (0–8), measures the degree of likelihood that there are sufficient components of key syndromes present to allow a diagnosis to be made. Community surveys using the same techniques have been carried out in Camberwell, UK; Edinburgh; the Outer Hebrides; Canberra, Australia; the Netherlands; Spain; Finland; and in two African villages (Bebbington et al 1981, 1989, Surtees et al

1986, Surtees & Sashidharan 1986, Brown & Harris 1978, Henderson et al 1979, Hodiamont et al 1987, Lehtinen et al 1990, Vazquez-Barquero et al 1986, Orley & Wing 1979.

Community studies of the 1980s

The previous experience and findings of the 1975 New Haven survey and the availability of the DIS paved the way for the launching in 1980 of the first large-scale epidemiological community survey of psychiatric disorder ever undertaken in the US (Regier et al 1984). The Epidemiological Catchment Area study involved over 18 000 community and institutional residents in five US sites. The availability of a diagnostic instrument suitable for use by lay interviewers and the interest in obtaining accurate rates of psychiatric disorders from community-based studies led to a proliferation of similar studies throughout the world. These studies were initiated in the 1980s and the results are still emerging as this chapter goes to press.

Table 8.1 Epidemiological community surveys of psychiatric disorders using DSM-III

Place	n	Age (years)	Investigator
USA – ECA	18572	18+	Weissman et al 1988a, b
New Haven	5034		
Baltimore	3481		
St Louis	3004		
Durham, NC	3921		
Los Angeles	3132		
Edmonton, Canada	3258	18+	Bland et al 1988
Puerto Rico	1551	17–64	Canino et al 1987
Florence, Italy	639	18+	Faravelli et al 1985
Seoul, Korea	5100	18–65	Lee et al 1987
Taiwan	11004	18+	Hwu et al 1989
Urban	5005		
Small towns	3004		
Rural villages	2995		
New Zealand	1498	18+	Joyce et al 1990

Table 8.1 shows the place, time, sample size and age of subjects in the recent community surveys using the DIS and DSM-III criteria. Published data are presented as available from these sites. It should be emphasized that these are all surveys of persons living

in the community. Institutional samples are not included. However, given the relatively low rate of chronic institutionalization for affective disorder, the focus on a community sample gives a reasonable picture of the prevalence of the disorders. The data on risk factors are derived from the epidemiological surveys cited or, where available, from new clinical studies that seem relevant.

In addition, the work begun by Wing in the 1970s using the PSE and ICD criteria continued. The result of seven studies will be described. The current studies are included in Table 8.2. Four of these studies used a two-phase design in which the initial sample was first screened. In the Canberra (Australia), Nijmegen (The Netherlands) and Santander (Spain) studies, the General Health Questionnaire (GHQ) was used as a screen. In the Camberwell (UK) studies, a short form of the PSE was used as a screen. The Finnish study was a longitudinal one-stage study. The Greek and Greek Cypriot studies were one-stage and were all carried out by clinicians. Table 8.2 also shows the number of subjects sampled in the stage 1 screening and the number interviewed with the PSE in stage 2.

BIPOLAR DISORDER

In this section we summarize findings for bipolar disorder from the recent studies. In succeeding sections we will deal similarly with major depression and with dysthymia.

Definition

The essential feature is a distinct period when the predominant mood is either elevated, expansive, or irritable; and when there are associated symptoms of the manic syndrome. These symptoms include hyperactivity, pressure of speech, flight of ideas, inflated self-esteem, decreased need for sleep, distractibility, and excessive involvement in activities that have a high potential for painful consequences which is not recognised.

The DSM-III criteria include a period of at least one week with the mood change and at least three of the additional associated features, without a mood-incongruent delusion or hallucination dominantly the clinical feature, outside the time of presence of the affective syndrome. The disorder should not be superimposed on either schizophrenia, schizophreniform disorder or a paranoid disorder.

For ICD-9 this would probably be equivalent to

Table 8.2 Recent epidemiological studies using PSE and ICD-9

Place	n Sampled	n interviewed 2nd stage	Age (years)	Investigator
Nijmegen Netherlands	3245	775	18–64	Hodiamont et al 1987
Camberwell UK	800	310	18–64	Bebbington et al 1981
Canberra Australia	756	170	18+	Henderson et al 1979
Santander Spain	1223	452	18+	Vazquez-Barquero et al 1986
Two districts Finland	747	—	30+	Lehtinen et al 1990
Athens Greece	487	—	18+	Mavreas & Bebbington 1988
Greek Cypriots in UK	285	—	18+	Mavreas & Bebbington 1988

manic and mixed affective psychosis (296. 1, 3) and M in the CATEGO class.

Rates

Table 8.3 shows the published 6-month annual and/or lifetime rates of bipolar disorder from six community surveys in the US; Puerto Rico; Edmonton, Canada; Florence, Italy; Taiwan; and Seoul, Korea. All the studies in Table 8.3 used the DIS and DSM-III criteria (refer to Table 8.1 for sample size). The consistency in rates is remarkable, especially given the fact that these rates are not adjusted for age or other demographic factors. The current and lifetime rates are close, possibly reflecting the fact that bipolar disorder is a chronic illness, although reporting artifact cannot be excluded. The 6-month rates per 100 range from 0.1 in Edmonton and Los Angeles to 1.2 in St Louis. The annual rates per 100 range from 0.03 in small towns of Taiwan to 1.7 in Florence, Italy. Possible contributions to this slightly higher rate in Florence are the small sample size and the fact that psychiatric hospitals were abolished in Italy in 1978. Therefore, those with bipolar illness may be better represented in the general community. In addition, in Florence the subjects' own physicians were the interviewers over the 2-month period, thereby conceivably promoting greater accuracy and/or quantity of information from the sample. The lifetime rates per 100 again are lowest in Taiwan (0.07 small towns, 0.1 rural villages and 0.16 in urban areas) and in Seoul, Korea (0.4). The highest rates per 100

Table 8.3 Prevalence rates per 100 for bipolar disorder based on community surveys using DIS and DSM-III diagnosis

Place	Rate/100* 6-month	1-year	Lifetime
USA-ECA	0.9	1.0	1.2
New Haven	1.1	1.3	1.6
Baltimore	0.9	0.9	1.2
St Louis	1.2	1.4	1.6
Durham, NC	0.6	0.6	0.7
Los Angeles	0.1	0.6	1.1
Edmonton, Canada	0.1	0.2	0.6
Puerto Rico	0.3	0	0.5
Florence, Italy	—	1.7	—
Seoul, Korea	—	—	0.4
Taiwan			
Urban	—	0.12	0.16
Small towns	—	0.03	0.07
Rural villages	—	0.10	0.10
New Zealand	—	—	—

*Rates rounded off to 1 decimal point in most cases

are found in the US (1.2, 5-site ECA total) and Puerto Rico (1.1). In general, at the time periods reported, the rates of bipolar disorder were lowest in Taiwan (particularly in small towns) and in Korea, followed by Puerto Rico and Piedmont, NC, where large, rural areas predominate. More detailed analyses were not published, but overall it is the similarities in the rates rather than their differences which are most striking.

Table 8.2 shows the sample sizes and ages and Table 8.4 shows the point prevalence rates per 100 in five studies using the PSE-ICD-9. The rates range from 0.08 to 0.8, close to the 6-month and 1-year rates in the DSM-III studies previously noted.

Table 8.4 Point prevalence rates per 100 for manic and mixed affective states based on community surveys using PSE, CATEGO and ICD-9

Place	Point prevalence rate/100
Nijmegen The Netherlands	0.1
Camberwell UK	0.8
Canberra Australia	0.4
Santander Spain	0.08
Finland	0.4

Interestingly, these rates of about 1% lifetime prevalence and lower for point prevalence are not too dissimilar from the morbidity risk rates of 0.6/100 and 0.9/100 in industrialized nations, extracted from studies using a variety of diagnostic methods and reported in the 1982 review (Boyd & Weissman 1982).

Risk factors

Sex ratios

In 1982, we noted that epidemiological data showed no significant sex differences in rates of bipolar disorder. These findings were consistent with emerging studies of relatives (Gershon et al 1987) and are consistent with reports from the 1980 surveys reviewed here. No significant sex differences in rates of bipolar disorder were found in studies reporting rates of bipolar disorder by sex (the US, ECA, Puerto Rico, Edmonton, Taiwan) and no mention is made of differences in rates in the other published data, or the numbers in the study were too small to interpret.

Age of onset

Bipolar illness, when compared with other affective disorders, seems to have an earlier onset and narrower period of risk. Modal age of onset by cross-national retrospective studies as of 1980 (Krauthammer & Klerman 1979) was about 30 years of age with significant decrease in first onset after 50 years (Clayton 1981). None of the new epidemiological studies reported have sampled adolescents. Despite anecdotal evidence since Kraepelin's day that mania commonly begins in adolescence, the notion that it can only rarely be diagnosed at that age has prevailed in the literature. Nevertheless, several clinical studies reported one-fourth to one-third of their cases to have had an onset of bipolar disorder prior to 20 years of age (Perris 1966, Winokur et al 1969, Loranger & Levine 1978). Since the 1982 edition of the book, Joyce and associates (1990) have noted many misdiagnoses of schizophrenia in hospitalized patients with bipolar disorder and found the modal age of onset in their patients to be 15–19 years of age. Akiskal et al (1985) found mean age of symptom onset to be 15.9 years among referred siblings and offspring of manic depressives. Large-scale DSM-III-based community studies of children and adolescents are only now being undertaken. These investigations may reveal greater adolescent onset of bipolar disorder that previously may have been misdiagnosed as character pathology, conduct disorder or, in the presence of psychotic features, as schizophrenia. Akiskal et al (1985), Gammon et al (1983) and others have rich anecdotal evidence for adolescent onset. More recent epidemiological studies corroborate an early age of onset of bipolar disorder. The ECA studies found a mean age of first onset to be 21 years, with a range from 18 years in Los Angeles to 26 years in Baltimore. The Edmonton, Canada, study found a median age of onset in the late teens, with few first onsets after 25 or before 10 years of age.

Somewhat related to observed earlier mean ages of onset for bipolar disorder is the apparently increasing lifetime prevalence in younger birth cohorts. Gershon et al (1987) first observed, among relatives of affectively ill probands, increasing rates of manic, schizoaffective and unipolar illness among those family members born after 1940. Most recently, in a study based on the 5-site ECA data, Lasch et al (1990) found an increasing lifetime prevalence of bipolar disorder in white men and women born since 1935. The implications of such secular changes in rates and possible artifactual explanations will be discussed later.

Socioeconomic status (SES)

A number of studies since Faris & Dunham's (1967)

landmark survey of a socioeconomic cross-section of Chicago have corroborated their finding of an association between higher social class and bipolar illness (Weissman & Myers 1978, Krauthammer & Klerman 1979). This subject has been reviewed by Bagley (1973), who points out that there are three possible explanations for the excess of manic depressive illness in the upper socioeconomic classes: 1) there may be a diagnostic bias such that patients from lower socioeconomic classes are not accurately diagnosed; 2) a particular type of personality may predispose certain individuals both to the disorder and to a rise in the social scale; and 3) the stresses of life in the upper socioeconomic classes or the stress of having moved up into such classes may predispose certain individuals to the disorder. Bagley finds that there is some evidence in the literature to support the first two hypotheses and indirect evidence to support the third.

In particular, higher rates of manic depression appear to prevail clinically among professional and/or highly educated men and women (Welner et al 1979, Woodruff et al 1971). Community surveys do not consistently find evidence for the increased risk of bipolar disorder in upper social classes. Weissman & Myers, in their 1978 New Haven study, found higher point prevalence rates of bipolar illness in the higher social classes. However, the ECA study, which had a considerably larger and more diverse sample, found no differential prevalence within occupation, income or education categories. Although the Puerto Rico study did not examine socioeconomic class *per se*, it did include educational level and found no significant differences for bipolar illness (Canino et al 1987). The association with sociodemographic factors could not be examined in the recent ICD studies for low prevalence disorders. These studies used two-stage samples and presented point prevalence rates so the resulting actual number of cases was low.

Race

There is no evidence from the ECA study that the rates of bipolar disorder are different between blacks and whites. Although several past studies have indicated greater bipolar prevalence among black males (Somervell et al 1989), these studies looked only at hospitalized patients and did not control for socioeconomic status. However, Williams' argument (1986) that *middle class* African-Americans are undersampled even in the ECA study, may be well founded since the socioeconomic class distribution of the races in the

sample was not directly addressed. Baltimore and Piedmont had, respectively, a 32% and 36.6% representation of blacks. St Louis oversampled blacks by design and New Haven's sample was 10% black. Another major ethnic sampling was of Hispanics, who comprised 57% of the Los Angeles sample (Burnam et al 1987, Karno et al 1987, 1989).

Somervell et al (1989) found no significant differences in rates for bipolar disorder by race in an extensive examination of the ECA data. Interestingly, the South Korean and Taiwan community surveys reported the lowest prevalence rates for bipolar disorder. Whether or not such a difference represents true diagnostic racial variability, artifacts of translation or cultural interpretation of behaviour is unclear.

Marital status

While some previous studies documented in the 1982 edition suggested that bipolar disorder was more common among single and divorced persons, other data were contradictory. The ECA data showed across sites that married persons had significantly lower rates of bipolar illness than divorced or never-married persons. There was an increasing rate of bipolar disorder among multiple divorced persons, possibly reflecting the consequences of the illness. Bland et al (1988) in Edmonton found no marital status effect.

Geographic area

The ECA sites from St Louis and Durham, NC, sampled rural as well as urban areas and found significantly higher 1-year rates of bipolar disorder in urban areas. A similar trend was found for 6-month prevalence in Puerto Rico (Canino et al 1987) and Taiwan (Hwu et al 1989).

Family history

While the epidemiological community studies did not assess family history, the familial nature of bipolar illness has been well established by several clinical studies and should be included as an important risk factor for bipolar disorder. Bipolar disorder is consistently increased in first-degree relatives of bipolar patients as compared with the relatives of patients with major depression or of normal controls. Cyclothymia, hyperthymia and major depression are also significantly elevated in relatives of bipolar patients.

Summary

Community-based rates per 100 for lifetime prevalence of bipolar disorder in the US are 0.7–1.6 (average 1.2). Cross-national DSM-III-based rates per 100 have ranged from lifetime risks of 0.16 and 0.41, respectively, in Taiwan and Korea to 0.5 in Puerto Rico, 0.6 in Canada and finally 1.7 (annual prevalence) in Italy. The point prevalence rates per 100 based on studies using ICD-9 range from 0.08–0.8. Again, it is the similarities rather than the differences in cross-cultural rates that are most notable. Bipolar rates are similar in men and women and are increased in divorced persons. There is a trend for increased risk in urban areas. There is little community-based evidence that higher socio-economic status is over-represented among persons with bipolar disorder.

The mean age of onset, reported in the past to be 28–30 years of age, is now 21 years, with many onsets in adolescence. There may have been secular changes in the rates of bipolar disorder, with rate increases and an earlier age of onset in the cohort born since 1935. Family history, although not assessed in the community surveys, remains one of the most important risk factors for bipolar disorder.

MAJOR DEPRESSION

Definition

The essential feature is either a dysphoric mood, usually depression, or loss of interest or pleasure in all or almost all usual activities and pastimes. This disturbance is prominent, relatively persistent and associated with other symptoms of the depressive syndrome. These symptoms include appetite disturbance, change in weight, sleep disturbance, psychomotor agitation or retardation, decreased energy, feelings of worthlessness or guilt, difficulty concentrating or thinking and thoughts of death or suicide or suicidal attempts.

The specific DSM-III criteria include dysphoric mood or loss of interest or pleasure in almost all activities, together with at least four of the associated symptoms present for at least 2 weeks. The clinical picture should not be dominated by a mood-incongruent delusion or hallucination outside the time when the affective syndrome is present. The condition should not be superimposed on either schizophrenia, schizophreniform disorder or a paranoid disorder. It should not be due to any organic mental disorder or uncomplicated bereavement.

For the ICD-9, major depression would probably be equivalent to manic-depressive disorder, depressive type (296.2) or neurotic depression (300.4), which are D, R, and N in the CATEGO classes.

Rates

Table 8.5 shows the 6-month, 1-year and lifetime rates per 100 as available in published reports. The ECA study across all five sites yielded a 6-month rate per 100 of 2.2 with a range of 1.5 in Durham to 2.8 in New Haven. 1-year prevalence in the ECA study was 2.7 with a range from 1.7 in Durham to 3.4 in New Haven. The annual rates are lower in Taiwan and higher in Florence (5.2) and in New Zealand (5.3); they are not reported in other sites.

Table 8.5 Prevalence rates per 100 for major depression based on community surveys using DIS and DSM-III diagnosis

Place	Rate/100*		
	6-month	1-year	Lifetime
USA – ECA	2.2	2.6	4.4
New Haven	2.8	3.4	5.8
Baltimore	1.7	1.9	2.9
St Louis	2.3	2.7	4.4
Durham, NC	1.5	1.7	3.5
Los Angeles	2.6	3.2	5.6
Edmonton, Canada	3.2	—	8.6
Puerto Rico	3.0	—	4.6
Florence, Italy	—	5.2	—
Seoul, Korea	—	—	3.4
Taiwan			
Urban	—	0.6	0.9
Small towns	—	1.1	1.7
Rural villages	—	0.8	1.0
New Zealand	5.3	5.3	12.6

*Rates rounded off to 1 decimal place in most cases

The lifetime rate per 100 in the ECA was 4.4, ranging from 2.9 in Baltimore to 5.8 in New Haven. These rates were similar to Puerto Rico's (4.6) and Seoul's (3.4). The rates are considerably higher in New Zealand (12.6) and in Edmonton, Canada (8.6). Taiwan, again, reports the lowest rates. The ECA study rates are significantly lower than the 1975 New Haven lifetime rate of 18 per 100 (Weissman & Myers 1978).

The RDC criteria used in the original New Haven study are not quite as exclusionary as those in the DSM-III; however, most of the discrepancy may be due to the relatively limited scope of probing for lifetime episodes allowed by the DIS as compared with the SADS. The differences could also be due to the 1975 sample, which was based on a follow-up and only included 511 persons. An obvious question beyond or perhaps related to that of cultural differences is whether some of these cross-national studies differ in *risk factor* distribution, which might explain the variation. It is of note, too, that most non-US studies sampled communities which were geographically and perhaps in other respects more homogeneous than did the ECA five-site study, which by design had diverse ethnic, racial and socioeconomic samples. Puerto Rico's data resembled the ECA results, with a 6-month prevalence of 3 per 100 and lifetime prevalence of 4.6 per 100.

In Taiwan, on the other hand, urban, small town and rural villages had by far the lowest rates obtained cross-nationally even though, on the basis of case criteria and measurement as well as sampling, these studies are comparable to the ECA and other cited surveys. It is possible that the Taiwanese either underreport symptoms in general, or do so selectively by diagnosis. Whereas substance abuse/dependence and then major depression are the most prevalent disorders in the ECA study, anxiety-related and psychophysiological disorders prevail in Taiwan, with major depression only fifth in prevalence. Moreover, although DSM-III diagnosed psychopathology in general is more prevalent in the US ECA study than in the samples from Taiwan, differences overall were not as great as for those of individual diagnostic categories.

The Korean study found the total lifetime prevalence per 100 of major depression to be 3.4, comparable to the lower end of the ECA five-site range. Unlike the Taiwan sample, in this more westernized country affective disorders in general were relatively prevalent, as in the US, at 5.4. However, as in Taiwan, this rate too was exceeded by anxiety-related disorders.

There is now limited incidence data from the ECA study (Eaton et al 1989). Incidence rates from community epidemiological surveys of psychiatric disorders are usually quite rare, since very large samples studied prospectively are required to generate estimates. However, the advantage of incidence studies in studying risk factors is well-known and makes them a potentially valuable tool for understanding. Overall annual incidence per 100 of first-onset major depression across four sites (New Haven was excluded) was 1.6 (Eaton et al 1989).

Table 8.6 shows the rates of depression from the ICD-9 studies. The rates per 100 are lowest in the Finnish study (4.6) and highest in the Greek study (7.4). The other studies show rates as follows: Nijmegen (5.4), Camberwell (7.1), Canberra (4.8), Santander (6.1). The ICD-9 studies have somewhat higher rates than those reported for the DSM-III studies. If only depressive psychosis and inhibited depression are included, the rates are comparable with the DSM-III studies for 6-month prevalence rates. Possibly neurotic depression is a more inclusive category and may overlap with dysthymia in DSM-III. Bebbington et al (1989) (not shown here) have estimated rates of minor depression. They have shown that the lifetime risk up to 65 years of age is quite high, 46% for men and 72% for women. These rates drop to 16% and 20% respectively when stricter criteria are used.

Table 8.6   Point prevalence rates per 100 for depression by sex based on community surveys using PSE, CATEGO (D, R N) and ICD-9 (296.2/300.4)

Place	Male	Female	Total
Nymegen Netherlands	4.3	7.7	5.4
Camberwell UK	4.9	9.2	7.1
Athens Greece	4.3	10.2	7.4
Greek Cypriots in Camberwell	4.2	7.1	5.6
Canberra Australia	4.3	7.7	6.1
Santander Spain	4.3	5.5	4.6
Two districts Finland	3.6	5.5	4.6
Edinburgh Scotland	—	4.3	—

Risk factors

For a complete review of the ECA data on sociodemographic factors and major depression, see Weissman et al 1988a, 1990.

Sex ratios

In marked contrast to bipolar disorder, the increased risk of major depression in women has been well-documented in clinical and epidemiological studies in the Western industrialized world. Weissman & Klerman (1977, 1985) reviewed the studies more than 10 years ago and concluded that this 'gender gap' was not simply an artefact of a tendency for women to report distress and/or seek help more readily than men. They pointed to the fact that even in community studies, the rates of major depression are higher in women than men.

Numerous explanations for this sex difference have been advanced and have been reviewed elsewhere (Weissman & Klerman 1977). The consistently higher rates of major depression in women than in men were found in the new community surveys (Table 8.7) and were noted in all the ICD-9 studies (Table 8.6). The sex ratios of females to males were about 2:1, with a range of 1.4:1 in urban areas of Taiwan to 2.7:1 in the US ECA. These sex-ratio differences were also consistent with the incidence data from four sites of the ECA, where the annual incidence was nearly twice as great in women than men.

Table 8.7 Rates of major depression by sex in community surveys using DIS and DSM-III diagnoses

	Lifetime rates/100		
Place	Female	Male	Sex ratios female/male
USA – ECA*	7.0	2.6	2.7
Edmonton	11.4	5.9	1.9
New Zealand	16.3	8.8	1.9
Taiwan			
Urban	1.0	0.7	1.4
Small towns	2.5	1.0	2.6
Rural villages	1.4	0.6	2.3
Seoul	4.1	2.6	1.6
Puerto Rico	5.5	3.5	1.6
	Annual incidence rate/100		
USA – ECA	1.98	1.10	1.8

*Four sites – New Haven excluded

In summary, high female-to-male ratios for major depression diagnosis are remarkably consistent across cultures and persistent over time. Moreover, the effect is strong enough to have prevailed over a highly variable history of epidemiological methods and sampling that have only relatively recently been systematized. There is a suggestion in several studies (further explored under the 'age' risk variable) of a decreasing sex difference in rates among those persons born in the last 30–40 years, although the finding and its significance are controversial and warrant further study. Finally, although it has been well established by widely available measures that more women than men are diagnosable as depressed, the reason for this finding remains unclear from an empirical standpoint.

Secular changes

Until recently the conventional wisdom has been that major depression increases with age. Studies thoughout the 1970s began to show that persons 18–44 years of age were at highest risk for all forms of depression. It was thought that men's risk peaked between 66 and 70 years of age, later than that for women (Charney & Weissman 1988). Most recent evidence indicates, however, that the rates for *both* sexes are higher at younger ages than previously recognized (including during childhood). Women and men 18–44 years of age in the ECA study had the highest 1-year prevalence. Similar findings were uncovered in a number of cross-national community studies (Blazer & Williams 1980). As might be expected, given this data, age of onset for both men and women has decreased as well, with a mean in the ECA studies of 27 years, roughly corroborated by recent studies in Edmonton, Canada and New Zealand.

What is counter-intuitive and argues against a simple age effect for major depression is the *decrease* in lifetime prevalence with age found in the ECA. Although not a universal finding (exceptions were Mexican Americans in the Los Angeles site of the ECA study, Puerto Rico and rural South Korea), it appears remarkably consistently across cultures that individuals born after the Second World War have higher lifetime risk than do those born prior to the Second World War, in spite of the former's younger age at sampling (Wickramaratne et al 1989, Klerman & Weissman 1989). A simple age effect might predict changes in period prevalence, incidence and/or age of onset, but cumulative lifetime risks should increase with age or at least flatten if older age is actually protective. The *drop* in lifetime risk with age is now seen in the studies from the US (ECA; for summary, see Klerman & Weissman 1989), Germany (Wittchen 1986), New Zealand (Joyce et al 1990,

Oakley-Brown et al in press), Canada (Bland et al 1988, Newman et al 1988) and perhaps urban Seoul (Lee et al 1987).

Arguments for one of a possible number of artefacts have arisen as well, especially a memory loss effect with increasing age. Though the latter remains at this time the hardest to refute, several studies fail to support a diminishing recall hypothesis (Farrer et al 1989, Lavori et al 1987), as does the simple fact that at least three historically non-industrialized cultures using the same diagnostic criteria and instruments did not exhibit increasing lifetime rates with age.

Other possible explanations for the effect include selective mortality and/or institutionalization, selective migration, changing diagnostic criteria, threshold changes in reporting among mental health professionals, and/or society at large and reporting bias of interviewees. These and other questions of artefact are reviewed extensively elsewhere (see Klerman & Weissman 1989).

Ample evidence exists for both period and birth-cohort effects, which are difficult to distinguish from each other. A *period* effect refers to rate changes associated with the period of time during which disease onset occurs. A *birth-cohort* effect refers to a changing rate associated with the period of time during which the proband or subject was born. Increasing lifetime morbidity and/or earlier age of onset for people of both sexes born since the 1930s have been noted by a number of investigators even prior to recent cross-national studies cited. Klerman & Weissman (1989) recognized a strong birth-cohort effect and earlier age of onset in both cross-national community and large scale family studies in the US. Similarly, Hagnell (1986) conducted the 25-year longitudinal follow-up of 2500 inhabitants of Lundby, Sweden, between 1947 and 1975. This had probably the best design for assessing temporal changes. They found an increase in risk for depression among both sexes in the cohorts born after 1937. Most pronounced, however, was the *10*-fold risk in lifetime rates for 20–39 year old males during the 1957–1972 period as compared with rates for the same age and sex during 1947–1957.

Evidence for a *period* effect has been found by Lavori et al (1987), who described both a post-1930 birth-cohort effect among siblings of depressed patients and a powerful 1965–1975 period effect for all birth cohorts. Wickramaratne et al (1989) analysed the ECA data closely and discovered a similar combination of birth-cohort (especially 1935–1945) and period (1960–1975) effects such that the latter effect, though by definition not age-specific, was most powerful in the 'at risk' birth cohort. These findings are consistent with other widely recognized temporal trends associated with depression, such as increased alcoholism, drug abuse and suicide, all of which have markedly increased, especially among young people and most particularly among young males born since the mid 1950s. The relatively short time-frames involved in these studies (i.e. too short for expressed phenotypes of widespread genetic changes to occur) implicate environmental mediation of the temporal rate changes. Environmental forces could be biological, historical, cultural or economic.

Whatever the exact nature of the environmental risk factors, they appear to have shifted recently such that more people, especially those born since the Second World War, have a higher risk of depression and an earlier age of onset. Interestingly, this trend is not seen in all cultures – e.g. Korea, Puerto Rico and Mexican Americans living in Los Angeles do not show the same extent of increase (Burnam et al 1987, Karno et al 1987).

Race – ethnicity

Overall, it was the similarities rather than the differences among racial groups in rates of major depression in the ECA that were the most striking (Somervell et al 1989). Cross-culturally, Puerto Rico did not significantly differ in rates of major depression from the ECA study, except for the absence of a birth-cohort effect (Canino et al 1987). On the other hand, the studies from South Korea (Lee et al 1987) and especially Taiwan (Hwu et al 1989) yielded lower rates of major depression than did the previously discussed Western surveys. The reasons for these differences are unclear. It should be noted that, although the ECA study sampled several ethnic/racial groups widely represented in the US and found few consistent differences, most of these groups are presumably less culturally or genetically distinct from the rest of the US population. The same problem, too, of separating racially or ethnically associated cultural distinctions from socioeconomic variables exists for major depression as it does in the previously discussed case of bipolar disorder, both in the US and cross-culturally. However, the potential artefact of socioeconomic *selection* is eliminated in these household probability samples as compared with studies restricted to clinical populations. The comparison between Greeks living in Athens and British Greek Cypriot immigrants living in Camberwell is especially noteworthy (Mavreas & Bebbington 1988). While there were higher rates of anxiety disorders among both Greek groups as compared with the Camberwell subjects, the rates of depression were quite comparable.

Socioeconomic status

The ECA study found no association between socioeconomic status and major depression, although the 1975 small-community survey by Weissman & Myers (1978) found current rates of major depression to be higher among lower social classes and lifetime rates higher among the upper classes. The authors hypothesized that this finding might have reflected greater persistence rather than frequency of disorder among the presumably less well-treated lower classes. Their study was confined to New Haven, whereas the present ECA study is both larger and more geographically heterogeneous. Although socioeconomic status *per se* had little effect, the rates of major depression were found to be lower among those who were employed and/or financially independent. The unemployed and those in public assistance had a threefold increased risk of major depression. The causal direction is unclear, however, since those with major depression are less likely to be capable of obtaining or maintaining employment; lack of employment, with or without public assistance, poses psychological stress that could contribute to developing or sustaining major depression. A study in Puerto Rico examined the relationship of major depression to educational level and found a non-significant trend for higher lifetime and 6-month rates among those with 7–11 years of education versus 0–6 years, 12–15 years or longer than 16 years. One might hypothesize that the 7–11 years category are those who 'dropped out' before completing high school and thereby added to their lives the stress of reduced employment and social options. Alternatively, there may be a shared vulnerability to not completing high school and to developing major depression. Of course, adolescents who are depressed may be less likely to finish high school. The group with less than 6 years of formal education is probably the currently oldest group who were not required by law to attend school at a time when education was a luxury.

Urban/rural residents

The studies from the US ECA, Puerto Rico, Taiwan and South Korea all examined this geographical distinction, and three found trends or significant differences. The exception was the study from Korea (Lee et al 1987), which found no difference in rates of major depression between urban and rural Seoul. The ECA study found significant urban versus rural rates of major depression in the two sites examined for this effect but in opposite directions. In Durham, NC (where rural areas sampled were outlying and isolated from the urban centre), there was more than twice the 1-year prevalence in the urban as compared with the rural areas. In St Louis, on the other hand (where the urban area is both substantially larger than Durham and is more transitionally connected via 'suburban sprawl' to the rural area), major depression was about 40% more prevalent in the 'rural' sample. Similarly, the Taiwanese 'small town' (versus 'rural village' or 'metropolitan Taipei') samples had trends towards greater major depression rates that for females were markedly significant (Hwu et al 1989). These authors hypothesized an effect in the more transitional small-town areas of greater instability, which was a result of conflict in values between the industrialized metropolitan area and traditional rural areas, thereby increasing the psychological stress on these people. Puerto Rico showed trends towards higher rates in 6-month and lifetime rates among urbanites as compared with rural dwellers, consistent with the Durham study. This urban versus rural variable, among others, may contribute to the rising rates of major depression observed over the last century if one hypothesizes greater stress in the world's increasingly urban and possibly less stable, transitional living environments.

Marital status

Powerful effects exerted on major depression rates by marital history were found in the ECA study *regardless of current status* and controlling for sex, age and race/ethnicity. Married and never-divorced persons had the lowest 1-year prevalence; those divorced or 'cohabiting' had the highest rates. However, persons never married (or cohabiting) had rates of major depression relatively close to the low rates for the continuously married persons. *Current* status is highly significant in its association between major depression and separation/divorce status – the latter carrying two to three times the risk of any other status. Edmonton, Canada, also reports similar findings, although never-married rates were exactly the same as those for continuously married persons. This apparent protective effect of continuous marriage may interact with gender as suggested under the 'sex' risk section, although the present study does control for sex. Perhaps in previous studies, in decades when divorce was less accessible or sanctioned, unhappy marriages were more prevalent and especially predisposed towards major depression among women as compared with men. In the ECA study in the 1980s, continuous marriages are certainly fewer and may reflect more satisfactory and reciprocal relationships than was the case in previous studies. These findings are consistent with Brown & Harris's report (1978) that women lacking a close, confiding, reciprocal relationship (e.g. trapped in unhappy marriages) are four times more likely than those who have such a relationship to develop major depression under stress. Again, causal inferences about the direction of the relationship between marital status and major depression are difficult, because major depression could predispose to marital difficulties and vice versa.

Family history

The possible contribution of genetics to affective disorder susceptibility has been suggested since the 1960s when differential clustering for bipolar and unipolar illness prompted subsequent division of depression into these two categories. Studies in the 1970s (Winokur & Morrison 1973, Winokur 1979) indicated a two- to threefold increased risk of major depression among first-degree relatives of probands with major depression as compared with relatives of normal controls. In addition, lifetime diagnosis of major depression was more than twice as likely among first-degree relatives of bipolar probands as compared with normal control relatives (Freimer & Weissman 1990, Gershon et al 1982).

Twin studies using DSM-III or RDC criteria, though few, have revealed 27% versus 12% concordance rates, respectively, among monozygotic and dizygotic twin probands with major depression. Of great diagnostic interest, the monozygotic concordance for major depression was almost the same for twins of bipolar disorder probands, although the reverse did not occur (Torgersen 1986). Studies such as these indicate genetic bases for major depression and also some overlap, as well as clear differentiation, between major depression and bipolar disorder (bipolar disorder concordance for monozygotic twins was 75%).

Genes probably play a role in the aetiology of major depression, although their role is not as great as in bipolar disorder. Moreover, although non-genetic factors seem to exert a comparatively greater role in

major depression, there is also evidence that a number of homogeneous subtypes of depression may be nested within this broad DSM-III diagnosis.

Summary

The rates of major depression are considerably higher than for bipolar disorder and more variable by site. The lifetime rate per 100 varies between 2.9 and 12.6 in the DSM-III studies. An exception to this range is the extremely low rate per 100 of 1–2 in Taipei, Taiwan, as was the case for bipolar illness. Prevalence rates, most notably lifetime prevalence rates, are substantially lower than those found in the 1975 New Haven study of major depression. As discussed, this reduced prevalence is most likely to be a function of the greater exclusion criteria of DSM-III versus RDC diagnoses and the lesser probing capability of the lay-administered DIS as compared with the SADS in obtaining lifelong history of symptoms. Furthermore, the sample size in 1975 was one-tenth that of the ECA and was restricted to an age range of 26 years and older and to one particular town. The point prevalence per 100 of major depression in the 1975 New Haven study (3.7) was, in fact, comparable to the ECA's New Haven 1-year prevalence per 100 (3.4). The point prevalence rates in the ICD-9 studies are higher (ranging from 4.6 per 100 to 7.7 per 100) than the DSM-III studies and are comparable when neurotic depression is excluded. In fact, Surtees & Sashidharan (1986) tested the comparability in rates in matched samples from the Edinburgh and the St Louis surveys and found similar rates of major depression.

A number of risk factors emerge from current community data. Female gender continues to be a clear risk factor according to almost all study sources. There also appears to be powerful evidence of both birth-cohort (post 1935–1945, depending on the study) and period (1960–1975) changes in rates of major depression. Cross-national data continue to accumulate for these effects. In addition (yet related) to decreasing lifetime rates with age, there is evidence of decreasing age of onset of major depression, which now averages around 27 years of age rather than the mid-30s.

Positive family history of major depression (or of bipolar disorder) is also a clear risk for major depression, although the effect is not as strong in the case of bipolar disorder.

Although there are less community data on race and ethnicity than for other variables, the ECA study shows few black/white differences in rates of major depression once social class and education are controlled. Asians, especially the Taiwanese, appear to have substantially lower rates of major depression, as well as other DSM-III disorder rates, than do Western populations.

The urban/rural variable may exert some impact on major depression by an as yet unclear mechanism. In several Western cases, urban dwellers have higher rates of major depression, although in Taiwan and in one US case transitional zones not usually sampled had the highest prevalence.

Socioeconomic status *per se* exerted no significant impact on rates in the ECA study, although in Puerto Rico and the U.S. respectively the specific variables of both higher level of education and being employed did appear protective against major depression.

Finally, the ECA study found both history of and current marital status to have a profound effect on rates of major depression. Specifically, continuously married persons had the lowest rates of major depression and divorced people had the highest rates, with never-married persons most resembling those who were married.

DYSTHYMIA

Definition

The essential feature is a chronic disturbance in mood involving either depressed mood or loss of interest or pleasure in all or almost all usual activities and pastimes, and associated symptoms, but not of sufficient severity and duration to meet the criteria for a major depressive episode. Dysthymia overlaps with depressive neurosis. The primary distinction between dysthymia and major depression is that the former is chronic but symptomatically less severe.

The specific DSM-III criteria include 2 years or more of depressive symptoms not reaching the criteria for major depression, with no more than a few months free of symptoms. During the depression there should be prominent depressed mood or loss of interest and pleasure, with at least three of 13 possible accompanying symptoms. If the disturbance is superimposed on a pre-existing mental disorder, such as obsessive-compulsive disorder or alcohol dependence, the depressed mood should be clearly distinguishable from the individual's usual mood.

Dysthymia may overlap with neurotic depression in ICD-9, but the latter also includes shorter, non-chronic episodes.

Rates

Rates for dysthymia *per se* are limited to lifetime prevalence, since by definition the disorder is chronic for at least 2 years. In the ECA study the overall dysthymia rate per 100 was 3, somewhat comparable to the earlier 'depressive personality' rate (Table 8.8). Of interest, almost half (42%) of those with dysthymia had also experienced an episode of major depression in their lifetime.

Table 8.8 Rates of dysthymia by sex in community surveys using DIS and DSM-III diagnoses

Place	Lifetime rates/100			Sex ratios female/male
	Female	Male	Total	
USA – ECA	4.1	2.2	3.0	1.9
New Haven	—	—	3.2	—
Baltimore	—	—	2.1	—
St Louis	—	—	3.8	—
Durham, NC	—	—	2.3	—
Los Angeles	—	—	4.2	—
Edmonton	5.2	2.2	3.7	2.4
Puerto Rico	7.6	1.6	4.7	4.8
Florence	—	—	2.3	—
Taiwan				
Urban	1.1	0.7	0.9	1.6
Small towns	1.6	1.4	1.5	1.1
Rural villages	1.4	0.6	0.9	2.6
Seoul	2.8	1.6	2.2	1.7

The rate per 100 of dysthymia varied from 2.1 in Baltimore to 4.2 in Los Angeles. In Edmonton, Canada (Bland et al 1988), overall prevalence was 3.7, much as in the US. Korea reports a rate of 2.2 per 100 and Italy (Faravelli & Incerpi 1985), a rate of 2.3 per 100 (given as 1-year prevalence). Puerto Rico had the highest rate, 4.7, due to a very high prevalence among women there. Again, as with all DSM-III disorders, Taiwan had the lowest rates per 100, which ranged among its three geographic regions from 0.92 in the city to 1.51 in the small towns. In spite of dysthymia being relatively less well defined and studied as compared with major depression or bipolar disorder, there exists considerable agreement among the limited studies cited on its prevalence, which lies between bipolar disorder and major depression, but appears to be closer to the high rates of major depression. As shown in Table 8.5, the point prevalence rates of neurotic depression in the ICD-9 are about 4 per 100 to 5.2 per 100, but it is unclear if this is equivalent to dysthymia.

Risk factors

For more detail on sociodemographic associations with dysthymia, see Weissman et al 1988a, b.

One might expect risk variables to be similar to those for major depression – especially the more robust ones such as gender – if the two disorders lie on a continuum of severity. In fact, there is clinical evidence that some dysthymia may, in part, be an incompletely resolved residuum or a prodromal state of major depression. However, in either of these cases one might expect a higher prevalence of dysthymia than major depression, which is not the case. Family studies appear to support not only some diagnostic overlap but also qualitative distinctiveness of these disorders.

Sex

The ECA study yielded about a 1.9:1 female-to-male ratio for dysthymia, slightly less than for major depression (Table 8.5). The female-to-male sex ratio was slightly higher in Edmonton, 2.4:1 and was considerably higher in Puerto Rico, 4.8:1. The Taiwan ratios also ranged from about 1.5:1 in the city to 2.5:1 in the villages. The sex ratio in Seoul, 1.7:1, was comparable to the US. In Taiwan, there was considerable variability, from 2.6:1 in rural villages through 1.6:1 in urban Taiwan to equal, 1.1:1, in small towns.

Age

Unlike major depression, the ECA study found that the rates of dysthymia increased with age but levelled off between 30 and 65 years of age and then decreased markedly. South Korea reports an increase in prevalence with age, but did not sample those over 65. Edmonton also found an increasing prevalence with age, except for after 65 years of age when, as in the ECA study, a steep drop-off occurs. The increase in prevalence with age serves to argue against a simple memory effect in the case of major depression, since one might expect the same effect for dysthymia. It may be that the chronic nature of dysthymia renders it more memorable than the more severe but shorter-lived major depression, although there is no evidence to indicate that this is the case. Puerto Rico revealed roughly the same rates in the 18–24 and 25–55 age

groups, indicating a probable *decrease* in risk in the 25–44-year-old age group compared with the 18–24-year-old category during which most of the onsets may have occurred. Prevalence then rose in the 45–64-year-old group, which was the maximum age sampled.

Race

Race comparisons were made only in the ECA study where, as in the case of major depression, there were no significant black/white differences in rates. In the case of dysthymia, however, Hispanic rates exceeded those of whites and blacks, consistent with Puerto Rico's relatively high dysthymia rate. Regarding the Asian studies, South Korea, a less historically isolated nation than Taiwan, again reported rates roughly comparable to those of Western nations, whereas Taiwan differed markedly in having lower figures.

Socioeconomic status

The ECA study found significantly higher dysthymia rates among 18–44-year-olds with an income of less than $20 000 a year as compared with those making more than $20 000 a year. However, income had little effect in the 45–64-year-olds or in the 65 and older group (Weissman et al 1988b).

Marital status

The ECA study found that dysthymia was more prevalent among all persons unmarried and under the age of 65 than among married people of the same age, with rates in the 45–65-year-old range being double those of comparable married persons. Edmonton also reported higher rates among divorced or widowed people as compared with married persons, although by far the lowest rates were among those never married. Ratios were 4:1 for divorced or widowed versus never-married, and 3:1 for married versus never-married. It must be remembered, though, that Edmonton's 18–24-year-old group had, as would be expected, the lowest lifetime prevalence; presumably this is also the most frequent age group in the never-married category. As with major depression, the direction of the relationship between marital status and depression is ambiguous.

Urban/rural

While the ECA has no reported data for dysthymia on urban versus rural differences, Taiwan, Korea and

Puerto Rico have. Urbanites in Korea showed a trend towards higher rates (2.4 per 100 versus 1.9 per 100) and those in Puerto Rico had significantly higher rates of dysthymia as compared with rural dwellers (5.5 per 100 versus 3.3 per 100). In Taiwan, on the other hand, urban and rural areas differed little but, as in the case rates of major depression, rates of dysthymia in the transitional small towns were relatively high (1.51 per 100 versus 0.92 per 100 and 0.94 per 100 in the urban and rural areas respectively).

Summary

Dysthymia, a milder but more chronic form of depression than major depression, appears to be somewhat less prevalent over a lifetime than major depression, with the exceptions of Puerto Rico and Taiwan, where lifetime risk for the two disorders is about equal. Puerto Rico's greater prevalence relative to other nations appears to be accounted for mainly by the high dysthymia rate among its women. Most other nations found a female-to-male ratio of roughly 2:1, consistent with, although slightly lower than, that found for major depression.

Race, marital status and geographical position carry similar risks for dysthymia as they do for major depression except for the trend in the ECA and the clearly higher rates in Puerto Rico for Hispanic prevalence. Asian groups compared with Western surveys as they did for major depression, with rates from South Korea resembling those of the West and rates from Taiwan being substantially lower. The ECA project found for dysthymia, unlike major depression, a significant inverse relationship between income and disorder, especially in younger persons. Finally, also unlike the case for major depression (or bipolar disorder), rates increased or levelled off with age until after 65 years of age, when compromised memory may well have accounted for the observed drop in lifetime prevalence.

THE ZURICH STUDIES

No review would be complete without a mention of the Zurich study, which provides longitudinal information on the epidemiology of affective disorders in a single cohort.

Angst & Dobler-Mikola (1984) followed a cohort 19–20 years of age, selected from the general population of Zurich, for 4 years (see Angst et al 1984 for review). General diagnostic schemes were used,

including RDC, DSM-III, Feighner and their own system, which required work impairment and symptoms thresholds and differed by sex. As expected, the rates varied by criteria used and the stricter criteria produced lower rates. They found a 1-year prevalence rate of 7 per 100 for major depression using DSM-III criteria and 0.75 per 100 for bipolar disorder. If fewer symptoms are required for males than females, then the sex difference disappears. In a more recent report, Angst noted the high prevalence of brief, recurrent episodes of depression (Angst et al 1990). This important sample of young adults is being followed longitudinally.

FUTURE DIRECTIONS

The application of structured diagnostic instruments to assess psychiatric disorders and their use in epidemiological studies of communities throughout the world have created the possibility of cross-national comparisons. However, it must be acknowledged that the American system of DSM-III or the forthcoming DSM-IV is not universally accepted. Under the framework of the World Health Organization and the Alcohol, Drug Abuse and Mental Health Administration Joint Project on Standardization of Diagnoses and Classification, Wing and a group of international investigators have developed a new system known as Schedules for Clinical Assessment in Neuropsychiatry (SCAN, Wing et al 1990). This system is being tested with the aim of developing a comprehensive procedure for clinical examination that is also capable of generating many of the categories of the *International Classification of Diseases*, 10th edn, and the *Diagnostic and Statistical Manual of Mental Disorders*, 3rd edn – revised.

SCAN is being field tested in 20 centres in 11 countries. The project's chief goal is to foster the development of techniques that can be used to study psychopathology across nations, regions and cultures so as to create the basis for collaborative studies that will examine the causes, risk factors, outcomes and consequences of mental disorders.

In a parallel development under the same sponsorship, Robins et al (1988) have developed the Composite International Diagnostic Interview (CIDI), based on the National Institute of Mental Health Diagnostic Interview Schedule. The interview is modified for international use in various ways and has adopted certain features of the ninth edition of the Present State Examination (PSE-9).

The two instruments are complementary in the sense that the CIDI is designed for use in large community surveys that necessitate the employment of lay interviewers, whereas SCAN can only be used in its full form by professionals already experienced in examining people with a range of psychiatric disorders. The availability of two diagnostic methods that bridge the major classification systems will further facilitate future cross-national comparative studies.

Lastly, it should be noted that none of the epidemiological studies mentioned included children, even though it is quite clear that many affective disorders first occur in adolescence and to a lesser extent in childhood. Currently, there is field testing of epidemiological methods applicable to children ongoing in several US centres in preparation for a large epidemiological study of children. When the next edition of this volume is published, this data should be available.

REFERENCES

Akiskal H S, Downs J, Jordan P, Watson S, Dougherty D, Pruitt D B 1985 Affective disorders in referred children and younger siblings of manic depressives. Archives of General Psychiatry 42: 996–1003

American Psychiatric Association 1987 Diagnostic and statistical manual of mental disorders, 3rd edn – revised. American Psychiatric Association Press, Washington, DC

Angst J, Dobler-Mikola 1984 The Zurich study: III. Diagnosis of depression. European Archives of Psychiatry and Neurological Science 234: 30–37

Angst J, Dobler-Mikola, Binder J 1984 The Zurich study: a prospective epidemiological study of depressive, neurotic and psychosomatic syndromes: I. Problem and methodology. European Archives Psychiatry and Neurological Science 234: 13–20

Angst J, Merikangas K, Scheidegger P, Wicki W 1990 Recurrent brief depression: a new subtype of affective disorder. Journal of Affective Disorders 19(2): 87–89

Bagley C 1973 Occupational status and symptoms of depression. Social Science and Medicine 7: 327–339

Bebbington P, Hurry J, Tennant C, Sturt E, Wing J K 1981 Epidemiology of mental disorders in Camberwell. Psychological Medicine 11: 561–579

Bebbington P, Katz R, McGuffin P, Tennant C, Hurry J 1989 The risk of minor depression before age 65: results from a community survey. Psychological Medicine 19: 393–400

Bland R C, Newman S C, Orn H (eds) 1988 Epidemiology of psychiatric disorders in Edmonton. Acta Psychiatrica Scandinavica 77 (suppl 338)

Blazer D, Williams C D 1980 Epidemiology of dysphoria and depression in an elderly population. American Journal of Psychiatry 137: 439–444

Boyd J H, Weissman M M 1982 Epidemiology. In: Paykel E S (ed) Handbook of affective disorders. Churchill Livingstone, Edinburgh, p 109–125

Brown G W, Harris T O 1978 Social origins of depression: a study of psychiatric disorder in women. Tavistock, London

Burnam M A, Hough R L, Escobar J I, Karno M 1987 Six-month prevalence of specific psychiatric disorders among Mexican Americans and non-hispanic whites in Los Angeles. Archives of General Psychiatry 44: 687–691

Canino G J, Bird H R, Shrout P E, Rubio-Stipec M, Bravo M, Martinez R, Sesman M, Guevara L M 1987 The prevalence of specific psychiatric disorders in Puerto Rico. Archives of General Psychiatry 44: 727–735

Charney E A, Weissman M M 1988 Epidemiology of depressive and manic syndromes. In: Georgotas A, Cancro R (eds) Depression and mania. Elsevier Press, New York p 45–74

Clayton P J 1981 The epidemiology of bipolar affective disorder. Compre psychiatry 22: 31–41

Cooper J E, Kendell R E, Gurland B J, Sharpe L, Copeland J R M, Simon R 1972 Psychiatric diagnosis in New York and London: a comparative study of mental hospital admissions. Maudsley Monograph No. 22. Oxford University Press, Oxford

Dohrenwend B P, Dohrenwend B S 1982 Perspectives on the past and future of psychiatric epidemiology. American Journal of Public Health 72: 1271–1277

Eaton W W, Kramer M, Anthony J C, Dryman A, Shapiro S, Locke B Z 1989 The incidence of specific DIS/DSM-III mental disorders: data from the NIMH Epidemiologic Catchment Area Program. Acta Psychiatrica Scandinavica 79: 163–178

Faravelli C, Incerpi G 1985 Epidemiology of affective disorders in Florence. Acta Psychiatrica Scandinavica 72: 331–333

Faris R E L, Dunham H W 1967 Mental disorders in urban areas: an ecological study of schizophrenia and other psychoses. University of Chicago Press, Chicago

Farrer L A, Florio L P, Bruce M L, Leaf P J, Weissman M M 1989 Reliability and consistency of self-reported age at onset of major depression. Journal of Psychiatric Research 23: 35–47

Feighner J P, Robins E, Guze S B, Woodruff R A, Winokur G, Munoz R 1972 Diagnostic criteria for use in psychiatric research. Archives of General Psychiatry 26: 57–63

Freimer N, Weissman M M 1990 The genetics of affective disorder. In: Deutsch S I, Weizman A, Weizman R (eds) Application of basic neuroscience to child psychiatry. Plenum Publishing Company, New York, p 285–296

Gammon G D, John K, Rothblum E D, Mullen K, Tischler G L, Weissman M M 1983 Use of a structured diagnostic interview to identify bipolar disorder in adolescent inpatients: frequency and manifestations of the disorder. American Journal of Psychiatry 140: 543–547

Gershon E S, Hamovit J, Guroff J J, Dibble E, Leckman J F, Sceery W, Targum S D, Nurnberger J I, Goldin L R, Bunney W E 1982 A family study of schizoaffective bipolar I, bipolar II, unipolar, and normal control probands. Archives General Psychiatry 39: 1157–1167

Gershon E, Hamovit J, Gurroff J, et al 1987 Birth-cohort changes in manic and depressive disorders in relatives of bipolar, and schizoaffective patients. Archives of General Psychiatry 44: 314–319

Hagnell O 1986 The 25-year follow-up of the Lundby study: incidence and risk of alcoholism, depression, and disorders of the senium. In: Barret, Rose (eds) Mental disorders in the community: findings from psychiatric epidemiology. Guilford Press, New York

Henderson S, Duncan-Jones P, Byrne D G, Scott R, Adcock S 1979 Psychiatric disorder in Canberra. Acta Psychiatrica Scandinavica 60: 355–374

Hollingshead A B, Redlich F D 1958 Social class and mental illness. John Wiley, New York

Hodiamont P, Peer N, Syben N 1987 Epidemiological aspects of psychiatric disorder in a Dutch health area. Psychological Medicine 17: 495–505

Hwu H-G, Yeh E-K, Chang L-Y 1989 Prevalence of psychiatric disorders in Taiwan defined by the Chinese Diagnostic Interview Schedule. Acta Psychiatrica Scandinavica 79: 136–147

Joyce P R, Oakley-Browne M A, Wells J E, Bushnell J A, Hornblow A R 1990 Birth cohort trends in major depression: increasing rates and earlier onset in New Zealand. Journal of Affective Disorders 18: 83–90

Karno M, Hough R L, Burnam M A, Escobar J I, Timbers D M, Santan F, Boyd J H 1987 Lifetime prevalence of specific psychiatric disorders among Mexican Americans and non-Hispanic whites in Los Angeles. Archives of General Psychiatry 44: 695–701

Karno M, Golding J M, Burnam M A, Hough R L, Escobar J I, Wells K M, Boyer R 1989 Anxiety disorders among Mexican Americans and non-Hispanic whites in Los Angeles. Journal of Nervous and Mental Disorders 177: 202–209

Klerman G L 1980 Overview of affective disorders In: Kaplan H J, Freedman A M, Sadock B J (eds) Comprehensive textbook of psychiatry, 3rd edn. Williams & Wilkins, Baltimore

Klerman G L, Weissman M M 1989 Increasing rates of depression. Journal of the American Medical Association 261: 2229–2235

Kraepelin E 1921 Manic depressive insanity and paranoia. E & S Livingstone, Edinburgh

Krauthammer C, Klerman G L 1979 The epidemiology of mania. In: Shopsin B (ed) Manic illness. Raven Press, New York, p 11–28

Lasch K, Weissman M M, Wickramaratne P J, Bruce M L 1990 Birth cohort changes in the rates of mania. Psychiatry Research 33: 31–37

Lavori P W, Klerman G L, Keller M B, Reich T, Rice J, Endicott J 1987 Age-period-cohort analysis of secular trends in onset of major depression: Findings in siblings of patients with major affective disorder. Journal Psychiatric Research: 23–36

Lee C-K, Han J-H, Choi J-O 1987 The epidemiological study of mental disorders in Korea (IX): alcoholism anxiety and depression. Seoul Journal of Psychiatry 12: 183–191

Lehtinen V, Lindholm T, Veijola J, Vaisanen E 1990 The prevalence of PSE-CATEGO disorders in a Finnish adult population cohort. Society for Psychiatry and Psychiatric Epidemiology 25: 187–192

Leighton D C, Harding J S, Macklin D B, MacMillan A M,

Leighton A H 1963 The character of danger. Basic Books, New York

Loranger A W, Levine P M 1978 Age at onset of bipolar affective illness. Archives of General Psychiatry 35: 1345–1348

Mavreas V G, Bebbington P E 1988 Greeks, British Greek Cypriots and Londoners: a comparison of morbidity. Psychological Medicine 18: 433–442

Myers J K, Weissman M M 1980 Screening for depression in a community sample: the use of a self-report scale to detect the depressive syndrome. American Journal of Psychiatry 137: 1081–1084

Newman S C, Bland R C, Orn H 1988 Morbidity risk of psychiatric disorders. Acta Psychiatrica Scandinavica 77: 50–56

Oakley-Browne M A, Joyce P R, Wells J E, Bushnell J A, Hornblow A R (in press) Six-month and other period prevalences of specific psychiatric disorders in the Christchurch urban area. Australian and New Zealand Journal of Psychiatry

Orley J, Wing J K 1979 Psychiatric disorders in two African villages. Archives of General Psychiatry 36: 513–520

Pasaminick B, Roberts D W, Lemkau P V, Krieger D E 1956 A survey of mental disease in an urban population. American Journal Public Health 47: 923–929

Perris C 1966 A study of bipolar (manic-depressive) and unipolar recurrent depressive psychoses. Acta Psychiatrica Scandinavica (suppl) 194

Regier D A, Myers J K, Kramer M, Robins L N, Blazer D G, Hough R L, Eaton W W, Locke B Z 1984 The NIMH Epidemiologic Catchment Area Program: historical context, major objectives, and study population characteristics. Archives of General Psychiatry 41: 934–941

Robins L N, Helzer J E, Croughan J, Ratcliff K S 1981 National Institute of Mental Health Diagnostic Interview Schedule. Archives of General Psychiatry 38: 381–389

Robins L N, Wing J, Wittchen H U, Helzer J E, Babor T F, Burke J, Farmer A, Jablenski A, Pickens R, Regier D A, Sartorius N, Towle L H 1988 The composite international diagnostic interview: an epidemiologic instrument suitable for use in conjunction with different diagnostic systems and in different cultures. Archives of General Psychiatry 45: 1069–1077

Somervell P D, Leaf P J, Weissman M M, Blazer D G, Bruce M L 1989 The prevalence of major depression in black and white adults in five United States communities. American Journal of Epidemiology 130: 725–735

Spitzer R L, Endicott J, Robins E 1978 Research diagnostic criteria. Biometrics Research Division, Evaluation Section, New York State Psychiatric Institute, New York

Srole L, Langner T S, Michael S T, Opler M K, Rennie T A C 1962 Mental health in the metropolis. McGraw-Hill, New York

Surtees P G, Sashidharan S P 1986 Psychiatric morbidity in two matched community samples: A comparison of rates and risks in Edinburgh and St Louis. Journal of Affective Disorders 10: 101–113

Surtees P G, Sashidharan S P, Dean C 1986 Affective disorder amongst women in the general population: a longitudinal study. British Journal of Psychiatry 148: 176–186

Torgersen S 1986 Genetic factors in moderately severe and

mild affective disorders. Archives of General Psychiatry 43: 222–226

Vazquez-Barquero J F, Diez-Manrique J F, Pena C, Quintanal G, Lopez L M 1986 Two stage design in a community survey. British Journal of Psychiatry 149: 88–97

Weissman M M, Klerman G L 1977 Sex differences in the epidemiology of depression. Archives of General Psychiatry 34: 98–111

Weissman M M, Klerman G L 1978 Epidemiology of mental disorders: Emerging trends in the US. Archives of General Psychiatry 35: 705–712

Weissman M M, Klerman G L 1985 Gender and depression. Trends in the neurosciences 8: 416–420

Weissman M M, Myers J K 1978 Affective disorders in a US urban community. Archives of General Psychiatry 35: 1304–1311

Weissman M M, Leaf P J, Tischler G L, Blazer D G, Karno M, Bruce M L, Florio L P 1988a Affective disorders in five United States communities. Psychological Medicine 18: 141–153

Weissman M M, Leaf P J, Bruce M L, Florio L 1988b The epidemiology of dysthymia in five communities: rates, risks, comorbidity, and treatment. American Journal of Psychiatry 145: 815–819

Weissman M M, Bruce M L, Leaf P J, Florio L P, Holzer C 1990 Affective disorders. In: Robins L, Regier D (eds) Affective disorders. Free Press New York p 53–81

Welner A, Marten S, Wochnick E, Davis M A, Fishman R, Clayton P J 1979 Psychiatric disorders among professional women. Archives of General Psychiatry 36: 169–173

Wickramaratne P J, Weissman M M, Leaf P J, Holford T R 1989 Age, period and cohort effects on the risk of major depression: results from five United States communities. Journal of Clinical Epidemiology 42: 333–343

Williams D H 1986 The epidemiology of mental illness in Afro-Americans. Hospital and Community Psychiatry 37: 42–49

Wing J K, Cooper J E, Sartorius N 1974 Measurement and classification of psychiatric symptoms: an instructional manual for the PSE and CATEGO program. Cambridge University Press, New York

Wing J K, Mann S A, Leff J P, Nixon J M 1978 The concept of 'case' in psychiatric population surveys. Psychological Medicine 8: 203–217

Wing J K, Babor T, Brugha T, Burke J, Cooper J E, Giel R, Jablenski A, Regier D, Sartorius N 1990 SCAN: Schedules for clinical assessment in neuropsychiatry. Archives of General Psychiatry 47: 589–592

Winokur G 1979 Unipolar depression: is it divisible into autonomous subtypes? Archives of General Psychiatry 36: 47–52

Winokur G, Morrison J. The Iowa 500: follow-up of 225 depressives. British Journal of Psychiatry 123: 543–548

Winokur G W, Clayton P J, Reich T 1973 Manic depressive illness. CV Mosby, St Louis

Wittchen H U 1986 Contribution of epidemiological data to the classification of anxiety disorders. In: Hand I, Wittchen H U (eds) Panic phobias. Springer Verlag, Berlin, p 18–27

Woodruff R A, Robins L N, Winokur G, Reich T 1971 Manic depressive illness and social achievement. Acta Psychiatrica Scandinavica 47: 237–249

World Health Organization 1978 Mental disorders: glossary and guide to their classification in accordance with the 9th revision of the International Classification of Diseases. WHO, Geneva

9. Genetics

John I. Nurnberger Jr   Elliot S. Gershon

Affective disorder is a broad and heterogeneous category of psychiatric illness. Its prevalence may range up to 20% of the population or more, depending on definition (Weissman & Myers; see also chapter 8 1978). The more severe types of affective disorder, such as bipolar illness, clearly run in families, and available evidence suggests that they are highly heritable. This appears to be considerably less true with the milder forms of depression.

Single-gene forms of bipolar disorder have been proposed for many years (e.g. Reich et al 1969). Initial evidence from DNA markers supported a single-gene form on chromosome 11 (Egeland et al 1987). A second gene was localized to the X-chromosome in other families (Baron et al 1987). However, neither of these findings has been consistently replicated. With the recent advances in mapping the entire human genome (Donis-Keller et al 1987), systematic scanning of the genome for affective illness genes has been undertaken at several centres. The strategy is to perform genetic linkage analyses in pedigrees containing multiple cases of illness, using appropriately located chromosomal linkage markers. No linkages have yet been reported from these studies. The alternate molecular strategy to linkage is association: specific genes are examined for alterations associated with illness. This strategy has been greatly aided by new methods of molecular scanning for differences in genomic sequences in many individuals (Rossiter & Caskey 1990).

Potential aetiological markers include induction of rapid eye movement (REM) sleep by cholinergic pharmacological agents, light suppression of melatonin and lithium ratio in red blood cells.

There is an increasing interest in studies of populations at high risk (on the basis of having an ill parent or sibling). These studies permit the testing of physiological hypotheses regarding the vulnerability to affective illness in populations free of the effects of the illness itself or of treatments for it. They also permit the assessment of the ability of a biological or clinical characteristic to *predict* the presence of illness or the course of illness over time.

We will first review results using the classical epidemiological genetic methods, then comment on the spectrum of affective illness and finally consider linkage and pathophysiological marker studies.

EPIDEMIOLOGICAL STUDIES

Family studies

Family studies in affective disorder have consistently demonstrated aggregation of illness in relatives (Table 9.1). The actual risk figures vary with the criteria used and probably many other factors (Gershon 1984). In a recent study at NIMH, 25% of relatives of bipolar probands were found to have bipolar or unipolar illness themselves, compared with 20% of relatives of unipolar probands and 7% of relatives of controls. In the same study 40% of the relatives of schizoaffective probands demonstrated affective illness at some point in their lives (age-corrected morbid risk data—Gershon et al 1982). These data demonstrate increased risk in relatives of patients; they also show that the various forms of affective illness appear to be related in a hierarchical way: relatives of schizoaffective probands may have schizoaffective illness themselves, but are more likely to have bipolar or unipolar illness. Ill relatives of bipolar probands have either bipolar or (more likely) unipolar illness (Fig. 9.1).

If pedigrees of affective patients are considered as a group, it has generally not been possible to fit single-gene models to them, as reviewed elsewhere (Nurnberger & Gershon 1984). Multifactorial models have been consistent with some data sets. These models imply multiple factors, genetic and/or environmental. An

Table 9.1 Lifetime prevalence of affective illness in first-degree relatives of patients and controls (adapted from Nurnberger et al 1986)

		Morbid risk %	
	Number at risk	Bipolar	Unipolar
Bipolar probands			
Perris 1966	627	10.2	0.5
Winokur & Clayton 1967	167	10.2	20.4
Goetzl et al 1974	212	2.8	13.7
Heltzer & Winokur 1974	151	4.6	10.6
Mendlewicz & Rainer 1974	606	17.7	22.4
James & Chapman 1975	239	6.4	13.2
Gershon et al 1975	341	3.8	8.7
Smeraldi et al 1977	172	5.8	7.1
Johnson & Leeman 1977	126	15.5	19.8
Pettersen 1977	472	3.6	7.2
Angst et al 1979, 1980	401	2.5	7.0
Taylor et al 1980	601	4.8	4.2
Gershon et al 1981, 1982	598 (572)*	8.0	14.9
Rice et al (1987)	567	10.4	23.1
Unipolar probands			
Perris 1966	684	0.3	6.4
Gershon et al 1975	96	2.1	14.2
Smeraldi et al 1977	185	0.6	8.0
Angst et al 1979, 1980	766	0.1	5.9
Taylor et al 1980	96	4.1	8.3
Weissman et al 1984b (severe)	242 (234)	2.1	17.5
Weissman et al 1984b (mild)	414 (396)	3.4	16.7
Gershon et al 1981, 1982	138 (133)	2.9	16.6
Rice et al 1987	1176	5.4	28.6
Normal probands			
Gershon et al 1975	518 (411)	0.2	0.7
Weissman et al 1984b	442 (427)	1.8	5.6
Gershon et al 1981, 1982	217 (208)	0.5	5.8

*Number at risk (corrected for age) for bipolar illness appears first in at-risk column; in parentheses is number at risk for unipolar illness when this is available separately.

alternative explanation is heterogeneity, i.e. single major genes are important in at least some families, but it is not the same gene in each family.

Heterogeneity is an emerging theme in consideration of the genetics of many psychiatric disorders. It is invoked to explain disparate results in schizophrenia and Alzheimer's disease as well as bipolar disorder. This explanation seems consistent with our knowledge of the genetics of other common diseases such as coronary artery disease, hypertension, epilepsy and diabetes. It is consistent, also, with our knowledge of the multiple possible origins of the *syndromes* of these disorders; that is, we know that many drugs and diseases may cause clinical manifestations identical to mania (Krauthammer & Klerman 1978) or depression (Wood et al 1988).

Age of onset may be useful in dividing affective illness into more genetically homogeneous subgroups. Early-onset probands have increased morbid risk of illness in relatives in some data sets (Weissman et al 1988, Strober et al 1988).

A birth-cohort effect has been observed in recent family studies: there is an increasing incidence of affective illness among persons born more recently (Klerman et al 1985). This appears to be true for schizoaffective and bipolar illness as well as unipolar (Gershon et al 1987b). It is true among relatives at risk to a greater degree than in the general population; this may be interpreted as a greater incidence of manifestation of illness among vulnerable persons, or (if vulnerability is single locus) greater penetrance.

Twin studies

Twin studies, as summarized over 50 years, show consistent evidence for heritability (Table 9.2). On average, monozygotic twin pairs show concordance 65% of the time and dizygotic twin pairs 14% of the time. Though the actual concordance figures vary widely (at least partially because of variation in diagnostic criteria), there is a consistent increased concordance in monozygotic as opposed to dizygotic twins. These figures are not age-corrected (though at least the Danish series reported by Bertelsen have passed through most of their life-span) and are reported as pairwise rather than probandwise concordance; thus they probably represent a conservative estimate of heritability. A representative statistic for heritability from twin studies is 59%, using the method of Holzinger (1929). This is comparable to the heritability of schizophrenia and also comparable to those for

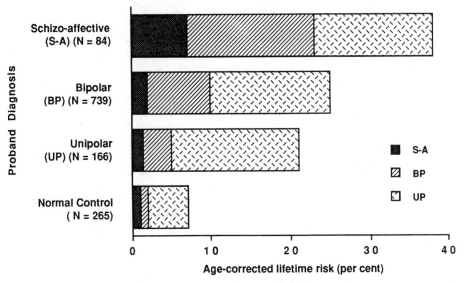

Fig. 9.1   Affective disorders in parents, siblings, adult offspring of probands, Bethesda, USA (Gershon et al 1982)

common diseases of other organ systems such as diabetes and hypertension. Evironmental influences may be related to age of onset, timing of onset of episodes and severity of course; however, the most important determinants of whether or not affective illness is manifest appear to be genetic.

The probands in twin studies include bipolar as well as unipolar patients. Bertelsen et al (1977) have shown that concordance in monozygotic twins increases with severity in this way: bipolar I probands 80% concordance; bipolar II probands 78% concor-

dance; unipolar probands with three or more episodes 59% concordance; unipolar probands with fewer than three episodes 33% concordance. This is consistent with the family study data noted above, which shows increased morbid risk of illness in relatives, rising with the severity of the diagnosis of the proband. Heritability for minor depression or neurotic/reactive depression has not been consistently demonstrable in twin studies (Torgersen 1986, Kendler et al 1987, Andrews et al 1990, Englund & Klein 1990, Torgersen 1990).

Table 9.2   Concordance rates for major affective disorder in monozygotic and dizygotic twins

Study	Monozygotic twins		Dizygotic twins	
	Concordant pairs total pairs	Concordance %	Concordant pairs total pairs	Concordance %
Luxenberger (1930)	3/4	75.0	0/13	0.0
Rosanoff et al (1935)	16/23	69.6	11/67	16.4
Slater (1953)	4/7	57.1	4/17	23.5
Kallman (1954)	25/27	92.6	13/55	23.6
Harvald & Hauge (1975)	10/15	66.7	2/40	5.0
Allen et al (1974)	5/15	33.3	0/34	0.0
Bertelsen (1979)	32/55	58.3	9/52	17.3
Torgersen (1986)	14/37	37.8	8/65	12.3
Totals	109/183	59.6%	47/343	13.7%

Adoption studies

Several adoption studies of affective illness have been performed. The results have been generally consistent with genetic hypotheses. Mendlewicz & Rainer (1977) report the largest set of bipolar probands (29), a group of control probands and a group of probands with poliomyelitis. The risk for affective disorder in the biological relatives of the bipolar probands was 31% as opposed to 2% in the relatives of the control probands. The risk in biological relatives of adopted bipolars was similar to the risk in relatives of bipolars who were not adopted (26%). Adoptive relatives did not show increased risk.

Two other adoption studies including a broader class of affective probands (Cadoret 1978, Wender et al 1986) showed evidence for genetic factors, but also possible environmental influences. In these studies adoptive relatives of affective probands had a tendency to excess affective illness themselves, compared with the adoptive relatives of controls. Von Knorring et al (1983) did not find concordance in psychopathology between adoptees and biological relatives when examining the records of 56 adoptees with depression (only five bipolar). Taken together, these data suggest that genetic factors are more clearly prominent in families with bipolar illness than in those without.

The affective disorder adoption studies also provide evidence for genetic factors in suicide. Biological relatives of adoptees with depression had a 15-fold increase in suicide in comparison with biological relatives of control adoptees (Wender et al 1986). A study by Schulsinger et al (1979) suggests that it is not only affective illness that confers a vulnerability to suicide, but that suicide itself may be 'heritable' independent of psychiatric diagnosis. This may be related to personality characteristics such as impulsivity, which in turn has been related to deficient central serotonergic neurotransmission clinically manifest in low cerebrospinal fluid 5-HIAA (Asberg et al 1986). Autopsy studies of central serotonin receptors in completed suicides are generally consistent with this view (Stanley et al 1986).

AFFECTIVE SPECTRUM

Major affective disorder clearly includes classic bipolar and unipolar disorders. As noted above, both bipolar and unipolar disorders are found in the relatives of bipolar probands but primarily unipolar disorders in the relatives of unipolars. This suggests that some unipolar illness is genetically related to bipolar illness and that some is not; however, we are unable at this time to distinguish the types on purely clinical grounds. Comments on other disorders follow.

Bipolar II disorders

Bipolar II disorder is defined by periods of depression plus hypomania without frank mania. Most investigators find that this disorder is genetically related to bipolar I and unipolar disorder. It is less clear that it is distinct in the sense of 'breeding true'. However there is some evidence in recent family studies for an excess of bipolar II illness in relatives of bipolar II probands (reviewed in Gershon et al 1987a). It has been demonstrated that bipolar II disorder tends to be a stable lifetime diagnosis (that is, patients do not frequently convert to bipolar I – Dunner et al 1976).

Rapid-cycling bipolar disorder

Rapid-cycling bipolar illness has been a subject of great theoretical and clinical interest. The entity was defined by Dunner & Fieve (1974) as including patients with four or more episodes per year, although individual patients have been described who have regular cycles of 48 hours. Rapid cyclers were found to be relatively resistant to lithium prophylaxis. A link with thyroid pathology has been proposed (Cowdry et al 1983, Bauer et al 1990). In some patients rapid cycling has been reported to be induced by tricyclic antidepressant treatment (Wehr & Goodwin 1979). Whether such patients are distinct from spontaneous rapid cyclers is controversial (Lewis & Winokur 1982, Angst 1985).

There is no evidence that genetic vulnerability to rapid-cycling bipolar illness is different from the genetic vulnerability to bipolarity alone. Dunner and colleagues (1977) reported family history data from rapid-cycling patients; 21 of 29 rapid-cycling patients had at least one affectively ill relative compared with 123 of 217 non-rapid-cyclers ($X^2 = 2.0$, NS). The number of relatives studied was too small to calculate meaningful morbid risk statistics. Since relatives were not directly interviewed we would expect an underestimate of illness frequency in both groups (Gershon & Guroff 1984).

In the NIMH series (Nurnberger et al 1988b), 29 out of 195 bipolar episodic schizoaffective patients were judged to be rapid cyclers (15%). 25 of the 29 were female (86%). The age-corrected morbid risk for major affective disorder was 23.5% in 179 relatives of rapid cyclers and 31.0% in 189 relatives of matched non-rapid cyclers ($X^2 = 2.6$, NS). The prevalence of rapid cycling itself was also not different in the two groups of relatives. Rapid cycling thus appears to arise from factors which are separable from the genetic vulnerability to bipolar illness and which do not lead to aggregation within families.

Unipolar mania

This entity includes bipolar I patients with no history of major depression. They tend to be male, are responsive to lithium and on further history or follow-up are usually found to have at least subclinical depressions. This group is not distinguishable from other bipolar I patients on the basis of family pattern of illness (Nurnberger et al 1979).

Seasonal affective disorder

Rosenthal et al (1985) have described patients with a pronounced seasonal pattern, usually with winter depressions and euthymia or hypomania during summer. This entity has not been well studied genetically.

Cyclothymia

This condition of repetitive high and low mood swings, generally not requiring clinical attention, is probably genetically related to bipolar disorder (Gershon et al 1982, Akiskal et al 1977).

Schizoaffective disorder

Patients with episodes of mood disorder with (RDC) psychotic symptoms are probably not different from those without in terms of risk of illness in family members (Rosenthal et al, 1980). Patients with episodes of mood-incongruent psychosis during depression or intermittent psychosis during euthymia (schizoaffective acute) have an increase in affective illness in relatives and an increase in schizophrenia in relatives (Gershon et al 1982). In the NIMH studies, this group has the highest genetic load (total risk for affective or schizophrenic illness in relatives) of any diagnostic category (Gershon et al 1988) and one suspects that they may carry genes for both disorders. Patients with chronic psychosis and superimposed episodes of mood disorder (schizoaffective chronic) also confer risk for both chronic psychosis and mood

disorder to relatives but have less overall genetic load (Table 9.3).

Schizophrenia

A number of studies include data on risk for bipolar illness in relatives of schizophrenics and vice versa. With the exception of Mendlewicz et al 1980, all studies have found that the risk of bipolar illness in relatives of schizophrenic probands was about 1% and that the risk of schizophrenic illness in relatives of bipolar probands was similarly about 1%. In each study where comparable data was obtained, the risk of homotypic illness was much greater (see Mendlewicz et al 1980, Baron et al 1982, Gershon et al 1988, Guze et al 1983, Frangos et al 1985 and Kendler et al 1985 for schizophrenic probands, Mendlewicz et al 1980, Baron et al 1982, Gershon et al 1982 and Rice et al 1987 for bipolar probands). However, some studies (including our own) have found an increase in depression in relatives of schizophrenic patients (Gershon et al 1988). This again suggests there are different types of depression on a genetic basis. It may be that some forms of schizophrenia spectrum disorder predispose to depression (or that the burden of coping with a schizophrenic relative brings on depression in some people).

The Kraepelinian dichotomy traditionally postulates clinical and genetic independence of manic-depressive illness and schizophrenia, although Kraepelin himself noted that the distinction in individual cases was often not clear-cut. The existence of schizoaffective disorder presents a challenge to this dichotomy, with its mixed clinical picture and increased morbid risks of both affective and schizophrenic disorders in relatives (Gershon et al 1988). Many of the dense pedigrees we have observed have both manic-depressive and schizophrenic individuals. Crow (1990) has proposed that the dichotomy is fundamentally in error, and that there is a single psychosis gene with a continuum of heritable expressions ranging between affective and schizophrenic syndromes. Other possibilities which could produce the clinical overlap in pedigrees include genetic heterogeneity, with at least one form producing both affective and schizophrenic clinical presentations, and multifactorial inheritance.

Dysthymia

Akiskal (1983) has suggested that this is a heterogeneous category including some unipolar depression

Table 9.3   Family studies of schizophrenia and schizoaffective disorder* (Gershon et al 1988)

Source, y	No. of relatives	Schizophrenia (chronic)	Schizophrenia (not chronic)	Schizoaffective (chronic)	Schizoaffective (not chronic)	Other psychosis†	Bipolar I and bipolar II	Unipolar
Angst et al 1979								
SA schizodominant	425	5.9‡	—	3.3§	—	—	5.8‖	—
SA affectdominant	416	4.6‡	—	2.9§	—	—	7.8‖	—
SA, with mania	539	5.9‡	—	4.1§	—	0.5	1.0	5.9
SA, without mania	336	4.2‡	—	1.2§	—	0	1.2	5.2
Mendlewicz et al 1980								
Schizophrenia	—	16.9‡	—	—	—	—	8.6‖	—
Schizoaffective	—	10.8‡	—	—	—	—	34.6‖	—
Bipolar	—	1.8‡	—	—	—	—	39.4‖	—
Unipolar	—	3.2‡	—	—	—	—	28.5‖	—
Baron et al 1982								
Schizophrenia	178.7	7.9	—	1.7¶	0#	—	0.6	4.5
SA mainly schizophrenic	73.2	4.1	—	0.7¶	0#	—	0	10.9
SA mainly affective	64.4	0	—	0¶	3.2#	—	1.6	26.5
Bipolar	135.2	0.7	—	0¶	1.5#	—	14.5	16.3
Unipolar	143.5	0	—	0.8¶	3.0#	—	2.2	17.7
Gershon et al 1982, 1988								
SA (acute)	69	4.9	0	1.6	5.8	3.2	11.7	16.4
Bipolar	738	0.3	0	0.1	1.6	0.6	7.2	14.9
Unipolar	165	0	0	0	0.7	4.4	2.9	16.7
Schizophrenia	108	3.1	0	0	5.0	3.1	1.3	14.7
SA (chronic)	129	1.7	0.8	2.5	0	6.7	8.8	9.3
Control	380	0.6	0	0	0.6	1.2	0.3	6.7
Abrams & Taylor 1983								
Schizophrenia	124.5	1.6	—	—	—	—	—	6.9**
Guze et al, 1983								
Schizophrenia	111	8.1	—	—	—	—	0	2.7
Unspecified psychosis	62	6.4	—	—	—	—	0	8.1
Other patients	1076	1.1	—	—	—	—	1.1	5.7
Frangos et al 1985								
Schizophrenia	572	3.3††	—	—	—	1.2	0.7‖	—
Control	694	0.6††	—	—	—	0.9	2.7‖	—
Kendler et al 1985								
Schizophrenia	723	3.7	0.1	1.4	—	3.4	1.2‡‡	6.0
Control	1056	0.2	0	0.1	—	0.3	0.3‡‡	7.6
Kendler et al 1986								
Schizophreniform	91	3.6	0	0	—	1.5	1.3‡‡	5.8
Schizoaffective	149	5.6	2.2	2.7	—	2.8	3.8‡‡	7.3
SA mainly schizophrenic	75	8.2	—	—	—	4.2	1.4‡‡	6.1
SA other or mainly affective	84	3.8	—	—	—	7.9	5.6‡‡	9.1

Table 9.3   Family studies of schizophrenia and schizoaffective disorder* — (Contd)

Source, y	No. of relatives	Morbid Risk in Relatives by Proband Diagnosis, %						
		Schizophrenia (chronic)	Schizophrenia (not chronic)	Schizoaffective (chronic)	Schizoaffective (not chronic)	Other psychosis†	Bipolar I and bipolar II	Unipolar
Rice et al 1987								
SA bipolar	139	0.7§§	—	0.7‖‖	0¶¶	—	9.4	23.0##
SA depressed	72	2.8§§	—	0‖‖	0¶¶	—	6.9	22.2##
Bipolar I	567	1.1§§	—	0.5‖‖	0.2¶¶	—	10.4	23.1##
Bipolar II	271	0.4§§	—	0.4‖‖	0¶¶	—	11.1	26.9##
Major depressive disorder	1176	0.3§§	—	0.2‖‖	0.3¶¶	—	5.4	28.6##

*SA indicates schizoaffective disorder

†Includes other psychiatric disorders requiring hospitalization

‡All schizophrenia

§All schizoaffective

‖All affective

¶Schizoaffective (mainly schizophrenic)

#Schizoaffective (mainly affective)

**Unipolar and bipolar

††'Definite' diagnoses

‡‡Bipolar I only

§§Schizophrenia (chronicity not specified)

‖‖Schizoaffective (bipolar)

¶¶Schizoaffective (depressed)

##Major depressive disorder

with residual symptoms and some characterologic depressive disorders. Definitive family studies remain to be performed. These disorders do not seem to aggregate in relatives of unipolar or bipolar patients (Gershon et al 1982).

Minor depression

Minor depressive episodes are no more likely to be found in the relatives of affective probands than in the relatives of controls, and thus are not part of the genetic spectrum of major affective disorder (Gershon et al 1982).

Other disorders

Borderline personality disorder

Available evidence from family studies (Loranger et al 1982, Baron et al 1985) suggests that affective disorder as well as borderline personality disorder aggregate in the families of probands with borderline characteristics themselves.

Eating disorders

Family studies of anorexia and bulimia have generally found excess affective illness in relatives. Our own study found risks for affective disorder in relatives of anorexics very similar to the risks in relatives of bipolar probands (Gershon et al 1984). An increase in eating disorders themselves was also found in relatives. A study in normal-weight bulimics did not find excess affective illness in relatives (Stern et al 1984) though a later NIMH series did (Kassett et al 1989). It is difficult to assemble a population of eating disorder probands who do not also have depression to test the relation of the two types of disorders further.

Attention-deficit disorder

Children with attention-deficit disorder appear to have increased depression in their relatives (Biederman et al 1987). The opposite has not been demonstrated (bipolar/unipolar probands have not been reported to have increased risk of attention-deficit disorder in their offspring). Again this suggests that the type of depression that is seen in relatives of those with other disorders may be distinct.

Alcoholism

Alcoholism is probably not genetically related to bipolar illness. Winokur (Winokur et al 1971) has assembled evidence that unipolar depressive patients with alcoholic or sociopathic relatives are distinct from those without (see review in Nurnberger & Gershon 1984).

LINKAGE AND ASSOCIATION STUDIES

Linkage

Despite the effort devoted to gene-mapping studies in bipolar illness, the studies to date have not yielded consistently reproducible linkages. With this perspective, we summarize the available reports of linkage and discuss the current state of genetic mapping methods relevant to these diseases.

Linkage has been reported to various loci, most notably on the X-chromosome, where the first positive reports were of linkage to colour-blindness (Reich et al 1969, Baron et al 1987). However, non-replications have also been reported in a sizeable series of pedigrees (Gershon et al 1979, Berrettini et al 1990). Also the reported linkage in some pedigrees to both colour-blindness *and* Xg (Mendlewicz & Fleiss 1974) must be incorrect, since Xg and colour-blindness are at opposite ends of the X chromosome. Recent re-analysis of the marker genotypes in these pedigrees suggests a systematic genotyping error in the original analysis, since Xg and colour-blindness are linked to *each other* in these data (Gershon 1991).

Risch & Baron (1982) re-analysed all the published data, using methods which allowed for multigenerational pedigrees and variable penetrance. They also tested for linkage in the presence of heterogeneity and concluded that, if all the reported pedigrees were pooled together, they were consistent with linkage with heterogeneity of bipolar disorder to colour-blindness, and no linkage to Xg. Since then the inconsistency among reports of linkage to the X-chromosome has persisted. Baron et al (1987) found linkage with no recombination of bipolar disorder with colour-blindness and glucose-6-phosphate dehydrogenase (on chromosomal region Xq28) in four Sephardic pedigrees but not in one Ashkenazi pedigree in Israel.

Mendlewicz et al (1987) found loose linkage in Belgium of bipolar disorder to factor IX (FIX), which is at Xq27, 30–35 cm from colour-blindness/G6PD. Berrettini et al (1990) *excluded* linkage in nine new US pedigrees to the Xq28 region, using DNA probes of three loci (F8, DXS52, DXS15). In the same pedigrees, Gejman et al (1990) found no linkage to FIX and to two loci between FIX and Xq28 (DXS98, DXS105).

Other linkages to bipolar illness have been reported, but the most recent evidence is not supportive. Egeland et al (1987) reported that, in an Amish pedigree in Pennsylvania, bipolar illness was linked to markers of 11p15. This has not been replicated in other pedigrees; furthermore, in extensions of the original Amish pedigree and in new cases in the original pedigree, the linkage did not hold up (Kelsoe et al 1989).

Linkage of HLA to bipolar and unipolar illness has been reported but several negative studies make this locus an unlikely candidate for affective disorder (reviewed by Gershon et al 1987a).

Association

Association refers to identification of a particular (molecular) characteristic more frequent in patients than controls; this represents an alternative molecular strategy to linkage, which identifies a chromosomal region (usually of many millions of base pairs) containing an illness gene. This alternative is particularly attractive for candidate gene hypotheses. Association may be due to linkage disequilibrium or to the identity of the associated region with the disease gene. The chromosomal region of linkage disequilibrium will generally be considerably smaller than the region within which linkage is detectable in pedigrees (see Bodmer 1986).

The statistical power of association studies (to detect an abnormality) is superior to that of linkage studies for very heterogeneous disorders (Gershon et al 1989). For well-characterized candidate genes, particularly those with known genomic sequences, association has become a preferred test for ruling in or out an aetiological role in illness.

Despite the statistical power of molecular association methods, they have not been successful in psychiatry. Some initial positive reports of associations of illness with restriction-fragment-length polymorphisms (RFLPs) (Blum et al 1990, Leboyer et al 1990) have not yet been confirmed by others (Korner et al 1990, Bolos et al 1990). The base pair sequence differences which determine an RFLP represent only a small fraction of the possible molecular sequence differences, and it is desirable to have scanning of the base pairs of an entire expressed gene and flanking sequences in a series of patients and controls.

Recent developments do allow screening of genomic sequences in a series of individuals much more efficiently than was previously possible (Rossiter & Caskey 1990). These methods include denaturing gradient gel electrophoresis (DGGE) of amplified genomic fragments from different individuals (Sheffield et al 1989, Kogan & Gitschier 1990, Traystman et al 1990) and genomic amplification with transcript sequencing (GAWTS) (Stoflet et al 1988, Bottema et al 1989). The amplifications are done by polymerase chain reaction (PCR). We expect these methods will be attempted with various neurotransmitter receptor molecules and other candidate genes in affective disorders.

PATHOPHYSIOLOGICAL MARKER STUDIES

Trait markers should: 1) separate patients from controls, even when patients are in the well state and medication free; 2) be heritable, based on twin studies or family studies; 3) be associated with illness within pedigrees: ie they should be found in ill relatives; they will also be found in some well relatives ('carriers') especially those who have not passed completely through the age of risk; ill relatives without the marker (presumed phenocopies) should not be found more often than the incidence of disorder within the general population; 4) separate high-risk from low-risk young people; that is, a) offspring of patients should show the trait more than offspring of controls, and b) within offspring at risk, the distribution of the trait should separate those at greater risk from those at lower risk (this requires validation by follow-up studies). These

Table 9.4 Current status of proposed genetic vulnerability markers for major affective disorders

Finding	Patient/control trait difference	Heritability	Pedigree Study	High-risk Study	Reference
Platelet MAO	Yes	Yes	Negative	No data	Rice et al 1984
CSF 5-HIAA	Unclear	Possibly	No data	No data	Van Praag & de Haan 1979 Oxenstierna et al 1986
Platelet α-adrenoceptor	Possibly	Yes	Possibly	No data	Siever et al 1984 Kafka et al 1980 Propping & Friedl 1983 Healy et al 1982 Garcia-Sevilla et al 1981, 1986 Wood and Coppen 1983 Daiguji et al 1981
Lymphoblast β-receptor	Possibly	Yes	Possibly	No data	Wright et al 1984 Berrettini et al 1987
Lithium erythrocyte/plasma ratio	Possibly	Yes	Negative	No data	Dorus et al 1979 1983 Shaughnessy et al 1985
Platelet binding [H^3] IMI	No	Possibly	No data	No data	Berrettini et al 1982 Mellerup et al 1982 Langer et al 1986 Suranyi-Cadotte et al 1982 Friedl & Propping 1984
Duarte PC 1 brain protein	Yes	Possibly	No data	No data	Comings 1979
Melatonin suppression by light	Yes	Possibly	No data	Yes	Lewy et al 1985 Nurnberger et al 1988a
Cholinergic REM induction	Yes	Yes	Yes	No data	(see Table 9.5)
Urinary tyramine excretion	Yes	No data	No data	No data	Bonham-Carter et al 1980
Electrodermal response	Yes	Yes	No data	Negative	Zahn et al 1989

and other clinical genetic strategies are discussed in more detail in Goldin et al 1986 and Gershon & Goldin 1986.

The quest for the physiological basis of genetic vulnerability to mood disorder has led in many different directions. Some of this work is summarized in Table 9.4. Most putative biological vulnerability markers have not passed the tests of heritability and association with illness within pedigrees. A discussion of some of the more notable work in this area follows:

Neurotransmitter receptor

Platelet alpha adrenoceptor density appears to be heritable and associated with illness but has not been studied in families (Kafka et al 1980, Propping & Friedl 1983). Beta-receptor density on lymphoblasts has been found to be reduced in bipolar patients in the work of Wright et al (1984), but only a few ill relatives have been studied. These also had decreased density, whereas well relatives did not. Our group, however, was unable to replicate this finding (Berrettini et al 1987).

Lithium transport

Dorus et al (1979, 1983) found that if erythrocyte plasma lithium ratio and affective illness are considered as a single trait, no combination of single-locus and multifactorial inheritance could describe this trait, but that if the psychiatric criterion was changed to 'ever hospitalized', a single locus genetic model would fit. These data, however, have a modest number of ill relatives evaluated for lithium transport, and no probands evaluated, so they cannot be accepted as a demonstration of segregation of lithium transport with illness in pedigrees. Waters et al (1983b), studying 73 individuals from 12 affective disorder families, found no segregation of affective illness with inhibition of lithium efflux by phloretin, which is thought to measure the same sodium–lithium countertransport system as the lithium erythrocyte-plasma ratio. Egeland et al (1984) found no segregation of lithium erythrocyte-plasma ratio with affective illness in a large Amish pedigree.

Cholinergic REM induction

Sleep disturbance is common in depression; one of the most consistent observations is the shortening of REM latency. REM may be induced in volunteer subjects by an injection of a small dose of physostigmine or arecoline during sleep. In a series of studies, bipolar patients have been shown to be more sensitive than controls to the REM inducing effects of arecoline, even when euthymic and off all medication. Further studies have shown that sensitivity to REM induction may be heritable and that it associates with affective disorder within pedigrees (Table 9.5). These studies suggest central muscarinic cholinergic supersensitivity in brainstem areas in bipolar illness. However, methodological issues require resolution, and the precise neurochemical and anatomical interpretation of these studies remains to be elucidated.

Light suppression of melatonin

Melatonin is secreted at high levels during the night and barely detectable levels during daytime. Night-time melatonin secretion may be suppressed by 500 lux light. Bipolar patients are more sensitive to this effect of light, even when euthymic and medication-free (Lewy et al 1985). This appears to be true of young people with a bipolar parent also, prior to any manifestation of illness in that group (Nurnberger et al 1988a). The studies of light sensitivity appear to reflect changes in the multisynaptic pathway from the retina to the pineal, perhaps at the level of the suprachiasmatic nucleus. The secretion of melatonin has not been demonstrated to have clear functional consequences in man so far. It is likely to be related, however, to the timing of multiple circadian processes which are disregulated in affective disorder.

HIGH-RISK STUDIES

Retrospective analysis of patients and controls is a poor strategy for determining predictors of illness. In clinical interviews of families, one often finds that there are as many hypotheses about the aetiology and onset of a condition as there are informants. Even the temporal order of events is subject to unconscious falsification. Methodological problems of such studies have been summarized elsewhere (Paykel 1982). Cross-sectional studies of offspring of patients compared with offspring of controls answer these objections. However, such studies do not allow the investigator to differentiate between predictors of illness and non-specific characteristics of life in a family with an ill person. High risk studies allow this differentiation. The high-risk strategy is equally important in confirming putative genetic markers for vulnerability to an illness (Goldin et al 1986). Examining markers in populations of ill patients versus controls is susceptible to errors because of 1) the

Table 9.5 Studies of cholinergic REM induction

Study	Drug	Subjects	Findings
Sitaram et al 1980	Arecoline HBr 0.5 mg	19 patients (remitted, BP and UP) 16 controls	Patients were more sensitive
	Arecoline HBr 1.0 mg	9 patients 10 controls	Patients were more sensitive
Sitaram et al 1981, 1982	Arecoline HBr 0.5 mg	7 acutely depressed patients 5 volunteers with personal or family history	Acutely depressed similar to remitted; at risk similar
Nurnberger et al 1983	Arecoline HBr 0.5 mg	7 monozygotic twin pairs	Twins concordant for REM induction time but not for baseline REM–REM interval
Berger et al 1983	Physostigmine 0.5 mg	45 patients 8 controls	No difference in REM induction time patients awakened more frequently
Dube et al 1985	Arecoline 0.5 mg	20 1° MDD 19 1° MDD 2° Anx 18 1° Anx 14 1° Anx 2° MDD 26 normal controls	1° MDD more sensitive than controls and 1° Anx
Jones et al	Arecoline 0.5 mg	53 depressed patients 17 psychiatric controls 20 normal controls	Endogenous depressives more sensitive
Krieg & Berger 1987	RS 86 1.5 mg orally	8 depressed patients 8 controls	Patients more sensitive (REM latency)
Sitaram et al 1987	Arecoline 0.5 mg	35 ill relatives 31 well relatives	Ill relatives more sensitive than well
Nurnberger et al 1989	Arecoline 0.5 mg	18 remitted bipolar patients 14 controls	Patients more sensitive

effects of the illness itself; and 2) the effects of treatment. Such errors might be false positives or false negatives (treatment effects, for instance, may obscure real group differences). Studying genetically vulnerable individuals who have not yet manifested illness avoids these pitfalls.

A number of investigators have examined offspring of manic-depressive patients in cross-sectional designs (Cytryn et al 1984, Decina et al 1983, Gaensbauer et al 1984, Gershon et al 1985, McNeil & Kaij 1979, McNeil et al 1983, Waters et al 1983a, Weissman et al 1984a, Winters et al 1981, Zahn-Waxler et al 1984).

Decina et al (1983) at the New York State Psychiatric Institute, studied 7- to 14-year old children of 18 bipolar manic-depressive parents compared with 18 control children screened to ensure negative family history. 16 of the index children received a DSM-III or RDC diagnosis by consensus of interviews blind to the family history; the index children also manifested more verbal-performance discrepancies on the WISC-R

(Wechsler Intelligence Scale for Children — Revised Version), a higher number of colour/movement responses on the Rorschach (consistent with a hypothesis about the relationship of colour responses to affect), and more left-handedness. These children are being followed prospectively. McNeil, Kaij and co-workers (McNeil & Kaij 1979, McNeil et al 1983) have described the initial phases of a long-term follow-up of 88 offspring of mothers with a history of non-organic psychosis (six subcategories); the study began during the pregnancy of the mother and the offspring are still quite young. Waters et al (1983a) studied 55 offspring of 17 bipolar patients and found 32% to have a major affective diagnosis and 13% to have minor depression. Perinatal and educational problems were associated with an early onset (and with low IQ) but not with absolute risk. No control group was studied. Cytryn et al (1984) compared 19 children of 13 bipolar or unipolar parents with 21 children of 15 normal parents (the children ranged in age from 5 to 15 years old.

Either 9 or 11 of the index families had more than one child depressed (depending on criteria) compared with 3 out of 13 control families ($p < 0.05$).

One set of studies examined a small number of infants and young children with a bipolar parent (Davenport et al 1984, Gaensbauer et al 1984, Zahn-Waxler et al 1984), finding evidence of social and affective disturbances. Weissman et al (1984a) performed a family history study of 194 children aged 6–18 years: 74 children of two ill parents, 60 children of one ill parent (unipolar), and 60 children of controls. Parents were interviewed, but the children were not directly examined. A significant relationship was found between parental illness and diagnoses in the children (for both depression and any psychiatric diagnosis, in particular attention-deficit disorder and separation anxiety). Additional predictors of risk in offspring were: early-onset illness in the proband; increased incidence of illness in the proband's first-degree relatives; and single, widowed or divorced marital status in the proband.

Gershon et al (1985) did not find a significant difference in affective diagnoses between 29 children of bipolar parents and 37 children of controls (the children ranged in age from 6–17 years old). There was an increase in all DSM-III diagnoses in the index group ($p < 0.05$, one tailed). The notable element of this study was the high rate of psychiatric diagnoses in control children (51%), although there was no evidence of increased morbid risk of affective illness in the control families. The authors suggested that the general incidence of psychiatric disorders in childhood might be underestimated.

Akiskal et al (1985) reported a 3-year follow-up study of offspring of affectively ill patients who presented for evaluation; about half the sample showed indications of bipolarity (including pharmacologically induced hypomania) during the follow-up period.

Depue et al (1981) reported the development and validation of a self-report instrument, the General Behavior Inventory (GBI), to measure subclinical hypomania and depression with the purpose of identifying persons at risk for bipolar mood disorder. This instrument was found to be capable of identifying subjects from a college population as 'cases' who would also meet RDC criteria for an affective disorder (Depue et al 1981). A 19-month follow-up study confirmed continued psychiatric impairment in these subjects (Klein & Depue 1984). Increased cortisol excretion has been reported in GBI cases (Depue et al 1985) as has slower recovery from stressful events. An increase in GBI-defined cyclothymia (Klein & Depue 1985) has been found in offspring of bipolar patients. However, it is not clear from the published reports of these studies whether the authors have identified a cyclothymic subgroup which is distinct from persons having more severe affective disorder or whether the various validation studies include abnormalities related to the presence of major depressives in their identified subgroup.

We have begun a long-term follow-up study of adolescent and young adult offspring of bipolar parents (Nurnberger et al 1988c). We studied 15- to 25-year olds because this is the decade of greatest increase in new cases of bipolar illness in data from the National Institutes of Mental Health (NIMH) family study (Gershon et al 1982). Probands were specified as bipolar (or episodic schizoaffective). The final group of controls comprised 39 unrelated persons; the 'one ill parent' group included 38 offspring from 23 families; the '1+ or 2 ill parents' group included 15 offspring from nine families. Excluding subjects with diagnoses that led to elimination of controls from the study, more offspring of patients than controls had a diagnosed Axis I disorder (25 of 40 as compared to 12 of 39; $X^2 = 6.76$, df = 2, $p < 0.01$); this is consistent with previous reports, although differences in ascertainment of the groups should be noted. During the course of a 2-year follow-up five high risk offspring developed major affective disorders as compared with none of the controls. The Sensation-Seeking Scale (Zuckerman, 1971, Zuckerman, 1985), in total score and in two subscales, differentiated the high-risk from the control group. The hypomania subscale on the GBI did likewise. Offspring of bipolar parents may be more prone to respond to dysphoric feeling states by 'disinhibitory' behavior. It may be that a combination of dysphoria and disinhibitory responses will serve as a predictive marker for major mood disorder; this hypothesis must be tested in follow up studies.

EMPIRICAL DATA FOR GENETIC COUNSELLING

Molecular genetic studies hold great promise in the future for families with affective disorder, particularly bipolar disorder. The availability of DNA markers would make genetic counselling for these disorders much more precise. Such counselling has already begun for families with Huntington's disease. At present, however, such markers are not clinically useful for affective disorder. This is also the case for aetiological markers. Consequently genetic counselling must be based on empirical risk figures.

Severe affective disorder affects about 7% of the population on a lifetime basis (about 5% unipolar and about 2% bipolar I and II) (Gershon et al 1982). Risk is increased to about 20% in first-degree relatives of unipolar patients and 25% in first-degree relatives of bipolar patients. It appears to be 25–40% in relatives of schizoaffective patients. The risk to offspring of two affectively ill parents is in excess of 50%. Overall risk figures appear to be rising in recent years, but more so in relatives of patients than in the general population (keeping at about a 3:1 ratio). Thus, for relatives born since 1940, risk in relatives of bipolar patients is probably 35% rather than 25%. Families with affectively ill members should educate themselves regarding the symptoms and treatment for the disorder since early recognition and intervention may prevent the social disruption consequent to these disorders. New methods presently available may elucidate genetic vulnerability markers and, ultimately, bring more specifically targeted treatment strategies.

ACKNOWLEDGMENT

Pablo V. Gejman MD contributed his molecular expertise and advice to this manuscript.

REFERENCES

Abrams R, Taylor MA 1983 The genetics of schizophrenia: A reassessment using modern criteria. American Journal of Psychiatry 140: 171–175

Akiskal H S 1983 Dysthymic disorder: psychopathology of proposed chronic depressive subtypes. American Journal of Psychiatry 140: 11–20

Akiskal H S Djenderedjian A H, Rosenthal R H 1977 Cyclothymic disorder: validating criteria for inclusion in the bipolar affective group. American Journal of Psychiatry 134: 1227–1233

Akiskal H S, Downs J, Jordan P, Watson S, Daugherty D, Pruitt D B 1985 Affective disorder in referred children and younger siblings of manic depressives. Mode of onset and prospective course. Archives General Psychiatry 42: 996–1003

Allen M G, Cohen S, Pollin W, Greenspan S I 1974 Affective illness in veteran twins: a diagnostic review. American Journal of Psychiatry 131: 1234–1239

Andrews G, Stewart G, Allen R, Henderson A S 1990 The genetics of six neurotic disorders: a twin study. Journal of Affective Disorders 19: 23–29

Angst J 1985 Switch from depression to mania – a record study over decades between 1920 and 1981. Psychopathology 18: 140–154

Angst J, Felder W, Lohmeyer B 1979 Schizoaffective disorders: results of a genetic investigation I. Journal of Affective Disorders 1: 139–153

Angst J, Felder W, Lohmeyer B 1979 Are schizoaffective psychoses heterogeneous? II. Results of a genetic investigation. Journal of Affective Disorders 1: 155–165

Angst J, Frey, R, Lohmeyer B, Zerben-Rudin E 1980 Bipolar manic depressive psychoses: results of a genetic investigation. Human Genetics 55: 237–254

Asberg M, Nordstrom P, Bendz-Traskman L 1986 Cerebrospinal fluid studies in suicide. In: Mann, Stanley (eds) Psychobiology of suicidal behavior. New York Academy of Sciences, New York, p 243–255

Baron M, Gruen R, Asnis L, Kane J 1982 Schizoaffective illness, schizophrenia and affective disorders: Morbidity risk and genetic transmission. Acta Psychiatrica Scandinavica 65: 253–262

Baron M, Gruen M A, Asnis M S, Lord S 1985 Familial transmission of schizotypal and borderline personality disorders. American Journal of Psychiatry 142: 927–933

Baron M, Risch N, Hamburger R, Mandel B, Kushner S, Newman M, Drumer D, Belmaker R H 1987 Genetic linkage between X-chromosome markers and bipolar affective illness. Nature 326: 289–292

Bauer M S, Whybrow P C, Winokur A 1990 Rapid cycling bipolar affective disorder. I. Association with grade I hypothyroidism. Archives of General Psychiatry 47: 427–432

Berger M, Lund R, Bronisch T, von Zerssen D 1983 REM latency in neurotic and endogenous depression and the cholinergic REM induction test. Psychiatry Research 10: 113–123

Berrettini W H, Nurnberger J I Jr, Post R M, Gershon E S 1982 Platelet 3H-imipramine binding in euthymic bipolar patients. Psychiatry Research 7: 215–219

Berrettini W H, Cappellari C B, Nurnberger J I Jr, Gershon E S 1987 Beta-adrenergic receptors on lymphoblasts. A study of manic-depressive illness. Neuropsychobiology 17: 15–18

Berrettini W H, Goldin L R, Gelernter J, Gejman P V, Gershon E S, Detera-Wadleigh S 1990 X-chromosome markers and manic-depressive illness. Rejection of linkage to $X_{gg}28$ in nine bipolar pedigrees. Archives of General Psychiatry 47: 366–373

Bertelsen A, Harvald B, Hauge M 1977 A Danish twin study of manic-depressive disorders. British Journal Psychiatry 130: 330–351

Biederman J, Munir K, Knee D, Armentano M, Autor S, Waternaux C, Tsuang M 1987 A family study of patients with attention deficit disorder and normal controls. Journal of Psychiatric Research 20: 263–274

Blum K, Noble E P, Sheridan P J, Montgomery A, Ritchie T, Jagadeeswaran P, Nogami H, Briggs A H, Cohn J B 1990 Allelic association of human dopamine D2 receptor gene in alcoholism. Journal of the American Medical Association 263: 2055–2060

Bodmer W F 1986. Human genetics: The molecular challenge. Cold Spring Harbor Symposia on Quantitative Biology 51: 1–13

Bolos A M, Dean M, Brown G L, Goldman D 1990 Population and pedigree studies rule out a widespread association between the dopamine D2 receptor gene and alcoholism. American Journal of Human Genetics 47: (0187) A49

Bonham-Carter S M, Reveley M A, Sandler M, Dewhurst J, Little B C, Hayworth J, Priest R G 1980 Decreased urinary output of conjugated tyramine is associated with lifetime vulnerability to depressive illness. Psychiatry Research 3: 13–22

Bottema C D, Koeberl D D, Sommer S S 1989 Direct carrier testing in 14 families with haemophilia b. Lancet 2: 526–529

Cadoret R J 1978 Evidence for genetic inheritance of primary affective disorder in adoptees. American Journal of Psychiatry 135: 463–466

Comings D E 1979 Pc 1 Duarte, a common polymorphism of a human brain protein, and its relationship to depressive disease and multiple sclerosis. Nature 227: 28–32

Cowdry R W, Wehr T A, Zis A P, Goodwin F K 1983 Thyroid abnormalities associated with rapid-cycling bipolar illness. Archives of General Psychiatry 40: 414–424

Crow T J 1990 The continuum of psychosis and its genetic origins – The sixty-fifth Maudsley lecture. British Journal of Psychiatry 156: 788–797

Crtryn L, McKnew D H, Zahn-Waxler C, Radke-Yarrow M, Gaensbauer T J, Harmon R J, Lamour M 1984 A developmental view of affective disturbances in the children of affectively ill parents. American Journal of Psychiatry 141: 219–222

Daiguji M, Meltzer Y H, Tong C, U'Pritchard D C, Young M, Kravitz H 1981 Alpha 2-adrenergic receptors in platelet membranes of depressed patients: no change in number or 3H-yohimbine affinity. Life Sciences 29: 2059–2064

Davenport Y B, Zahn-Waxler C, Adland M L, Mayfield A 1984 Early child-rearing practices in families with a manic-depressive parent. American Journal of Psychiatry 141: 230–235

Decina P, Kestenbaum C J, Farber S, Kron L, Gargan M, Seckeim H A, Fieve R R 1983 Clinical and psychological assessment of children of bipolar probands. American Journal of Psychiatry 140: 548–553

Depue R A, Slater J F, Wolfstetter-Kausch H, Klein D, Goplerud E, Farr D 1981 A behavioral paradigm for identifying persons at risk for bipolar depressive disorder: A conceptual framework and five validation studies. Journal of Abnormal Psychology Monographs 90: 381–437

Depue R A, Kleiman R M, Davis P, Hutchinson M, Krauss S P 1985 The behavioral high-risk paradigm and bipolar affective disorder, VIII. Serum free cortisol in nonpatient cyclothymic subjects selected by the general behavior inventory. American Journal of Psychiatry 142: 175–181

Donis-Keller H, Green P, Helms C, Cartinhour S, Weiffenbach B, Stephens K, Keith T P, Bowden D W, Smith D R, Lander E S 1987 A genetic linkage map of the human genome. Cell 51: 319–337

Dorus E, Pandey G N, Shaughnessey R, Davis J M 1979 Low platelet monoamine oxidase activity, high red blood cell lithium ratio, and affective disorders: a multivariate assessment of genetic vulnerability to affective disorder. Biological Psychiatry 14: 989–994

Dorus E, Cox N J, Gibbon R D, Shaughnessy R, Pandey G N, Cloninger C R 1983 Lithium ion transport and affective disorders within families of bipolar patients. Archives of General Psychology 40: 545–552

Dube S, Kumar N, Ettedgui E, Pohl R, Jones D, Sitaram N 1985 Cholinergic REM induction response; separation of anxiety and depression. Biological Psychiatry 20: 408–418

Dunner D L, Fieve R R 1974 Clinical factors in lithium carbonate prophylaxis failure. Archives of General Psychiatry 30: 229–233

Dunner D L, Fleiss J L, Fieve R R 1976 The course of development of mania in patients with recurrent depression. American Journal of Psychiatry 133: 905–908

Dunner D L, Patrick V, Fieve R R 1977 Rapid cycling manic depressive patients. Comprehensive Psychiatry 18: 561

Egeland J, Frazer A, Kidd K 1984. Affective disorders among the Amish. III. Na-Li counterflow and COMT in bipolar pedigrees. American Journal of Psychiatry 141: 1049–1054

Egeland J A, Gerhard D S, Pauls D L, Sussex J N, Kidd K K, Allen C R, Hostetter A M, Housman D E 1987 Nature 325: 783–787

Englund S A, Klein D N 1990 The genetics of neurotic-reactive depression: a reanalysis of Shapiro's (1970) twin study using diagnostic criteria. Journal of Affective Disorders 18: 247–252

Frangos E, Althanassenas G, Tsitourides S, Karsanou N, Alexandrakou P 1985 Prevalence of DSM-III schizophrenia among the first-degree relatives of schizophrenic probands. Acta Psychiatrica Scandinavica 72: 382–386

Friedl W, Propping P 1984 3H-imipramine binding in human platelets, a study in normal twins. Psychiatry Research 11: 279–285

Gaensbauer T J, Harmon R J, Cytryn L, McKnew D H 1984 Social and affective development in infants with a manic-depressive parent. American Journal of Psychiatry 141: 223–229

Garcia-Sevilla J A, Zis A P, Hollingsworth M A, Greden J F, Smith C B 1981 Platelet alpha 2-adrenergic receptors in major depressive disorder. Binding of tritiated clonidine before and after tricyclic antidepressant drug treatment. Archives of General Psychiatry 38: 1327–1333

Garcia-Sevilla J, Guimon J, Garcia-Vallejo P, Fuster M J 1986 Biochemical and functional evidence of supersensitive platelet alpha 2-adrenoceptors in major affective disorder. Effect of long-term lithium carbonate treatment. Archives of General Psychiatry 43: 51–57

Gejman P V, Detera-Wadleigh S, Martinez M M, Berrettini W D, Goldin L R, Gelernter J, Hsieh W T, Gershon E S 1990 Manic depressive illness not linked to factor IX region in an independent series of pedigrees. Genomics 8: 648–655

Gershon E S 1984 Letter to the editor: What is the familial morbid risk of major depression? Archives of General Psychiatry 41: 103–105

Gershon E S 1991 Marker genotyping errors in old data on X-linkage in bipolar illness. Biological Psychiatry in press

Gershon E S, Guroff J J 1984 Information from relatives: diagnosis of affective disorders. Archives of General Psychiatry 41: 173–184

Gershon E S, Baron M, Leckman J F 1975 Genetic models of the transmission of affective disorders. Journal of Psychiatric Research 12: 301–317

Gershon E S, Targum S D, Matthysse S, Bunney W E Jr 1979 Color blindness not closely linked to bipolar illness. Archives of General Psychiatry 36: 1423–1434

Gershon E S, Goldin L R, Weissman M M, Nurnberger J I Jr 1981 Family and genetic studies of affective disorders in the Eastern United States: A provisional summary. In: Perris C, Struwe G, Jansson B (eds) Biological psychiatry. Elsevier, Amsterdam, p 157–162

Gershon E S, Hamovit J, Guroff J J, Dibble E, Leckman J F, Sceery W, Targum S D, Nurnberger J I Jr, Goldin L R, Bunney W E Jr 1982 A family study of schizoaffective, bipolar I, bipolar II, unipolar, and normal control probands. Archives of General Psychiatry 39: 1157–1167

Gershon E S, Schreiber J L, Hamovit J R, Dibble E D, Kaye E, Nurnberger J I Jr, Andersen A E, Ebert M 1984 Clinical findings in patients with anorexia nervosa and affective illness in their relatives. American Journal of Psychiatry 141: 1419–1422

Gershon E S, McKnew D, Cytryn L, Hamovit J, Schreiber J, Hibbs E, Pellegrini D 1985 Diagnosis in school-age children of bipolar affective disorder patients and normal controls. Journal of Affective Disorders 8: 283–291

Gershon E S, Goldin L R 1986 Clinical methods in psychiatric genetics; I. Robustness of genetic marker investigative strategies. Acta Psychiatrica Scandinavica 74:113–118

Gershon E S, Berrettini W, Nurnberger J I Jr, Goldin L R 1987a Genetics of affective illness. In: Meltzer H Y (ed) Psychopharmacology: A Third Generation of Progress. Raven Press, New York, p 481–491

Gershon E S, Hamovit J H, Guroff J J, Nurnberger J I Jr, 1987b Birth-cohort changes in manic and depressive disorders in relatives of bipolar and schizoaffective patients. Archives of General Psychiatry 44: 314–319

Gershon E S, DeLisi L E, Hamovit J, Nurnberger J I Jr, Maxwell M E, Schreiber J, Dauphinais D, Dingman C W II, Guroff J J 1988 A controlled family study of chronic psychoses: Schizophrenia and schizoaffective disorder. Archives of General Psychiatry, 45: 328–336

Gershon E S, Martinez M, Goldin L, Gelernter J, Silver J 1989 Detection of marker associations with a dominant disease gene in genetically complex and heterogeneous diseases. American Journal of Human Genetics 45: 578–585

Goetzl V, Green R, Whybrow P, Jackson R 1974. X-linkage revisited: A further family study of manic depressive illness. Archives of General Psychiatry 31: 665–673

Goldin L R, Nurnberger J I Jr, Gershon E S 1986 Clinical methods in psychiatric genetics II – The high risk approach. Acta Psychiatrica Scandinavica 74: 119–128

Guze S B, Cloninger C R, Martin R L, Clayton P J 1983 A follow-up and family study of schizophrenia. Archives of General Psychiatry 40: 1273–1276

Harvald B, Hauge M 1975. In: Neal J V, Shaw M W, Shull W J (eds) Genetics and the epidemiology of chronic diseases. PHS Publication No. 1163. US DHEW, Washington, DC, p 61–76

Healy D, Carney P A, Leonard B E 1982 Monoamine-related markers of depression: changes following treatment. Journal of Psychiatric Research 17: 251–260

Helzer J E, Winokur G 1974 A family interview study of male manic-depressives. Archives of General Psychiatry 31: 73–77

Holzinger K J 1929 The relative effect of nature and nurture influences on twin differences. Journal of Educational Psychology 20: 241

James N M, Chapman C J 1975 A genetic study of bipolar affective disorder. British Journal of Psychiatry 126: 449–456

Johnson G F S, Leeman M M 1977 Analysis of familial factors in bipolar affective illness. Archives of General Psychiatry 34: 1074–1083

Jones D, Kelwala S, Bell J, Dube S, Jackson E, Sitaram N 1985 Cholinergic REM sleep induction response correlation with endogenous major depressive subtype. Psychiatry Research 14: 99–110

Kafka M S, van Kammen D P, Kleinman J E, Nurnberger J I Jr, Siever L J, Uhde, T W, Polinsky R J 1980 Alpha-adrenergic receptor function in schizophrenia, affective disorders and some neurological diseases. Communications in Psychopharmacology 4: 477–486

Kallman F 1954 In: Hoch P H, Zubin J(eds) Depression. Grune & Stratton, New York, p1–24

Kassett J A, Gershon E S, Maxwell M E, Guroff J J, Kazuba D M, Smith A L, Brandt H A, Jimerson D C 1989 Psychiatric disorders in the first-degree relatives of probands with bulimia nervosa. American Journal of Psychiatry 146: 1468–1471

Kelsoe J R, Ginns E I, Egeland J A, Gerhard D S, Goldstein A M, Bale S J, Pauls D L, Long R T, Kidd K K, Conte G 1989 Re-evaluation of the linkage relationship between chromosome 11p loci and the gene for bipolar affective disorder in the Old Order Amish. Nature 342: 238–243

Kendler K S, Gruenberg A M, Tsuang M T 1985 Psychiatric illness in first-degree relatives of schizophrenic and surgical control patients. Archives of General Psychiatry 42: 770–779

Kendler K S, Gruenberg A M, Tsuang M T 1986 A DSM-III family study of nonschizophrenic psychotic disorders. American Journal of Psychiatry 143: 1098–1105

Kendler K S, Heath A, Martin N G, Eaves L J 1987 Symptoms of anxiety and symptoms of depression: same genes, different environments? Archives of General Psychiatry 44: 451–457

Klein D N, Depue R A 1984 Continued impairment in persons at risk for bipolar affective disorder: Results of a 19-month follow-up study. Journal of Abnormal Psychology 93: 345–347

Klein D N, Depue R A 1985 Obsessional personality traits and risk for bipolar affective disorder: an off-spring study. Journal of Abnormal Psychology 94: 291–297

Klerman G L, Lavori P W, Rice J, Reich T, Endicott J, Andreasen N C, Keller M B, Hirschfield P M A 1985 Birth-cohort trends in rates of major depressive disorder among relatives of patients with affective disorder. Archives of General Psychiatry 42: 689–695

Kogan S, Gitschier J 1990 Mutations and a polymorphism in the factor VIII gene discovered by denaturing gradient gel electrophoresis. Proceedings of the National Academy of Sciences of the USA 87: 2092–2096

Korner J, Fritze J, Propping P 1990 RFLP alleles at the tyrosine hydroxylase locus: No association found to affective disorders. Psychiatry Research 32: 275–280

Krauthammer C, Klerman G L 1978 Secondary mania: Manic syndromes associated with antecedent physical illness or drugs. Archives of General Psychiatry 35: 1333–1339

Kreig J C, Berger M 1987 REM sleep and cortisol response to the cholinergic challenge with RS 86 in normals and depressives. Acta Psychiatrica Scandinavica 76: 600–602

Langer S Z, Gazlin A M, Lee C R, Shoemaker H 1986 In: Porter R, Brock G, Clark S, eds Antidepressants and Receptor Function. John Wiley, Chichester, p 3–29

Leboyer M, Malafosse A, Boularand S, Campion D, Gheysen F, Samolyk, Henriksson B, Denise E, DesLauriers A, Lepine J P, Zarifian E, Clerget-Darpoux F, Mallet J 1990 Tyrosine hydroxylase polymorphisms associated with manic-depressive illness. Lancet 335: 1219

Lewy A J, Nurnberger J I Jr, Wehr T A, Pack D, Berker L E, Powell R L, Newsome D A 1985 Supersensitivity to light: possible trait marker for manic-depressive illness. American Journal of Psychiatry 142: 725–727

Lewis J L, Winokur G 1982 The induction of mania. A natural history study with controls. Archives of General Psychiatry 39: 303–310

Loranger A W, Oldham J M, Elaine H T 1982 Familial transmission of DSM-III borderline personality disorder. Archives of General Psychiatry 39: 795–799

Luxenberger H 1930 Psychiatrisch-neurologische Zwillingspathologie. Zentralblatt für die gesamte Neurologie und Psychiatrie 14: 145–180

McNeil T J, Kaij L 1979 Etiological relevance of comparisons of high-risk and low-risk groups. Acta Psychiatrica Scandinavica 59: 545–560

McNeil T F, Kaij L, Malmquist-Larsson A, Naslund B, Persson-Blennow I, McNeil N, Blennow G 1983 Offspring of women with nonorganic psychoses. Development of a longitudinal study of children at high risk. Acta Psychiatrica Scandinavica 68: 234–250

Mellerup E T, Plenge P, Rosenberg R 1982 3H-imipramine binding sites in platelets from psychiatric patients. Psychiatry Research 7: 221–227

Mendlewicz J, Fleiss J L 1974 Linkage studies with X-chromosome markers in bipolar (manic-depressive) and unipolar (depressive) illness. Biological Psychiatry 9: 261–294

Mendlewicz J, Rainer J D 1974 Morbidity risk and genetic transmission in manic depressive illness. American Journal of Human Genetics 26: 692–701

Mendlewicz J, Rainer J D 1977 Adoption study supporting genetic transmission in manic-depressive illness. Nature 368: 327–329

Mendlewicz J, Linkowsky P, Wilmotte J 1980 Relationship between schizoaffective illness and affective disorders or schizophrenia: Morbidity risk and genetic transmission. Journal of Affective Disorders 2: 289–302

Mendlewicz J, Simon P, Sevy S, Charon F, Brocas H, Legros S, Vassart G 1987 Polymorphic DNA marker on X chromosome and manic depression. Lancet 1: 1230–1232

Nurnberger J I Jr, Roose S P, Dunner D L, Fieve R R 1979 Unipolar mania; a distinct clinical entity? American Journal of Psychiatry 136: 1420–1423

Nurnberger J I Jr, Sitaram N, Gershon E S, Gillin J C 1983 A twin study of cholinergic REM induction. Biological Psychiatry 18: 1161–1165

Nurnberger J I Jr, Gershon E S 1984 Genetics of affective disorders. In: Post R M, Ballenger J C eds Neurobiology of Mood Disorder. Williams & Wilkins, Baltimore, p 76–101

Nurnberger J I Jr, Goldin L R, Gershon E S 1986 Genetics of psychiatric disorders. In: Winokur G, Clayton P J (eds) The medical basis of psychiatry. W B Sanders, p 486–521

Nurnberger J I Jr, Berrettini W, Tamarkin L, Hamovit J, Norton J, Gershon E 1988a Supersensitivity to melatonin suppression by light in young people at high risk for affective disorder: a preliminary report. Neuropsychopharmacology 1: 217–223

Nurnberger J I Jr, Guroff J J, Hamovit J, Berrettini W, Gershon E 1988b A family study of rapid-cycling bipolar illness. Journal of Affective Disorders 15: 87–91

Nurnberger J I Jr, Hamovit J, Hibbs E D, Pellegrini D, Guroff J J, Maxwell M E, Smith A, Gershon E S 1988c A high risk study of primary affective disorder: selection of subjects, initial assessment, and 1- to 2-year follow-up. In: (Dunner D L, Gershon E S, Barrett J E (eds) Relatives of Risk for Mental Disorder. Raven Press, New York

Nurnberger J I Jr, Berrettini W, Mendelson W, Sack D, Gershon E S 1989 Measuring cholinergic sensitivity: I. Arecoline effects in bipolar patients. Biological Psychiatry 25: 610–617

Oxenstierna G, Edman G, Iselius L, Oreland L, Ross S B, Sedvall G 1986 Concentrations of monoamine metabolites in the cerebrospinal fluid of twins and unrelated individuals—a genetic study. Journal of Psychiatric Research 20: 19–29

Paykel E S 1982 Life events and early environment. In: Paykel E S (ed) Handbook of Affective Disorders. Churchill Livingstone, Edinburgh, p146–161

Perris C 1986 A study of bipolar (manic-depressive) and unipolar recurrent depressive psychoses. Acta Psychiatrica Scandinavica (suppl) 194: 15–44

Pettersen U 1977 Manic depressive illness: a clinical social and genetic study. Acta Psychiatrica Scandinavica (suppl) 269: 1–93

Propping P, Friedl W 1983 Genetic control of adrenergic receptors on human platelets. A twin study. Human Genetics 64:105–109

Reich T, Clayton P J, Winokur G 1969 Family history studies: V. The genetics of mania. America Journal of Psychiatry 125: 1358–1369

Rice J, McGuffin P, Goldin L R, Shaskan E G, Gershon E S 1984 Platelet monoamine oxidase (MAO) activity: evidence for a single major locus. American Journal of Human Genetics 36: 36–43

Rice J, Reich T, Andreasen N C, Endicott J, Van Eerdewegh M, Fisherman R, Hirschfield R M A, Klerman G L 1987 The familial transmission of bipolar illness. Archives of General Psychiatry 44: 441–447

Risch N, Baron M 1982 X-linkage and genetic heterogeneity in bipolar-related major affective illness; reanalysis of linkage data. Analysis of Human Genetics 46: 153–1166

Rosanoff A J, Handy L, Plesset I R 1935 The etiology of manic-depressive syndromes with special reference to their occurrence in twins. American Journal of Psychiatry 91: 725–762

Rosenthal N E, Rosenthal L N, Stallone F, Dunner D L, Fieve R R 1980 Toward the validation of RDC schizoaffective disorder. Archives of General Psychiatry 37: 804–810

Rosenthal N E, Sack D A, Carpenter C J, Parry B L, Mendelson W B, Wehr T A 1985 Antidepressant effects of light in seasonal affective disorder. American Journal of Psychiatry 142: 163–170

Rossiter B J, Caskey C T 1990 Molecular scanning methods of mutation detection. Journal of Biological Chemistry 265: 12753–12756

Schulsinger F, Kety S S, Rosenthal D, Wender P H 1979 A family study of suicide. In: Schou M, Stromgren E (eds) Origin prevention and treatment of affective disorders. Academic Press, London p 277–287

Shaughnessy R, Greene S C, Pandey G N, Dorus E 1985. Red-cell lithium transport and affective disorders in a multigeneration pedigree: evidence for genetic transmission of affective disorders. Biological Psychiatry 20: 451–460

Sheffield V C, Cox D R, Lerman L S, Myers R M 1989 Attachment of a 40-base-pair g+c-rich sequence (gc-clamp) to genomic DNA fragments by the polymerase chain reaction results in improved detection of single-base changes. Proceedings of the National Academy of Sciences of the USA 86: 232–236

Siever L J, Kafka M S, Targum S, Lake C R 1984 Platelet alpha-adrenergic binding and biochemical responsiveness in depressed patients and controls. Psychiatry Research 11: 287–302

Sitaram N, Nurnberger J I Jr, Gershon E S, Gillin J C 1980 Faster cholinergic REM sleep induction in euthymic patients with primary affective illness. Science 208: 200–202

Sitaram N, Moore A M, Vanskiver C, Blendy J, Nurnberger J I Jr, Gershon E S, Gillin J C 1981 In: Pepeu G, Ladinsky H (eds) Advances in behavioral biology: cholinergic mechanisms. Plenum Press, New York, p 947–962

Sitaram N, Nurnberger J I Jr, Gershon E S, Gillin J C 1982 Cholinergic regulation of mood and REM sleep: potential model and marker of vulnerability to affective disorder. American Journal of Psychiatry 139: 571–576

Sitaram N, Dube S, Keshavan M, Davies A, Reynal P 1987 The association of supersensitive cholinergic REM-induction and affective illness within pedigrees. Journal of Psychiatric Research 21: 487–497

Slater E 1953 Psychotic and neurotic illness in twins. Medical Research Council Special Report Series No. 278, Her Majesty's Stationery Office, London

Smeraldi E, Negri F, Melica A M 1977 A genetic study of affective disorder. Acta Psychiatrica Scandinavica 56: 382–398

Stanley M J, Mann J J, Cohen L S 1986 Serotonin and serotonergic receptors in suicide. In: Mann, Stanley (eds) Psychobiology of suicidal behavior. New York Academy of Sciences, New York, 487: 122–127

Stern S L, Dixon K N, Nemzer E, Lake M D, Sansone R A, Smeltzer D J, Lantz S, Schrier S S 1984 Affective disorder in the families of women with normal weight bulimia. American Journal of Psychiatry 141: 1224–1227

Stoflet E S, Koeberl D D, Sarkar G, Sommer S S 1988 Genomic amplification with transcript sequencing. Science 239: 491–494

Strober M, Morrell W, Burroughs J, Lampert C, Danforth H, Freeman R 1988 A family study of bipolar I disorder in adolescence: Early onset of symptoms linked to increased familial loading and lithium resistance. Journal of Affective Disorders 15: 255–268

Suranyi-Cadotte B E, Wood P L, Vasavan N P, Schwartz G 1982 Normalization of platelet [3H] imipramine binding in depressed patients during remission. European Journal of Pharmacology 85: 357–358

Taylor M A, Abrams R, Hayman M A 1980 The classification of affective disorders: a reassessment of the bipolar-unipolar dichotomy. Journal of Affective Disorders 2: 95–109

Torgersen S 1986 Genetic factors in moderately severe and mild affective disorders. Archives of General Psychiatry 43: 222–226

Torgersen S 1990 Comorbidity of major depression and anxiety disorders in twin pairs. American Journal of Psychiatry 147: 1199–1202

Traystman M D, Higuchi M, Kasper C K, Antonarakis S E, Kazazian H H Jr 1990 Use of denaturing gradient gel electrophoresis to detect point mutations in the factor VIII gene. Genomics 6: 293–301

Van Praag H M, de Haan S 1979 Central serotonin metabolism and frequency of depression. Psychiatry Research 1: 219–224

von Knorring A L, Cloninger C R, Bohman M, Sigvardsson S 1983 An adoption study of depressive disorders and substance abuse. Archives of General Psychiatry 40: 943–950

Waters B, Marchenko I, Smiley D 1983a Affective disorder, paranatal and educational factors in the offspring of bipolar manic-depressives. Canadian Journal of Psychiatry 28: 527–531

Waters B, Thakkar J, Lapierre Y 1983b Erythrocyte lithium transport variables as a marker for manic-depressive disorder. Neuropsychobiology 9: 94–98

Wehr T A, Goodwin F K 1979 Rapid cycling in manic-depressives induced by tricyclic antidepressants. Archives of General Psychiatry 36: 555–559

Weissman M M, Myers J K 1978 Affective disorders in a US urban community: the use of research diagnostic criteria in an epidemiological survey. Archives of General Psychiatry 35: 1304–1311

Weissman M M, Prusoff B A, Gammon G D, Merikangas K R, Leckman J F, Kidd K K 1984a Psychopathology in the children (ages 6–18) of depressed and normal parents. Journal of the American Academy of Child Psychology 23: 78–84

Weissman M M, Gershon E S, Kidd K K, Prusoff B A, Leckman J F, Dibble E, Hamovit J, Thompson W D, Pauls D L, Guroff J J 1984b Psychiatric disorders in the relatives of probands with affective disorder. Archives of General Psychiatry 41: 13–21

Weissman M M, Warner V, Wickramaratne P, Prusoff B A 1988 Early-onset major depression in parents and their children. Journal of Affective Disorders 15: 269–277

Wender H, Kety S S, Rosenthal D, Schulsinger F, Ortmann J, Lunde I 1986 Psychiatric disorders in the biological and adoptive families of adopted individuals with affective disorders. Archives of General Psychiatry 43: 923–929

Winokur G, Clayton P 1967 Family history studies: I. Two types of affective disorders separated according to genetic and clinical factors. In: Recent Advances in Biological Psychiatry. Plenum Press, New York, ch 9: 35–50

Winokur G, Cadoret R, Dorzab J Baker M 1971 Depressive disease – a genetic study. Archives of General Psychiatry 24: 135–144

Winters K C, Stone A A, Weintraub S, Neale J M 1981 Cognitive and attentional deficits in children vulnerable to psychopathology. Journal of Abnormal Child Psychology 94: 435–453

Wood K, Coppen A 1983 Prophylactic lithium treatment of patients with affective disorders is associated with decreased platelet [3H] dihydroergocryptine binding. Journal of Affective Disorders 5: 253–258

Wood K A, Harris M J, Morreale A, Rizos A L 1988 Drug-induced psychosis and depression in the elderly. Psychiatric Clinics of North America 11: 167–193

Wright A F, Loudon J B, Hampson M E, Crichton D N, Steel C M 1984 Beta-adrenoceptor binding defector in lymphoblastoid cell lines from manic-depressive subjects. Clinical Neuropharmacology (suppl 1) 7: 194–195

Zahn T P, Nurnberger J I Jr, Berrettini W H 1989 Electrodermal activity in young adults at genetic risk for affective disorder. Archives of General Psychiatry 46: 1120–1124

Zahn-Waxler C, McKnew D H, Cummings E M, Davenport Y B, Radke-Yarrow M 1984 Problem behaviors and peer interactions of young children with a manic-depressive parent. American Journal of Psychiatry 141: 236–240

Zuckerman M 1971 Dimensions of sensation seeking. Journal of Consulting and Clinical Psychology 36: 45–52

Zuckerman M 1985 Sensation seeking, mania, and monoamines. Neuropsychobiology 13: 121–128

10. Life events and social stress

Eugene S. Paykel *Zafra Cooper*

This chapter will review evidence concerning the effects of the social environment on the development, maintenance and relapse of affective disorders. We will distinguish two main aspects: life events, which represent recent major changes in the environment, and social support, one aspect of the supportive or stressful qualities of the environment not linked to recent change.

Since the 1960s there has been a large volume of systematic research on the role of recent life events in psychiatric disorder. The life event literature now clearly indicates that the risk of depression is considerably increased following stressful life events, but that there are many other causative and modifying factors. More recently the focus of interest has moved to other aspects of the social environment, particularly social support. The literature is less extensive, but it has grown rapidly. It is clear that poor social support is associated with depression but the explanation of the association is not yet fully worked out.

THEORETICAL AND METHODOLOGICAL ISSUES

The nature of life events and social support

Many discussions of life events do not define the term. In this chapter, by life events we mean a change in the external environment which occurs sufficiently rapidly to be approximately dated. This involves several elements: change, something which is relatively abrupt rather than slow, and something which involves the external environment, usually the social environment. An event should be external and potentially verifiable. A change which is solely subjective, such as the realization that one's job bores one, may have a personal reality, but is not an event. There is one exception: the development of a personal physical illness is usually accepted as a life event since, although an internal change, it is externally verifiable, and its personal implications are similar to those of major changes in the social environment.

Similarly, few investigators of social support have provided a conceptual definition which could be used to develop precise measures. Some published definitions are circular, using the word 'support' in the definition without defining it.

Among more satisfactory definitions Cobb (1976) defined social support as information leading the subject to believe that he is cared for and loved, is esteemed and valued and belongs to a social network of communication and mutual obligation. This definition focusses only on emotional support but, in a later paper, Cobb (1979) offered descriptions of other kinds of support which included instrumental support, active support and material support. House (1981) suggested that social support involved emotional concern, instrumental aid, information, and appraisal (information relevant to self evaluation).

There is some consensus that social support is multidimensional. Thoits (1985) suggests that it refers to helpful functions performed for an individual by significant others, such as family members, friends, co-workers, relatives and neighbours. The functions may include: socio-emotional aid, such as demonstration of love, caring, esteem, value empathy, sympathy, and/or group belonging; instrumental aid, such as actions and materials that enable fulfilment of everyday responsibilities and obligations; informational aid, which refers to communications such as advice, personal feedback and job information.

Measurement issues

Three issues are of particular importance in guiding the development of useful measures of life events and social support.

The first is the reliability of retrospective information. It is a greater problem for life events, since life events by their very nature have to be reported retrospectively. The inherent inaccuracies of recall over fairly long periods may lead to events being forgotten, or to others being reported which have occurred outside the study period. In addition, events may be over-reported or exaggerated by people who experience subsequent psychiatric disorder, in an attempt to explain the disorder in terms of previous life stress.

It is difficult to design studies which are truly prospective regarding life event information but easier to do so for social support. Nonetheless, a large proportion of published social support studies measure support retrospectively, and the same issues apply.

The second issue is that of objective reality versus perception. Psychiatric disorder leads to distorted perceptions of all sorts of events and social situations: for instance, the depressive may, as a result of self-blame, exaggerate a minor life event occurrence. Disorder may, in addition, lead to an 'effort after meaning' to explain its occurrence in terms of prior life stress. In the assessment of social support, objective availability and subjective perception may differ considerably. Which of the two is more important for disorder is an empirical question, and they should not be confounded. Careful interviewing is needed to establish the reality.

The third issue concerns the origins of circumstances in the social environment. They are not necessarily externally engendered. The depressive may lose his job or become isolated due to illness-induced incapacity, or to personality inadequacy. Two methodological precautions can deal with this. First, one can date symptom onset and only consider occurrences preceding it. Secondly, the judgment of independence of life events introduced by Brown et al (1973a) can be used. Detailed circumstances of an occurrence are examined to establish the likelihood of external origin. The problems are greater for social support, since support is not a datable event and occurs over a period of time. Many studies of social support are cross-sectional rather than longitudinal and predictive. It is not easy to be certain that one is measuring support at a specific time before onset of disorder. In addition, independence is difficult to unravel for social support and this had rarely been attempted. Independence of disorder may be established but it appears likely that personality characteristics contribute greatly to development and maintenance of social networks, in a way which is inextricably entangled.

Measures

The earliest studies of life events and psychiatric disorder used pencil and paper self-report checklists (Holmes & Rahe 1967). Although at the time such questionnaires represented a considerable advance in method, it is now clear that they cannot satisfactorily resolve the problems summarized above. Questionnaires do not enable full definitions to be given of what is to count as a rateable event. Without such definitions, which are often complex, the borderlines of a life event such as a marital argument can be very uncertain. Information is prone to retrospective unreliability and reality cannot be separated from perception.

These difficulties led to the development of semi-structured interview schedules which allow the interviewer to obtain more detailed information about the circumstances of the subject's life. Two such interviews are the Bedford College Life Events and Difficulties Schedule (LEDS) (Brown & Harris 1978) and the Interview for Recent Life Events (Paykel 1983). Both interviews allow detailed timing of events, so that attention can be focussed on a specific period prior to disorder, and have procedures for quantification of stress and exclusion of events probably due to illness. A review of studies of reliability and validity (Paykel 1983) has shown adequate performance for interviews of this kind, with rather lower figures for self-report questionnaires.

There is no generally accepted measure of social support, despite the development of numerous self-report questionnaires (Blazer 1983, Waring & Patton 1984, Billings & Moos 1985) and the existence of some interview methods of assessment (Brown & Harris 1978, Brown et al 1986, Henderson 1981). Self-report questionnaires may be adequate for assessing subjective perception but they are not able to assess objective availability or quality of support. To obtain accurate information on so complex a topic it is necessary to use investigator-based interviews. Issues of reliability and validity are at present of greater concern for social support than for life events.

Assessments of social support vary in the extent to which they measure a range of aspects of social support. Many studies measure only one aspect, for example the presence of an intimate confiding relationship with a spouse or lover (Brown & Harris 1978). Others measure some composite which does not allow the various aspects of support to be separated (Andrews et al 1978, Lin et al 1979, Aneshensel & Stone 1982). Some combine subjective and objective support

(Billings & Moos 1985, Flaherty et al 1983, Hallstrom 1986); others measure these separately (Brugha et al 1990, Henderson 1981); while others measure only objectively defined support (Brown & Prudo 1981, Campbell et al 1983). Studies vary too as to whether they only measure close support (Brown & Harris 1978) or include also the notion of diffuse support (Surtees 1980, Henderson 1981). A few investigators have assessed multiple dimensions (Parry & Shapiro 1986, Ullah et al 1985).

Depressive samples

Sampling also requires attention. Depression is common in the general population and in such circumstances selection factors may distort the characteristics of those who receive psychiatric treatment. On the other hand, depression in the general population may be milder and different in quality to depression in those receiving psychiatric care (Sireling et al 1985). Such depressions might be more understandable and more closely linked with social stress or support (Bebbington et al 1981). There is some safety in only drawing conclusions regarding clinical disorder from findings in clinical groups. The life event literature is sufficiently extensive for this to be possible, but there are not yet sufficient social support studies for reviews to focus predominantly on them.

For social support, there has recently been some interest in sex differences (Brugha et al 1990, Salokangas et al 1988, Emmerson et al 1989). It may be that certain types of support are more significant for women than for men, or that the way social support exerts its protective function is different in men and women.

RECENT LIFE EVENTS

Life events and onset of depression

There have been many studies of life events and onset of depressive episodes. Table 10.1 summarizes findings of 27 published retrospective controlled comparisons of psychiatrically treated depressed patients, one employing two comparison groups. 16 studies, from USA, England, Eire, Italy, Spain, Poland, The Netherlands, Kenya and India, employed general population controls, including two studies of elderly patients (Murphy 1982, Emmerson et al 1989). All found more events reported prior to depressive onset, although in one study, with small numbers, the differ-

ence did not reach significance. Two studies compared depressives with medical patient controls. Both found more events reported by depressed patients but the differences were not very striking or clearly attributable to causes rather than effects of depression. Medical patients may experience events due to illness, and more medical disorders may be contributed to by life stress.

Comparisons of depressed patients and other psychiatric patients are also summarized in the table. Depressives have been found to report more events than schizophrenics, indicating in the retrospective frame greater causative effects. In one study (Leff & Vaughn 1980) differences for independent events were suggestive but not significant and there was no difference for undesirable events. Two additional studies not shown in the table failed to find differences between depressives and schizophrenics, but life event methodologies were limited (Eisler & Polak 1971, Lahniers & White 1976). A third study (Harder et al 1980) did not clearly separate depressives and other neurotics.

Some comparisons with mixed psychiatric patients have also suggested that life event effects are greater in depression, but these results are not consistent. On the other hand, three comparisons of suicide attempters with depressed patients found more events in suicide attempters. Suicide attempters, the majority of whom take overdoses, tend to be young and often do not show the depressive syndrome. Other studies comparing these patient groups with general population controls indicate that the largest patient-control differences are for suicide attempts, with much smaller effects for schizophrenia, and that depression is intermediate (Paykel & Cooper 1991).

All studies in Table 10.1 were of disorder sufficiently severe to present to psychiatrists. One study (Bebbington et al 1981) found greater life events in depressed people in the community than in outpatients. Although this may be the case, the findings in Table 10.1 also make it clear that events are implicated in major disorder presenting to psychiatrists.

Some other studies using different designs or samples are not shown in the table. In a study using patients as their own controls, event rates in depressed patients dropped on follow-up but not fully to general population levels (Paykel 1974). A small study found depressed pathological gamblers to have experienced more life events, especially undesirable events and exits, in the 6 months before onset of depression than in normal controls (Roy et al 1988). One study has shown heroin addicts with secondary depression to have more stressful events than those without depression (Prusoff

Table 10.1   Controlled comparisons of life events and onset of clinical depression

Nature of controls	Author	Excess any events	Excess separations	Excess other types of events
General population	Paykel et al 1969	Yes	Yes	Various, especially undesirable events
	Thompson & Hendrie 1972	Yes	Not reported	More stress overall
	Cadoret et al 1972	Suggestive	Suggestive	Not reported
	Brown et al 1973b	Yes	Not reported	Markedly and moderately threatening events
	Fava et al 1981	Yes	Yes	Undesirable, negative impact
	Vadher & Ndetei 1981	Yes	Yes	Suggestive only
	Chatterjee et al 1981	Yes	Yes	Health, interpersonal
	Bebbington et al 1981	Yes, males only	Not reported	Events of severe and moderate threat
	Murphy 1982	Yes	Suggestive	Health
	Billings et al 1983	Yes	Yes	Various negative events
	Faravelli & Ambonetti 1983	Yes	Not reported	Undesirable, exit and severe
	Bidzinska 1984	Yes	No	Marital and family conflicts, work overload, failures
	Roy et al 1985	Yes	No	Undesirable events
	Brugha & Conroy 1985	Yes	Not reported	Undesirable, threatening. Not independent, uncontrolled
	Ezquiaga et al 1987	Yes	Not reported	Threatening, independent
	Emmerson et al 1989	Yes	Not reported	Severely threatening
	Cornelis et al 1989	Yes	No	Undesirable, higher stress
Medical patients	Forrest et al 1965	Yes, weak	No	Social factors
	Hudgens et al 1967	Yes, weak	No	Moves, interpersonal discord
Other psychiatric patients	*Schizophrenics*			
	Beck & Worthen 1972	Yes	Suggestive	Events of higher rated hazard
	Brown et al 1973b	Yes	Not reported	Events/moderate and marked threat over longer time
	Jacobs et al 1974	Yes	Yes	Undesirable, health financial interpersonal discord
	Leff & Vaughn 1980	Suggestive	Not reported	Not for undesirable events
	Suicide attempters			
	Paykel et al 1975	Fewer events in depressives	No	Fewer events in depressives, especially undesirable, upsetting
	Slater & Depue 1981	Fewer events in depressives	No. Fewer exits	Fewer independent events
	Cohen-Sandler et al 1982	Fewer events in depressives	Fewer deaths, separations	Casenote study in children
	Mixed psychiatric patients			
	Sethi 1964	Yes	Yes	Not reported
	Levi et al 1966	Yes	Yes	Not reported
	Malmquist 1970	No	No	No
	Uhlenhuth & Paykel 1973	No	No	No

et al 1977) while another study obtained similar findings for depressed compared with non-depressed schizophrenic patients (Roy et al 1983), as did a questionnaire study of secondarily depressed and non-depressed alcoholics (Fowler et al 1980). A follow-up study of addicts found events to be associated with continuing depression, failure of recovery and also failure of abstinence (Kosten et al 1983, 1986).

Goodyer and colleagues studied effects of life events in children attending a child psychiatry clinic (Goodyer et al 1985, 1987). In comparison with community controls, children had experienced more events of severe negative impact in the 12 months before onset. These effects were apparent in four diagnostic groups: conduct disorder, severe mood disorder, mild mood disorder and neurotic disorder. Marital/family and accident/illness events appeared to be more important for conduct disorder and mild mood disorder, and exit events for severe mood disorder. The effects extended across the full year, but tended to be more marked in the immediate preceding 16 weeks. In a further study in a new sample (Goodyer et al 1990), events and poor friendships exerted independent effects and showed an additive interaction. Prepubertally, the effects of poor friendships were the same in anxiety and in depressive disorders, but postpubertally poor friendships were more strongly associated with anxiety disorders.

Epidemiological studies have also been used to study effects of life events. Since the literature on patient groups is extensive, the epidemiological literature will not be reviewed in detail. Among studies showing association of life events and minor psychiatric disorder are those of Myers et al (1971), Dohrenwend (1973a,b), Uhlenhuth et al (1974) and Bebbington et al (1988). The important studies by Brown and colleagues, which have also predominantly been based on community samples, are reviewed in later sections.

Types of life event

A specific hypothesis would suggest that depression and only depression is induced by certain types of events. Most prominent in the literature is the role of loss. The concept of loss is somewhat diffuse, including interpersonal separations and deaths, loss of self esteem and other kinds of loss.

Interpersonal losses of various kinds have received the most study. Findings from the studies are summarized in Table 10.1. 21 studies have reported specifically on recent separations. In 11, depressed patients reported more separations than the control groups, which included both general population and other psychiatric patients, suggesting some specificity. There was no excess over medical patients. Two studies not only found exit events related to depression but also found that their converse, entrance events, were not (Paykel et al 1969, Fava et al 1981). However, one study (Slater & Depue 1981) found that primary depressed patients making a suicide attempt had experienced more exits than those who did not, indicating a greater relationship to the attempt.

Also common in the studies are arguments and discord with various key interpersonal figures. They may involve threat of separation. Blows to the self esteem and failures have not usually been explicitly reported, but are probably also common. As can be seen from the table, a wide variety of events is involved. In general the studies suggest only weak specificity. There is some relationship between depression and interpersonal losses, but these also precede other disorders, and many depressions are not preceded by them. The strongest relationship appears when events are categorized in rather broad terms such as 'threatening' or undesirable. This extends well beyond interpersonal loss.

Brown and colleagues in recent studies of women in the community have refined their original use of the broad concept of threat and investigated specific qualities of events (Brown et al 1986, 1988). 'Matching' events arising out of long-term difficulties were found to be associated with development of depression below case level, and 'fresh start' events implying hope of a better future, with recovery from chronic depression of greater than 12 months duration.

Whether different types of events are involved in anxiety and depression is not clear. Uhlenhuth & Paykel (1973) found no difference in amount or type of life event stress between predominantly depressed and anxious patients in a mixed neurotic sample. Barrett (1979), in a similar study in symptomatic volunteers, found more exit events and undesirable events in depressed patients but it was not clear whether this simply reflected a general excess of stressful types of events in depressed people. Finlay-Jones & Brown (1981) in general practice patients found more 'loss' events preceding depression and 'danger' events preceding anxiety. Goodyer et al (1990) did not find life event patterns to distinguish children who were depressed from those who were anxious.

Some specific events have received individual study. Parkes (1964) in a retrospective study found increased bereavement in psychiatric patients, particularly those who were depressed, compared with expected figures. Birtchnell (1970a,b) found recent death of a parent (excluding the most recent year) more common in admissions to a psychiatric hospital than in general population controls. There were no differences between depressed and non-depressed patients but the incidence of death of a parent was higher in severely depressed patients than moderately depressed. In a subsequent study using a larger case register sample, patient-control differences were most marked for depressed patients, and for loss of a parent of opposite sex to the patient (Birtchnell 1975).

Studies of hysterectomy and depression were reviewed in a previous edition of this Handbook (Paykel 1982), as were studies of the association of depression with carcinoma. The latter association may reflect metabolic effects rather than psychosocial ones. The evidence for hysterectomy was equivocal 10 years ago; now there has been one good study which indicates that hysterectomy leads to amelioration rather than worsening of psychiatric symptoms (Gath et al 1982).

One circumstance which has received more study is that of childbirth. Here hormonal effects as well as social stress might be important. For depression, particularly milder episodes, additional stressful life events appear to be a strongly associated factor (Paykel et al 1980, O'Hara et al 1984, Cooper & Stein 1989, Martin et al 1989). This suggests that social stress is important. In contrast, major postpartum psychoses do not appear to be associated with stressful life events (Dowlatshahi & Paykel 1990, Brockington et al 1990). Most of the studies of milder depression do not directly address the question as to whether rates are raised overall compared to non-puerperal women, as would be expected if childbirth itself were pathogenic. A few recent studies have suggested that rates are only a little increased (Cooper et al 1988, Cox et al 1989), again different to the markedly raised rates for postpartum psychoses (Kendell et al 1987).

Difficulties

One form of chronic stress included in the work of Brown and colleagues has been 'difficulties', defined as problems which last at least for 4 weeks. In most studies using their methods, difficulties have been amalgamated with life events as 'provoking agents' rather than analysed separately, and the findings are therefore discussed here. In the original study by Brown & Harris (1978), difficulties (other than health) which were rated high on threat and had lasted more than 2 years were associated with increased depression. The effect was manifested in the absence of severe events, but presence of both events and difficulties resulted in little increase of depression above that for either one singly. In a recent study, Emmerson et al (1989) found no increased rates for difficulties, which were rare in their comparatively affluent elderly Australian sample. Such vulnerability factors as lack of a confiding relationship, which have featured prominently in these studies, could also be regarded as difficulties: the distinction between them appears based on whether effects on depression were found to be direct or only to occur in the presence of life events.

Endogenous depression

A further issue involves the distinction between endogenous or psychotic and neurotic depression. A proportion of depressive episodes are not preceded by life events: probably around 30% in the controlled studies. However, as the term is usually employed, endogenous depressions are also regarded as showing a specific symptom pattern including greater severity, psychomotor retardation or agitation, sometimes depressive delusions, early morning wakening, diurnal variation with morning worsening (Rosenthal & Klerman 1966).

Several recent studies using careful life event methods have shown that life events and symptom pattern are only weakly related. Paykel (1984) found that when symptoms and life event information were collected by different raters, the two showed only a low correlation, although in the predicted direction. In another study (Paykel 1979) a simple clinical judgment as to whether the depression was precipitated was found to be unrelated to symptom pattern. In a third study (Paykel et al 1984), using separate interviewers, again only a very weak relationship between life stress and symptom pattern was found, reaching significance only when persisting problems at the time of presentation were examined, rather than life events at onset.

Brown et al (1979) found that psychotic and neurotic depressives showed little difference in the proportions whose illnesses had been preceded by a severe event or major difficulty. When the depressions were divided into those with and without a provoking agent, relatively few individual symptoms distinguished them. Benjaminsen (1981), Katschnig & Berner (1984) and Monroe et al (1985) compared neurotic and non-neurotic depressives and found little difference regarding stressful events. Matussek & Neuner (1981), using a lengthy and probing interview, found differences between neurotic and endogenous depression only for separations from an important partner. Contrary to expectation, Dolan et al (1985) found antecedent life events to be associated with more severe rather than less severe illness, and Brugha & Conroy (1985) found greater patient-control life event differences for CATEGO R (retarded or endogenous) than for N (neurotic) depressives.

Bebbington et al (1981) in a small study did find fewer life events in patients with endogenous symptom pattern, but found little evidence of this in a larger sample (Bebbington et al 1988). Roy et al (1985) found that neurotic depressives had significantly more life events than endogenous depressives and the excess of events found over normal controls was due only to the neurotic subjects.

Overall, it would appear that life events bear only a weak relationship to symptom pattern, and that the latter is predominantly determined by some other mechanism.

Bipolar manic depressive disorder

One group which has not yet been adequately studied is that of bipolar disorder. Four studies have examined mania. Ambelas (1979) found that manic patients had four times as many stressful life events in the 4 weeks preceding admission as a surgical control group. Information on manic subjects was mainly based on case notes, but most of the events listed did appear to be independent, and they were mainly unpleasant in character. Loss events were present twice as often as threat events and bereavement was found in five out of 14 cases. Kennedy et al (1983) looked at the 4 months before onset in manic patients, using both a matched control group and patients as their own controls. They found a twofold increase in life events during the 4-month period. The within-patient control comparison was used to test whether or not these patients might have more life events in any 4-month period, for reasons such as personality traits, but this was not found to be the case. A third recent report which may have overlapped in samples with Ambelas (1979) gave similar findings, with a much more marked effect for first attacks (Ambelas 1987). However, Sclare & Creed (1990) found no difference in rates of independent life events in manics over 30 weeks before onset and the same subjects in a period after recovery.

A study in a lithium clinic found that mood fluctuations in treated manic depressives were not stress-related (Hall et al 1977). It is possible therefore that a major life crisis may contribute to the onset of a disorder for which subsequent attacks are much more biologically determined. However, Aronson & Shukla (1987) found a sudden peak of relapses in bipolar disorder in a lithium clinic shortly after a hurricane, a clearly independent event. One study (Glassner & Haldipur 1983) found more evidence of stressful life events in bipolars with onset over the age of 20 than under, suggesting that constitutional factors might be more important in the latter.

Mania is a disorder producing increased activity and disinhibition, and readily leading to new dependent events such as job changes, financial problems from overspending, arguments and disruptions of old relationships and initiation of new ones. Particular care therefore needs to be taken to define independent events in such studies.

Life events and outcome of depression

In recent years, the relationship between life events and outcome of depression has come under investigation. Several studies have examined events at onset, really one aspect of endogenous and reactive depression. In short term studies of 4–6 weeks outcome, Lloyd et al (1981) found that presence of life events at onset had no influence, Rowan et al (1982, unpublished analyses) found a weak trend for outcome to be worse where a major life event had occurred but Reno & Halaris (1990) found more independent events in responders to desipramine than in non-responders. In a follow-up of cases identified in a community survey, Tennant et al (1981) found better outcome where a threatening event had occurred before onset.

In longer follow-ups of 6-9 months, Parker et al (1988) found in neurotic depressives that break-up of an intimate relationship in the preceding year was associated with good outcome at 6 and 20 weeks. Other life events did not predict outcome. Monroe et al (1985) found that more onset events predicted a better outcome over 3–9 months, with the effect being particularly evident for patients with endogenous symptoms.

In a 1-year follow-up of elderly depressives (Murphy 1983), life events at onset did not predict outcome. In a somewhat different retrospective study, Billings & Moos (1984) compared depressives with either a recurrent or non-recurrent illness. A comparable proportion of each were found to have experienced life events at onset.

Events concurrent with treatment might be expected to have greater effects. In the short-term study cited earlier, Lloyd et al (1981) found that patients who had a poor outcome after 4 weeks were more likely to have experienced undesirable events, physical illnesses, illnesses in family members and events outside the patient's control. Rowan et al (1982) found that events occurring during a 6-week treatment period had no significant effect on outcome, but few major independent events occurred. Tennant et al (1981) in a study of community cases, found that remission was more likely over a one month period in the presence of a 'neutralizing' event, defined as an event which caused minimal threat but which counteracted the effect of an earlier threatening event or difficulty.

Five studies have examined concurrent events over follow-up periods of between 3 and 9 months. Surtees (1980) found that greater event stress was associated with worse outcome. Paykel & Tanner (1976), in a drug continuation study in women, found that relapse was associated with undesirable life events. These relapses appeared to be separate from those related to drug withdrawal. Monroe et al (1985) failed to find outcome influenced by concurrent events. Reno & Halaris (1990) found somewhat paradoxical relationships, with greater event stress associated with better response but difficulties associated with relapse, but in both cases findings applied only to perceived rather than independently rated stress. Hickie & colleagues (Hickie 1990) found that break-up of a dysfunctional relationship was associated with a better outcome.

Among longer-term follow-up studies in patients, Murphy (1983) and Giel et al (1978) both found worse outcome where threatening events had occurred. In women in the community, Brown et al (1988) found recovery from chronic depression preceded by reduction in ongoing difficulties and occurrence of events implying a fresh start towards a better future. In a 7-year follow-up Wittchen (1987) found events over the whole period excluding the last year, and particularly loss events, to predict worse outcome. However, in a 12-month follow-up of a small sample of patients on maintenance therapy Mendlewicz et al (1986) found no overall effect of life events on relapse, although there was a non-significant association with bereavement.

The picture emerging from these studies is that life events at onset do not greatly affect outcome, although there is a weak trend to better outcome where there have been antecedent events. However, where events occur concurrently with treatment, negative events lead to worse outcome, and neutralizing events to better outcome.

Prospective studies and magnitude of effect

An excellent strategy for examining the proportions of subjects affected adversely by an event, and also effects of modifying factors, is the prospective study in which all subjects undergoing a specific event are followed up. Among a number of events which have been studied in this manner are bereavement (see chapter 39), loss of employment (Kasl et al 1975), mastectomy (Maguire et al 1978) and effects of other physical illnesses.

Such studies indicate that, while many subjects undergo considerable distress, relatively few develop overt clinical depression and even fewer seek psychiatric help. Clayton's studies of bereavement are instructive. Among 40 bereaved subjects followed up (Clayton et al 1968), the majority developed depressed mood, sleep disturbance and crying, but ideas of guilt and suicidal thoughts were uncommon. Although 25% consulted a physician for symptoms related to grief, only one subject saw a psychiatrist. In a second study of a new sample, 35% showed symptoms of depression after one month, 17% after a year, but none saw a psychiatrist (Bornstein et al 1973).

Such studies form a useful balance to case-control studies, which ignore base rates for events and disorder in the general population. The majority of events experienced by depressives, although stressful, are not of catastrophic magnitude. They are not uncommon in the general population and are often experienced without overt disorder following. Paykel (1974) attempted a hypothetical calculation which suggested that less than 10% of exit events were followed by clinical depression.

There have been several attempts to quantify the causative effect. Brown et al (1973b) used the concept of 'brought forward time': an estimate of the average time from an onset brought about by an event to the time a spontaneous onset would have occurred if no event were present. They concluded that the effect was large in magnitude and formative for depression but smaller and only triggering for schizophrenia.

Paykel (1978) used an epidemiological measure, the relative risk, or ratio of the rate of disease among those exposed to a causative factor to the rate among those not exposed. This can be applied to the control studies using an approximation, relative odds. In selected published studies, the risk of developing depression in the 6 months after the most stressful classes of events was found to be approximately 6:1, falling off rapidly with time after the event. The relative risks for schizophrenia were much lower, at only 2–3 over 6 months, but for suicide attempts they were higher.

Cooke (1987) has used an alternative epidemiological measure, the population attributable risk, expressed as a percentage. This is an estimate of the proportion of disorder caused by life events, and is most easily applied to epidemiological general population studies. Applying this to a number of published studies of depression he obtained values ranging from 29–69%, but mainly around 40%.

Relative and attributable risks of this magnitude indicate effects which are important, but not exclusive. They suggest disorders with multifactorial causation, in which any single factor may account for only a relatively small proportion of the variance. Although events are important, a large part in determining whether an event is followed by disorder must be attributed to other modifying factors. There may be a whole host of these, both genetic and environmental, ranging from biochemical through personality and coping mechanisms to social experiences, early or recent.

SOCIAL SUPPORT

Social support and life events

In interpreting the rapidly growing literature on psychiatric disorder and social support, some specific additional issues of method arise regarding the relationship between support and life events. The first involves separating the two. Life events such as divorce, death of a spouse or marriage may result in loss or gain of social support, and changes in support may alter the likelihood of the occurrence of life events. Champion (1990), in an analysis of published studies, found a positive relationship between lack of intimacy and occurrence of adversity. These problems can best be overcome with longitudinal data, using independent measures of support, life events and disorder at various points in time.

A further complicating issue about claims for the aetiological role of social support is the debate about whether the role of social support is direct or indirect. Two different views have been proposed, and both have gained some support from the literature. The so-called buffering hypothesis proposes that lack of social support only increases the risk of subsequent disorder in the face of adversity, so that support serves as a

protective buffer between adverse life events and subsequent disorder (Alloway & Bebbington 1987, Thoits 1982, Cohen & Wills 1985). The alternative view is that lack of social support increases the risk of disorder irrespective of the presence of other life stress (Cohen & Wills 1985, Aneshensel & Stone 1982). This claim about the direct role of social support has been termed the main effect hypothesis. A considerable impetus to application of these ideas in depression came from the seminal study of Brown & Harris (1978) which found an event buffering role for absence of vulnerability factors related to social support in women.

A much debated question has been the appropriate statistical model to test for a buffering effect. The term buffering may describe at least two kinds of interaction effect, a multiplicative interaction or an additive one. Often it is assumed that interaction in this area is synonymous with a statistical interaction effect as determined by most traditional multivariate analyses. This interaction is multiplicative and is the most extreme type of interaction whereby one variable multiplies the effect of the other. There are other forms of synergistic effects whereby one variable potentiates another and adds to its effect, but the magnitude does not amount to multiplication. This is called an additive interaction. Neither model of buffering is exclusively correct. Rutter (1983) has argued persuasively that the choice of a method of analysis should depend on the hypothesized mechanisms of interaction. Another strategy is to test both additive and multiplicative concepts of buffering, stating clearly the model one is testing (Paykel et al 1980, Costello 1982, Solomon & Bromet 1982).

Cross-sectional studies

Table 10.2 summarizes 24 recent cross-sectional studies of social support. Life events were also assessed in all but eight of the studies. Some of these studies made use of a naturally occurring stressful event such as unemployment, retirement or the nuclear accident at Three Mile Island (Ullah et al 1985, Salokangas et al 1988, Solomon & Bromet 1982). Most of the studies investigated social support in community samples, but some used patients. The samples investigated were mainly of mixed sex, but some studies were confined to women (Brown & Harris 1978, Brown & Prudo 1981, Solomon & Bromet 1982, Campbell 1983). Two studies (Lin et al 1979, Andrews et al 1978) investigated the dependent variable, mental state or psychological functioning, by questionnaire only, but most studies used a semi-structured interview, in particular

Table 10.2 Cross-sectional studies of social support and affective disorders

Authors	n	Sex	Dependent variable	Questionnaire/ interview	Quest/ interview period	Time period	Social support measure content	Life events	Result
Community samples									
Andrews et al 1978	863	Mixed	GHQ74	Q	Q	Not specified	Postal survey Crisis support Neighbourhood interaction Community participation	Questionnaire 2–13 months prior to survey	Relationship between social support and impairment independent of life event stress
Brown & Harris 1978	458	Women	Judgement of caseness based on PSE	I		12 months prior to onset? – not specified	LEDS – intimacy	LEDS year before interview	Lack of social support, increased vulnerability to disorder in presence of life events.
Lin et al 1979	170	Mixed	Self-report symptom scale	Q		Not specified	Scale of interaction and involvement with neighbours and community and social adjustment	Holmes & Rahe scale 6 months prior to interview	Relationship between events and illness and between social support and absence of illness – no interaction or buffering.
Paykel et al 1980	120	Women postpartum	Clinical Interview for Depression	I		Not specified	Support from husband	Interview for recent life events prior $10\frac{1}{2}$ months	Poor support vulnerability factor in presence of stressful life event.
Brown & Prudo 1981	335	Women	Judgement of caseness based on PSE	I		12 months prior to onset?	LEDS – intimacy; social integration	LEDS 12 months prior to interview	Provoking agent plus lack of intimacy, 3 children <14 and regular churchgoing increase risk of depression
Solomon & Bromet 1982	435	Women	Mental state RDC for depression and anxiety SAD-S	I		Not specified	Social network interview – intimacy	Three Mile Island incident and life event scale 12 months prior to interview	No confidant; association with increased affective disorder in those who had experienced stress
Aneshensel & Stone 1982	1000	Mixed	Current depressive symptomatology especially depressed mood	I		Not specified	Number of close relationships; perceived social support	Life events in past year; perceived strain	Life events and strain associated with depression Close relationships and perceived support negatively related to depression. Effects direct – no interaction.

Study	N	Group	Disorder measure		Support measure		Time period	Life events	Findings
Costello 1982	449	Women	PSE Mental state	I	LEDS – intimacy	I	Not specified	LEDS 12 months prior to interview	Lack of intimacy increased risk of depression. Severe events and difficulties associated with depression. No interactions
Campbell et al 1983	110	Women	Mental state PSE	I	LEDS – intimacy	I	Not specified	LEDS 12 months prior to interview	Lack of confiding relationship increased risk of disorder in face of provoking agent
Ullah et al 1985	1150	Mixed 17-year-olds	GHQ Zung scale depression and anxiety	I	Support – information emotional instrumental social contacts	I	Not specified	Not assessed but all subjects unemployed	Only lack of instrumental support associated with psychological distress. Only partial support for stress buffering
Bebbington et al 1984	310	Mixed	Mental state PSE	I	LEDS – intimacy	I	Not specified	LEDS 10 months before onset or interview	Lack of confidant associated with disorder. No confirmation for vulnerability model. No interaction with events.
Hallstrom 1986	800	Women	Mental state DSM III	I	Intimacy – assumed not present in never married, divorced, widowed, as well as those who reported lack of intimacy	I	No period specified	Interview covering 10 defined stressors 1 year prior to onset	Lack of intimacy increased risk of depression without provoking agent
Parry & Shapiro 1986	193	Women	Mental state PSE	I	Instrumental support Expressive support Intimacy	I	Some aspects 7 days prior to interview	LEDS 12 months prior to interview	Life events and support have independent effects on distress. No interactions
Friedman et al 1988	4913	Mixed	Major depressive disorder – DIS	I	Social contacts social activities satisfaction with work	I	2 weeks prior to interview	Not assessed	Poorer intimate relationships for those currently depressed vs past disorder, other disorder and no disorder

Table 10.2 Cross-sectional studies of social support and affective disorders — *(contd)*

Authors	n	Sex	Dependent variable	Questionnaire/ interview	Social support measure content	Quest/ interview	Time period	Life events	Result
Salokangas et al 1988	389	Mixed	GHQ	Q & I	Married intimate vs married non-intimate vs unmarried non-intimate	I	Not specified	Not formally assessed: about to retire or retired	Married intimate > nonmarried intimate > non-intimate in terms of lack of depressive symptoms gender differences
Birchnell 1988	50	Women	Mental state PSE	I	Social integration; presence of close friend	I	Not specified	Not assessed	Those with fewer friends had higher scores on PSE
Patient samples									
Henderson et al 1978	50	Mixed	GHQ PSE	I	Social Interactions Schedule	I	Week prior to interview	Life events schedule	Patients had fewer good friends and fewer contacts outside home than controls. No difference in life events.
Leff & Vaughn 1980	30	Mixed	Mental state PSE	I	CFI expressed emotion – measure of criticism of close relative, usually spouse	I	Present level of EE	Brown & Birley schedule 3 months prior to onset	Combination of threatening life event and high EE more susceptible to depression
Murphy 1982	119 (168 controls)	Mixed	PSE mental state	I	LEDS – intimacy	I	Not specified 12 months prior to onset	LEDS 12 months prior to onset or prior to interview	Severe event without intimacy increased risk of depression
Brugha et al 1982	50	Mixed	PSE mental state	I	Social Interactions Schedule. Size of network. Number of social contacts. Quality of social interactions	I	Past week	Not assessed	Patient < contacts close relatives, good friends than controls
Flaherty et al 1983	44	Mixed	HRSD SAS – self report Marital and familial functioning	I	Social support network – support received from 5 closest members	Q	Not specified	Schedule of recent events for last years	Patients with high social support better scores on HRSD. No effect for life events
Roy & Kennedy 1984	72	Mixed	GHQ – short psychiatric interview	Q & I	Marital interview (Quinton)	I	Year before onset of depression	Not assessed	Lack of good marital relationship associated with depression

| Merikangas et al 1985 | 45 | Mixed | RDC for major depression | I | Self report marital questionnaire | Q | Measured after recovery from acute episode | Not measured | Marriages of depressed patients worse in all areas than controls |
| Emmerson et al 1989 | 186 | Depressed patients $n = 101$ Community residents $n = 85$ mixed | DSM III at least 4 weeks | I | ISSI and LEDS modified intimacy | I | Not specified 12 months prior to onset? | LEDS 12 months prior to onset | Lack of confiding relationship associated with depression in men but not women. No association of life events with depression |

the PSE. Other studies required subjects to meet well-recognized diagnostic criteria such as DSMIII or RDC without specifying exactly what form the interview took (Hallstrom 1986, Emmerson et al 1989).

Measures of social support varied rather more than the measurement of mental state. Approximately half the studies measured intimacy of some form or other, while others measured degree of social integration (Brown & Prudo 1981), community participation (Andrews et al 1978, Lin et al 1979), size of social network (Brugha et al 1982, Aneshensel & Stone 1982), availability of good friends (Birtchnell 1988). The study of Vaughn & Leff (1976) assessed expressed emotion rather than social support. Expressed emotion involves the quality of close family relationships and in depression, since the subjects tend to be married and middle-aged, the relative assessed is usually the spouse and the main component is the number of critical comments made, although warmth and positive remarks are also measured. Thus it measures the quality of a key intimate relationship. Most studies have not measured the range of different aspects of social support, but a few (e.g. Parry & Shapiro 1986, Ullah et al 1985) did include a variety of dimensions. Three studies (Andrews et al 1978, Flaherty et al 1983, Merikangas et al 1985) measured social support by questionnaire only. The issue of whether studies measured perceived or objective support is not so clear, since although most studies employed interviews, many did not state explicitly whether they assessed objective support, nor what precautions might have been taken to establish this.

Only six studies (Henderson et al 1978, Leff & Vaughn 1980, Brugha et al 1982, Roy & Kennedy 1984, Merikangas et al 1985, Friedman et al 1988) specified precisely the time period over which social support was being measured and in all but two studies (Roy & Kennedy 1984, Merikangas et al 1985) this period was more or less contemporaneous with the time of the assessment of mental state. More importantly, no attempt was made to establish the temporal relationships between social support and the onset of depression. One study assessed social support a year before the onset of depression (Roy & Kennedy 1984) and one assessed it after recovery from an acute episode (Merikangas et al 1985). For most studies it is not clear whether the level of social support found is a function of current mental state, a result of previous life stress, a pre-existing vulnerability factor or a causal factor in its own right.

In drawing conclusions from these studies, caution is

needed because of these issues and their cross-sectional nature. There is clearly an association between lack of social support broadly defined and psychological distress or disorder, although this relationship is not necessarily aetiological. The relationship appears to hold good in both community and patient samples and in both female and mixed samples. Two studies reported sex differences. In the study by Salokangas et al (1988) the effect of having a close friend seemed to depend on sex of subject, although effects of intimate relationships did not. Friendship was associated with a less than average symptom level in men who were not married, while it was associated with a high level of symptoms in women. The authors' interpretation was that women had the ability to retain close friends despite psychiatric difficulties. Emmerson et al (1989) found a confiding relationship to be associated with depression in men, but not in women.

The majority of these studies did not support the stress buffering view of social support, but found independent effects for social support and life events (Andrews et al 1978, Henderson et al 1978, Lin et al 1979, Aneshensel & Stone 1982, Flaherty et al 1983, Bebbington et al 1984, Hallstrom 1986, Parry & Shapiro 1986, Emmerson et al 1989). On the other hand, at least seven studies produced support for some form of the Brown & Harris vulnerability model (Brown & Harris 1978, Paykel et al 1980, Leff & Vaughn 1980, Brown & Prudo 1981, Murphy 1982, Solomon & Bromet 1982, Campbell et al 1983). It may be that there is both an independent effect and some increased amplification of the effect of events. The majority of studies did not test both multiplicative and additive models of interaction.

Longitudinal studies

There are far fewer longitudinal than cross-sectional studies of social support. The studies fall into two categories: those which measure social support prior to onset and its subsequent role in onset (Henderson 1981, Bolton & Oatley 1987, Brown et al 1986) and those that relate social support at the time of disorder to subsequent outcome (e.g. Waring & Patton 1984, Miller et al 1987, George et al 1989, Brugha et al 1990). Although this latter strategy allows the identification of factors which may predict persistence, remission, recovery or relapse of disorder, it does not necessarily elucidate factors that produce onset.

As can be seen from Table 10.3, the studies divide almost equally between community and patient studies.

The research strategy has usually been to attempt to identify those aspects of social support at the time when the individual is depressed which predict the subsequent outcome of the depression. In general, in both kinds of samples, lack of social support while individuals are depressed has been found to predict subsequent poor outcome. Only three studies, all using community samples (Henderson 1981, Bolton & Oatley 1987, Brown et al 1986), were truly prospective in that they identified deficiencies in social support prior to the onset of disorder and related these to subsequent disorder. Two of these (Brown et al 1986, Bolton & Oatley 1987) found evidence of a buffering or interactive effect of social support, while the third provided some evidence for direct effects. The Henderson study found the strongest effects for perceived support rather than objective support while the Brown study found the strongest relationship between support in a crisis, retrospectively assessed, and subsequent onset.

In general, these longitudinal studies have investigated a range of different concepts of social support measured in a variety of ways. Most studies have investigated intimacy or close support in some form but other dimensions of support such as social integration and expressed emotion have also been assessed.

Two studies investigated women exclusively (Brown et al 1986, Miller et al 1987), while all others included both sexes. Only Brugha et al (1990) reported sex differences. In women the significant predictors of recovery were found to be the number of primary group members named and contacted and satisfaction with social support. In men, on the other hand, negative social interaction with members of the primary group and living as married were associated with recovery.

The results of these studies generally confirm the view that poor or absent social support at the time of disorder is related to subsequent course. There is also some suggestion that deficient social support may be an independent causal factor in producing disorder, but there is less support for this. In particular, no longitudinal studies have investigated whether absence of social support predicts development of depressive disorder sufficient to present for psychiatric treatment. The evidence for a stress buffering effect of social support is less strong.

THE FUTURE OF SOCIAL STRESS RESEARCH IN DEPRESSION

After 20 years the general outlines of the relationship

between life events and depression are now well established. Life events precede and contribute to a substantial proportion of depressions and to some other disorders. Type of life event is only weakly related to type of disorder: those events which are more generally stressful are also more likely to produce disorder. Some disorders are more strongly associated with life events than others. Depression is one of these, with the possible exception of bipolar disorder. Life events make only a partial contribution and it is clear that many factors contribute to aetiology, even in the individual case. Stress may interact with personality, cognitive style, genes, social support and neurochemical mechanisms. The basic descriptive work in life events has been completed, and the field needs to move towards exploration of underlying mechanisms and interactions with other factors.

In the area of social support findings are less definitive, but there have now been many studies. A smaller proportion of the studies has been carried out in patient samples and much of the work which depends on community samples still requires confirmation in patient groups, in severely depressed inpatients and in bipolars. There is clearly an association between poor social support and depression. Both life-event stress-buffering and independent effects of social support have been demonstrated and both probably apply. The origins and mechanisms of the association between social support and depression, and the degree to which it is causative, are not yet clear. This is partly because longitudinal designs have not yet been sufficiently exploited, and are difficult to apply to onset. While the independence of social support from disorder can be established, there is still a complex interrelationship between personality, capacity to forge social ties and the amount of social support available.

It is useful to consider requirements for future studies of social support. Psychiatric status should be established by a standard interview in which well-defined symptoms are assessed, and patient samples should be more extensively used. Onset of disorder should be rated as accurately as possible. Social support should be clearly defined and a valid and reliable interview method of assessing it should be used. In order to establish the exact role of support in onset and maintenance of disorder, careful attention must be paid to the timing of the assessment of support. To test an onset theory, social support should be assessed independently of disorder and prior to its onset. It may be possible to achieve this using retrospective assessment techniques, but ideally a prospective study along the lines reported

Table 10.3 Longitudinal studies of social support and affective disorders

Authors	n	Sex	Dependent variable	Quest/ interview	Social support measure content	Quest/ interview	Life events	Assessment points	Result
Community samples									
Myers et al 1975 Eaton 1978 (reanalysis)	720	Mixed	Psychiatric disorder Gurin index	I	Not clearly specified Social integration	I	Life crises not clearly specified	Initial 2-year follow-up	Those with high symptom levels and few life events were less integrated in community than those with few symptoms and many life events
Henderson 1981	323	Mixed	CHQ – 30 item	Q	ISSI Close bonds and diffuse ties	I	List of recent experiences interview for adverse events	4 waves at 4-month intervals	Deficiencies in personal relationships and perceived inadequacy associated with development of neurotic symptoms under adversity
Blazer 1983	331	Mixed	18-item depression scale	Q	Duke questionnaire	Q	Not assessed	Initial assessment; 30 month follow up	Depression at time I associated with improvement of social support at time II
Parker & Blignault 1985	66	Mixed	Zung depression scale PSE	Q & I	Social relationships; intimacy	I	LEDS	Initial assessment; 6-week follow-up; 20-week follow-up	Improvement at 6 and 20 weeks predicted by break up of intimate relationship in preceding 12 months
Brown et al 1986	400	Women	Caseness based on PSE	I	Intimacy SESS	I	LEDS	Initial assessment; 1-year follow-up	Negative evaluation of self and other indices of lack of support from a core tie at first interview were associated with increased risk of subsequent depression once a stressor occurred. Lack of support from core tie at time of crisis particularly highly associated with increased risk

Study	N	Sample	Depression measure	I/Q	Social support measure	I/Q	Life stress measure	Timing	Findings
Miller et al 1987	415	Women	Psychiatric assessment schedule	I	Social support interview	I	LEDS	Initial assessment; 6-month follow-up; 1-year follow-up	Impaired relationships went with continuing illness
Bolton & Oatley 1987	49	Men (unemployed)	Beck Depression Inventory	Q	Semi-structured interview. Quantity of social interaction, emotional support, material assistance, evenings out	I	Recent unemployment Social Readjustment Rating Scale	Initial assessment; 6–8-month follow-up	Depression scores at follow up higher for those who remained unemployed and who had little social contact prior to being unemployed

Patient samples

Study	N	Sample	Depression measure	I/Q	Social support measure	I/Q	Life stress measure	Timing	Findings
Vaughn & Leff 1976	32	Depressed Mixed	Relapse of depression PSE	I	Level of critical comments of relative usually spouse	I	Not assessed	EE measured at index episode	Level of EE in key relative at index episode predicted subsequent relapse of depression
Surtees 1980	80	Depressed Mixed	HRSD semi-structured version	I	Support – close and diffuse	I	LEDS	Index episode 28-week follow-up	Social support conferred partial immunity against recurrence of symptoms
Waring & Patton 1984	75	Depressed Mixed	BDI GHQ	Q	Waring intimacy questionnaire	Q	Not assessed	Index episode 1-month follow-up	Patients with lowest levels of intimacy failed to improve at 1-month follow-up
Billings & Moos 1985	424	Depressed Mixed	Depression severity on rating scale: employment, self-esteem, etc	Q by postal survey	Supportive aspects of family social resources, stress at work, number of friends, network contacts and close relationships	Q	Life stress by questionnaire	At treatment intake; 12-month follow-up	Life stress and social resources related to functioning at follow up
George et al 1989	150	Depressed Mixed	CES-D Depression Scale	I	Duke social support index	I	19-item life event checklist	Index episode 6–32 months later	Size of network and subjective social support predictors of depressive symptoms at follow-up
Brugha et al 1990	130	Depressed Mixed	PSE	I	IMSR – social network and support contacts and quality	I	Adversity measure	Index episode 4-month follow-up	Recovery associated with social support gender differences

by Brown et al (1986) should be undertaken. Frequent serial assessments of support and disorder would allow changes in support to be related to onset and subsequent maintenance of disorder.

Interactions of life stress with factors other than social support have received relatively little study. Interactions with personality and cognitive factors have been studied in laboratory situations but need further exploration outside this setting. It could be, for instance, that obsessional personalities are vulnerable to events involving major changes of life patterns, and work failures are Achilles' heels for Type As, but there is little overt evidence.

Perhaps the greatest gap lies in relationships between psychosocial and biological factors, including underlying neurobiological mechanisms. Social events make their impacts through psychological perceptions and these have their substrates and concomitants in brain function.

In the area of interaction with genetics, Patrick et al (1978) hypothesized that depressives ought to show an inverse relationship between presence of life events and the degree of family history loading at onset of the first episode of bipolar disorder. Assessing this retrospect-

ively, they failed to find it. McGuffin et al (1988), in a recent careful study in unipolar cases, obtained similar findings. In this study life events as well as depression appeared to be familial.

Calloway et al (1984a,b), in the neuroendocrine field, found no relationship between the presence of life events and dexamethasone non-suppression, but presence of difficulties on Brown's interview was associated with blunted TSH response to TRH. Few other studies have employed social-stress measures with biological markers, either state- or trait-related.

Interactions of life events, and particularly those with social support, may also have practical implications. Many of the events implicated in disorder are of a type over which the individual and the clinician have no control, and which would require major changes in the structure of society to avoid. Others are inevitable consequences of the life cycle. However, social support may be amenable to therapeutic intervention. Modifying levels of social support in an attempt to prevent or ameliorate disorder offers both an experimental method of demonstrating aetiological effects of support and an approach to treatment and prophylaxis.

REFERENCES

Alloway R, Bebbington P E 1987 The buffer theory of social support: a review of the literature. Psychological Medicine 17: 91–108

Ambelas A 1979 Psychologically stressful events in the precipitation of manic episodes. British Journal of Psychiatry 135: 15–21

Ambelas A 1987 Life events and mania. A special relationship? British Journal of Psychiatry 150: 235–240

Andrews G, Tennant C, Hewson D Schonell M 1978 The relation of social factors to physical and psychiatric illness. American Journal of Epidemiology 108: 27–35

Aneshensel C S, Stone J D 1982 Stress and depression: a test of the buffering model of social support. Archives of General Psychiatry 39: 1392–1396

Aronson T A, Shukla S 1987 Life events and relapse in bipolar disorder: the impact of a catastrophic event. Acta Psychiatrica Scandinavica 75: 571–576

Barrett J E 1979 The relationship of life events to onset of neurotic disorders. In: Barrett J E (ed) Stress and mental disorder. Raven Press, New York, p 87–109

Bebbington P E, Tennant C, Hurry J 1981 Adversity and the nature of psychiatric disorder in the community. Journal of Affective Disorders 3: 345–366

Bebbington P E, Sturt E, Tennant C, Hurry J 1984 Misfortune and resilience: a replication of the work of Brown and Harris. Psychological Medicine 14: 347–363

Bebbington P E, Hurry J, Tennant C 1988 Adversity and the symptoms of depression. International Journal of Social Psychiatry. 34(3): 163–171

Beck J C, Worthen K 1972 Precipitating stress, crisis theory and hospitalization in schizophrenia and depression. Archives of General Psychiatry 26: 123–129

Benjaminsen S 1981 Stressful life events preceding the onset of neurotic depression. Psychological Medicine 11: 369–378

Bidzinska E J 1984 Stress factors in affective diseases. British Journal of Psychiatry 144: 161–166

Billings A G, Moos R H 1984 Chronic and nonchronic unipolar depression. The differential role of environment stressors and resources. Journal of Nervous Disease 172: 65–75

Billings A G, Moos R H 1985 Psychosocial processes of remission in unipolar depression: comparing depressed patients with matched community controls. Journal of Consulting and Clinical Psychology 53: 314–325

Billings A G, Cronkite R C, Moos R H 1983 Social-environment factors in unipolar depression: comparisons of depressed patients and nondepressed controls. Journal of Abnormal Psychology 92(2): 119–133

Birtchnell J 1970a The relationship between attempted suicide, depression and parent death. British Journal of Psychiatry 116: 307–313

Birtchnell J 1970b Depression in relation to early and recent parent death. British Journal of Psychiatry 116: 299–306

Birtchnell J 1975 Psychiatric breakdown following recent

parent death. British Journal of Medical Psychology 48: 379–390

Birtchnell J 1988 Depression and life circumstances: a study of young, married women on a London housing estate. Social Psychiatry and Psychiatric Epidemiology 23: 240–246

Blazer D G 1983 Impact of late-life depression on the social network. American Journal of Psychiatry 140: 162–166

Bolton W, Oatley K 1987 A longitudinal study of social support and depression in unemployed men. Psychological Medicine 17: 453–460

Bornstein P E, Clayton P J, Halikas J A, Maurice W L, Robins E 1973 The depression of widowhood after thirteen months. British Journal of Psychiatry 122: 561–566

Brockington I F, Martin C, Brown G W, Goldberg D, Margison F 1990 Stress and puerperal psychosis. British Journal of Psychiatry 157: 331–334

Brown G W, Birley J L T, 1968 Crises and life changes and the onset of schizophrenia. Journal of Health and Social Behaviour 9: 203–214

Brown G W, Harris T 1978 The social origins of depression: a study of psychiatric disorder in women. Tavistock, London

Brown G W, Prudo R 1981 Psychiatric disorder in a rural and an urban population: aetiology of depression. Psychological Medicine 11: 581–599

Brown G W, Sklair F, Harris T O, Birley J L T 1973a Life-events and psychiatric disorders. Part 1. Some methodological issues. Psychological Medicine 3: 74–87

Brown G W, Harris T O, Peto J 1973b Life events and psychiatric disorders. Part 2. Nature of causal link. Psychological Medicine 3: 159–176

Brown G W, NiBhrolchain M, Harris T O 1979 Psychotic and neurotic depression. Part 3. Aetiological and background factors. Journal of Affective Disorders 1: 195–211

Brown G W, Andrews B, Harris T, Adler Z, Bridge L 1986 Social support, self-esteem and depression. Psychological Medicine 16: 813–831

Brown G W, Adler Z, Bifulco A 1988 Life events, difficulties and recovery from chronic depression. British Journal of Psychiatry 152: 487–498

Brugha T S, Conroy R 1985 Categories of depression: reported life events in a controlled design. British Journal of Psychiatry 147: 641–646

Brugha T S, Conroy R, Walsh N, Delaney W, O'Hanlon J, Dondero E, Daly L, Hickey N et al 1982 Social networks, attachments and support in minor affective disorders: a replication. British Journal of Psychiatry 141: 249–255

Brugha T S, Bebbington B, MacCarthy B, Potter J, Sturt E, Wykes T, 1987 Social networks, social support and the type of depressive illness. Acta Psychiatrica Scandinavica 76: 664–673

Brugha T S, Bebbington P E, MacCarthy B, Sturt E, Wykes T, Potter J 1990 Gender, social support and recovery from depressive disorders: a prospective clinical study. Psychological Medicine 20: 147–156

Cadoret R J, Winokur G, Dorzab J, Baker M 1972 Depressive disease: life events and onset of illness. Archives of General Psychiatry 26: 133–136

Calloway S P, Dolan R J, Fonagy P, De Souza V F A,

Wakeling A 1984a Endocrine changes and clinical profiles in depression. 1. The dexamethasone suppression test. Psychological Medicine 14: 744–758

Calloway S P, Dolan R J, Fonagy P, De Souza V F A, Wakeling A 1984b Endocrine changes and clinical profiles in depression. 2. The thyrotropin-releasing hormone test. Psychological Medicine 14: 759–765

Campbell E A 1983 Depression in women: the role of life events, social factors and psychological vulnerability. Unpublished D Phil thesis, University of Oxford

Campbell E, Cope S, Teasdale J 1983 Social factors and affective disorder: an investigation of Brown and Harris's model. British Journal of Psychiatry 143: 548–553

Champion L 1990 The relationship between social vulnerability and the occurrence of severely threatening life events. Psychological Medicine 20: 157–161

Chatterjee R N, Mukherjee S P, Nandi D N 1981 Life events and depression. Indian Journal of Psychiatry 23: 333–337

Clayton P, Desmarais L, Winokur G 1968 A study of normal bereavement. American Journal of Psychiatry 125: 168–178

Cobb S 1976 Social support as a moderator of life stress. Psychosomatic Medicine 38: 300–315

Cobb S 1979 Social support and health through the life course. In: Riley M W (ed) Aging from birth to death: interdisciplinary perspectives. American Association for the Advancement of Science, Washington D C, p 147–188

Cohen S, Wills T A 1985 Stress, social support and the buffering hypothesis. Psychological Bulletin 98: 310–357

Cohen-Sandler R, Berman A L, King R A 1982 Life stress and symptomatology: determinants of suicidal behaviour in children. Journal of the American Academy of Child Psychiatry 21: 178–186

Cooke D J 1987 The significance of life events as a cause of psychological and physical disorder. In: Cooper B (ed) Psychiatric epidemiology. Croom Helm, New York p 67–80

Cooper P J, Stein A 1989 Life events and postnatal depression: the Oxford study. In: Cox J L, Paykel E S, Page M L (eds) Childbirth as a life event. Duphar Medical Relations, Southampton

Cooper P J, Campbell E A, Day A, Kennerley H, Bond A 1988 Non-psychotic psychiatric disorder after childbirth. A prospective study of prevalence, incidence, course and nature. British Journal of Psychiatry 152: 799–806

Cornelis C M, Ameling E H, de Jonghe F 1989 Life events and social network in relation to the onset of depression. A controlled study. Acta Psychiatrica Scandinavica 88: 174–179

Costello C G 1982 Social factors associated with depression: a retrospective community study. Psychological Medicine 12: 329–339

Cox J L, Paykel E S, Page M L 1989 Current approaches: childbirth as a life event. Duphar Medical Relations, Southampton.

Dohrenwend B S 1973a Life events as stressors: a methodological inquiry. Journal of Health and Social Behaviour 14: 167–175

Dohrenwend B S 1973b Social status and stressful life events. Journal of Personality and Social Psychology 28: 225–235

Dolan R J, Calloway S P, Fonagy P, De Souza F V A, Wakeling A 1985 Life events, depression and hypothalamic-pituitary-adrenal axis function. British Journal of Psychiatry 147: 429–433

Dowlatshahi D, Paykel E S 1990 Life events and social stress in puerperal psychoses: absence of effect. Psychological Medicine 20: 655–662

Eaton W W 1978 Life events, social supports, and psychiatric symptoms: a re-analysis of the New Haven data. Journal of Health and Social Behavior 19: 230–234

Eisler R M, Polak P R 1971 Social stress and psychiatric disorder. Journal of Nervous and Mental Disease 153: 227–233

Emmerson J P, Burvill P W, Finlay-Jones R, Hall W 1989 Life events, life difficulties and confiding relationships in depressed elderly. British Journal of Psychiatry 155: 787–792

Ezquiaga E, Gutierrez J L A, Lopez A G 1987 Psychosocial factors and episode number in depression. Journal of Affective Disorders 12: 135–138

Faravelli C, Ambonetti A 1983 Assessment of life events in depressive disorders. A comparison of three methods. Social Psychiatry 18: 51–56

Fava G A, Munari F, Pasvan L, Kellner R 1981 Life events and depression. A replication. Journal of Affective Disorders 3: 159–165

Finlay-Jones R, Brown G W 1981 Types of stressful life event and the onset of anxiety and depressive disorders. Psychological Medicine 11: 803–815

Flaherty J, Gaviria M, Black E 1983 The role of social support in the functioning of patients with unipolar depression. American Journal of Psychiatry 140: 473–476

Forrest A D, Fraser R H, Priest R G 1965 Environmental factors in depressive illness. British Journal of Psychiatry 111: 243–253

Fowler R C, Liskow B I, Tanna V L 1980 Alcoholism, depression and life events. Journal of Affective Disorders 2: 127–135

Friedman L, Weissman M M, Leaf P J, Bruce M L 1988 Social functioning in community residents with depression and other psychiatric disorders: results of the New Haven Epidemiologic Catchment Area Study. Journal of Affective Disorders 15: 103–112

Gath D, Cooper P, Day A 1982 Hysterectomy and psychiatric disorder: I. Levels of psychiatric morbidity before and after hysterectomy. British Journal of Psychiatry 140: 335–350

George L K, Blazer D G, Hughes D C, Fowler N 1989 Social support and outcome of major depression. British Journal of Psychiatry 154: 478–485

Giel R, Ten Horn GHMM, Ormel J, Schudel WJ, Wiersma O 1978 Mental illness, neuroticism and life events in a Dutch village sample: a follow-up. Psychological Medicine 8: 235–243

Glassner B, Haldipur C V G 1983 Life events and early and late onset of bipolar disorder. American Journal of Psychiatry 140: 215–217

Goodyer I, Kolvin I, Gatzanis S 1985 Recent undesirable life events and psychiatric disorder in childhood and adolescence. British Journal of Psychiatry 147: 517–523

Goodyer I M, Kolvin I, Gatzanis S 1987 The impact of recent undesirable life events on psychiatric disorders in childhood and adolescence. British Journal of Psychiatry 151: 179–184

Goodyer I, Wright C, Altham P 1990 The friendships and recent life events of anxious and depressed school-age children. British Journal of Psychiatry 156: 689–698

Hall K S, Dunner D L, Zeller G, Fieve R R 1977 Bipolar illness: a prospective study of life events. Comprehensive Psychiatry 18: 497–502

Hallstrom T 1986 Social origins of major depression: the role of provoking agents and vulnerability factors. Acta Psychiatrica Scandinavica 73: 383–389

Harder D W, Strauss J S, Kokes R F, Ritzler B A, Gift T E 1980 Life events and psychopathology severity among first psychiatric admissions. Journal of Abnormal Psychology 89: 165–180

Henderson S 1981 Social relationships, adversity and neurosis: an analysis of prospective observations. British Journal of Psychiatry 138: 391–398

Henderson S, Duncan-Jones P, McAuley H, Ritchie K 1978 The patient's primary group. British Journal of Psychiatry 132: 74–86

Hickie I B 1990 Interpersonal relationships and depressive disorders. M D thesis, University of New South Wales

Holmes T H, Rahe R H 1967 The social readjustment rating scale. Journal of Psychosomatic Research 11: 213–218

House J S 1981 Work stress and social support. Addison-Wesley, Reading, M A

Hudgens R W, Morrison J R, Barchha R 1967 Life events and onset of primary affective disorders. A study of 40 hospitalised patients and 40 controls. Archives of General Psychiatry 16: 134–145

Jacobs S C, Prusoff B A, Paykel E S 1974 Recent life events in schizophrenia and depression. Psychological Medicine 4: 444–453

Kaplan B H, Cassel J C, Gore S 1977 Social support and health. Medical Care 15: 47–58

Kasl S V, Gore S, Cobb S 1975 The experience of losing a job: Reported changes in health, symptoms and illness behaviour. Psychosomatic Medicine 37: 106–122

Katschnig H, Berner P 1984 The poly-diagnostic approach in psychiatric research. In: Proceedings of the International Conference on Diagnosis and Classification of Mental Disorder and Alcohol and Drug Related Problems (Copenhagen, 13–17 April 1982). World Health Organization, Geneva

Kendell R E, Chalmers J C, Platz C 1987 Epidemiology of puerperal psychoses. British Journal of Psychiatry 150: 662–673

Kennedy S, Thompson R, Stancer H C, Roy A, Persad E 1983 Life events precipitating mania. British Journal of Psychiatry 142: 398–403

Kosten T R, Rounsaville B J, Kleber H D 1983 Relationship of depression to psychosocial stressors in heroin addicts. Journal of Nervous and Mental Disease 171: 97–104

Kosten T R, Rounsaville B J, Kleber H D 1986 A 2.5-year follow-up of depression, life crises, and treatment effects on abstinence among opioid addicts. Archives of General Psychiatry 43: 733–738

Lahniers C E, White K 1976 Changes in environmental life events and their relationship to psychiatric hospital admissions. Journal of Nervous and Mental Disease 163: 154–158

Leff JP, Vaughn C 1980 The interaction of life events and relatives' expressed emotion in schizophrenia and depressive neurosis. British Journal of Psychiatry 136: 146–153

Levi L D, Fales C H, Stein M, Sharp V H 1966 Separation and attempted suicide. Archives of General Psychiatry 15: 158–165

Lin N, Ensel W, Simeone R, Kuo W 1979 Social support, stressful life events and illness: a model for an empirical test. Journal of Health and Social Behaviour 20: 108–119

Lloyd C, Zisook S, Click M, Jaffe K E 1981 Life events and response to antidepressants. Journal of Human Stress 7: 2–15

Maguire G P, Lee E G, Bevington D J, Kuchemann C S, Crabtree R J, Cornell C E 1978 Psychiatric problems in the first year after mastectomy. British Medical Journal 1: 963–965

Malmquist C P 1970 Depression and object loss in psychiatric admissions. American Journal of Psychiatry 126: 1782–1787

Martin C J, Brown G W, Goldberg D P, Brockington I F 1989 Psychosocial stress and puerperal depression. Journal of Affective Disorders 16: 283–293

Matussek P, Neuner R 1981 Loss events preceding endogenous and neurotic depressions. Acta Psychiatrica Scandinavica 64: 340–350

McGuffin P, Katz R, Bebbington P 1988 The Camberwell Collaborative Depression Study. III. Depression and adversity in the relatives of depressed probands. British Journal of Psychiatry 152: 775–782

Mendlewicz J, Charon F, Linkowski P 1986 Life events and the dexamethasone suppression test in affective illness. Journal of Affective Disorders 10: 203–206

Merikangas K R, Prusoff B A, Kupfer D J, Frank E 1985 Marital adjustment in major depression. Journal of Affective Disorders 9: 5–11

Miller P McC, Ingham J G, Kreitman N B, Surtees P G, Sashidharan S P 1987 Life events and other factors implicated in onset and remission of psychiatric illness in women. Journal of Affective Disorders 12: 73–88

Monroe S M, Thase M E, Hersen M, Himmelhoch J M, Bellack A S 1985 Life events and the endogenous-nonendogenous distinction in the treatment and posttreatment course of depression. Comprehensive Psychiatry 26(2): 175–186

Murphy E 1982 Social origins of depression in old age. British Journal of Psychiatry 141: 135–142

Murphy E 1983 The prognosis of depression in old age. British Journal of Psychiatry 142: 111–119

Myers J K, Lindenthal J J, Pepper M P 1971 Life events and psychiatric impairment. Journal of Nervous and Mental Diseases 152: 149–157

Myers J K, Lindenthal J J, Pepper M P 1975 Life events, social integration and psychiatric symptomatology. Journal of Health and Social Behavior 16: 421–427

O'Hara M W, Nennaber D J, Zekoski E M 1984 Prospective study of post partum depression. Prevalence, course and predictive factors. Journal of Abnormal Psychology 93(2): 158–171

Parker G, Blignault I 1985 Psychosocial predictors of outcome in subjects with untreated depressive disorder. Journal of Affective Disorders 8: 73–81

Parker G, Blignault I, Manicavasagar V 1988 Neurotic depression: delineation of symptom profiles and their relation to outcome. British Journal of Psychiatry 152: 15–23

Parkes C M 1964 Recent bereavement as a cause of mental illness. British Journal of Psychiatry 110: 198–204

Parry G, Shapiro D A 1986 Social support and life events in working-class women: stress buffering or independent effects? Archives of General Psychiatry 43: 315–323

Patrick V, Dunner D L, Fieve R R 1978 Life events and primary affective illness. Acta Psychiatrica Scandinavica 58: 48–55

Paykel E S 1974 Life stress and psychiatric disorder: application of the clinical approach. In: Dohrenwend B S, Dohrenwend B P (eds) Stressful life events: their nature and effects. John Wiley, New York, p 135–149

Paykel E S 1978 Contribution of life events to causation of psychiatric illness. Psychological Medicine 8: 245–253

Paykel E S 1979 Recent life events in the development of the depressive disorders: implications for the effects of stress Academic Press, New York, p 245–262

Paykel E S 1982 Life events and early environment. In: Paykel E S (ed) Handbook of affective disorders. Churchill Livingstone, Edinburgh, p 146–161

Paykel E S 1983 Methodological aspects of life events research. Journal of Psychosomatic Research 27: 341–352

Paykel E S 1984 Life events, social support and clinical psychiatric disorder. In: Sarason I G, Sarason B R (eds) Social support: theory, research and applications. NATO ASI Series, p 321–347

Paykel E S, Cooper Z C (1991) Recent life events and psychiatric illness. In: Seva A (ed) European handbook of psychiatry and mental health. University Press of Zaragoza, Zaragoza, Spain, p 350–363

Paykel E S, Tanner J 1976 Life events, depressive relapse and maintenance treatment. Psychological Medicine 6: 481–485

Paykel E S, Myers J K, Dienelt M N 1969 Life events and depression: a controlled study. Archives of General Psychiatry 21: 753–760

Paykel E S, Prusoff B A, Myers J K 1975 Suicide attempts and recent life events: a controlled comparison. Archives of General Psychiatry 32: 327–333

Paykel E S, Emms E M, Fletcher J, Rassaby E S 1980 Life events and social support in puerperal depression. British Journal of Psychiatry 136: 339–346

Paykel E S, Rao B M, Taylor C M 1984 Life stress and symptom pattern in out-patient depression. Psychological Medicine 14: 559–568

Prusoff B, Thompson W D, Sholomskas D, Riordan C 1977 Psychosocial stressors and depression among former heroin-dependent patients maintained on methadone. Journal of Nervous and Mental Disease 165: 57–63

Reno R M, Halaris A E 1990 The relationship between life stress and depression in an endogenous sample. Comprehensive Psychiatry 31(1): 25–33

Rosenthal S H, Klerman G L 1966 Content and consistency in the endogenous depressive pattern. British Journal of Psychiatry 112: 471–484

Rowan P R, Paykel E S, Parker R R 1982 Phenelzine and amitriptyline: effects on symptoms of neurotic depression. British Journal of Psychiatry 140: 475–483

Roy A, Kennedy S 1984 Risk factors for depression in Canadians. Canadian Journal of Psychiatry 29: 11–13

Roy A, Thompson R, Kennedy S 1983 Depression in chronic schizophrenia. British Journal of Psychiatry 142: 465–470

Roy A, Breier A, Doran A R, Pickar D 1985 Life events in depression. Relationship to subtypes. Journal of Affective Disorders 9: 143–148

Roy A, Custer R, Lorenz V, Linoila M 1988 Depressed pathological gamblers. Acta Psychiatrica Scandinavica 77: 163–165

Rutter M 1983 Statistical and personal interactions: facets and perspectives. In: Magnusson D, Allen V (eds) Human development: an interactional perspective. Academic Press, London

Salokangas R K R, Mattila V, Joukamaa M 1988 Intimacy and mental disorder in late middle age. Acta Psychiatrica Scandinavica 78: 555–560

Sclare P, Creed F 1990 Life events and the onset of mania. British Journal of Psychiatry 156: 508–514

Sethi B B 1964 Relationship of separation to depression. Archives of General Psychiatry 10: 186–195

Sireling L I, Freeling P, Paykel E S, Rao B M 1985 Depression in general practice: clinical features and comparison with out-patients. British Journal of Psychiatry 147: 119–126

Slater J, Depue R A 1981 The contribution of environmental events and social support to serious suicide attempts in primary depressive disorder. Journal of Abnormal Psychology 90: 275–285

Solomon Z, Bromet E 1982 The role of social factors in affective disorder: an assessment of the vulnerability model of Brown and his colleagues. Psychological Medicine 12: 123–130

Surtees P G 1980 Social support, residual adversity and depressive outcome. Social Psychiatry 15: 71–80

Tennant C, Bebbington P, Hurry J 1981 The short-term outcome of neurotic disorders in the community: the relation of remission to clinical factors and to 'neutralizing' life events. British Journal of Psychiatry 139: 213–220

Thoits P A 1982 Conceptual, methodological and theoretical problems in studying social support as a buffer against life stress. Journal of Health and Social Behavior 23: 145–159

Thoits P A 1985 Social support processes and psychological well-being: theoretical possibilities. In: Sarason I G, Sarason B (eds) Social support: theory, research and applications. Martinus Nijhof, The Hague

Thompson K C, Hendrie H C 1972 Environmental stress in primary depressive illness. Archives of General Psychiatry 26: 130–132

Uhlenhuth E H, Paykel E S 1973 Symptom configuration and life events. Archives of General Psychiatry 28: 743–748

Uhlenhuth E H, Lipman R S, Balter M B, Stern M 1974 Symptom intensity and life stress in the city. Archives of General Psychiatry 31: 759–764

Ullah P, Banks M, Warr P 1985 Social support, social pressures and psychological distress during unemployment. Psychological Medicine 15: 283–295

Vadher A, Ndetei D M 1981 Life events and depression in a Kenyan setting. British Journal of Psychiatry 139: 134–149

Vaughn C E, Leff J P 1976 The influence of family and social factors on the course of psychiatric illness. British Journal of Psychiatry 129: 125–137

Waring E M, Patton D 1984 Marital intimacy and depression. British Journal of Psychiatry 145: 641–644

Wittchen H U 1987 Chronic difficulties and life events in the long-term course of affective and anxiety disorders: results from the Munich follow-up study. In: Angermeyer M C (ed) From social class to social stress. Springer, Berlin, p 176–196

11. Early environment

Gordon Parker

PARENTAL RISK FACTORS TO ADULT DEPRESSION

On theoretical grounds, a number of early environmental factors might dispose a child to subsequent depression, including family, socioeconomic and cultural variables. Early parent — child relationships and parenting behaviours have been held as central determinants of later psychopathology, with the underlying 'parental deprivation' hypothesis being subjected to detailed empirical research. The absence of a parallel literature for other theoretically relevant early environmental factors makes sensible explication difficult. This chapter will therefore focus on the research literature evaluating parental deprivation as a risk factor for adult depression.

According to Mendelson (1974), 'from the days of Abraham through Klein to Jacobson', analysts have expressed a recurring theme 'that adult depressive illnesses recapitulate early infantile parathymias or disappointments', with lack of gratification from the mother-figure inducing a susceptibility to frustration by lack of later 'love objects', the recipients then regressing to a state of depression. After reviewing psychoanalytic views about developmental factors, Mendelson nevertheless concluded that much analytic theorizing had been doctrinaire, quite lacking in legitimate doubt, inadequate in diagnostic delineation of depressive types, based on small samples and replete with overgeneralization and reification – concerns that are relevant in any review of the early parental environment experienced by depressives.

The early history of the parental deprivation hypothesis is well described and requires only a brief note. While the psychoanalysts derived their concepts from historical reconstructions based on the reports of adults, Bowlby developed his views using primary data based on observations of very young children. He subsequently published a WHO monograph (Bowlby 1951) arguing that infants and children required warm, intimate and continuous relationships with their mothers to ensure mental health, initiating the utilitarian 'maternal deprivation' debate.

Rutter (1972) was clearly concerned about the broadness of the proposition. He noted that, while 'different types of deprivation (perceptual, social, biological and psychological) tend to accompany one another', progress is unlikely until the basic variables underlying the concept of 'maternal deprivation' are differentiated and the separate effects of each specified. Bowlby's later writings provide a useful framework for explication. After reviewing the tenets of attachment theory, Bowlby (1977) stated that care-givers (parents) have two roles: firstly, 'to be available and responsive as and when wanted and, secondly, to intervene judiciously should the child . . . be heading for trouble'. By contrast, Bowlby described 'pathogenic parenting' as involving: 1) 'parents being persistently unresponsive to the child's care-eliciting behaviour and/or actively disparaging and rejecting'; 2) discontinuities of parenting; or 3) parents 'inverting the normal relationship' by exerting pressure on the child to act as an attachment figure to the parent. Such theorizing is consistent with oft-put vignettes of the characteristics of the parents of subjects with psychiatric (particularly neurotic) and other disorders. These attributes (i.e. lack of care, overprotection) have been encapsulated in terms such as the 'asthmatogenic' and 'schizophrenogenic' parent, and were even implicated as determinants of depression in the classic seventeenth century text on melancholia by Burton (see Hunter & Macalpine 1963, p 94). Bowlby's postulates thus encouraged empirical research assessing the impact of discontinuities in parenting ('parental loss') and the relevance of anomalous parenting ('parental style'). Each broad topic will now be considered.

PARENTAL LOSS

While there is no dispute that loss of a parent is associated with acute distress in a child (Raphael 1983), it remains unclear whether loss *per se* disposes to depression in adulthood. Although a link is accepted in many texts, such a conclusion may reflect prominent studies with positive findings. For instance, Brown et al (1977) argued that loss of mother before the age of 11 years was associated with a greater risk of adult depression, and judged that a direct causal effect was likely. Further, they reported that past loss by death was associated with psychotic-like depressive symptoms (and their severity), while other types of past loss were associated with neurotic-type depressive symptoms and their severity, and concluded that 'these associations probably reflect direct causal links'. There is an immediate problem in drawing conclusions from such studies, as 'loss' in the Brown study included death and separation, with 'death' including death of a husband, a sibling or a child (including stillbirths) as well as parental death.

A synthesis of review papers examining the 'parental loss' proposition captures the variable interpretations over an extended period. Granville-Grossman (1968) concluded that 'no consistent evidence has been found in the studies cited on parental deprivation... to support the view that early environment is of aetiological importance in the affective disorders'. Rutter (1972) considered the evidence to be somewhat contradictory but concluded that 'depressive disorders during adult life may be particularly common when a parent has died during the person's adolescence'. Heinicke (1973) held that the childhood experience of parental death was associated with a greater incidence of depression, attempts at suicide and a severer form of depression. Becker (1974) concluded that 'there is no consistent, substantial evidence for a relationship between early parental loss *per se* and either predisposition to depression or severity of depressive episode'. Tennant et al (1980) concluded that if potential confounding effects are taken into account, there is a non-existent or negligible long-term psychopathological effect. Similarly, Richards & Dyson (1982) commented that, in relation to separation, 'if effects exist they must be relatively weak or the studies would have been able to demonstrate them much more consistently'. A key difficulty resides in varying definitions of 'loss'. To clarify this issue, relevant parental loss research will be sub-divided into two sections: parental death and parental separation.

Parental death as a risk factor to depression

Some 60 research studies were screened to select those that reached minimal criteria for addressing, directly or in part, the key proposition. Studies were excluded for the following reasons: 1) the sample comprised children; 2) 'death' included others than parents; 3) 'death' was aggregated with other loss or separation experiences; 4) global measures of 'caseness' were used, so that non-depressive conditions were included; 5) no measure of 'depression' was described; 6) dimensional state measures of depression were used to define adult depression – thus limiting consideration to studies assessing current, recent or lifetime depression; and 7) there was either no control group or the control group was categorically inappropriate.

Considerable latitude was allowed in accepting studies that failed to control for a set of reasonable variables in such an inquiry (i.e. sex, social class, age – when parental bereavement is increased during times such as war – and parental age, non-hospital patients); as well as studies that failed to specify the 'type' of depression, when parental death might have selective relevance to either melancholic or non-melancholic disorders. Table 11.1 lists the ten studies that met basic criteria. Only three demonstrated a significantly increased rate of parental bereavement and the rates in the two earliest tabled studies were significant because of extremely high early bereavement rates (35–41%) in the depressives, certainly far higher than bereavement rates in other depressive samples, suggesting the possibility of referral biases. Thus, it would appear reasonable to suggest that there is neither strong nor consistent data supporting a link between parental death and adult depression, at least in treated depressives. As the listed studies were of depressed patients, any link (if it had been demonstrated) might lie between parental death and depressed patient 'status' (i.e. help-seeking) rather than with depression *per se*. This last issue may be pursued further by examining 'community depressives'. Several studies are of relevance.

Birtchnell (1980) sub-sampled a psychiatric case register, deriving 160 women whose mother had died before the patient reached 11 years, contrasted with 80 'control' women whose natural parents had not died before the subjects were 26 years, with groups matched by decade of birth. If parental death disposes to depression, a differential depression rate across the groups would be expected. Instead, Birtchnell estimated 67% of the mother-bereaved versus 74% of the 'controls' to

Table 11.1   Selected controlled studies examining adult depression rates in parent-bereaved subjects

| Authors | Depressives | | Control | | Results |
	Sample	Bereavement Rate	Group	Bereavement Rate (%)	Hypothesis: parental death in childhood is significantly associated with depression in adulthood
Brown 1961	216 depressed outpatients	41% before 15 years	General practice patients Census	20 17	Yes
Forrest et al 1965	158 inpatient and outpatient depressives	35% before 15 years	58 general hospital patients	17	Yes
Pitts et al 1965	366 depressed inpatients	Not formally reported	General hospital controls	Not formally reported	No
Hopkinson & Reed 1966	200 manic depressive inpatients	19% before 15 years	Brown's general practice patients Brown's census data	20 17	No
Dennehy 1966	361 inpatient depressives	17% had father die, 11% had mother die before 15 years	Census for fathers Census for mothers	12 6	Yes
Munro 1966	153 inpatient depressives	22% before 16 years	General hospital out-patients	20	No
Hudgens et al 1967	34 depressives & 6 manics (hospitalized)	15% before 14 years	General hospital patients	17	No
Birthchnell 1972	2699 depressives on register	11% before 10 years	General population sample	8	No
Roy 1983	300 neurotic depressives	13% before 17 years 9% before 11 years	General hospital patients	11 7	No
Favarelli et al 1986	100 with major depression 118 outpatient depressives	12% before 10 years 9% before 10 years	Hospital employees	9	No

have had a depressive disorder. Hallstrom (1987) examined a Swedish population sample, and contrasted 60 women having a current or recent major depressive episode with 400 women negative for depression. Parental death before 17 years was calculated at 18% in each group, so that parental death was not over-represented in the depressives.

Two British studies require closer examination. Harris et al (1986) derived a female sample from two Walthamstow general practices, but with decision rules to over-select those initially affirming parental loss in childhood. Respondents were interviewed as 'cases' or 'non-cases' of depression using the Present State Examination. For those reporting maternal and paternal deaths in the first 17 years, the case rates of

depression in the preceding 12 months were 22% and 8% respectively, compared to a case rate of 4% in those not reporting early parental death (or any other parental loss). The comparison group was somewhat optimized in that members experienced no 'losses'. If we compare rates of depression in those who experienced early parental death with the remainder, then the comparative current depression rates are 22% versus 14% (for exposure or no exposure to maternal death) and 8% versus 15% for exposure and non-exposure to paternal death, suggesting rather similar rates of current depression amongst those contrasted for one specific event—early parental bereavement or none. A second study by the same group (Bifulco et al 1987) used a similar design, studying women in Islington.

Depression in the 12 months before interview was reported by 14% of those whose mother had died before 17 years and by 13% reporting paternal bereavement, contrasting with a 15% rate for those who had experienced no parental loss (death or separation) and an 18% rate for the total sample of 395 women.

While these two studies concluded that 'loss of a mother before the age of 17' is associated with clinical depression, it is clear that when examined specifically, current depression does not appear to be over-represented in those reporting early parental death. The authors proceeded to delineate the more important 'loss' risk factors (such as lack of parental care) that will be considered shortly.

Overall, the studies offer little support for the proposed relationship between parental loss by death in childhood and depression in adulthood and so clarify variable conclusions reached in previous reviews. Tennant et al (1980) noted that 'where experimental and control samples were most rigorously matched, no association was found between childhood parental bereavement and depression in later life', while Crook & Eliot (1980) also came to a similar conclusion. Consequences of parental bereavement may well be influential, but remain to be explicated. Speculation by Birtchnell (1980) that 'the actual death of a parent is undoubtedly disturbing but does not cause lasting harm, and that any ill effects that do follow are related to inadequate mothering subsequent to loss' appears appropriate and will be considered in the next section.

Parental separation as a risk factor for adult depression

A dozen studies examining parental 'separation' (not due to death) were reviewed in preparing this chapter. Definitions of separation were frequently broad. Unlike contextual ratings of adult life events, parental 'separation' in childhood or adolescence has rarely been quantified in terms of severity and salience, thus failing to respect the reality that separations may be permanent, transient, developmental (e.g. boarding school attendance), ameliorated by on-going contact (e.g. telephone) or even desired, and that they may be modified or reversed by a variety of events. Equivalence of 'loss' following 'separation' is generally assumed. Ratings are also problematic when the realities of obtaining valid data for retrospective events are considered. More significant, however, was the notable concentration on the event per se in the published literature and the frequent failure to consider higher order variables (i.e. where the antecedents and consequences of the separation may be more influential than separation *per se*).

The potential for inconsistencies in research findings is well illustrated by considering the effects of variable definitions of 'separation'. For instance, Roy (1983) (see Table 11.1) studied the relationship between parental death and adult depression in a matched controlled clinical study of 300 neurotic depressives. No significant differences were found and it was concluded that the experience of parental death in childhood was not, in itself, a risk factor for neurotic depression. Recognizing that examination of loss by death is likely to exclude those experiencing loss through permanent separation (not due to death), Roy (1985), in a matched controlled study of 300 non-endogenous depressives, found early permanent separation before both 11 and 17 years to affect risks for adult depression. In almost all cases, permanent separation was due to a permanent break-up of the parents' marriage. The majority of the reviewed studies demonstrated or suggested a link between parental separation and adult depression. On the basis of such findings, Tennant (1988) concluded that 'in those studies where loss seemed to predict depression, the effect can largely be attributed to prolonged separations from parents, which are most often due to divorce'.

Once again, if depressives in treatment are more likely to report separation from parents, is separation a risk factor to disorder itself? Thus, Tennant et al (1981) considered whether parental loss might dispose to 'symptomatic disorder' (or psychiatric caseness) in adulthood and/or to 'psychiatric illness behaviour' (i.e. patient status). As required for such an inquiry, they assessed a community sample (in Camberwell, London). They distinguished between parental death and parent-child separation. There was no clear evidence that early death of mother or father disposed either to adult psychiatric morbidity or to help-seeking behaviour. While parent-child separation (i.e. 'abnormal' separation experience of more than a week) was not linked with adult psychiatric 'caseness', it was associated with increased psychiatric service utilization. The authors therefore favoured a link whereby parent-child separation influenced the development of illness behaviour.

Further 'process' studies require consideration. Parker & Manicavasagar (1986) studied 79 women whose mothers had died when they were aged 8–12 years and whose fathers had subsequently remarried. The most consistent predictor of adult depression was low social class, a finding compatible with studies showing a poorer outcome for adult bereavement in lower social class subjects, where ongoing economic restrictions and related privations might act as mediating or determining variables. Subsidiary analyses were therefore undertaken, establishing that lower social class subjects were more likely to report poor or inadequate replacement mothering, to score their fathers and stepmothers more deviantly on the Parental Bonding Instrument (PBI), and to report less support from their husbands. Other variables associated with adult depression in the whole sample were bereavement circumstances (i.e. sudden death of the mother), family support being perceived as deficient in the immediate post-bereavement phase, a longer delay before the stepmother assumed a maternal role and the judgment of any replacement mother-figure as being inadequate. The picture that emerges from this study is of a diathesis being established by a host of post-bereavement circumstances but with a common feature of impaired parental support. Low social class must be suspected of exerting a pathoplastic effect by shaping an ecology of adverse environments.

Tennant (1988) reviewed a number of studies showing that certain separation experiences (e.g. evacuation during the Second World War, parents at work, school-effected separations) were not associated with increased morbidity, while prolonged separations due to marital problems and parental illness were associated, before proposing that 'family discord' disposed to adult psychopathology, particularly depression. Tennant cautioned against parental 'divorce' being accepted simplistically as a risk factor, noting the independent effects of (poor) pre-separation parenting as well as post-divorce relationships between children and parents, after accepting that 'poor parenting' undoubtedly causes psychological morbidity both in childhood and in later life. Tennant's summary comments are worth quoting: 'With parent-child separations, only those occurring in relation to family discord, such as divorce, appear to have any long-term impact. Even those data are brittle when one considers that crucial confounding variables (such as parental psychopathology and the family and social environment before separation) have never been adequately controlled.'

Thus, while we cannot conclude that prolonged parental separation is not a causal risk factor to adult depression, the research evidence (in moving beyond estimating baldly the role of parental loss as a global risk factor) suggests several higher-order effects in explaining any link between parental loss and adult depression. Research on the behaviour of parents is now reviewed as a logical extension of this proposition.

PARENTAL STYLE

Numerous multivariate studies (see Roe & Siegelman 1963, Parker et al 1979, Arrindell et al 1986), have refined central constructs underlying parental attitudes and behaviours. A principal dimension of 'care' has been generated consistently (with parents ranging from caring to indifferent and/or rejecting). The next most consistently generated dimension has been variably termed 'overprotection' or 'control' (with parents ranging from being overprotective, controlling and encouraging of dependency, to being encouraging of their child's progressive independence, autonomy and socialization). A broad research hypothesis emerges: that experience of high levels of controlling behaviour together with low levels of parental care result in an increased risk in adulthood of developing neurotic disorders, particularly depression.

As noted at the beginning of this chapter, both parental overprotection and deficiencies in parental care have been held by a number of theorists to predispose to adult depression. In addition to Bowlby and a number of analysts, behaviourists (e.g. Liberman & Raskin 1971) and cognitive therapists (e.g. Beck 1967) have articulated mechanisms by which such 'pathogenic' characteristics might operate. We shall focus first, however, on evidence assessing or refining the proposition.

Measures of parenting are clearly problematic, since retrospective self-reports may not correspond to earlier 'actual' parenting and parenting may change over different stages of child and adolescent development. Again, causal postulates must be closely examined when associations are capable of non-causal explanations. For instance, genetic factors may determine both parental style and depression in the recipient, creating spurious associations. Again, certain characteristics in the child may elicit deviant or unsatisfactory parenting, also creating non-causal links between reports of parenting and depression in the recipient.

In terms of measures, Gerlsma et al (1990) recently reviewed 14 factor-analytically-derived measures of parental style, and concluded that only three met basic psychometric criteria – the CRPBI (Schaefer 1965), which is completed by children, and the PBI (Parker et al 1979) and EMBU (Perris et al 1980), which are completed retrospectively by adults. There are a number of studies examining the extent to which depressives report anomalous earlier parenting on those two latter measures, with several now reviewed.

The PBI (Parental Bonding Instrument) requires subjects to score parents and generates scale scores for care and protection. Additionally, each parent can be allocated to one of four broad parental styles, including high care/low protection ('optimal parenting') and low care/high protection ('affectionless control').

Seven studies have now been reported in non-clinical groups (see Parker 1983a for separate studies of university students, twins and adoptees, as well as Howard 1981, Parker & Hadzi-Pavlovic 1984, Richman & Flaherty 1986, Merskey et al 1987), examining for links between PBI scores and (generally) trait depression scores. Consistent associations, although not always significant, have been reported linking higher depression levels with low parental care and with parental overprotection.

There are now a number of studies examining PBI scores returned by clinical depressives. Importantly, studies of separate depressive disorders indicate that PBI findings vary in relation to broad depressive type, suggesting some specificity to the parental deprivation hypothesis. Case-control studies examining the categorical 'melancholic' depressive 'type', have shown no evidence of earlier anomalous parenting being overrepresented. Specifically, Parker (1979) assessed patients with bipolar depressive illness, whose PBI scores were contrasted with age and sex-matched routine general practice attenders. No significant PBI differences were established. A replication study by Joyce (1984), in New Zealand, of bipolar depressives and general practice controls, gave similar findings. One unipolar depressive group has been studied (Parker et al 1987), with endogenous depressives also returning similar PBI scores to age and sex-matched controls.

By contrast, several case-control studies of neurotic depressives in Australia (Parker 1979, 1983b, Parker et al 1987 and Hickie et al 1990a) have consistently established anomalous PBI scores (i.e. low care/high protection) to be overrepresented. An effect of sex of parent with sex of child was noted in one (Parker 1983b), with females reporting more anomalous parenting from mothers and males more anomalous parenting from fathers, while a discriminant function analysis established that low paternal and maternal care were the two strongest discriminators between the depressives and controls. In a predominantly neurotic/reactive depressive group (in that four-fifths were judged as non-melancholic) of 37 outpatient depressives attending the

Yale Depression Research Unit (Plantes et al 1988), the finding was replicated with significantly less parental care and greater parental protection being reported by the patients in comparison to US controls.

The EMBU (Egna Minnen Betraffande Uppfostran or 'my memories of upbringing') measure was developed by Swedish researchers (Perris et al 1980), and was initially designed to assess more than a dozen *a priori* parental constructs, while subsequent research (Arrindell et al 1986) has proposed a two-factor EMBU model of parental style, with scales labelled 'care' and 'protection' as for the PBI. The similarity between the PBI and the EMBU in terms of identifying central dimensions of 'care' and 'protection' through independent research is noteworthy.

Several EMBU studies have now been reported. Perris et al (1986) contrasted scores returned by a diagnostically heterogeneous group of 141 recovered depressives (unipolar, bipolar, neurotic-reactive and unspecified subjects) with scores provided by a control group of 180 subjects, and focused on three EMBU factors. The unipolars reported less 'emotional rejection' (both parents), less 'emotional warmth' (both parents) and less maternal 'overprotection', while the 'unspecified' depressives reported less 'emotional warmth' from each parent. For the depressives to report both less rejection and less warmth appears paradoxical, but such a result could reflect a general age response bias, with older subjects tending not to affirm items – an interpretation supported by an association between age and EMBU scores.

Importantly, this study failed to find any differences between the 'neurotic-reactive' depressives and controls, a finding at variance with the PBI studies. In an earlier study, Perris et al (1985) studied 54 bipolar and 52 unipolar Italian depressives, matched against an Italian EMBU data bank of 200 subjects. Both the unipolar and bipolar depressives scored their parents significantly lower on 'emotional warmth', but no differences were established on the 'rejection' and 'overprotection' scales. Although the authors interpreted their findings as compatible with the PBI studies, there are some differences. These may reflect the differing strategies or may indicate that associations are less clear than suggested by the PBI findings.

Gerlsma et al (1990) have recently reported a meta-analysis of the published literature examining perceived parental rearing practices in depressed and anxious patients, reviewing a number of studies already noted here. In comparison to anxiety disorders, where they judged that there was a 'consistent picture' of a parental style marked by 'affectionless control', a similar trend for those with depressive disorders was held to be 'in the same direction but somewhat less consistent'. Any attenuated trend may well represent the extent to which 'melancholic' depressives have been included in some samples if, as the PBI research suggests, anomalous parenting is not relevant to that depressive type.

Assuming that depressives with the non-melancholic or non-endogenous type are more likely to report anomalous earlier parenting, several non-causal postulates require rejection before any causal 'parental deprivation' hypothesis can be supported. Several such explanations will now be considered.

1. Anomalous parental reports as a consequence of depressed mood

As depression is associated with, if not defined by, a negative judgemental set, it is possible that depressed subjects might score their parents negatively, merely as a consequence of having a depressed mood. Parker (1981) and Plantes et al (1988) examined that possibility by having clinical depressives score their parents on the PBI when depressed and, secondly, when recovered or significantly improved. Both found no statistically significant difference in PBI scores when subjects were depressed and when they had improved. In a nonclinical sample of post-partum subjects, Gotlib et al (1988) established for three separate sub-groups (i.e. those initially depressed, then remitted; those depressed on both occasions of testing; and those not depressed on either occasion of testing) that PBI scores 'were remarkably stable over time'. As, in all studies where examined, anomalous PBI scores persisted in the neurotic/reactive depressives upon recovery, we can conclude that PBI-derived reports of parental dysfunction are not merely a consequence of depressed mood influencing reporting. The fact that the PBI appears to be robust to any effects of a depressed mood is noteworthy, given the frequency with which depressed mood is cited as a seemingly insurmountable methodological limitation to life events research in general and to data derived retrospectively in particular.

2. Anomalous parental reports as a consequence of personality style or response bias

As a variant of the first postulate, this proposition concedes the possibility that neurotic/reactive depressives may return anomalous scores as a consequence of personality style – whereby they seek to blame others, be critical of others or otherwise reflect a general 'plaintive set'. With regard to the PBI, two strategies have addressed this issue in part. Firstly, on the assumption that a personality style of 'neuroticism' may reflect a 'plaintive set' bias, links between higher depression levels and PBI scale scores were examined before and after partialling out subjects' scores on the Eysenck Personality Inventory 'neuroticism' scale in a nonclinical group (Parker 1979). Neuroticism levels did not then appear to determine the general associations between PBI scores and depression levels to any significant degree.

An alternative strategy has been used which assumes that, if such a response bias exists, subjects should score all important interpersonal relationships under the influence of that bias. The Intimate Bond Measure or IBM was developed as a self-report measure of fundamental interpersonal components underlying adult intimate relationships (Wilhelm & Parker 1988), and has 'care' and 'control' scales approximating to the PBI scales. If a general response or perceptual bias exists whereby neurotic depressives tend to judge others as uncaring and overprotective or controlling, we would anticipate associations between the relevant care and control/overprotection scales of the two measures. Two studies have examined for links (Hickie et al 1990a, b) and found little support for that proposition. Thus, anomalous PBI scores returned by neurotic depressives do not appear determined by a general response bias to rate interpersonal relationships negatively or positively.

3. A spurious association determined by a common genetic variable

Associations between PBI scores and 'neurotic' depression could reflect a genetic influence (e.g. 'neuroticism'), which might both cause a parent to be overprotective and uncaring as well as cause depression in the child, with the link between the two outcome variables spuriously suggesting a causal process. That postulate has been investigated by having adoptees score their adopting parents on the PBI (Parker 1982). Support for the 'genetic determinant' hypothesis would require non-existent links between PBI scores for adopting parents and depression scores. Higher trait depression scores in the adoptees were strongly associated with low parental care and high parental protection (as in previous studies of non-clinical subjects). In fact, the associations tended to be stronger than the previously studied samples whose members scored their biological parents. Thus, findings from that study suggest that a genetic explanation is unlikely, although such a research strategy has not been applied in clinical depressive groups.

4. Might anomalous parenting merely dispose to help-seeking rather than depression in the recipient?

Mackinnon et al (1989) suggested that any association between neurotic depression and earlier anomalous parenting might be restricted to those who seek help, become psychiatric patients and are therefore 'cases' in the case-control studies. Thus, parental anomalies might dispose more to a sense of help-seeking than to depression and therefore, when examined in patient samples, create or inflate a non-existent or weak link with depressive 'caseness'. This explanation appears unlikely when, as noted earlier, PBI scores have been shown to be linked with trait depression levels in non-clinical groups.

One necessary strategy for examining this postulate is to study community samples or subjects not selected by referral for psychiatric treatment. Two published studies have produced variable findings. Mackinnon et al (1989) failed to demonstrate the expected anomalous PBI scores in community depressives. By contrast, Birtchnell (1988) screened women attending their general practitioner and established that the 'depressives' reported significantly less maternal care and greater maternal protection, with similar trends for fathers. A third study, more strictly community-based, is of interest. In the Christchurch, New Zealand, Psychiatric Epidemiology Study (Wells et al 1989), 1498 subjects chosen by probability sampling were interviewed in their homes, with women aged 18–44 years being over-sampled. Members of a reinterview sample (90 chosen randomly and 74 females who met DSM criteria for major depression in the previous year) were requested to complete the PBI measure. While results are as yet unpublished, Joyce (personal communication) has provided data showing that the depressives scored both parents as significantly less caring and as significantly more protective than the random sample with depressives excluded. In this community-generated sample, and with depression defined on a 'case' basis, the quantified case-control differences were similar in degree to those reported earlier in clinical groups. The selection strategy, with an emphasis on deriving depressive 'cases', suggests that PBI differences for clinically diagnosed depressives are unlikely to be merely a reflection of a help-seeking bias.

5. Anomalous parenting as a consequence of pre-morbid characteristics

On theoretical grounds, it is conceivable that those with a 'depressive temperament' in childhood might elicit an anomalous parental response. Kagan et al (1987) have suggested that behavioural inhibition (evidenced by shyness and fearfulness in infancy and caution and introversion in childhood) is a risk factor to psychopathology. Personality has also been examined as a risk factor to depression and, while most studies have been retrospective, there is the clear suggestion that a shy, anxious, dependent, interpersonally sensitive and neurotic personality style disposes to depression in adulthood (Boyce 1990). Thus, it is important to explore whether such pre-morbid characteristics might elicit 'affectionless control'. One limited study has been reported (Parker 1981) of a non-clinical group with mothers interviewed about their child's early characteristics (especially shyness, timidity and independence) and with the children (then young adults) scoring their mothers on the PBI. The study showed that, when such childhood characteristics were controlled for, PBI care and overprotection scores remained linked with depression levels in the children. More sophisticated studies are required, however, to exclude and/or to quantify such a contribution.

6. Validity of self-report measures

Again the focus is on the PBI to consider another possible limitation to research of the parental deprivation hypothesis – any reliance on self-report measures. While the PBI was designed to reflect a combination of innumerable parental attitudes and behaviours, thus assuming some constancy in care and protection levels over quite distinct phases of childhood and adolescence, it is likely that the measure focuses on perceptions 'of later childhood and early adolescence' (Mackinnon et al 1989). We need then to know the extent to which PBI scores are a valid measure of both 'perceived' and of 'actual' parenting over time. If, as it appears, neurotic depressives perceive their parents as significantly more likely to evidence 'affectionless control', and if the PBI measures only perceived parenting, then there may be no causal link between 'actual' anomalous parenting and depression in adulthood. This concern has encouraged a number of studies of the properties of the PBI (see Parker 1989) with validity strategies including a cross-over sibling study (with siblings scoring for themselves and for their sibling on the basis of their observations), studies of MZ and DZ twins and comparison of scores returned at semi-structured interview of parents with PBI scores returned by their children. Such studies cannot be conclusive, because construct validity can never be proved absolutely, but they have suggested that the PBI meets acceptable validity criteria both as a measure of perceived and of actual parenting style.

Gerlsma et al (1990) noted that 'no matter how ingenious the research designed to establish validity of retrospective data, the most compelling proof would come from prospective studies'. In that regard, some studies are worth noting. Richman & Flaherty (1986) had students complete PBI scales on entry to medical school and assessed their mood state 7 months later. Low parental care and high parental protection assessed at baseline were associated with higher depression levels at follow-up. In a multiple regression analysis (with baseline depression and personality variables such as dependency and low self-esteem controlled), low paternal care and high maternal protection remained significant predictors of depression severity at follow-up. Gotlib et al (1988) reported that the level of PBI care assessed in women in the postnatal period was predictive of the level of depression 30 months later and noted how low PBI care scores differentiated those who remained depressed from those who had remitted at·that follow-up.

In summary, while a number of non-causal explanations of links between 'affectionless control' and neurotic/reactive depressive disorder which have been examined are not supported, a causal process cannot be claimed by default. Speculation about that proposition will be examined shortly.

AN INTEGRATION

Until now we have formally considered 'parental loss' and 'parental style' as relatively independent categories. But, as already indicated, research suggests that it might be more useful to pursue the proposition that, if parental loss disposes to adult depression, it does so more as a consequence of deficits in parenting before and/or after the loss. Pre-loss deficits might be a consequence of individual parental characteristics (e.g. psychopathology including formal mental illness, incapacity to 'bond' resulting in parenting and marital difficulties) or of the parental dyad (e.g. marital discord). Post-loss deficits (e.g. a reduced social and parental network, a depressed remaining parent, socioeconomic privation) would be expected, if only

because of the extra stress necessarily faced by a single (let alone separated) parent.

An important recent study by Brier et al (1988) is of relevance here. The authors studied 90 adult volunteers who had experienced parental loss in childhood, subdivided on the basis of the presence (77%) or absence (23%) of major psychiatric disorder (PD) in the volunteers. The PD-positive group scored as having a poorer overall quality of home life and poorer personal adaptation during childhood subsequent to the loss, with subjects being highly likely to report a non-supportive relationship with the surviving parent. The total score on the Home Life and Personal Adaptation Scale was the single most powerful predictor of adult psychopathology. Accepting earlier PBI studies that 'inadequate parenting, irrespective of early loss, is associated with the development of depressive illness in adulthood', the authors suggested that in cases of parental loss, the chance of inadequate parenting is increased because of the grief, anxiety and depression experienced by the surviving parent. An important negative finding was that those with and without adult psychopathology did not differ in a first-degree family history of psychiatric disorder, suggesting that genetic factors were not determining adult psychopathology. While the authors favoured the postulate that adult psychopathology was increased by the post-loss quality of home life, one alternative explanation requires consideration in replication studies – that characteristics of the loss may establish an immediate diathesis to adult psychopathology in some subjects, and that such a diathesis may be independent of post-loss family characteristics.

Two British studies (Harris et al 1986, Bifulco et al 1987) established that parental loss per se did not predict depression when post-loss parental care was taken into account. The first (Walthamstow) study has been noted earlier. While analysis of the quality of care was difficult, because of complicated patterns and changes over time, a 'post-loss lack of care' index was derived, with parameters of 'high indifference' and 'low control' corresponding to the PBI parental style of 'affectionless control'. Various analyses established that it was the 'lack of care' rather than the loss of mother itself which was of importance. Thus, the earlier view put by the same research team (Brown et al 1977) – that associations between past loss and later depression 'probably reflect direct causal links' is now modified to conclude that 'loss' *per se* is largely irrelevant as a direct factor, but that it may interact with the more likely direct factor (deficient parental care).

Two other variables require consideration: marital discord and psychopathology in the parents. It is possible that these might predispose the child directly or indirectly to future depression. One empirical study is worth noting. Fendrich et al (1990) studied 220 children (aged 6–23 years) at high or low risk for major depression by virtue of the presence or absence of major depression in the parents, since it had been previously established that children of depressed parents are at increased risk for depression (Weissman et al 1987). They found that children of depressed parents were more likely to be exposed to all five defined family risk factors (i.e. poor marital adjustment, parent-child discord, low family cohesion, affectionless control and parental divorce) and were more likely to receive a lifetime psychiatric diagnosis (76% versus 57%). The lifetime chance of major depression was significantly predicted by two factors – low family cohesion and parental 'affectionless control' – but only in those with a low family risk (i.e. neither parent depressed). Thus the authors concluded that the risk of psychopathology for children of depressed parents is not additionally increased by family risk factors, with the deleterious effects of these risk factors being limited to children of non-depressed parents. Additionally, they suggested that if the 'increased risk for children of depressed parents for depression is indicative of a genetic pathway, the increased risk for children of being in disharmonious family environments may be indicative of an environmental pathway'. The authors noted the limitations of such cross-sectional research and of the measures, but the study is important in suggesting the complexities that are involved in explicating genetic and environmental risk factors, their independence or inter-relationship, and in highlighting the necessity to resolve antecedent – consequence issues. As such complex research is in its infancy, our capacity to synthesize meaningful pathways is extremely limited, but it does appear that family environmental factors may differ in their relevance across those 'at risk' and 'not at risk' because of genetic and/or familial factors.

PATHWAYS

The studies so far reviewed find strong evidence for the central role of a lack of adequate parental care as a key developmental risk factor to adult depression, whether insufficient care reflects a personal style in the parents or is a consequence of parental separation, marital discord, socioeconomic privation or other factors. As Harris et al (1986) note, the 'focus of enquiry should now move . . . to a detailed exploration of how lack of care in childhood can have an impact many years later'.

Most analytic writers have, in varying ways, held that a lack of parental care fixates the individual to feelings of helplessness, engenders feelings of inferiority and self-disparagement and makes the recipient more vulnerable to frustration or deprivation by subsequent 'love subjects'. Bowlby (1977) suggested that such parental deprivation engendered 'anxious attachment', with the child being anxious, insecure and overdependent and, under stress, disposed to develop neurotic symptoms, particularly depression. The PBI research (and to a lesser extent the EMBU research), implicating 'affectionless control' to the later onset of non-melancholic depression, had encouraged speculation (Parker 1983a) that care and protection anomalies exert their influence in different ways. Specifically, decrements in care may result in a child being vulnerable as a consequence of a low intrinsic level of self-esteem and self-worth. Similarly, Perris (1988) has theorized that dysfunctional parental attitudes promote 'dysfunctional self-schema' in the child as well as 'systematic cognitive distortions', with each consequence increasing vulnerability to life stressors. By contrast, parental overprotection may contribute by delaying the usual socialization process and, by restricting the graduated tasks that promote competence and autonomy, make the individual vulnerable when handling independent tasks or social stressors.

Brown et al (1986) have developed a complex model based on results from their Walthamstow and Islington studies, whereby loss of a mother (in association with an ongoing insufficiency of parental care, together with low social class) induces a sense of helplessness and a particular style of attachment and increases the chance of exposure to provoking factors, with the resulting decrements in mastery and self-esteem disposing the individual to depression. Such models require close consideration.

An indirect way of assessing mediating variables is by examining influences on continuity and discontinuity in development. Two studies are of relevance here. Quinton et al (1984) undertook a prospective study of 94 girls reared in an institution following a breakdown in parenting, who were contrasted with a general population group of 51 girls. The institution-raised women were more severely dysfunctional in psychosocial terms and were much more likely to be rated as 'poor' parents in adulthood, suggesting continuity in development to the extent of a 'cycle of transmitted deprivation'. But a minority of the institutional women were not poor parents, and the researchers considered possible determinants of the well-recognized finding that parental deprivation is not always associated with a poor outcome. Findings suggested that a 'spouse's good qualities exerted a powerful ameliorating effect leading to good parenting', and the researchers established that this effect was not due to assortative mating, whereby non-deviant women might have selected more optimally functioning husbands. Thus, adult dysfunction is not necessarily set by the end of a childhood lacking in optimal parenting, and the authors noted that conditions in adult life may 'facilitate or impede adaptive psychosocial functioning', with a caring adult intimate relationship exerting a powerful protective effect.

Similar findings emerged in a study by Parker & Hadzi-Pavlovic (1984). Women whose mothers had died in childhood and whose fathers had remarried were studied, with lifetime depressive episodes together with state and trait depression levels being assessed. Sequences of parenting (i.e. high/low PBI care from fathers and stepmothers) and marital affection (i.e. high/low care) were examined. Those who experienced 'low care' from all three 'carers' (father, stepmother and husband) scored 30% higher on the state and 77% higher on the trait depression measures than those who experienced 'high care' within each relationship. Those who experienced 'high care' from each parent-figure and then 'low care' from their husband had high depression levels, only slightly less than those experiencing low care from all figures. The converse effect was demonstrated for those experiencing low parental care and subsequent high spouse care. After excluding response bias determinants, the authors concluded that results favoured a discontinuity model whereby 'close affectional ties in adult life may modify the effects of

parental deprivation'. These two studies are important in suggesting that intimate relations (effected by parents or spouses) dispose to, or protect the individual from depression by influencing self-esteem.

As noted earlier, several studies (Hickie et al 1990a, b) have examined for links between parental and spouse measures of care and control. Significant associations could occur as a consequence of a response bias (with subjects scoring both relationships in a similar way because of personality style and other influences) or a developmental diathesis, whereby subjects may seek partners with interpersonal characteristics akin to their parents. In both studies, general associations were not found, apart from recipients of extreme deprivation in parental care scoring their partner as extremely deficient in care. If these findings are valid in reflecting actual interpersonal characteristics, then we can draw two important conclusions about the parental deprivation hypothesis.

Firstly, low parental care may both dispose to depression in adulthood directly and indirectly, in that those exposed to gross decrements in care may be locked into a cycle of ongoing deprivation and be more inclined to expose themselves to a variety of 'depressogenic' experiences. Secondly, the 'continuity hypothesis' requires considerable qualification, in that compensating or mitigating factors such as adequate substitute parental care and subsequent care from others in close interpersonal relationships may modify any diathesis (be it protective or predisposing) to adult depressive experience. As adult intimate relationships appear to modify considerably any early trajectory established by parental deprivation – as presumably do other self-esteem modifying variables (e.g. gainful employment) – it is hardly surprising that evidence in support of any direct association between certain parental deprivation experiences and adult depression has been so variable across the many reported studies.

REFERENCES

Arrindell W A, Perris C, Perris H, Eisemann M, Van Der Ende J, Von Knorring L 1986 Cross-national invariance of dimensions of parental rearing behaviour: comparisons of psychometric data of Swedish depressives and healthy subjects with Dutch target ratings on the EMBU. British Journal of Psychiatry 148: 305–309

Beck A T 1967 Depression. Staples Press, London

Becker J 1974 Depression: theory and research. Winston, Washington, DC

Bifulco A T, Brown G W, Harris T O 1987 Childhood loss of parent, lack of adequate parental care and adult

depression: a replication. Journal of Affective Disorders 12: 115–128

Birtchnell J 1972 Early parent death and psychiatric diagnosis. Social Psychiatry 7: 202–210

Birtchnell J 1980 Women whose mothers died in childhood: an outcome study. Psychological Medicine 10: 699–713

Birtchnell J 1988 Depression and family relationships. A study of young, married women on a London housing estate. British Journal of Psychiatry 153: 758–769

Bowlby J 1951 Maternal care and mental health. World Health Organization, Geneva

Bowlby J 1977 The making and breaking of affectional bonds. British Journal of Psychiatry 130: 201–210

Boyce P 1990 High interpersonal sensitivity as a vulnerability risk factor to neurotic depression. Unpublished MD thesis, University of New South Wales

Brier A, Kelsoe J R, Kirwin P D, Beller S A, Wolkowitz D P 1988 Early parental loss and development of adult psychopathology. Archives of General Psychiary 45: 987–993

Brown F 1961 Depression and childhood bereavement. Journal of Mental Science 8: 754–777

Brown G W, Harris T, Copeland J R 1977 Depression and loss. British Journal of Psychiatry 130: 1–18

Brown G W, Harris T O, Bifulco A 1986 Long-term effects of early loss of parent. In: Rutter M, Izard C E, Read P B (eds) Depression in young people: developmental and clinical perspectives. Guildford Press, New York

Crook T, Eliot J 1980 Parental death during childhood and adult depression: A critical review of the literature. Psychological Bulletin 87: 252–259

Dennehy C 1966 Childhood bereavement and psychiatric illness. British Journal of Psychiatry 212: 1049–1069

Favarelli C, Sacchetti E, Ambonetti A, Conte G, Pallanti S, Vita A 1986 Early life events and affective disorder revisited. British Journal of Psychiatry 148: 288–295

Fendrich M, Warner V, Weissman M M 1990 Family risk factors, parental depression and childhood psychopathology. Developmental Psychology 26: 40–50

Forrest A D, Fraser R H, Priest R G 1965 Environmental factors in depressive illness. British Journal of Psychiatry 111: 243–253

Gerlsma C, Emmelkamp P M G, Arrindell W A 1990 Anxiety, depression and perception of early parenting: a meta-analysis. Clinical Psychology Review 10: 251–277

Gotlib I H, Mount J H, Cordy N I, Whiffen V E 1988 Depression and perceptions of early parenting: a longitudinal investigation. British Journal of Psychiatry 152: 24–27

Granville-Grossman K L 1968 The early development in affective disorder in recent developments in affective disorders. British Journal of Psychiatry Special Publication No. 2

Hallstrom T 1987 The relationships of childhood socio-demographic factors and early parental loss to major depression in adult life. Acta Psychiatrica Scandinavica 75: 212–216

Harris T, Brown G W, Bifulco A 1986 Loss of parent in childhood and adult psychiatric disorder: the role of lack of adequate parental care. Psychological Medicine 16: 641–659

Heinicke C M 1973 Parental deprivation in early childhood In: Scott J P, Senay E C (eds) Separation and depression. Clinical and research aspects. American Association for the Advancement of Science, Maryland

Hickie I, Wilhelm K, Parker G, Boyce P, Madzi-Pavlovic D, Brodaty H, Mitchell P 1990a Perceived dysfunctional intimate relationships: a specific association with the non-melancholic depressive type. Journal of Affective Disorders 19: 99–107

Hickie I, Parker G, Wilhelm K, Tennant C 1990b Perceived interpersonal risk factors non-endogenous depression. Psychological Medicine 21: 399–412

Hopkinson G, Reed G F 1966 Bereavement in childhood and depressive psychosis. British Journal of Psychiatry 112: 459–463

Howard J 1981 The expression and possible origins of depression in male adolescent delinquents. Australia and New Zealand Journal of Psychiatry 15: 311–318

Hudgens R W, Morrison J R, Barchha R G 1967 Life events and onset of primary affective disorders: a study of 40 hospitalised patients and 40 controls. Archives of General Psychiatry 16: 134–145

Hunter R, Macalpine I 1963 Three hundred years of psychiatry. Oxford University Press, London

Joyce P R 1984 Parental bonding in bipolar affective disorder. Journal of Affective Disorders 7: 319–324

Kagan J, Reznick J S, Sividman N 1987 The physiology and psychology of behavioral inhibition in children. Child Development 51: 660–680

Liberman R P, Raskin D E 1971 Depression: a behavioral formulation. Archives of General Psychiatry 24: 515–523

Mackinnon A J, Henderson A S, Scott R, Duncan-Jones P 1989 The parental bonding instrument (PBI): an epidemiological study in a general population sample. Psychological Medicine 19: 1023–1034

Mendelson M 1974 Psychoanalytic concepts of depression. Spectrum, New York

Merskey H, Lau C L, Russell E S et al 1987 Screening for psychiatric morbidity. The pattern of psychological illness and premorbid characteristics in four chronic pain populations. Pain 30: 141–157

Munro A 1966 Parental deprivation in depressive patients. British Journal of Psychiatry 112: 443–457

Parker G 1979 Parental characteristics in relation to depressive disorders. British Journal of Psychiatry 134: 138–147

Parker G 1981 Parental reports of depressives: an investigation of several explanations. Journal of Affective Disorders 3: 131–140

Parker G 1982 Parental representations and affective symptoms: examination for an hereditary link. British Journal of Medical Psychology 55: 57–61

Parker G 1983a Parental overprotection: a risk factor in psychosocial development. Grune & Stratton, New York

Parker G 1983b Parental 'affectionless control' as an antecedent to adult depression. Archives of General Psychiatry 48: 956–960

Parker G 1989 The parental bonding instrument: psychometric properties reviewed. Psychiatric Developments 4: 317–335

Parker G, Hadzi-Pavlovic D 1984 Modification of levels of depression in mother-bereaved women by parental and marital relationships. Psychological Medicine 14: 125–135

Parker G, Manicavasagar V 1986 Childhood bereavement circumstances associated with adult depression. British Journal of Medical Psychology 59: 387–391

Parker G, Tupling H, Brown L B 1979 A parental bonding instrument. British Journal of Medical Psychology 52: 1–10

Parker G, Kiloh L, Hayward L 1987 Parental representations of neurotic and endogenous depressives. Journal of Affective Disorders 13: 75–82

Perris C 1988 A theoretical framework for linking the experience of dysfunctional parental rearing attitudes with manifest psychopathology. Acta Psychiatrica Scandinavica 78: (suppl 344) 93–109

Perris C, Jacobsson L, Lindstrom H, Von Knorring L, Perris H 1980 Development of a new inventory for assessing memories of parental rearing behaviour. Acta Psychiatrica Scandinavica 61: 265–274

Perris C, Maj M, Perris H, Eisemann M 1985 Perceived parental rearing behaviour in unipolar and bipolar depressed patients: a verification study in an Italian sample. Acta Psychiatrica Scandinavica 72: 172–175

Perris C, Arrindell W A, Perris H, Eisemann J, Van der Ende J, Von Knorring L 1986a Perceived depriving parental rearing and depression. British Journal of Psychiatry 148: 170–175

Pitts F N, Meyer J, Brooks M, Winokur G 1965 Adult psychiatric illness assessed for childhood parental loss and psychiatric illness in family members – a study of 748 patients and 250 controls. American Journal of Psychiatry 121 (suppl): i-x

Plantes M M, Prusoff B A, Brennan J, Parker G 1988 Parental representations of depressed outpatients from a US sample. Journal of Affective Disorders 15: 149–155

Quinton D, Rutter M, Liddle C 1984 Institutional rearing, parental difficulties and marital support. Psychological Medicine 14: 107–124

Raphael B 1983 The anatomy of bereavement. Basic Books, New York

Richards M P M, Dyson M 1982 Separation, divorce and the development of children: a review. DHSS, London

Richman J A, Flaherty J A 1986 Childhood relationships, adult coping resources and depression. Social Science and Medicine 23: 709–716

Roe A, Siegelman M 1963 A parent – child relations questionnaire. Child Development 34: 355–369

Roy A 1983 Early parental death and adult depression. Psychological Medicine 13: 861–865

Roy A 1985 Early parental separation and adult depression. Archives of General Psychiatry 42: 987–991

Rutter M 1972 Maternal deprivation reassessed. Penguin, Harmondsworth

Schaefer E S 1965 A configurational analysis of children's reports of parent behavior. Journal of Consulting Psychology 29: 552–557

Tennant C 1988 Parental loss in childhood: its effect in adult life. Archives of General Psychiatry 45: 1045–1050

Tennant C, Bebbington P, Hurry J 1980 Parental death in childhood and risk of adult depressive disorders. Psychological Medicine 10: 289–299

Tennant C, Smith A, Bebbington P, Hurry J 1981 Parental loss in childhood: relationship to adult psychiatric impairment and contact with psychiatric services. Archives of General Psychiatry 38: 309–314

Weissman M M, Gammon G D, John K et al 1987 Children of depressed parents: increased psychopathology and early onset of major depression. Archives of General Psychiatry 44: 847–853

Wells J E, Bushnell J A, Hornblow A R, Joyce P R, Oakley-Browne M A 1989 Christchurch psychiatric epidemiology study, Part 1: methodology and lifetime prevalence for specific psychiatric disorders. Australian and New Zealand Journal of Psychiatry 23: 315–326

Wilhelm K, Parker G 1988 The development of a measure of intimate bonds. Psychological Medicine 18: 225–234

12. Personality

Robert M. A. Hirschfeld   M. Tracie Shea

INTRODUCTION

Clinical theorists have described a relationship between personality and depression since the time of Hippocrates and Aristotle. However, empirical research on this relationship has been carried out only in the last two decades. This chapter will summarize the research literature relevant to personality and depression within the context of the rich conceptual history relating these two important domains of human experience.

MODELS

There are four major models of the relationship between personality and depression: predisposition, complication, spectrum and pathoplasty. Each of these models has a theoretical rationale and has implications for theory and for clinical practice. A brief overview for each model follows.

The predispositional (or 'vulnerability') model

This concept refers to the notion that certain personality characteristics are antecedent to depression and render the individual vulnerable to depression under certain conditions. This approach has predominated both in theory and research. It has been particularly attractive because it provides an aetiological explanation for depression in a given individual and provides a context to deal with and explain the interaction of an individual with the environment.

The theoretical issues involved in personality as a predisposition have been addressed in several reviews, including those of Klerman & Hirschfeld (1988) and Akiskal and colleagues (1983). The trait most associated in the clinical literature with predisposition to depression is undue interpersonal dependency, an

excessive need for reassurance, support and attention from other people (Hirschfeld et al 1976, 1977, Chodoff 1972, Birtchnell 1984). Cognitive psychologists have also addressed this issue, principally in the learned helplessness and cognitive theories of depression (Alloy & Abramson 1988).

Cloninger (1987) has proposed a theory of heritable personality traits with specific neurobiological bases. The theory relates interpersonal and behavioural functioning with neurotransmitter and other brain activity. He proposes three basic dimensions, those of novelty seeking, harm avoidance and reward dependence, for which he has demonstrated evidence of independence. The theory relates some types of depression, particularly non-autonomous depression, to individuals who have high reward dependence, high harm avoidance and high novelty seeking.

The complication model

This model proposes the reverse of the predispositional model. According to the complication approach, one consequence of the experience of a clinical depression is personality change, particularly when the episode is severe and protracted. Thus, the experience and the devastation of a depression may lead to and cause changes in personality in terms of an individual's perception of himself or herself and his/her style of interacting with other people. For example, pessimism and dependency may become permanent features of personality following multiple depressive episodes.

The spectrum model

This model focuses on the relationship between temperamental or constitutional aspects of personality and affective disorders. According to this view, whose proponents include Kraepelin, Kretschmer and more recently Akiskal, certain personality characteristics may be considered milder manifestations of affective disorders, with both representing expressions of the same underlying genetic endowment or liability. Thus, certain behavioural patterns such as cyclothymia are viewed as a continuum blending at one end with normality and corresponding at the other to the full-blown depressive syndrome. The liability may be expressed as a 'depressive character' including pessimism, moodiness, passivity, negativity and low energy.

The pathoplasty model

This proposes that personality characteristics influence the symptomatic expression and course of the depressive episode but are not aetiological or involved in the pathogenesis of depression. Thus certain personality 'types' may be associated with specific depressive symptom profiles, such as a histrionic personality with more hostile, angry, complaining symptoms during the depressive episode.

The pathoplasty hypothesis has not received much attention in the decade since the work of Paykel et al (1976), who demonstrated that patients with more neurotic symptoms showed more evidence of an oral dependency and less obsessionality, whereas patients with histrionic personalities tended to be less severely ill with more hostility.

IMPEDIMENTS TO RESEARCH

There are several methodological impediments to testing a hypothesis about the relationship between personality and depression. Chief among these is the confounding of state and trait. Other issues include assessment methods for personality, dimensional versus categorical approaches to personality, the heterogeneity of depression and the timing of assessments.

The state/trait issue

It has been well documented that, when depressed, patients do not provide valid reports of their premorbid functioning. Indeed, even partially recovered patients hold distorted views of themselves and their situation (Hirschfeld & Klerman 1979, 1983, Liebowitz et al 1979, Reich et al 1987, Joffe & Regan 1988, Coppen & Metcalfe 1965, Ingraham 1966, Kerr et al 1970,

Bianchi & Ferguson 1977). For example, in a longitudinal study of a large sample of patients with depression (Hirschfeld & Klerman 1983), patients completed self-report personality batteries first during their depressive episodes and again following a complete recovery from the episode one year later. When the scores were compared, it was clear that clinical state markedly influenced scores on the personality scales assessing emotional strength, interpersonal dependency, and extroversion. Despite the fact that the patients had been instructed to respond to items according to their 'usual self', they reported more pathology when depressed.

These findings raise questions about the validity of theories or data regarding premorbid personality and depression based on observations made while patients are depressed. One important consequence of the patient's distortions is that the clinician may also make erroneous judgments about the personality, because the clinician views the patient's personality through the eyes and thoughts of the patient while depressed.

Self-report measures of personality disorders have been shown to be influenced by anxiety (Mavissakalian & Hamann 1988) and depression (Joffe & Regan 1988). In addition the presence of depression has been shown to affect not only self report, but also clinical assessments of personality disorders (Shea 1989). In all cases the direction of change is toward more normal personality following recovery from the Axis I disorder. Some recent work suggests that structured interviews may be less affected by the depressed state (Pfohl et al 1990).

Assessment methods for personality

The assessment of personality has a long tradition in academic psychology, particularly in the quantitative techniques of psychometrics and the application of multivariate statistics and computer technology in the past several decades. There are many scales for assessment of individual personality traits and newly developed techniques for the evaluation of personality types.

The assessment of personality *disorders*, as distinct from personality *traits*, has only recently received attention. The creation of the DSM-III Axis II provided a major stimulus to the development of quantitative techniques of diagnosing the specific personality disorders. The attempt was made in DSM-III to define personality disorders primarily on descriptive and behavioural features, and to avoid inferences regarding unconscious mental processes, genetic background, or other presumed aetiological factors. The reliability and validity of personality disorders assessment is an area of much current research. In the last decade a number of structured interviews, such as the Structured Interview for DSM-III Personality (SIDP) (Pfohl et al 1983) and the Personality Disorder Examination (PDE) (Loranger et al 1984) have been developed.

Dimensional versus categorical approaches

The conception of personality traits ranging smoothly from normal to abnormal contrasts sharply with the categorical (or typological) approach to personality disorders. In general the advocates of the dimensional approach come from psychometrics and psychology, while categorical or typological approaches are more often used by psychiatrists and other clinicians. Both the ICD and the DSM approaches utilize a typological or categorical approach to personality disorder definition.

Heterogeneity of depression

Heterogeneity of patient samples represents another problem which affects both replicability and generalizability of findings. Although there is reasonable agreement on homogeneity among patients and families with bipolar disorder, there is little agreement about homogeneity of unipolar disorders. Unipolar depression is usually considered to encompass a variety of illnesses with different aetiologies and treatments; it is not clear whether hypotheses relating personality and depression are relevant to all forms of depression or only to specific subtypes. Therefore, different findings from different studies of depressed patients may be hard to integrate because of diagnostic heterogeneity.

Timing of assessments

Personality ratings obtained from patients who have fully recovered may not reflect premorbid personality, since personality traits may have been affected by the depressive episode (i.e. the complication hypothesis). The only way to circumvent this issue is to conduct a prospective study (i.e. to make assessments in a large group of people with no history of psychiatric illness and follow them for an extended period). This is obviously difficult to accomplish from a feasibility point

of view, and there have been relatively few such investigations.

STUDIES OF PERSONALITY TRAITS AND DEPRESSION

During the 1970s and early 1980s a number of investigators used structured interviews to diagnose psychiatric disorders in clinical samples, waited until patients had fully recovered from their depressive illness and then measured personality using objective self-report instruments. These studies (Kendell & Discipio 1968, Liebowitz et al 1979, Beck et al 1980, Hirschfeld & Klerman 1979, Perris 1971, Murray & Blackburn 1974, Donnelly et al 1976), in general showed moderate introversion among unipolar depressed patients and 'normal' levels of neuroticism. However, no studies addressed interpersonal dependency, the personality feature most described in the clinical literature as predispositional for depression. Therefore, the Interpersonal Dependency Inventory was developed (Hirschfeld et al 1977) and was subsequently included in the NIMH Psychobiology of Depression Collaborative Research Program.

In this study, 17 personality scales were divided into four clusters of emotional strength, interpersonal dependency, extroversion and miscellaneous. The most marked difference in personality between assessments of patients completed after full recovery from depression and of a never psychiatrically ill comparison group was in the emotional strength cluster. Patients who had recovered from either unipolar or bipolar depression were characterized by less emotional strength, more moodiness and less ability to cope with stress (Hirschfeld et al 1986, 1983). Recovered patients had significantly higher levels of interpersonal dependency than did controls.

In the extroversion/introversion cluster there were some unexpected findings. Both bipolar and unipolar recovered women were significantly more introverted than were the comparison group. Among the men, only the unipolar men were significantly introverted. The bipolar recovered men evidenced only normal levels of extroversion, not supporting the notion of the extraverted, perhaps 'hypomanic' personality.

Personality may also be associated with speed of recovery from depression. Frank and colleagues (1987) found that personality scores assessed following recovery differed between groups divided on rapidity of response to tricyclic antidepressant medication and interpersonal psychotherapy. Normal (or 'rapid') responders (who showed a clear-cut remission of symptoms within 8 weeks and who have remained well for a subsequent 8 weeks) were compared with 'slow' responders (who achieved remission after 8 but before 16 weeks). The rapid/normal responders had significantly higher levels of emotional strength and stability and were less interpersonally dependent. The two groups did not differ on extroversion scores.

Premorbid assessment of personality

Truly premorbid assessments of personality require identification of a large pool of high-risk subjects early enough in life so that they can be assessed prior to their first episode of depression, and require follow-up, usually for several years.

In the NIMH Psychobiology Study, 438 first-degree relatives and/or spouses of probands and/or family study control subjects had no history or current mental disorder at the time that they were first evaluated and completed personality assessments. During an interim 6-year period, 29 of these people suffered a first episode of major depression. This group of 29 subjects was compared with a group of 370 subjects who continued to be free of any mental disorder at the second 6-year follow-up evaluation.

Among the young adults, aged 17–30, there were no significant differences on any of the 17 self-report personality assessments between those who subsequently became depressed and those who remained free of any psychiatric disorder. However, among the adults, aged 31–41, several differences emerged. Among the emotional strength cluster, those who subsequently suffered their first episode of major depression were characterized as being more neurotic, less emotionally stable and less resilient. In addition, those who were to suffer their first onset were more interpersonally dependent than those who remained free of illness. Overall the differences, even among the 31–41-year-old group, were less than those with the post-recovery patients on nearly all variables where there were differences.

The personality scores obtained from the first onset group, even among the 31–41-year-old adults, were considerably more healthy than those obtained from patients who had recovered from either unipolar or bipolar depression. This difference between the relatives and patients may mean that not only does depression influence personality assessments *during* an illness, but also the depression may result in personality changes *after recovery*. An alternate explanation is that the difference in personality scores may reflect differ-

ences in severity of illness present in the patients as compared to that in the relatives.

The personality features found to be predictive of first onset of major depression do not have well-established theoretical relevance to depression and may not be specific to depression. Rather they appear to serve as non-specific vulnerability factors for mental illnesses in general. In support of this observation is a study by Reich and colleagues (1987), who found very similar personality profiles in samples of patients recovered from panic disorder when compared with recovered depressives. Both recovered groups showed significantly less emotional strength and significantly more interpersonal dependency than controls. The groups did not differ from one another on any of these measures.

The lack of differences with the comparison group in the young adult age group and the differences with the comparison group for the 31–41-year-old group raises several questions. Do the personalities of never-ill subjects improve as they age, or do those of the subjects experiencing a first onset get worse? Is the change in predictive power due to a cohort effect?

Definitive answers are not yet available, but the data do suggest that even in those subjects without a history of mental illness, there is a decrease in some variables, particularly those of emotional strength and dependency, between age groups. In addition, the younger individuals who would experience their first episode were slightly less interpersonally dependent than older subjects who were to experience their first episode.

The data suggest that there are strong maturational effects in emotional strength. Thus over time subjects in the never-ill group seemed to grow emotionally stronger, whereas those in the first-onset group did not.

Nonetheless, all of the emotional strength scores in the first-onset relatives indicated substantially better emotional strength and resiliency in the relatives than in the recovered patients.

A study by Angst & Clayton (1986) assessed personality factors in a sample of 6315 19-year-old conscripts in the Swiss Army in 1971. Personality assessment was obtained by the Freiburg Personality Inventory, a 212-item German self-report inventory whose nine primary factors measure nervousness, aggressivity, depressiveness, excitability, even temper, striving for dominance, inhibition and frankness. A follow-up diagnostic assessment 12 years later disclosed 16 cases of bipolar disorder and 19 cases of unipolar disorder on the basis of retrospective medical record interviews. Compared with controls, subjects with unipolar disorder were premorbidly more aggressive and autonomically labile. The increase in autonomic lability is similar to the differences in neuroticism that were found in the NIMH Psychobiology Study.

Personality predictors of depression may be changing. The personality features predicting depression may be consistent and valid for a particular cohort, but the personality and other predictors of depression for successive generations may be somewhat different. A powerful temporal effect indicative of a mixture of both cohort and period factors has been demonstrated for depressive disorders, particularly since the Second World War. It may be that there is an interaction between birth cohorts and personality factors among adults born just before and during the Second World War, which may no longer be true. This lack of influence of personality factors in the younger segment may be due to more powerful and over-riding influence of other risk factors such as family loading for major depressive disorder.

PERSONALITY DISORDERS

Overview

While earlier research investigating the relationship between personality and depression focused on personality *traits*, more recently there has been a shift towards investigations of the relationship between pathological personality, or personality *disorders*, and depression. These include investigations of the influence of personality disorders on outcome and course of depression, investigations of various 'spectrum' models based on presence or absence of pathological personality features, and family studies of personality disorders and affective disorders.

Personality features have long been associated with attempts to define meaningful subtypes of affective disorder. One example of this concept is the old notion of 'neurotic' depression, believed to have 'psychological' causes and to be associated with more 'neurotic' personality traits than 'endogenous' depression (Klerman et al 1979). This approach to subtyping depression on the basis of personality features begins with the assumption that there are at least two different forms of depression which are distinguishable by the presence or absence of certain personality features. This approach also assumes that the depression occurring in the presence of certain personality features has a different aetiology. Other models do not assume that

the depressive disorder in patients with and without personality disturbance is a different disorder. Personality disorder and depressive disorder may be viewed as caused by independent factors (genetic and/or environmental), or as manifestations of the same underlying cause.

Spectrum models

Several spectrum models relevant to personality disorders and affective disorders have been proposed. Winokur's concept of *'depressive spectrum disease'* is based on the use of familial patterns to define subtypes of depressive disorders. 'Depressive spectrum disease' is defined by the presence of alcoholism and/or antisocial personality in first-degree relatives of unipolar depressives; these disorders are believed to form a spectrum with depression. 'Pure depressive disease', in contrast, is defined by the absence of alcoholism and antisocial personality in relatives. A more restrictive definition of pure depressive disease requires the presence of a history of depression in the relatives. Patients with depression and no family history are classified by Winokur as 'sporadic' or 'nonfamilial depression'.

Characteristics associated by Winokur with depressive spectrum disease include earlier age of onset of depression, female gender, personality problems and difficulties (particularly more frequent divorce and separation), lifelong irritability, a more variable illness and less chronicity.

Other investigators have attempted to replicate Winokur's findings. Some have found the expected differences in personality variables (Van Valkenburg et al 1977); others have not (Andreasen & Winokur 1979). Neither of these studies found differences in age of onset. Van Valkenburg and colleagues (1977) found course differences consistent with Winokur's predictions. Biological differences have been more consistently reported, particularly more frequent dexamethasone non-suppression in pure depressive disease when compared to depressive spectrum disease (see chapter 3). Differences have also been found in EEG sleep recordings and insulin insensitivity (Lewis & Winokur 1983).

Akiskal and colleagues (1981) have identified a similar subset of depressed patients (*character spectrum disorder*), on the basis of chronic characterological problems rather than a specific family history. These patients usually have hysteroid-antisocial features and irritable dysphoria, normal REM latency and a normal level of dexamethasone suppression. They often are substance abusers, are resistant to somatic therapies, have a family history of alcoholism or sociopathy and tend to be non-responsive to somatic therapies. Akiskal proposes that these patients have a closer affinity to patients with alcoholism, sociopathy and somatization than to those with a primary affective disorder. This subgroup of character spectrum disorders is clearly similar to Winokur's subtype of depressive spectrum disease.

Findings from other studies investigating differences between depressed patients with and without a personality disorder have tended to support Winokur's and Akiskal's subtypes, (i.e. patients with personality disorders resemble the spectrum subtypes). Depressed patients with personality disorders have been found to have a younger age of onset of depression, more frequent separation and divorce, poorer response to treatment and more familial alcoholism and sociopathy (Pfohl et al 1984, Black et al 1988, Reich & Troughton 1988, Shea et al 1987). In contrast to Winokur's findings of a more favourable course for depressive spectrum, these more recent studies have found that depressed patients with personality disorders have a *worse* outcome than those without personality disorders. Some studies (Pfohl et al 1984, Black et al 1988) have also found depressed patients with personality disorders to be characterized by less frequent dexamethasone non-suppression, compared to patients with depression alone.

Akiskal distinguishes the character spectrum group from another subgroup of affective disorder patients with secondary personality disorders. This latter group (*cyclothymic – bipolar II spectrum*) consists of atypical, chronic and complicated forms of affective disorder with *secondary* personality dysfunction. Akiskal proposes that these 'subaffective' disorders represent genetically attenuated cyclothymic forms of bipolar illness. A crucial distinction from character spectrum disorder is that the personality disturbances (i.e. relationship instability and marital failure, promiscuous behaviour, alcohol and drug use) in these patients, which are often the most visible clinical features, are viewed as an integral part of the affective psychopathology. In this model, the affective disorder, which occurs on a spectrum, is genetically transmitted and the personality disturbance is a *consequence* of the affective disorder.

The cyclothymic — bipolar relationship is another example of the spectrum hypothesis. While not generally considered to be a personality disorder, cyclothymia has a number of attributes that are similar to personality disorders, such as early onset and an enduring pattern of behaviour. This model has been investigated by Depue and colleagues (1985) and Klein & Depue (1984).

In summary, there is support for the existence of a subtype of affective disorder characterized by personality disturbance, which may be associated with an increased familial rate of alcoholism and/or antisocial personality. This subtype has also been shown to differ from other forms of affective disorder on variables of phenomenology, course, biology and treatment response, with varying degrees of consistency. The use of the term spectrum implies that affective disorder in these patients is related (familially and/or genetically) to alcoholism and antisocial personality as manifestations of the same underlying disorder. This group of patients is distinguished from another group of patients with personality disturbance who are believed to be on a cyclothymic – bipolar II continuum, and from a subgroup of depressive disorder patients *without* personality disturbance or a family history of personality disturbance or alcoholism.

Family studies of borderline personality disorder and depression

A number of studies have reported familial rates of personality disorder and/or depressive disorder in probands with borderline personality disorder (Docherty et al 1986). In general, these studies have supported a link between borderline personality disorder and depressive disorder. First-degree relatives of borderline personality disorder probands have been found to be at high risk for major depression (Baron et al 1985, Loranger et al 1982, Pope et al 1983, Akiskal et al 1985, Zanarini et al 1988). These findings are qualified by the fact that two of the three studies that differentiated between borderline personality disorders with and without comorbid depression found the relatives of 'pure' borderline personality disorders to be at lower risk for depression than those of borderline personality disorders with a history of depression (Pope et al 1983, Zanarini et al 1988). The borderline personality disorder sample studied by Baron and colleagues (1985) did not, however, have comorbid depression.

While this research suggests a link between borderline personality disorder and affective disorder, it is not clear whether: 1) the link is associated with a subtype of borderline personality disorder (i.e. borderline personality disorders with comorbid depressive disorder); or

2) the link is associated with a subtype of depressive disorder. With regard to the latter point, a recent study by Coryell & Zimmerman (1989) compared rates of personality disorder in first-degree relatives of probands with non-psychotic major depression, psychotic major depression, schizophrenia or no DSM-III psychiatric disorder. They did not find an increase of borderline personality disorder among relatives of patients with major depression, but did find a significant increase in cluster B ('dramatic-erratic') personality disorders in the relatives of patients with nonmelancholic depression and normal dexamethasone suppression. This finding suggests a more specific link between cluster B personality disorders and a *subtype* of depression, and could be interpreted as supporting the spectrum or phenocopy models.

THE INTERFACE BETWEEN PERSONALITY AND DEPRESSION – DEPRESSIVE PERSONALITY DISORDER

Is a disorder at the juncture between personality and depression, that of depressive personality disorder?

Depressive personality has a rich theoretical and clinical tradition (Phillips et al 1990). Kraepelin (1921) wrote, 'the depressive temperament is characterized by a permanent, gloomy, emotional stress in all the experiences of life'. He described patients with persistent gloominess, joylessness, anxiety and a predominantly depressed, despondent and despairing mood. Such patients were also serious, burdened, guilt-ridden, self-reproaching, self-denying and lacking in self-confidence.

This viewpoint was further developed by other German psychiatrists, including Kretschmer (1925) and Schneider (1958). Schneider's description of the symptoms of depressive psychopathy included: 1) gloomy, pessimistic, serious and incapable of relaxation; 2) quiet; 3) sceptical; 4) worrying; 5) duty-bound; and 6) self-doubting.

These were further refined by Akiskal, who modified slightly the Schneiderian criteria to include hypersomnolence and low energy (Akiskal 1989). On the basis of his clinical experience and research, Akiskal found that this group of patients has a positive family history of unipolar or bipolar mood disorder, are responsive to tricyclic antidepressants and have a shortened REM latency similar to patients with major depression. He argues strongly for separating these patients, whom he considers part of the affective spectrum, from a variety of other patients with chronic depression who are

characterized by mixed personality disorders, often with a family history of alcoholism and antisocial personality, as described above.

Psychoanalytical formulations of depressive character have emphasized low self-esteem, self-deprivation and self-denial to the point of masochism (Berliner 1966, Mendelson 1974, Simons 1986, Kernberg 1987). A disturbed early childhood experience and object loss are emphasized in the development of the disorder. In the official nomenclatures, the International Classification of Disease (ICD) of the World Health Organization and the Diagnostic and Statistical Manual (DSM) of the American Psychiatric Association, depressive personality was subsumed under depressive neuroses in earlier editions and under dysthymia in more recent ones. A major problem with this approach is that these diagnostic categories are over-inclusive in terms of composite illnesses. For example, the term 'neurotic depression' has been described as having at least six separate meanings (Klerman et al 1979).

An attempt to integrate several different theoretical streams has been proposed by a group working on a proposal for the depressive personality disorder for DSM-IV (Hirschfeld et al 1990). In this scheme, the core feature of depressive personality disorder would be excessive negative and pessimistic beliefs about oneself and other people. Although there may be overlaps with features of other axis II personality disorders, each can be distinguished conceptually by the proposed core pathology. These other personality disorders include self-defeating, borderline, obsessive-compulsive and passive-aggressive personality disorders.

The core concept in self-defeating personality disorder is a tendency towards victimization and suffering. This concept involves an active role on the part of the individual in producing and maintaining this suffering. In contrast, the individual with depressive personality disorder experiences unhappiness and dissatisfaction but does not seek situations to reinforce this. His/her dysphoria and unhappiness are less tied to specific situations.

The overlap between borderline personality disorder and depressive personality disorder is in the area of dysphoria and negative feelings toward other people. Borderline mood is characterized by instability with a tendency to dysphoria as well as irritability or anxiety, whereas the depressive personality disorder is characterized by fairly persistent dysphoria. In terms of self-concept, a person with borderline personality disorder feels emptiness and boredom in contrast to someone with depressive personality disorder who has chronic low self-esteem and feelings of inadequacy and worthlessness. Thus the person suffering from borderline personality disorder is struggling with the absence of a clear sense of self, which is not the case for the person suffering from depressive personality disorder.

The essential core features of an individual with obsessive-compulsive personality disorder are tendencies to be withholding and controlling, in contrast to the unhappy, negativistic and critical nature of those individuals suffering from depressive personality disorder.

The negativism of a person with passive-aggressive personality disorder is directed toward other people who have some authority or influence over him/her, and not toward other people in general. The negativism is related to his/her subordinate role. This issue is irrelevant to the person with depressive personality disorder. In this case, negativism is more generally directed, and does not necessarily increase in the presence of people making demands on the person. Also, the person with depressive personality disorder is not necessarily obstructive towards other people.

Table 12.1   Proposed criteria for depressive personality disorder

1. Tendency to dysphoria, dejection, gloominess, cheerlessness, joylessness

2. Prominent self-concepts of inadequacy, worthlessness and low self-esteem

3. Critical, blaming, derogatory and punitive toward oneself, and prone to guilt

4. Brooding and given to worry

5. Negativistic, critical and judgmental towards others

6. Pessimistic

Depressive personality disorder is also distinguished from mood disorders in that the core concept and key diagnostic criteria are not primarily affective but rather cognitive and temperamental. This does not mean to imply that it is not possible to have both the depressive personality disorder and an affective disorder in the same individual. Indeed it may be common. However, it is possible to have one without the other and the disorders emphasize different characteristics. Mood disorders emphasize the dysphoric disturbances and associated affective symptomatology, whereas in depressive personality disorder it is the long-standing, early onset, cognitive and temperamental attributes which pervade all aspects of life, especially interper-

sonal interactions. The criteria (see Table 12.1) are refinements of the Kraepelinian, Schneiderian and Akiskalian criteria for depressive temperament and criteria from cognitive psychology.

The relationship of this complex of symptoms with that of mood disorders is currently a topic of empirical research.

CONCLUSION

Research over the past two decades has helped to answer several important questions about the relationship between personality and depression. These are summarized below.

1. Personality factors appear to have a non-specific effect on vulnerability to depression. People who have recovered fully from major depression in general are less emotionally strong, less resilient, less able to cope with stress, more moody and more introverted than those without a history of psychiatric illness. These personality qualities are not strongly associated theoretically with pathogenesis of depression. They have also been identified in patients who have recovered from other psychiatric illnesses, including anxiety disorders. Interpersonal dependency is also moderately increased in patients who have recovered from depression and is a more specific risk factor.

2. In an investigation of personality assessments made prior to the first onset of depression no differences were found between those who went on to suffer depression and those who remained psychiatrically well in a young adult age group (ages 17–30). Among adults aged 31–41 differences were found that were consistent with those of the recovered patients, but were much more modest in degree. This may be due to a change in psychosocial risk factors over time.

3. The relationship of personality disorders and depression is currently a subject of great clinical and research interest. Of particular interest is the spectrum notion, in which some personality disorders, particularly borderline, histrionic, and avoidant, may be related genetically to mood disorders, similar to cyclothymia and bipolar disorder.

4. Whether there is a depressive personality disorder is a controversial subject. Clinical theorists have described a syndrome of depressive temperament and disorder characterized by dejection, gloominess, inadequacy and negativity toward oneself and other people. Many researchers, particularly those with experience in mood disorders, consider this syndrome to be subsumed under the mood disorder rubric. Future empirical research is essential to resolve this question.

ACKNOWLEDGMENT

The authors would like to express their thanks and appreciation to Ms Kathleen Talbot, whose assistance in the preparation of this manuscript was invaluable.

REFERENCES

Akiskal H S 1989 Validating affective personality types. In: Robins L, Barrett J (eds) The validity of psychiatric diagnosis. Raven Press New York, p 217–227

Akiskal H S, King D, Rosenthal T L, Robinson D, Scott-Strauss A 1981 Chronic depression: Part I. Clinical and familial characteristics in 137 probands. Journal of Affective Disorders 3: 297–315

Akiskal H S, Hirschfeld R M A, Yervanian B I 1983 The relationship of personality to affective disorders: a critical review. Archives of General Psychiatry 40: 801–810

Akiskal H S, Chen S E, Davis G C, Puzantian V R, Kashgarian M, Bolinger J M 1985 Borderline: an adjective in search of a noun. Journal of Clinical Psychiatry 46: 41–48

Alloy L B, Abramson L Y 1988 Depressive realism: four theoretical perspectives. In: Alloy L B (ed) Cognitive process in depression. Guildford Press, New York, p 223–264

Andreasen N C, Winokur G 1979 Secondary depression: familial clinical, and research perspectives. American Journal of Psychiatry 136: 62–66

Angst J, Clayton P 1986 Premorbid personality of depressive, bipolar, and schizophrenic patients with special reference to suicidal issues. Comprehensive Psychiatry 27: 511–532

Baron M, Gruen R, Rainer J D, Kane J 1985 A family study of schizophrenic and normal control probands: implications for the spectrum concept of schizophrenia. American Journal of Psychiatry 142: 447–455

Beck P, Shapiro R W, Sihm F, Nielsen B M, Sorensen B, Rafaelsen O J 1980 Personality in unipolar and bipolar manic—melancholic patients. Acta Psychiatrica Scandinavica 62: 245–257

Berliner B 1966 Psychodynamics of the depressive character. Psychoanalytic Forum 1: 244–251

Bianchi G N, Ferguson D M 1977 The effect of mental state on MPI scores. British Journal of Psychiatry 131: 306–309

Birchnell J 1984 Dependence and its relationship to depression. British Journal of Medical Psychology 57: 215–225

Black D W, Bells S, Hulbert J, Nasrallah A 1988 The importance of Axis II patients with major depression: a controlled study. Journal of Affective Disorders 14: 115–122

Chodoff P, 1972 The depressive personality: a review. Archives of General Psychiatry 27: 666–673

Cloninger C R 1987 A systematic method for clinical description and classification of personality variants: a proposal. Archives of General Psychiatry 44: 573–588

Coppen A, Metcalfe M 1965 Effect of a depressive illness on MPI scores. British Journal of Psychiatry 111: 236–239

Coryell W H, Zimmerman M 1989 Personality disorders in families of depressed, schizophrenic, and never ill probands. American Journal of Psychiatry 146: 496–502

Depue R A, Klerman R M, Davis P, Hutinson M, Krauss S P 1985 The behavioral high-risk paradigm and bipolar affective disorder, VIII: serum free cortisol in GBI-selected nonpatient cyclothymes. American Journal of Psychiatry 142: 175–181

Docherty J P, Fiester S F, Shea M T 1986 Syndrome diagnosis and personality disorder. In: Frances A J, Hales R E (eds) American Psychiatric Association Annual Review of Psychiatry 5: 315–355

Donnelly E F, Murray G E, Goodwin F K 1976 Cross-sectional and longitudinal comparisons of bipolar and unipolar depressed groups on the MMPI. Journal of Consulting and Clinical Psychology 44: 233–237

Frank E, Kupfer D J, Jacob M, Jerrett D 1987 Personality features and response to acute treatment in recurrent depression. Journal of Personality Disorders 1: 14–26

Hirschfeld R M A, Klerman G L 1979 Personality attributes and affective disorders. American Journal of Psychiatry 136: 67–70

Hirschfeld R M A, Klerman G L 1983 Personality and depression: empirical findings. Archives of General Psychiatry 40: 993–998

Hirschfeld R M A, Klerman G L, Chodoff P, Korchin S, Barrett J 1976 Dependency – self-esteem – clinical depression. Journal of the American Academy of Psychoanalysis 4 (3): 373–388

Hirschfeld R M A, Klerman G L, Gough H G et al 1977 A measure of interpersonal dependency. Journal of Personality Assessment 41: 610–618

Hirschfeld R M A, Klerman G L, Clayton P J, Keller M B, McDonald-Scott P, Larkin B H 1983 Assessing personality: effects of the depressive state on trait measurement. American Journal of Psychiatry 140: 695–699

Hirschfeld R M A, Klerman G L, Keller M B, Andreasen N C, Clayton P J 1986 Personality of recovered patients with bipolar affective disorder. Journal of Affective Disorders 11: 81–89

Hirschfeld R M A, Shea M T, Gunderson J G, Phillips K A 1990 Proposal for a depressive personality disorder (DSM-IV work group on personality disorders)

Ingraham J G 1966 Changes in MPI scores in neurotic patients: a three year follow-up. British Journal of Psychiatry 112: 931–939

Joffe R T, Regan J J 1988 Personality and depression. Journal of Psychiatric Research 22: 279–286

Kendell R E, Discipio W J, 1968 Eysenck personality inventory scores of patients with depressive illness. British Journal of Psychiatry 114: 767–70

Kernberg O 1987 Clinical dimensions of masochism. In: Glick R A, Meyers D I (eds) Masochism: current and therapeutic contributions. Analytic Press, Hillsdale, p 576

Kerr T A, Schapira K, Roth M 1970 The relationship between the Maudsley Personality Inventory and the course of affective disorders. British Journal of Psychiatry 116: 11–19

Klein D N, Depue R A 1984 Continued impairment in persons at risk for bipolar affective disorder: results of a 19 month follow-up study. Journal of Abnormal Psychology 93: 345–347

Klerman G L, Hirschfeld R M A, 1988 Personality as a vulnerability factor: with special attention to clinical depression. In: Henderson, Burrows (eds) Handbook of social psychiatry. Elsevier, Amsterdam, p 41–53

Klerman G L, Endicott J, Spitzer R, Hirschfeld R M A 1979 Neurotic depressions: a systematic analysis of multiple criteria and meanings. American Journal of Psychiatry 136: 57–61

Kraepelin E 1921 Manic depressive illness and paranoia. E & S Livingstone, Edinburgh

Kretschmer E 1925 Physique and character. Harcourt Brace Jovanovich, New York

Lewis D A, Winokur G 1983 The familial classification of primary unipolar depression: biological validation of distinct subtypes. Comprehensive Psychiatry 24: 495–501

Liebowitz M R, Stallone F, Dunner D L, Fieve R F 1979 Personality features of patients with primary affective disorders. Acta Psychiatrica Scandinavica 60: 214–244

Loranger A W, Oldham J M, Tulis E H 1982 Familial transmission of DSM III borderline personality disorder. Archives of General Psychiatry 39: 795–799

Loranger A W, Oldham J M, Russakoff L M, et al 1984 Personality disorders examination: a structural interview for making DSM-III Axis II and ICD-9 Diagnoses (PDE). New York Hospital-Cornell Medical Center, Winchester Division, White Plains, NY

Mavissakalian M, Hamann M 1988 Correlates of DSM III personality disorder in panic disorder and agoraphobia. Comprehensive Psychiatry 29: 344–535

Mendelson M 1974 Psychoanalytic concepts of depression. Halsted Press, New York

Murray L G, Blackburn I M 1974 Personality differences in patients with depressive illness and anxiety neurosis. Acta Psychiatrica Scandinavica 50: 183–191

Paykel E S, Klerman G L, Prusoff B A 1976 Personality and symptom patterns in depression. British Journal of Psychiatry 129: 327–334

Perris C 1971 Personality patterns in patients with affective disorders. Acta Psychiatrica Scandinavica 221: 43–51

Pfohl B, Stangl D, Zimmerman M, 1983 Structured interview for DSM III personality (SIDP). Department of Psychiatry, University of Iowa College of Medicine, Iowa City, IO

Pfohl B, Stangl D, Zimmerman M 1984 The implications of DSM III personality disorders for patients with major depression. Journal of Affective Disorders 7: 309–18

Pfohl B, Black D W, Noyes R, Coryell W H, Barrash J 1990 Axis I/II comorbidity findings: implications for validity. In: Oldham J M (ed) Axis II: New perspectives on validity. American Psychiatric Association Press, Washington, DC

Phillips K A, Gunderson J G, Hirschfeld R M A, Smith L E 1990 A review of the depressive personality. American Journal of Psychiatry 147: 830–837

Pope H G, Jonas J M, Hudson J I, Cohen B M, Gunderson J G 1983 The validity of DSM-III borderline personality disorders. Archives of General Pscyhiatry 40: 23–30

Reich J, Noyes R, Troughton E 1988 Comparison of DSM-III personality disorders in recovered depressed and panic disorder patients. Journal of Nervous and Mental Disease 176: 300–304

Reich J, Hirschfeld R M A, Coryell W H, O'Gorman T 1987 State and personality in depressed and panic patients. American Journal of Psychiatry 144: 181–187

Schneider K 1958 Psychopathic personalities. In: Depressive psychopaths (trans M W Hamilton) Cassell, London, p 79–84

Simons R C 1986 Psychoanalytic contributions to psychiatric nosology: forms of masochistic behavior. Journal of the American Psychoanalytic Association 35: 583–608

Shea M T 1989 Influence of symptomatic state on assessment of personality disorders. Paper presented at the annual meeting of the Society for Psychotherapy Research, Toronto, Canada

Shea M T, Glass O R, Pilkonis P A, Watkins J, Docherty J P 1987 Frequency and implications of personality disorders in a sample of depressed outpatients. Journal of Personality Disorders 1: 27–42

Van Valkenburg C, Lowry M, Winokur G, Cadoret R 1977 Depression spectrum disease versus pure depressive disease. American Journal of Psychiatry 165 (5): 341–347

Zanarini M C, Gunderson J G, Marino M F, Schwartz E O, Frankenburg F R 1988 DSM-III disorders in the families of borderline outpatients. Journal of Personality Disorders 2: 293–302

13. Psychodynamics

Myer Mendelson

FREUD

The psychodynamic understanding of depression has evolved parallel to the development of psychoanalytic theory in general, although this understanding has naturally not always remained precisely in step with the general theory to which it was related.

One of Freud's earliest conceptions of neurotic illness was that of anxiety and neurasthenia as 'actual neuroses'. In this early model—one, however, that he stubbornly adhered to for much of his career—neurotic illnesses were conceptualized as transformed libido, excessively or inadequately discharged. In his adoption of this model, Freud was pre-eminently the 'biologist of the mind' that Sulloway (1979) labelled him.

It was with this model in mind that Freud (1893) first theorized about melancholia in some early drafts of unpublished papers that he sent to his friend Fliess in Berlin. Freud was never more Victorian than when he confidently expatiated on the pathological consequences of masturbation. 'I am now asserting that *every* neurasthenia is sexual' (italics in the original) and neurasthenia, he felt, was caused by excessive and abnormal sexual discharge through masturbation, resulting in sexual anaesthesia and weakness. Freud saw 'striking connections' between this sexual anaesthesia and melancholia. 'Everything that provokes anaesthesia encouraged the generation of melancholia . . . melancholia is generated as an intensification of neurasthenia through masturbation'. (Freud 1895)

In 1917, Freud published his classic paper *Mourning and Melancholia*. Since he acknowledged that melancholia 'takes on various clinical forms the grouping together of which into a single unity does not seem to be established with certainty; and (that) some of these forms suggest somatic rather than psychogenic affections' and since his material was limited to only a few cases 'whose psychogenic nature was indisputable',

he cautiously claimed no general validity for his findings.

He was careful to define what he meant by melancholia, the distinguishing features of which, he noted, were a 'profoundly painful dejection, cessation of interest in the outside world, loss of the capacity to love, inhibition of all activity, and a lowering of the self-regarding feelings to a degree that finds utterances in self-reproaches and self-revilings, and culminates in a delusional expectation of punishment'. In short, this was a picture of a depressive psychosis.

He observed that melancholia, like mourning, occurs after the loss of a loved object, either actually by death or emotionally by rejection or after 'the loss of some abstraction which has taken place of one, such as one's country, liberty, an ideal, and so on'.

Freud directed attention to the loss of self-esteem in melancholia. The patient reproaches himself, castigates himself and vilifies himself. Freud is willing to agree that the patient 'really is as lacking in interest and as incapable of love and achievement as he says'. Furthermore, he wryly acknowledges that when the patient describes himself in such derogatory terms 'it may be so, so far as we know, that he has come pretty near to understanding himself'. He, however, sardonically wonders 'why a man has to be ill before he can be accessible to a truth of this kind'.

In his attempt to understand the melancholic's psychological stituation, Freud notes that 'in him one part of the ego sets itself over against the other, judges it critically and, as it were, takes it as its object'. He identifies this part of the ego, this 'critical agency' with the conscience.

Then Freud goes on to make his classic observation: 'If one listens patiently to a patient's many and various self-accusations, one cannot in the end avoid the impression that often the most violent of them are hardly at all applicable to the patient himself, but that with insignificant modifications they do fit someone else, someone whom the patient loves or has loved or should love'. In other words, the patient is actually accusing and complaining not of himself but of the lost loved object.

Freud was indicating that, in melancholic patients, the lost object becomes identified with the ego by a process of incorporation or introjection and that the hostility that was felt for the rejecting or disappointing object becomes experienced as directed against the ego, with which the object is now identified.

Freud explained the different responses of the mourner and the melancholic to object loss by postulating the omnipresence of ambivalence in the love relationships of the potential melancholic. He theorised that, after the loss of the object and its introjection, the hostile part of the ambivalence which had been felt toward the object manifests itself in the hatred and sadism which is discharged against the ego (and its introjected object) in self-reproaches and self-vilification. He visualized 'each single struggle of ambivalence' as loosening 'the fixation of the libido to the object by disparaging it, denigrating it and, even as it were, killing it'.

Mourning and Melancholia was written at a time when Freud was interested in exploring the libidinal vicissitudes that he associated with the phenomenon of narcissism. He considered that melancholia can only occur when the object-choice has been established on a narcissistic basis so that the libido becomes withdrawn from the object to the ego with which the ego has become identified. As Freud viewed it, 'this substitution of identification for object-love is an important mechanism in the narcissistic affections.'

At this time, Freud still viewed identification as a pathological process which occurred when the lost object, initially chosen on a narcissistic basis, was taken into the ego 'in accordance with the oral or cannibalistic phase of libidinal development'. It was only much later in the evolution of psychoanalytic theory that fantasies of incorporation, oral or otherwise, were differentiated from processes of introjection and identification.

As I noted above, Freud believed that some forms of melancholia appeared somatic rather than psychological in origin. And even in psychogenic melancholia he discerned some constitutional features. He believed that the melancholic's ambivalence might be constitutional, that it might be an element of every relation in which the individual participated. And he considered the diurnal variation that is found in melancholia to be somatic in nature and not explainable psychologically.

ABRAHAM

The next contribution to the theory of depression was greatly influenced by Freud's (1905) observations on infantile sexuality. Freud had described a number of erogenous zones or portions of skin or mucous membrane, the stimulation of which produced pleasurable feelings of a sensual quality. The first pregenital phase of psychosexual development was, according to Freud, the oral phase. Since this primary stage of physical gratification was associated with the act of sucking and taking nourishment, Freud conferred upon it the rather evocative adjective 'cannibalistic'.

Abraham (1916) repeated an earlier notion that the lack of their accustomed sexual gratification made many neurotics depressed and he went on to observe that these patients often resorted to oral gratification (e.g. eating sweets or drinking milk) to prevent the onset of depression or to relieve it once it had occurred. He cited many clinical examples of this use of oral eroticism. Abraham had observed (1911) that melancholic patients mourn for their lost capacity to love. They then, according to him, regress to this earlier phase of sexual development in which gratification is obtained by oral means. Abraham postulated that in addition to, or instead of, the overt manifestations of such a regression, the melancholic unconsciously directs upon his love object the wish to devour or to incorporate it, a wish or a fantasy that is coloured by the depressive's repressed hostility. Thus, actually, the patient wishes to destroy and demolish his object by incorporating it. Abraham felt that these unconscious cannibalistic wishes, of which he provided many clinical examples, explained the patient's loss of appetite 'as though complete abstention from food could alone keep him from carrying out his repressed impulses'.

In his next contribution to the study of depression, Abraham (1924) held that all of the following factors were essential in the psychogenesis of melancholia:

1. A constitutional, inherited intensification of oral erotism, i.e. an increased capacity to experience pleasure in the oral zone.

2. As a result of this constitutional intensification, a special psychosexual fixation at the oral level, leading to intensified needs and consequently intensified frustrations associated with the acts of sucking, eating, drinking, kissing, etc.

3. Early and repeated disappointments in childhood such as the shattering discovery that one is not the mother's favourite or, even worse, that one is not loved at all.

4. The occurrence of such a disappointment pre-oedipally, i.e. prior to the time when one's love for the mother and rivalry with the father have been resolved. Abraham postulated that this pre-oedipal timing might account for the permanent association of libidinal and hostile feelings.

5. The repetition of this disappointment later in life. Abraham believed that the melancholic's 'subsequent disappointments derive their importance from being representations of his original one (and that) the whole sum of his anger is ultimately directed against one single person – against the person, that is, whoh he had been most fond of as a child and who had then ceased to occupy this position in his life'.

Abraham furthermore believed that the melancholic was distinguished from the obsessional, whom otherwise, he felt, he resembled so much, by regressing to the anal-expulsive phase (in which the object is given up) rather than to the anal-retentive phase in which the obsessional still clings to his object.

Considering Abraham's preoccupation with the unconscious libidinal and sadistic activity of the gastrointestinal tract, Blanco's comment (1941) that Abraham seems to think of melancholia as a kind of mental indigestion appears not too far off the mark. He seems to have thought of the melancholic's love-object as something to gratify the intensified needs of his oral zone, as something to be sucked perpetually and unprotestingly while retaining it and controlling it in an anal way. If it turned out to be disappointing, he conceptualized it as being cannibalistically incorporated and then sadistically battered and assaulted until, ceasing to retain its qualities as a love-object, it is then disdainfully rejected and excreted.

RADO

In 1923, Freud published *The Ego and the Id*, in which he delineated the structural model of pyschoanalysis with its three psychic 'structures', the id, the ego and the superego.

It was in the context of this advance in theory that Rado (1928) made the next important contribution to the theory of depression.

Although by no means disregarding the instinctual vicissitudes that characterized Abraham's picture of the melancholic, Rado added a psychological dimension that added depth and richness to Abraham's essentially semi-visceral formulation of melancholia. Rado brought into central focus the role of self-esteem in the problem of melancholia, a concept that had certainly not been neglected previously but had not occupied the centre of the stage as it was destined to do from then on.

Rather than focusing on the depressive's constitutional intensification of oral erotism, Rado directed attention to the depressive's 'intensely strong craving for narcissistic gratification'. He compared the depressive to a young child whose self-esteem is overwhelmingly dependent on the love and approval of his parents rather than on his own achievements and activities. He saw the depressive exhibiting a marked intolerance for the disappointments and trivial offences that the more secure individual can disregard. The depressive, as Rado viewed him, 'is most happy when living in an atmosphere permeated with libido'.

Rado described a sequence of events that ensues if the love-object withdraws his love. As Rado viewed the consequences of such a withdrawal or rejection, based on the domineering and autocratic behaviour of the depressive towards his love-object, the patient reacts with bitterness and anger. It is only when this 'rebellion' fails, that the patient resorts to 'a fresh weapon (the last weapon)' to win back the love that is lost.

When a child angers his parents, punishment and repentance win back their love for him. Gradually, as the parent-figures are incorporated into the superego, guilt and reparation take place on the psychic plane without the imposition of parental punishment. The child has, as it were, rewon the affection of his parents, his internalized parents or his superego, by the punishment that was intrapsychically administered, i.e. by his guilt. His ego thus becomes the object of punishment by his superego which represents at one and the same time the internalization of both his judging and his loving parents. The guilt thus serves to reduce the tension between the ego and the superego and self-esteem is restored. Thus the sequence: guilt, atonement and forgiveness.

Rado visualized a similar process in melancholia. The 'good' aspect of the love-object, the latest representation of the parent-figures, is introjected into the superego. The 'bad' component of the rejecting love-object is incorporated into the ego and 'becomes the victim of the sadistic tendency now emanating from the superego' until finally, the punishment being complete, 'the ego . . . heaves a sigh of relief and with every sign of blissful transport unites itself with the "good object".

Thus, in this drama of expiation, Rado ignored the element of constitution and instead emphasized the pyschological predisposition. He expanded the concept of narcissism, emphasizing the precarious self-esteem of the melancholic and his craving for external narcissistic supplies. He saw the self-reproaches of the melancholic as an expiation designed to win back the love of his introjected love object, now identified with his superego.

GERO

In a fascinating, detailed study of the analyses of two depressives, Gero (1936) was able to demonstrate clinically the underlying intense narcissistic craving, the intolerance of frustrations, the consequent rage and hostility and the introjection of the love-object in these two patients. From his case material he disputed the universality of the obsessional character structure in depression. But most importantly, Gero pointed out that the importance of orality in depression extended far beyond the satisfaction of the eroticism of the oral zone. 'The essentially oral pleasure is only one factor in the experience satisfying the infant's need for warmth, touch, love and care.' With a more sophisticated grasp of the importance of object-relations, he was able to anticipate theorists such as Fairbairn (1952), Guntrip (1961) and Kernberg (1976) when he pointed out that 'the need to be touched, to be warmed, calls for an object. Even with the infant these demands are directed toward an object.' He thus expanded the concept of orality in a sense that represents the current usage of the term since it now refers to the yearning for love, warmth and approval as well as to the pleasurable stimulation of the oral zone. It was in this more general sense of affection, dependency and gratification that Gero agreed with Abraham and Rado that 'oral erotism is the favourite fixation point of the depressive'.

BIBRING

By the early 1950s, increasing doubts had been expressed about the universal validity of the classical psychoanalytic formulations. Helene Deutsch (1932), Rado (1951) and Gero (1953) had begun to raise questions about whether significant psychodynamic differences existed in different depressive syndromes. And indeed these questions were very pertinent. Whether the formulations derived mainly from a small number of manic-depressive patients were as applicable to agitated involutional depressive psychoses or the lonely, 'empty' depressed states found in schizoid patients or to listless, apathetic post-viral depressions as they were to the retarded, cyclical depressions of the manic-depressive type was not at all obvious.

Two clinicians and theorists, Bibring and Edith Jacobson, proceeded to modify the theory of depression to take into consideration these challenging new questions and observations. They agreed that depressive illness was essentially an affective state characterized by a loss of self-esteem. Bibring (1953), however, struck some interesting new notes.

First of all, unlike Rado—and Fenichel (1945)—he did not see all depressions as attempts at reparation, as despairing efforts to extract the needed 'supplies' from external objects or the superego. Indeed, he saw the reparative attempts, when they were present, as reactions to the depressive loss of self-esteem.

Secondly, in contrast to other writers who emphasized the oral fixations of the depressive, Bibring, while acknowledging the great frequency of oral fixations in the predisposition to depression and of the orally dependent type among those so predisposed, appealed to clinical experience to establish his thesis that self-esteem may be lowered in ways other than by the frustration of the need for affection and love. He argued that self-esteem can be decreased and depression induced by the frustration of other narcissistic aspirations. Among them, he referred to 'the wish to be good, not to be resentful, hostile, defiant, but to be loving, not to be dirty, but to be clean, etc.' which he associated not with the oral but with the anal phase; and 'the wish to be strong, superior, great, secure, not to be weak and insecure' which he linked to fixations at the phallic phase of psychosexual development.

He believed that the frustration of any of these wishes would lead to a feeling of helplessness and to a decrease of self-esteem. Thus Bibring succeeded in indicating that all depressive reactions had something in common, namely a fall in self-esteem, without at the same time denying that depressed states exhibit a complexity and multiplicity of forms.

Bibring, like Freud, Rado and others, tended to personify and reify the term 'ego', as when he referred to 'the collapse of the self-esteem of the ego, since it feels unable to live up to its aspirations' or when he spoke of 'the ego's awareness of its helplessness' or when he referred to the ego as the 'seat' of depression. In *Mourning and Melancholia* Freud had used the terms 'ego' and 'self' interchangeably, but in 1923, he gave the ego its current conceptual structural status by noting that 'in every individual there is a coherent organization of mental processes which we call his ego'. By 1933, Freud was warning against the dangers of anthropomorphism and reification, as have many others since (Freud 1933). Brierley (1951) noted that the temptation to personify is insidious. Beres (1956) warned that the concept of the ego is a working concept and that the risk of personifying it must be avoided. In 1962, he was even more explicit about the danger of referring to the psychic structures as if they had spatial location (Beres 1962). He disapproved of locutions implying the presence of fantasies, affects or other contents 'in' the ego or id which, he reminded us, were theoretical constructs. He insisted that 'they do not have existence in space'. Others, Holt (1967), Grossman & Simon (1969) and Schafer (1970), have also been prominent in the battle against personification and anthropomorphism.

Apart from his persistent tendency to personify the ego, however, Bibring introduced a concept that was praised by many discriminating theorists, and, as recently as 1975, was utilized by Anthony (1975) in a thoughtful review of the subject of depression in children. This concept was that of depression as an 'ego-psychological phenomenon, a state of the ego, an affective state'.

Bibring argued that because depression is an affective illness, the ego is therefore the seat of depression, in line with Freud's reference to the ego as the seat of anxiety. This reference to the ego as the 'seat' of either anxiety or depression is a clear example of reification. If we are to speak logically and coherently, we have to say that it is *the person* and not the ego that is depressed.

Furthermore, according to Bibring, 'depression is primarily not determined by a conflict between the ego on the one hand, and the id, or the superego, or the environment on the other hand, but stems primarily from a tension within the ego itself, from an inner-systemic "conflict"'.

This concept served to underscore the point that not all depressions were characterized by guilt – i.e. by intersystemic tension. This picture of depression won enthusiastic approval from writers such as Rapaport (1959), Mahler (1966) and Rubinfine (1968) but was criticized as only partially valid by Jacobson (1971). It was my contention in a review of the subject (Mendelson 1974) that this issue was neither valid nor invalid, but rather a pseudo-issue that represented a red herring in the theorizing about depression.

It seems clear that, properly understood, the term

'ego', like the terms 'superego' and 'id', are ordering abstractions, theoretical devices to classify data according to semi-arbitrary but clinically useful categories. They are not mutually exclusive structures which do or do not 'contain' affects, defences or self-representations.

What Bibring did accomplish, which represents his major contribution to the evolution of the psychoanalytic theory of depression, was to conceptualize self-esteem in terms broader than had prevailed when he wrote his paper. He went beyond the stereotyped theoretical fixation on external narcissistic supplies on the one hand and hate and guilt on the other hand. He broadened the concept of self-esteem in a clinically useful way that was to be surpassed only by Jacobson. And it is as a clinical contribution rather than a theoretical one that Bibring's paper deserves to be remembered. His attempt to clothe his astute clinical observations in theoretical terms unfortunately contributed to two decades of conceptual confusion about depression as an ego phenomenon.

JACOBSON

Jacobson's contribution to the understanding of depression was related to her theoretical model of the development of the self and the object world. Her writings are of great significance in providing a theoretical substructure for two themes that were to preoccupy psychoanalytic theorists throughout the 1970s and the 1980s, the self and object relations. The very title of her 1964 book, *The Self and the Object World*, adumbrated some of the directions in which psychoanalytic theory was to move in the next 25 years. She wrote this book and her book on depression (Jacobson 1971) under the influence of Hartman's contributions to ego psychology.

Jacobson utilized Hartmann's (1950) important distinction between the terms 'self' and 'the ego'. As they both used these terms – and their usage has become incorporated into contemporary analytical theory – the 'self' refers to one's own person as distinguished from others, whereas 'the ego' refers to one of the structures of the psychic apparatus. Hartmann, and after him, Jacobson, adopted the terms 'self-representation' or 'self-image' to refer to the 'endopsychic representation of our bodily and mental self'. In addition, the analogous terms 'object-representation' and 'object-image' were used to stand for the endopsychic representations of person-or thing-objects.

In their conceptualization, the self-and object-representations, part of what Sandler & Rosenblatt (1962) were later to refer to as the 'inner representational world', became cathected with libidinal or aggressive energy in degrees that are reflections of the individual's developmental vicissitudes. A predominantly libidinal cathexis of the self-image, as Jacobson viewed it, produced high self-esteem, whereas a largely aggressively cathected self-representation produced low self-esteem and perhaps depression.

Jacobson considered that the infant goes through a period of learning to tolerate his ambivalence. This learning process is characterized by 'constant cathectic shifts and changes' in which libido and aggression are continuously turned from the self to the love-object and back again, or from one object to another. Frequent fusions and separations of the self- and object-images occur in this phase. Sometimes one image is cathected only with libido, while all the aggression is directed to another one. This will go on until ambivalence can be tolerated and distinct images can be cathected with mixtures of both love and hate.

Jacobson conceptualized one's self-image as being first not a firm unit but as consisting early in life of an ever-fluctuating series of changing self-images derived from the infant's early unstable perceptions of himself and of those objects or part-objects (such as the breast) with which he comes in contact. Under favourable circumstances, the self-image gradually becomes integrated into a relatively stable, consistent, firm endopsychic representation of himself and becomes readily distinguished from the internal representations of objects.

Expressed clinically, the child begins to acquire a firm sense of his own identity and becomes able to differentiate himself from other people. Furthermore, under favourable developmental circumstances, his self-representation becomes optimally libidinally cathected. In a family setting of loving parents and tolerable frustrations, the child develops an optimal level of self-esteem and self-confidence and a reduced predisposition to depression.

If the child is less fortunate, he may acquire a poorly integrated, aggressively cathected and less adequately differentiated self-image. Expressed in clinical terms, he may, depending on his developmental vicissitudes, develop problems of identity or a tendency to experience low self-esteem which, in turn, predisposes him to depression; or, more seriously, he may develop difficulties in distinguishing himself from others, with possible psychotic problems of depressive, paranoid or schizophrenic type.

Jacobson (1953, 1954, 1971) considered that loss of self-esteem (or in other words, feelings of inferiority, weakness, impoverishment or helplessness) represents 'the central psychological problems of depression'. All the factors that can be included among the determinants of self-esteem, therefore, can also be considered as having important relevance for depression.

Among these determinants are:

1. The self-representations. Pathological development of the self-representations, for any reason, will, of course, have an important effect on the self-esteem. As an example of this, one might point to the effect of a devalued or distorted body image on self-esteem (e.g. Mendelson 1964, Mendelson & Stunkard 1964, Peto 1972). The individual's actual abilities, talents and achievements also naturally affect his developing self-esteem.

2. The superego. The parental standards, prohibitions and demands are gradually internalized and comprise the basis of the self-critical superego functions. If developmental vicissitudes endow the child with a primitive or archaic superego which reflects its unmodified, unmodulated fantasy-influenced perceptions of parental expectations in early childhood, then the patient's self-esteem is proportionately vulnerable and he is correspondingly more predisposed to depression.

3. The ego ideal. The more within reach this is, the more prone it is to stimulate attempts to live up to it and thus to enhance self-esteem. The more unrealistic and grandiose one's expectations of oneself happen to be, the more likely it is that self-esteem will suffer and that depression will ensue. According to Annie Reich (1953), who paid particular attention to the study of the ego ideal, 'an over-grandiose ego ideal—combined, as it not infrequently is, with inadequate talents and insufficient ego strength—leads to intolerable inner conflicts and feelings of insufficiency'.

4. The self-critical ego functions. With the maturation of the ego and the increasing ability to discriminate between the reasonable and the unreasonable, our concepts of value and our actions are considerably modified. The more mature the self-critical ego functions are, the more tempered and realistic will be our idealism and expectations and goals.

Jacobson indicated the broad base of her concept of self-esteem by indicating that success or failure, good or bad health, affection and love or neglect and dislike from the earliest or the most current love-objects all have an effect on self-esteem and thus on depression.

In this way, Jacobson made room in her conceptual model for a wide variety of determinants of self-esteem and depression and did so largely in the terminology of ego psychology rather than in the more simplistic framework of Bibring who, while referring to depression as an ego phenomenon, nevertheless used psychosexual fixation points as his major explanatory device.

With the refinement of conceptualization characteristic of her theoretical model, Jacobson was able to explain Freud's formulation of regressive identification in melancholia in a more sophisticated way. She conceived of such an identification occurring when the boundaries of the self- and object-representations dissolve away and result in a fusion of these previously separate images. When this type of regression occurs, the target of the patient's hostility – the disappointing object representation – becomes fused with and indistinguishable from the self-representation. Thus the self-vilification and the self-reproaches follow. But the process of dissolution of boundaries between self- and object-images is, by definition, a psychotic process and the resulting depression is therefore psychotic as in fact was the melancholia that Freud defined and described in his classic paper. But it will be remembered that Freud explicitly denied 'any claim of general validity' for his formulation. Nevertheless, by a strange fate, this type of regressive identification, involving as it does what is referred to loosely as the dissolution of ego boundaries, the essence of a psychotic process, became for many clinicians the model for all depressive reactions.

AGGRESSION, PSYCHIC ENERGY AND SELF-ESTEEM

Ever since Freud wrote *Mourning and Melancholia*, aggression and depression have been linked in psychoanalytic theory. Jacobson (1953), for example, in a footnote on Bibring's view of depression, stated quite firmly that 'whereas he refuses to ascribe the central part in the pathology of depression to aggression and its vicissitudes, I am convinced, on clinical and theoretical grounds, that this view is correct'. Since so much in the psychoanalytic theory of depression has to do with the theme of aggression in depression let us examine this issue more carefully.

As we have just seem, Freud's model of the role of aggression in melancholia was derived from a study of psychotic depression. And even then, there are many psychotic depressions that do not involve self-vilification and self-depreciation and thus do not conform to Freud's formulation. Nevertheless, Jacobson saw aggression as a universal feature in depression. What did she mean by this?

In her use of the term 'aggression', Jacobson did not mean by it, or did not mean by it exclusively, aggressive or hostile feelings. As I noted in an extended evaluation of the concept of aggression (Mendelson 1974), Jacobson, to a large extent, conceptualized aggression as psychic energy. When Jacobson insisted that aggression is central in depression, what she meant was that low self-esteem is caused by the cathexis of the self-representation with aggressive psychic energy. So, by definition, aggression (i.e. aggressive psychic energy, not aggressive feelings or behaviour) must always be present in depression.

But the concept of psychic energy has been subjected to much criticism by, among others, Apfelbaum (1965), Beres (1965), Waelder (1966), Schafer (1968), Rosenblatt & Thickstun (1970) and Applegarth (1971); and more recently, and more warily by Gill (1977), Applegarth (1977), Swanson (1977) and others. The debate did not cease in the eighties but became much more desultory. Gill (1988) once again entered into the fray against metapsychology. From the other side was heard Opatow's (1989) heart-felt cry of woe: 'I have felt astonishment and sometimes despair, at recent challenges to the Freudian concept of the instinctual drive'. Some writers argue that the concept of psychic energy is vulnerable to criticism because of its vitalistic character; some, because of the use that is made of it for tautological pseudo-explanations that tend to block off further inquiry by seeming to provide an explanation. Other writers reject the concept of psychic energy because of its absolute incompatibility with present-day neurophysiology. And still others have criticized the concept because it lends itself to a kind of linguistic confusion to which even sophisticated theorists who prize conceptual clarity fall victim. The very name of this concept, 'psychic energy', invites endless comparisons and confusion with physical energy. The name and nature of this concept are thus misleading and breed scientific mischief and seemingly interminable debates about its value and significance. Gedo (1979), in his revision of psychoanalytic theory, dismissed the concept without even bothering to argue about it: 'I have become persuaded that neither a literal nor a metaphorical interpretation of the concept of psychic energy is epistemologically tenable; in other words, to retain scientific respectability, psychoanalysis must decisively reject all of the constructs within its theory based (even in part) on energy assumptions'.

What are we to think then, of Jacobson's position on the central importance in depression of aggression and its vicissitudes? To depict the self-image as cathected with aggressive energy is not equivalent to explaining the cause of low self-esteem. It is just another way of saying that self-esteem is low. It is tautological, not explanatory: it says the same thing in different language. And it exquisitely represents the chief danger that so many have referred to in using energic terminology. Its metaphoric quality soon becomes forgotten and it assumes existential properties in the minds of its users. It misleads the writer into thinking he has understood the cause of a phenomenon and, therefore, produces premature closure.

The cause of low self-esteem had to do not with the vicissitudes of psychic energy but, as Jacobson so discerningly observed, with a number of important variables, including early deprivation, deficiencies in the individual's actual talents or abilities and his expectations of himself, realistic or unrealistic, both in the moral sphere and in the sphere of his effectiveness. In addition, there are biochemical and pharmacological variables that appear to be correlated with low self-esteem and with depressive illness – but that goes far beyond the scope of this chapter.

OTHER VIEWS OF DEPRESSIVE PREDISPOSITION

Low self-esteem, as we have seen, has been widely regarded not only as a manifestation of depression, but as constituting an important predisposition to depression. However, there have been other ways of viewing the psychological predisposition to depressive illness.

Abraham wrote of primal disappointments at the oral level as predisposing to depression. Melanie Klein (1934, 1940) visualized the predisposition to depression as stemming not from particular early disappointments or traumatic experiences, but from the very quality of the mother – infant relationship. Leaning heavily on a terminology involving introjected 'good' and 'bad' objects, she essentially maintained that until the infant can become confident of love, despite his rage, every frustration, every removal of the breast, every absence of the mother is interpreted by him as a loss of a good object, a loss which is due to his own destructive fantasies and which is accompanied by feelings of sadness, guilt and regret. Klein believed that every infant goes through this 'depressive position', this complex of 'feelings of sorrow for the loved objects, the fear of losing them and the longing to regain them' until he becomes more fully assured of his mother's love for him.

Those children who are so unfortunate as not to meet with sufficient love for this to happen, or whose reality testing is insufficiently developed to disprove these anxieties, who have never succeeded in securely installing their good objects within themselves and who, consequently, never feel sufficiently loved are presumed by Klein to be always predisposed to return to the depressive position, to feelings of loss and sorrow and guilt and lack of self-esteem. In other words, they are particularly liable to depressive episodes.

This theory of the universal 'depressive position' that is believed by Klein to be the central anxiety situation in human development, bears some resemblance to, but is by no means identical with, Benedek's (1956, 1975) 'depressive constellation' and Mahler's (1966) 'basic depressive mood'.

Sandler & Joffe (1965) also described an early depressive reaction that they viewed as a precursor to later depression. They felt that the feeling of low self-esteem, so widely regarded as central to depressive illness, basic and nuclear as it might appear at first glance, was actually too complex and elaborate to do justice to the elemental affective core of depression. They then dissected out of the concept of self-esteem an even more fundamental biological affective state which was referred to initially (Sandler 1960) as the 'feeling of safety' but which they later (Sandler & Joffe 1965) labelled 'an ideal state of well-being'.

In the attainment of this ideal state of well-being, Sandler & Joffe saw the role of the love-object as being that of a 'vehicle'. When the object is lost, what occurs is not only the actual loss of the object, but the loss of that affective state of well-being for which the object was so instrumental or, in the writers' term, 'the vehicle'. They visualized the loss of this state of well-being as resulting in psychic pain. They conceived of this psychic pain as occurring when there was a discrepancy, for whatever reason, between the actual state of an individual and his ideal state of well-being. They considered that psychic pain could exist even prior to the time when cognitions or self-representations developed. They did not equate depression with this psychic pain, since they felt that there were a variety of possible reactions to this pain. It is only when these measures, such as acting out, drugs or alcohol, are not resorted to or when they fail and lead to helplessness that the depressive reaction ensues.

It is worthy of note that neither Bibring, who focussed on the depressive's failure to attain highly valued aspirations, nor Sandler and his colleagues, who interested themselves in the discrepancies between the actual and ideal states of individuals, regarded these failures or discrepancies as constituting the essence of depression. In both cases, it is the helplessness that is felt in the face of these circumstances that defines for them the depressive reaction.

Beck (e.g. 1967, 1970), on the basis of extensive empirical studies, postulated an alternative model of predisposition to depression. He, too, avoided the term 'self-esteem' because of its complex mixture of affective and cognitive components but, unlike Sandler & Joffe, he singled out the latter for closer study. His work on the cognitive elements in self-esteem led him to take the theoretical step of postulating an aetiological primacy for cognitive distortions in depression. Thus, for him, negative self-concepts and other cognitions lead to low self-esteem, which constitutes the core of depressive illness, although he too views depression as a complex phenomenon involving biological as well as cognitive elements.

OBJECT RELATIONS

Whether conceptualized as self-esteem or as the affective state of well-being, these desirable psychological and affective states have been described as coming about – or at least initiated – by early relations between the infant and growing child and his primary love objects. Thus, theories about the psychological predisposition to depression have focused almost, but not entirely (see Brenner 1979), on early pregenital object-relations. This was usually done implicitly and descriptively, without the theoretical models that were used being labelled as 'object-relations theory', which still tended to have a Fairbairnian rather than an orthodox psychoanalytic flavour. In her study of the determinants of self-esteem, Jacobson used the language of the ego psychology that had been inaugurated by Anna Freud (1936) and by Hartmann (1939). However, her metapsychology was not only characterized by structural and economic terminology. She also made generous use of concepts such as 'self-images' and 'object-representations', 'introjection', 'projection', 'the self' and 'the object world'; concepts which have come to represent some of the chief code words of the new object-relations theory. Thus, Jacobson represents an important transitional position in the evolution of psychonalytic theory.

The concept of object-relations has been implied in psychoanalytic writing on depression since Freud wrote *Mourning and Melancholia*. However, it was Kernberg who, as far back as 1968, began to conceptualize his formulations explicitly in terms involving object-relations theory. This approach, as he visualized it, encompassed such issues as the integration and differentiation of self- and object-representations, the depth and stability of relationships with others, and the tolerance of feelings of ambivalence, guilt, separation and depressive affect.

Historically, as Kernberg (1976, p111–136) and Friedman (1975) have indicated, Melanie Klein (1934) may be considered to have introduced the focus on object-relations, although her ideas were so controversial that they failed to become integrated into the mainstream of psychoanalytic thought.

Fairbairn (1952), influenced by Klein, outlined a theory of psychoanalysis that was explicitly formulated around object-relations instead of instinctual drives. His contention that libido was object-seeking and not pleasure-seeking represented the polemical battle-cry of disagreement with classical Freudian psychoanalysis. Nevertheless, with his attention to internalized relations, with his concept of an inner world of objects established by processes of introjection and splitting and with his emphasis on early mother-child relationships, his ideas began to bear some resemblance to, though they were very far from identical with, theorists in the other camp.

Concurrently and subsequently, Balint (e.g. 1968), Winnicott (1958, 1965) and Mahler (1968) were publishing observations on early development which could easily and perhaps best be encompassed within an object-relations model. It was Kernberg, however, who most explicitly accomplished the incorporation of object-relations theory into the mainstream of psychoanalytic thinking in a series of works (Kernberg 1975, 1976) on borderline and narcissistic personalities.

In this chapter, however, our focus of interest is depression. One might naturally ask then 'What light does object-relations theory shed on depressive illness?'

It will be recalled that Jacobson, in her consideration of the determinants of self-esteem and of depression, outlined the development of self- and object-representations and discussed the conditions for their integration and their differentiation from one another and also for their pathological fusion in depressive and other psychotic decompensations. Kernberg (1976, p 57) explicitly labels as object-relations theory that aspect of psychoanalytic metapsychology which concerns itself with the development of self- and object-images as 'reflections of the original infant—mother relationship and its later development into dyadic, triangular, and multiple internal and external interpersonal relationship'. As he views it (Kernberg 1976, p 58) object-relations theory 'transcends any psychoanalytic school or group and represents a general psychoanalytic development to which authors of very different orientations have contributed significantly'.

He, like Jacobson, outlines a model for the development of an integrated, stable 'internal representational world' (Sandler & Rosenblatt 1962) of object relationships out of an initial amorphous mass of fluctuating, diffuse, undifferentiated self-object images characterized by unmodulated primitive affects.

It will be remembered that Jacobson conceptualized self-esteem in the language of instinctual drives and psychic energy as the libidinal or aggressive cathexis of the self-image. In the evolution of psychoanalytic theory, Kernberg comes at a point where he carefully tries to balance the claims of affects and drives. He speaks of basic units of 1) self-images, 2) object-images and 3) 'affect dispositions' which colour these images with pleasurable or unpleasurable affective tones, but, paying due respect to the concept of psychic energy, he rounds out his discussion (Kernberg 1976, p 64) of the development of object-relations with the observation that these affects of pleasure or unpleasure 'actualize respectively, libidinal and aggressive drive derivatives'.

Sandler & Sandler (1978), in an interesting contribution to the topic of object-relationships and affects, however, dispute this way of explaining the affective tone of self- and object-images. For them, affects are simply subjective feeling-states, either pleasurable or unpleasurable. Harking back to an earlier paper (Joffe & Sandler 1967), they dismiss psychic energy with the observation that 'it is increasingly clear that conceiving of an object relationship as the energic investment of an object is inadequate and simplistic'. As they see it, wish-fulfilment is a much more useful way of visualizing object-relationships. They, like Kernberg, think of object-relations not in isolation, but in units which they characterize as wishes. 'In psychological terms, every wish involves a self-representation, object-representation and the representation of the interaction between them'.

As they view it, each partner in every relationship, at any given time 'has a role for the other and negotiates with the other in order to get him or her to respond in a particular way'. This occurs not only between people, but also in fantasy, in the inner representational world. And to those who are familiar with Joseph Sandler's views, it will come as no surprise that these wishes are often 'motivated by the need to restore feelings of well-being and safety', the absence of which may produce the sequence of pain, depressive response and depressive illness.

Thus, the Sandlers make explicit, in the theoretical context of object-relations, the intricate and subtle negotiations that go on interpersonally and intrapsychically in order to gratify needs and wishes that maintain or restore that core of well-being that is so important an element in self-esteem and so essential in warding off depression.

From a later, more balanced and comprehensive perspective, the Sandlers were able to declare, with Fairbairn's insistence in mind, that libido was object-seeking and not pleasure-seeking, that 'the traditional distinction between the search for objects on the one hand and the search for wish-fulfilment or need-satisfaction on the other fades into insignificance. *The two can be regarded as being essentially the same*' (italics in the original).

Furthermore, their view that much of our life – though not, of course, all – 'is involved in the concealed repetition of early object relationships in one form or another' allows us to understand concepts such as primal disappointments or the depressive position from a more revealing perspective.

OTHER ASPECTS OF DEPRESSION

We have been discussing the psychological predisposition to depressive illness in the latter part of this chapter. The papers on depression written during the last decade have not provided any enhanced understanding of depression. Although Leo Stone (1986) insists on the pre-eminent importance of an archaic characterological core in depressive illness, these articles (Chodoff 1972, Stone 1986, Milrod 1988) tend to emphasize, to paraphrase a comment by Akiskal (1985), one or another *mélange* of traits such as orality, guilt and aggression. Many other papers are so esoteric, abstract or idiosyncratic that they have failed to win general acceptance.

Most psychoanalytic papers on depression tend to ignore the increasingly refined diagnostic understanding of depressive illness proceeding in the general psychiatric literature and best represented by the work of Akiskal and his group (e.g. Akiskal 1985).

Apart from the occasional fleeting reference to 'the biology and pharmacology of depression' (Stone 1986), the psychoanalytic literature mostly ignored the psychobiology of depression. There was no debate or dialogue. There were instead two ongoing monologues each addressed to a different audience. At least, this was generally the case until 1980, when the issue suddenly passed from the decorous pages of academic journals and exploded into a legal battle.

A white male physician had been admitted to a prestigious private hospital with a very severe depression. He was treated for 'a narcissistic personality disorder' which was believed to be at the core of his depression. He received individual psychotherapy 4 days a week for 7 months during which time he lost 40 pounds, experienced severe insomnia and had such marked psychomotor agitation that his feet became swollen and blistered, requiring medical attention. After 7 months his family arranged for his transfer to another private psychiatric hospital where he was treated with antidepressants and quickly recovered.

Several years later, in 1982, the patient sued the hospital which had withheld medications, claiming that because he had not been treated with antidepressants he had 'lost a lucrative medical practice, his standing in the medical community, and custody of two of his children' (Klerman 1990). In a hearing before a Health Care Arbitration Panel, the plaintiff had the benefit of a large number of expert witnesses including Drs Gerald Klerman, Donald Klein, Frank Ayd and Bernard Carroll. The panel found for the plaintiff. Before any legal action could be taken, however, the case was settled out of court, so that it does not represent a legal precedent.

In a mixed legal and psychoanalytic critique of Klerman's review of the implications of this case, Alan Stone (1990) argued for a psychodynamic rather than a biological perspective on the matter of treatment of depressed patients. However, in a humanitarian spirit he conceded that 'I would have insisted on "biological treatment in the face of obvious psychotic deterioration"'. It should be noted that Stone is writing as an interested observer in the case. He was not involved in the treatment of the patient. If the symptoms became too severe he would intervene with antidepressants.

He seems to ignore or misunderstand the issue: that the patient suffered from what most contemporary clinicians regard as a diagnostic entity, an affective illness rather than a collection of symptoms. This has been demonstrated by phenomenological, descriptive, familial, genetic, electroencephalographic and other studies. It has also been demonstrated that many of the premorbid temperaments and personality structures are themselves subclinical forms of the full-blown affective illness (e.g. Akiskal 1984).

Even Cooper (1985), a past president of the American Psychoanalytic Association, acknowledged that 'as psychoanalysts we should welcome any scientific knowledge that removes from our primary care illnesses which we cannot successfully treat by the methods of our profession because the etiology lies elsewhere. . . . Psychoanalysis is a powerful instrument for research and treatment but not if it is applied to the wrong patient population.'

As we have seen, many writers have emphasized that depressive illness is a complex psychophysiological disorder of which depressive affect is only one, not even universally present, element. Sleep disturbances, diurnal variation of symptoms, agitation or psychomotor retardation, impairment of concentration, loss of appetite, libido and of interest in usual pursuits, somatic pains or sensations, anxiety and peculiar, qualitatively distinct feelings in one's head all may be found in patients who are sick with a depressive illness.

Jacobson (1971) explicitly indicated that she concerned herself only with that aspect of the psychosomatic illness that we call depression which can be understood psychologically, implying that hers was by no means a comprehensive perspective on depression. However, some additional views have been expressed that carry this conservative reservation to more extreme lengths. Basch (1975) has announced flatly that 'the depressive syndrome is a mental illness, but not necessarily a psychological illness'. And Wolpert (1975), in the same vein, believes that bipolar depression (but not neurotic and not, for some reason, unipolar depression) 'is basically a physiological illness with psychological consequences'. Harking back to an old concept of Freud's, he expresses the view that manic-depressive illness is an 'actual neurosis', genetically determined, in which the symptoms have no psychological meaning but are instead entirely somatic in their nature.

It is only in the last 15 years that psychoanalytic attention has begun gradually to shift to inherited biological aspects of affective illness. The pure psychoanalytical approach has met its greatest challenge in the sphere of the affective illnesses.

REFERENCES

Abraham K 1911 Notes on the psychoanalytic investigation and treatment of manic-depressive insanity and allied conditions. In: Selected papers on psycho-analysis (1927). Hogarth Press, London, p 137–156

Abraham K 1916 The first pregenital stage of the libido. In: Selected papers on psycho-analysis (1927). Hogarth Press, London, p 248–279

Abraham K 1924 A short study of the development of the libido, viewed in the light of mental disorders. In: Selected papers on psycho-analysis (1927). Hogarth Press, London, p 418–502

Akiskal H S 1984 Characterological manifestations of affective disorders: toward a new conceptualization. Integrative Psychiatry 2: 83–88

Akiskal H S 1985 Interaction of biologic and psychologic factors in the origin of depressive disorders. Acta Psychiatrica Scandinavica (suppl 319) 71: 131–139

Anthony E J 1975 Childhood depression. In: Anthony E J, Benedek T (eds) Depression and human existence, Little, Brown, Boston p 231–277

Apfelbaum B 1965 Ego psychology, psychic energy and the hazards of quantitative explanations in psychoanalytic theory. International Journal of Psycho-Analysis 46, 168–182

Applegarth A 1971 Comments on aspects of the theory of psychic energy. Journal of the American Psychoanalytic Association 19: 379–416

Applegarth A 1977 Psychic energy reconsidered – discussion. Journal of the American Psychoanalytic Association 25: 599–633

Balint M 1968 The basic fault. Tavistock Publications, London

Basch M F 1975 Toward a theory that encompasses depression: a revision of existing causal hypotheses in psychoanalysis. In: Anthony E J, Benedek T (eds) Depression and human existence. Little, Brown, Boston p 485–534

Beck A T 1967 Depression: clinical, experimental and theoretical aspects. Paul B Hoeber, New York

Beck A T 1970 The core problem in depression: the cognitive triad. Science and Psychoanalysis 17: 47–55

Benedek T 1956 Toward the biology of the depressive constellation. Journal of the American Psychoanalytic Association 4: 389–427

Benedek T 1975 Ambivalence and the depressive constellation in the self. In: Anthony E J, Benedek T (eds) Depression and human existence. Little Brown, Boston, p 143–167

Beres D 1956 Ego deviation and the concept of schizophrenia. Psychoanalytic study of the child 11: 164–235

Beres D 1962 The unconscious fantasy. Psychoanalytic Quarterly 31: 309–328

Beres D 1965 Structure and function in psychoanalysis. International Journal of Psycho-Analysis 46: 53–63

Bibring E 1953 The mechanism of depression. In Greenacre P (ed) Affective disorders. International Universities Press, New York, p 14–47

Blanco I M 1941 On introjection and the process of psychic metabolism. International Journal of Psycho-Analysis 46: 53–63

Brenner C 1979 Depressive affect, anxiety, and psychic conflict in the phallic-oedipal phase. Psychoanalytic Quarterly 48: 177–197

Brierley M 1951 Trends in psychoanalysis. Hogarth Press, London

Chodoff P 1972 The depressive personality. Archives of General Psychiatry 27: 666–673

Cooper A M 1985 Will neurobiology influence psychoanalysis? American Journal of Psychiatry 142: 1395–1402

Deutsch H 1932 Psychoanalysis of the neuroses. Hogarth Press, London, ch XI

Fairbairn W R D 1952 Psychoanalytic studies of the personality. Tavistock Publications, London

Fenichel O 1945 The psychoanalytic theory of neurosis. Norton, New York

Freud S 1893 Draft B. The aetiology of the neuroses. Standard Edition, Vol 1 (1950). Hogarth Press, London, p 178–184

Freud S 1895 Draft G. Melancholia. Standard Edition, Vol 1 (1950). Hogarth Press, London, p 200–206

Freud S 1905 Three essays on the theory of sexuality. Standard Edition, Vol 7 (1953). Hogarth Press, London, p 130–243

Freud S 1917 Mourning and melancholia. Standard Edition, Vol 14 (1957). Hogarth Press, London, p 243–258

Freud S 1923 The ego and the id. Standard Edition, Vol 19 (1961). Hogarth Press, London, p 12–66

Freud S 1933 An Outline of psycho-analysis. Standard Edition, Vol 22 (1964). Hogarth Press, London, p 7–182

Freud A 1936 The ego and the mechanisms of defense. International Universities Press (1946), New York

Friedman L J 1975 Current psychoanalytic object relations theory and its clinical implications. International Journal of Psycho-Analysis 56: 137–146

Gedo J E 1979 Beyond interpretation. International Universities Press: New York

Gero G 1936 The construction of depression. International Journal of Psycho-Analysis 17: 423–461

Gero G 1953 An equivalent of depression: anorexia. In: Greenacre P (ed) Affective disorders. International Universities Press, New York, p 117–139

Gill M M 1977 Psychic energy reconsidered – discussion. Journal of the American Psychoanalytic Association 25: 581–597

Gill M M 1988 Metapsychology revisited. Annual of Psychoanalysis 16: 35–48

Grossman W J, Simon B 1969 Anthropomorphism: motive, meaning and causality in psychoanalytic theory. Psychoanalytic Study in the Child 24: 79–111

Guntrip H 1961 Personality structure and human interaction. Hogarth Press, London

Hartmann H 1939 Ego psychology and the problem of adaptation (1958). International Universities Press, New York

Hartmann H 1950 Comments on the psychoanalytic theory of the ego. Psychoanalytic Study of the Child 5: 74–96

Holt R R 1967 Beyond vitalism and mechanism: Freud's concept of psychic energy. In: Masserman J H (ed) Science and psychoanalysis, Grune & Stratton, New York, p 1–41

Jacobson E 1953 Contribution to the metapsychology of cyclothymic depression. In: Greenacre P (ed) Affective disorders. International Universities Press, New York, p 49–83

Jacobson E 1954 The self and the object world: vicissitudes of their infantile cathexes and their influence on ideational and affective development. Psychoanalytic Study of the Child 9: 75–127

Jacobson E 1964 The self and the object world. International Press, New York

Jacobson E 1971 Depression. International Universities Press, New York

Joffe W G, Sandler J 1967 Some conceptual problems involved in the consideration of disorders of narcissism. Journal of Child Psychotherapy 2: 56–66

Kernberg O 1968 The treatment of patients with borderline personality organization. In: Borderline conditions and pathological narcissism (1975). Jason Aronson, New York, p 69–109

Kernberg O 1975 Borderline conditions and pathological narcissism. Jason Aronson, New York

Kernberg O F 1976 Object-relations theory and clinical psychoanalysis. Jason Aronson, New York

Klein M 1934 A contribution to the psychogenesis of manic-depressive states. In: Contributions to psychoanalysis, 1921–1945 (1948). Hogarth Press, London, p 282–310

Klein M 1940 Mourning and its relation to manic-depressive states. In: Contributions to psycho-analysis, 1921–1945 (1948). Hogarth Press, London, p 311–338

Klerman S L 1990 The psychiatric patient's right to effective treatment: implications of Osheroff vs. Chestnut Lodge. American Journal of Psychiatry 147: 409–418

Mahler M G 1966 Notes on the development of basic moods: the depressive affect. In: Loewenstein R M, Newman L M, Schur M, Solnit A H (eds) Psychoanalysis – a general psychology. International Universities Press, New York, p 152–168

Mahler M S 1968 On human symbiosis and the vicissitudes of individuation. Vol 1. Infantile psychosis. International Universities Press, New York

Mendelson M 1964 Psychological aspects of obesity. Medical Clinics of North America 48: 1373–1385

Mendelson M 1974 Psychoanalytic concepts of depression. Spectrum Publications, New York, ch VIII

Mendelson M, Stunkard A J 1964 Obesity and the body image (abstract). Psychosomatic Medicine 26: 638

Milrod D 1988 A current view of the psychoanalytic theory of depression. Psychoanalytic Study of the Child 43: 83–100

Opatow B 1989 Drive theory and the metapsychology of experience. International Journal of Psycho-Analysis 79: 645–660

Peto A 1972 Body image and depression. International Journal of Psycho-Analysis 53: 259–263

Rado S 1928 The problem of melancholia. International Journal of Psycho-Analysis 9: 420–438

Rado S 1951 Psychodynamics of depression from the etiologic point of view. Psychosomatic Medicine 13: 51–55

Rapaport D 1959 Edward Bibring's theory of depression. In Gill M M (ed) The collected papers of David Rapaport. Basic Books, New York, p 758–773

Reich A 1953 Narcissistic object choice of women. Journal of the American Psychoanalytic Association 1: 22–44

Rosenblatt A D, Thickstun J T 1970 A study of the concept of psychic energy. International Journal of Psycho-Analysis 51: 265–278

Rubinfine D L 1968 Notes on a theory of depression. Psychoanalytic Quaterly 37: 400–417

Sandler J 1960 The background of safety. International Journal of Psycho-Analysis 41: 352–356

Sandler J, Joffe W G 1965 Notes on childhood depression. International Journal of Psycho-Analysis 46: 88–96

Sandler J, Rosenblatt J 1962 The concept of the representational world. Psychoanalytic Study of the Child 18: 128–145

Sandler J, Sandler A M 1978 On the development of object relations and affects. International Journal of Psycho-Analysis 59: 285–296

Schafer R 1968 Aspects of Internalization. International Universities Press, New York

Schafer R 1970 An overview of Heinz Hartmann's contribution to psychoanalysis. International Journal of Psycho-Analysis 51: 425–446

Stone L 1986 Psychoanalytic observations on the pathology of depressive illness: selected spheres of ambiguity or disagreement. Journal of the American Psychoanalytic Association 34: 329–362

Stone A A 1990 Law, science, and psychiatric malpractice: a response to Klerman's indictment of psychoanalytic psychiatry. American Journal of Psychiatry 147: 419–427

Sulloway F J 1979 Freud, biologist of the mind. Basic Books, New York

Swanson D R 1977 A critique of psychic energy as an explanatory concept. Journal of the American Psychoanalytic Association 25: 603–633

Waelder R 1966 Adaptational view ignores 'drive'. International Journal of Psychiatry 2: 569–575

Winnicott D W 1958 Collected papers. Basic Books, New York

Winnicott D W 1965 The maturational processes and the facilitating environment. International Universities Press, New York

Wolpert E A 1975 Manic-depressive illness as an actual neurosis. In: Anthony E J, Benedek T (eds) Depression and human existence. Little, Brown, Boston, p 199–221

14. Animal models

William T. McKinney

The creation of animal models for the study of affective disorders is a relatively recent development in the field of psychiatry. However, in recent years there has been a significant expansion in the types of animal paradigms that are being used for affective disorders and an increasing realization of their value among a range of approaches to studying the disorders. There have been a number of review articles on this topic in the last several years (McKinney 1989, 1988, Willner 1990, Katz 1981a).

Historically, part of the difficulty with animal models for any clinical disorder has been a tendency for premature clinical labelling. Animals have been subjected to a variety of experimental situations and the resulting behaviours have been labelled as depression, anxiety, neurasthenia and so forth. Such labelling has usually been based solely on the behaviours produced and their apparent similarity to the behaviours exhibited by humans with a given clinical condition. The important ethological principle that two different species can exhibit similar overt behaviours for quite different underlying reasons has frequently been ignored. This laxity in labelling has often alienated clinicians, who have failed to see the similarities between conditions used to produce abnormal behaviour in many animals and those which were thought to predispose to human psychopathology.

At the outset of this chapter it should be said that there is no such thing as a comprehensive animal model for depression or mania or for that matter, any psychiatric syndrome. Furthermore, it is unlikely that there will ever be one. To start one's research with this as a fundamental goal is misguided. The field of animal modelling research needs to begin to ask the proper questions and the recognition of this has been an increasingly important development in the field. Animal models are basically experimental preparations which are developed in one species for studying

phenomena occurring in another species. The concept of animal models involves the development of a variety of experimental paradigms in animals which might be used to study specific questions about human depression, rather than the production of a 'depressed' or 'manic' animal.

Certain paradigms will be more suitable to studying certain aspects of affective disorders in animals and other paradigms will be more suitable for other aspects. If this principle seems self-obvious, it has not always been so. The field has been plagued by countless arguments about which animal model is 'best'. Which animal model is 'best' depends on the questions that one wants to investigate, and there is no universally 'best' model. For example, if one's primary interest is in developing animal paradigms that have high empirical or predictive validity and which will enable the screening for potential antidepressant drugs in a cost-effective manner, one set of approaches might be used. On the other hand, if one is interested in studying the mechanisms by which early experience translates into developmentally-based vulnerability to reaction to later stressors, a quite different approach is indicated.

RATIONALE FOR THE USE OF ANIMAL MODELS IN DEPRESSION RESEARCH

As mentioned previously, animal models are basically experimental preparations which are developed in one species for the purpose of studying specific aspects of the human illness. They should not be viewed as replicas of human depression in its entirety. There will inevitably be important differences and the study of both similarities and differences is important. One might ask the question: Why have animal models in the first place, rather than doing all the necessary studies in humans? One answer to this question is that many of the studies one would like to do concerning depression cannot be done in humans. For example, it is possible by using animal preparations to control inducing conditions precisely and to study the behavioural and neurobiological effects on both a short- and a long-term basis. In relation to depression, prospective studies which examine the effects of developmental events on both behaviour and neurobiology can be done much more easily in animals. In this context one can study much more easily the interaction among variables, that is, how altered neurobiological functioning might affect the behavioural reactions to stress and vice versa.

Mechanistic studies are more feasible in certain animal species. For example, more direct and potentially more detailed neurobiological studies can be done in certain types of animal preparations and these may relate well to many clinical studies in affective disorders.

It is possible in animal experiments to focus on specific behaviour patterns and study their origins, pathophysiology and treatment responsiveness rather than dealing with global syndromes. For example, anhedonia can be studied in animal models (Willner 1990).

Animal models have played an important role in the preclinical development of antidepressant drugs and in helping our understanding of the mechanism of action of drugs. This has been done in ways that would have been impossible in human studies.

Animal models can also be used to understand the mechanism of established treatment techniques, e.g. why do certain drugs work in depression and others do not?

KINDS OF ANIMAL MODELS

Several authors have categorized the general kinds of animal models (McKinney 1988, Willner 1990, McKinney, 1989). Different authors use different terms, but they can basically be conceptualized in the following four categories:

1. Those models developed to mimic a specific sign or symptom of the human disorder (behavioural similarity models)
2. Those developed to evaluate aetiological theories of psychopathology (theory driven models)
3. Those developed with the primary purpose of studying underlying mechanisms (mechanistic models)
4. Those developed to permit preclinical evaluation of treatment methods (empirical validity models)

There is obvious overlap among these categories and models, but the reason for having them is the importance of maintaining clarity about the primary purpose of developing experimental paradigms in the first place, because the approaches to be utilized and the evaluation of these approaches could be quite different.

Behavioural similarity models

These models are designed to simulate the specific signs or symptoms of human affective disorders. The major purpose in developing these models is not to evaluate specific aetiological theories or to develop new drugs; rather, one tries to produce behaviours which are as similar as possible to those seen in human depression. Thus, the validity of the model is in terms of how closely one approximates human depression from a phenomenological standpoint.

Theory driven models

In these models one attempts to develop an animal paradigm to evaluate a specific theory of affective disorders. The idea is to operationalize the theory and to develop paradigms that will enable one to evaluate it. These types of models can enable the prospective evaluation of specific inducing conditions where hypotheses have been generated from clinical studies of humans.

Models designed to study underlying mechanisms

Some would say this is the major goal for the development of animal models in the first place, i.e. the improved understanding of the pathophysiology of disease processes. This utilization of animal models is relatively new and what the field is struggling with now is which types of animal preparation lend themselves to what types of mechanistic study. For example, not all animal models lend themselves easily to molecular and submolecular mechanistic studies and one should be careful not to equate mechanisms with only these types of approaches. One cannot necessarily transpose techniques of mechanism studies, even from one species to another, and the development of which types of mechanistic study can be used on what species is an area that is unsettled and highly controversial at the present time.

Empirically valid models

These types of animal preparations have perhaps the

longest history in the field and have mainly involved the use of animal preparations to develop antidepressant drugs. In an ideal empirically valid model, all drugs which work in the animal preparation will work in human affective disorders and vice versa. In other words, there should be no false positives and no false negatives. This 100% correspondence between the effects of the drug in the animal model and in a clinical condition is rarely, if ever, met although there are a number of animal models with high empirical validity. A word of caution is in order in this regard. The fact that an animal preparation has high empirical validity does not establish it as 'valid' on other grounds.

HISTORY OF THE ANIMAL MODELLING FIELD

Some historical perspective is important in understanding the field of animal models as they relate to psychopathology in general. This section will be brief and reference is made to additional sources for more detail. Pavlov (1941) is often said to be the originator of research on animal modelling of human psychopathology. Without going into the details of his work, perhaps of central importance is that it represented one of the first moves away from a correlational method of behavioural analysis to an experimental study of psychopathology. Pavlov was followed by a number of other workers (Gantt 1971, Liddell 1947, Masserman 1943, Hebb 1947) and the principles that resulted from these lines of work have been reviewed (McKinney 1989).

With regard to depression and affective disorders, the history of the field dates back to at least 1928, when Tinkelpaugh (1928) reported the case of a young rhesus monkey who developed significant behavioural changes following separation from a female monkey with whom he had lived by himself for about 3 years. These changes were seen following separation and again when he was allowed to see this monkey. The changes described included agitation, anorexia, social withdrawal and self mutilation. Several workers, notably Yerkes & Yerkes (1929), have described how newly captured gorillas had a high death rate and have attributed this to the loss of familiar surroundings. Others have described behavioural changes resembling depression in chimpanzees who have lost their mothers and there have been a number of other scattered clinical case reports in the literature in which animals are described as exhibiting something resembling human depression. Such syndromes have been described in natural and semi-naturalistic settings, as well as in experimental laboratories.

The more serious scientific development in the field of animal modelling of depression dates to the reports of Senay (1966), who originally presented the concept of animal models for human depression and reported a study using separation of German shepherd dogs from the investigator as the independent variable. He reported a decrease in object seeking and an increase in avoidance behaviours but, interestingly, found that these changes were significantly influenced by each animal's preseparation temperament. The changes persisted until reunion with the investigator 2 months after separation. Work in this area was not developed further until several years later when McKinney & Bunney (1969) wrote a paper outlining the history of this field and suggested criteria and alternatives for developing animal models for depression. At that time, investigators from several laboratories were concurrently doing mother–infant separation studies in several non-human primate species. Concomitant with this mother–infant separation research was the development of experimental work involving 'learned helplessness'.

These lines of investigation, combined with the development in recent years of more refined induction techniques, have provided impetus for the creation and use of animal models for depression. The remainder of this chapter will briefly summarize the work with regard to several of the major animal models of affective disorders. In the case of most of these models the literature is by now quite large and justice cannot be done to it in a review chapter such as this. However, key references are provided for each of the models.

LEARNED HELPLESSNESS MODEL (UNCONTROLLABILITY MODELS)

One approach to the creation of animal models of depression has been termed 'learned helplessness' (Seligman 1973, 1976, Seligman & Maier 1967). For many clinicians, 'hopelessness' and 'helplessness' represent some of the core features of severe human depression. For instance, Beck (1967) proposed a 'cognitive triad' in depression which involves negative conception of the self, negative interpretations of one's experiences, and a negative view of the future. This triad is sometimes reflected in feelings of helplessness and hopelessness. Depressed patients often describe such feelings and think that nothing they do matters and that they have no control over what happens to them. 'Learned helplessness' is an operational construct which Seligman and associates used to refer to a stable behaviour pattern characterized by failure to initiate responses to escape traumatic events and failure to learn that one's own responses can be instrumental in terminating noxious stimuli.

Their basic experimental paradigm consisted of two phases. During the first phase, the animal undergoes repeated noxious stimulation and at the same time is prevented from engaging in any activities that would bring relief from such stimulation, i.e. it cannot escape. For instance, a dog is subjected to electrical shock while strapped in a pavlovian harness so that no response on its part can terminate this shock. During the second phase, the animal is unharnessed when exposed to the noxious stimulation, thereby providing it with the opportunity to evade or escape the shock. Normally, an unharnessed dog that has not previously experienced an inescapable shock would immediately jump the barrier that separates the electrified grid from the non-electrified section of the shuttle box. Exposure to prior multiple sessions of inescapable aversive stimuli impairs the animal's adaptive responding in future situations where escape from aversive stimuli is possible. While in the shuttlebox, the dog seems to 'give up', in as much as it accepts the highly traumatic shock experience. This 'learned helplessness' state can be reversed by forcibly moving the animal to the non-electrified section of the shuttlebox and is also treatable with tricyclic antidepressants.

Thus, a situation exists where a dog 'learns' that no response on its part can alter its circumstances, i.e. 'hopelessness' and 'helplessness' and then 'relearns' (therapy) that its actions can affect its fate. In the view of Seligman and others, learned helplessness parallels clinical depression in which an individual feels loss of control over the reinforcers in the environment. Negative expectations about the effectiveness of one's efforts in bringing about the control of one's own environment lead to passivity and diminished initiation of responses. This theory has had considerable heuristic value and has stimulated a large literature. For example, an entire issue of the *Journal of Abnormal Psychology* (1978) was devoted to the topic of 'learned helplessness' as a model for depression. Its application to human depression is a subject of considerable controversy.

For example, an alternative explanation for the behavioural phenomena observed by Seligman has taken the form of the 'motor activation deficit' theory (Weiss et al 1970, 1976, Miller 1972, Weiss 1968). This hypothesis basically states that changes seen in such experiments are caused by disturbances of noradrenaline in certain brain regions and that if these neurochemical changes can be prevented by prior pharmacological treatment the behavioural effects do not occur. There are now considerable data from a systematic series of studies to show that these behavioural changes in the learned-helplessness-type paradigm are caused by significant depletion of noradrenaline in the locus ceruleus region of the brain (Weiss & Goodman 1984). Based on the above work and additional data, it has been argued that the uncontrollability effects can be completely explained in neurochemical terms and that it is not necessary to invoke any cognitive or learning concepts implied by the term learned helplessness.

There is other exciting work going on in the uncontrollability area that relates mainly to the interface between the behavioural state and underlying neurochemical substrates. In addition to the work by Weiss's group mentioned previously, other groups have been involved in studying the neurochemical substrates of uncontrollability models (Anisman & Zacharko 1982, Anisman et al 1979). Work by Petty & Sherman (1980, 1981a, b) has highlighted the neurochemical substrates of the learned helplessness paradigm and more recent work by Henn et al (1985) has shown that specific alterations in hippocampal beta-receptors occur with the development of helplessness-type behaviour.

PROPOSED PHARMACOLOGICAL MODELS FOR DEPRESSION

Historically the most prevalent drug model used for depression has been the reserpine model. The effectiveness of various antidepressants and many new drugs has been evaluated on the basis of their ability to reverse reserpine-induced 'depression' in the laboratory. This is an example of a model which is empirically valid when used to screen drugs, but which may bear little relationship to the depressive illness itself. More recently, a much larger number of pharmacological models have been suggested and Porsolt (1983) provides an overview of these.

One particular behavioural screening test which has received considerable publicity and has been presented as bearing a close relationship to the clinical phenomenon of depression has been developed by Porsolt et al (1977, Porsolt 1981) and is called the

Behavioural Despair Test. There are a number of derivative tests which are very similar to this basic approach. This is a test based on the observation that rats, when forced to swim in a restricted space from which they cannot escape, will eventually cease apparent attempts to escape and become immobile except for small movements necessary to keep their heads above water. It has been suggested that this characteristic behavioural immobility reflects a state of 'despair' in the rat and it has been shown that this immobility is reduced by administration of a variety of agents therapeutically effective in depression. Porsolt (1981) also reports data to indicate that the reduction of immobility by antidepressant treatments can be disassociated from more stimulative effects on locomotor activity. Thus, the theoretical rationale of this test as stated by Willner (1990) derives entirely from its supposed relationship to learned helplessness and has a considerable degree of predictive validity. A number of modifications of the behavioural despair procedure have been developed with the most significant being the 'tail suspension test'. In this test, mice are suspended by the tail and show struggling followed by immobility similar to that found in forced swimming tests. Antidepressants at very low doses have been shown to increase the duration of mobility and to increase the power.

SEPARATION MODELS

These models are based on the theoretical concept that humans and other animal species are in their most stable condition when they have secure social attachment systems and that disruption of these systems is very stressful. The result of such disruptions is a development of grief reactions and, in some vulnerable individuals, these can serve as a risk factor for the development of clinical depressions. The reaction to separations is obviously influenced by many variables, including developmental, social and biological ones. Determining the influence of these variables and how they might interact with each other has been extremely difficult in humans and investigators have used animal paradigms to begin to study the behavioural and, more recently, the neurobiological effects of separation. In general, studies of mother–infant separation in primates are of two basic types. The first and by far the largest group of studies consists of research which experimentally separates the mother and infant in order to investigate the characteristics of the mother–infant relationship. Such studies have centred on the

behaviour of both mother and infant prior to, during and following a brief separation, or separations. While interpretation of data gathered in such studies may include reference to human mother – infant relationships, their focus has been on the assessment of the dyadic relationship of the monkeys rather than on the individual behaviour of one or the other. The second group consists of studies which have been conducted for the explicit purpose of 'modelling' human depressive disorders. These studies are much more limited in number than the mother–infant dyad studies and tend to involve permanent separations from mother, observational assessment of primarily the infant's behaviour and assessment of biochemical or biophysiological variables in addition to behaviour alterations.

The first report of mother – infant separation in primates was that of Jensen & Tolman (1962). These investigators separated two pig-tailed macaque infants aged 5 and 7 months from their mothers and then reunited the subjects with their own or the other subject's mother. They reported the separations as being highly stressful and accompanied by loud distress vocalizations and arousal. Further, they found development of own-mother-specific behavioural patterns in both subjects across repeated presentations of mothers. Mother–infant interactive behaviours were reported to increase dramatically within own mother – infant pairs across separations.

A number of other investigators subsequently have studied mother – infant separation in several primate species. For example, Seay et al (1962) separated rhesus macaques from their mothers at the ages of 5.5–7 months. These investigators, in agreement with Jensen & Tolman (1962), reported that separation was a highly traumatic event for both mothers and infants. The authors interpreted their data as being consistent with Bowlby's (1960) theory of primary separation anxiety and for the first time described the 'protest – despair' stages in non-human primate subjects. The 'protest' stage consists of disorientated scampering, high-pitched screeching and a general increase in activity levels. The 'despair' stage is characterized by decreased activity, vocalization, food and water intake, withdrawal and sometimes death. Reite & Short (1978) have demonstrated that this latter stage in *Macaca nemestrina* (pig-tailed macaque) infants is accompanied by sleep EEG changes closely resembling those in human depression. Rhesus macaque infants who are undergoing the protest stage following maternal separation show an elevation of the enzymes involved in catecholamine synthesis as well as serotonin levels in the hypothalamus (Breese et al 1973). Data are not yet available for brain amine function during the despair stage of mother–infant separation.

A number of parameters have been found to influence the response to maternal separation. These include the age at which the separation occurs, the nature of the preseparation relationship, the housing conditions during the separation and the length of separation, along with many others.

One variable which has been found to be quite important is that of species. For example, Rosenblum & Kaufman (1968) have reported strikingly different responses to maternal separation in four pig-tailed macaques and five bonnet macaques. Pig-tailed infants initially showed protest to separation and then decreased activity and withdrawal from social interactions. After the despair phase, the subjects gradually became more active and showed more interest in their environment, though they never fully recovered from the despair phase. Upon reunion, mother–infant affiliative behaviour increased dramatically over preseparation levels, a phenomenon which persisted for up to 3 weeks after the reunion. By contrast, bonnet infants did not exhibit profound despair behaviour. While some degree of protest was found, the reaction was much less intense than that shown by the pig-tailed infants. The authors ascribed these differences to basic social behaviour dissimilarities between the two species. While pig-tailed macaques show specificity of mother–infant dyadic relationships, bonnet macaques exhibit a social orientation which is much more flexible and relaxed in terms of mother relationships. Bonnet infants, after the first 3 months of life, spend much more time interacting with animals other than their own mothers than do pig-tailed infants. During separation, it became clear that the bonnet infants established mothering relationships with 'aunts' in their social group, whereas pig-tailed infants were essentially unaccepted by other adult females in the group. So powerful was the substitute mothering in the bonnet animals that one of the five subjects never re-established a maternal relationship with its own mother but instead remained in close behavioural interaction with the substitute mother. Since the original study it was found that a depressive episode similar to that seen in rhesus infants could be produced in a bonnet infant if all conspecifics were removed from a mixed species living pen area (Kaufman & Stynes 1978).

Intensive studies on rhesus macaque mother–infant separations have been done by Hinde and his colleagues (Hinde & Davies 1972, Hinde et al 1966, Hinde & White 1974). Typically, their research has involved group-living subjects, with maternal separation accomplished in most cases by removal of the mother from the group for short periods of time. They confirm the existence of the 'protest–despair' stage with variations depending on the methodology used. In addition, they have suggested that infants contribute more to proximity of the dyad prior to separation. They have also found that preseparation levels of some behaviours are predictive of the levels of the same behaviours following separation. Furthermore, sex of the infant is suggested as an influencing variable, with males possibly being more severely affected by the separation than females. Of special interest in the Hinde studies is the documentation that early maternal separation experience has long-term effects several years later, even without any intervening separations. For example, infants who undergo early maternal separation and are then, several years laters, exposed to open field testing respond quite differently from animals who have not experienced early separation. They are much more tentative with their open field exploration and much more hesitant to explore.

The reaction to maternal separation not only involves behavioural effects but also major neurobiological changes. These include sleep changes, along with heart rate and body temperature changes (Reite 1977, Reite et al 1974, 1981a, 1982). Significant sleep changes which have been reported to occur during maternal separation include increased sleep latency, more frequent arousals, less total sleep and a disruption of REM sleep. As referred to above, other studies have examined neurochemical effects in rhesus monkey infants in the protest stage (Breese et al 1973). The effects of maternal separation on the cortisol response have been examined in squirrel monkeys (Coe et al 1978, Levine et al 1978, Smotherman et al 1979, Vogt & Levine 1980, Levine et al 1977). Brief separations from the mother or from a surrogate produce a marked increase in the pituitary-adrenal response. There are also data to suggest that separation affects the immune system (Coe et al 1985, Reite et al 1981b).

Peer separation studies

Bowden & McKinney (1972) and Suomi et al (1970) have proposed peer–peer separation as another approach to studying separation responses in primates. A number of studies have established the peer separation paradigm as a means for reliably inducing a protest–despair reaction, the nature and magnitude of which are dependent on variables which can be controlled by the investigator. Present data indicate that peer separation can produce a reliably predictable and stable separation response over repeated separations and thus it is possible to use repeated measures and repeated treatments and crossover designs. A number of variables have been found to influence the response to peer separation. The behavioural effects following peer separation have been shown to be both treatable and preventable by imipramine (Suomi et al 1978), thus adding further evidence to support peer–peer separation as a reasonable approach to developing animal models of depression. Using the repeated separation paradigm, studies have also been done of the interaction between the status of neurotransmitter systems and behavioural responses (Kraemer & McKinney 1979, Kraemer et al 1984). This kind of approach has involved studying the interactive effect between various drugs which affect neurotransmitter systems and the effects of such drugs on experimental peer–peer separations. This represents an example of a way in which animals can be used to study systematically the interaction among these two sets of variables in a controlled manner. Monkeys treated with alphamethylparatyrosine (AMPT), which is an inhibitor of noradrenaline and dopamine synthesis, show a more severe response to separation while on low doses of this drug. They are on such low dosages that no behavioural effects can be seen when the animals are unstressed and living in a stable social group. In other words, in this type of animal preparation, it is possible to sort out in a systematic way how the depressive response to peer separation is influenced by drugs. Specifically, AMPT increases huddling and decreases locomotion during separation. Similar studies have been conducted utilizing parachlorophenylalanine (PCPA) and fusaric acid (FA). PCPA did not have differential effects on behaviour dependent on social housing condition and therefore did not appear to potentiate the peer separation despair response at any dose despite the fact that drug treatment did, at a high enough dose level, produce some despair-like behaviour in both social and separation settings. However, fusaric acid had effects that were virtually opposite to those of AMPT and similar to imipramine in that it increased locomotion and decreased huddling in the separation condition without having any significant effects in the social housing condition.

CHRONIC STRESS MODELS

This approach to developing animal models has been developed largely in rodents by Katz and associates (Katz 1981a, b, 1982, Katz et al 1981a, b, 1982, Katz & Hersh 1981, Roth & Katz 1981). In this paradigm rats are subjected to an unpredictable chronic stress regimen. These stressors are typically administered over a period of several weeks and then the animals are tested in an open field setting in which they show lowered open field activity and a failure to manifest the activation normally seen after an acute stress. The decreased exploratory behaviours are reversed by electroconvulsive treatment and a variety of drugs including MAO inhibitors and tricyclic antidepressants.

CHANGES IN DOMINANCE HIERARCHY

Another type of proposed model is based on the importance of a dominance hierarchy in most nonhuman societies (Price 1967, Price & Sloman 1987). In this paradigm it has been postulated that changes in the stability in the dominance arrangement can produce behavioural alteration, and specifically that depression may be associated with falling in dominance hierarchy and mania with elevation. Gardner (1982) has, in this context, proposed an evolutionary perspective on manic-depressive disorders. Key experiments in understanding of dominance hierarchies is also being conducted by McGuire and Raleigh (Raleigh 1986, Raleigh et al 1988, Brammer et al 1989). These latter sets of studies provide important data regarding the relationship between social status and neurotransmitter systems, and how alterations in either of these affects the other.

ANIMAL MODELS FOR MANIA

Although most of the work in animal models of affective disorders has been directed toward depression there has been some work relevant to mania. The reader is referred to several review articles for further detail regarding this topic (Harrison-Read 1981, Mamelak 1978, Murphy 1977, Petty & Sherman 1981b). The major induction techniques utilized in producing animal models of mania involve amphetamine-induced hyperactivity, morphine activation, other drug-induced hyperactivity, 6-hydroxydopamine models and more evolutionarily-based models.

ACKNOWLEDGMENT

Portions of the research reported herein, as well as the writing of this chapter, were supported by research grants from NIMH (MH-21982), NICHD (10570) and by the Wisconsin Psychiatric Research Institute, the Department of Veterans Affairs and the John D. and Catherine T. MacArthur Foundation Mental Health Research Network I (Psychobiology of Depression and Other Affective Disorders).

REFERENCES

Anisman H, Zacharko R M 1982 Depression: The predisposing influence of stress. Behavioural and Brain Science 5: 89–137

Anisman J, Grimmer L, Irwin J, Remington G, Sklan L S 1979 Escape performance after inescapable shock in select bred lines of mice: response maintenance and catecholamine. Journal of Comparative and Physiological Psychology 93: 229–241

Beck A 1967 Depression: clinical, experimental and theoretical aspects. Harper & Row, New York

Bowden D M, McKinney W T 1972 Behavioural effects of peer separation, isolation and reunion on adolescent male rhesus monkeys. Developmental Psychobiology 5: 353–362

Bowlby J 1960 Grief and mourning in infancy and early childhood. Psychoanalytic Study of the Child 15: 9–52

Brammer G L, Raleigh M J, McGuire M T 1989 Serotonin type 2 receptors mediate the serotonin influence on social behaviours in vervet monkeys. American Journal of Primatology 18: 155

Breese G P, Smith R D, Mueller R A et al 1973 Induction of adrenal catecholamine-synthesizing enzymes following mother—infant separation. Nature: New Biology 246: 94–96

Coe C L, Mendoza S P, Smotherman W P, Levine S 1978 Mother—infant attachment in the squirrel monkey: adrenal response to separation. Behavioural Biology 22: 256–263

Coe C, Wiener S, Rosenberg L, Levine S 1985 Endocrine and immune responses to separation and maternal loss in nonhuman primates. In: Reite M, Field T (eds) The biology of social attachment. Academic Press, New York

Gantt W H 1971 Experimental basis for neurotic behaviour. In: Kimmel H D (ed) Experimental basis for neurotic behaviour. Academic Press, New York, p 33–47

Gardner R 1982 Mechanisms in manic-depressive disorder: an evolutionary model. Archives of General Psychiatry 39: 1430–1441

Harrison-Read P E 1981 Behavioural studies with lithium in rats: Implications for animal models of mania and depression. In: Radhey L, Singa L (eds) Neuroendocrine regulation and altered behaviour. Plenum Press, New York, p 223–262

Hebb D O 1947 Spontaneous neurosis in chipanzees: theoretical relations with clinical and experimental phenomena. Psychosomatic Medicine 9: 3–16

Henn F A, Johnson A, Edwards E 1985 Melancholia in rodents: neurobiology and pharmacology. Psychopharmacology Bulletin 21: 443–446

Hinde R A, Davies L M 1972 Changes in mother-infant relationship after separation in rhesus monkeys. Nature 239: 41–42

Hinde R A, White L E 1974 Dynamics of a relationship: rhesus mother–infant ventro–ventral contact. Journal of Comparative and Physiological Psychology 86: 8–23

Hinde R A, Spencer-Booth Y, Bruce M 1966 Effects of 6-day maternal deprivation on rhesus monkey infants. Nature 210: 1021–1023

Jensen G D, Tolman C W 1962 Mother–infant relationship in the monkey, *Macaca nemistrina*: The effect of brief separation and mother–infant specificity. Journal of Comparative and Physiological Psychology 55: 131–136

Journal of Abnormal Psychology 1978, 87: whole issue

Katz R J 1981a Animal models and human depressive disorders. Neuroscience and Biobehavioural reviews 5: 231–246

Katz R J 1981b Animal model of depression: Effects of electroconvulsive shock therapy. Neuroscience and Biobehavioural Reviews R: 273–279

Katz R J 1982 Animal model of depression: pharmacological sensitivity of a hedonic effect. Pharmacology, Biochemistry, and Behaviour 16: 965–969

Katz R J, Hersh S 1981 Amitriptyline and scopolamine in an animal model of depression. Neuroscience and Biobehavioural Reviews 5: 265–273

Katz R J, Roth K A, Carroll R J 1981a Acute and chronic stress effects on open field activity in the rat: Implications for a model of depression. Neuroscience and Biobehavioural Reviews 5: 247–253

Katz R J, Roth K A, Schmaltz K 1981b Amphetamine and tranylcypromine in an animal model of depression: pharmacological specificity of the reversal effect. Neuroscience and Biobehavioural Reviews 5: 259–265

Katz R J, Roth K A, Mefford I A, Carroll B J, Barchas J 1982 The chronically stressed rat—a novel animal model of endogenomorphic depression. In: Proceedings of the Third World Congress of Biological Psychiatry, Stockholm, Sweden

Kaufman C, Stynes A J 1978 Depression can be induced in a bonnet macaque infant. Psychosomatic Medicine 40: 71–75

Kraemer G W, McKinney W T 1979 Interactions of pharmacological agents which alter biogenic amine metabolism and depression. Journal of Affective Disorders 1: 33–54

Kraemer G W, Ebert M H, Lake R C, McKinney W T 1984 Cerebrospinal fluid measures of neurotransmitter changes associated with pharmacological alteration of the despair response to social separation in rhesus monkeys. Psychiatry Research 11: 303–315

Levine S, Mendoza S P, Coe C L, Smotherman W P, Kaplan J 1977 The pituitary-adrenal response as an indication of attachment in mother and infant squirrel monkeys. American Society of Primatologists, Washington, D C

Levine S, Coe C L, Smotherman W P 1978 Prolonged cortisol elevation in the infant squirrel monkey after reunion with mother. Physiology and Behaviour 20: 7–10

Liddell H S 1947 The experimental neurosis. Annual Review of Physiology 9: 569–580

McKinney W T 1988 Models of mental disorders. Plenum Publishing, New York

McKinney W T 1989 Basis of development of animal models

in psychiatry: an overview. In: Koob G F, Ehlers C L, Kupfer D J (eds) Animal models of depression. Birkhauser, Basel

McKinney W T, Bunney W E 1969 Animal model of depression, I. Review of evidence: implications for research. Archives of General Psychiatry 21: 240–248

Mamelak M 1978 An amphetamine model of manic depressive illness. International Pharmacopsychiatry 13: 193–208

Masserman J H 1943 Behaviour and Neurosis: an experimental psychoanalytic approach to psychobiologic principles. University of Chicago Press, Chicago

Miller N E 1972 Interactions between learned and physical factors in mental illness. Seminars in Psychiatry 4: 239–254

Murphy D L 1977 Animal models for mania. In: Hanin I, Usdin E (eds) Animal models in psychiatry and neurology. Pergamon Press, New York, p 211–223

Pavlov I P 1941 Conditional reflexes and psychiatry. International Publishers, New York

Petty F, Sherman A D 1980 Regional aspects of the prevention of learned helplessness by Desipramine. Life Sciences 26: 1447–1452

Petty F, Sherman A D 1981a GABAergic modulation of learned helplessness. Pharmacology Biochemistry, and Behaviour 15: 567–570

Petty F, Sherman A D 1981b A pharmacologically pertinent animal model of mania. Journal of Affective Disorders 3: 381–387

Porsolt R D 1981 Behavioural despair. In: Enma S J, Malick J B, Richelson E (eds) Antidepressants: neurochemical, behavioural and clinical perspectives. Raven Press, New York, p122–139

Porsolt R D 1983 Pharmacological models of depression. In: Angst J (ed) The origins of depression: current concepts and approaches. Springer-Verlag, Berlin

Porsolt R D, Anton G, Blavet N, Jalfre M 1977 Depression: a new animal model sensitive to antidepressant treatments. Nature 21: 730–732

Price J 1967 The dominance hierarchy and the evolution of mental illness. Lancet 2: 243–246

Price J S, Sloman L 1987 Depression as yielding behaviour: An animal model based on Schjelderup-Ebbe's pecking order. Ethology and Sociobiology 8: 85S–98S

Raleigh M J 1986 Social constraints, dominance rank, and monoaminergic function in vervet monkeys. American Journal of Primatology 10: 424

Raleigh M J, Brammer G L, McGuire M T 1988 CSF 5-HIAA, male dominance, and aggression in vervet monkeys. American Journal of Primatology 14: 437

Reite M 1977 Maternal separation in monkey infants: A model of depression. In: Hanin I, Usdin E (eds) Animal models in psychiatry and neurology. Pergamon Press, New York, p 127–139

Reite M, Short R A 1978 Nocturnal sleep in separated monkey infants. Archives of General Psychiatry 35: 1247–1253

Reite M, Kaufman I C, Pauley J D, Stynes A J 1974 Depression in infant monkeys: physiological correlates. Psychosomatic Medicine 36: 363–367

Reite M, Short R, Seiler C, Pauley J D 1981a Attachment, loss and depression. Journal of Child Psychology and Psychiatry 22: 141–169

Reite M, Harbeck, Hoffman A 1981b Altered cellular immune response following peer separation. Life Sciences 29: 1133–1136

Reite M, Seiler C, Crowley T J, Hydinger-MacDonald M, Short R 1982 Circadian rhythm changes following maternal separation. Chronobiologia 9: 1–11

Rosenblum L A, Kaufman I C 1968 Variations in infant development and response to maternal loss in monkeys. American Journal of Orthopsychiatry 83: 418–426

Roth K A, Katz R J 1981 Further studies on a novel animal model of depression: therapeutic effects of a tricyclic antidepressant. Neuroscience and Biobehavioural Reviews 5: 253–259

Seay B M, Hansen E, Harlow H F 1962 Mother—infant separation in monkeys. Journal of Child Psychology and Psychiatry 3: 123–132

Seligman M E P 1973 Fall into helplessness. Psychology Today 7: 43–48

Seligman M E P 1976 Reversal of performance deficits and perceptual deficits in learned helplessness and depression. Journal of Abnormal Psychology 85: 11–26

Seligman M E P, Maier S F 1967 Failure to escape traumatic shock. Journal of Experimental Psychology 74: 1–9

Senay E C 1966 Toward an animal model of depression: a study of separation behaviour in dogs. Journal of Psychiatric Research 4: 65–71

Smotherman W P, Hunt L E, McGinnis L M, Levine S 1979 Mother–infant separation in group living rhesus macaques: a hormonal analysis. Developmental Psychobiology 12: 211–217

Suomi S, Harlow H, Domek C 1970 Effects of repetitive infant—infant separations of young monkeys. Journal of Abnormal Psychology 76: 161–172

Suomi S J, Seaman S F, Lewis J K, Delizio R D, McKinney W T 1978 Effects of imipramine treatment of separation induced social disorders in rhesus monkeys. Archives of General Psychiatry 35: 321–325

Tinkelpaugh O L 1928 The self mutilation of a male macaque rhesus monkey. Journal of Mammalogy 9: 293–300

Vogt J L, Levine S 1980 Response of mother and infant squirrel monkeys to separation and disturbance. Physiology and Behaviour 24: 829–832

Weiss J M 1968 Effects of coping responses on stress. Journal of Comparative and Physiological Psychology 65: 251–260

Weiss J M, Stone E A, Hanell N 1970 Coping behaviour and brain norepinephrine level in rats. Journal of Comparative and Physiological Psychology 72: 153–160

Weiss J M, Glazer H I, Pohorecky L A 1976 Coping behaviour and neurochemical changes in rats: an alternative explanation for the original 'learned helplessness' experiments. In: Serban G, King A (eds) Animal models in human psychobiology. Plenum Press, New York

Weiss J M, Goodman P A 1984 Neurochemical mechanisms underlying stress induced depression. In: McCabe P, Schneiderman N (eds) Stress and coping, vol 1. Lawrence Erlbaum, New Jersey

Willner P 1990 Animal models of depression: an overview. Pharmacology and Therapeutics 45: 425–455

Yerkes R M, Yerkes A W 1929 The great apes. Yale University Press, New Haven, Connecticut

15. Neurochemistry

Pedro L. Delgado   Lawrence H. Price   George R. Heninger
Dennis S. Charney

Over the past 10 years, an increased understanding of the biological effects of antidepressant treatments has emerged. Partly because of this, the number of effective treatments for depression and mania has begun to increase. Understanding of the neurochemical aspects of affective disorders should further aid in the development of new treatments and clarify the reasons for treatment failures and for the temporal delay in action of most antidepressant treatments.

As basic knowledge of central nervous system (CNS) function emerged, the first biological hypotheses of the pathophysiology of affective disorders and of the mechanism of antidepressant action were proposed. This process was stimulated primarily by the fortuitous discovery of several effective antidepressant medications in the early 1950s.

The first major hypotheses of the pathophysiology of depression and of antidepressant action were the catecholamine (Schildkraut 1964, Bunney & Davis 1965) and indoleamine (Coppen 1967) deficiency hypotheses. However, after extensive efforts to do so, these hypotheses have only been partially supported (Heninger et al 1990) and as increased understanding has emerged of the complex regulation of neurotransmitter synthesis, release, pre- and postsynaptic receptors, the interaction of receptors with second and third messenger systems and ultimately of the effects of these receptor interactions on gene expression, the early hypotheses have been modified (Charney et al 1990).

BIOLOGICAL HYPOTHESES OF AFFECTIVE DISORDERS AND ANTIDEPRESSANT ACTION

The catecholamine deficiency hypothesis of depression was based on the observation that many antidepressant drugs increased synaptic concentrations of noradrenaline (NA) while the catecholamine depleting drug reserpine seemed to cause depression-like symptoms (Schildkraut 1965, Bunney & Davis 1965). This hypothesis postulated that depression was due to a deficiency and mania an excess of brain noradrenaline. The indoleamine hypothesis postulated that a deficit of brain serotonin (5-HT) was responsible for depression since drugs which increased synaptic 5-HT such as monoamine oxidase (MAO) inhibitors or 5-HT precursors such as 5-hydroxytryptophan (5-HTP) and L-tryptophan (TRP) relieved depression (Coppen 1967, Lapin & Oxenkrug 1969, Murphy et al 1978).

However, these hypotheses have not accounted for the lack of immediate efficacy of antidepressant treatments, given the rapid effect of various antidepressants on increasing synaptic NA and 5-HT concentrations. Further, deficiencies of NA or 5-HT or their metabolites in cerebrospinal fluid, blood or urine have not been consistently demonstrated in depressed patients despite intensive efforts to do so (Charney et al 1981b). A subgroup of depressed patients with a history of impulsivity or suicide do appear to have decreased cerebrospinal fluid (CSF) levels of the primary metabolite of 5-HT, 5-hydroxyindoleacetic acid (5-HIAA). However, decreased cerebrospinal fluid 5-HIAA is found in other diagnoses as well (Åsberg et al 1987, Roy et al 1990).

Most effective antidepressant medications (except bupropion) and electroconvulsive therapy have profound effects on catecholamine and indoleamine neurotransmitter systems (Carlsson & Lindqvist 1978, Charney et al 1981b). As new data emerged that alterations in the function of CNS neurotransmitter systems could occur by changes in the sensitivity of presynaptic and postsynaptic receptors, without an alteration in the amount of the neurotransmitter itself, the deficiency hypotheses were modified and the 'receptor sensitivity hypothesis' of antidepressant action was proposed. This hypothesis stated that the delayed therapeutic effects of antidepressant treatment were related to time-dependent alterations in catecholamine and indoleamine receptor sensitivity and implied that the pathophysiology of depression may be more related to abnormal regulation of receptor sensitivity than to deficiencies of a neurotransmitter (Charney et al 1981b).

A similar view, the 'dysregulation hypothesis', was subsequently expressed by Siever & Davis. The dysregulation hypothesis proposed that in affective disorders, regulatory or homeostatic mechanisms controlling neurotransmitter function were dysregulated and that effective pharmacologic agents restore normal regulation to these systems (Siever & Davis 1985).

The dysregulation and receptor-sensitivity hypotheses were proposed because of the failure of previous studies to identify clear evidence of catecholamine or indoleamine deficiencies in depressed patients and in the context of continuing evidence that catecholamines and or indoleamine neurotransmitters were involved in affective disorders and antidepressant action. For example, selective 5-HT (fluoxetine) and NA (desipramine) reuptake inhibitors have been clearly demonstrated to be effective antidepressant agents and 5-HT$_{1A}$ partial agonists may likewise have antidepressant properties (Robinson et al 1990). The dysregulation and receptor-sensitivity hypotheses went beyond neurotransmitter content and proposed that functional deficiencies in neurotransmission could occur with normal neurotransmitter content.

The receptor-sensitivity hypothesis is predominantly a hypothesis of antidepressant action while the dysregulation hypothesis is primarily a hypothesis of pathophysiology. These may be quite separate questions which are not mutually exclusive. That is, a patient with a dysregulated neurotransmitter system may respond to a drug that, by altering receptor sensitivity, regulates the functional state of that neurotransmitter system.

Figure 15.1, using a 5-HT neurone as an example, depicts some of the possible sites at which such dysfunction and the therapeutic action of antidepressants might occur. Genetically, environmentally or possibly traumatically acquired dysfunction at one of many presynaptic or postsynaptic sites could lead to an overall 'dysregulation' of neurotransmission which would have very similar or identical functional and behavioural consequences. Antidepressants could act at one or more of these sites to restabilize neurotransmission. Similar examples could be detailed for each CNS neurotransmitter system.

BIOLOGICAL HETEROGENEITY IN THE PATHOPHYSIOLOGY OF AFFECTIVE DISORDERS: IMPLICATIONS FOR NEUROCHEMICAL INVESTIGATIONS

It is currently believed that depression is a biologically heterogeneous disorder. It would he highly unlikely, given the great deal of redundancy of function and interaction among CNS neurotransmitter systems, that only one type of abnormality, whether inherited or environmentally caused, was responsible for all forms of major depression, dysthymia, cyclothymia and bipolar disorders. In fact, it is known that certain types of cerebral infarct (Robinson & Chait 1985), hypothyroidism (Sachar 1973), some of the porphyrias, acquired immune deficiency syndrome (Perry 1990) and numerous types of drugs can cause very similar or indistinguishable symptoms as are found in affective disorders of unknown aetiology. Mania can likewise be caused by a host of drugs and pathological conditions (Larson & Richelson 1988).

Heterogeneity of affective disorders could occur at multiple levels. This includes both heterogeneity of aetiology as well as of pathophysiology, each of which could occur at a neuroanatomical and/or neurochemical level. For example, Figure 15.1 depicts how multiple abnormalities could affect the functioning of a 5-HT neurone (aetiological heterogeneity), leading to the same overall dysfunction of 5-HT neurotransmission. However, given the great deal of interaction and interdependence among neurotransmitter systems in the CNS, it is possible that dysfunction of one of several neurotransmitter systems (pathophysiological heterogeneity) could lead to similar behavioural manifestations. Each of these dysfunctional neurotransmitter systems could likewise have multiple types of abnormalities which have led to the dysfunction.

The possible aetiological and pathophysiological heterogeneity underlying affective disorders makes interpretation of studies attempting to identify neurochemical abnormalities in patients with these disorders complicated. One prediction from the concept of heterogeneity is that antidepressant drugs which are selective for one neurotransmitter system may not be effective in all patients with dysfunction of that neurotransmitter system. For example, an antidepressant which blocked 5-HT reuptake might be more likely to be effective in a patient with postsynaptic 5-HT dysfunction than in a patient with a presynaptic abnor-

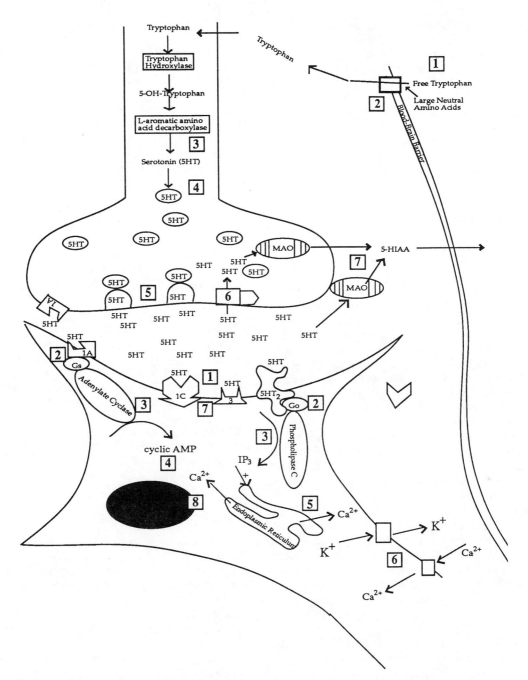

Fig. 15.1   Schematic representation of serotonergic neuron and possible sites of biological abnormalities in affective disorder patients and sites of antidepressant action. **Presynaptic factors**: 1. Plasma level of precursor; 2. Uptake of precursor; 3. Transmitter synthesis; 4. Transmitter storage; 5. Transmitter release; 6. Transmitter reuptake; 7. Transmitter degradation. **Postsynaptic factors**: 1. Receptor binding; 2. Receptor-G-protein coupling; 3. Second messenger system; 4. Protein phosphorylation; 5. Calcium release; 6. Ion channels; 7. Regulation of receptor function; 8. Gene expression

MAO: Monoamine oxidase; 5-HIAA: 5-hydroxyindoleacetic acid

mality which impaired the release or synthesis of 5-HT. Likewise, in a patient with an inability to regulate receptor sensitivity effectively, it might be predicted that a 5-HT reuptake inhibitor would be unable to induce the same 5-HT receptor sensitivity changes which it did in 'normal' laboratory animals, and thus be rendered ineffective.

Thus, it is important to keep these considerations in mind when assessing the results of biological studies in affective disorders. Type II errors are likely and abnormal results of neurochemistry tests may not be an accurate predictor of treatment response.

THE 5-HT SYSTEM

Evaluation of biological studies of the 5-HT system requires some understanding of the organization of this system in the CNS. 5-HT neurones innervate large portions of the CNS and appear to modulate behaviour (Aghajanian 1981, Aghajanian et al 1987). 5-HT cell bodies originate from a relatively localized area of the brainstem located within the raphe nuclei (Dahlstrom & Fuxe 1964). The 5-HT cell bodies within the raphe nuclei are subdivided into nine groups (B1–B9). Most of the ascending projections of these 5-HT nuclei come from the dorsal raphe (B7), the median raphe (B8) and the B9 cell groups (Kuhar et al 1971, Parent et al 1981).

Ascending 5-HT cell bodies project to distinct and separate brain regions and are organized in a topographical fashion which has functional significance. Interestingly, 5-HT nerve terminals appear to be composed of two distinct classes with different morphology, pharmacological and probably functional properties (Molliver 1987, Blier et al 1990b). Nerve fibres from the dorsal raphe have a fine morphology, with small granular varicosities and a greater degree of responsiveness to 5-HT_{1A} agonists, while fibres from the median raphe are coarse, with large spherical varicosities, and demonstrate a reduced level of responsiveness to 5-HT_{1A} agonists (Blier et al 1990b).

There are at least five distinct subtypes of 5-HT receptors in humans. These receptor subtypes have been designated 5-HT_{1A}, 5-HT_{1C}, 5-HT_{1D}, 5-HT_2 and 5-HT_3 (Peroutka 1988, Gonzalez-Heydrich & Peroutka 1990). The anatomic localization of 5-HT receptor subtypes appears to follow a pattern which is closely related to the pattern of differing types of nerve terminals and most likely also has functional significance (Molliver 1987, Blier et al 1990b).

Preclinical studies of the 5-HT system

The 5-HT system has been the most intensively studied neurotransmitter system in relation to the biology of depression and the mechanism of antidepressant action. The emphasis on 5-HT has been maintained primarily because of results from studies investigating the mechanism of antidepressant action (Heninger & Charney 1987). The most intriguing of these studies have been electrophysiological studies in laboratory animals suggesting that most antidepressant drugs and electroconvulsive therapy enhance neurotransmission across 5-HT synapses after long-term but not short-term administration (de Montigny & Blier 1984, Fuxe et al 1984, Blier et al 1990a). Antidepressants may cause an enhancement of 5-HT function through different mechanisms. Tricyclic antidepressant drugs and ECT appear to sensitize postsynaptic neurones to the effects of 5-HT, while monoamine oxidase inhibitors (MAOI) enhance availability of 5-HT and 5-HT reuptake inhibitors desensitize presynaptic inhibitory 5-HT autoreceptors (Blier at al 1990a).

Other preclinical studies in laboratory animals demonstrate that the 5-HT system is involved in the regulation of many of the types of physiological process which form the core of the symptoms of depression. The behaviours regulated by the 5-HT system in laboratory animals include a wide variety of physiological processes including appetite, sleep, sexual function, pain sensitivity, body temperature and circadian rhythms (Meltzer & Lowy 1987).

Clinical studies of 5-HT function

TRP and 5-HIAA in body fluids

Levels of L-tryptophan (TRP), the precursor of 5-HT synthesis, and 5-HIAA, the principal metabolite of 5-HT, have been extensively studied in various body fluids of psychiatric patients and healthy subjects. Some of these data suggest that a subset of depressed patients have lower levels of plasma TRP and another, possibly different subgroup, have lower cerebrospinal fluid levels of 5-HIAA, thus lending partial support to the original indoleamine-deficiency hypothesis (Coppen 1967).

Decreased plasma free and/or total TRP levels (Coppen et al 1973, Coppen & Wood 1978, Shaw et al 1978), or a decreased ratio of TRP to competing large neutral amino acids (LNAA; DeMyer et al 1981, Joseph et al 1984, Maes et al 1987, Cowen et al 1989b) have been reported in some drug-free depressed patients compared to healthy controls. However, not all studies have confirmed these findings (Riley & Shaw 1976, Curzon 1979, Møller et al 1979).

Further, several methodological issues have to be resolved before these findings can be adequately assessed. For instance, it is unclear whether decreased plasma TRP is primary or secondary to the depressed state, since various factors can influence plasma TRP levels. Glucocorticoids, tricyclic antidepressants, salicylates and a variety of other drugs can increase the activity of the enzyme tryptophan pyrrolase and shunt TRP away from the 5-HT synthetic pathway and towards the production of quinolinic acid, thus lowering plasma TRP levels (Morgan & Badawy 1989, see Badawy 1977 for a review). An example of this effect was reported by Maes et al (1990) who noted that a single dose of 1 mg dexamethasone reduced fasting total plasma TRP by 21%.

Other factors which can influence plasma TRP levels are related to dietary intake. A weight-reducing diet over a 3-week period lowers plasma TRP levels (Anderson et al 1989). Both weight loss and elevations of cortisol are common in depression and most studies investigating plasma TRP in depression have not controlled for these variables.

TRP has also been measured in the lumbar and ventricular CSF of depressed patients, with conflicting results. Lumbar CSF levels of TRP have been reported as being low (Coppen et al 1972) and normal (Ashcroft et al 1973, Banki et al 1981), while ventricular CSF TRP has been reported as being low compared to neurological controls (Bridges et al 1976).

Studies of CSF TRP levels are difficult to interpret. Not only are the variables described above for plasma tryptophan operant, but the potential effect of factors which can influence the uptake of TRP into the brain are also of concern. For example, beta-adrenergic agonists increase brain levels of TRP and other LNAA while decreasing plasma TRP and LNAA, possibly by affecting the uptake mechanism for LNAA into the CNS (Eriksson & Carlsson 1988).

In spite of the inability to ascertain the reasons for diminished plasma or CSF TRP, the findings are inherently interesting. Modest decreases in plasma TRP levels (15–25% decrease) have been shown to alter neuroendocrine indices of CNS 5-HT function in healthy humans, especially women (Delgado et al 1989, Anderson et al 1989). Therefore, diminished plasma TRP over an extended period of time could conceivably lead to behavioural effects in some humans. Diminished precursor availability could cause,

predispose to or exacerbate depression in some patients.

An extensive literature exists on the relationship of CSF levels of the 5-HT metabolite 5-HIAA to depression, impulsivity, aggression and suicide. The results of these studies have recently been reviewed (Åsberg et al 1987, Meltzer & Lowy 1987, Roy et al 1990). In brief, most authors conclude that a subgroup of depressed patients (35%) fall into a low CSF 5-HIAA group and that patients with low CSF 5-HIAA are more prone to impulsive, violent suicide. This finding has not been restricted to patients with depression but is also present in patients with other psychiatric illnesses (arsonists, some alcoholics and some schizophrenics) who are suicidal or impulsive (Åsberg et al 1987, Roy et al 1990).

5-HT depletion

Parachlorophenylalanine (PCPA) is a tryptophan hydroxylase inhibitor. It reduces the content of 5-HT by blocking the rate-limiting step in its synthesis (Koe & Weissman 1966). In non-psychiatric patients with 5-HT-producing carcinoid tumours PCPA acutely leads to a variety of behavioural changes such as lethargy, irritability, anxiety, depression and psychosis, although many patients demonstrate little behavioural change (Carpenter 1970).

Two clinical studies published in the 1970s reported that PCPA appeared rapidly to reverse the antidepressant effects of both imipramine (Shopsin et al 1975) and tranylcypromine (Shopsin et al 1976) within 24 hours in patients with major depression. These studies have been criticized because of the lack of placebo control and the small number of patients studied. No direct attempts at replication have been reported, although our group has replicated the finding using the plasma TRP depletion paradigm (see below).

Plasma tryptophan depletion

Depletion of TRP, an essential amino acid and precursor of 5-HT, through dietary methods, specifically reduces brain 5-HT function (Fernstrom 1977, Curzon 1981, Young et al 1989, Moja et al 1989). Ingestion of TRP-free amino acid mixtures in vervet monkeys decreases plasma TRP and CSF TRP and 5-HIAA with no change in CSF tyrosine, homovallinic acid (HVA) or 3-methoxy-4-hydroxyphenylethylene glycol (MHPG) (Young et al 1989). Ingestion of TRP-free amino acid mixtures in laboratory animals leads to extremely rapid changes in both plasma TRP and brain 5-HT with maximal reductions of brain 5-HT occurring within 2 hours of ingestion of the TRP-free mixture (Young et al 1989, Moja et al 1989).

TRP-free or low-TRP diets administered to healthy humans cause reductions of plasma TRP levels (Rose et al 1954, Young et al 1969, 1971, Delgado et al 1989). Rapid plasma TRP depletion (by 70–80% within 5 hours following ingestion of the TRP-free amino acid load) causes decreased concentration and an increased reporting of negative mood states in healthy males (Young et al 1985, Smith et al 1987).

We have studied a combination of a 1-day low-TRP diet followed by a TRP-depleting amino acid drink in depressed patients in a double-blind, placebo-controlled, crossover fashion. Drug-free, symptomatic depressed patients did not worsen or improve on the day of the TRP depletion, but 35% of these patients demonstrated a clinically apparent but transient (24–48 hours) decrease in Hamilton Depression Scale (HDRS) score on return to normal TRP intake *the day after* the test (Delgado et al 1990a).

However, depressed patients who had achieved a clinical remission after 4–6 weeks of antidepressant treatment experienced a transient depressive relapse within 4 hours of the TRP depletion procedure with gradual (48–72 h) return to remitted state on return to normal TRP intake (Delgado et al 1990b).

Table 15.1 depicts the relationship of antidepressant type to depressive relapse in 38 remitted patients studied with the TRP depletion to date. While 13/14 patients responding to fluvoxamine, fluoxetine or a MAOI relapsed, only 2/11 patients responding to desipramine relapsed. The relapse rate during the non-TRP-depleting control drink is 0/38.

These data suggest that some antidepressant treatments (fluvoxamine, fluoxetine and MAOIs) may be dependent on CNS 5-HT availability for their therapeutic effects while other antidepressant treatments such as desipramine may be relatively less dependent on 5-HT availability. This data suggests that antidepressants may mediate their therapeutic effects through different mechanisms.

What is perhaps even more intriguing is that the drug-free depressed patients did not worsen during the TRP-depleted state, as predicted, but rather improved on the day following the test, a totally unexpected result. This implies that while enhancement of 5-HT function is necessary for maintaining an antidepressant response, the 5-HT system may be modulating some

other neurotransmitter system or brain region which is critically important in the pathophysiology of depression.

Table 15.1 Depressive relapse during tryptophan depletion in relation to antidepressant type

Antidepressant type	No. relapses/total no. patients tested	relapse (%)
Desipramine	2/11	18
Fluoxetine	2/2	100
Fluvoxamine	5/6	83
Monoamine oxidase inhibitors	6/6	100
Desipramine+lithium	1/3	33
Fluvoxamine+lithium	2/3	67
Fluoxetine+thioridazine	0/1	0
Amphetamine	1/1	100
Bupropion	0/2	0
Nortriptyline	1/2	50
Imipramine	1/1	100

Total: 22/38

Platelet 5-HT uptake

Platelet membranes contain secondary carrier systems for the uptake of 5-HT. This carrier system is saturable, energy, temperature and Na^+-dependent and is inhibited by ouabain and specific uptake inhibitors. The 5-HT transporter in platelets is thought to be similar to or identical with that found in the CNS (see Marcusson & Ross 1990 for review).

Most studies have found the uptake of radiolabelled 5-HT by platelets to be decreased in drug-free depressed patients compared to healthy controls (Pare et al 1974, Tuomisto 1974, Tuomisto et al 1979, Tuomisto & Tukiainen 1976, Coppen et al 1978, Rausch et al 1982, Ehsanullah 1980, Ross et al 1980, Meltzer et al 1981, Wood et al 1983, Goodnick & Meltzer 1984, Healy & Leonard 1987).

It remains controversial whether manic patients have normal (Meagher et al 1990) or decreased (Meltzer et al 1981) platelet 5-HT uptake. It is also unclear whether decreased platelet 5-HT uptake is a state or trait marker for depression.

Decreased platelet 5-HT uptake in depressed patients appears related to a decrease in the V_{max} as opposed to a decrease in the rate of uptake (K_m). This suggests that a noncompetitive type of inhibition is responsible. However, the decreased V_{max} may not be related to decreased number of uptake sites since there is no correlation between platelet 5-HT uptake and ^{3}H-imipramine labelling of the actual uptake sites in any patient group or in healthy subjects (Wood et al 1983, Meltzer & Lowy 1987). The finding seems unrelated to previous antidepressant treatment time, since antidepressant treatment with 5-HT reuptake inhibitors decreases platelet 5-HT uptake in a competitive fashion, decreasing the K_m without altering the V_{max} (Marsden et al 1987, Schlake et al 1989).

^{3}H-imipramine binding

The 5-HT uptake site on human platelets has undergone extensive investigation with several radioligands. ^{3}H-imipramine has been the most commonly utilized probe. Initial studies reported marked decreases in the number of 5-HT uptake sites labelled by ^{3}H-imipramine (Briley et al 1980). Since then considerable controversy has ensued, with numerous studies confirming this finding and many not. Two carefully designed recent studies involving large numbers of drug-free depressed patients and controls have failed to identify differences in platelet ^{3}H-imipramine binding between depressed patients (or diagnostic subtypes of depressed patients) and healthy subjects (Bech et al 1988, Theodorou et al 1989, Healy et al 1990). Given the large number of patients and the great deal of attention to methodological detail in the two most recent studies (Theodorou et al 1989, Healy et al 1990), it seems unlikely that abnormalities of platelet ^{3}H-imipramine binding exist in most depressed patients.

5-HT reuptake sites, as labelled by ^{3}H-imipramine, have been found to be reduced in the frontal cortex of suicide victims (Stanley et al 1982) and the hippocampus and occipital cortex of depressed patients (Perry et al 1983). However, serious questions about the methodology have been raised, confounding the interpretation of these postmortem studies (Marcusson & Ross 1990).

5-HT$_2$ receptor binding

5-HT$_2$ receptors are located on postsynaptic neurones innervated by 5-HT containing nerve terminals in the CNS as well as on blood platelet membranes. Another strategy utilized to assess the status of the 5-HT system has been the direct measurement of 5-HT$_2$ receptors in postmortem brains and peripheral tissues of depressed patients.

5-HT$_2$ receptor binding has been reported by most investigators to be increased in the brains of some depressed patients (McKeith et al 1987) and suicide victims (Stanley & Mann 1983, Mann et al 1986, Arora & Meltzer 1989a, Arango et al 1990) compared to brains of normals matched for age, sex and time to autopsy. However, not all investigators have found differences in 5-HT$_2$ receptor binding in the brains of depressed patients and suicide victims compared to non-depressed controls (Owen et al 1983, Cheetham et al 1988).

5-HT$_2$ receptors are also localized on whole human platelets (MacBride et al 1983, Geaney et al 1984). Platelet 5-HT$_2$ receptors have been reported to be increased in depressed patients (Biegon et al 1987, 1990b, Arora & Meltzer 1989b, Pandey et al 1990) and suicidal soldiers (Biegon et al 1990a) compared to healthy subjects. Further, the increased 5-HT$_2$ receptor binding was reported to return to normal levels after successful antidepressant treatment (Biegon et al 1987, 1990b). Interestingly, 5-HT$_2$ receptor binding normalized in 11 depressed patients who had a successful treatment response to maprotiline, while in four treatment nonresponders 5-HT$_2$ receptor binding did not change or increased further (Biegon et al 1990b). However, in a similar study assessing change in 5-HT$_2$ receptor binding following antidepressant treatment, Pandey et al found no normalization following successful treatment (treatment drug not specified) and no differences between responders and nonresponders (Pandey et al 1990).

As with brain 5-HT$_2$ receptor binding, not all investigators have detected differences in platelet 5-HT$_2$ receptor binding in depressed patients compared to nondepressed controls (Cowen et al 1987, MacBride et al 1987). However MacBride et al did detect an increase in 5-HT$_2$ receptors in those depressed patients who had made suicide attempts (MacBride et al 1987).

Neuroendocrine studies of 5-HT function

Neuroendocrine measures of CNS 5-HT function have been extensively utilized to assess the involvement of the 5-HT system in depression and antidepressant action. Increased 5-HT activity leads to an enhanced release of several hormones, including the pituitary hormones prolactin, adrenocorticotrophic hormone (ACTH) and growth hormone, as well as the peripherally released hormones cortisol and renin. Hormonal studies are also discussed in chapters 16 and 17, from the standpoint of specific neuroendocrine systems.

One of the most studied of the neuroendocrine measures has been the hormone response to the intravenous administration of the 5-HT precursor TRP. Intravenous TRP reliably enhances the release of prolactin and less reliably increases the release of growth hormone and ACTH in humans (Charney et al 1982a, Winokur et al 1986). The prolactin response to intravenous TRP is thought to be due to the stimulation of 5-HT_1 receptors by 5-HT, although the nature of the contribution from 5-HT_2 receptors remains controversial (Charig et al 1986, Idzikowski et al 1987, Heninger et al 1989, Price et al 1990).

The prolactin (Heninger et al 1984, Cowen & Charig 1987, Deakin et al 1990) and growth hormone (Cowen & Charig 1987, Deakin et al 1990) responses to intravenous TRP infusion are blunted in depressed patients when compared to healthy controls.

While cortisol responds poorly to TRP infusion when administered in the morning (Winokur et al 1986), afternoon infusion of TRP gives more consistent ACTH and cortisol responses and these responses are blunted in drug-free, euthymic bipolar patients when compared to healthy subjects, although no differences in prolactin or growth hormone have been observed (Nurnberger et al 1989b).

Another 5-HT precursor, 5-HTP, has also been studied in depression but the results are difficult to interpret because 5-HTP is metabolized into 5-HT both intraneuronally and extraneuronally and may act as a false transmitter in non-serotonergic neurones (Fuxe et al 1971, Ng et al 1972). Further, 5-HTP may have direct actions on cortisol release at the level of the adrenal gland (Van de Kar et al 1985).

5-HTP leads to an increase in plasma ACTH and cortisol but has no effect on prolactin (Meltzer et al 1984). This is in contrast to the neuroendocrine profile seen with most other 5-HT agonists, which cause the release of prolactin. The cortisol response to 5-HTP is increased in depressed patients compared to controls (Meltzer et al 1984).

Prolactin responses to the 5-HT releasing and 5-HT reuptake blocking drug fenfluramine have been found to be blunted in some depressed patients when compared to healthy subjects (Siever et al 1984b, Coccaro et al 1989), although these responses have been inconsistent and some studies have found no difference between healthy subjects and depressed patients (Asnis et al 1988, Weizman et al 1988). Mitchell & Smythe have recently reported that, while the peak increase in prolactin was decreased in endogenous depressed patients following fenfluramine, this apparent 'blunting' was accounted for by covarying for baseline levels both of prolactin and cortisol (Mitchell & Smythe 1990). The cortisol response to fenfluramine in depressed patients has been reported as no different (Asnis et al 1988, Mitchell & Smythe 1990) or reduced (Weizman et al 1988) when compared to controls.

Clomipramine is a highly potent and selective 5-HT reuptake inhibitor but is metabolized into a desmethylated metabolite which has significant effects on blocking the reuptake of NA. By using an intravenous infusion of clomipramine, investigators have hoped to diminish the metabolism into the desmethylated metabolite and thus increase the selectivity of this test towards the 5-HT system (Golden et al 1989). Intravenous infusion of clomipramine leads to an increased release of prolactin, growth hormone, ACTH and cortisol in healthy subjects (Golden et al 1989, 1990). The prolactin response to intravenous clomipramine is blunted and the growth hormone response is exaggerated in depressed patients compared to healthy subjects (Golden et al 1990).

Neuroendocrine responses to the non-selective postsynaptic 5-HT receptor agonist MCPP, a metabolite of the antidepressant trazodone, include an increase in the release of prolactin, cortisol and growth hormone in healthy humans (Mueller et al 1985, Charney et al 1987, Murphy et al 1989, Kahn et al 1990a). The prolactin response to MCPP is not different between depressed patients and healthy controls (Kahn et al 1990b, Price et al unpublished data), although depressed patients have an exaggerated physical symptom response compared to healthy subjects (Kahn et al 1990b).

Drugs belonging to the azaspirodecanedione family (buspirone, ipsapirone, gepirone and tandospirone) have recently been developed which demonstrate high partial agonist affinity for the 5-HT_{IA} receptor. These compounds are currently being investigated as possible antidepressants. The hormone responses to 5-HT agonists are thought to be related to partial agonist activity of these drugs on postsynaptic 5-HT_{IA} receptors and the hypothermic response is thought to be mediated through presynaptic 5-HT_{IA} activity (Cowen et al 1990, Lesch et al 1990a). Ipsapirone is the only drug in this class whose neuroendocrine profile has been studied in depressed patients. It causes a decrease in body temperature in healthy subjects and this response is blunted in depressed patients (Lesch et al 1990a).

In none of the above studies with indirect acting 5-HT agonists such as TRP, 5-HTP or fenfluramine, or

Table 15.2 Neuroendocrine abnormalities of the serotoninergic system in depressed patients compared with healthy subjects and effects of antidepressant treatments

Receptor subtype/location	Stimulus	Response	Type of abnormality in patients	Effect of ADT	Type of ADT
Presynaptic and postsynaptic 5-HT$_1$	Tryptophan	⇑Prolactin	Blunted response	Increase response	Desipramine Amitriptyline Fluvoxamine Clomipramine MAOI Lithium Carbamazepine
				No effect	Mianserin Bupropion Trazodone
	Fenfluramine	⇑Prolactin	Blunted response	Increase response	TCA ECT
Presynaptic 5-HT$_{1A}$	Ipsapirone	⇓Temperature	Blunted response	Further blunting	Amitriptyline
Postsynaptic 5-HT$_1$/5-HT$_2$	MCPP	⇑Prolactin	None	Not tested	
	5-HTP	⇑Cortisol	Increased response	Normalize Increase further	TCA MAOI

ADT: antidepressant treatment; MAOI: monoamine oxidase inhibitors;
TCA: tricyclic antidepressants; ECT: electroconvulsive therapy;
MCPP: m-clorophenylpiperazine; 5-HTP: 5-hydroxytryptophan

5-HT reuptake inhibitors such as intravenous clomipramine, or direct acting 5-HT agonists such as MCPP and ipsapirone, have there been any significant changes in mood in drug-free depressed patients. Table 15.2 summarizes the neuroendocrine abnormalities of 5-HT function reported in affective disorder patients.

Effects of antidepressant treatment on neuroendocrine measures of 5-HT function

Long-term treatment with the antidepressant drugs desipramine, amitriptyline, fluvoxamine, MAOIs, clomipramine, carbamazepine and lithium enhance the prolactin response to intravenous TRP infusion (Charney et al 1984a, Price et al 1985, 1989a,b, Anderson & Cowen 1986, Cowen 1988, Cowen et al 1989a, Elphick et al 1990), but the atypical antidepressants bupropion, mianserin and trazodone have no effect (Cowen et al 1989a, Price et al 1989b). However, in none of the above studies is the degree of enhancement of the prolactin response correlated with treatment outcome.

The increased cortisol response to 5-HTP is attenuated after tricyclic antidepressant treatment (nortripty-line, imipramine, desipramine) but increased further by lithium when compared to the drug-free state (Meltzer & Lowy 1987).

The prolactin response to fenfluramine is enhanced after chronic antidepressant treatment with lithium (Muhlbauer 1984, Muhlbauer & Muller-Oerlinghausen 1985) and imipramine (Shapira et al 1989, 1990). These data are similar to those obtained for the enhanced prolactin response to TRP infusion (Price et al 1990). Further, the prolactin response to fenfluramine has been reported to be enhanced after electroconvulsive treatment (Shapira et al 1990).

In healthy subjects the prolactin response to intravenous clomipramine is enhanced after 3–4 days of lithium treatment, while the cortisol response is unchanged (McCance et al 1989).

Chronic treatment with amitriptyline further impaired the ipsapirone-mediated hypothermic response in depressed patients (Lesch et al 1990b). These findings suggest that depressed patients may have abnormalities of presynaptic 5-HT$_{1A}$ receptor function or of presynaptic 5-HT function apart from the sensitivity of 5-HT$_{1A}$ receptors. This could involve mechanisms regulating cell firing, transmitter release or synthesis. The effects of chronic antidepressant treatment on the temperature response are consistent with the preclinical studies suggesting that 5-HT$_{1A}$ agonists decrease presynaptic 5-HT$_{1A}$ receptor sensitivity in laboratory animals (Blier et al 1990a,b).

5-HT function in affective disorders

An impressive amount of data suggests that presynaptic 5-HT dysfunction may be present in some depressed patients and that most antidepressant medications enhance 5-HT function. This data is summarized in Tables 15.2 and 15.3. The data suggesting that some drug-free depressed patients have impaired presynaptic 5-HT dysfunction includes the findings of lower plasma TRP levels, reduced CSF 5-HIAA, decreased platelet 5-HT uptake, a blunted prolactin response to TRP and fenfluramine, as well as the preliminary report of a blunted hypothermic response to the 5-HT$_{1A}$ partial agonist ipsapirone. That the blunted prolactin response to TRP and fenfluramine is due to presynaptic dysfunction is suggested by the normal prolactin response to the postsynaptic 5-HT agonist MCPP.

Table 15.3 Abnormalities of 5-HT function in affective disorder patients which have been replicated in independent studies.

Decreased plasma tryptophan

Decreased CSF 5-HIAA

Decreased platelet 5-HT uptake

Increased 5-HT$_2$ receptor binding in:
— platelets
— cortex of suicides

Decreased ^{3}H-imipramine binding in:
— platelets (two large recent non-replications)
— frontal cortex and hippocampus

Decreased prolactin response to:
— intravenous tryptophan
— oral fenfluramine

Decreased hypothermic response to ipsapirone

Depressive relapse after rapid tryptophan depletion in antidepressant-treated depressed patients

It was unexpected to find that lowering 5-HT content through plasma TRP depletion does not seem to worsen a depressed state in drug-free depressed patients. This suggests that, if presynaptic 5-HT dysfunction is present in some depressed patients, either 5-HT function is already inhibited or decreased

5-HT function only predisposes to the state of depression but does not directly cause it.

That a diminished level of 5-HT function is not the immediate cause of the depressed state is suggested by the absence of clear-cut depressive symptoms in carcinoid patients treated with PCPA and the lack of immediate antidepressant response in drug-free depressed patients during testing with intravenous TRP and 5-HTP, or oral fenfluramine and postsynaptic 5-HT agonists. Even massive increases in 5-HT release, as caused by the combination of TRP and a MAOI, do not rapidly alleviate depression, rather the acute response (as is often the case with fenfluramine and potent 5-HT reuptake inhibitors) is nausea and clonic movements (Price et al 1985). Further, decreased CSF levels of 5-HIAA seem more related to impulsivity and aggression than to depression.

On the other hand, considerable data suggests that enhancement of 5-HT neurotransmission may be one mechanism of antidepressant action. The enhanced prolactin response to TRP and fenfluramine in depressed patients after antidepressant treatment suggests this. Further, interfering with 5-HT function by lowering 5-HT content through TRP depletion or synthesis inhibition with PCPA transiently reverses antidepressant response.

The above data suggest that enhanced synaptic transmission through the 5-HT system may initiate a series of events which lead to an antidepressant response in some patients and that interfering with 5-HT synthesis once the antidepressant response has commenced will rapidly reverse the antidepressant response. However, the fact that drugs which rapidly increase 5-HT transmission do not lead to even a transient mood improvement acutely would suggest that while enhanced 5-HT neurotransmission may set into motion a series of events which results in an antidepressant response, the functional activity of the 5-HT system is not directly causing the depressed mood or reversing the depressed mood, but rather influencing some other system or brain area which is.

THE NORADRENALINE (NA) SYSTEM

Most NA cell bodies originate from the locus ceruleus in the dorsal pons (Redmond 1987). These cell bodies project to most brain regions and, like 5-HT neurones, seem to exert a modulatory effect on their target site. Not all NA-containing nerve terminals in the cortex make synaptic contact with the local cortical neurones; rather, some of these neurones release NA in a manner similar to that through which hormones are secreted, and thus have generalized effects on other CNS regions (Woodward et al 1979). Locus ceruleus neurones are not uniform and demonstrate a laminar distribution and at least four distinct cell types (Chan-Palay & Asan 1989). There is a natural loss of locus ceruleus neurones with aging, and recent morphological studies suggest that this loss of cell bodies can range from 30–40%. In a recent morphological study of locus ceruleus neuronal loss with aging it was noted that the subject with the greatest loss (55%) was a woman with a history of chronic depression without dementia (Chan-Palay & Asan 1989).

The locus ceruleus is exquisitely sensitive to novel stimuli. It appears to modulate levels of arousal and has been postulated to be involved in opiate and alcohol withdrawal states, anxiety disorders and depression (Charney & Redmond 1983, Redmond 1987). Locus ceruleus neurones receive inputs from many different neurotransmitter systems and the firing rate and sensitivity to other incoming stimuli is regulated by these other neurotransmitter systems. These modulating systems include inhibitory input from the 5-HT, opioid, gamma-amino-butyric-acid (GABA), dopamine DA and glycine systems and excitatory input from the corticotrophin releasing hormone (CRH), methylxanthine, glutamate, substance P and muscarinic cholinergic systems (Redmond 1987, Charney et al 1990 for review). Another regulatory mechanism is through an inhibitory presynaptic alpha$_2$ adrenoreceptor which, when stimulated, decreases the firing rate of locus ceruleus neurones.

Traditionally, adrenergic receptors have been classified as being either of the alpha- or beta-adrenergic subtype and each of these subtypes has two secondary subtypes (alpha$_1$, alpha$_2$, beta$_1$, beta$_2$). Recent pharmacological, radioligand binding and molecular biology data suggest that a new classification scheme is in order (Bylund 1988). This new classification divides adrenergic receptors into three groups based on the G-protein coupling utilized by that receptor. The three groups are the beta-adrenergic subtype (G$_s$ coupled; beta$_1$, beta$_2$), the alpha$_2$-adrenergic subtype (Gi coupled; alpha$_{2a}$, alpha$_{2b}$, alpha$_{2c}$), and the alpha$_1$-adrenergic subtype (Gx coupled; alpha$_{1a}$, alpha$_{1b}$) (Bylund 1988). Most clinical studies to date have not assessed the results of their studies in this new light.

Abnormalities of NA function have long been suspected in affective disorders (Schildkraut 1965, Bunney & Davis 1965). The NA deficiency hypothesis of depression was based on the observation that the catecholamine-depleting drug reserpine caused symptoms similar to depression in some individuals, and MAOIs and tricyclic antidepressants led to an enhanced synaptic availability of NA. As new knowledge regarding the processes regulating neurotransmitter synthesis, release and receptor activation have emerged, the original catecholamine deficiency hypothesis has been replaced by the previously described receptor sensitivity (Charney et al 1981b) and dysregulation (Siever & Davis 1985) hypotheses.

Preclinical studies of the NA system

Most of the evidence for an involvement of the NA system in depression comes from investigations of the mechanism of action of antidepressant drugs. The most significant finding from this type of study is the ability of numerous antidepressant treatments to decrease the density of the beta-adrenergic receptor. Long-term treatment with tricyclic antidepressants, MAOIs, trazodone, iprindole and ECT, but not selective 5-HT reuptake inhibitors, bupropion, mianserin and nomifensine decreases beta-adrenoreceptor binding in laboratory animals (Heninger et al 1990). Increases in alpha$_1$-adrenoreceptor binding have also been reported for many antidepressants and decreases in alpha$_2$-adrenoreceptor binding have been reported for some antidepressants, but these findings have been much less consistent than for beta-adrenoreceptors (see Charney et al 1981b, Heninger & Charney 1987, for review).

Electrophysiological studies in laboratory animals find that MAOIs produce an immediate decrease in the firing rate of the locus ceruleus and this decrease persists with long-term treatment (Blier et al 1986). This suggests that the changes in locus ceruleus firing rate are not sufficient for an antidepressant response to MAOIs.

Clinical studies of NA function

NA metabolites

The relationship of NA and metabolites of NA in plasma, CSF and urine has received a great deal of attention and numerous reviews have been written (Zis & Goodwin 1982, Siever 1987, Kindler & Lerer 1990). The literature on this topic is extensive and numerous contradictory reports have been published.

Overall, CSF, plasma and urine measurements of NA and its primary metabolite, MHPG, in unipolar and bipolar affective disorder patients have revealed no convincing patterns or differences from healthy subjects. It is possible that patients with affective disorders may have an increased variability in plasma NA and MHPG compared to other groups (Siever et al 1986, Siever 1987).

NA depletion

The synthesis of NA and DA can be reduced by administration of the tryrosine hydroxylase inhibitor, alpha-methyl-para-tyrosine (AMPT). AMPT has been studied in a variety of non-psychiatric disorders and in general causes sedation, anxiety, tremor, diarrhoea, galactorrhoea and rebound insomnia after drug discontinuation (Engelman et al 1968). Even after administration over several months AMPT does not seem to cause depressive symptoms (Engelman et al 1968). AMPT has been reported in open trials to decrease craving for opiates and amphetamines (Pozuelo 1976), decrease tic movements in Tourette's syndrome (Sweet et al 1974), reduce oral tardive dyskinesia (Gerlach & Thorsen 1976) and potentiate antipsychotic efficacy in schizophrenia (Carlsson et al 1972).

AMPT may have more behavioural effects in individuals with affective disorders than in other persons. In an open treatment trial of AMPT in patients with essential hypertension, six of 20 hypertensive patients had a history of a previous depressive episode. Three of these six became agitated on AMPT, requiring drug discontinuation (Engelman et al 1968). In a double-blind trial, AMPT reduced manic symptoms in five of seven bipolar patients in the manic phase but two had an increase in manic symptoms (Brodie et al 1970, Bunney et al 1971). In the same study, three of four psychotically depressed patients became more depressed after AMPT treatment (Brodie et al 1970, Bunney et al 1971). In three depressed patients having had a therapeutic response to imipramine, AMPT had no significant effect on the antidepressant response (Shopsin et al 1975).

Another method of NA depletion is with the dopamine-beta-hydroxylase (DBH) inhibitor fusaric acid. Fusaric acid has been administered to hypertensive subjects with no reports of any significant CNS effects (Suda et al 1969). Fusaric acid administered to manic patients, in doses which could reduce plasma DBH activity by >90% and significantly lower CSF MHPG, did not reduce manic symptoms but increased psychosis ratings in bipolar manic patients (Sack & Goodwin 1974). Fusaric acid has been reported to decrease craving and psychological withdrawal in an open trial in amphetamine abusers (Pozuelo 1976). Fusaric acid has not been studied in depression.

NA receptor binding and function

The awareness that many antidepressants had significant effects on adrenergic receptor sensitivity in laboratory animals prompted investigation of these receptors in humans. Peripheral alpha$_2$- and beta-adrenergic receptors are present on blood cells and have been studied in patients with affective disorders.

Peripheral alpha$_2$-adrenergic receptors located on blood platelets have been extensively investigated with a variety of radiolabelled alpha$_2$-adrenergic receptor agonist and antagonist probes. This literature has recently been reviewed (Piletz et al 1986, Katona et al 1987).

Platelet alpha$_2$-adrenergic receptor number as measured by ^{3}H-clonidine (Garcia-Sevilla et al 1981), ^{3}H-dihydroergocryptine (Siever et al 1984a), ^{3}H-adrenaline (Garcia-Sevilla et al 1987), ^{3}H-para-aminoclonidine (Piletz et al 1990) have been reported to be increased compared to healthy subjects. However, other studies utilizing ^{3}H-clonidine (Georgotas et al 1987), ^{3}H-dihydroergocryptine (Wood & Coppen 1982), ^{3}H-yohimbine and ^{3}H-rauwolscine (Siever 1987) have revealed no significant difference between healthy subjects and depressed patients.

It has recently been argued that abnormalities of platelet alpha$_2$-adrenergic receptors involve an increase in the high affinity agonist state of the receptor and only drugs which are likely to label this high affinity state will demonstrate the abnormality (Garcia-Sevilla et al 1986, 1990, Piletz et al 1990). It is postulated that this explains the reasons for the lack of uniform difference in alpha$_2$-adrenergic receptor number between depressed patients and healthy subjects as measured by ^{3}H-yohimbine and other related alkaloids, compared to the more positive results reported for agonists (Garcia-Sevilla et al 1986).

Studies of peripheral alpha$_2$-adrenergic receptor responsiveness have been used to assess the above conflicting results in receptor number. However, these studies have also been contradictory, with some studies noting no difference between patients and controls and other studies noting a blunted cyclic adenosine monophosphate (cAMP) response (see Siever 1987, Kindler & Lerer 1990 for reviews).

In a recent attempt to further elucidate the relationship of platelet alpha$_2$-adrenergic receptor number to physiological responsiveness, Garcia-Sevilla et al

(1990) have investigated the alpha$_2$-adrenergic receptor-mediated inhibition of platelet adenylate cyclase and induction of platelet aggregation. They found evidence of hypersensitive responses to alpha$_2$-adrenergic receptor agonists in drug-free depressed patients which were desensitized following long-term antidepressant treatment (Garcia-Sevilla et al 1990).

There is one report of increased cortical ^{3}H-clonidine binding in the brains of suicide victims compared to sudden death controls (Meana & Garcia-Sevilla 1987).

Beta-adrenergic receptors are present on blood lymphocytes. Measurement of these receptors has also yielded mixed results, with some authors reporting decreased numbers (Extein et al 1979) and others reporting no difference (Cooper et al 1985, Mann et al 1985) between depressed patients and healthy subjects. On the other hand, the cyclic adenosine monophosphate (cAMP) response to stimulation of beta-adrenergic receptors by beta-adrenergic agonists has led to consistent reports of a blunted response in depressed patients when compared to healthy subjects (Extein et al 1979, Pandey et al 1979, 1985, Mann et al 1985, Ebstein et al 1988). Interestingly, there is a dissociation between plasma NA levels and the affinity of agonists for the beta-adrenergic receptor in depressed patients (Buckholtz et al 1988), in contrast to the normal association between agonist affinity and plasma NA levels seen in non-depressed populations (Feldman et al 1983).

Beta-adrenergic receptors have also been studied in the human CNS. The anatomic distribution of beta-adrenergic receptors has been determined in the human brain through homogenate binding and autoradiographic techniques (Enna et al 1977, Pazos et al 1982). Several studies have examined these receptors in the postmortem brains of depressed patients and individuals who have committed suicide. The results from these studies have been mixed, with some investigators reporting no difference from controls in beta-adrenergic receptor density (Crow et al 1984, Meyerson et al 1982). More recent studies utilizing 'drug- and pathology-free' brains and investigating the regional distribution of beta-adrenergic receptors have consistently identified increased beta-adrenergic receptor density in the brains of suicides (Mann et al 1986, Biegon & Israeli 1988, Arango et al 1990).

Table 15.4 Neuroendocrine abnormalities of the noradrenergic system in depressed patients and effects of antidepressant treatments

Receptor subtype/location	Stimulus	Response	Type of abnormality in patients	Effect of ADT	Type of ADT
Postsynaptic alpha$_2$-adrenergic	Clonidine	⇑Growth hormone	Blunted response	None	Desipramine Amitriptyline Mianserin Trazodone MAOI
	Guanfacine	⇑Growth hormone	None	Not tested	
	Desipramine	⇑Growth hormone	Blunted response	Not tested	
Postsynaptic alpha$_1$-adrenergic	Amphetamine	⇑Cortisol	Blunted response	None	TCA ECT
Postsynaptic beta-adrenergic	Diurnal Variation	⇑Melatonin	Blunted response	Increase response	Desipramine MAOI
	Artificial Light	⇓Melatonin	Blunted	Not tested	
Presynaptic alpha$_2$-adrenergic	Desipramine	⇑MHPG	None	Not tested	
	Yohimbine	⇑MHPG	None	Not tested	

ADT: antidepressant treatment; MAOI: monoamine oxidase inhibitors;
TCA: tricyclic antidepressants; ECT: electroconvulsive therapy;
MHPG: 3-methoxy-4-hydroxy-phenethylglycol

Neuroendocrine studies of NA function

The vast majority of neuroendocrine challenge studies of the NA system in depression have involved investigations of alpha$_2$-adrenergic receptor responsiveness. The neuroendocrine abnormalities of the NA system are summarized in Table 15.4. Both presynaptic and postsynaptic alpha$_2$-adrenergic receptors are present in the CNS. Stimulation of postsynaptic alpha$_2$-adrenergic receptors causes an increased release of growth hormone (Lal et al 1975). The release of growth hormone by alpha$_2$-adrenergic receptor agonists is thought to be mediated by the activation of postsynaptic alpha$_2$-adrenergic receptors within the hypothalamus exerting a stimulatory effect on the secretion of growth hormone releasing hormone (GHRH; Frohman & Jansson 1986). However, factors other than adrenergic receptor activation exert an effect on the growth hormone response to clonidine such that depletion of both 5-HT and NA leads to a weaker growth hormone response to clonidine than depletion of NA alone in rats (Soderpalm et al 1987).

Stimulation of presynaptic alpha$_2$-adrenergic receptors causes a decrease in the firing rate of the locus ceruleus and a decrease in sympathetic outflow (Leckman et al 1981). The decrease in sympathetic outflow through the inhibition of the locus ceruleus firing rate is thought to be significantly reflected by a decrease in plasma levels of the primary metabolite of NA, MHPG (Leckman et al 1981).

Clonidine, an alpha$_2$-adrenergic receptor agonist, causes an increase in the secretion of growth hormone, feelings of sedation, a decrease in the secretion of MHPG and a decrease in blood pressure in humans (Lal et al 1975, Matussek et al 1980). In an impressive number of replication studies, the growth hormone response to both oral and intravenous clonidine has consistently been found to be blunted in depressed patients compared to healthy controls (Matussek et al 1980, Checkley et al 1981, 1984, Siever et al 1982a, Charney et al 1982b, Boyer et al 1982, Ansseau et al 1984, 1988) (see also ch. 16). However, studies with low-dose oral clonidine (Katona et al 1986) and low-dose intravenous clonidine (Dolan & Calloway 1986) have not found a difference in the growth hormone response between patients and controls. The blood pressure and MHPG changes have been more variable with most studies failing to find significant differences (Heninger et al 1990).

Another slightly more selective alpha$_2$-adrenergic receptor agonist, guanfacine, causes an increase in the secretion of growth hormone which is not different in depressed patients compared to healthy controls (Eriksson et al 1988). The reasons for the inconsistency between the growth hormone response to clonidine and guanfacine is not clear, although clonidine, as a partial agonist, may be more likely to uncover a functional defect in alpha$_2$-adrenergic receptor responsiveness than the full agonist, guafacine (Eriksson et al 1988). Further, issues of endogenous versus non-endogenous subtype, dose and other alpha$_2$-adrenergic receptor subtypes may also be responsible.

Considerable variability in the amount of growth hormone released in response to clonidine exists across both patients and healthy subjects. In an attempt to investigate the underlying reasons for this variability, Eriksson et al measured the growth hormone response to guanfacine as well as to GHRH in the same subjects. If the mechanisms underlying the variability were related to differences in alpha$_2$-adrenoreceptor sensitivity, then the growth hormone response to guanfacine should be different to the response to GHRH. They found a significant correlation between the growth hormone responses to these two agents, suggesting that the variability of the growth hormone response might be due to factors other than alpha$_2$-adrenergic receptor responsiveness (Eriksson et al 1988).

Yohimbine, an alpha$_2$-adrenergic receptor antagonist, increases the firing rate of the locus ceruleus, with a resultant increase in sympathetic outflow (Redmond 1987). Oral and intravenous yohimbine increases MHPG and blood pressure in healthy human subjects (Charney et al 1982d, Goldberg et al 1986). Depressed patients demonstrate an increased cortisol and blood pressure response to intravenous yohimbine compared to healthy subjects, while the plasma MHPG is not significantly different between the two groups of subjects (Heninger et al 1988).

Amphetamine causes release and blocks reuptake of both NA and DA. It has been used as a neuroendocrine challenge probe of both the NA and DA systems, with growth hormone and cortisol used to assess the response. The growth hormone response is thought to be due to DA stimulation of DA$_2$ receptors and NA stimulation of postsynaptic alpha$_2$-adrenergic receptors. The cortisol response is thought to be mediated by NA stimulation of postsynaptic alpha$_1$-adrenergic receptors.

Neuroendocrine challenge studies with amphetamine have reported a blunted growth hormone response in depressed patients compared to healthy subjects (Langer et al 1975, 1976, Arato et al 1983). The blunted growth hormone response was seen only in endogenously depressed patients (Langer et al 1975, 1976). However, questions regarding the interpretations of the blunted growth hormone response have been raised because of the 'normal' blunting of this response after the menopause and the presence of more postmenopausal women in the patient groups than in the control groups in most studies (Matussek 1988). Studies investigating the growth hormone response to amphetamine in postmenopausal endogenous depressed patients (and two male endogenous depressive patients) and matched controls have reported no difference in this hormone response (Halbreich et al 1982).

Nurnberger et al (1982) have studied the neuroendocrine effects of amphetamine in 'well state' bipolar twins and matched healthy twins in an effort to distinguish state and trait variables in the neuroendocrine, biochemical, physiological and behavioural responses to amphetamine. While there were no patient/control differences in any of the measures, the behavioural 'excitation' and pre-treatment levels of plasma MHPG, prolactin and growth hormone were significantly correlated between the twins, although plasma amphetamine level, cortisol and blood pressure and heart rate were discordant.

The cortisol response to methylamphetamine in depressed patients before and after recovery was reported to be lower in the depressive phase compared to the recovered phase (Checkley & Crammer 1977). Attempts to identify diagnostic subtypes of depression using this measure appear to support the distinction between endogenous and non-endogenous forms of depression. When compared to reactive depressive and other non-depressed psychiatric patients, the cortisol response to methylamphetamine was blunted only in endogenous depressives (Checkley 1979). In a larger replication using dextroamphetamine, the cortisol response to this NA and DA releasing agent was also found to be diminished in endogenously depressed patients compared to healthy controls (Sachar et al 1980, 1985). However when the cortisol response to dextroamphetamine was assessed at 8 a.m. rather than the 4 p.m. time used in the previous studies (Checkley & Crammer 1977, Checkley 1979, Sachar et al 1980, 1985), no difference was noted between depressed patients and healthy subjects (Feinberg et al 1981).

Desipramine is a tricyclic antidepressant which is relatively selective as a NA reuptake inhibitor, but with significant anticholinergic and antihistaminic effects as well. Single oral doses of desipramine cause a dose-dependent increase in growth hormone, cortisol (Laakmann et al 1977, 1986) and MHPG (Charney et al 1981a). The growth hormone response to desipramine is blocked by the non-selective alpha-adrenergic antagonist phentolamine and the alpha$_2$-adrenergic antagonist yohimbine and potentiated by the non-selective beta-adrenergic antagonist propranolol, while the selective alpha$_1$-adrenergic antagonist prazosin has no effect, suggesting that at least the growth hormone response to desipramine is mediated by stimulation of postsynaptic alpha$_2$-adrenergic receptors (Laakmann et al 1977).

The growth hormone response to desipramine has been reported to be blunted in pre-menopausal female endogenous depressives (Meesters et al 1985) and male endogenous depressives (Laakmann et al 1986) compared to healthy subjects. The cortisol response to desipramine has also been reported to be blunted in endogenous depressed patients (Asnis et al 1986).

Nocturnal melatonin secretion is mediated by direct stimulation of beta-adrenergic receptors by NA released from NA neurones (Brownstein & Axelrod 1974). In humans, treatment with the beta-adrenergic receptor antagonist propranolol blocks night time melatonin secretion (Hanssen et al 1977). Environmental light treatment also decreases nocturnal melatonin secretion (Lewy et al 1980) and this is thought to be due to a decrease in NA neurotransmission induced by bright light (Brownstein & Axelrod 1974, Frazer et al 1986).

The night time increase in melatonin secretion is blunted in depressed patients compared to healthy subjects (Wetterberg 1983, Frazer et al 1986).

Effects of antidepressant treatment on neuroendocrine measures of NA function

Long-term antidepressant treatment with desipramine, amitriptyline, clorgyline, trazodone or mianserin (Charney et al 1981c, 1982c, Charney & Redmond 1983, 1984b, Siever et al 1982b, Price et al 1986) has no effect on the growth hormone response to clonidine. Short-term treatment with lithium tends to normalize a blunted growth hormone response to clonidine in both depressives and controls while causing a blunted response in those healthy controls who had normal responses prior to lithium (Brambilla et al 1988).

Long-term treatment with desipramine and amitriptyline (Charney et al 1981a, 1981b, 1981c, 1982c) but not trazodone or mianserin (Charney et al 1984b, Price et al 1986) blocks the decrease in plasma

MHPG and blood pressure caused by clonidine. This effect is thought to be due to antidepressant-induced decreased presynaptic alpha$_2$-adrenergic receptor sensitivity.

The cortisol response to methylamphetamine or dextroamphetamine is not affected by tricyclic antidepressant treatment or electroconvulsive therapy (Checkley 1979, Sachar et al 1980).

Treatment with desipramine (Cowen et al 1985) clorgyline and tranylcypromine (Murphy et al 1986) elevate plasma melatonin levels, presumably by increasing NA neurotransmission. However, this is unexpected, since chronic antidepressant treatment decreases beta-adrenergic receptor function (Heninger et al 1990). It is interesting to note that one week of desipramine treatment in healthy subjects increases melatonin secretion but after 3 weeks of treatment this response returns to pretreatment levels (Cowen et al 1985).

NA function in affective disorders

Studies of NA function in affective disorder patients have suggested that postsynaptic abnormalities may be present in some depressed patients. Tables 15.4 and 15.5 summarize this data. Measures of postsynaptic NA activity suggest that there is a functional blunting of the responsiveness of hypothalamic alpha$_1$- and alpha$_2$-adrenergic receptors and lymphocyte beta-adrenergic receptors. While abnormalities have been identified in drug-free depressed patients, most antidepressant treatments have not consistently modified measures of NA function. However, CNS beta-adrenergic receptors have not been studied.

Table 15.5 Abnormalities of NA function in affective disorder patients which have been replicated in independent studies

Increased α_2-adrenergic receptor binding in platelets

Decreased cAMP response to beta-adrenergic receptor agonists in platelets

Increased β-adrenergic receptors in brains of suicide victims

Decreased growth hormone response to clonidine, amphetamine and desipramine

Decreased cortisol response to methylamphetamine

Decreased nighttime melatonin secretion

Presynaptic dysregulation of the NA system has not been identified. The lack of difference in the CSF, plasma and urinary measures of NA function, as well as the lack of difference in the MHPG, blood pressure and sedative responses to desipramine between healthy subjects and depressed patients, suggests relatively normal presynaptic NA activity. The failure to identify a difference between healthy subjects and depressed patients in the behavioural response to yohimbine adds further support to this conclusion.

The most consistent finding in regard to possible postsynaptic adrenergic dysfunction is the blunted growth hormone response to clonidine in drug-free depressed patients. The blunted growth hormone response to desipramine further supports the idea of a postsynaptic alpha$_2$-adrenergic defect. Moreover, the failure to identify significant patient/control differences in the growth hormone response to the DA agonist apomorphine suggests that this abnormality may be specific to the NA system and not related to abnormalities in GNRH regulation of growth hormone. Likewise, since the growth hormone response to amphetamine is most likely to be mediated via the stimulation of postsynaptic DA as well as alpha$_2$-adrenergic receptors, it is not surprising to see no patient/control difference using this probe. Still unexplained is the failure to identify differences between depressed patients and healthy subjects using the more selective alpha$_2$-adrenergic agonist guanfacine. This finding needs replication.

Confusing this issue are the contradictory results obtained in studies of platelet alpha$_2$-adrenergic receptors. These studies suggest that some depressed patients have hypersensitive platelet alpha$_2$-adrenergic receptors. This is in sharp contrast with the blunted growth hormone response to clonidine in depressed patients. However, platelet alpha$_2$-adrenergic receptors may well be regulated differently from those in the CNS.

Another postsynaptic abnormality is the blunted cortisol response to amphetamine and desipramine. The cortisol response to NA agonists is thought to reflect activation of postsynaptic alpha$_1$-adrenergic receptors. The blunting of this response is presumably mediated through hypothalamic corticotropin releasing hormone (CRH) secretion, although direct effects on the adrenal gland have not been excluded. However, no relationship between the cortisol response to either desipramine or amphetamine and to dexamethasone non-suppression has been found.

Assessment of postsynaptic beta-adrenergic receptor function in peripheral lymphocytes suggests that an abnormality may exist beyond the receptor level. The blunted nocturnal melatonin surge in depressed patients and the fact that depressed patients maintain an enhanced night time melatonin surge after long-term desipramine treatment while healthy subjects demonstrate a return to baseline melatonin levels after long-term desipramine treatment suggests possible differences in beta-adrenergic receptor regulation between healthy subjects and depressed patients.

Wachtel (1989) has recently postulated that a dysregulation of neuronal second messenger function is involved in the aetiology of affective disorders. This hypothesis suggests that in depression there is an imbalance of the major second messenger systems in the CNS resulting from diminished adenylate cyclase pathway activity and increased phospholipase C pathway activity, and in mania the reverse (Wachtel 1989). This hypothesis is primarily based on the observed dysfunction of lymphocyte beta-adrenergic receptor function.

A considerable amount of neurochemical data does not fully support a second messenger imbalance hypothesis (e.g. normal growth hormone responses to guanfacine, no abnormality in platelet alpha$_2$-adrenergic receptor activity, lack of widespread dysfunction in all neurotransmitter systems utilizing the same second messenger). However, the observation that most of the identified abnormalities reported for the NA system are postsynaptic would suggest that an abnormality of some aspect of postsynaptic adrenergic receptor coupling to G-proteins or second or third messenger systems may be involved.

Overall it appears that postsynaptic abnormalities in alpha$_1$-and alpha$_2$-adrenergic receptor function may exist in some depressed patients but antidepressant treatments do not have consistent effects on neurochemical measures of NA function. Further, treatment with the tyrosine hydroxylase inhibitor AMPT did not reverse antidepressant response to imipramine in a small number of patients and AMPT does not lead to depressive symptoms in non-psychiatric patients (Carpenter 1970, Shopsin et al 1975). These data suggest that the NA system may be involved in depression, but that changes in NA activity are not a common mechanism of action of antidepressant treatments. However, it is not possible to exclude the possibility that specific antidepressant medications may in part or in whole mediate their therapeutic effects by altering NA activity.

THE CHOLINERGIC SYSTEM

Acetylcholine (ACh) was the first neurotransmitter to be identified. Even so, research on the behavioural aspects of the CNS cholinergic systems has lagged behind our understanding of the behavioural aspects of the NA, 5-HT and DA systems. This appears to have been due primarily to the extensive involvement of the cholinergic mechanisms in the regulation of the parasympathetic nervous system and in the regulation of voluntary movement, which made difficult and tended to obscure research on the behavioural effects of ACh (Bartus et al 1987).

New evidence suggests that, like other neurotransmitter receptor systems, multiple subtypes of the muscarinic cholinergic receptors may exist. At least two subtypes of muscarinic cholinergic receptor designated as M_1 and M_2, with each utilizing a different G-protein second messenger system, have been identified (Avissar & Schreiber 1989). Up to five subtypes of the human muscarinic receptor (M_1, M_2, M_3, M_4, M_5) have now been cloned (Bonner et al 1987). While stimulation of the M_1, M_3 and M_5 receptors caused an increase in phosphoinositol turnover, stimulation of the M_2 subtype did not, suggesting that the M_2 receptor may be associated with another second messenger system (Pepitoni et al 1990). Selective agonists and antagonists for these receptors have only recently been developed and studied.

The cholinergic hypothesis of depression and mania (Janowski et al 1972) was postulated in the context of data which documented significant anticholinergic properties of most antidepressant drugs and of the mood-altering properties of cholinomimetics and anticholinergics in both healthy subjects and affective disorder patients (see Janowski & Risch 1987, Dilsaver & Coffman 1989 for reviews). The cholinergic hypothesis states that excess cholinergic activity is involved in depression and that mania is due to an imbalance between the NA (increased) and cholinergic (decreased) systems (Janowski et al 1972).

Clinical studies of cholinergic function

Some cholinomimetic drugs appear to cause behavioural depression in healthy humans (E1-Yousef et al 1973), unlike the modest behavioural effects of DA, NA and 5-HT agonists. Organophosphate insecticides (Gershon & Shaw 1961) and physostigmine (Janowski et al 1982), both drugs which greatly enhance CNS cholinergic activity by interfering with the enzyme acetylcholinesterase, lead to behavioural depression in some healthy humans and patients with affective disorders. The non-selective muscarinic cholinergic agonist arecoline exacerbates depressive symptoms in depressed patients (Nurnberger et al 1983, Risch et al 1982). However, the orally-administered M_1 agonist RS-86 did not induce depressive symptoms in healthy subjects, drug-free depressed patients or drug-free remitted affective disorder patients (Berger et al 1989). Furthermore, although early reports of RS-86 rapidly reducing manic symptoms were promising (Berger et al 1986), a subsequent negative report (van Berkestijn et al 1990) casts doubt on the antimanic effects of this drug. Other reports of other cholinomimetic drugs having antimanic properties have been criticized because of the non-specific anergic state induced by some cholinomimetics (Carroll et al 1973).

Some anticholinergic drugs have been abused. Along with euphoria, some of these drugs cause psychedelic-like effects (Lawry 1977, Wilcox 1983). Qualitatively however, the euphoria-producing effects of anticholinergics (Bolin 1960) do not appear as closely related to mania as are the euphoria-producing effects of the NA and DA releasers cocaine and amphetamine.

Cholinomimetic drugs elevate adrenocorticotrophic hormone (ACTH), cortisol and beta-endorphin secretion in humans (Janowski & Risch 1987). Physostigmine infusions cause increases in ACTH, cortisol and beta-endorphin (Risch et al 1982). Physostigmine reverses the normal suppression of cortisol by dexamethasone in healthy subjects (Carroll et al 1980, Doerr & Berger 1983). Furthermore, depressed patients demonstrate an enhanced release of ACTH and beta-endorphin in response to physostigmine compared to healthy subjects (Risch 1982).

A strategy utilized to assess the cholinergic system in affective disorder patients has been the use of cholinergic agonists to induce rapid eye movement (REM) sleep. CNS cholinergic activity is increased during REM sleep (Hobson et al 1986). Cholinergic agonists such as physostigmine and arecoline, when infused 20 minutes following the termination of the first REM period, shorten the time to the onset of the next REM period in humans (Sitaram et al 1976, Sitaram et al 1980).

The induction of REM sleep by cholinomimetics is more rapid in unipolar and bipolar depressed patients compared to healthy subjects (Sitaram et al 1980, Sitaram & Gillin 1980, Nurnberger et al 1989a, Berger et al 1989). Shortened REM induction by cholinomimetics is also present in drug-free, euthymic unipolar and bipolar patients, suggesting that it is a trait marker for affective disorders (Sitaram et al 1981, Gillen et al 1982, Nurnberger et al 1989a).

However, Berger et al (1989) have reported no difference in REM induction between healthy subjects and euthymic (seven unipolar and two bipolar) affective disorder patients who were drug-free from 4 months to 6 years prior to testing with the cholinergic M_1 receptor agonist RS-86. In the same study, Berger et al found significantly shorter REM induction times for patients currently suffering from a major depressive episode when compared to healthy subjects. These results call into question whether shortened REM induction by cholinomimetics is a state or trait marker.

There are significant technical issues to be considered and resolved in the REM induction studies. One issue is the relationship of muscarinic receptor subtypes in REM sleep induction. Physostigmine causes stimulation of both muscarinic and nicotinic receptors, and arecoline has effects on multiple muscarinic cholinergic receptor subtypes. Both drugs cause considerable side effects due to their peripheral effects and both drugs have to be administered intravenously because of their short half-lives.

Cholinergic function in affective disorders

In comparison to the amount of data available on the 5-HT and NA systems, relatively little data exists on the neurochemistry of the cholinergic system in affective disorders. This lack of data is striking given the consistent reports of major acute effects of cholinomimetic and anticholinergic drugs on mood and the consistent lack of demonstrable acute effects of 5-HT and NA agonists and antagonists on mood.

Some cholinomimetic drugs have depressogenic effects. It is not clear whether these effects are mediated through interactions with other neurotransmitter systems, and whether they are mediated through the muscarinic or nicotinic systems. It is also not clear whether these depressogenic effects are any more likely in depressed patients than healthy controls.

Whether anticholinergic drugs have antidepressant properties also remains unclear. While it is often claimed that anticholinergic drugs are antidepressant (Janowski & Risch 1987, Dilsaver & Coffman 1989), there is surprisingly little published data to support these claims. It has been the lack of treatment data, in spite of available drugs with which to test the cholinergic hypothesis, which has served as one of the most significant criticisms of this hypothesis.

The neuroendocrine effects of some cholinomimetic drugs on hypothalamic–pituitary–adrenal (HPA) function in healthy subjects appears to mimic the alterations seen in some depressed patients. However, relatively little has been done towards further understanding of these phenomena and the enhanced ACTH and beta-endorphin release in response to physostigmine in depressed patients has not been further studied to date. Also, the receptor types and subtypes mediating the behavioural and neuroendocrine effects of cholinomimetic drugs remains to be elucidated.

The shortened time to induction of REM sleep by cholinergic agonists is an extremely interesting finding which adds considerable support to the hypothesis that postsynaptic muscarinic cholinergic supersensitivity exists in some depressed patients. The behavioural and neurochemical data available on the role of cholinergic mechanisms in affective disorders is tantalizing and deserves much more attention than it has currently been given. Selective agonists and antagonists for muscarinic cholinergic receptor subtypes may further help to provide new avenues for study and antagonists for these receptor subtypes may be evaluated as potential antidepressants.

THE DOPAMINERGIC SYSTEM

Dopaminergic cell bodies located in the ventral mesencephalon form the majority of DA cell bodies and project widely throughout the CNS. These cell bodies give rise to the nigro-striatal, mesocortical and mesolimbic DA projections. These projections and others arising from the ventral mesencephalon are diverse and complexly regulated. A great degree of anatomical and functional overlap exists between these projections as well as a surprising degree of heterogeneity and uniqueness. The heterogeneity appears to be related to the diversity of nerve terminal systems, feedback loops, enzyme composition, co-released peptides and differences in autoreceptor sensitivity within different target brain regions (see Roth et al 1987 for review).

Dopaminergic cell bodies projecting to the hypothalamus and pituitary arise from a different brain region and are referred to as the tuberoinfundibular (TIDA) and tuberohypophysial (THDA) neurones. These cell bodies arise primarily from the arcuate nucleus. The THDA neurones project ventrally to the neurointerme-

diate lobe of the pituitary and the TIDA neurones project to the hypothalamus and the hypothalamic-hypophysial portal system (Moore 1987). Dopaminergic TIDA projections are involved in the tonic inhibition of prolactin secretion as well as stimulating the release of growth hormone.

Some investigators have hypothesized that dysfunction of DA neurotransmission may be involved in depression and especially in mania (Jimerson 1987). This hypothesis is based on the observations that some DA agonists, such as L-DOPA, amphetamine, methylphenidate and bromocriptine, have been associated with the development of mania and that DA antagonists are efficacious in the treatment of mania. Further, medications such as bupropion and nomifensine, both of which enhance DA activity, are effective antidepressants.

However, none of the above drugs are specific DA agonists and antagonists and most have pronounced effects on the NA system. Antidepressant trials with more selective DA agonists such as piribedil, while apparently efficacious in some patients, have on the whole been disappointing. Further, cocaine, which has some of the most potent effects on the release of DA, appears not to be efficacious in most depressed patients (Post et al 1974), although this may only apply to a subset of depressed patients since many dysthymic patients and mildly depressed patients report improvement of depression early on in the use of cocaine, with the subsequent development of more dysphoric reactions over time (personal observations).

Clinical studies of dopaminergic function in affective disorders

Neuroendocrine challenge strategies designed to assess DA function in depressed patients have used the prolactin and growth hormone responses to direct and indirect DA agonists as measures of DA tone. It is worth noting that considerable evidence supports the observations that the TIDA and THDA DA neurones are regulated differently and may not provide an accurate index of the functional state of the mesolimbic or mesocortical DA projections (Moore 1987, Jimerson 1987).

Apomorphine is a direct acting postsynaptic and presynaptic DA_2 receptor agonist. Apomorphine leads to an increase in the secretion of growth hormone, ACTH, cortisol, beta-endorphin and a decrease in the secretion of prolactin in humans (Brown et al 1979, Jezova & Vigas 1988). Limiting factors in the use of apomorphine have been the occurrence of nausea, which itself could confound results by causing indirect effects on the release of hormones and the fact that decreasing levels of prolactin, which is already released only in small amounts, is difficult.

Neuroendocrine responses to apomorphine have been studied in depression and for the most part no difference in the suppression of prolactin or the increased release of growth hormone between healthy subjects and depressed patients has been identified (Willner 1983, Jimerson 1987). Electroconvulsive therapy has been reported to enhance the growth hormone response to apomorphine in depressed patients and amitriptyline appears to blunt the growth hormone response in both healthy subjects and depressed patients to a similar degree (Balldin et al 1982, Costain et al 1982, Cowen et al 1984).

The neuroendocrine effects of amphetamine have been reviewed in the preceding section on assessment of NA function and have produced mixed results, with some studies reporting a blunted growth hormone response and others reporting no difference between depressed patients and controls (see Jimerson 1987, Matussek 1988 for reviews).

More interesting is the rapid but transient improvement in mood in some depressed patients after acute administration of amphetamine (Fawcet & Siomopoulos 1971, Joyce 1985). Although it has been suggested that the pretreatment improvement of mood following amphetamine in depressed patients predicts subsequent antidepressant response (Fawcet & Siomopoulos 1971), this has not been fully verified or aggressively followed up.

L-DOPA is the immediate precursor for the synthesis of NA and DA. L-DOPA has also been used to assess DA and NA activity in depression, although, as for amphetamine, it cannot be established with certainty which neurotransmitter is responsible for the neuroendocrine profile. For the most part, the growth hormone and prolactin responses to L-DOPA and bromocriptine in depressed patients have been found to be no different than for healthy subjects (see Jimerson 1987, for review).

Dopaminergic function in affective disorders

As described above, neurochemical abnormalities of the DA system have not been established in depression. While mixed DA/NA releasing agents such as amphetamine, methylphenidate and cocaine appear to cause an elevation of mood and even mania-like states in healthy subjects and mood elevation in some depressed patients, this does not appear to be related to any neuroendocrine abnormalities in depression.

The lack of neuroendocrine abnormalities of the DA system in depression may be because of the distinct nature of the regulation of the TIDA and THDA neurones, but suggests that abnormalities of DA function may not be involved in most forms of depression. Further evidence in support of this view is the lack of depressogenic effect of DA antagonists in either healthy subjects or depressed patients. However, the antidepressant medications nomifensine and bupropion may in fact be mediating their therapeutic effects through the DA system and may indicate that a subgroup of depressed patients may have abnormalities of the DA system.

NEUROPEPTIDES

Within the past 10–15 years an increasing number of peptides previously thought to exist only outside the brain have been localized in the CNS. Many peptides such as CRH, somatostatin, beta-endorphin, ACTH, thyrotropin releasing hormone (TRH), arginine vasopressin, oxytocin, vasoactive intestinal polypeptide (VIP), cholecystokinin (CCK), substance P, neuropeptide Y and galanin have been localized in the mammalian CNS and many of these neuropeptides are co-localized and co-released with classical neurotransmitters such as NA, 5-HT, DA and ACh. In some situations there is more than one neuropeptide colocalized with a classical neurotransmitter. An example of this is the co-localization of TRH and substance P with 5-HT in some raphe neurons (Johansson et al 1981).

Data on this topic are increasing exponentially and promise to alter our current hypotheses of brain function dramatically. For example, many neuropeptides modulate the activity of the co-localized classical transmitter. In rat brain, neuropeptide Y and galanin both modulate NA release from NA nerve terminals where these peptides are co-released, but have no effect on NA release in brain areas where the peptides are not naturally found (Goldstein & Deutch 1989).

Opioids

Opioid peptides and various opiate receptor agonists and antagonists have pronounced effects on behaviour and on the release of pituitary and adrenal hormones. After the discovery of endogenously occurring opioid peptides (Pert & Snyder 1973) and the characterization of opiate receptors, the uncovering of some of the behavioural effects of the opioid peptides and the involvement of these substances in 'stress' responses in laboratory animals, a heightened level of interest ensued in the neuroendocrine effects of opioid peptides and other opiates (Gold et al 1988).

Numerous investigations of the effects of opioid agonists on mood in depressed and manic patients have been conducted. While initial results were promising, subsequent placebo-controlled trials have revealed no significant antidepressive effects of many synthetic and natural opioids (see Berger & Nemeroff 1987 for review).

Neuroendocrine effects of opiates have also been investigated in humans. These include investigations assessing the effects of methadone (Gold et al 1980) and beta-endorphin (Catlin et al 1980) on plasma cortisol levels, and morphine and methadone on plasma prolactin (Extein et al 1980). While most (Extein et al 1980, Judd et al 1982, Robertson et al 1984), but not all (Zis et al 1985a) investigators have found a blunted prolactin response to morphine and methadone in depressed patients compared to healthy controls, the prolactin response to the specific mu-opiate receptor agonist fentanyl was not different from controls (Matussek & Hoehe 1989) and the cortisol response to morphine has been variable with a subgroup of depressed patients demonstrating an 'escape' of the suppression of cortisol by these opiates (Zis et al 1985b,c, Banki & Arato 1987, Zis 1988). In these studies many of the patients with an 'escape' of suppression of cortisol also had abnormal dexamethasone suppression tests (Zis 1988).

The neuroendocrine profiles of opiate antagonists have also been investigated in depressed patients and although robust increases in cortisol have been noted these are not different from those found in healthy subjects (Zis 1988 for review).

A blunted prolactin response to morphine and methadone has been the only consistently identified neuroendocrine abnormality of the opioid system in depressed patients. However, the neuroendocrine effects of opiates may be mediated through catecholamine and indoleamine neurotransmitter systems. For example, opiate-induced increases in growth hormone secretion may be mediated via changes in the NA system (Koenig et al 1980, Eriksson et al 1981) and possibly the histaminergic and cholinergic systems (Penalva et al 1983) and increases in prolactin secretion may be mediated through the DA

(Grandison & Guidotti 1977, Tolis et al 1978) and/or serotonergic (Spampinato et al 1979) systems. This makes interpretation of the blunted prolactin response to opiate agonists difficult since blunting of the prolactin response to various 5-HT probes is a consistently replicated finding in depressed patients (Heninger et al 1990). It is interesting that in some studies the euphoric response to fentanyl is blunted in depressed patients compared to healthy controls (Matussek & Hoehe 1989).

CRH

Abnormalities of the HPA axis have been some of the most studied biological abnormalities in depression (see also ch. 17). There has been extensive research into the preclinical and clinical aspects of HPA function because of the abnormal cortisol response to stress, and to the synthetic steroid dexamethasone, seen in many depressed patients (Carroll et al 1968, 1976, 1981). Cortisol production by the adrenal cortex is stimulated primarily by the hormone ACTH, whose release is in turn stimulated primarily by corticotrophin releasing hormone (CRH) and vasopressin and inhibited by glucocorticoids. CRH secretion is enhanced by 5-HT, NA and cholinergic inputs and is diminished by GABA and glucocorticoids (Holsboer 1989). CRH further feeds back to the locus ceruleus and increases its firing rate.

Abnormal levels of basal cortisol in depression and stressful situations were identified almost 30 years ago (Gibbons 1964, Mason et al 1965). Shortly after this, Carroll reported the lack of normal suppression of cortisol following an oral dose of the synthetic corticosteroid dexamethasone (Carroll et al 1968). Although the sensitivity of the dexamethasone suppression test (DST) for diagnosing depression is not adequate, and only tentative predictive validity for the DST has been established (Carroll et al 1981), the abnormal lack of normal suppression of plasma cortisol in depressed patients has continued to be replicated. Given the current level of understanding of the regulation of the HPA axis, considerable research is now being focused on attempting to understand the pathophysiology which underlies DST non-suppression in depressed patients.

Since the identification and synthesis of CRH in the early 1980s (Vale et al 1981, Speiss et al 1981, Shibahara et al 1983), it has become available as a neuroendocrine probe of HPA activity. The ACTH response to CRH infusion is blunted in depressed patients compared to controls (Holsboer et al 1984) but cortisol release is exaggerated and the cortisol response to CRH is therefore not different between depressed patients and healthy subjects (Holsboer 1989). Furthermore, the blunting of the ACTH response is reversed when cortisol biosynthesis is blocked by metyrapone, suggesting that the blunting of the ACTH response is caused in part by feedback inhibition of ACTH release by circulating cortisol (Von Bardeleben et al 1988). Based on the above it has been hypothesized that the reasons for hypercortisolism in depression are related to hypersecretion of CRH (Holsboer 1989).

Recent investigations measuring CSF levels of CRH in depressed patients add support to this hypothesis, in that depressed patients have been found to have elevated CSF levels of CRH compared to healthy subjects and non-depressed psychiatric patients (Nemeroff et al 1984, Banki et al 1987, Widerlöv et al 1988a). However, the specificity of these findings is unclear since both elevated CSF levels of CRH and a blunted ACTH response to CRH are found in other disorders (Taylor & Fishman 1988).

Reduced binding sites for CRH have recently been measured in the frontal cortex of suicide victims (Nemeroff et al 1988). This data as well as the findings of increased CSF CRH and the blunted ACTH response to CRH suggest that CRH is hypersecreted in depression and this hypersecretion of CRH leads to a compensatory downregulation of CRH receptors in the frontal cortex and hypothalamus (Nemeroff et al 1988).

Somatostatin

Somatostatin is a tetradecapeptide which was first isolated and characterized in the early 1970s (Brazeau et al 1973). Initially, somatostatin was identified in relationship to its effect of inhibiting the release of growth hormone (somatotropin). Somatostatin is found in significant concentrations in the hypothalamus, amygdala and nucleus accumbens in human brain. Somatostatin receptors are localized in the deep layers of the cortex, cingulate cortex, claustrum, the locus ceruleus and the limbic system (Vecsei & Widerlöv 1988).

Somatostatin is involved in the regulation of a variety of behaviours and vegetative functions in animals, which had led to the hypothesis that it is involved in affective disorders. Somatostatin is involved in the regulation of slow wave sleep and REM sleep, food consumption, locomotor activity, analgesia and learning (Rubinow et al 1988). It is also involved in the regulation of a variety of other hormones and neurotransmitters including TRH, insulin, glucagon, CCK, secretin, motilin, calcitonin, parathyroid hormone, DA, NA, 5-HT and ACh (see Vecsei & Widerlöv 1988, Rubinow et al 1988 for reviews).

Compared to healthy subjects, depressed patients have been noted to have decreased CSF levels of somatostatin (Gerner & Yamada 1982, Rubinow et al 1983). While this finding has now been replicated in six other studies, it is not specific to depressed patients, since decreased somatostatin has been found in Parkinson's disease, Alzheimer's disease, multiple sclerosis and senile dementia (see Rubinow et al 1988, Vecsei & Widerlöv 1988 for reviews).

Neuropeptide Y

Neuropeptide Y is a 36 amino acid peptide localized primarily in the forebrain within the CNS. The majority of neuropeptide Y neurones are short interneurones. Neuropeptide Y is also found co-localized with NA, somatostatin, GABA and galanin (de Quidt & Emson 1986). Neuropeptide Y has effects on pituitary hormone release, autonomic function and various behaviours in laboratory animals which have been suggested to be indicative of its possible involvement in affective disorders (Widerlöv et al 1988b).

Neuropeptide Y levels in the cortex are increased by the antidepressant drugs imipramine and zimelidine (Heilig et al 1988) as well as by ECT (Stenfors et al 1989, Wahlestedt et al 1990). Neuropeptide Y administration has been reported to exert anxiolytic/sedative effects in rats (Heilig et al 1988). Neuropeptide Y levels have been found to be reduced in the CSF of patients with major depression (Widerlöv et al 1986, 1988b, 1989) and a negative correlation exists between neuropeptide Y levels and ratings of anxiety in depressed patients (Widerlöv et al 1989).

COMMENT

Since the first biological hypotheses of the pathophysiology of affective disorders were proposed 25 years ago (Schildkraut 1965, Bunney & Davis 1965, Coppen 1967, Janowski et al 1972) considerable progress has been made in understanding the neuropharmacology and neurophysiology of CNS function. This increased knowledge has in part led to new hypotheses of the pathophysiology of affective disorders and of the mechanism of antidepressant action (Charney et al

1981b, 1990, Siever & Davis 1985). It has also led to the awareness that symptoms such as depressed mood, and other core symptoms of affective disorders such as alterations in appetite, sleep and libido, may be caused by alterations in the function of more than one CNS neurotransmitter system. Because of this knowledge the concept of pathophysiological heterogeneity within affective disorders has begun to evolve.

Brain neurotransmitter systems interact with each other and modulate each other's function. For example, NA denervation prevents tricyclic antidepressants from causing a sensitization of forebrain neurons to 5-HT in laboratory animals (Gravel & de Montigny 1987). Lesions of the 5-HT system increase low agonist affinity beta-adrenergic receptor density (Gillespie et al 1988). Depletion of both NA and DA results in a greater blunting of the growth hormone response to clonidine in rats than depletion of NA alone (Soderpalm et al 1987). Long-term treatment with the beta-adrenergic agonist clenbuterol causes an increase in 5-HT_{1A} receptors in mouse brain (Frances et al 1987).

The 'classical' neurotransmitter systems such as the NA, DA and 5-HT systems are organized in highly complex and specialized fashions. Each of these neurotransmitter systems includes discrete subsystems which are organized in a topographical fashion and have differing neuropharmacology and neurophysiology. Many of these subsystems include subsystem-specific interactions with selective receptor subtypes, differing neurone morphology and differences in co-localized neuropeptides. The function of these systems is further modulated by neuropeptides such as CRH, somatostatin, neuropeptide Y and the opioid peptides.

The complexity of the regulation of CNS function described above impacts greatly on any formulation of the possible pathophysiology of affective disorders and the mechanism of antidepressant action. These data highlight the possibility of pathophysiological heterogeneity. Moreover, it is entirely possible that the mechanism of antidepressant action is also heterogeneous and is possibly not correcting the underlying deficit in affective states. In fact, many treatments in medicine involve groups of heterogeneous treatments which restore normal function by re-establishing a critical homeostatic balance rather than by correcting the underlying condition directly. Examples of this include treatments for cardiac arrhythmias, hypertension, heart failure, colitis, diarrhoea, headache, autoimmune disorders and many other conditions. Given these possibilities, it is important to conceptualize the pathophysiology of

affective disorders as not only being heterogeneous, but possibly being separate from the locus of antidepressant action.

Pathophysiology of affective disorders

A common pathophysiology of depression has not been identified. Abnormal presynaptic 5-HT, postsynaptic NA and postsynaptic cholinergic system function, as well as increased CSF CRH and decreased CSF somatostatin and neuropeptide Y levels, have been reported and replicated in drug-free depressed patients in separate studies. None of these abnormalities are present in all depressed patients, even when endogenous, melancholic or bipolar subtypes are distinguished. These abnormalities have not had predictive validity for course of illness, diagnostic subtype or treatment response. However, as discussed previously, underlying biological heterogeneity may obscure attempts to establish the validity of neurochemical abnormalities through outcome measures.

It is not known whether the abnormalities cited above are the representation of different underlying causes or whether they are a result of interactions between neurotransmitter systems. Given the degree of interaction between neurotransmitter systems described above, it is possible that some of the identified abnormalities in affective disorder patients may be secondary to dysfunction of another system. For example, since CRH influences the firing rate of the locus ceruleus, excessive CRH production would also be likely to cause abnormal responses to drugs which alter locus ceruleus activity. Until the interactions between different neurotransmitter systems and the differences in regulation within neurotransmitter systems are taken into account it cannot be determined whether the abnormalities described above are secondary to abnormalities of another system or whether they represent biological subtypes of affective disorders.

Mechanism of antidepressant action

The original hypotheses of antidepressant action were derived from data obtained from in vitro and in vivo studies of the acute effects of tricyclic antidepressants and monoamine oxidase inhibitors on catecholamine and indoleamine neurotransmission. These early hypotheses were closely linked to the deficiency hypotheses of affective disorders (Schildkraut 1965, Bunney & Davis 1965, Coppen 1967). However, the original deficiency hypotheses have not been supported and considerable evidence suggests that it is unlikely that a catecholamine or indoleamine deficiency is involved in depression. The temporal delay in therapeutic action of antidepressants is also not accounted for by these hypotheses.

More recent attempts to understand antidepressant action in light of the temporal delay in therapeutic effect have focused on adaptive changes in the NA and 5-HT systems after long-term treatment. The receptor-sensitivity hypothesis was one of the first examples of this (Charney et al 1981b). This hypothesis argues that adaptive changes in receptor sensitivity account for the temporal delay in antidepressant action.

The 5-HT hypothesis, as expressed by de Montigny and colleagues (Blier et al 1990a), argues that the receptor sensitivity alterations within the 5-HT system which occur after long-term antidepressant treatment lead to an enhancement of 5-HT neurotransmission. They posit that it is this enhancement of 5-HT neurotransmission which leads to the antidepressant response.

In reviewing the literature on this topic derived from human studies, a great deal of data, mostly from neuroendocrine studies, suggests that many antidepressant medications and electroconvulsive therapy enhance 5-HT neurotransmission after long-term treatment. Rapidly interfering with 5-HT synthesis transiently reverses antidepressant response in two thirds of recently remitted depressed patients (Shopsin et al 1975, 1976, Delgado et al 1990b). However, evidence of enhanced 5-HT function is not correlated with successful antidepressant treatment. These data suggest that enhancement of 5-HT neurotransmission may be necessary but not sufficient to achieve and maintain an antidepressant response to many antidepressant treatments.

Given the abnormalities reported in drug-free affective disorder patients, surprisingly few effects common to most antidepressants have been noted in clinical studies of the NA, DA and ACh systems. In a small number of imipramine-remitted patients catecholamine depletion with the tyrosine hydroxylase inhibitor AMPT was without effect (Shopsin et al 1975). The antidepressant effects of some antidepressants such as desipramine and bupropion, as predicted by their pharmacological profiles, may be less dependent on 5-HT for their therapeutic effects (Delgado et al 1990b).

At this stage it must be said that a unitary mechanism of antidepressant action has not been identified. Simply increasing synaptic concentrations of catecholamines or indoleamines does not rapidly reverse depression in most depressed patients (see Charney et al 1981b, 1990 for review). The 5-HT receptor sensitivity hypothesis (Blier et al 1990a) would predict that, since the alterations in the 5-HT system which are thought to underlie antidepressant action lead to an enhancement of 5-HT neurotransmission, then any procedure which enhances 5-HT neurotransmission should be rapidly antidepressant. This is not the case. Furthermore, rapidly lowering 5-HT through TRP depletion in drug-free depressed patients does not uniformly worsen depression (Delgado et al 1990b).

As described within the section on 5-HT, it is perhaps more likely that 5-HT (and possibly other neurotransmitter systems) are influencing another system which is involved in antidepressant action. Given the relationships of the 5-HT system to other neurotransmitter systems, this might entail a critical balance between 5-HT and NA, DA or ACh, or some effects on neuropeptide content. 5-HT neurones directly modulate the function of several cortical interneurones, including those containing neuropeptide Y. Given the recent reports of increased neuropeptide Y concentrations following antidepressant medications (Heilig et al 1988) and ECT (Stenfors et al 1989, Wahlestedt et al 1990) in laboratory animals, it may be that changes in neuropeptide Y or other neuropeptides such as CRH may underlie successful antidepressant response.

Implications for future studies

The relationships of the 5-HT, DA, NA and ACh systems to each other and to regulatory neuropeptides need much more assessment. Future studies should begin to look beyond the catecholamine and indoleamine transmitters and to assess co-released transmitters and neuropeptides as well as incorporating the concepts of neural networks. Much more research on the role of neuropeptides in normal CNS function and affective illness is critical. Brain imaging with positron emission tomography and single photon emission tomography, combined with pharmacological challenge studies, may provide a better response measure than hormones or metabolites. More specific probes of neurotransmitter receptors and second and third messenger function must be developed. It will be necessary to identify the biological subtypes of affective syndromes in order to make fundamental advances in the discovery of new treatments and outcome predictors.

REFERENCES

Aghajanian G K 1981 The modulatory role of serotonin at multiple receptors in the brain. In: Jacobs B L, Gelperin A (eds) Serotonin neurotransmission and behaviour. MIT Press, Cambridge, MA, p 156–185

Aghajanian G K, Sprouse J S, Rassmussen K 1987 Physiology of midbrain serotonin system. In: Meltzer H Y (ed) Psychopharmacology: the third generation of progress. Raven Press, New York, p 141–150

Anderson I M, Cowen P J 1986 Clomipramine enhances prolactin and growth hormone responses to L-tryptophan. Psychopharmacology 89: 131–133

Anderson I M, Crooks W S, Gartside S E, Parry-Billings M, Newsholme E A, Cowen P J 1989 Effect of moderate weight loss on prolactin responses in normal female volunteers. Psychiatry Research 29: 161–167

Ansseau M, Scheyvaerts M, Doumont A, Poirrier R, Legros J J, Franck G 1984 Concurrent use of REM latency, dexamethasone suppression, clonidine, and apomorphine tests as biological markers of endogenous depression: a pilot study. Psychiatry Research 12: 261–272

Ansseau M, Von Frenckell, Cerfontaine R et al 1988 Blunted response of growth hormone to clonidine and apomorphine in endogenous depression. British Journal of Psychiatry 153: 65–71

Arango V, Ernsberger P, Marzuk P M et al 1990 Autoradiographic demonstration of increased serotonin 5-HT_2 and β-adrenergic receptor binding sites in the brain of suicide victims. Archives of General Psychiatry 47: 1038–1047

Arato M, Rihmer Z, Banki C M, Grof P 1983 The relationships of neuroendocrine tests in endogenous depression. Progress in Neuro-Pharmacology and Biological Psychiatry 7: 715–718

Arora R C, Meltzer H Y 1989a Serotonergic measures in the brains of suicide victims: 5-HT_2 binding sites in the frontal cortex of suicide victims and control subjects. American Journal of Psychiatry 146: 730–736

Arora R C, Meltzer H Y 1989b Increased serotonin-2 (5-HT_2) receptor-binding as measured by (^{3}H)-Ilysergic acid diethylamine (^{3}H-LSD) in the blood-platelets of depressed patients. Life Sciences 44: 725–734

Åsberg M, Schalling D, Traskman-Bendz L, Wagner A 1987 Psychobiology of suicide, impulsivity, and related phenomena. In: Meltzer H Y (ed) Psychopharmacology: the third generation of progress. Raven Press, New York, p 655–668

Ashcroft G W, Blackburn I M, Eccleston D et al 1973 Changes on recovery in the concentrations of tryptophan and the biogenic amine metabolites in the cerebrospinal fluid of patients with affective illness. Psychological Medicine 3: 319–325

Asnis G M, Lemus C Z, Halbreich U 1986 The desipramine cortisol test - a selective noradrenergic challenge (relationship to other cortisol tests in depressives and normals). Psychopharmacology Bulletin 22: 571–578

Asnis G M, Eisenberg J, van Praag H M, Lemus C Z, Freidman H, Miller A 1988 The neuroendocrine response to fenfluramine in depressives and normal controls. Biological Psychiatry 24: 117–120

Avissar S, Schreiber G 1989 Muscarinic receptor subclassification and G-proteins: significance for lithium action in affective disorders and for the treatment of the extrapyramidal side effects of neuroleptics. Biological Psychiatry 26: 113–130

Badawy A A-B 1977 Minireview: the functions and regulation of tryptophan pyrrolase. Life Sciences 21: 755–768

Balldin J, Granerus A K, Lindstedt G, Modigh K, Walinder J 1982 Neuroendocrine evidence for increased responsiveness of dopamine receptors in humans following electroconvulsive therapy. Psychopharmacology 76: 371–376

Banki C M, Arato M 1987 Multiple hormonal responses to morphine: relationship to diagnosis and dexamethasone suppression. Psychoneuroendocrinology 12: 3–11

Banki C M, Molnar G, Fekete I 1981 Correlation of individual symptoms and other clinical variables with cerebrospinal fluid amine metabolites and tryptophan in depression. Archiv für Psychiatrie und Nervenkrankheitten 229: 345–353

Banki C M, Bissette G, Arato M, O'Connor L, Nemeroff M S, Nemeroff C B 1987 CSF corticotropin-releasing factor-like immunoreactivity in depression and schizophrenia. American Journal of Psychiatry 144: 873–877

Bartus R T, Dean R L, Flicker C 1987 Cholinergic psychopharmacology: an integration of human and animal research on memory. In: Meltzer H Y (ed) Psychopharmacology: the third generation of progress. Raven Press, New York, p 219–232

Bech P, Eplov L, Gastpar M et al 1988 WHO pilot study on the validity of imipramine binding in affective disorders: trait versus state characteristics. Pharmacopsychiatry 21: 147–150

Berger P A, Nemeroff C B 1987 Opioid peptides in affective disorders. In: Meltzer H Y (ed) Psychopharmacology: the third generation of progress. Raven Press, New York, p 637–646

Berger M, Krieg JC, Rummler R et al 1986 The treatment of mania with the cholinomimetic drug RS 86. Pharmacopsychiatry 19: 326–327

Berger M, Riemann D, Hochli D, Spiegel R 1989 The cholinergic rapid eye movement sleep induction test with RS-86. Archives of General Psychiatry 46: 421–428

Biegon A, Israeli M 1988 Regionally selective increases in β-adrenergic receptor density in the brains of suicide victims. Brain Research 442: 199–203

Biegon A, Weizman A, Karp L, Ram A, Tiano S, Wolff M 1987 Serotonin 5-HT_2 receptor binding on blood platelets – a peripheral marker for depression? Life Sciences 41: 2485–2492

Biegon A, Essa N, Israeli M, Elizur A, Bruch S, Bar-Nathan A A 1990a Serotonin 5-HT_2 receptor binding on blood platelets as a state dependent marker in major affective disorder. Psychopharmacology 102: 73–75

Beigon A, Grinspoon A, Blumenfeld B, Bleich A, Apter A, Mester R 1990b Increased serotonin 5-HT_2 receptor binding on blood platelets of suicidal men. Psychopharmacology 100: 165–167

Blier P, de Montigny C, Azzaro AJ 1986 Modification of serotonergic and noradrenergic neurotransmissions by repeated administration of monoamine oxidase inhibitors: electrophysiological studies in the rat central nervous system. Journal of Pharmacology and Experimental Therapeutics 237: 987–994

Blier P, de Montigny, Chaput Y 1990a A role for the serotonin system in the mechanism of action of antidepressant treatments: preclinical evidence. Journal of Clinical Psychiatry 51(4,suppl): 14–20

Blier P, Serrano A, Scatton B 1990b Differential responsiveness of the rat dorsal and medican raphe 5-HT systems to 5-HT$_1$ receptor agonists and p-chloroamphetamine. Synapse 5: 120–133

Bolin R R 1960 Psychiatric manifestations of Artane toxicity. Journal of Nervous and Mental Disorders 131: 256–259

Bonner R L, Buckley N J, Young A C, Brann M R 1987 Identification of a family of muscarinic acetycholine receptor genes. Science 237: 527–532

Boyer P, Schaub C, Pichot P 1982 Growth hormone response to clonidine test in depressive states. Neuroendocrinology Letters 4: 178

Brambilla F, Catalano M, Lucca A, Smeraldi E 1988 Effect of lithium treatment on the growth hormone-clonidine test in affective disorders. European Journal of Clinical Pharmacology 35: 601–605

Brazeau P, Vale W, Burgus R et al 1973 Hypothalamic polypeptide that inhibits the secretion of immunoreactive pituitary growth hormone. Science 179: 77–79

Bridges P C, Bartlett J R, Sepping P, Kantamaneni B D, Curzon G 1976 Precursors and metabolites of 5-hydroxytryptamine and dopamine in the ventricular cerebrospinal fluid of psychiatric patients. Psychological Medicine 6: 399–405

Briley M, Raisman R, Sechter D, Zarifian E, Langer S Z 1980 ^{3}H-imipramine binding in human platelets: a new biochemical parameter in depression. Neuropharmacology 19: 1209–1210

Brodie H K H, Murphy D L, Goodwin F K, Bunney W E 1970 Catecholamines and mania: the effect of alpha-methyl-para-tyrosine on manic behaviour and catecholamine metabolism. Clinical Pharmacology and Therapeutics 12: 218–224

Brown G M, Freind W C, Chambers J W 1979 Neuropharmacology of hypothalamic-pituitary regulation. In: Tolis G, Labrie F, Martin J B, Naftolin F (eds) Clinical neuroendocrinology. A pathophysiological approach, Raven Press, New York, p 47–81

Brownstein M, Axelrod J 1974 Pineal gland: 24-hour rhythm in norepinephrine turnover. Science 184: 163–165

Buckholtz N S, Davies A O, Rudorfer M V, Golden R N, Potter W Z 1988 Lymphocyte beta adrenergic receptor function versus catecholamines in depression. Biological Psychiatry 24: 451–457

Bunney W E Jr Davis J M 1965 Norepinephrine in depressive reactions: a review. Archives of General Psychiatry 13: 483–494

Bunney W E Jr, Brodie H K H, Murphy D L, Goodwin F K 1971 Studies of alpha-methyl-para-tyrosine, L-dopa, and L-tryptophan in depression and mania. American Journal of Psychiatry 127: 872–881

Bylund D B 1988 Subtypes of α_2-adrenoreceptors: pharmacological and molecular biological evidence converge. Trends in the Pharmacological Sciences 9: 356–361

Carlsson A, Lindqvist M 1978 Effects of antidepressant

agents on the synthesis of monoamines. Journal of Neural Transmission 43: 73–91

Carlsson A, Persoon T, Roose B-E, Walinder J 1972 Potentiation of phenothiazines by α-methyltyrosine in treatment of chronic schizophrenia. Journal of Neural Transmission 33: 83–90

Carpenter W T 1970 Serotonin now: clinical implications of inhibiting its synthesis with para-chlorophenylalanine. Annals of Internal Medicine 73: 607–629

Carroll B J, Martin F I, Davies B M 1968 Resistance to suppression by dexamethasone of plasma 11-OHCS levels in severe depressive illness. British Medical Journal 3: 285–287

Carroll B J, Frazer A, Schless A, Mendels J 1973 Cholinergic reversal of manic symptoms. Lancet 1: 427–428

Carroll B J, Curtis G C, Mendels J 1976 Neuroendocrine regulation in depression: I. Limbic system-adrenalcortical dysfunction. Archives of General Psychiatry 33: 1039–1044

Carroll B J, Greden J F, Haskett R et al 1980 Neurotransmitter studies of neuroendocrine pathology in depression. Acta Psychiatrica Scandinavica (suppl 280) 61: 183–199

Carroll B J, Feinberg M, Greden J F et al 1981 A specific laboratory test for the diagnosis of melancholia: standardization, validation, and clinical utility. Archives of General Psychiatry 38: 15–22

Catlin D H, Poland R E, Gorelick D A et al 1980 Intravenous infusion of beta-endorphin increases serum prolactin, but not growth hormone or cortisol, in depressed subjects and withdrawing methadone addicts. Journal of Clinical Endocrinology and Metabolism 50: 1021–1025

Chan-Palay V, Asan E 1989 Quantitation of catecholamine neurons in the locus coeruleus in human brains of normal young and older adults and in depression. Journal of Comparative Neurology 287: 357–372

Charig E M, Anderson I M, Robinson J M et al 1986 L-tryptophan and prolactin release: Evidence for 5HT$_1$ and 5-HT$_2$ receptors. Human Psychopharmacology 1: 93–97

Charney D S, Redmond D E 1983 Neurobiological mechanisms in human anxiety: evidence supporting central noradrenergic hyperactivity. Neuropharmacology 22(12B): 1531–1536

Charney D S, Heninger G R, Sternberg D E, Roth R H 1981a Plasma MHPG in depression: effects of acute and chronic desipramine treatment. Psychiatry Research 5: 217–229

Charney D S, Menekes D B, Heninger G R 1981b Receptor sensitivity and the mechanism of action of antidepressant treatment. Archives of General Psychiatry 38: 1160–1180

Charney D S, Heninger G R, Sternberg D E et al 1981c Presynaptic adrenergic receptor sensitivity in depression: the effect of long-term desipramine treatment. Archives of General Psychiatry 38: 1334–1340

Charney D S, Heninger G R, Renhard J F, Sternberg D E, Hafstead K M 1982a Effect of intravenous L-tryptophan on prolactin and growth hormone and mood in healthy subjects. Psychopharmacology 77: 217–222

Charney D S, Heninger G R, Sternberg D E, Hafstead K M, Giddings S, Landis H 1982b Adrenergic receptor sensitivity in depression: effects of clonidine in depressed patients and healthy subjects. Archives of General Psychiatry 39: 290–294

Charney D S, Heninger G R, Sternberg D E 1982c Failure of chronic antidepressant treatment to alter growth hormone response to clonidine. Psychiatry Research 7: 135–138

Charney D S, Heninger G R, Sternberg D E 1982d Assessment of α_2 adrenergic autoreceptor function in humans: Effects of oral yohimbine. Life Sciences 30: 2033–2041

Charney D S, Heninger G R, Sternberg D E 1984a Serotonin function and the mechanism of action of antidepressant treatment. Archives of General Psychiatry 41: 359–365

Charney D S, Heninger G R, Sternberg D E 1984b The effect of mianserin on alpha-2-adrenergic receptor function in depressed patients. British Journal of Psychiatry 144: 407–416

Charney D S, Woods S W, Goodman W K, Heninger G R 1987 Serotonin function in anxiety: II. Effects of the serotonin agonist m-CPP in panic disorder patients and healthy subjects. Psychopharmacology 92: 14–24

Charney D S, Southwick S M, Delgado P L, Krystal J H 1990 Current status of the receptor sensitivity hypothesis of antidepressant action: Implications for the treatment of severe depression. In: Amsterdam J D (ed) Pharmacotherapy of depression. Marcel Dekker, Basel p 13–34

Checkley S A 1979 Corticosteroid and growth hormone responses to methylamphetamine in depressive illness. Psychological Medicine 9: 107–115

Checkley S A, Crammer J L 1977 Hormone responses to methylamphetamine in depression: a new approach to the noradrenaline depletion hypothesis. British Journal of Psychiatry 131: 582–586

Checkley S A, Slade A P, Shur E 1981 Growth hormone and other responses to clonidine in patients with endogenous depression. British Journal of Psychiatry 138: 51–55

Checkley S A, Glass I B, Thompson C, Corn T, Robinson P 1984 The GH response to clonidine in endogenous as compared to reactive depression. Psychological Medicine 14: 773–777

Cheetham S C, Crompton M R, Katona C L E, Horton R W 1988 Brain 5-HT$_2$ receptor binding in depressed and suicide victims. Brain Research 443: 272–280

Coccaro E F, Siever L J, Klar H M et al 1989 Serotonergic studies in patients with affective disorders: correlates with suicidal and impulsive aggressive behaviour. Archives of General Psychiatry 46: 587–599

Cooper S J, Kelly J G, King D J 1985 Adrenergic receptors in depression: effects of electroconvulsive therapy. British Journal of Psychiatry 147: 23–29

Coppen A 1967 The biochemistry of affective disorders. British Journal of Psychiatry 113: 1237–1264

Coppen A, Wood K 1978 Tryptophan and depressive illness. Psychology and Medicine 8: 49–57

Coppen A, Brooksbank B W, Peet M 1972 Tryptophan concentration in the cerebrospinal fluid of depressive patients. Lancet 1: 1393

Coppen A, Eccleston E G, Peet M 1973 Total and free tryptophan concentration in the plasma of depressive patients. Lancet 2: 60–63

Coppen A, Swade C, Wood K 1978 Platelet 5-hydroxytryptamine accumulation in depressive illness. Clinica Chimica Acta 87: 165–168

Costain D W, Cowen P J, Gelder M G, Grahame-Smith D G 1982 Electroconvulsive therapy and the brain: Evidence for increased dopamine-mediated responses. Lancet 2: 400–404

Cowen P J, Charig E M 1987 Neuroendocrine responses to tryptophan in major depression. Archives of General Psychiatry 44: 958–966

Cowen P J 1988 Prolactin response to tryptophan during mianserin treatment. American Journal of Psychiatry 145: 740–741

Cowen P J, Braddock L E, Gosden B 1984 The effect of amitriptyline treatment on the growth hormone response to apomorphine. Psychopharmacology 83: 378–379

Cowen P J, Green A R, Grahame-Smith D G, Braddock L E 1985 Plasma melatonin during desmethylimipramine treatment: evidence for changes in noradrenergic transmission. British Journal of Psychiatry 19: 799–805

Cowen P J, Charig E M, Fraser S, Elliot J M 1987 Platelet 5-HT receptor binding during depressive illness and tricyclic antidepressant treatment. Journal of Affective Disorders 13: 45–50

Cowen P J, McCance S L, Cohen P R et al 1989a Lithium increases 5-HT-mediated neuroendocrine responses in tricyclic resistant depression. Psychopharmacology 99: 230–232

Cowen P J, Parry-Billings M, Newsholme E A 1989b Decreased plasma tryptophan levels in major depression. Journal of Affective Disorders 16: 27–31

Cowen P J, Anderson I M, Grahame-Smith D G 1990 Neuroendocrine effects of azapirones. Journal of Clinical Psychopharmacology 10(suppl 3):21S–25S.

Crow T J, Cros A J, Cooper S J et al 1984 Neurotransmitter receptors and monoamine metabolites in the brains of patients with Alzheimer-type dementia and depression, and suicides. Neuropharmacology 23: 1561–1569

Curzon G 1979 Relationships between plasma, CSF and brain tryptophan. Journal of Neural Transmission 15(suppl): 93–105

Curzon G 1981 Influence of plasma tryptophan on brain 5-HT synthesis and serotonergic activity. In Haber B, Gabay S (eds) Serotonin: current aspects of neurochemistry and function. Plenum Press, New York, p 207–219

Dahlstrom A, Fuxe K 1964 Evidence for the existence of monoamine-containing neurons in the central nervous system: I Demonstration of monoamines in cell bodies of brain neurons. Acta Physiologica Scandinavica 62(suppl 232): 1–55

Deakin J F W, Pennell I, Upadhyaya A J, Lofthouse R 1990 A neuroendocrine study of 5-HT function in depression: evidence for biological mechanisms of endogenous and psychosocial causation. Psychopharmacology 101: 85–92

Delgado P L, Charney D S, Price L H, Landis H, Heninger G R 1989 Neuroendocrine and behavioural effects of dietary tryptophan restriction in healthy subjects. Life Sciences 45: 2323–2332

Delgado P L, Charney D S, Price L H, Aghajanian G K, Heninger G R 1990a Rapid tryptophan depletion alters mood in depression. American Psychiatric Association 143rd Annual Meeting, New York, NY. New Research Abstract 184

Delgado P L, Charney D S, Price L H, Aghajanian G K, Landis H, Heninger G R 1990b Serotonin function and the mechanism of antidepressant action: Reversal of antidepressant induced remission by rapid depletion of plasma tryptophan. Archives of General Psychiatry 47: 411–418

de Montigny C, Blier P 1984 Effects of antidepressant treatment on 5-HT neurotransmission: electrophysiological and clinical studies. Advances in Biochemical Psychopharmacology 39: 223–240

DeMyer M K, Shea P A, Hendrie H C, Yoshimura N N 1981 Plasma tryptophan and five other amino acids in depressed and normal subjects. Archives of General Psychiatry 38: 642–646

de Quit M E, Emson P C 1986 Distribution of neuropeptide Y (NPY)-like immunoreactivity in the rat central nervous system. II. Immunohistochemical analysis. Neuroscience 18: 545–618

Doerr P, Berger M 1983 Physostigmine-induced escape from dexamethasone in normal subjects. Biological Psychiatry 18: 261–268

Dilsaver S C, Coffman J A 1989 Cholinergic hypothesis of depression: a reappraisal. Journal of Clinical Psychopharmacology 9: 173–179

Dolan R J, Calloway S P 1986 The human growth hormone response to clonidine: relationship to clinical and neuroendocrine profile in depression. American Journal of Psychiatry 143: 772–774

Ebstein R P, Lerer B, Shapira B, Shemesh Z, Moscovich E D G, Kindler S 1988 Cyclic AMP second messenger amplification in depression. British Journal of Psychiatry 152: 665–669

Ehsanullah R S B 1980 Uptake of 5-hydroxytryptamine and dopamine into platelets from depressed patients and normal subjects – influence of clomipramine, desmethylclomipramine, and maprotiline. Postgraduate Medical Journal (suppl 1): 31–35

Elphick M, Yang J, Cowen P J 1990 Effects of carbamazepine on dopamine-and serotonin-mediated neuroendocrine responses. Archives of General Psychiatry 47: 135–140

El-Yousef M K, Janowski D S, Davis J M, Rosenblatt J E 1973 Induction of severe depression by physostigmine in marijuana intoxicated individuals. British Journal of Addition 68: 321–325

Enna S J, Bennet J P, Bylund D B et al 1977 Neurotransmitter receptor binding: regional distribution in human brain. Journal of Neurochemistry 28: 233–236

Engelman K, Horwitz D, Jequier E, Sjoerdsma A 1968 Biochemical and pharmacologic effects of α-methyltyrosine in man. Journal of Clinical Investigation 47: 577–594

Eriksson E, Balldin J, Lindstedt G, Modigh K 1988 Growth hormone response to the alpha$_2$-adrenoreceptor agonist guanfacine and to growth hormone releasing hormone in depressed patients and controls. Psychiatry Research 26: 59–67

Eriksson E, Eden S, Modigh K 1981 Importance of norepinephrine α$_2$-receptor activation for morphine-induced rat growth hormone secretion. Neuroendocrinology 33: 91–96

Eriksson T, Carlsson A 1988 β-adrenergic control of brain uptake of large neutral amino acids. Life Sciences 42: 1583–1589

Extein I, Tallman J, Smith C C, Goodwin F K 1979 Changes in lymphocyte beta-adrenergic receptors in depression and mania. Psychiatry Research 1: 191–197

Extein I, Pottash A L C, Gold M S, Sweeney D R, Martin D M, Goodwin F K 1980 Deficient prolactin response to morphine in depressed patients. American Journal of Psychiatry 137: 845–846

Fawcet J, Siomopoulos V 1971 Dextroamphetamine response as a possible predictor of improvement with tricyclic therapy in depression. Archives of General Psychiatry 25: 244–247

Feldman R D, Limbird L E, Nadeau J, Fitzgerald G A, Robertson D, Wood A J J 1983 Dynamic regulation of lymphocyte beta adrenergic receptor-agonist interactions by physiological changes in circulating catecholamines. Journal of Clinical Investigation 72: 164–170

Feinberg M, Greden J F, Carroll B J 1981 The effect of amphetamine on plasma cortisol in patients with endogenous and nonendogenous depression. Psychoneuroendocrinology 6: 355–357

Fernstrom J D 1977 Effects of the diet on brain neurotransmitters. Metabolism 26: 207–223

Frances H, Bulach C, Simon P, Fillion M, Fillion G 1987 Chronic beta-adrenergic stimulation increases in mice the sensitivity to methysergide and the number of cerebral high affinity serotonin binding sites (5-HT-1). Journal of Neural Transmission 67: 215–224

Frazer A, Brown R, Kocsis J et al 1986 Patterns of melatonin rhythms in depression. Journal of Neural Transmission 21 (suppl): 269–290

Frohman L A, Jansson J-O 1986 Growth hormone releasing hormone. Endocrine Reviews 7: 223–253

Fuxe K, Butcher L L, Engel J 1971 D,L-5-hydroxytryptophan-induced changes in central monoamine neurons after peripheral decarboxylase inhibition. Journal of Pharmacy and Pharmacology 23: 420–424

Fuxe K, Ogren S, Benfenati F, Agnati L 1984 Central 5-HT neurons as targets for antidepressant drug actions: differential modulation of 5-HT receptor populations in the central nervous system of the rat. Advances in Biochemical Psychopharmacology 39: 271–284

García-Sevilla J A, Zis A P, Hollongsworth P J, Greden J F, Smith C B 1981 Platelet alpha-2 adrenergic receptors in major depressive disorder: binding of tritiated clonidine before and after tricyclic antidepressant drug treatment. Archives of General Psychiatry 38: 1327–1333

García-Sevilla J A, Guimón P, García-Vallejo P, Fuster M J 1986 Biochemical and functional evidence of supersensitive platelet α$_2$-adrenoreceptors in major affective disorder: effect of long-term lithium carbonate treatment. Archives of General Psychiatry 43: 51–57

García-Sevilla J A, Udina C, Fuster M J, Alvárez E, Casas M 1987 Enhanced binding of [^{3}H] (-)adrenaline to platelets of depressed patients with melancholia: effect of long-term clomipramine treatment. Acta Psychiatrica Scandinavica 75: 150–157

García-Sevilla J A, Padró D, Giralt T, Guimón J, Areso P 1990 α$_2$-Adrenoreceptor-mediated inhibition of platelet adenylate cyclase and induction of aggregation in major depression: effect of long-term cyclic antidepressant drug treatment. Archives of General Psychiatry 47: 125–132

Geaney D P, Schacter M J, Elliot J M, Grahame-Smith D G 1984 Characterization of 3H-Iysergic acid diethylamide binding to 5-hydroxytryptamine receptor on human platelet membranes. European Journal of Pharmacology 97: 87–93

Georgotas A, Schweitzer J, McCue R E, Armour M, Friedhoff A J 1987 Clinical and treatment effects on ^{3}H-clonidine and ^{3}H-imipramine binding in elderly depressed patients. Life Sciences 40: 2137–2143

Gerlach J, Thorsen K 1976 The movement pattern of oral tardive dyskinesia in relation to anticholinergic and antidopaminergic treatment. International Pharmacopsychiatry 11: 1–7

Gerner R H, Yamada T 1982 Altered neuropeptide concentrations in cerebrospinal fluid of psychiatric patients. Brain Research 238: 298–302

Gershon S, Shaw F H 1961 Psychiatric sequelae of chronic organophosphorus insecticides. Lancet 1: 1371–1374

Gibbons J L 1964 Cortisol secretion rate in depressive illness. Archives of General Psychiatry 10: 572

Gillen J C, Sitaram N, Mendelson W B 1982 Acetylcholine, sleep, and depression. Human Neurobiology 1: 211–219

Gillespie D D, Manier D H, Sanders-Bush E, Sulser F 1988 The serotonergic/noradrenergic-link in brain, II: role of serotonin in the regulation of beta adrenoreceptors in the low agonist affinity conformation. Journal of Pharmacology and Experimental Therapeutics 244: 154–159

Gold P W, Extein I, Pickar D, Rebar R, Ross R, Goodwin F K 1980 Suppression of plasma cortisol in depressed patients by acute intravenous methadone infusion. American Journal of Psychiatry 137: 862–863

Gold P W, Goodwin F K, Chrousos G P 1988 Clinical and biochemical manifestations of depression: relation to the neurobiology of stress (Part II). New England Journal of Medicine 319: 413–420

Goldberg M R, Jackson R V, Krakau J, Island D P, Robertson D 1986 Influence of yohimbine on release of anterior pituitary hormones. Life Sciences 39: 395–398

Golden R N, Hsiao J, Lane E, Hicks R, Rogers S, Potter W Z 1989 The effects of intravenous clomipramine on neurohormones in normal subjects. Journal of Clinical Endocrinology and Metabolism 68: 632–637

Golden R N, Hsiao J K, Lane E et al 1990 Abnormal neuroendocrine responsivity to acute i.v. clomipramine challenge in depressed patients. Psychiatry Research 31: 39–47

Goldstein M, Deutch A Y 1989 The inhibitory actions of NPY and galanin on ^{3}H-norepinephrine release in the central nervous system: relation to a proposed heirarchy of neuronal coexistence. In: Mutt V et al (eds) Neuropeptide Y. Raven Press, New York, p 153–162

Gonzalez-Heydrich J, Peroutka S J 1990 Serotonin receptor and reuptake sites: pharmacological significance. Journal of Clinical Psychiatry 51(suppl 4): 5–12

Goodnick P J, Meltzer H Y 1984 Neurochemical changes during discontinuation of lithium prophylaxis. II. Alterations in serotonin function. Biological Psychiatry 19: 891–898

Grandison L, Guidotti A 1977 Regulation of prolactin release by endogenous opiates. Nature 270: 357–359

Gravel P, de Montigny C 1987 Noradrenergic denervation

prevents sensitization of rat forebrain neurons to serotonin by tricyclic antidepressant treatment Synapse 1: 233–239

Halbreich U, Sachar E J, Asnis G M et al 1982 Growth hormone response to dextroamphetamine in depressed patients and normal subjects. Archives of General Psychiatry 39: 189–192

Hanssen T, Heyden T, Sundberg I, Wetterberg L 1977 Effect of propranolol on serum prolactin (letter) Lancet 2: 309–310

Healy D, Leonard B E 1987 Monoamine transport in depression: kinetics and dynamics. Journal of Affective Disorders 12: 91–103

Healey D, Theodorou A E, Whitehouse A M et al 1990 ^{3}H-imipramine binding to previously frozen platelet membranes from depressed patients, before and after treatment. British Journal of Psychiatry 157: 208–215

Heilig M, Wahlestedt C, Ekman R, Widerlöv E 1988 Antidepressant drugs increase the concentration of neuropeptide Y (NPY)-like immunoreactivity in the rat brain. European Journal of Pharmacology 147: 465–467

Heninger G R, Charney D S 1987 Mechanism of action of antidepressant treatments: Implications for the etiology and treatment of depressive disorders. In: Meltzer H Y (ed) Psychopharmacology: the third generation of progress. Raven Press, New York, p 535–544

Heninger G R, Charney D S, Sternberg D E 1984 Serotonergic function in depression: prolactin response to intravenous tryptophan in depressed patients and healthy subjects. Archives of General Psychiatry 41: 398–402

Heninger G R, Charney D S, Price LH 1988 Alpha-2-adrenergic receptor sensitivity in depression: The plasma MHPG, behavioural, and cardiovascular response to yohimbine. Archives of General Psychiatry 45: 165–175

Heninger G R, Charney D S, Price L H, Delgado P L, Woods S, Goodman W 1989 Effects of serotonergic agonists on neuroendocrine response of rhesus monkeys and patients with depression and anxiety disorders. In: Dahl S G, L F Gram (eds) Clinical pharmacology in psychiatry. Psychopharmacology Series 7. Springer-Verlag, Berlin, p 95–104

Heninger G R, Charney D S, Delgado P L 1990 Neurobiology of treatments for refractory depression. In: Tasman A, Goldfinger S M, Kaufman C A (eds), Review of psychiatry, vol. 9 American Psychiatric Press, Washington, D C, p 33–58

Hobson J A, Lydic R, Baghdoyan H A 1986 Evolving concepts of sleep cycle generation: from brain centers to neuronal populations. Behavioural Brain Science 9: 371–448

Holsboer F 1989 Psychiatric implications of altered limbic-hypothalamic-pituitary-adrenocortical activity. European Archives of Psychiatry Neurological Science 238: 302–322

Holsboer F, Bardeleben U von, Gerken A, Stella G K, Muller O A 1984 Blunted corticotropin and normal cortisol response to human corticotropin-releasing factor (h-CRF) in depression. New England Journal of Medicine 311: 1127

Idzikowski C, Cowen P J, Nutt D, Mills F J 1987 The effects of chronic ritanserin treatment on sleep and the neuroendocrine response to L-tryptophan. Psychopharmacology 93: 416–420

Janowski D S, Risch S C 1987 Role of acetylcholine mechanisms in the affective disorders. In: Meltzer H Y (ed)

Psychopharmacology: the third generation of progress. Raven Press, New York, p 527–533

Janowski D S, El-Yousef M K, Davis J M, Sekerke H J 1972 A cholinergic adrenergic hypothesis of mania and depression. Lancet 2: 632–635

Janowski D S, Risch S C, Judd L L, Parker D C, Kalin N H, Huey L Y 1982 Behavioural effects of physostigmine in affective disorder patients. In: Clayton P J, Bennett J R (eds) Treatment of depression. Raven Press, New York

Jezova D, Vigas M 1988 Apomorphine injection stimulates β-endorphin, adrenocorticotropin, and cortisol release in healthy men. Psychoneuroendocrinology 13: 479–485

Jimerson D C 1987 The role of dopamine mechanisms in the affective disorders. In: Meltzer H Y (ed) Psychopharmacology: the third generation of progress. Raven Press, New York, p 505–511

Johansson O, Hokfelt T, Pernow B et al 1981 Immunohistochemical support for three putative transmitters in one neuron: coexistence of 5-hydroxytryptamine, substance P- and thyrotropin releasing hormone-like immunoreactivity in medullary neurons projecting to the spinal cord. Neuroscience 6: 1857–1881

Joseph M S, Brewerton T D, Reus V I, Stebbins G T 1984 Plasma L-tryptophan/neutral amino acid ratio and dexamethasone suppression in depression. Psychiatry Research 11: 185–192

Joyce P R 1985 Mood response to methylphenidate and dexamethasone suppression test as predictors of treatment response to zimelidine and lithium in major depression. Biological Psychiatry 20: 598–604

Judd L L, Risch S C, Parker D C, Janowski D S, Segal D S, Huey L Y 1982 Blunted prolactin response. A neuroendocrine abnormality manifested by depressed patients. Archives of General Psychiatry 39: 1413–1416

Kahn R S, Wetzler S, Asnis G M, Kling M A, Suckow R F, van Praag H M 1990a Effects of m-chlorophenylpiperazine in normal subjects: a dose-response study. Psychopharmacology 100: 339–344

Kahn R S, Wetzler S, Asnis G M, Papolos D, van Praag H M 1990b Serotonin receptor sensitivity in major depression. Biological Psychiatry 28: 358–362

Katona C L E, Theodorou A E, Davies S L et al 1986 Platelet binding and neuroendocrine responses in depression. In: Deakin J F W (ed) The biology of depression. Gaskell, London, p 121–136

Katona C L E, Theodorou A E, Horton R W 1987 Alpha$_2$ adrenoreceptors in depression. Psychiatric Developments 2: 129–149

Kindler S, Lerer B 1990 Norepinephrine and depression: a reappraisal. In Pohl R, Gershon S (eds) The biologic basis of psychiatric treatment. Progress in Basic and Clinical Pharmacology 3. Karger, Basel, p 120–141

Kow B K, Weissman A 1966 P-chlorophenylalanine: a specific depletion of brain serotonin. Journal of Pharmacology and Experimental Therapeutics 154: 499–516

Koenig J, Mayfield M A, Coppings R J, McCann S M, Krulich L 1980 Role of central nervous system neurotransmitters in mediating the effects of morphine on growth hormone and prolactin secretion in the rat. Brain Research 197: 453–468

Kuhar M J, Roth R H, Aghajanian G K 1971 Selective reduction of tryptophan hydroxylase activity in the rat

forebrain after midbrain raphe lesions. Brain Research 35: 167–176

Laakmann G, Schumacher G, Benkert O, v on Werder K 1977 Stimulation of growth hormone secretion by desimipramine and chlorimipramine in man. Journal of Clinical Endocrinology and Metabolism 44: 1010–1013

Laakmann G, Zygan K, Schoen H W et al 1986 Effects of receptor blockers (methysergide, propranolol, phentolamine, yohimbine, and prazosin) on the desimipramine-induced pituitary hormone stimulation in humans. Part I: Growth hormone. Psychoneuroendocrinology 11: 447–461

Lal S, Tolis G, Martin J B, Brown G M, Guyda H 1975 Effect of clonidine on growth hormone, prolactin, leutinizing hormone, follicle-stimulating hormone, and thyroid-stimulating hormone in the serum of normal men. Journal of Clinical Endocrinology and Metabolism 41: 827–832

Langer G, Heinze G, Reim B, Matussek N 1975 Growth hormone response to d-amphetamine in normal controls and depressive patients. Neuroscience Letters 1: 185–189

Langer G, Heinze G, Reim B, Matussek N 1976 Reduced growth hormone response to amphetamine in endogenous depressive patients. Archives of General Psychiatry 33: 1471–1475

Lapin I P, Oxenkrug G F 1969 Intensification of the central serotonergic processes as a possible determinant of the thymoleptic effect. Lancet 1: 132–136

Larson E W, Richelson E 1988 Organic causes of mania. Mayo Clinic Proceedings 63: 906–912

Lawry T P 1977 Trihexphenidyl abuse. American Journal of Psychiatry 134: 1315

Leckman J F, Redmond D E, Heninger G R 1981 Effects of oral clonidine on plasma 3-methoxy-4-hydroxy-phenethylglycol (MHPG) in man: preliminary report. Life Sciences 26: 2179–2185

Lesch K P, Mayer S, Disselkamp-Tietze J, Hoh A, Schoenhammer G, Schulte H M 1990a Subsensitivity of the 5-hydroxytryptamine$_{1A}$ (5-HT$_{1A}$) receptor mediated hypothermic response to ipsapirone in unipolar depression. Life Sciences 46: 1271–1277

Lesch K P, Disselkamp-Tietze J, Schmidtke A 1990b 5-HT$_{1A}$ receptor function in depression: effect of chronic amitriptyline treatment. Journal of Neural Transmission 80: 157–161

Lewy A J, Wehr, T A, Goodwin F K, Newsome D A, Markey S P 1980 Light suppresses melatonin secretion in humans. Science 210: 1267–1269

MacBride P A, Mann J J, McEwen B, Beigon A 1983 Characterization of serotonin binding sites on human platelets. Life Sciences 33: 2033–2041

MacBride P A, Mann J J, Polley J J, Wiley A J, Sweeney J A 1987 Assessment of binding indices and physiological responsiveness of the 5-HT$_2$ receptor on human platelets. Life Sciences 40: 1799–1809

McCance S L, Cohen P R, Cowen P J 1989 Lithium increases 5-HT-mediated prolactin release. Psychopharmacology 99: 276–281

McKeith I G, Marshall E F, Ferrier I N et al 1987 5-HT receptor binding in postmortum brain from patients with affective disorders. Journal of Affective Disorders 13: 67–74

Maes M, Ruyter M, Hobin P, Suy E 1987 Relationship between the dexamethasone suppression test and the L-tryptophan/competing amino acid ratio in depression. Psychiatry Research 21: 323–335

Maes M, Schotte C, Scharpe S, Martin M, Blockx P 1990 The effect of glucocorticoids on the availability of L-tryptophan and tyrosine in the plasma of depressed patients. Journal of Affective Disorders 18: 121–127

Mann J J, Brown R P, Halper J P et al 1985 Reduced sensitivity of lymphocyte beta-adrenergic receptors in patients with endogenous depression and psychomotor agitation. New England Journal of Medicine 313: 715–720

Mann J J, Stanley M, McBride P A, McEwen B S 1986 Increased serotonin$_2$ and β-adrenergic receptor binding in the frontal cortices of suicide victims. Archives of General Psychiatry 43: 954–959

Marcusson J O, Ross S B 1990 Binding of some antidepressants to the 5-hydroxytryptamine transporter in brain and platelets. Psychopharmacology 102: 145–155

Marsden C A, Tyrer P, Casey P, Sievewright N 1987 Changes in whole blood 5-hydroxytryptamine (5-HT) and platelet 5-HT uptake during treatment with paroxetine, a selective 5-HT uptake inhibitor. Journal of Psychopharmacology 1: 244–250

Mason J, Sachar E J, Fishman J, Hamburg D, Handlon J 1965 Corticosteroid responses to hospital admission. Archives of General Psychiatry 13: 1

Matussek N, Ackenheil M, Hippius H et al 1980 Effects of clonidine on growth hormone release in psychiatric patients and controls. Psychiatry Research 2: 25–36

Matussek N 1988 Catecholamines and mood: neuroendocrine aspects. Current Topics in Neuroendocrinology 8: 145–182

Matussek N, Hoehe M 1989 Investigations with the specific μ-opiate receptor agonist, fentanyl in depressive patients: growth hormone, prolactin, cortisol, noradrenaline and euphoric responses. Neuropsychobiology 21: 1–8

Meagher J B, O'Halloran A, Carney P A, Leonard B E 1990 Changes in platelet 5-hydroxytryptamine uptake in mania. Journal of Affective Disorders 19: 919–196

Meana J J, Garcia-Sevilla J A 1987 Increased alpha$_2$ adrenoreceptor density in the frontal cortex of depressed suicide victims. Journal of Neural Transmission 70: 377–381

Meesters P, Kerkhofs M, Charles G, Decoster C, Vanderelst M, Mendlewicz J 1985 Growth hormone response after desipramine in depressive illness. European Archives of Psychiatry and Neurological Science 235: 140–142

Meltzer H Y, Lowy M T 1987 The serotonin hypothesis of depression. In: Meltzer H Y (ed) Psychopharmacology: the third generation of progress. Raven Press, New York, p 513–526

Meltzer H Y, Ramesh C A, Arora R C, Baber R, Tricou B J 1981 Serotonin uptake in blood platelets of psychiatric patients. Archives of General Psychiatry 38: 1322–1326

Meltzer H Y, Umberkoman-Wiita B, Robertson A, Tricou B J, Lowy M, Perline R 1984 Effect of 5-hydroxytryptophan on serum cortisol in major affective disorders. Archives of General Psychiatry 41: 366–374

Meyerson A S, Rauh C E, Abel M S, Coupet Y, Lippa A S, Rauh C E, Beer B 1982 Human brain receptor alterations in suicide victims. Pharmacology, Biochemistry and Behaviour 17: 159–163

Mitchell P, Smythe G 1990 Hormonal responses to fenfluramine in depressed and control subjects. Journal of Affective Disorders 19: 43–51

Moja E A, Cipollo P, Castoldi D, Tofanetti O 1989 Dose-response decrease in plasma tryptophan and in brain tryptophan and serotonin after tryptophan-free amino acid mixtures in rats. Life Sciences 44: 971–976

Møller S E, Kirk L, Honore P 1979 Free and total plasma tryptophan in endogenous depression. Journal of Affective Disorders 1: 69–76

Molliver M E 1987 Serotonergic neuronal systems: What their anatomic organization tells us about function. Journal of Clinical Psychopharmacology 7: 3S–23S

Moore K E 1987 Hypothalamic dopaminergic neuronal systems. In Meltzer H Y (ed.) Psychopharmacology: the third generation of progress. Raven Press, New York, p 127–139

Morgan C J, Badawy A A-B 1989 Effects of a suppression test dose of dexamethasone on tryptophan metabolism and disposition in the rat. Biological Psychiatry 25: 360–362

Mueller E A, Murphy D L, Sunderland T 1985 Neuroendocrine effects of m-chlorophenylpiperazine, a serotonin agonist, in humans. Journal of. Clinical Endocrinology and Metabolism. 61: 1179–1184

Muhlbauer H D 1984 The influence of fenfluramine stimulation on prolactin plasma levels in lithium long-term-treated manic-depressive patients and healthy subjects. Pharmacopsychiatry 17: 191–193

Muhlbauer H D, Muller-Oerlinghausen B 1985 Fenfluramine stimulation of serum cortisol in patients with major affective disorders and healthy controls: further evidence for a central serotonergic action of lithium in man. Journal of Neural Transmission 61: 81–94

Murphy D L, Cambell I, Costa J L 1978 Current status of the indoleamine hypothesis of the affective disorders. In: Lipton M A, DiMascio A, Killam K F (eds) Psychopharmacology: a generation of progress. Raven Press, New York, p 1235–1247

Murphy D L, Tamarkin L, Sunderland T, Garrick N A, Cohen R M 1986 Human plasma melatonin is elevated during treatment with the monoamine oxidase inhibitors clorgyline and tranylcypromine but not deprenyl. Psychiatry Research 17: 119–127

Murphy D L, Mueller E A, Hill J L, Tolliver T J, Jacobsen F M 1989 Comparative anxiogenic, neuroendocrine, and other physiologic effects of m-chlorophenylpiperazine given intravenously or orally to healthy volunteers. Psychopharmacology 98: 275–282

Nemeroff C B, Widerlov E, Bissette G et al 1984 Elevated concentrations of corticotropin-releasing factor-like immunoreactivity in depressed patients. Science 226: 1342–1344

Nemeroff C B, Owens M J, Bissette G, Andorn A C, Stanley M 1988 Reduced corticotropin releasing factor binding sites in the frontal cortex of suicide victims. Archives of General Psychiatry 45: 577–579

Ng L K Y, Chase T N, Colburn R W, Kopin I J 1972 Release of ^{3}H-dopamine by L-5-hydroxytryptophan. Brain Research 45: 499–505

Nurnberger J I Jr, Gershon E S, Jimerson D C et al 1982 Behavioural, biochemical and neuroendocrine responses to amphetamine in normal twins and 'well state' bipolar patients. Psychoneuroendocrinology 7: 163–176

Nurnberger J I Jr, Jimerson D C, Simmons-Alling S et al 1983 Behavioural, physiological, and neuroendocrine responses to arecoline in normal twins and 'well state' bipolar patients. Psychiatry Research 9: 191–200

Nurnberger J I Jr, Berrettini W, Mendelson W, Sack D, Gershon E S 1989a Measuring cholinergic sensitivity: I. Arecoline effects in bipolar patients. Biological Psychiatry 25: 610–617

Nurnberger J I Jr, Berrettini W, Simmons-Alling S, Lawrence D, Brittain H 1989b Blunted ACTH and cortisol response to afternoon tryptophan infusion in euthymic bipolar patients. Psychiatry Research 31: 57–67

Owen F, Cross A J, Crow T J et al 1983 Brain 5-HT$_2$ receptors and suicide (letter). Lancet 2: 1256

Pandey G N, Dysken M W, Garver D L, Davis J M 1979 Beta-adrenergic receptor function in affective illness. American Journal of Psychiatry 136: 675–678

Pandey G N, Sudershan P, Davis J M 1985 Beta adrenergic receptor functon in depression and the effect of antidepressant drugs. Acta Pharmacologica et Toxicologica 56(suppl 1): 66–79

Pandey G N, Pandey S C, Janicak P G, Marks R C, Davis J M 1990 Platelet serotonin-2 receptor binding sites in depression and suicide. Biological Psychiatry 28: 215–222

Pare C M B, Trenchard A, Turner P 1974 5-hydroxytryptamine in depression. Advances in Biochemical Psychopharmacology 11: 275–279

Parent A, Descarries L, Beaudet A 1981 Organization of ascending serotonin neurons in the adult rat brain. A radioautographic study after intraventricular administration of [^{3}H]5-hydroxytryptamine. Nueroscience 6: 115–138

Pazos A, Probst A, Palacios J M 1982 β-adrenoreceptor subtypes in the human brain: autoradiographic localization. Brain Research 358: 324–328

Penalva A, Villanueuva L, Casanueva F, Cavagnini F, Gomez-Pan A, Muller E E 1983 Cholinergic and histaminergic involvement in the growth hormone releasing effect of an enkephalin analogue FK 33824 in man. Psychopharmacology 80: 120–124

Pepitoni S, Borkowski J, Mallon R, McQuade R D 1990 Expression of 5 human muscarinic receptor subtypes in HeLa cells. Society for Neuroscience, 20th Annual Meeting, Abstract 92.18, Part I, p 204

Peroutka S J 1988 5-hydroxytryptamine receptor subtypes: molecular, biochemical and physiological characterization. Trends in the Neurosciences 11: 496–500

Perry S W 1990 Organic mental disorders caused by HIV: update on early diagnosis and treatment. American Journal of Psychiatry 147: 696–710

Perry E K, Marshall E F, Blessed G, Tomlinson B E, Perry R H 1983 Decreased imipramine binding in the brains of patients with depressive illness. British Journal of Psychiatry 142: 188–192

Pert C B, Snyder S H 1973 Opiate receptor: demonstration in nervous tissue. Science 179: 1011–1014

Piletz J E, Schubert D S P, Halaris A 1986 Evaluation of studies on platelet alpha$_2$ adrenoreceptors in depressive illness. Life Sciences 39: 1589–1616

Piletz J E, Halaris A, Saran A, Marler M 1990 Elevated ^{3}H-para-aminoclonidine binding to platelet purified plasma membranes from depressed patients. Neuropsychopharmacology 3: 201–210

Post R M, Kopin J, Goodwin F K 1974 The effects of cocaine on depressed patients. American Journal of Psychiatry 131: 511–517

Pozuelo J 1976 Suppression of craving and withdrawal in humans addicted to narcotics or amphetamines by administration of alpha-methyl-para-tyrosine (AMPT) and 5-butylpicolinic acid (fusaric acid) Cleveland Clinic Quarterly 43: 89–94

Price L H, Charney D S, Heninger G R 1985 Effects of tranylcypromine treatment on neuroendocrine, behavioural and autonomic response to tryptophan in depressed patients. Life Sciences 37: 809–818

Price L H, Charney D S, Heninger G R 1986 Effects of trazodone treatment on alpha-2-adrenoreceptor function in depressed patients. Psychopharmacology 89: 38–44

Price L H, Charney D S, Delgado P L, Heninger G R 1989a Lithium treatment and serotonergic function: neuroendocrine, behavioural, and physiologic responses to intravenous L-tryptophan in affective disorder patients. Archives of General Psychiatry 46: 13–19

Price L H, Charney D S, Delgado P L, Heninger G R 1989b Effects of desipramine and fluvoxamine treatment on the prolactin response to L-tryptophan: a test of the serotonergic function enhancement hypothesis of depression. Archives of General Psychiatry 46: 625–631

Price L H, Charney D S, Delgado P L et al 1990 Clinical data on the role of serotonin in the mechanism(s) of action of antidepressant drugs. Journal of Clinical Psychiatry 51(4 suppl): 44–50

Rausch J L, Shah N S, Burch E A Donald A G 1982 Platelet serotonin uptake in depressed patients: circadian effect. Biological Psychiatry 17: 121–123

Redmond D E 1987 Studies of the nucleus locus coeruleus in monkeys and hypotheses for neuropsychopharmacology. In: Meltzer H Y (ed) Psychopharmacology: the third generation of progress. Raven Press, New York, p 967–975

Riley C J, Shaw D M 1976 Total and nonbound tryptophan in unipolar illness. Lancet 2: 1249

Risch S C 1982 Beta-endorphin hypersecretion in depression: possible cholinergic mechanism. Biological Psychiatry 17: 1071–1079

Risch S C, Janowski D S, Judd L J et al 1982 Correlated cholinomimetic-stimulated beta-endorphin and prolactin release in humans. Peptides 3: 319–322

Robertson A G, Jackman H, Meltzer H Y 1984 Prolactin response to morphine in depression. Psychiatry Research 11: 353–364

Robinson R G, Chait R M 1985 Emotional correlates of structural brain injury with particular emphasis on post-stroke mood disorders. Critical Reviews in Clinical Neurobiology 1(4): 285–318

Robinson D S, Rickels K, Feighner J et al 1990 Clinical effects of the 5-HT$_{1A}$ partial agonists in depression: a composite analysis of buspirone in the treatment of depression. Journal of Clinical Psychopharmacology 10(3 suppl): 67S–76S

Rose W C, Haines W J, Warner D T 1954 The amino acid requirements of man. Journal of Biological Chemistry 206(1): 421–430

Ross S B, Aperia B, Beck-Friis J, Jansa S, Wetterberg L, Aberg A 1980 Inhibition of 5-hydroxytryptamine uptake in human platelets by antidepressant agents in vivo. Psychopharmacology 67: 1–7

Roth R H, Wolf M E, Deutch A Y 1987 Neurochemistry of midbrain dopamine systems. In: Meltzer H Y (ed) Psychopharmacology: the third generation of progress. Raven Press, New York, p 81–94

Roy A, Virkkunen M, Linnoila M 1990 Serotonin in suicide, violence, and alcoholism. In: Coccaro E F, Murphy D L (eds) Serotonin in major psychiatric disorders. American Psychiatric Press, Washington, DC, p 187–208

Rubinow D R, Gold P W, Post R M et al 1983 CSF somatostatin in affective illness. Archives of General Psychiatry 40: 409–412

Rubinow D R, Davis C L, Post R M 1988 Somatostatin in neuropsychiatric disorders. Progress in Neuro-Psychopharmacology and Biological Psychiatry 12: S137–S155

Sachar E J 1973 Endocrine factors in psychopathological states. In: Mendels J (ed) Biological psychiatry. John Wiley, New York, p 175–197

Sachar E J, Asnis G, Nathan R S, Halbreich U, Tabrizi M A, Halpern F S 1980 Dextroamphetamine and cortisol in depression. Archives of General Psychiatry 37: 55–757

Sachar E J, Puig-Antich J, Ryan N D et al 1985 Three tests of cortisol secretion in adult endogenous depression. Acta Psychiatrica Scandinavica 71: 1–8

Sack R L, Goodwin F K 1974 Inhibition of dopamine-β-hydroxylase in manic patients. A clinical trial with fusaric acid. Archives of General Psychiatry 31: 649–654

Schildkraut J J 1965 The catecholamine hypothesis of affective disorders: a review of supporting evidence. American. Journal of Psychiatry 122: 509–522

Schlake H-P, Kuhs H, Rolf L H et al 1989 Platelet 5-HT transport in depressed patients under double-blind treatment with paroxetine versus amitryptline. Acta Psychiatrica Scandinavica 80(suppl 350): 149–151

Shapira B, Reiss A, Kaiser N, Kindler S, Lerer B 1989 Effect of imipramine treatment on the prolactin response to fenfluramine and placebo challenge in depressed patients. Journal of Affective Disorders 16: 1–4

Shapira B, Lerer B, Litchenberg P, Kindler S, Calev A 1990 Serotonergic responsivity in major depression. American Psychiatric Association 143rd Annual Meeting, New York, NY, New Research Abstract 413

Shaw D M, Tidmarsh S F, Johnson A L, Michalakeas A C, Riely G T, Blazek R, Francis A F 1978 Multicompartmental analysis of amino acids: II. Tryptophan in affective disorders. Psychological Medicine 8: 487–494

Shibahara S, Morimoto Y, Furutani Y et al 1983 Isolation and sequence analysis of the human corticotropin-releasing factor precursor gene. EMBO Journal 2: 775–779

Shopsin B, Gershon S, Goldstein M, Friedman E, Wilk S 1975 Use of synthesis inhibitors in defining a role for biogenic amines during imipramine treatment in depressed patients. Psychopharmacology Communications 1: 239–249

Shopsin B, Friedman E, Gershon S 1976 Parachlorophenylalanine reversal of tranylcypromine effects in depressed patients. Archives of General Psychiatry 33: 811–891

Siever L J 1987 Role of noradrenergic mechanisms in the etiology of the affective disorders. In: Meltzer HY (ed) Psychopharmacology: the third generation of progress. Raven Press, New York, p 493–504

Siever L J, Davis K L 1985 Overview: toward a dysregulation hypothesis of depression. American Journal of Psychiatry 142: 1017–1031

Siever L J, Uhde T W, Insel T R, Roy B F, Murphy D L 1982b Growth hormone response to clonidine unchanged by chronic clorgyline treatment. Psychiatry Research 7: 139–144

Siever L J, Kafka M S, Insel T R, Lake C R, Murphy D C 1984a Effect of clorgyline administration on human platelet alpha-adrenergic receptor binding and platelet cyclic AMP responses. Psychiatry Research 9: 37–44

Siever L J, Murphy D L, Slater S, de la Vega E, Lipper S 1984b Plasma prolactin changes following fenfluramine in depressed patients compared to controls: an evaluation of central serotonergic responsivity in depression. Life Sciences 34: 1029–1039

Siever L J, Uhde T W, Jimerson D L, Lake C R, Kopin I J, Murphy D L 1986 Indices of noradrenergic output in depression. Psychiatry Research 19: 59–73

Siever L J, Uhde T W, Silberman E K et al 1982a Growth hormone response to clonidine as a probe of noradrenergic receptor responsiveness in affective disorder patients and controls. Psychiatry Research 6: 171–183

Siteram N, Gillin J C 1980 Development and use of probes of the CNS in man: evidence of cholinergic abnormality in primary affective illness. Biological Psychiatry 15: 925–955

Sitaram N, Wyatt R J, Dawson S, Gillin J C 1976 REM sleep induction by physostigmine infusion during sleep. Science 191: 1281–1283

Sitaram N, Nurnberger J I, Gershon E S, Gillin J C 1980 Faster cholinergic REM sleep induction in euthymic patients with primary affective illness. Science 208: 200–202

Sitaram N, Moore A M, Vanskiver C et al 1981 Hypersensitive cholinergic functioning in primary affective illness. In: Pepeu G (ed) Cholinergic mechanisms. Raven Press, New York, p 947–962

Smith S E, Pihl R O, Young S W, Ervin F R 1987 A test of possible cognitive and environmental influences on the mood lowering effect of tryptophan depletion in normal males. Psychopharmacology 91: 451–457

Soderpalm B, Andersson L, Carlsson M, Modigh K, Eriksson E 1987 Serotonergic influence on the growth hormone response to clonidine in the rat. Journal of Neural Transmission 69: 105–114

Spampinato S, Locatelli V, Cocchi D et al 1979 Serotonin in the prolactin-releasing effect of opioid peptides. Endocrinology 105: 163–170

Speiss J, Rivier J, Rivier C, Vale W 1981 Primary structure of corticotropin-releasing factor from ovine hypothalamus. Proceedings of the National Academy of Sciences of the USA 78: 6517–6521

Stanley M, Mann J J 1983 Increased serotonin-2 binding sites in frontal cortex of suicide victims. Lancet 1: 214–216

Stanley M, Virgilio J, Gershon S 1982 Tritiated imipramine binding sites are decreased in the cortex of suicides. Science 216: 1337–1339

Stenfors C, Theordorsson E, Mathe A A 1989 Effect of repeated electroconvulsive treatment on regional concentrations of tachykinins, neurotensin, vasoactive intestinal polypeptide, neuropeptide Y, and galanin in rat brain. Journal of Neuroscience Research 24: 445–450

Suda H, Takeuchi T, Nagatsu T et al 1969 Inhibition of dopamine-β-hydroxylase by 5-akylpicolinic acid and their hypotensive effects. Chemistry and Pharmacy Bullitin 17: 2377

Sweet R D, Bruun R, Shapiro E, Shapira A K 1974 Presynaptic catecholamine antagonists as treatment for Tourette syndrome. Archives of General Psychiatry 31: 857–861

Taylor A L, Fishman L M 1988 Corticotropin-releasing hormone. New England Journal of Medicine 319: 213–222

Theodorou A E, Katona C L E, Davies S L et al 1989 ^{3}H-imipramine binding to freshly prepared platelet membranes in depression. Psychiatry Research 29: 87–103

Tolis G, Dent R, Gupta H 1978 Opiates, prolactin and the dopamine receptor. Journal of Clinical Endocrinology and Metabolism 47: 200–203

Tuomisto J 1974 A new model for studying 5-HT uptake by blood platelets: a re-evaluation of tricyclic antidepressants as uptake inhibitors. Journal of Pharmacy and Pharmacology 26: 92–100

Tuomisto J, Tukiainen E 1976 Depressed uptake of 5-hydroxytryptamine in blood platelets from depressed patients. Nature 262: 596–598

Tuomisto J, Tukiainen E, Ahlfors U G 1979 Decreased uptake of 5-hydroxytryptamine in blood platelets from depressed patients with endogenous depression. Psychopharmacology 65: 141–147

Vale W, Spiess, Rivier C, Rivier J 1981 Characterization of a 41-residue ovine hypothalamic peptide that stimulates secrétion of corticotropin and beta endorphin. Science 213: 1394–1397

Van Berkestijn H, Mulder-Hajonides van der Meulen L, Flentge F, Dols L, van den Hoofdakker R 1990 RS-86 in manic disorder. Biological Psychiatry 27: 109–112

Van de Kar L D, Karteszi M, Bethea C L, Ganong W F 1985 Serotonergic stimulation of prolactin and corticosterone secretion is mediated by different pathways from the mediobasal hypothalamus. Neuroendocrinology 41: 380–384

Von Bardeleben U, Stalla G K, Muller O A, Holsboer F 1988 Blunting of ACTH response to human CRF in depressed patients is avoided by metyrapone pretreatment. Biological Psychiatry 24: 782–786

Vecsei L, Widerlöv E 1988 Brain and CSF somatostatin concentrations in patients with psychiatric or neurological illness: An overview. Acta Psychiatrica Scandinavica 78: 657–667

Wachtel H 1989 Dysbalance of neuronal second messenger function in the aetiology of affective disorders: a pathophysiological concept hypothesising defects beyond first messenger receptors, Journal of Neural Transmission 75: 21–29

Wahlstedt C, Blendy J A, Kellar K J, Heilig M, Widerlöv E, Ekman R 1990 Electroconvulsive shocks increase the concentration of neocortical and hippocampal neuropeptide Y (NPY)-like immunoreactivity in the rat. Brain Research 507: 65–68

Weizman A, Mark M, Gil-Ad I, Tyano S, Laron Z 1988 Plasma cortisol, prolactin, growth hormone and immunoreactive β-endorphin response to fenfluramine challenge in depressed patients. Clinical Neuropharmacology 11: 250–256

Wetterberg L 1983 The relationship between the pineal gland and the pituitary-adrenal-axis in health, endocrine, and psychiatric conditions. Psychoneuroendocrinology 8: 75–80

Widerlöv E, Wahlestedt C, Håkanson R, Ekman R 1986 Altered brain neuropeptide function in psychiatric illness-with special emphasis on NPY and CRF in major depression. Clinical Neuropharmacology 9(suppl 4): 572–574

Widerlöv E, Bissette G, Nemeroff C B 1988a Monoamine metabolites, corticotropin releasing factor and somatostatin as CSF markers in depressed patients. Journal of Affective Disorders 14: 99–107

Widerlöv E, Lindstrom L H, Wahlestedt C, Ekman R 1988b Neuropeptide Y and peptide YY as possible cerebrospinal markers for major depression and schizophrenia, respectively. Journal of Psychiatric Research 22: 69–79

Widerlöv E, Heilig M, Ekman R, Wahlestedt C 1989 Neuropeptide Y- possible involvement in depression and anxiety. In: Mutt V, Fuxe K, Hokefelt T (eds) Nobel Conference on NPY. Raven Press, New York, p 331–342

Wilcox J A 1983 Psychoactive properties of benztropine and trihexphenidyl. Journal of Psychoactive Drugs 15: 319–321

Willner P 1983 Dopamine and depression: a review of recent evidence. III. The effects of antidepressant treatments. Brain Research Reviews 6: 237–246

Winokur A, Lindberg N D, Lucki I, Phillips J, Amsterdam J D 1986 Hormonal and behavioural effects associated with intravenous L-tryptophan administration. Psychopharmacology 88: 213–219

Wood K, Coppen A 1982 Alpha₂ adrenergic receptors in depression. Lancet 1: 1121–1122

Wood P L, Suranyi-Cadotte B E, Nair N P V, LaFaille F, Schwartz G 1983 Lack of association between ^{3}H-imipramine binding sites and uptake of serotonin in control, depressed, and schizophrenic patients. Neuropharmacology 22: 1211–1214

Woodward D J, Moises H C, Waterhouse B D, Hoffer B J, Freedman R 1979 Modulating actions of norepinephrine in the central nervous system. Federation Proceedings 38: 2109–2116

Young V R, Hussein M A, Murray E, Scrimshaw N S 1969 Tryptophan intake, spacing of meals, and diurnal fluctuations of plasma tryptophan in men. American Journal of Clinical Nutrition 22: 1563–1567

Young V R, Hussein M A, Murray E, Scrimshaw N S 1971 Plasma tryptophan response curve and its relation to tryptophan requirements in young adult men. Journal of Nutrition 101: 45–60

Young S N, Smith S E, Pihl R, Ervin F R 1985 Tryptophan depletion causes a rapid lowering of mood in normal males. Psychopharmacology 87: 173–177

Young S N, Ervin F R, Pihl R O, Finn P 1989 Biochemical

aspects of tryptophan depletion in primates. Psychopharmacology 98: 508–511

Zis A P 1988 Opiodergic regulation of hypothalamo-pituitary-adrenal function in depression and Cushing's disease: an interim report. Psychoneuroendocrinology 13: 419–430

Zis A, Goodwin F K 1982 The amine hypothesis. In: Paykel E (ed) Handbook of affective disorders. Guilford Press, New York, p 175–190

Zis A P, Haskett R F, Albala A A, Carroll B J, Lohr N E 1985a Prolactin response to morphine in depression. Biological Psychiatry 20: 287–292

Zis A P, Haskett R F, Albala A A, Carroll B J Lohr N E 1985b Cortisol escape from morphine suppression. Psychiatry Research 15: 91–95

Zis A P, Haskett R F, Albala A A, Carroll B J Lohr N E 1985c Opioid regulation of hypothalamic-pituitary-adrenal function in depression. Archives of General Psychiatry 42: 383–386

16. Neuroendocrinology

Stuart Checkley

In biological psychiatry it is necessary to distinguish between aetiology, pathogenesis and the mechanism of action of effective treatments. Aetiology refers to the genetic and environmental factors which predispose an individual towards developing a specific illness. Pathogenesis refers to the biological processes which underlie the state of the illness. It is quite possible that different systems in different parts of the brain are involved in aetiology and pathogenesis and it is equally possible that therapeutic drug action involves quite separate systems again. This chapter will review neuroendocrine studies of the aetiology and pathogenesis of depression and will briefly look at neuroendocrine studies of the mechanism of action of antidepressant drugs.

NEUROENDOCRINE STUDIES OF THE AETIOLOGY OF DEPRESSION

The principal aetiological factors behind depressive illness are genetic predisposition, environmental stress and the interaction between the two. The biology of stress is a large subject and it is not certain how it results in the triggering of depression in predisposed individuals. However adrenal steroids are released in response to stress and steroid hormones are known to regulate the expression of genes: it has therefore been argued (Checkley 1991) that life events may interact with genetic predisposition through the genomic actions of stress-sensitive steroid hormones. In this section the possibility will be discussed that the aetiological effects of Cushing's syndrome, myxoedema and the postpartum state are also mediated by the genomic effects of hormones.

Cushing's syndrome

Symptoms of depression were included in the earliest descriptions of Cushing's syndrome (Cushing 1932) and subsequent studies using standardized diagnostic interviews have shown that depression is seen in roughly half of all patients with Cushing's syndrome (Jeffcoate et al 1979, Cohen 1980, Kelly et al 1980).

When Cushing's syndrome is corrected the associated depression is alleviated in most although not all cases (Jeffcoate et al 1979, Kelly et al 1983). This provides some evidence that the Cushing's syndrome triggered the depression rather than the depression triggering the Cushing's syndrome. Cushing's disease is the commonest form of Cushing's syndrome and is due to the autonomous production of ACTH, which results in high plasma concentrations of ACTH and cortisol. In adrenal carcinoma the autonomous production of corticosteroids suppresses the production of ACTH. The fact that depression is seen in adrenal carcinoma (Kelly et al 1980) suggests that it is the cortisol rather than the ACTH which causes depression. The same conclusion can be drawn from the fact that in Nelson's syndrome the high ACTH but absent corticosteroid levels which occur are not associated with depression (Kelly et al 1980). Further evidence for this conclusion comes from the observation that metyrapone, which inhibits the synthesis of cortisol, has an antidepressant effect in Cushing's syndrome even though ACTH levels rise under those circumstances (Jeffcoate et al 1979). For all of these reasons it would appear to be the corticosteroids which trigger the onset of depression. How might they do it?

Corticosteroids bind to two classes of receptor in the brain: type I receptors, which preferentially bind mineralocorticoids and the naturally occurring corticosteroids, and type II receptors, which preferentially bind the synthetic glucocorticoids such as dexamethasone (Reul & de Kloet 1986). The development of learned helplessness in animals depends upon the activation of type II receptors and can be prevented by pretreatment with selective type II antagonists (de Kloet et al 1988).

When type II antagonists can be given to man it will be possible to test the hypothesis that depression in Cushing's syndrome results from the activation of type II corticosteroids.

Interaction between thyroid hormones and mood

Frank psychosis has long been known to co-exist with myxoedema (Clinical Society of London 1888) and, in more recent studies, depression and cognitive defects have been the most common abnormalities. In most early cases thyroid replacement corrects the psychiatric abnormality, suggesting that the two are causally related (Whybrow et al 1969). Although thyrotoxicosis has been reported in association with manic depressive illness the association may have been due to chance as patients have been described with multiple and unrelated episodes of thyrotoxicosis and manic depressive illness (Checkley 1978). A more convincing example of an effect of thyroid hormones on mood is the ability of triiodothyronine to potentiate the effect of tricyclic antidepressants in patients with endogenous depression (Goodwin et al 1982).

The mechanisms by which thyroid hormones affect mood is not known. However thyroid hormones exert most of their biological effects at the gene and so it is possible that such a genomic action explains their effects upon mood.

Puerperal psychosis

Whereas bereavement may cause a fourfold increase in the incidence of depression, childbirth is followed by a 20-fold increase in the likelihood of psychosis over the ensuing months (Kendell et al 1987). Most of these psychoses are affective disorders (Meltzer & Kumar 1985), but whether this dramatic increase in the incidence of psychosis is due to endocrine or psychological factors is not known. However in an ongoing study we have found that adverse life events are associated with an increased incidence of unipolar depression but not of bipolar affective disorders, in the postpartum period (Marks, Wieck, Checkley and Kumar unpublished data). A biochemical basis may therefore be needed to explain the triggering of bipolar affective disorder in the postpartum period.

Plasma and, presumably, brain concentrations of the sex steroids oestrogen and progesterone fall 100-fold in the first postpartum week (Willcox et al 1980). For the

following reasons these changes are the most likely endocrine trigger for affective psychosis:

1) The change in sex steroids is much greater than those in any other hormone in the postpartum period.
2) As sex steroids are lipid-soluble, changes in plasma are associated with similar changes in brain.
3) Changes in brain levels will be detected by sex steroid receptors in limbic forebrain regions (Koch & Ehret 1989) and gene expression in these brain regions will be modified as a result (Beato 1989).
4) The fact that postpartum psychosis sometimes relapses with the onset of the first menstrual period postpartum is also consistent with a steroidal aetiology (Brockington et al 1988).
5) So too is a preliminary report that postpartum psychosis can be prevented by treatment with oestrogen and testosterone (Hamilton 1982).

Changes in brain oestrogen receptors have been found in animals studied postpartum (Koch & Ehret 1989) and we have found neuroendocrine evidence of similar changes in man (Bearn et al 1990). The oestrogen-sensitive neurophysin (ESN) response to ethinyl oestradiol depends on the stimulation of central oestrogen receptors: the response is reduced in the first 2 weeks postpartum at the time of greatest risk for the development of postpartum psychosis (Bearn et al 1990).

If oestrogen withdrawal triggers the onset of postpartum psychosis it would be most likely to do so by sensitizing central dopaminergic systems (Cookson 1982). In women with a previous history of postpartum psychosis we have found that enhanced growth hormone (GH) responses to the dopamine agonist apomorphine on the fourth day postpartum predict the subsequent development of bipolar (but not unipolar) affective illness (Weick et al 1989).

From these clinical studies it would seem likely that, whereas psychosocial factors may influence the incidence of unipolar affective disorder in the postpartum period, endocrine factors may be more important in the triggering of bipolar affective disorder. The hypothesis that bipolar affective disorder is triggered by the effects of sex steroid withdrawal on central dopamine function is supported by our recent data.

NEUROENDOCRINE STUDIES OF THE PATHOGENESIS OF DEPRESSION

In this section will be discussed those neuroendocrine

studies which have shed most light on the neurochemical changes in depression. The hypersecretion of corticotrophin releasing hormone (CRH) is described by Holsboer (Chapter 17) and will not be discussed further. This section is restricted to changes in the secretion of growth hormone, prolactin, thyroid hormones and in the biological rhythms which influence the secretion of these and other hormones.

Growth hormone

Growth hormone (GH) secretion in depression

In Figure 16.1 are shown the principal hormonal factors which influence GH secretion in man and in Figure 16.2 the principal neurotransmitters (Checkley 1980, Dieguez et al 1987)

Healthy resting adults normally only secrete GH at the time of the first episode of slow-wave sleep. In depression the sleep GH secretion has been reported to be normal (Rubin et al 1990) reduced or advanced (Mendlewicz et al 1985). Total GH secretion may be normal (Rubin et al 1990) reduced or phase increased (Mendlewicz et al 1985).

GH responses to clonidine

The GH response to the alpha$_2$ agonist clonidine has been found to be reduced in most although not all studies of patients with endogenous depression (Matussek et al 1980, Checkley et al 1981, Siever et al 1982, Lechin et al 1985, Dolan & Calloway 1986,

Horton et al 1986, Ansseau et al 1988, Lesch et al 1988b, Amsterdam et al 1989). Some of the reports of reduced GH responses could be due to the use of drug-free periods of no more than 3 weeks: these are known to be inadequate (Corn et al 1984b). Other studies have used much longer wash-out periods.

In three studies reduced GH responses to clonidine have also been reported in recovered depressives (Siever et al 1986, Mitchell et al 1988, Matussek 1988).

GH responses to desipramine

Although not studied in as much detail as the GH response to clonidine, reduced GH responses to desipramine have also been reported in depressed patients (Laakmann 1980, Calil et al 1984, Meesters et al 1985, Ryan et al 1988). Since the GH response to desipramine is blocked by alpha$_2$ antagonists (Laakmann et al 1986) it is reasonable to assume that it involves the same central alpha$_2$-adrenoceptors as does the GH response to clonidine. However, the GH response to another alpha$_2$ agonist, guanfacine, has been reported to be normal in patients with endogenous depression (Eriksson et al 1988) and this paradoxical finding calls for further study.

GH responses to apomorphine

Although most studies have reported normal GH responses to apomorphine in endogenous depression

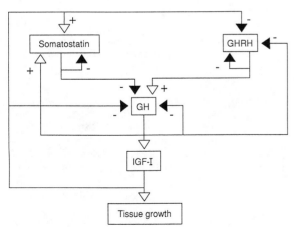

Fig. 16.1 Hormonal control of growth hormone (GH) secretion in man
GHRH = growth hormone releasing hormone; IGF - I = insulin like growth factor I (also called somatostatin C)
For references see Dieguez et al 1987

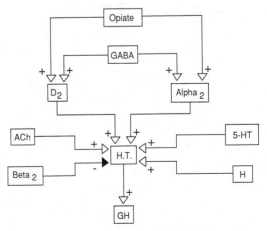

Fig. 16.2 Neurotransmitter control of GH secretion in man. D$_2$ = dopamine D$_2$ receptor; ACh = acetylcholine; H = histamine; H.T. = hypothalamus
For references see Checkley 1980 and Dieguez et al 1987

(Frazer 1975, Casper et al 1977, Corn et al 1984a, Jimerson et al 1984, Meltzer et al 1984), one of the best controlled studies (Ansseau et al 1988) reported reduced responses.

GH responses to growth hormone releasing hormone (GHRH)

Lesch has reported in detail on two samples of depressed patients both of whom have had reduced GH responses to GHRH. In one sample plasma somatomedin C concentrations were raised (Lesch et al 1988b) and significant correlations were found between GH responses to GHRH and the GH response to clonidine (Lesch et al 1988b). In the other sample plasma concentrations of insulin-like growth factor I (IGF-I) were raised and again reduced GH responses to GHRH were found (Lesch et al 1988a).

Neuhauser & Laakmann (1988) have also reported reduced GH responses to GHRH but others have reported normal responses (Eriksson et al 1988, Krishnan et al 1988, Thomas et al 1989). The negative studies were large and well conducted and it is not at present clear why there is disagreement concerning the GH responses to apomorphine and GHRH in depression.

GH secretion in depression: conclusions

1) The GH responses to clonidine and desipramine are reduced in depressed patients, particularly in those with endogenous depression. This finding is not specific to depression, being found also in obsessive compulsive disorder, agoraphobia and chronic schizophrenia.

2) Some but not all of these findings could be due to insufficiently long drug-free wash-out periods.

3) As the GH responses to clonidine and desipramine all involve the stimulation of alpha$_2$-adrenoceptors and as both are reduced in depression it is possible that there is a defect at central alpha$_2$-adrenoceptors in the neuroendocrine system. However, normal responses to guanfacine have been found in one study (Eriksson et al 1988).

4) In some of these studies significant correlations have been reported in depressed patients between the size of the GH response to GHRH and the size of the GH response to clonidine (Lesch et al 1988b) and to desipramine (Neuhauser & Laakmann 1988). It is therefore possible that the reduced GH responses to alpha$_2$-adrenoceptor stimulation are due to a generalized failure in the responsiveness of GH secretion to GHRH.

5) Raised plasma concentrations of insulin-like growth factor I (IGF-I) have been reported in depression and as these levels correlated with the size of the GH response to GHRH (Lesch et al 1988a) it is possible that raised IGF-I levels restrain GH responses to GHRH and other stimuli in depression. Reports of raised plasma concentrations of IGF-I would be consistent with GH hypersecretion but this is not consistently found in depressed patients (Rubin et al 1990). Raised plasma concentrations of IGF-I would, if replicated, explain the various reports of reduced GH secretion in depression but the cause of IGF-I hypersecretion remains unknown.

Prolactin secretion in depression

The principal influences on prolactin secretion in man are shown in Figure 16.3. The various components of this system have been investigated in depression in the following ways.

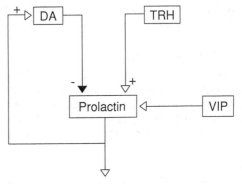

Fig 16.3   Control of prolactin secretion in man
DA = dopamine; TRH = thyrotropin releasing hormone; VIP = vasoactive intestinal polypeptide

1. 24-hour secretion of prolactin

The most recent and best controlled studies of prolactin secretion report normal values in depressed patients (Jarrett et al 1987, Unden et al 1987, Baumgartner et al 1988, Linkowski et al 1988, Rubin et al 1989).

2. The prolaction response to thyrotrophin releasing hormone (TRH)

TRH is a hypothalamic hormone which stimulates the pituitary secretion of prolactin: the prolactin response to TRH may be normal in depression (Zis et al 1986,

Unden et al 1987, Baumgartner et al 1988, Roy & Pickar 1988, Rubin et al 1989).

3. Prolactin responses to dopamine agonist or antagonist drugs

Dopamine is thought to be the hypothalamic hormone which inhibits prolactin secretion. The prolactin response to the dopamine agonists apomorphine (Jimerson et al 1984, Meltzer et al 1984), piribedil (Joffe et al 1986) and methylphenidate (Joyce et al 1986) are normal in depression. However, the prolactin response to the dopamine antagonist metoclopramide (Joyce et al 1987) is increased, at least in bipolar patients.

The prolactin response to sulpiride is probably normal in unipolar depression (Kaneko et al 1986). Thus in unipolar depression basal prolactin secretion is probably normal, as is the response of prolactin to manipulation of the hypothalamic hormones TRH and dopamine.

Tryptophan is the natural precursor of 5-hydroxytryptamine (5-HT) and the best studied neuroendocrine probe of 5-HT function is the prolactin response to tryptophan. This response in man is increased by the 5-HT uptake inhibitor clomipramine (Anderson & Cowen 1986); it is reduced by the non-selective 5-HT antagonist methysergide (McCance et al 1987) but it is unchanged by selective $5-HT_2$ and $5-HT_3$ antagonists (Charig et al 1986). For these reasons the prolactin response to tryptophan is thought to depend upon the stimulation of one or more classes of $5-HT_1$-receptors.

The fact that the prolactin response to tryptophan is reduced in depressed patients (Heninger et al 1984, Cowen & Charig 1987) can therefore be interpreted as evidence of altered 5-HT receptor function.

The same conclusion can be drawn from the findings in depression of reduced prolactin responses to fenfluramine (Siever et al 1984, Weizman et al 1988, Coccaro et al 1989, Mitchell & Smythe 1990) and to clomipramine (Golden et al 1990).

Prolactin responses to opiate agonists

Reduced prolactin responses to the stimulation of opiate receptors have been reported in some (Extein et al 1980, Robertson et al 1984, Banki & Arato 1987) but not all (Zis et al 1985, Frecska et al 1989, Matussek & Hoehe 1989) studies of depressed patients. However the effects of opiates on prolactin are mediated through dopamine and 5-HT (Muller & Nistico 1989) and so any reduced prolactin response to opiate drugs in depression could be explained by a 5-HT defect. Indeed, virtually all of the changes in prolactin secretion in unipolar depression can at present be explained by a defect in central 5-HT neurotransmission.

Depression and changes in the hypothalamic–pituitary–thyroid axis

Control of the hypothalamic–pituitary–thyroid (HRT) axis is shown in Figure 16.4. Depression is associated with changes at each point in the axis.

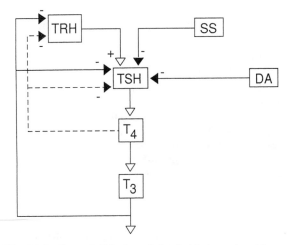

Fig. 16.4 Control of the hypothalamic–pituitary–thyroid axis in man
TRH = thyrotropin releasing hormone; SS = somatostatin; TSH = thyroid stimulating hormone or thyrotropin; DA = dopamine; T_4 = thyroxin which is metabolized to T_3 = triiodothyronin

1) CSF concentrations of thyrotropin releasing hormone (TRH) are raised in some depressed patients (Banki et al 1988).

2) Plasma concentrations of thyroid stimulating hormone (TSH) are reduced in depression (Rubin et al 1987).

3) The TSH response to TRH is reduced in depressed patients (Loosen et al 1987).

4) Plasma concentrations of thyroxine (T4) and triiodothyromine (T3) are reduced in some depressed patients (see below).

5) Increased titres of antithyroid antibodies are found in about a fifth of all depressed patients (see below).

Antithyroid antibodies

The incidence of detectable antimicrosomal and antithyroglobulin antibodies in depressed patients may be double that in the general population (Nemeroff et al 1985, Haggerty et al 1987). However, as most patients with such abnormal antibody titres have normal thyroid function it is hard to relate this abnormality to the other thyroid abnormalities in depression.

Plasma concentrations of thyroxine (T4) and triiodothyromine (T3)

Small reductions in plasma concentrations of T3 have been reported in most of the recent and better controlled studies of thyroid function in depression (Kjellman et al 1983, Sternbach et al 1985, Rubin et al 1987, Rao et al 1989, Rupprecht et al 1989, Wang & Shin 1989).

As plasma concentrations of free T4 and indirect measures of this are usually normal, the low T3 levels could be due to a reduced metabolic conversion of T4 to T3. Such changes have been described in fasted healthy volunteers and in patients with anorexia nervosa. Further studies are needed, but at present it would seem that weight loss might explain low plasma concentrations of T3 in depression.

Plasma concentrations of TSH

The measurement of basal TSH concentration is difficult as baseline values are close to the sensitivity of most of the available assays. This may explain why reduced plasma concentrations of TSH have only been found in those studies which assayed the results of multiple baseline estimations (Rubin et al 1987). As T3 inhibits the secretion of TRH it is presumably the case that the depressed individuals with low TSH levels are different from the patients with low T3 levels.

The TSH response to TRH

Some 40 published studies have reported a small reduction in the TSH response to TRH in depression. The finding is by no means specific to depression and has also been reported, though less convincingly, in other psychiatric conditions including alcoholism and schizophrenia (Loosen 1987).

TSH treatment is known to 'downregulate' the TRH receptors which mediate the TSH response to TRH (Winokur et al 1983) and, as there is evidence of increased TRH production in depression (Banki et al 1988), this increased secretion of TRH is one possible explanation of the reduced TSH response to TRH.

Cerebrospinal fluid concentrations of TRH in depression

Increased cerebrospinal fluid concentrations of TRH have been found in two studies of endogenous depression (Kierkegaard et al 1979, Banki et al 1988). It cannot be assumed that TRH levels in lumbar CSF are an indication of TRH hypersecretion into the hypothalamic pituitary portal veins.

Conclusions

Relatively small changes have been reported at all points in the hypothalamic pituitary thyroid axis in depression. In some patients:

1) TRH secretion may be increased
2) plasma TSH concentrations are reduced
3) the TSH response to TRH is reduced
4) plasma T3 concentrations are reduced
5) titres of antithyroid antibodies are elevated.

Of these changes, 2) and 3) are causally inter-related and both may be a consequence of 1) although that is not certain. Change 4) could be due to change 5) but could not possibly be related to changes 1)–3). At least two and possibly four separate pathogenetic processes are operative, presumably in different patients. No large well controlled study has investigated 1)–5) in the same patients: clearly this needs to be done.

Neuroendocrine rhythms and depression

The suprachiasmatic nuclei of the hypothalamus contain an endogenous biological rhythm which is apparent even when the nuclei are surgically isolated from the rest of the brain (Turek 1985). The organization of most circadian rhythms depends upon the integrity of these nuclei (Hastings & Herbert 1986). For these reasons it is thought that the suprachiasmatic nuclei are the locus of the master clock which controls neuroendocrine and other biological rhythms.

Circadian rhythms have been described for the hormones ACTH, cortisol and melatonin. 24 hour rhythms have also been described for TSH, prolactin and GH, although in the case of this second group of hormones secretion is linked to the sleep – wake cycle and not to an independent rhythm (Van Cauter 1989).

Studies of neuroendocrine rhythms in depression have recently been reviewed in detail (Checkley 1989). The main conclusions of that review are as follows:

1) The amplitude of ACTH and cortisol secretion is elevated in depression. The onset of HPA activation is phase-advanced in patients with hypercortisolaemia but the offset of HPA activation is equally phase-delayed. The evidence for a phase delay of the entire ACTH/cortisol rhythm is not convincing.

2) The amplitude of the melatonin rhythm may be reduced in depression although this is controversial (Thompson et al 1988). There is some evidence of phase shift of the melatonin rhythm.

In some studies of depressed patients the nocturnal secretion of GH, prolactin and TSH has been found to be disrupted. Such disruption could however be due to the disturbed sleep–wake cycles of these patients and to the fact that the secretion of these three hormones is coupled to sleep.

In summary, neuroendocrine rhythms function impressively well in depressed patients.

The pathogenesis of depression is unlikely to involve a primary disturbance of the suprachiasmatic nuclei: the primary disturbance may, however, be very close to the suprachiasmatic nuclei since depression is more readily entrained to circadian and circannual rhythms than is any other psychiatric or medical disorder (Checkley 1989):

1) 48-hour cycling affective disorders maintain their periodicity under free running conditions. (Dirlich et al 1981): this phenomenon has not been described in the case of other psychiatric illnesses.

2) The diurnal variations of mood in depression may be coupled to the endogenous cortisol rhythm (von Zerssen et al 1985).

3) The regularity of 4 a.m. mood switches in rapid-cycling manic depressives also implies a coupling to a biological clock (Checkley 1989).

4) Seasonal rhythms are more evident in manic depressive disorder than in other psychiatric illness (Checkley 1989).

NEUROENDOCRINE STUDIES OF THE MECHANISM OF ACTION OF ANTIDEPRESSANT DRUGS

For the last 10 years the study of the neuropharmacology of antidepressant drugs has been dominated by the possibility that their therapeutic effects are due to adaptive changes at monoamine receptors. In animals there is strong evidence that chronic treatment with antidepressant drugs results in reduced responsiveness of $beta_1$-, $alpha_2$-, $5\text{-}HT_{1a}$- and $5\text{-}HT_2$-receptors and in an increased responsiveness of $alpha_1$- and dopamine D_2-receptors (Stephenson 1990, Willner 1990). What is not clear is:

1) whether any of these changes occurs in man
2) whether they are functionally significant
3) whether they are causally related to antidepressant response.

Neuroendocrinology has so far provided the most definitive answers to the first two of these questions: the third has yet to be tested.

Neuroendocrine evidence that antidepressant drugs downregulate alpha₂-adrenoceptors

Neuroendocrine evidence that antidepressant drugs downregulate $alpha_2$-adrenoceptors

The GH response to clonidine is a neuroendocrine marker of the responsiveness of hypothalamic $alpha_2$-adrenoceptors (Checkley et al 1986). When depressed patients and healthy volunteers are treated with desipramine for one week the GH response to clonidine is increased possibly due to an increased availability of noradrenaline. With further treatment this initial effect becomes attenuated (Glass et al 1982, Corn et al 1984b). In animals the GH response to clonidine is increased by chronic treatment with the $alpha_2$ antagonist yohimbine and reduced by chronic treatment with clonidine and with imipramine (Eriksson et al 1982). Taken together these studies strongly suggest that the attenuation of the GH response to clonidine by chronic antidepressant treatment in man is due to adaptive change at $alpha_2$-adrenoceptors.

Neuroendocrine evidence that noradrenergic neurotransmission is increased by chronic treatment with antidepressant drugs

The secretion of the pineal hormone melatonin is controlled by a noradrenergic innervation which has pre-junction $alpha_2$-adrenoceptors and postjunctional $alpha_1$- and $beta_1$-adrenoceptors (Klein 1985). The same receptors have been shown to influence the secretion of melatonin in man (Checkley & Palazidou 1988). It follows that the secretion of melatonin is a measure of the net output of this system (Fig. 16.5). If antidepressant treatment results in a net increase in noradrenergic neurotransmission then the secretion of melatonin will be increased.

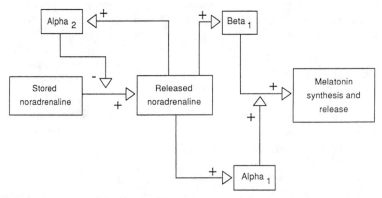

Fig. 16.5 The role of prejunctional alpha$_2$-adrenoceptors and of post-junctional alpha$_1$- and beta$_1$-adrenoceptors in the control of melatonin secretion in man
For references see Checkley & Palazidou 1988

Just such an increase has been found in most studies of the effect of antidepressant treatment on melatonin secretion (Thompson et al 1985, Murphy et al 1986, Sack & Lewy 1986, Bearn et al 1988). Two groups reported a non-significant trend towards an increase (Cowen et al 1985, Frazer et al 1986) but no group has reported that melatonin secretion in man is reduced by chronic treatment with antidepressant drugs. It cannot be assumed that the brain and the pineal react similarly to antidepressants (Fuller & Perry 1977) but, within the pineal gland, noradrenergic neurotransmission is increased by chronic treatment with antidepressant drugs in man.

Though studied in less detail, similar conclusions can be drawn from the effects of antidepressant drugs on the prolactin response to tryptophan. This neuroendocrine marker of 5-HT neurotransmission is also increased when patients are treated with antidepressant drugs for 3 weeks (Charney et al 1984). Whether this change is due to weight change requires further investigation (Cowen et al 1990).

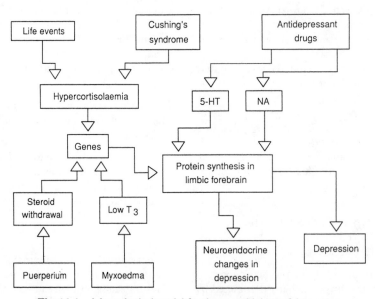

Fig. 16.6 A hypothetical model for the neurobiology of depression

SYNTHESIS

Thus far the neuroendocrine studies of the aetiology, pathogenesis and therapeutics of depression have been discussed separately. Their conclusions can each be summarized in the form of testable hypotheses:

i) that the influences of steroid and thyroid hormones on mood are genomically mediated

ii) that in depression there is a disturbance of hypothalamic function which may either be a disturbance of peptide (CRH, GHRH, TRH) and/or of monoamine (noradrenaline and 5-HT) function

iii) that antidepressant treatments increase monoaminergic neurotransmission.

Whether or not these separate approaches to the neurobiology can be integrated in a unity model is less certain. Given in Figure 16.5 is a speculative model which seeks to integrate these different biological processes. At the left-hand side of the figure are the aetiological factors which are seen to modify protein synthesis in limbic forebrain by genomic action. The pathogenesis of depression lies in this protein synthesis and the neuroendocrinology of depression is one of its consequences. Antidepressant treatments acting through monoamine systems may directly modify the synthesis of these proteins.

REFERENCES

Agren H, Lundqvist G 1984 Low levels of somatostatin in human CSF mark depressive episodes. Psychoneuroendocrinology 9: 233–248

Amsterdam J D, Maisling G, Skolnick B, Berwish N, Winokur A 1989 Multiple hormone responses to clonidine administration in depressed patients and healthy volunteers. Biological Psychiatry 26: 265–278

Anderson I M, Cowen P J 1986 Clomipramine enhances the prolactin responses to L-tryptophan. British Journal of Clinical Pharmacology 22: 216

Ansseau M, Von Frenckell R, Cerfontaine J L, Papart P, Franck G, Timsit-Berthier M, Geenen V, Legros J J 1988 Blunted response of growth hormone to clonidine and apomorphine in endogenous depression. British Journal of Psychiaty 153: 65–71

Banki C M, Arato M 1987 Multiple hormonal responses to morphine: relationship to diagnosis and dexamethasone suppression. Psychoneuroendocrinology 12: 3–11

Banki C M, Bissette G, Arato M, Nemeroff C B 1988 Elevation of immunoreactive CSF TRH in depressed patients. American Journal of Psychiatry 145: 1526–1531

Baumgartner A, Graf K J, Kurten I 1988 Prolactin in patients with major depressive disorder and in healthy subjects. 1. Cross-sectional study of basal and post-TRH and post-dexamethasone prolactin levels. Biological Psychiatry 24: 249–267

Bearn J A, Treasure J, Murphy M, Franey C, Arendt J, Wheeler M, Checkley S A 1988 A Study of sulpha-toxymelatonin excretion and gonadotrophin status during weight gain in anorexia nervosa. British Journal of Psychiatry 152: 372–376

Bearn J A, Fairhall K M, Robinson I F, Lightman S, Checkley S A 1990 Changes in a proposed new neuroendocrine marker of oestrogen receptor function in post-partum women. Psychological Medicine 30: 779–784

Beato M 1989 Gene regulation by steroid hormones. Cell 56: 335–344

Brockington I F, Kelly A, Hall P, Deakin W 1988 Premenstrual relapse of puerperal psychosis. Journal of Affective Disorders 14: 287–292

Calil H M, Lesieur P, Gold P W, Brown G M, Zavadil A P,

Potter W Z 1984 Hormonal responses to zimelidine and desipramine in depressed patients. Psychiatry Research 13: 231–242

Caspar R C, Davis J M, Pandey G N, Garver D, Dekirmenjian H 1977 Neuroendocrine and amine studies in affective illness. Psychoneuroendocrinology 2: 105–114

Charig E M, Anderson I M, Robinson J M, Nutt D J, Cowen P J 1986 L-tryptophan and prolactin release: evidence for interaction between 5-HT$_1$ and 5-HT$_2$ receptors. Human Psychopharmacology 1: 93–97

Charney D S, Heninger G R, Sternberg D E 1984 Serotonin function and mechanism of action of antidepressant treatment. Archives of General Psychiatry 359–365

Checkley S A 1978 Thyrotoxicosis and the course of manic-depressive illness. British Journal of Psychiatry 133: 219–223

Checkley S A 1980 Neuroendocrine test of monoamine function in man: a review of basic theory and its application to the study of depressive illness. Psychological Medicine 10: 35–53

Checkley S A 1989 The relationship between biological rhythms and the affective disorders. In: Arendt J, Minors D S, Waterhouse J M (eds) Biological rhythms in clinical practice, p 160–183

Checkley S A 1990 Neuroendocrine effects of psychotropic drugs. Baillière's Clinical Endocrinology and Metabolism 5: 15–34

Checkley S A 1991 Neuroendocrine mechanisms and the precipitation of depression by life events. British Journal of Psychiatry (in press)

Checkley S A, Palazidou E 1988 Melatonin and antidepressant drugs: clinical pharmacology. In: Miles A, Philbrick D R S, Thompson C (eds) Melatonin clinical perspectives. Oxford University Press, Oxford, p 190–204

Checkley S A, Slade A P, Shur E 1981 Growth hormone and other responses to clonidine in patients with endogenous depression. British Journal of Psychiatry 138: 51–55

Checkley S A, Corn T H, Glass I B, Burton S W, Burke C A 1986 The responsiveness of central alpha$_2$ adrenoceptors in depression. In: Deakin J F W (ed) The biology of depression. Gaskell Publications, London, p 100–120

Clinical Society of London 1888 Report on myxoedema. Transactions of the Clinical Society of London 21 (suppl) 18

Coccaro E F, Siever L J, Klar H M, Maurer G, Cochrane K, Cooper T B, Mohs R C, Davis K L 1989 Serotonergic studies in patients with affective and personality disorders. Correlates with suicidal and impulsive aggressive behaviour. Archives of General Psychiatry 46: 587–599

Cohen S I 1980 Cushing's syndrome: a psychiatric study of 29 patients. British Journal of Psychiatry 136: 120–124

Cookson J 1982 Post-partum psychosis, dopamine and oestrogens. Lancet 2: 672

Corn T H, Hale A S, Thompson C, Bridges P K, Checkley S A 1984a A comparison of the growth hormone response to clonidine and apomorphine in the same patients with endogenous depression. British Journal of Psychiatry 144 636–639

Corn T H, Honig A, Thompson C, Checkley S A 1984b Effects of desipramine treatment upon central adrenoceptor function in normal subjects. British Journal of Psychiatry 144: 139–145

Cowen P J, Charig E M 1987 Neuroendocrine responses to intravenous tryptophan in major depression. Archives of General Psychiatry 44: 958–966

Cowen P J, Green A R, Graham-Smith D G, Braddock L E 1985 Plasma melatonin during desmethylimipramine treatment: evidence for changes in noradrenergic transmission. British Journal of Clinical Pharmacology 19: 799–805

Cowen P J, McCance S L, Gelder M G, Graham-Smith D G 1990 Effect of amitriptyline on endocrine responses to intravenous tryptophan. Psychiatry Research 31: 201–208

Cushing H 1932 The basophil adenomas of the pituitary body and their clinical manifestations (pituitary basophilism) Bulletin of the Johns Hopkins Hospital 50: 137–195

De Kloet E R, De Kock S, Schild V, Veldhuis H D 1988 Antiglucocorticoid RU38486 attenuates retention of a behaviour and disinhibits the hypothalamic-pituitary and adrenal axis at different brain sites. Neuroendocrinology 27: 109–115

Dieguez C, Page M D, Scanlon M F 1987 Growth hormone neuroregulation and its alteration in disease states. Clinical Endocrinology 27: 109–143

Dirlich G, Kammerloher A, Schulz H, Lund R, Doerr P, Von Zerssen D 1981 Temporal co-ordination of rest-activity cycle. Body temperature, urinary free cortisol and mood in a patient with 48-hour unipolar depressive cycles in clinical and time-cue-free environments. Biological Psychiatry 16: 163–179

Dolan R J, Calloway S P 1986 The human growth hormone response to clonidine: relationship to clinical and neuroendocrine profile in depression. American Journal of Psychiatry 143: 772–774

Eriksson E, Eden S, Modigh K 1982 Up- and down-regulation of central postsynaptic alpha$_2$ adrenoceptors reflected in G H response to clonidine in the reserpine treated rat. Psychopharmacology 77: 327

Eriksson E, Balldin J, Linstedt G, Modigh K 1988 Growth hormone responses to the alpha$_2$ adrenoceptors agonist guanfacine and to growth hormone releasing hormone in depressed patients and controls. Psychiatry Research 26: 59–67

Extein I, Pottash A L C, Gold M S, Sweeney D R, Martin D M, Goodwin F K 1980 Deficient prolactin response to morphine in depressed patients. American Journal of Psychiatry 137: 845–846

Frazer A 1975 Adrenergic responses in depression: implications for a receptor defect. In: Mendels J (ed) Biological psychiatry. John Wiley, New York, p 7–26

Frazer A, Brown R, Kocsis J, Caroff S, Amsterdam J, Winokur A, Sweeney J, Stokes P 1986 Patterns of melatonin rhythms in depression. Journal of Neural Transmission (suppl 21): 269–290

Frecska E, Arato M, Banki C M, Mohari K, Perenyi A, Bagdy G, Fekete M I 1989 Prolactin response to fentanyl in depression. Biological Psychiatry 25: 692–696

Fuller R W, Perry K W 1977 Increase of pineal norepinephrine concentration in rats by desipramine but not fluoxetine: implication concerning the specificity of these uptake inhibitors. Journal of Pharmacy and Pharmacology 29: 710–711

Glass I B, Checkley S A, Shur E, Dowling S 1982 The effect of desipramine upon central adrenergic functions in depressed patients. British Journal of Psychiatry 141: 327–376

Golden R N, Markey S P, Risby E D, Rudorfer M V, Cowdry R W, Potter W Z 1988 Antidepressants reduce whole blood norepinephrine turnover while enhancing 6-hydroxymelatonin output. Archives of General Psychiatry 45: 150–154

Golden R N, Hsiao J K, Lane E, Ekstrom D, Rogers S, Hicks S, Potter W Z 1990 Abnormal neuroendocrine responses to acute i.v. clomipramine challenge in depressed patients. Psychiatry Research 31: 39–47

Goodwin F K, Prange A J, Post R M, Muscettola G, Lipton M A 1982 Potentiation of antidepressant effects by L-triiodothyronine in tricyclic nonresponders. American Journal of Psychiatry 139(1): 34–38

Haggerty J J Jr, Simon J S, Evans D L, Nemeroff C B 1987 Relationship of serum TSH concentration and antithyroid antibodies to diagnosis and DST response in psychiatric inpatients. American Journal of Psychiatry 144: 1491–1493

Hamilton J A 1982 The identity of post-partum psychosis. In: Brockington I F, Kumar R (eds) Motherhood and mental illness. Academic Press, London, p 1–17

Hastings M H, Herbert J 1986 Endocrine rhythms. In: Lightman S L, Everitt B J (eds) Neuroendocrinology. Blackwell Scientific Publications, Oxford, p 49–102

Heninger G, Charney D S, Sternberg D E 1984 Serotonergic function in depression. Prolactin response to intravenous tryptophan in depressed patients and healthy subjects. Archives of General Psychiatry 41: 398–402

Horton R W, Katona C L E, Theodorou A E, Hale A S, Davies S L, Tunnicliffe C, Yamaguchi Y, Paykel E S, Kelly J S 1986 Platelet radioligand binding and neuroendocrine challenge tests in depression. In: Paykel E S (ed) Antidepressants and receptor functions. John Wiley, Chichester, p 78–83

Jarrett J B, Miewald J M, Fedorka I B, Coble P, Kupfer D J, Greenhouse J B 1987 Prolactin secretion during sleep: a comparison between depressed patients and healthy control subjects. Biological Psychiatry 22: 1216–1226

Jeffcoate W, Silverstone J, Edwards C, Besser G M 1979 Psychiatric manifestations of Cushing's syndrome: response to lowering of plasma cortisol. Quarterly Journal of Medicine 48: 465–472

Jimerson D C, Cutler N R, Post R M, Rey A, Gold P W, Brown G M, Bunney W E Jr 1984 Neuroendocrine responses to apomorphine in depressed patients and healthy control subjects. Psychiatry Research 13: 1–12

Joffe R T, Post R M, Ballenger J C, Rebar R, Rakita R, Gold P W 1986 Neuroendocrine effects of the dopamine agonist piribedil in depressed patients. Clinical Neuropharmacology 9: 448–455

Joyce R P, Donald R A, Nicholls M G, Livesey J H, Abbott R M 1986 Endocrine and behavioural responses to methylphenidate in depression. Psychological Medicine 16: 531–540

Joyce P R, Donal R A, Livesey J H, Abbott R M 1987 The prolactin response to metoclopramide is increased in depression and in euthymic rapid cycling bipolar patients. Biological Psychiatry 22: 508–512

Kaneko Y, Yamamoto Y, Kitamura Y, Sakai M, Nagasaki T, Nakajima K 1986 Effect of sulpiride on plasma prolactin in healthy volunteers and depressed patients. Neuropsychobiology 15: 155–159

Kelly W F, Checkley S A, Bender D A 1980 Cushing's syndrome, tryptophan and depression. British Journal of Psychiatry 142: 16–19

Kelly W F, Checkley S A, Bender D A, Mashiter K 1983 Cushing's Syndrome and depression – a prospective study of 26 patients. British Journal of Psychiatry 142: 16–19

Kendell R E, Chalmers J C, Platz C 1987 Epidemiology of puerperal psychosis. British Journal of Psychiatry 150: 662–673

Kierkegaard C, Faber J, Hummer C 1979 Increased levels of TRH in cerebrospinal fluid from patients with endogenous depression. Psychoneuroendocrinology 4: 227–235

Kjellman B F, Ljunggren J G, Beck-Friis J, Wetterberg L 1983 Reverse T3 levels in affective disorders. Psychiatry Research 10: 1–9

Klein D C 1985 Photoneural regulation of the mammalian pineal gland. In: Short R (ed) Photoperiodism, melatonin and the pineal. CIBA Foundation Symposium 117. Pitman, London, p 38–56

Koch M, Ehret G 1989 Immunocytochemical localization and quantitation of oestrogen-binding cells in the male and female (virgin, pregnant, lactating) mouse brain. Brain Research 489: 101–112

Krishnan K R, Manepalli A N, Ritchie J C, Rayasam K, Melville M L, Daughtry G, Thorner M O, Rivier J E, Vale W W, Nemeroff C B 1988 Growth hormone-releasing factor stimulation test in depression. American Journal of Psychiatry 145: 90–92

Laakmann G 1980 Beeinflussung der Hypophysenvorderlappen-Hormonsekretion durch Antidepressiva bei gesunden Probanden, neurotisch und endogen depressiven Patienten. Nervenartz 51: 725–732

Laakmann G, Zygan K, Schoen H W, Weiss A, Wittman M, Meissner R, Blaschke D 1986 Effect of receptor blockers (methysergide, propranolol, phentolamine, yohimbine and prazosin) on desipramine induced pituitary hormone stimulation in humans – I. Growth hormone. Psychoneuroendocrinology 2: 447–461

Lechin F, Van der Dijs B, Jakubowicz D, Camero R E, Villa S, Arocha L, Lechin A E 1985 Effects of clonidine on blood pressure, noradrenaline, cortisol, growth hormone and prolactin plasma levels in high and low intestinal tone depressed patients. Neuroendocrinology 41: 156–162

Lesch K P, Rupprecht R, Muller U, Pfuller H, Beckmann H 1988a Insulin-like growth factor I in depressed patients and controls. Acta Psychiatrica Scandinavica 78: 684–688

Lesch K P, Laux G, Erb A, Pfuller H, Beckmann H 1988b Growth hormone (GH) responses to GH-releasing hormone in depression: correlation with GH release following clonidine. Psychiatry Research 25: 301–310

Linkowski P, Van Cauter E, L'Hermite Baleriaux M, Kerkhofs M, Hubain P, L'Hermite M, Mendlewicz J 1989 The 24 hour profile of plasma prolactin in men with major endogenous depressive illness. Archives of General Psychiatry 46: 813–819

Loosen P T 1987 The TRH stimulation test in psychiatric disorders: a review. In: Nemeroff C B, Loosen P T (eds) Handbook of clinical psychoneuroendocrinology. John Wiley, Chichester, p 336–360

Loosen P T, Garbutt J C, Prange A J 1987 Evaluation of the diagnostic utility of the TRH-induced response in psychiatric disorders. Pharmacopsychiatry 20: 90–95

McCance S L, Cowen P J, Waller H, Graham-Smith D G 1987 The effect of metergoline and endocrine responses to L-tryptophan. Journal of Psychopharmacology 2: 90–94

Matussek N 1988 Catecholamines and mood: neuroendocrine aspects. In: Ganten D, Pfaff D (eds) Current topics in neuroendocrinology. Springer-Verlag, Berlin, p 141–182

Matussek N, Hoehe M 1989 Investigations with the specific mu-opiate receptor agonist fentanyl in depressive patients: growth hormone, prolactin, cortisol, noradrenaline and euphoric responses. Neuropsychobiology 21: 1–8

Matussek N, Ackenheil M, Hippius H, Muller F, Schroder H T, Schultes H, Wasilewski B 1980 Effect of clonidine on growth hormone release in psychiatric patients and controls. Psychiatry Research 2: 25–36

Meesters P, Kerkhofs M, Charles G, Decoster C, Vanderelst M, Mendlewicz J 1985 Growth hormone release after desipramine in depressive illness. European Archives of Psychiatry and the Neurological Sciences 235: 140–142

Meltzer E S, Kumar R 1985 Puerperal mental illness, clinical features and classification: a study of 142 mother-and-baby admissions. British Journal of Psychiatry 147: 647–654

Meltzer H Y, Kolakowska T, Fang V S, Fogg L, Robertson A, Lewine R, Strahilevitz M, Busch D 1984 Growth hormone and prolactin response to apomorphine in schizophrenia and the major affective disorders. Relation to duration of illness and depressive symptoms. Archives of General Psychiatry 41: 512–519

Mendlewicz J, Linkowski P, Kerkhofs M, Desmedt D, Golstein J, Copinschi G, Van Cauter E 1985 Diurnal hypersecretion of growth hormone in depression. Journal of Clinical Endocrinology and Metabolism 60: 505–512

Mitchell P B, Smythe G 1990 Hormonal responses to fenfluramine in depressed and control subjects. Journal of Affective Disorders 19: 43–51

Mitchell P B, Bearn J A, Corn T H, Checkley S A 1988 Growth hormone response to clonidine after recovery in patients with endogenous depression. British Journal of Psychiatry 152: 34–38

Mulller E E, Nistico G 1989 Brain messengers and the pituitary. Academic Press, San Diego, CA

Murphy D L, Tamarkin L, Sunderland T, Garrick N A, Cohen R M 1986 Human plasma melatonin is elevated during treatment with monoamine oxidase inhibitors clorgyline and tranylcypromine but not deprenyl. Psychiatry Research 17: 119–127

Nemeroff C B, Simon J S, Haggerty J J Jr, Evans D L 1985 Antithyroid antibodies in depressed patients. American Journal of Psychiatry 142: 840–843

Neuhauser H, Laakmann G 1988 Stimulation of growth hormone by GHRH as compared to DMI in depressed patients. Pharmacopsychiatry 21: 443–444

Rao M L, Vartzopoulos D, Fels K 1989 Thyroid function in anxious and depressed patients. Pharmacopsychiatry 22: 66–70

Reul J M H M, De Kloet E R 1986 Anatomical resolution of two types of corticosterone receptor sites in rat brain with in vitro autoradiography and computerized image analysis. Journal of Steroid Biochemistry 24: 269–272

Robertson A G, Jackman H, Meltzer H Y 1984 Prolactin response to morphine in depression. Psychiatry Research 11: 353–364

Roy A, Pickar D 1988 TRH-induced prolactin release in unipolar depressed patients and controls. Journal of Psychiatry Research 22: 221–225

Rubin R T, Poland R E, Lesser I M, Martin D J 1987 Neuroendocrine aspects of primary endogenous depression. IV. Pituitary-thyroid axis activity in patients and matched control subjects. Psychoneuroendocrinology 12: 333–347

Rubin R T, Poland R E, Lesser I M, Martin D L 1989 Neuroendocrine aspects of primary endogenous depression. V. Serum prolactin measures in patients and matched control subjects. Biological Psychiatry 25: 4–21

Rubin R T, Poland R E, Lesser I M 1990 Neuroendocrine aspects of primary endogenous depression. X. Serum growth hormone measures in patients and matched controls subjects. Biological Psychiatry 27: 1065–1082

Rupprecht R, Rupprecht C, Rupprecht M, Noder M, Mahlstedt J 1989 Triiodothyronine, thyroxine, and TSH response to dexamethasone in depressed patients and normal controls. Biological Psychiatry 25: 22–32

Ryan N C, Puig Antich J, Rabinovich H, Ambrosini P, Robinson D, Nelson B, Novacenko H 1988 Growth hormone response to desmethylimipramine in depressed and suicidal adolescents. Journal of Affective Disorders 15: 323–337

Sack R L, Lewy A J 1986 Desmethylimipramine treatment increases melatonin production in humans. Biological Psychiatry 21: 406–409

Siever L J, Uhde T W, Silberman E K, Jimerson D C, Aloi J A, Post R M, Murphy D L 1982 Growth hormone response to clonidine as a probe of noradrenergic receptor responsiveness in affective disorder patients and controls. Psychiatry Research 6: 171–183

Siever L J, Murphy D L, Slater S, de La Vega E, Lipper S 1984 Plasma prolactin changes following fenfluramine in depressed patients compared to controls: an evaluation of central serotonergic responsivity in depression. Life Sciences 34: 1029–1039

Siever L J, Coccaro E F, Benjamin E, Rubinstein K, Davis K L 1986 Adrenergic and serotonergic receptor responsiveness. In: Paykel E S (ed) Antidepressants and receptor function. John Wiley, Chichester, p 148–163

Sternbach H A, Gwirtsman H E, Gerner R H, Hershman J, Pekary E 1985 The TRH stimulation test and reverse T3 in depression. Journal of Affective Disorders 8: 267–270

Stephenson J D 1990 Neuropharmacological studies of the serotonergic system. International Review of Psychiatry 2: 157–179

Thomas R, Beer R, Harris B, John R, Scanlon M 1989 GH responses to growth hormone releasing factor in depression. Journal of Affective Disorders 16: 133–137

Thompson C, Mezey G, Corn T, Franey C, English J, Arendt J, Checkley S A 1985 The effect of desipramine upon melatonin and cortisol secretion in depressed and normal subjects. British Journal of Psychiatry 147: 389–393

Thompson C, Franey C, Arendt J, Checkley S A 1988 A comparison of melatonin secretion in depressed patients and normal subjects. British Journal of Psychiatry 147: 389–393

Turek F W 1985 Circadian neural rhythms in mammals. Annual Review of Physiology 47: 49–64

Unden F, Ljunggren J G, Kjellman B F, Beck-Frijs J, Wetterberg L 1987 Unaltered 24h serum PRL levels and PRL response to TRH in contrast to decreased 24h serum TSH levels and TSH response to TRH in major depressive disorder. Acta Psychiatrica Scandinavica 75: 131–138

Van Cauter E 1989 Endocrine rhythms. In Arendt J, Minors D S, Waterhouse J M (eds) Biological rhythms in clinical practice. John Wright, London, p 23–50

Von Zerssen D, Barthelmes H, Dirlich G, Doerr P, Enrich H N, Von Lindern L, Lund R, Pirke K M 1985 Circadian rhythms in endogenous depression. Psychiatry Research 16: 51–63

Wang S Y, Shin S J 1989 Alterations in thyroid function tests in major depression. Taiwan I Hsueh Hui Tsa Chih 88: 143–147

Weick A, Hirst A D, Kumar R, Checkley S A, Campbell I C 1989 The growth hormone response to the dopamine agonist apomorphine is enhanced in women at high risk of puerperal psychosis. British Journal of Clinical Pharmacology 28: 748–749

Weizman A, Mark M, Gil Ad I, Tyano S, Laron Z 1988 Plasma cortisol, prolactin, growth hormone and immunoreactive β-endorphin response to fenfluramine challenge in depressed patients. Clinical Neuropharmocology 11: 250–256

Whybrow P, Prange A, Tredway C 1969 Mental changes accompanying thyroid gland dysfunction. Archives of General Psychiatry 20: 48–62

Willcox D L, Yovich J L, McColm S C, Phillips 1985 Progesterone, cortisol and oestradiol in the initiation of human parturition: partitioning between free and bound hormone in plasma. British Journal of Obstetrics and Gynaecolocy 92: 65–71

Willner P 1990 The role of slow changes in catecholamine receptor function in the action of antidepressant drugs. International Review of Psychiatry 2: 141–156

Winokur A, Amsterdam J D, Oler J, Mendels J, Snyder P J, Caroff S N, Brunswick D J 1983 Multiple hormonal responses to protirelin (TRH) in depressed patients. Archives of General Psychiatry 40: 525–531

Zis A P, Haskett R F, Albala A A, Carroll B J, Lohr N E 1985 Prolactin responses to morphine in depression. Biological Psychiatry 20: 287–292

Zis A P, Albala A, Haskett R F, Carroll B J, Lohr N 1986 Prolactin responses to TRH in depression. Journal of Psychiatric Research 20: 77–82

17. The hypothalamic–pituitary–adrenocortical system

Florian Holsboer

In patients with increased plasma levels of endogenous or exogenous corticosteroids two principal types of psychopathology have been identified: 1) affective syndromes and 2) cognitive impairment. Sometimes elevated levels of circulating corticosteroids due to drug administration or as part of Cushing's disease are associated with severe psychopathology, cross-sectionally indistinguishable from major depression, including melancholia with psychotic features. These psychic disturbances usually resolve after successful surgical removal of the adenomas which are hypersecreting ACTH or cortisol. A recent study by Haskett (1985) showed that affective syndromes usually preceded the endocrine diagnosis by 6–36 months, while complete resolution of psychopathology took up to 6 months after removal of abnormal endocrine tissue. Earlier investigations by Starkman & Schteingart (1981) revealed associations between the severity of psychiatric dysfunction and plasma ACTH and cortisol concentrations. More specific behavioural impairments have been reported in neuropsychological and sleep-EEG studies, largely corresponding to the characteristic changes found in major depression (for review see Fava et al 1987).

While behavioural changes resulting from endocrine lesions have long been recognized, the association between affective illness and changes in hypothalamic–pituitary–adrenal (HPA) regulation has only been appreciated much more recently. Today the accumulated evidence suggests that altered HPA activity as detected by dynamic function tests is directly involved in the pathogenesis of depressive syndromes (for review see Holsboer 1989).

HPA CORRELATES OF DEPRESSION

Baseline measures

Approximately 50–60% of patients presenting with major depressive disorder have distinct changes in their ACTH and cortisol secretory activity, which can be shown by measuring cortisol, corticotropin (ACTH) and corticotropin-releasing hormone (CRH) in plasma, urine and cerebrospinal fluid. Halbreich et al (1985) showed that cortisol secretory profiles of depressives resulted in mean 24-hour plasma cortisol levels that were significantly elevated when compared to controls. Linkowsky et al (1985) and Mortola et al (1987) studied the pulsatile activity and circadian rhythmicity of ACTH in relation to cortisol. These studies demonstrated that in depression the number of ACTH pulses was increased, while for cortisol it was not the number but the amount of cortisol released per burst which was increased. More recent studies in controls have documented a linear relationship between the magnitudes of ACTH and cortisol pulses (Krishnan et al 1990). However, the degree of temporal coincidence between ACTH and cortisol pulses was found to be variable (Follenius et al 1987, Krishnan et al 1990). The occurrence of ACTH pulses without changes in plasma cortisol concentrations and of cortisol peaks with no observable change in plasma ACTH raises the possibility that mechanisms other than ACTH may be involved in regulating cortisol secretion (Fehm et al 1984). Sympathetic innervation of the adrenal cortex and adrenogenic humoral factors, which act independently of the pituitary and are probably derived from the immune systems, may also be involved (Holsboer et al 1988a).

The concurrence of increased ACTH burst frequency and enhanced cortisol secretory amplitude among depressives is probably a secondary consequence of hypersensitivity of the adrenal glands which occurs in these patients (Amsterdam et al 1983). This hypersensitivity may develop after prolonged overexposure to ACTH, which is a trophic hormone and renders the gland hyperplastic. Two lines of research support this interpretation: 1) Following synthetic ACTH infusions to depressives with or without dexamethasone pretreatment the plasma cortisol surges have been found to be more pronounced among depressives and dexamethasone non-suppressors than in controls or dexamethasone suppressors (Amsterdam et al 1983, Gerken & Holsboer 1986, Jaeckle et al 1987); 2) enlarged adrenal size has been demonstrated in a group of depressives by computed X-ray tomography (Amsterdam et al 1987). These radiological data, which are surrounded by indications of pituitary enlargement in depression (Doraiswamy et al 1990) must be considered as preliminary since no confirmatory studies are yet available.

The Dexamethasone suppression test (DST)

After administration of a small dose (1–2 mg) of the long-acting synthetic steroid dexamethasone at 23.00 h to normal subjects, plasma cortisol levels remain suppressed throughout the following day. A large number of studies has shown that depressives frequently escape from this suppressive effect of dexamethasone (Rubin et al 1987). Many studies have explored the clinical utility of the DST as a laboratory aid to establish a reliable diagnosis. While initially some investigators claimed that nonsuppression of cortisol by dexamethasone would specifically indicate presence of the endogenous or melancholic subtype of major depression (Carroll et al 1981), there is now agreement that the test is not useful as a differential diagnostic aid (e.g. Holsboer et al 1986c). This is rendered more difficult by several recent changes in official diagnostic classifications. Additional confusion over the physiological validity arose after we found that non-suppressed plasma cortisol levels following dexamethasone were associated with lower plasma concentrations of the test drug (Holsboer 1983, Holsboer et al 1984a). However, studies of early biophase kinetics and studies comparing drug distribution after oral and intravenous dexamethasone administration among depressed suppressors and non-suppressors have shown that the outcome of the DST is not simply an artifact of the bioavailability of the test drug (Holsboer et al 1986a, Wiedemann & Holsboer 1990).

To date the most promising application of the DST remains its use as a state marker, which can be applied longitudinally to follow-up treatment response. Depressives who initially have elevated plasma cortisol levels after dexamethasone gradually normalize on the test during successful antidepressant treatment. Those patients who remain DST non-suppressors despite improvement of psychopathology are at risk of impending relapse into depression (Holsboer et al 1982, 1983, Greden et al 1983, Grunhaus et al 1987, Charles et al 1989, Coryell 1990). This time pattern, in which neuroendocrine alterations precede depressive psychopathology and normalize prior to full remission of psychopathology, strongly resembles the situation in patients with Cushing's syndrome (Haskett 1985).

While most of the data suggest that increased baseline levels of ACTH and cortisol and their inadequate suppression by dexamethasone correspond with severity of depression a clear-cut correlation between patterns of depressive psychopathology and HPA disturbance has not yet been identified. Instead of syndromes or diagnoses being contrasted with HPA measures, the latter should be considered as one of the symptoms of the clinical phenotype. Similarly, in other branches of medicine not all symptoms need to be specific to the disease, but they may be still considered informative as long as they provide valuable feedback information for the therapist.

Relationship of HPA overactivity to sleep

Sleep is one facet of human behaviour that can be objectively registered and analyzed by means of polygraphic recording. Since sleep disturbances are among the more prominent symptoms of depression several studies have attempted to explore whether or not changes in sleep architecture interact with altered HPA activity measures. Cortisol, the hormonal end point of HPA activity, has been shown to reduce the amount of sleep time spent in the rapid eye movement period, while the amount of slow-wave sleep increases (Born et al 1987). Since slow-wave sleep is most frequently decreased in depressives, concurrent hypercortisolaemia in these patients would oppose the illness-related reduction in slow-wave sleep. As illustrated in Figure 17.1, the major force driving hypercortisolaemia is increased hypothalamic production and secretion of CRH, which stimulates ACTH secretion from the anterior pituitary into the peripheral circulation. The latter hormone activates production and release of cortisol and other corticosteroids from the adrenocortical gland.

We tested whether human (h)CRH had any effect upon human sleep by injecting this neuropeptide into healthy controls in pulsatile fashion around the time of sleep onset (Holsboer et al 1988b). In keeping with

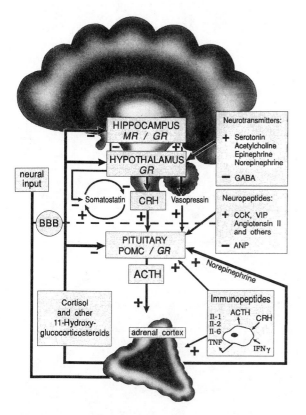

Fig. 17.1 External cognitive (e.g. psychosocial stressor) or non-cognitive (e.g. infective) stimuli and emotional disturbances arising from brain dysfunctions that underly affective syndromes or panic anxiety all activate various brain areas, which finally use the hypothalamus as a relay station to translate the brain activity pattern into changes of autonomic system function and hormonal secretion. While CRH is the permissive key hormone activating the HPA system many other transmitters and peptides serve to modulate dynamically the secretory activity of pituitary corticotrophic cells. At each level immunopeptides including interleukins derived from glia tissue (not shown in this figure) are involved in the regulatory circuits
MR = mineralocorticosteroid receptor; GR = glucocorticosteroid receptor; CRH = corticotropin releasing hormone; CCK = cholecystokinin; VIP = vasointestinal peptide; ANP = atrial natriuretic peptide; BBB = blood–brain barrier; ACTH = corticotropin; IFN-γ = interferon gamma; IL1,2,6 = interleukin 1,2,6; TNF = tumour necrosis factor

studies performed by Ehlers et al (1986), who administered the neuropeptide centrally in rats, we observed that hCRH reduced the amount of slow-wave sleep, decreased the nocturnal growth hormone surge and enhanced HPA activity, thus mimicking some of the

sleep–endocrine symptoms of depression (Steiger et al 1989, Jarrett et al 1990). In order to sort out the effects of ACTH and cortisol we studied the fragment ACTH(4–9), which is behaviourally active in a similar way to ACTH but is devoid of adrenogenic effects. We found that this peptide decreased both sleep efficiency and slow-wave sleep, which further suggests that several hypothalamic pituitary peptide hormones that are involved in central adaptation to stress may affect sleep in an opposite direction to glucocorticosteroids (Steiger et al in press). In affective illness the disturbance of slow-wave sleep that is frequently observed is probably a net effect of hypersecreted neuropeptides from the hypothalamic – pituitary system and of peripherally secreted adrenocortical hormones. After recovery from psychopathology, the HPA axis usually normalizes, while other endocrine alterations and sleep changes can persist over considerable time periods (Steiger et al 1989, Jarrett et al 1990). Whether or not the persistence of neurobiological changes increases the risk of a patient relapsing into a further depressive episode is subject to investigation.

PATHOPHYSIOLOGY OF EXAGGERATED HPA ACTIVITY IN DEPRESSION

Corticotropin releasing hormone (CRH)

Normal controls, when exposed to a stressor, respond with elevated ACTH and cortisol as part of their internal mechanisms of adaptation, established to match external demands. Among healthy individuals termination of stress exposure is always followed by a return of stress hormone levels to baseline. As mentioned above, depressives hypersecrete ACTH and cortisol throughout the 24-hour cycle, in the absence of any external stimuli (Fig. 17.2).

The presence of a hypothalamic neuropeptide controlling ACTH secretion was predicted by Harris more than 40 years ago. However, it took until 1981 for CRH to be isolated from ovine hypothalami (Vale et al 1981). The detection and sequencing of the gene coding for human CRH at chromosome 8 (Shibahara et al 1983) was immediately followed by many studies on human stress physiology and disorders associated with HPA pathophysiology.

The first series of reports utilizing human (h)CRH in depressives revealed a blunted ACTH response after i.v. administration of a test dose of hCRH (Holsboer et

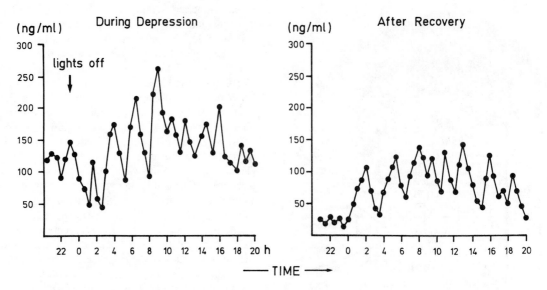

Fig. 17.2 The baseline cortisol pattern of a 52-year-old female patient with major depression reveals an increased amount of plasma cortisol released per secretory burst, in comparison to the secretory pattern after full recovery from the affective disorder. In aggregate, the mean amount of cortisol secreted per day is 81 ± 25 ng/ml in depressives, while the corresponding value in healthy controls is 64 ± 19 ng/ml. These values were reported by Halbreich et al (1985), who studied patients with a mean age of 42.5 ± 15.1 years.

al 1984b, 1986b, 1987a). The baseline cortisol secretion prior to hCRH stimulation was significantly higher in depressives and inversely related to the amount of ACTH produced by stimulation (see Fig. 17.3). We further observed that the cortisol responses among depressives were indistinguishable from those of controls, despite significantly lower ACTH release. This points toward a hypersensitive adrenal cortex resulting from long-term overexposure to ACTH, confirming conclusions drawn from ACTH and cortisol profiles at baseline and after ACTH challenges. Furthermore, pre-treatment of depressives with metyrapone, which suppresses cortisol biosynthesis, was found to result in normalized ACTH release after hCRH stimulation (von Bardeleben et al 1988). From these data we concluded that elevated circulating cortisol was the main but not the sole abnormality preventing adequate ACTH response via negative feedback. Therefore, exaggerated secretory activity of corticotrophic and adrenocortical cells must be related to a suprapituitary abnormality. This interpretation is consistent with our earlier studies applying ovine CRH (Holsboer 1983, Holsboer et al 1984c, 1985) and similar studies using the ovine heterologue by

Amsterdam et al (1987) and by Gold et al (1984, 1986).

In addition to baseline hypercortisolism, other mechanisms which might account for blunted ACTH response to CRH must be considered. Among these possibilities are altered processing and storage of ACTH precursors, desensitized CRH receptors at pituitary corticotrophs and alternative processing of proopiomelanocortin (POMC), the precursor of ACTH and beta-endorphin. For example, Rupprecht et al (1989) recently reported a dissociation of ACTH and beta-endorphin responses after CRH stimulation in depression. Young et al (1990a) applied a low dose ovine CRH challenge to depressives and controls and measured beta-endorphin, beta-lipotropin and cortisol in order to obtain information on the acute feedback regulation and actual CRH receptor sensitivity. They found a decreased total beta-endorphin and beta-lipotropin response and a normal adrenal cortisol response in depressives, which agrees with our original studies measuring ACTH and cortisol after human CRH. The beta-endorphin response pattern was found to be biphasic, showing an initial rapid release of beta-endorphin preceding the cortisol surge and a second

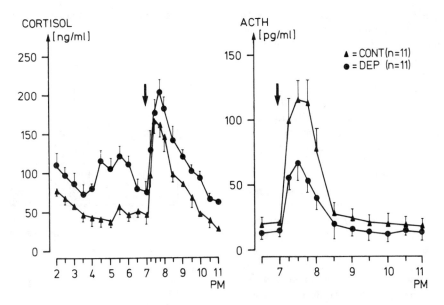

Fig. 17.3 Patients with elevated plasma cortisol levels at baseline (left) show significantly blunted ACTH release (right) following an intravenous test dose of 100 μg CRH at 19:00 hours. Note that despite decreased ACTH secretion depressives have plasma cortisol surges that are indistinguishable from normal controls. This finding suggests that among depressives with hypercortisolism several adaptive changes at each level of the brain—pituitary—adrenal system have occurred that result in an altered pituitary corticotroph response pattern to CRH, changes in feedback regulation and increased adrenocortical sensitivity (from Holsboer et al 1986b)

period of beta-endorphin increase while cortisol was elevated but stable. This pattern is consistent with the concept of two separate feedback phases (Keller Wood & Dallman 1985): 1) an early termination of corticotrophin secretion during the time of rapidly increasing corticosteroid levels; and 2) a silent period in corticosteroid feedback while high adrenocortical hormone levels are still increasing at a much slower rate than during the period immediately after stimulation. This important clinical study confirms conclusions drawn from animal investigations (Young & Akil 1985) and our work from combined dexamethasone-hCRH challenges among depressives — that, in addition to resting cortisol levels and adrenal hypersensitivity, it is also necessary to consider corticosteroid-receptor-mediated feedback mechanisms in the hypothalamic – pituitary system.

In agreement with the notion that overactive central CRH neurons are involved in depression with hypercortisolism are the studies of Nemeroff and colleagues. These investigators measured CRH in the cerebrospinal fluid and found elevated levels of this

peptide in depression (Nemeroff et al 1984). While it must be noted that CRH levels in the cerebrospinal fluid do not necessarily reflect CRH in the pituitary portal system, this observation agrees with a study showing that CRH receptors were downregulated in the frontal cortex of suicide victims, which is best explained by central overproduction of CRH (Nemeroff et al 1988).

The combined dexamethasone–CRH challenge test

In normal controls increasing dosages of dexamethasone result in a dose dependent decrease of the measurable amount of ACTH produced on hCRH stimulation (see Fig. 17.4). This would agree with the negative feedback effect of corticosteroids, restraining the stimulatory effect of CRH at the pituitary level. In depressives one would predict that, due to the elevated levels of endogenous corticosteroids, even lower dexamethasone dosages would suffice to prevent

ACTH release following CRH. Against expectation, however, we found that dexamethasone premedication enhanced pituitary responsiveness in depression instead of suppressing it (Holsboer et al 1987b, von Bardeleben & Holsboer 1989, 1991) (Fig. 17.5). We suspect that the adaptive responses of the binary corticosteroid receptor system in the brain is involved in this phenomenon (de Kloet 1991). Specifically, the differential binding properties of dexamethasone and endogenous corticosteroids at pituitary and brain receptors may account for the effects. In contrast to cortisol and other naturally occurring corticosteroids, dexamethasone does not bind to corticosteroid-binding globulin, which is present in the pituitary but not in the brain. Therefore, glucocorticoid receptor binding of dexamethasone predominates at the pituitary, depriving mineralocorticoid (MR, type I) and glucocorticoid (GR, type II) receptors in the brain of their natural ligands, an effect which is most probably not fully compensated by the synthetic test drug (Reul et al 1987).

This may not affect healthy normocortisolaemic controls, but only hypercortisolaemic depressives, whose brain glucocorticoid receptors are downregulated in response to prolonged overexposure to endogenous glucocorticosteroids (Sapolsky et al 1988). Since one of the major neuroendocrine functions of glucocorticoid receptors is to mediate negative feedback in response to elevated plasma corticosteroid levels, their downregulation would impede their capacity to shut off hypercortisolism. At the pituitary level CRH does not act alone, but is regulated dynamically by other neuropeptides, primarily vasopressin (see Fig. 17.1), and we postulate that the above finding is due to inadequate suppression of vasopressin secondary to impaired capacity of glucocorticoid receptors mediating the effects of dexamethasone. This notion is supported by animal studies, which have shown that AVP concentrations in hypophyseal portal blood react most sensitively to minor changes of circulating corticosteroids (Fink et al 1988). In order to test this hypothesis in humans we applied saline, hCRH, vasopressin and a combination of both neuropeptides to healthy controls after premedication with dexamethasone (von Bardeleben et al 1985). We observed that only the combination of both peptides was able to induce plasma cortisol and ACTH release during dexamethasone suppression (Fig. 17.6). Whether vasopressin or other neuropeptides are involved in synergizing the ACTH-releasing effect of CRH in dexamethasone premedicated depressives will require

investigation after the availability of specific neuropeptide antagonists.

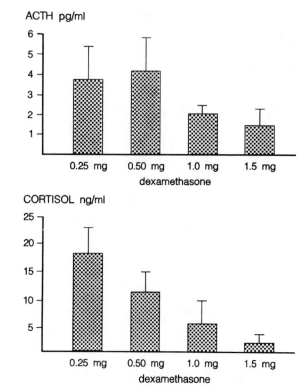

Fig. 17.4 Increasing dosages (0.25 mg, 0.5 mg, 1.0 mg, 1.5 mg) of dexamethasone administered at 23:00 hours to seven healthy controls in randomized order resulted in decreased amounts of released ACTH and cortisol after hCRH injection at 15:00 hours the following day. The corresponding areas under time-course curves that were registered following hCRH were: 0.25 mg dexamethasone: cortisol, 18.4 ± 4.1 mg $\times$ min $\times$ 1000/ml (AUC) ACTH, 3.9 ± 1.6 pg $\times$ min $\times$ 1000/ml; 0.5 mg dexamethasone: cortisol, 11.4 ± 2.6 AUC, ACTH, 4.1 ± 2.0 AUC; 1.0 mg dexamethasone: cortisol, 6.4 ± 3.3 AUC, ACTH, 2.2 ± 0.5 AUC; 1.5 mg dexamethasone: cortisol, 2.3 ± 1.4 AUC, ACTH, 1.5 ± 1.0 AUC (from von Bardeleben et al unpublished)

The occurrence of exaggerated cortisol and ACTH responses to a combined dexamethasone — hCRH challenge test is most pronounced during depression. After treatment and resolution of depressive psychopathology the phenomenon gradually disappears (Holsboer et al 1987b, Holsboer-Trachsler 1991). However, with increasing age the process of normalization is prolonged and frequently incomplete (Heuser

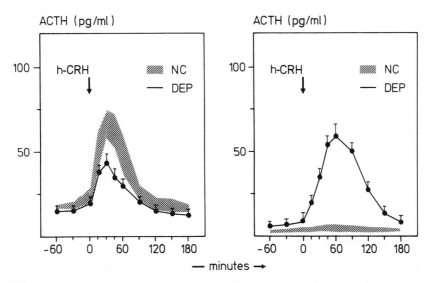

Fig. 17.5 Premedication of normal controls with 1.5 mg dexamethasone prevents the activation of HPA hormones following hCRH. Depressed patients show a paradoxical rise of cortisol and ACTH in the combined dexamethasone-CRH challenge indicating changes at the glucocorticosteroid receptor level (from von Bardeleben & Holsboer 1989, and unpublished data)

et al 1991). Long-term follow-up studies have revealed that a substantial proportion of patients who are assessed as remitted by psychometric evaluations still show elevated cortisol levels in the combined dexamethasone–hCRH test. During a depressive episode a large variety of homeostatic changes occur, leading to long-term changes in neuroendocrine regulation which we have called 'neuroendocrine scars'. These prevent the use of neuroendocrine findings during symptom-free intervals of recurrent depressives as trait markers. In order to clarify whether exaggerated cortisol responses among remitted patients were trait markers or 'scars' we created a high-risk group by selecting never-mentally-ill first-degree relatives from families with a high loading for depression (Krieg et al 1990). We observed that within this high-risk population a markedly higher proportion presented with aberrant HPA function as disclosed by altered cortisol response following a combined dexamethasone–hCRH challenge. However, at present we have only provisional evidence that premorbid HPA abnormalities in individuals who have never been mentally ill identify increased vulnerability for depression. Clarification of this issue requires extensive prospective studies among members of high-risk families, and such studies are currently in progress at the Max Planck Institute of Psychiatry in Munich.

ADAPTATION TO STRESS AND THE AGING PROCESS

The physiological aging process is often aggravated by a past and recent history of stressful experiences that have excessively activated neural and humoral adaptive mechanisms. As people age, the amount of stress accumulates and may impair neuroendocrine responses to further stressors. This interferes with the capability of the elderly to cope with perturbations such as loss of a spouse and social support, or physical illness. Clinical studies have shown that prolonged severe stress such as combat experience in war veterans may impair adequate responses to exogenous CRH (Smith et al 1989). In patients who have experienced repeated episodes of major depression, the amount of cortisol released in response to a combined dexamethasone – hCRH test has been found to increase with age (von Bardeleben & Holsboer 1991). Such an association is absent among controls. Similarly, baseline cortisol increases with increasing age among depressives, but not among controls (Halbreich et al 1984). If anything,

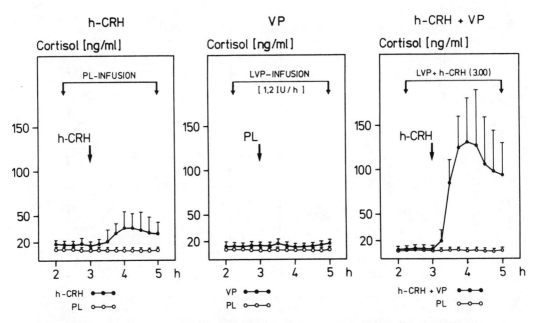

Fig. 17.6 In normal controls neither CRH nor vasopressin (VP) are capable of overriding the HPA suppressive effect of 1.5 mg dexamethasone. A simultaneous administration of both peptides (vasopressin as a continuous low dosed 1.2 IE/h infusion and hCRH as a 100 µg bolus) provokes a significant escape from dexamethasone suppression (from von Bardeleben et al 1985)

healthy aged controls show evidence of diminished sensitivity of corticotrophic cells or higher regulatory centres involved in ACTH regulation to the negative feedback effect of glucocorticoids (Pavlov et al 1986).

In order to explore the effect of episodic hypercortisolism upon age-related neuroendocrine changes, Heuser et al (1991) studied elderly endurance athletes who were in good physical and psychological health. In this sample the combined dexamethasone-hCRH test was applied to pick up subtle changes in negative feedback neuroregulation. The major finding of this study was that pretreatment with dexamethasone failed to suppress release both of ACTH and cortisol following CRH to the extent that it suppressed secretion of these hormones in sedentary controls. In fact, the hormonal profiles of runners resembled those of depressives, suggesting that similar regulatory changes had occurred. Which of the different levels involved in the negative feedback are involved in these changes is not yet clear. Chronic stress in rats results in decreased sensitivity to glucocorticosteroid feedback action (Young & Akil 1985, Young et al 1990b). In addition, hCRH receptors at the pituitary, but not at brain sites, are desensitized in response to elevated corticosteroid

levels (Hauger et al 1987). Since vasopressin synergizes with the effect of CRH on pituitary corticotrophs, we have suggested that the exaggerated response to CRH in dexamethasone-pretreated individuals is caused by elevated endogenous vasopressin secretion (von Bardeleben & Holsboer 1989, 1991; Heuser et al 1991). This interpretation is supported by findings of Fliers et al (1985) showing signs of increased activity of hypothalamic vasopressin neurones in aged human postmortem brains.

Of particular interest in this context are studies by Sapolsky and his colleagues (1985, 1986) testing two hypotheses: 1) whether aging is associated with disturbed hormonal responsiveness to stress; and 2) whether chronic stress accelerates neuronal loss in the hippocampus and eventually also in other brain areas. Sapolsky et al (1985) showed that, in contrast to young rats, aged animals fail to normalize stress-induced adrenocortical hypersecretion rapidly after termination of stress exposure. This finding is associated with a reduced number of glucocorticosteroid receptors in aged rats and can be mimicked by prolonged glucocorticosteroid exposure or chronic stress, which may lead not only to glucocorticoid receptor downregulation but also to hippocampal neuron loss, most pronouncedly in the CA3 area. Whether the proposed acceleration of brain aging by excessive glucocorticosteroid secretion is also relevant for human physiology is not yet proven. Data obtained with functional neuroendocrine tests such as the dexamethason – hCRH test in depressives or aged runners are in support of this hypothesis, but other mechanisms may be equally important (Eldridge et al 1989). Whether or not neuroendocrine commonalities between aging and depression point to a close neurobiological relationship is unknown. However, it is beyond debate that depression has an accelerating effect upon various physiological changes associated with the aging process (von Bardeleben & Holsboer 1991).

HPA ACTIVITY AND THE BRAIN—IMMUNO-ENDOCRINE SYSTEM

The central nervous system responds to external cognitive stimuli by individually altering its neuronal activity patterns and by secreting various neuropeptides, which control the pituitary gland. In a similar way the immune system surveys the outside world and coordinates adaptation to non-cognitive stressors, partly by secreting peptides that affect other tissues. With ongoing progress in brain research and immunology neuroscientists have become increasingly aware of the many functional analogies between the two systems, which may derive from their common need to deal with unfamiliar environmental stimuli and their possession of appropriate memories. Neuroanatomical studies have shown that the thymus gland, in which various immune cells differentiate, receives autonomic nerve fibres originating from the brain stem (Bulloch 1985). A direct pseudosynaptic relationship between nerve terminals among fields of lymphocytes which possess specific receptors for neurotransmitters, neuropeptides and corticosteroids has also been detected (Felten et al 1987). This enables immune cells to respond to humoral and neural signals from the brain. More recent research has shown bidirectionality of both systems, since immune cells and organs can influence central nervous activity (Besedovsky et al 1983). In this two-way communication, hormones of the HPA axis play a key role. As shown by Besedovsky & del Rey (1989) virus-induced activation of the HPA system is mediated by interleukin-1β (IL-1β), a cytokine produced predominantly by activated monocytes and macrophages but also by microglia cells. The effect of IL-1β involves stimulation of CRH from the paraventricular nucleus of the hypothalamus (Sapolsky et al 1987, Berkenbosch et al 1987), an area in the limbic brain that is densely innervated by IL-1β immunoreactive fibres (Breder et al 1988).

We are only at the very beginning of an understanding of the interaction between these peptides. In response to cognitive stress, such as an examination under time pressure, alertness is maximal, while non-cognitive stress, such as infection or tumour growth, renders the body tired, making one fall asleep. Both conditions are associated with elevated ACTH and glucocorticoids. Infusions of IL-1β directly into the rat brain enhance slow-wave sleep (Tobler et al 1984), thus helping to restore bodily integrity, while CRH reduces slow-wave sleep in animals and humans (Ehlers et al 1986, Holsboer et al 1988b). Therefore, in infection IL-1β appears to be the primary force for adequate adaptation, while under psychological stress CRH predominates. Both peptides act in concert to activate ACTH and cortisol and both are under negative feedback control by glucocorticoids (Lee et al 1988). This negative feedback loop also affects the differentiation and function of the monocyte-macrophage cell line (Baybutt & Holsboer 1990). In addition to these links some evidence of a bidirectional communication between the immune cells and peripheral endocrine glands has been demonstrated (for review see Blalock 1989). Smith et al (1990) showed that splenic lymphocytes from mice are capable of synthesizing a truncated ACTH epitope containing 25 amino acids whose sequence is identical to the amino-terminal end of pituitary ACTH, and which has the full endocrine activity. Another example is the finding that interferon-γ activates the adrenal cortex in healthy humans, without activating the pituitary corticotrophs (Holsboer et al 1988a).

Given this evidence of a brain–immunoendocrine network, the question arises as to what extent HPA overactivity in patients with affective disorders may impair their immune function, thus increasing their risk of cancer and infectious disease. While data exist indicating that some psychosocial stressors may be related to malignant breast disease in women (Cooper et al 1989), a causal connection between depressive symptoms and cancer morbidity remains unproven (Zonderman et al 1989). Alterations of immunity have been shown not to be a general phenomenon of major depression. However, an association between severity of depression, increasing age and impaired immune function has been reported (Schleifer et al 1989). Since HPA abnormality in depressives is accelerated by increasing age and severity (Halbreich et al 1985, von

Bardeleben & Holsboer 1991), it is likely that a causal relationship exists between attenuated immune function and depression in the elderly. More refined techniques than mitogen stimulation or cell counting need to be employed to investigate whether hypercortisolaemic depressives have changes in the immune system that are clinically relevant.

As long as no data are available to reject such a possibility any condition with excessive HPA activity must be considered as potentially harmful, since a large body of literature from basic research supports such a possibility. Sternberg & Wilder (1989) for example, concluded from their studies with an experimental model for arthritis that defective HPA-axis responses to inflammatory or immune mediators may increase susceptibility to inflammatory-autoimmune disease. Other investigations have shown that CRH, which may possibly be overproduced in major depression, reduces natural cytotoxicity, important in killing tumour and virally infected cells (Irwin et al 1989). Finally, replica-

tion of the human immunodeficiency virus in monocytes which harbour the virus (Markham et al 1986), and of the malignant human papilloma virus (HPV 16), is enhanced by glucocorticoids (Pater et al 1988).

In this context therapeutic strategies aimed at producing better coping with stressful life situations may act in part through their HPA deactivation. Such interventions should occur in the early states of disease, while the neuroendocrine alterations are still subtle (Villette et al 1990). If the immune system is severely compromised the contribution of improved coping styles and the concurrent neuroendocrine HPA changes could at best decelerate but not cure the disease process, although some psychic healers might argue otherwise.

HPA REGULATION IN STRESS, PANIC AND ANXIETY DISORDER

When CRH is administered into the cerebral ventricles

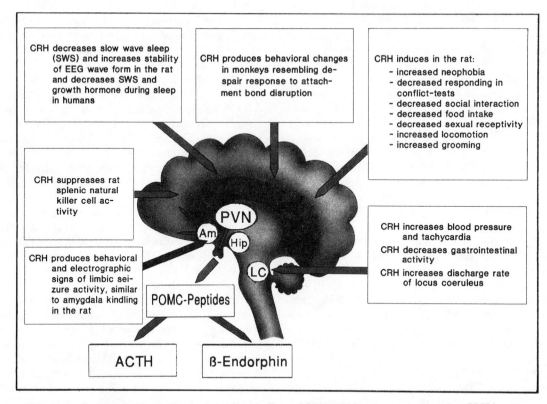

Fig. 17.7 Summary of non-endocrine behavioural effects of CRH, which supports the view that CRH is an important component in neuromediation of behavioural adaptation to stress. If CRH overproduction cannot be counterregulated by corticosteroids, depressive symptomatology may result

of the rat brain it produces not only secretion of pituitary adrenocortical hormones, but also behavioural changes indicative of enhanced fear in a novel open field, the acoustic startle test, social interaction tests and in operant conflict and conditioned emotional response paradigms (for review see Dunn & Berridge 1990). These locomotor activating and anxiogenic effects of CRH are independent of its endocrine effects and are consistent with its widespread distribution in the CNS, including brain areas not involved in neuroendocrine regulation (Swanson et al 1983). Together with other behavioural changes, such as increased heart rate, inhibited food consumption, disturbed sleep and decreased sexual receptivity, CRH is now viewed as a major coordinator of adaptive responses to cognitively perceived stressful situations. In hypersecretion CRH may act as a neurohormonal transmitter, mediating at least some of the nonendocrine symptoms of human depression (see Fig. 17.7). This view is supported by our finding that sleep EEG and sleep-associated changes in hormonal secretion characteristic of depression can be mimicked by CRH administration to healthy human controls (Holsboer et al 1988a).

This hypothesis is in line with the observation that benzodiazepines may reduce circulating levels of ACTH and cortisol, while inverse agonists stimulate them (Insel et al 1984). Recently, Calogero et al (1988) have reported that the benzodiazepine alprazolam attenuates stimulated CRH release from isolated rat hypothalami. Also Owens et al (1989) have found that benzodiazepines prevent the release of CRH from the median eminence. Interestingly, the CRH content of the locus ceruleus (LC) decreased after treatment with benzodiazepines. This brain-stem nucleus is of particular interest for two reasons: 1) its activity has repeatedly been implicated in stress responses, fear and arousal functions; and 2) CRH-containing neurones are located in close proximity to noradrenergic neurones in the LC (Swanson et al 1983). A strong functional interaction is also supported by the increases of LC-firing rates observed after CRH injections into this area and the increases of CRH concentrations found in the LC in response to stress. These stress-responsive CRH surges are reduced by the anxiolytic drug alprazolam, and the effect of alprazolam in deactivating CRH neurons can be blocked by benzodiazepine antagonists (Owens et al 1989). All these data suggest that panic and anxiety disorders are precipitated by a rapidly progressing dysregulation between CRH neurones and noradrenergic neurones at the LC. This

would result in a positive feedback circuit, which would result temporarily in explosive neuronal LC-CRH disinhibition, mutually triggering panic anxiety and a variety of LC- and HPA-related autonomic and endocrine changes.

This rather speculative hypothesis is supported by the observed suppression of CRH activity by benzodiazepines and by in vivo electrophysiology in rats, but it needs to be strengthened by neuroendocrine measurements during spontaneous panic attacks in humans. While such data are not at present available, two recent studies applying CRH to patients with panic disorders support the idea of episodic CRH bursts. Roy-Byrne et al (1986) and workers in our laboratory (Holsboer et al 1987c) found that ACTH responses following an ovine or human CRH probe were blunted (Fig. 17.8). In the study by Roy-Byrne baseline cortisol levels were elevated, probably due to the preceding insertion of the intravenous catheter and resulting anticipatory anxiety. In our study population we inserted the catheter 5 hours prior to CRH challenge and used a 'through-the-wall' technique leaving all manipulations unrecognized by the patients. Our finding of diminished ACTH response after hCRH in the absence of hypercortisolism suggests desensitized CRH receptors at anterior pituitary corticotrophs. These receptor changes are probably due to excessive overexposure to hypothalamic CRH as part of the complex symptom pattern during recurrent panic attacks.

It must be noted that the reported absence of elevated HPA measures during lactate-induced panic attacks does not question this hypothesis. Lactate infusions induce a significant osmotic and volume load, enhancing atrial natriuretic peptide secretion, which acts as a functional vasopressin antagonist (Dayanithi & Antoni 1990). Since vasopressin is the most important dynamic factor potentiating the effect of CRH at the pituitary level, blockade of its action during the lactate paradigm would reduce the endocrine effect of CRH to release ACTH. Thus, even if lactate-induced panic attacks were driven by central CRH, the counterregulatory mechanisms at the pituitary would compensate its peripheral endocrine effect.

EFFECTS OF HYPERCORTISOLISM AT THE CELLULAR AND MOLECULAR LEVEL

Genomic effects of corticosteroids

It has been mentioned in the beginning of this chapter that corticosteroids can precipitate a host of

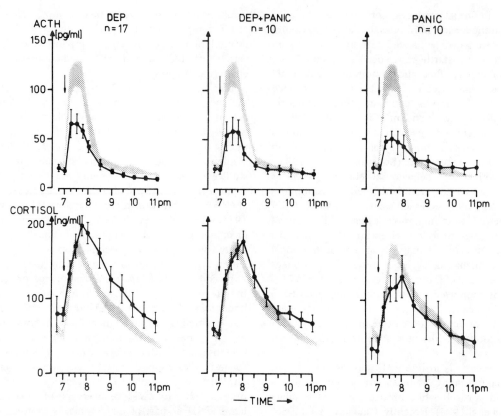

Fig. 17.8   Three patient samples with depression, panic disorder or a combination thereof all responded with decreased ACTH release following hCRH. Note that this proves true also for subjects with pure panic disorder, who were normocortisolaemic at baseline. This indicates a defect in these patients at the CRH receptor level, possibly secondary to excessive episodic CRH release associated with panic attacks (from Holsboer et al 1987c)

behavioural effects. At the cellular level physiological responses of brain neurones to corticosteroids are triggered by binding of the hormones to specific high affinity (K_D~1 nM) cytoplasmic receptors. These receptors, when not bound to ligands, are believed to be heteromers composed of a single steroid and DNA-binding subunit and two 90 kiloDalton heatshock proteins (Hsp-90). After penetration of the glucocorticoid into the cell it binds to the receptor, forming a nonactivated complex. The dissociation of the Hsp-90 subunit from the receptor activates the glucocorticoid-receptor complex by uncovering its DNA binding domain (Mendel et al 1986, Catelli et al 1985). The resultant conformational changes of the GC–GR complex confer increased affinity for high-affinity receptor sites in the chromatin (Fig. 17.9). Regulatory elements to which the activated GR binds have been

identified in many genes, including not only those which regulate the HPA system but also a host of other genes, encoding proteins that are directly or indirectly involved in mediation of behaviour.

Since most evidence points to excessive activity of CRH neurons as one possible mediator of behavioural changes in depression and panic anxiety, it is of particular concern as to why, in contrast to physiological stress responses, elevated corticosteroids fail fully to control CRH production by negative feedback regulation in these pathological conditions. To study the mechanism by which glucocorticoids decrease transcription of the CRH gene we transfected a mouse anterior pituitary cell line (AtT20) with a chimeric gene, containing the hCRH gene promotor fused to the bacterial chloramphenicol acetyltransferase (CAT) 'reporter'-gene. We observed that cAMP-induced gene

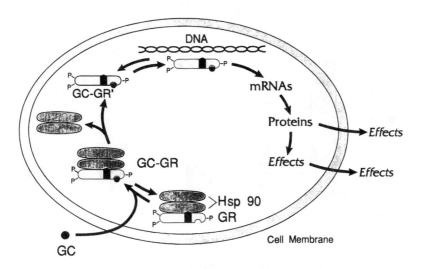

Fig. 17.9   After passive entry through the periplasmatic membrane, glucocorticoids bind to their specific receptors, which are localized within the cytoplasmic compartment as long as their specific ligand is absent. The receptors are known to be heteromeric structures containing only one steroid-binding polypeptide per complex, which is associated with other cellular components, most notably two heat shock proteins (Hsp90) monomers. These 90 kiloDalton proteins are believed to cover the DNA-binding site. The status of this and other polypeptide components of the receptor is not firmly established. Transformation to DNA binding ability occurs concurrently with the dissociation of Hsp90 and other cellular components from the steroid-bearing polypeptide. This released activated form may then translocate to the cell nucleus, where it acts as a transcriptional factor by binding to specific regulatory DNA sequences in the promotor regions of corticosteroid regulated genes. Steroids with low or completely missing affinity to the homone binding site fail to regulate hormone sensitive genes (see Fig. 17.10). The glucocorticoid antagonist RU 38486 binds with high affinity to the receptor. However, unlike agonists, it is believed to prevent dissociation of Hsp90 and other components of the inactive heteromer and hence its transformation into the active form, thus inhibiting nuclear receptor translocation. Hsp90 may also play another, more active role in glucocorticoid regulated transcription processes (modified from Munck & Mendel 1991)

transcription was repressed by dexamethasone, suggesting that glucocorticosteroids exert negative feedback at least in part via interaction with an AMP-responsive element at the 5'-flanking region (Phi Van et al 1990) (Fig. 17.10). These data support two different models of how activated GRs may repress gene transcription: 1) GR inhibition of target genes by protein–protein interaction; and 2) competition for specific DNA binding sites between additional positive transcription factors and the receptors.

Elucidation of the exact mechanism by which the GC–GR complex exerts negative feedback regulation at the level of the CRH gene will provide an in-depth understanding of how stressful external stimuli are translated into molecular events at the genomic level. In addition, from a full elucidation of the concerted action by which transformed GRs and other so far unidentified transcription factors accomplish regulation of the CRH gene, we hope to delineate a research strategy for molecular genetics of affective disorders, which would be more focused than are the conflicting linkage studies available at present (see ch. 9).

From recent studies by Pepin et al (1989) provisional evidence has emerged that antidepressants are involved in mechanisms of molecular HPA regulation. These investigators showed that the GR gene promotor is activated by several tricyclic antidepressants. They also found GRmRNA to be increased by desipramine and suggested that this effect was not mediated by

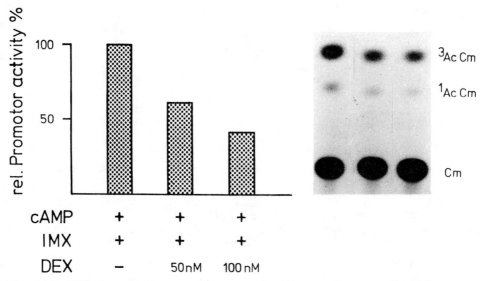

Fig. 17.10 CRH-gene promotor activity is increased by a cyclic-AMP analog and a phosphodiesterase inhibitor (IMX). The promotor is linked to a gene, coding for an enzyme that acetylates chloramphenicol (chloramphenicolacetyltransferase, CAT). The activity of the promotor is measured by the amount of chloramphenicol acetylation under various experimental conditions. As illustrated, the activity of the CRH genepromotor can be reduced by dexamethasone in a dose-dependent mode (Phi Van et al 1990)

monoamine reuptake, but rather by an action at the GR gene promotor or at other transcription factors involved. If it proves true that antidepressants enhance the feedback sensitivity by stimulating GR synthesis, this would provide better understanding of the mechanisms that account for gradual normalization of HPA alteration during successful antidepressant treatment (Holsboer et al 1982, 1983, 1987b, Greden et al 1983, Gerken et al 1985, Holsboer-Trachsler et al 1991).

Membrane effects of corticosteroids and neurosteroids

By applying corticosteroids directly to specific neurones immediate changes in their firing frequency can be observed (Hua & Chen 1989). These rapid effects result from a direct action of the steroid hormones on the plasma membrane, either by changing the lipid environment of the receptors, modifying the fluidity of the surrounding cell membrane, or through specific steroid-binding sites.

The best documented interaction between a steroid and a neurotransmitter receptor is the modification of the GABA$_A$–benzodiazepine (BDZ) receptor complex by the A-ring reduced metabolites of progesterone (3α-hydroxy-5α-pregnane-20-one; 3α-OHDHP) and

tetrahydrodeoxycorticosterone (5α-pregnane-3α, 21-diol-2-one; 3α-THDOC). Low concentrations of these derivatives (10^{-8} M), which are believed to be inactive at intracellular steroid receptors, potentiate the actions of GABA at the GABA$_A$–BDZ receptor complex. The effects of 3α-OH-DHP and 3α-THDOC resemble the effects of barbiturates, as both steroids increase the number of high-affinity GABA$_A$-recognition sites, enhance the affinity of BDZ sites and potentiate the actions of GABA on membrane currents by enhancing chloride channel conductance (Gee et al 1988). The latter effect is most probably achieved by a prolonged opening of the chloride channel. However, effects upon the frequency of channel openings may also play a role. Unlike effects with barbiturates, a reciprocal positive cooperativity between GABA- and steroid-binding sites has been found: steroids potentiate the binding of GABA and GABA, in turn, enhances the effects of steroids.

Seeburg and colleagues have recently demonstrated that various molecular forms of GABA$_A$ receptors can be studied by transient expression of cDNAs for various subunits of the GABA$_A$ receptor complex in human embryonic kidney cells (Pritchett et al 1988, 1989). From these studies emerged the existence of six alpha-subunits, three beta-subunits and two gamma-subunits from which GABA$_A$-receptors can be composed.

Coexpression of alpha- or beta-subunits together with a gamma$_2$-subunit is required for the positive or negative allosteric modulation of GABA-evoked chloride currents by either anxiolytic benzodiazepines or beta-carboline derivatives, which act as anxiogenic inverse BDZ agonists in the primate experiment.

The steroids 3α-OH-DHP or 3α-THDOC potentiate GABA$_A$ responses even in the absence of the gamma$_2$-subunit. Unlike BDZs these steroids also have a direct effect upon the GABA-gated chloride channel, at least in micromolar concentrations. The direct action of these steroids has been observed in the absence of GABA and can be blocked by bicuculline, a GABA-receptor antagonist (Fig. 17.11). This prompted Puia et al (1990) to suggest that steroid effects are elicited in close vicinity to the GABA recognition site. The GABA$_A$-modulating effects of this class of steroids are not limited to 3α-OHDHP and 3α-THDOC. Nanomolar concentrations of glucocorticoids enhance neuronal excitability, lowering the threshold for seizures (Majewska 1987).

Recently, another class of steroid which also modulates activity of GABA$_A$-receptors has been identified. These hormones, dehydroepiandrosterone, its precursor pregnenolone (pregn-5-ene-3β, 20α-diol) and their sulphated forms, were termed neurosteroids, because their precursor can be synthesized in primary cultures of rat glial cells (Jung-Testas et al 1989). Electrophysiological studies suggest that pregnenolone sulphate inhibits GABA-generated currents in isolated cortical neurones, thus behaving as an allosteric GABA$_A$-receptor antagonist (Majewska et al 1988). Neurosteroids such as dehydroepiandrosterone reduce neuronal and glial cell death and may improve learning in mice (Coleman 1988, Barrett-Connor et al 1986), while 3α-THDOC appears to enhance sleep and probably acts as an endogenous anxiolytic (Mendelson et al 1987).

The physiological significance of these findings is difficult to assess. To date, it appears that endogenous steroids derived from adrenal cortex or central tissues are potent modulators of the GABA$_A$–BDZ receptor complex, and may exceed the effects of benzodiazepines. Consequently, the physiological effectiveness of benzodiazepines or other ligands of the GABA$_A$–BDZ receptor complex may be determined by the neuroendocrine status of the patient. This might explain why severely depressed patients, whose HPA system is excessively active, frequently tolerate high dosages of benzodiazepines. Future research will show whether steroids derived from the adrenal corticosteroid family will give a lead for the development of a new class of drugs that can be of use in treating psychiatric syndromes in a similar way to the benzodi-

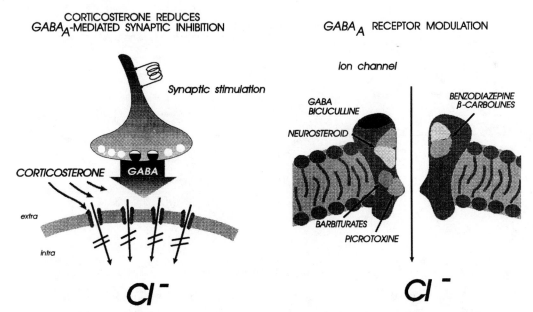

Fig. 17.11 Corticosteroids, and particularly metabolites derived from corticosterone precursors such as 3αTHDOC, 3αDHP or dehydroepiandrosterone, act through binding sites at the GABA$_A$—BDZ receptor complex to modulate chloride conductance.

azepines, but without the intrinsic risk of tolerance and dependence.

FUTURE RESEARCH STRATEGIES

As this review illustrates, studies of HPA activity in affective disorders must cover the whole range from clinical evaluation to animal experiments and investigations at the cellular and genomic level. Concerted clinical research is needed to study under which emotional conditions changes in humoral homeostasis occur that may trigger genes carrying noxious information. Within this investigative framework evaluation of temperament, life style, daily hassles and acute psychic trauma, which may burden an illness-prone individual and trigger or accelerate the disease process, is as indispensable as animal research studies. The latter must include rodents and primates, with application of acute or chronic stress paradigms during different segments of their life-span. In this dialogue between nature and nurture glucocorticoids serve as mediators between environmental psychosocial stressors and the level of cellular and genomic response. This research strategy renders artefactual any dichotomy between systemic physiology and mechanistic approaches of cell and molecular biology.

Family studies leave little doubt that almost all psychiatric disorders, including affective illness, have a specific genetic background, but their exact mode of transmission remains obscure. That is because genes do not act alone, but need to be regulated, and hormones are most important for this purpose (Fig. 17.12). The neuroendocrine system of human beings reacts individually to external stimuli and the degree of the stress hormone response is largely determined not only by the blueprint carried in genes but also by the specific life history. If the meaning of an external event is recognized as stressful it finally translates in the hypothalamus into activation of the HPA system, leading to elevation of plasma glucocorticosteroids. These hormones turn on a complex machinery to regulate genes, whose end products (proteins) may act in a certain yet unknown pattern to promote or prevent the pathophysiology that underlies affective disorders. Deciphering how genes that code for suspected proteins are regulated, and which alteration in protein synthesis accounts for dysregulation of these genes, will give us a lead for a more focused genetic research in psychiatry. If an aberrant protein is identified one may go back to the genomic DNA and mRNA, then map the position at the genome and use this information for linkage studies in affected pedigrees. This approach has several

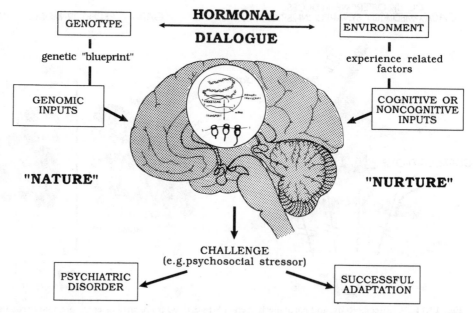

Fig. 17.12   Hormones are the brain's major tool to respond at neural circuitries and at cellular and molecular levels to events in the outside world.

advantages, particularly if one disbelieves in the presence of a single major gene responsible for a complex disorder such as depression.

A further conclusion from the present status of HPA investigations in affectively ill patients is that the field requires urgently a diagnostic classification which allows incorporation of laboratory findings. The rapid proliferation of new diagnostic schemes admittedly

camouflages our ignorance of underlying pathophysiology. Absence of objective biological markers will perpetuate the problem of defining clinical phenotypes with the necessary validity. In the author's view these indices can only be derived from progress in pathophysiology and at present the neuroendocrinology of the HPA system appears to be the most promising source for the urgently required laboratory markers.

REFERENCES

Amsterdam J D, Winokur A, Abelman E, Lucki I, Richels K 1983 Cosyntropin (ACTH alpha 1–24) stimulation test in depressed patients and healthy subjects. American Journal of Psychiatry 140: 907–912

Amsterdam J D, Maislin G, Winokur A, Kling M, Gold P 1987 Pituitary and adrenocortical responses to the ovine corticotropin-releasing hormone in depressed patients and healthy volunteers. Archives of General Psychiatry 44: 775–781

Barrett-Connor E, Khaw K T, Yen S S C 1986 A prospective study of dehydroepiandrosterone sulfate, mortality and cardiovascular disease. New England Journal of Medicine 315: 1519–1524

Baybutt H N, Holsboer F 1990 Inhibition of macrophage differentiation and function by cortisol. Endocrinology 127: 476–480

Berkenbosch F, van Oers J, del Rey A, Tilders F, Besedovsky H 1987 Corticotropin-releasing factor-producing neurons in the rat activated by interleukin-1. Science 238: 524–526

Besedovsky H, del Rey A 1989 Mechanism of virus-induced stimulation of the hypothalamus-pituitary-adrenal axis. Journal of Steroid Biochemistry 34: 235–239

Besedovsky H, del Rey A, Sorkin E, da Prada M, Burri R, Honegger C 1983 The immune response evokes changes in brain noradrenergic neurons. Science 221: 564–566

Blalock J E 1989 A molecular basis for bidirectional communication between the immune and neuroendocrine systems. Physiological Reviews 69: 1–27

Born J, Zwick A, Roth G, Fehm-Wolfsdorf G, Fehm H L 1987 Differential effects of hydrocortisone, fluocortolone, and aldosterone on nocturnal sleep in humans. Acta Endocrinologica 116: 129–137

Breder C D, Dinarello C A, Saper C B 1988 Interleukin-1 immunoreactive innervation of the human hypothalamus. Science 240: 321–324

Bulloch K 1985 Neuroanatomy of lymphoid tissue: a review. In: Guillemin R, Cohn M, Melnechuk T (eds) Neural modulation of immunity. Raven Press, New York, p 111–141

Calogero A E, Gallucci W T, Tomai T P, Loriaux D L, Chrousos G P, Gold P W 1988 Inhibition of corticotropin releasing hormone secretion by GABA A and GABA B receptor action in vitro: clinical implications. In: D'Agata R, Chrousos G P (eds) Recent advances in adrenal regulation and function. Raven Press, New York, p 279–284

Carroll B J, Feinberg M, Greden J F, Tarika J, Albala A A, Haskett R F, James N, Kronfold Z, Lohr N, Steiner M, De

Vigne J P, Young E 1981 A specific laboratory test for the diagnosis of melancholia. Archives of General Psychiatry 38: 15–22

Catelli M G, Binart N, Jung-Testas I, Renoir J M, Baulieu E E, Feramisco J R, Welch W J 1985 The common 90-kd protein component of non-transformed '8S' steroid receptors is a heat shock protein. European Molecular Biology Organization Journal 4: 3131–3135

Charles G A, Schittecatte M, Rush A J, Panzer M, Wilmotte J 1989 Persistent cortisol non-suppression after clinical recovery predicts symptomatic relapse in unipolar depression. Journal of Affective Disorders 17: 271–278

Coleman D L 1988 Therapeutic effects of dehydroepiandrosterone (DHEA) and its metabolites in obese-hyperglycemic mutant mice. Program of Clinical and Biological Research 265: 161–175

Cooper C L, Cooper R, Faragher E B 1989 Incidence and perception of psychosocial stress: the relationship with breast cancer. Psychological Medicine 19: 415–422

Coryell W 1990 DST abnormality as a predictor of course in major depression. Journal of Affective Disorders 19: 163–169

Dayanithi G, Antoni F A 1990 Atriopeptins are potent inhibitors of ACTH secretion by rat anterior pituitary cells in vitro: involvement of the atrial natriuretic factor receptor domain of membrane-bound guanylyl cyclase. Journal of Endocrinology 125: 39–44

de Kloet R E 1991 Brain corticosteroid receptor balance and homeostatic control. Frontiers in Neuroendocrinoloy 12: 95–165

Doraiswamy M, Lurie S, Figiel G, Husain M, Boyko O, Nemeroff C B, Krishnan R R 1990 Pituitary enlargement in depression. Biological Psychiatry, Supplement 27: 256

Dunn A J, Berridge C W 1990 Physiological and behavioural responses to corticotropin-releasing-factor administration: is CRF a mediator of anxiety or stress responses? Brain Research Reviews 15: 71–100

Ehlers C L, Reed T K, Heriksen S J 1986 Effects of corticotropin-releasing factor and growth hormone-releasing factor on sleep and activity in rats. Neuroendocrinology 42: 467–474

Eldridge J C, Brodish A, Kute T E, Landfield P W 1989 Apparent age-related resistance of type II hippocampal corticosteroid receptors to down-regulation during chronic escape training. Journal of Neuroscience 9: 3237–3242

Fava G A, Sonino N, Murray A M 1987 Major depression associated with endocrine disease. Psychiatric Developments 4: 321–348

Fehm H L, Klein E, Holl R, Voigt K H 1984 Evidence for extrapituitary mechanisms in the regulation of cortisol secretion in man. Journal of Clinical Endocrinology and Metabolism 58: 410–414

Felten D L, Felten S Y, Bellinger D L, Carlson S L, Ackerman K D, Madden K S, Olschowka J A, Livnat S 1987 Noradrenergic sympathetic interactions with the immune system structure and function. Immunological Review 100: 225–260

Fink G, Robinson I C A F, Tannahill L A 1988 Effects of adrenalectomy and glucocorticoids on the peptides CRF-41, AVP and oxytocin in rat hypophysial portal blood. Journal of Physiology 401: 329–345

Fliers E, Swaab D F, Pool C W, Vewer R W H 1985 The vasopressin and oxytocin neurons in the human supraoptic and paraventricular nucleus; changes with aging and in senile dementia. Brain Research 352: 45–53

Follenius M, Simon C, Brandenberger G, Lenzi P 1987 Ultradian plasma corticotropin and cortisol rhythms. Time series analysis. Journal of Endocrinological Investigations 10: 261–266

Gee K W, Bolger M B, Brinton R E, Coirini H, McEwen B S 1988 Steroid modulation of the chloride ionophore in rat brain: structure-activity requirements, regional dependence and mechanism of action. Journal of Pharmacology and Experimental Therapeutics 246: 803–812

Gerken A, Maier W, Holsboer F 1985 Weekly monitoring of dexamethasone suppression response in depression: its relationship to change of body weight and psychopathology. Psychoneuroendocrinology 10: 261–271

Gerken A, Holsboer F 1986 Cortisol and corticosterone response after syn-corticotropin in relationship to dexamethasone suppressibility of cortisol. Psychoneuroendocrinology 11: 185–194

Gold P W, Chrousos G, Kellner C, Post R, Roy A, Augerinos P, Shulte H, Oldfield E, Loriaux D L 1984 Psychiatric implications of basic and clinical studies with corticotropin-releasing factor. American Journal of Psychiatry 141: 619–627

Gold P W, Loriaux D L, Roy A, Kling M A, Clabrese J R, Kellner C H, Nieman L K, Post R M, Pickar D, Gallucci W, Augerinos P, Paul S, Oldfield E H, Cutler G B Jr, Chrousos G P 1986 Responses to corticotropin-releasing hormone in the hypercortisolism of depression and Cushing's disease. Pathophysiologic and diagnostic implications. New England Journal of Medicine 314: 1329–1335

Greden J F, Gardner R, King D, Grunhaus L, Carroll B J, Kronfold Z 1983 Dexamethasone suppression tests in antidepressant treatment of melancholia – the process of normalization and test-retest reproducibility. Archives of General Psychiatry 40: 493–500

Grunhaus L, Zelnik T, Albala A A, Rabin D, Haskett R F, Zis A P, Greden J F 1987 Serial dexamethasone suppression tests in depressed patients treated only with electroconvulsive therapy. Journal of Affective Disorders 13: 233–240

Halbreich U, Asnis G M, Zumoff B, Nathan R S, Shindledecker R 1984 Effect of age and sex on cortisol secretion in depressives and normals. Psychiatry Research 13: 221–229

Halbreich U, Asnis G M, Shindledecker R 1985 Cortisol secretion in endogenous depression. Archives of General Psychiatry 42: 904–908

Haskett R 1985 Diagnostic categorization of psychotic disturbance in Cushing's syndrome. American Journal of Psychiatry 142: 911–916

Hauger R L, Millan M A, Catt K J, Aguilera G 1987 Differential regulation of brain and pituitary corticotropin-releasing factor receptors by corticosterone. Endocrinology 120: 1527–1533

Heuser I, Wark H J, Keul J, Holsboer F 1991 Altered pituitary-adrenocortical function in elderly endurance athletes. Journal of Clinical Endocrinology and Metabolism (in press)

Holsboer F 1983 Prediction of clinical course by dexamethasone suppression test (DST) response in depressed patients – physiological and clinical construct validity of the DST. Pharmacopsychiatry 16: 186–191

Holsboer F 1989 Psychiatric implications of altered limbic-hypothalamic-pituitary-adrenocortical activity. European Archives of Psychiatry and Neurological Science 238: 302–322

Holsboer F, Liebl R, Hofschuster E 1982 Repeated dexamethasone suppression test during depressive illness. Normalization of test result compared with clinical improvement. Journal of Affective Disorders 4: 93–101

Holsboer F, Steiger A, Maier W 1983 Four cases of reversion to abnormal dexamethasone suppression test response as indicator of clinical relapse: a preliminary report. Biological Psychiatry 18: 911–916

Holsboer F, Haak D, Gerken A, Vecsei P 1984a Plasma dexamethasone concentrations and differential glucocorticoid suppression response of cortisol and corticosterone in depressives and controls. Biological Psychiatry 19: 281–291

Holsboer F, von Bardeleben U, Gerken A, Stalla G K, Müller O A 1984b Blunted corticotropin and normal cortisol response to human corticotropin-releasing factor in (h-CRF) in depression. New England Journal of Medicine 311: 1127

Holsboer F, Müller O A, Doerr H G, Sippell W G, Stalla G K, Gerken A, Steiger A, Boll E, Benkert O 1984c ACTH and multisteroid responses to corticotropin-releasing factor in depressive illness: relationship to multisteroid responses after ACTH stimulation and dexamethasone suppression. Psychoneuroendocrinology 9: 147–160

Holsboer F, Gerken A, Stalla G K, Müller O A 1985 ACTH, cortisol and corticosterone output after ovine corticotropin-releasing factor challenge during depression and after recovery. Biological Psychiatry 20: 276–286

Holsboer F, Wiedemann K, Boll E 1986a Shortened dexamethasone half-life in depressed dexamethasone nonsuppressors. Archives of General Psychiatry 43: 813–815

Holsboer F, Gerken A, von Bardeleben U, Grimm W, Beyer H, Müller O A, Stalla G K 1986b Human corticotropin-releasing hormone in depression. Biological Psychiatry 21: 601–611

Holsboer F, Philipp M, Steiger A, Gerken A 1986c Multisteroid analysis after DST in depressed patients – a controlled study. Journal of Affective Disorders 10: 241–249

Holsboer F, Gerken A, Stalla G K, Müller O A 1987a
Blunted aldosterone and ACTH release after human CRH
administration in depressed patients. American Journal of
Psychiatry 144: 229–231

Holsboer F, von Bardeleben U, Wiedemann K, Müller O A,
Stalla G K 1987b Serial assessment of corticotropin-
releasing hormone response after dexamethasone in
depression – implications for pathophysiology of DST
nonsuppression. Biological Psychiatry 22: 228–234

Holsboer F, von Bardeleben U, Buller R, Heuser I, Steiger A
1987c Stimulation response to corticotropin-releasing
hormone (CRH) in patients with depression, alcoholism
and panic disorder. Hormone and Metabolic Research 16:
80–88

Holsboer F, Stalla G K, von Bardeleben U, Hammann K,
Müller H, Müller O A 1988a Acute adrenocortical
stimulation by recombinant gamma interferon in human
controls. Life Sciences 42: 1–5

Holsboer F, von Bardeleben U, Steiger A 1988b Effects of
intravenous corticotropin-releasing hormone upon sleep-
related growth hormone surge and sleep-EEG in man.
Neuroendocrinology 48: 62–68

Holsboer-Trachsler E, Stohler R, Hatzinger M 1991
Repeated administration of the combined dexamethasone-
hCRH stimulation test during treatment of depression.
Psychiatry Research (in press)

Hua S Y, Chen Y Z 1989 Membrane receptor-mediated
electrophysiological effects of glucocorticoid on mammalian
neurons. Endocrinology 124: 687–691

Insel T R, Ninan P T, Aloi J, Jimerson D C, Skolnick P,
Paul S M 1984 A benzodiazepine receptor mediated
model of anxiety. Archives of General Psychiatry 41:
741–750

Irwin M, Jones L, Britton K, Hauger R L 1989 Central
corticotropin releasing factor reduces natural cytotoxicity.
Neuropsychopharmacology 2: 281–284

Jaeckle R S, Kathol R G, Lopez J F, Meller W H, Krummel S
J 1987 Enhanced adrenal sensitivity to exogenous
ACTH$_{1-24}$ stimulation in major depression: relationship to
dexamethasone suppression test results. Archives of
General Psychiatry 44: 233–240

Jarrett D B, Miewald J M, Kupfer D J 1990 Recurrent
depression is associated with a persistent reduction in sleep-
ralated growth hormone secretion. Archives of General
Psychiatry 47: 113–118

Jung-Testas I, Hu Z Y, Baulieu E E, Robel P 1989
Neurosteroids: biosynthesis of pregnenolone and
progesterone in primary cultures of rat glial cells.
Endocrinology 125: 2083–2091

Keller Wood M E, Dallman M F 1985 Corticosteroid
inhibition of ACTH secretion. Endocrine Review 5:
1–24

Krieg J C, Lauer C, Hermle L, von Bardeleben U, Pollmächer
T, Holsboer F 1990 Psychometric, polysomnographic, and
neuroendocrine measures in subjects at high risk for
psychiatric disorders: preliminary results.
Neuropsychobiology 23: 57–67

Krishnan K R R, Ritchie J C, Saunders W, Wilson W,
Nemeroff C B, Carroll B J 1990 Nocturnal and early
morning secretion of ACTH and cortisol in humans.
Biological Psychiatry 38: 47–57

Lee S W, Tsou A P, Chan H, Thomas J, Petrie K, Eugui E M,

Allison A C 1988 Glucocorticoids selectively inhibit the
transcription of the interleukin 1β gene and decrease the
stability of interleukin 1β mRNA. Proceedings of the
National Academy of Sciences of the USA 85: 1204–1208

Linkowski P, Mendlewicz J, LeClerq R, Brasseur M,
Hubain P, Goldstein J, Copinschi G, Van Cauter E 1985
The 24-hour profile of ACTH and cortisol in major
depressive illness. Journal of Clinical Endocrinology and
Metabolism 61: 429–438

Majewska M D 1987 Antagonist-type interaction of
glucocorticoids with the GABA receptor-coupled chloride
channel. Brain Research 418: 377–382

Majewska M D, Mienville J M, Vicini S 1988 Neurosteroid
pregnenolone sulfate antagonizes electrophysiological
responses to GABA in neurons. Neuroscience Letters 90:
279–284

Markham P, Salahuddin S, Veren K, Orndoff S, Gallo R 1986
Hydrocortisone and some other hormones enhance the
expression of HTLV-III. International Journal of Cancer
37: 67–72

Mendel D B, Bodwell J E, Gametchu B, Harrison R W,
Munck A 1986 Molybdate-stabilized nonactivated
glucocorticoid-receptor complexes contain a 90-kDa non-
steroid-binding phosphoprotein that is lost on activation.
Journal of Biological Chemistry 261: 3758–3763

Mendelson W B, Martin J V, Perlis M, Wagner R, Majewska
M D, Paul S M 1987 Sleep induction by an adrenal steroid
in the rat. Psychopharmacology 93: 226–229

Mortola J F, Liu J H, Gillin J C, Rasmussen D D, Yen S S C
1987 Pulsatile rhythms of adrenocorticotrophin (ACTH)
and cortisol in women with endogenous depression:
evidence for increased ACTH pulse frequency. Journal of
Endocrinology and Metabolism 65: 962–968

Munck A, Mendel D B 1991 Glucocorticoid receptors and
actions. American Review of Respiratory Disease (in press)

Nemeroff C B, Widerlöv E, Bissette G, Wallcus H, Karlsson I,
Eklund K, Kilts C S, Loosen P T, Vale W 1984 Elevated
concentrations of CSF corticotropin-releasing factor-like
immunoreactivity in depressed patients. Science 226:
1342–1344

Nemeroff C B, Owens M J, Bissett G, Andorn A C,
Stanley M 1988 Reduced corticotropin releasing factor
binding sites in the frontal cortex of suicide victims.
Archives of General Psychiatry 45: 577–579

Owens M J, Bissette G, Nemeroff C B 1989 Acute effects of
alprazolam and adinazolam on the concentrations of
corticotropin-releasing factor in the rat brain. Synapse 4:
196–202

Pater M M, Hughes G A, Hyslop D E, Nakshatri H, Pater A
1988 Glucocorticoid-dependent oncogenic transformation
by type 16 but not type 11 human papilloma virus DNA.
Nature 335: 832–835

Pavlov E P, Harman S M, Chrousos G P, Loriaux D L,
Blackman M R 1986 Responses of plasma
adrenocorticotropin, cortisol, and dehydroepiandrosterone
to ovine corticotropin-releasing hormone in healthy aging
men. Journal of Clinical Endocrinology and Metabolism
62: 767–772

Pepin M C, Beaulieu S, Barden N 1989 Antidepressants
regulate glucocorticoid receptor messenger RNA
concentrations in primary neuronal cultures. Molecular
Brain Research 6: 77–83

Phi Van L, Spengler D, Holsböer F 1990 Glucocorticoid repression of cAMP dependent hCRH gene promoter activity in a transfected mouse anterior pituitary cell line. Endocrinology 127: 1412–1418

Pritchett D B, Sontheimer H, Gorman C M, Kettenmann H, Seeburg P H, Schofield P R 1988 Transient expression shows ligand gating and allosteric potentiation of GABA$_A$ receptor subunits. Science 242: 1306–1308

Pritchett D B, Sontheimer H, Shivers B, Ymer S, Kettenmann H, Shofield P R, Seeburg P H 1989 Importance of a novel GABA$_A$ receptor subunit for benzodiazepine pharmacology. Nature 338: 582–585

Puia G, Santi M R, Vicini S, Pritchett D B, Purdy R H, Paul S M, Seeburg P H, Gosta E 1990 Neurosteroids act on recombinant human GABA$_A$ receptor. Neuron 4: 759–765

Reul J M, van den Bosch F R, de Kloet E R 1987 Relative occupation of type-I and type-II corticosteroid receptors in rat brain following stress and dexamethasone treatment: functional implications. Journal of Endocrinology 115: 459–467

Roy-Byrne P P, Uhde T W, Post R M, Gallucci W, Chrousos G P, Gold P W 1986 The corticotropin-releasing hormone stimulation test in patients with panic disorder. American Journal of Psychiatry 143: 896–899

Rubin R T, Poland R E, Lesser I M, Winston R A, Blodgett A L N 1987 Neuroendocrine aspects of primary endogenous depression. Archives of General Psychiatry 44: 328–2336

Rupprecht R, Lesch K P, Müller U, Beck G, Beckmann H, Schulte H M 1989 Blunted adrenocorticotropin but normal β-endorphin release after depression. Journal of Clinical Endocrinology and Metabolism 69: 600–603

Sapolsky R M, Krey L C, McEwen B S 1985 Prolonged glucocorticoid exposure reduces hippocampal neuron number: implications for aging. Journal of Neuroscience 5: 1222–1227

Sapolsky R M, Krey L C, McEwen B S 1986 The neuroendocrinology of stress and aging: the glucocorticoid cascade hypothesis. Endocrine Review 7: 284–304

Sapolsky R M, Rivier C, Yamamoto G, Plotsky P, Vale W 1987 Interleukin-1 stimulates the secretion of hypothalamic corticotropin-releasing factor. Science 238: 522–524

Sapolsky R M, Packan D R, Vale W W 1988 Glucocorticoid toxicity in the hippocampus: in vitro demonstration. Brain Research 453: 367–371

Schleifer S J, Keller S E, Bond R N, Cohen J, Stein M 1989 Major depressive disorder and immunity. Archives of General Psychiatry 46: 81–87

Shibahara S, Morimoto Y, Furutani Y, Notake M, Takahashi H, Shimizu S, Horikawa S, Numa S 1983 Isolation and sequence analysis of the human corticotropin-releasing factor precursor gene. Embo Journal 2: 775–779

Smith M A, Davidson J, Ritchie J C, Kudler H, Lipper S, Chappell P, Nemeroff C B 1989 The corticotropin-releasing hormone test in patients with posttraumatic stress disorder. Biological Psychiatry 26: 349–355

Smith E M, Galin F S, LeBoeuf R D, Coppenhaver D H, Harbour D V, Blalock J E 1990 Nucleotide and amino acid sequence of lymphocyte-derived corticotropin: endotoxin induction of a truncated peptide. Proceedings of the National Academy of Sciences 87: 1057–1060

Starkman M N, Schteingart D E 1981 Neuropsychiatric manifestations of patients with Cushing's Syndrome. Archives of General Psychiatry 141: 215–219

Steiger A, von Bardeleben U, Herth T, Holsboer F 1989 Sleep EEG and nocturnal secretion of cortisol and growth hormone in male patients with endogenous depression before treatment and after recovery. Journal of Affective Disorders 16: 189–195

Steiger A, Guldner J, Knisatscheck H, Lauer C, Rothe B, Holsboer F 1991 Effects of synthetic ACTH (i-9) fragment on sleep-EEG and nocturnal secretion of cortisol and growth hormone peptides (in press)

Sternberg E M, Wilder R L 1989 The role of the hypothalamic-pituitary-adrenal axis in an experimental model of arthritis. Psychoneuroendocrinimmunology 2: 102–108

Swanson L W, Sawchenko P E, Rivier J, Vale W W 1983 Organization of ovine corticotropin-releasing factor immunoreactive cells and fibers in the rat brain. An immunohistochemical study. Neuroendocrinology 36: 165–186

Tobler I, Borbély A A, Shwyzer M, Fontana A 1984 Interleukin-1 derived from astrocytes enhances slow wave activity in sleep EEG of the rat. European Journal of Pharmacology 104: 191–192

Vale W, Spiess J, Rivier C, Rivier J 1981 Characterization of a 41-residue ovine hypothalamic peptide that stimulates secretion of corticotropin and β-endorphin. Science 213: 1394–1397

Villette J M, Bourin P, Doinel C, Mansour I, Fiet J, Boudou P, Dreux C, Roue R, Deord M, Levi F 1990 Circadian variations in plasma levels of hypophyseal, adrenocortical and testicular hormones in men infected with human immunodeficiency virus. Journal of Clinical Endocrinology and Metabolism 70: 572–577

von Bardeleben U, Holsboer F 1989 Cortisol response to a combined dexamethasone-human corticotropin-releasing hormone challenge in patients with depression. Journal of Neuroendocrinology 1: 485–488

von Bardeleben U, Holsboer F 1991 Effect of age on the cortisol reponse to human CRH in depressed patients pretreated with dexamethasone. Biological Psychiatry 29: 1042–1050

von Bardeleben U, Holsboer F, Stalla G K, Müller O A 1985 Combined administration of human corticotropin-releasing factor and lysine vasopressin induces cortisol escape from dexamethasone suppression in healthy subjects. Life Sciences 37: 1613–1618

von Bardeleben U, Stalla G K, Müller O A, Holsboer F 1988 Blunting of ACTH response to human CRH in depressed patients is avoided by metyrapone pretreatment. Biological Psychiatry 24: 782–786

Wiedemann K, Holsboer F 1990 The effect of dexamethasone dosage upon plasma cortisol and dexamethasone during DST. Journal of Affective Disorders 19: 133–137

Young E A, Akil H 1985 Corticotropin releasing factor stimulation of ACTH and β-endorphin release: Effects of acute and chronic stress. Endocrinology 117: 23–30

Young E A, Watson S J, Kotun J, Haskett R F, Grunhaus L, Murphy-Weinberg V, Vale W, Rivier J, Akil H 1990a β-lipotropin-β-endorphin response to low-dose ovine corticotropin releasing factor in endogenous depression. Archives of General Psychiatry 47: 449–457

Young E A, Akana S, Dallman M F 1990b Decreased sensitivity to glucocorticoid fast feedback in chronically stressed rats. Neuroendocrinology 51: 536–542

Zonderman, A B, Costa P T, McCrae R R 1989 Depression as a risk of cancer morbidity and mortality in a nationally representative sample. Journal of American Medicine Association 262: 1191–1195

18. Neuropsychology and imaging

Trevor W. Robbins   Eileen M. Joyce   Barbara J. Sahakian

Until quite recently it was thought that even severe depression was associated with only minor impairments in psychological test performance (e.g. Friedman 1964). However, the comprehensive and important review by Miller (1975) did much to dispel this impression. He surveyed the evidence that both severe and mild forms of depression were associated with deficits on cognitive, motor, perceptual and communication tasks. Within the cognitive domain, he considered general intellectual impairment and speed, visuospatial ability, memory and learning, cognitive distortions regarding reinforcement contingencies and the passage of time, abstract thought and aspects of language. His major conclusions were that depressives of all subtypes exhibited deficits in each of the domains reviewed. However, although the degree of depression was generally related to the magnitude of the cognitive deficit there was little evidence of differentiation among subtypes. Where differences were evident it was generally found that the more severe forms of depression (i.e. major depressive disorders) were impaired whereas the milder forms were not. There was also little evidence of quantitative or qualitative differences from schizophrenia. Thus, there was no *characteristic* profile of cognitive changes in depression. 15 years after Miller's review, with the growth of more sophisticated theories in cognitive psychology, it is perhaps timely to consider whether this conclusion can be challenged.

A different approach to the study of mood and cognition has been to consider the psychological deficits in depression in the context of neurobiology. Prominent hypotheses are that the cognitive impairments in depression are similar to those produced by dysfunction of the non-dominant hemisphere (Flor-Henry 1976) or to those characteristic of so-called subcortical or fronto-subcortical dementia (Albert et al 1974). Both of these accounts emphasize the similarity of the cognitive deficits of depression to those resulting from forms of generally irreversible brain dysfunction that are not necessarily linked with depression. Rapid advances in measuring central nervous system function directly, using neuroimaging, promise to add a new dimension to the resolution of these possibilities (Schwartz et al 1987). Such techniques potentially have a special utility in the study of depressive disorders, where there is often no evidence of discrete structural lesions, but where there may be important changes in neurotransmitter function.

MEMORY AND LEARNING

Depressed patients often complain of difficulties with attention and concentration, especially when trying to learn or remember. Consequently, it is not surprising that much activity has been directed at understanding memory and learning deficits in depression. As in many other studies of the pathology of memory, research has been driven by the current theoretical vogue; correspondingly, there has been a shift from global structural models which postulate different memory stores to explanations of memory in terms of stages and forms of processing.

Stages of processing

Research in the 1960s and 1970s was dominated by the 'modal', two-stage theories of memory suggesting separate stores for short-term (primary) and long-term (secondary) memory and serial processes of registration, encoding, rehearsal, consolidation and retrieval of memory traces (see Atkinson & Shiffrin 1968). Cronholm & Ottosson (1961) concluded that unipolar patients with 'endogenous depression' showed deficits in 'learning' as indexed by immediate and delayed reproduction of various forms of stimulus material, although the forgetting decrements between the two tests were similar to those of controls. Sternberg & Jarvik (1976) found similar results in a comparable group of 'endogenous' depressed patients, but thought that impaired performance on immediate reproduction tests reflected registration or short-term memory deficits and unimpaired retention (computed from the difference between immediate and delayed reproduction) indicated intact long-term memory.

The interpretation of a selective impairment in short-term memory has not always been confirmed. For example, studying serial learning and free recall in a group of unipolar and bipolar patients as a function of clinical state, Henry et al (1971, 1973) found no differences between more and less depressed phases on the first trial of the serial learning task, suggesting that depression was not associated with impairments in short-term memory. However, as in the earlier studies, there was a significant deficit in learning in both unipolar and bipolar depressives on later trials of this task, and free recall was also impaired in the unipolar cases (who happened to be more depressed in this study).

Perhaps the most comprehensive study of memory in depressed patients from a perspective of stages of processing has been that of Corwin et al (1990a). These authors tested a group of medication-free patients with major depressive disorder and age-, sex-, and IQ-matched controls, using a battery of memory tasks with different requirements, including tests selective for short- and long-term memory and aspects of remote memory. Whereas simple measures of short-term memory store, such as Forward Digit Span, showed no significant differences between groups, three other indices with more stringent demands (Backward Digit Span, Bushke Recall Failure and Bushke Storage) were sensitive to deficits in the depressed group. This pattern of sensitivity was also shown over different forms of memory testing, in terms of both modality (e.g. verbal versus visual) and task requirements (e.g. implicit versus explicit memory tasks), suggesting that the depressed group did not have specific problems at a particular stage of memory storage. Rather, they experienced difficulties in memory that were related more to the overall processing requirements, as inferred from the relative difficulty of the tasks used, and irrespective of the precise memory stage.

Encoding processes

An early, but durable, hypothesis of the nature of the memory loss in depression was of impaired encoding

processes. Weingartner et al (1981a) showed that depressed patients appeared to use weak or incomplete encoding strategies to organize and transform events to be remembered; when structure or organization was provided the deficit was reversed. Although Weingartner subsequently supported an alternative hypothesis (see below), recent studies have continued to support the deficient encoding hypothesis (Golinkoff & Sweeney 1989). Williams & Scott (1988) also found evidence of shallow encoding (and possibly retrieval) strategies in their study of autobiographical memory. Depressed patients were less *specific* in their memories, especially for positive events, but also for negative ones. Watts & Cooper (1989) found that depressed patients fail to show the usual superior recall of central aspects of stories, possibly a related effect. In contrast, they showed an ability to use imagery as a memory aid equivalent to that of controls. The latter is a relatively automatic process, whereas the failure to use structure to organize stories probably reflects an impairment of encoding.

The specificity of these aspects of memory dysfunction is unclear, since few direct comparisons of memory loss in depression with other forms of amnesia have been reported. However, Squire & Zouzounis (1988) have compared self-ratings of memory dysfunction in depressed inpatients, a subgroup of which had received electroconvulsive therapy (ECT), and patients with Korsakoff's syndrome or amnesia secondary to anoxia, all roughly matched for degree of memory impairment. The results showed that the memory deficits experienced in depression and amnesia were distinguishable using these techniques. The depressed patients, prior to receiving ECT, showed equivalent levels of impairment across all of the questions, which included ratings for functions as varied as memory for remote events, memory for things read or seen recently on television and general alertness and attention. In contrast, the amnesic subjects reported considerably more problems on some ratings than others, a pattern resembling that seen in the depressed patients after ECT.

Effortful versus automatic cognitive processing

Rather than assuming that memory dysfunction in the depressed reflects impaired memory stores, several authors have hypothesized that the deficits occur in processes that transcend the divide between short- and long-term memory. An influential distinction has been that between cognitive operations that require 'effort' or cognitive capacity (for example, by requiring selective attention or sustained attention) and processes that can be accomplished automatically (Hasher & Zacks 1979). It can be argued that monitoring the frequency of an event or remembering incidental features requires only automatic memory processing, whereas the free recall of information is effortful. Weingartner and colleagues have pointed out that there is a continuum of effort required for different types of memory performance; recognition requiring less effort than free (i.e. unstructured) recall, which in turn requires less effort than serial recall (i.e. in a precise temporal sequence), which in turn requires less effort than speeded serial recall (see Weingartner & Silberman 1982). The hypothesis of Weingartner et al is that depressed patients have especial difficulty with *effortful* processing, which may extend to non-mnemonic functions.

Evidence for this hypothesis was obtained in a mixed group of seven unipolar and three bipolar patients, some of whom were not medicated at the time of testing (Roy-Byrne et al 1986). Deficits emerged in the depressed group when they were required to remember 32 concrete noun pairs (e.g. table/flower), but not when they were required to recall the type of comparative judgment they had made about the word pairs (e.g. about their size, value or weight). In a second test, the patients were unimpaired in remembering whether a word had been presented once or twice, but were deficient in free recall. Another experiment examined the relationship between the severity of depression, cognitive performance and the ability to sustain motor effort in hospitalized depressed patients (Cohen et al 1982). The patients had difficulty remembering three-letter trigrams, particularly after long delays and when depressed mood was intense. The latter was also highly ($r = -0.72$, $p < 0.01$) correlated with sustained motor effort, as measured with a standard hand grip dynamometer.

In further studies, Weingartner and colleagues have confirmed other predictions of the hypothesis; that recall is more sensitive to the deficit in depression than the less effortful recognition of stimulus material (see Weingartner & Silberman 1982; but see Watts & Sharrock 1987 for failures to find differential effects of cued and uncued recall); and that conceptual tasks with high information loads or stringent temporal deadlines are similarly discriminating (Silberman et al 1983b). Further evaluation of the hypothesis raises three main questions: (1) how specific are the effects in psychological terms? (2) how restricted are they to depression? (3) what are their neural or neurochemical correlates?

Many of the impairments that might be ascribed to loss of cognitive effort can also be considered in theoretically far less ambitious terms; for example, other interpretations of cognitive effort may reduce it to constructs of motivation or arousal. But manipulations of motivation do not necessarily benefit cognitive performance in the depressed, even though they may enhance speed of responding to the same degree as in normal subjects (Richards & Ruff 1989). Furthermore, various conditions that are thought to enhance arousal in normal subjects do not necessarily affect tasks thought to reflect cognitive effort (see Strupp et al 1986).

Alternatively, it can be asked whether the distinction between automatic and effortful tasks is anything other than a variation in level of *task difficulty*. Corwin et al (1990a) referred to the neutral dimension of task difficulty rather than cognitive effort as the crucial determinant of impairments in depression. In short, those tests which are most difficult are also the most discriminating in separating patients from controls. It is then questionable whether the cognitive effort hypothesis has any additional explanatory power. One way of testing this would be to compare the effects of varying levels of difficulty independently within the effortful and automatic domains. This has not been done explicitly. A study by Silberman et al (1983a) did in fact report greater deficits in the *easier* of two free recall conditions, suggesting that task difficulty could not be the complete explanation. But this result also provides problems for the effort hypothesis because free recall is an effortful task, and so one would have expected difficulty level within this domain to be related to the depressive deficit. Golinkoff & Sweeney (1989) interpreted a lack of interaction of task difficulty with depression in recall and recognition memory performance to reflect basic memory impairments in depression (specifically in encoding) rather than a general inability to allocate cognitive effort to more demanding tasks. Consistent with the cognitive effort hypothesis, these authors found that frequency monitoring was not impaired in a group of patients with major depression but, against this account, recognition memory was impaired as well as recall (see also Wolfe et al 1987), and this pattern of memory dysfunction was also found (though to a lesser degree) in a control group of patients with personality disorder. This study represents the most serious challenge to the cognitive effort hypothesis.

Another way of testing the task difficulty hypothesis would be to search for double dissociations of cognitive and automatic processing, perhaps across different patient groups. These are daunting problems, especially because deficient effortful processing probably occurs in other patient groups, including Parkinson's disease (Weingartner et al 1984), schizophrenia (Gjerde 1983) and dementia of the Alzheimer type (Jorm 1986). On the other hand, it has been claimed that patients with dementia of the Alzheimer type are impaired in both automatic and effortful aspects of memory function (Strauss et al 1985, Tariot & Weingartner 1986) and patients with anorexia nervosa exhibit deficits in automatic, rather than effortful, processing (Strupp et al 1986).

In neural terms, the value of the effortful—automatic dimension would be enhanced if 'effort' could be tied to the operation of specific neural regions or neurotransmitter projections. This is a theoretically interesting conundrum. Does effort reflect the operation of specific neural networks (e.g. efferent control of cortical activity by the frontal cortex) or of neurotransmitter systems of subcortical origin that innervate telencephalic regions? There is evidence that central catecholaminergic activity is related to cognitive effort. For example, the level of CSF 3-methoxy-4-hydroxyphenyl glycol (MHPG), the major CNS metabolite of noradrenaline, was significantly related to the facilitation of cognitive performance following d-amphetamine administration in depressed patients (Reus et al 1979). The presence of effortful processing deficits in patients with Parkinson's disease is consistent with a catecholaminergic substrate and several studies have shown beneficial effects of L-DOPA on memory functions that can be construed as reflecting effortful processing. Thus, Newman et al (1984) found that L-DOPA facilitated free recall, without affecting frequency monitoring or category fluency ('semantic memory') in elderly volunteers, whereas Henry et al (1973) and Murphy & Henry (1972) had much earlier reported beneficial effects of L-DOPA on serial learning and free recall in depressed patients. These effects are of considerable interest when it is realized that there were apparently no effects of L-DOPA on reaction time and that the facilitatory effects of cholinergic drugs may also be distinct in nature (Newman et al 1984).

Only further research will allow us to decide if cognitive effort or a related notion is a useful concept for explaining the nature of the intellectual deficit in depression.

Response biases and hedonic memory deficits in depression

A rather different approach to uncovering the nature of memory dysfunction in depression is to consider selective changes that are characteristic of the disorder. For example, there is evidence that 1) depressed subjects have a conservative response bias (e.g. tending to say 'no' more frequently than 'yes' in tests of recognition memory, when uncertain of the correct answer); and 2) depressed subjects have a selective memory deficit for material of positive affective tone.

Conservative response bias

Miller & Lewis (1977) were among the first investigators to report conservative bias in depressed patients. They compared groups of elderly, heterogeneous depressive and demented patients with normal controls and an apparently clear qualitative difference was obtained between the groups in visual recognition memory. Signal detection analyses of the *discriminative sensitivity* of the performance d' and the *response criterion*, β, suggested that, whereas the demented patients showed significant reductions in d', compared with both the depressed and control groups, the depressed patients exhibited increases in β in the direction of a more conservative criterion. This pattern of results suggested that the memory deficit in depression was more a function of decisional or strategic processes than poor memory *per se*. This basic result has been repeated several times (Zuroff et al 1983, Dunbar & Lishman 1984, Corwin et al 1990a), but nevertheless there is some controversy about its generality (Silberman et al 1983a, Watts et al 1987, Snodgrass & Corwin 1988, Corwin et al 1990b).

Selective deficits for positive affective material

It has long been suspected that depressed patients have more difficulty retrieving pleasant material than negatively-toned information (Meltzer 1930), findings consistent with the later notion of *negative set* in depression (Beck 1967). These early indications were confirmed in studies by Lishman (1972a, b, Lloyd & Lishman 1975), using more modern methodology. Experimental studies have shown that depressed patients inaccurately remember receiving more punishment and less positive reinforcement (Gotlib 1981), recall more negative than positive self-rated words (Bradley & Mathews 1983), more negative than positive themes in stories (Breslow et al 1981) and are quicker to respond to negative than positive cues in tests of autobiographical memory (Williams & Scott 1988). The selective memory impairment for positive material has also been shown to be mood-state dependent, both in clinically depressed patients (Clark & Teasdale 1982) and in normal subjects induced into a depressed mood (Teasdale & Fogarty 1979, see Johnson & Magaro 1987 for a review of the more wide-ranging question of the relationship between mood and memory). The selective effects are also task-dependent. For example, McDowall (1984) found that depressed patients recalled more unpleasant than pleasant words in a free recall task, but not in a pleasantness rating task.

The mechanisms underlying this selective deficit for positive material have proved to be more difficult to identify. The *salience* of the two types of memory material may differ between the control and patient groups and, alternatively, mood-congruent material (negative, of course, in depression) may receive more selective attention. Finally, unpleasant memories may *decay more slowly* in the depressed, showing an opposite pattern to normal (Holmes 1970). Nothing is known about the neural and neurochemical substrates of the selective memory deficit, but the analogy of mood with neurochemical state-dependency of memory may eventually form the basis of a satisfactory explanation.

Attentional and executive factors in memory

Memory failures in depression are often related to the subjective complaint of poor concentration and reduced attention was one of the subjective ratings which most distinguished depressives from amnesics in the study by Squire & Zouzounis (1988) reviewed above. Firm evidence for this association of memory failure and attentional deficit is provided by Corwin et al (1990a), who found that the concentration difficulty item on the Montgomery—Åsberg Depression Rating Scale was strongly and linearly related with memory performance, in contrast to other items rating psychomotor retardation and loss of interest. The lay term 'concentration', of course, is somewhat vague in its relationship to psychological processes, especially as two different phenomenological lapses of concentration have been identified, 'mind-wandering' and 'blanking' (Watts et al 1988). The former is reliably associated with poor memory for prose in depressed patients, whereas the latter is more closely connected to impairments in a test of planning, the 'Tower of London' task. This suggests that memory functions in depression may be particularly susceptible to competing thoughts (see also Sternberg & Jarvik 1976) but that not all of the

performance deficits in depression can be attributed to this factor.

Watts et al (1988) interpreted their results in terms of Shallice's (1982) model of the regulation of attention by a hypothetical Supervisor, which has been compared with a part of the influential Working Memory model of Baddeley (1986) called the Central Executive. This component of working memory refers to the processes by which attentional resources are allocated to task performance so that its various cognitive component processes are co-ordinated efficiently. In neural terms it corresponds most closely to frontal lobe function. There may well be gains in looking to these novel theories in order to understand the cognitive deficits in depression. There are preliminary indications that the depressed subjects do not exhibit specific impairments in the short-term memory 'satellite' systems of the Working Memory model, such as the Articulatory Loop (verbal rehearsal) and the Visuo-Spatial Sketchpad (imagery), but are deficient in the Central Executive. Thus, Barnard & Teasdale (1991) report preliminary results that show mutual interference in depressed patients between the production of thoughts or images and performance on tasks that require continuous monitoring and control. Silberman et al (1983b) similarly report that while logic, memory and attention seemed intact in depressed patients at an elementary level, their inability to co-ordinate these functions in a complex task was at the core of their thinking disorder. Perhaps the altered decisional response biases and selective memory functions, as well as the deficiencies in 'effortful processing' and encoding strategies, all reflect impaired functioning of the Central Executive in depression.

State versus trait factors and the effects of treatment

The evidence from studies of memory function before and after treatment, on balance, suggests that amelioration of depression is accompanied by a reduction in cognitive deficits. Learning was improved in unipolar patients treated with imipramine (Sternberg & Jarvik 1976) or ECT (Cronholm & Ottosson 1961) and euthymic bipolar patients taking lithium improved on tests of verbal and non-verbal recall (Calev et al 1986). These beneficial actions occur even though the therapeutic agents themselves sometimes have deleterious effects on other aspects of mnemonic performance (Calev et al 1989). For example, ECT *worsens* forgetting on retention tests (Cronholm & Ottosson 1961) and produces a pattern of subjective memory loss quite distinct from that seen in depression itself (Squire & Zouzounis 1988, Calev et al 1989). These results would seem to suggest that many of the cognitive deficits in memory and learning are indeed related to state rather than trait factors. This is supported by some of the results of Corwin et al (1990a), who showed that performance on the easier tasks was related to severity of depression. However, the deficits on difficult tasks were *not* obviously related to the severity of depression, suggesting that they may act as trait markers.

LATERALIZED COGNITIVE DYSFUNCTION

The possibility that the cognitive deficits in depression reflect right (non-dominant) hemisphere dysfunction is part of a wider controversy, beyond the scope of this chapter, concerning a special role for the right hemisphere in affect (Flor-Henry 1976, 1983, Silberman & Weingartner 1986, Wexler 1980). This conclusion has variously depended upon interpreting psychophysiological measures, relating patterns of neuropsychological deficits to abnormal right hemisphere function and inferring alterations in cerebral dominance from perceptual asymmetries in depressed patients.

Neuropsychological test performance

The claim that depressed patients exhibit more deficits in visuospatial than verbal tasks implies right (non-dominant) hemisphere dysfunction (Flor-Henry 1976, 1983, Goldstein et al 1977), although this conclusion is controversial (see Silberman & Weingartner 1986). More recent studies have provided only limited support for a selective right hemisphere deficit. For example, Richards & Ruff (1989), using a battery of tasks, found that only some of the visuospatial tests differentiated unmedicated depressed patients from controls. Robertson & Taylor (1985) found that non-verbal 'holistic functioning' was more impaired than verbal function in prisoners with affective disorder, regardless of subtype. Many of the tests used in these studies had already been shown to be sensitive to lesions of the right temporal lobes and Silberman et al (1983b) also found a pattern of errors in depressed subjects resembling that of patients with right temporal lobectomies. Abrams & Taylor (1987), however, found little evidence to support a selective right temporal lobe deficit in their study of depressed patients of the melancholic subtype. Rather, they characterized the neuropsychological profile as 'bifrontal-right parietal'.

Other investigators have not found a pattern of cognitive dysfunction in depression that can be related specifically to the non-dominant, right hemisphere (see Silberman & Weingartner 1986 for review). There is also some evidence that when task difficulty is matched, the difference between performance on verbal and non-verbal memory tasks in depressed patients disappears (Calev et al 1986, Corwin et al 1990a). Even if non-verbal tasks are considered more sensitive to depression, from the evidence already reviewed, it is clear that the right hemisphere dysfunction is, at best, only relative to other deficits that one would expect to be mediated by the left hemisphere.

Perceptual asymmetry

Studies using dichotic listening tasks have identified abnormal perceptual asymmetry in patients with depressive disorders (see Bruder 1988, for a review). Evidence for right hemisphere dysfunction has been found using musical stimuli, clicks or complex tones in dichotic listening tasks in several studies, as generally evidenced by the loss of the left-ear/right hemisphere advantage in depressed patients (e.g. Bruder et al 1981, 1989, Berger-Gross et al 1985). The results are less clear for verbal dichotic tasks. For example, groups of bipolar depressed patients showed a supranormally large right ear advantage (Lishman et al 1978, Bruder et al 1989), whereas unipolar depressive patients have been reported to show either *no* advantage for dichotic verbal material (Johnson & Crockett 1982, Moscovitch et al 1981) or a supranormal right ear advantage (Bruder et al 1989).

The suggestion that the laterality effects depend upon the subtype of depression was supported in the study by Bruder et al (1989) which also examined visual field asymmetries in depressed subjects using tachistoscopic presentations of verbal and visual material. The right visual field/left hemisphere advantage was retained for syllables in bipolars with a trend for a decrease in this advantage in unipolar depressives. In contrast, schizophrenics showed a left visual field advantage on the same task (Gur 1978). For dots, the converse left visual field/right hemisphere advantage was lost for the bipolar, but not the unipolar, group.

Depressed patients have also been shown to have atypical lateralized biases in the perception of emotional chimeric faces (Jaeger et al 1987), a task previously used to test the hypothesis of hemispheric specialization for the emotions in normals. Subjects are required to make a judgment as to which of two chimeric faces shows most emotion. Although both the controls and a group of unipolar depressives showed a significant right field/left hemisphere bias, it was significantly less lateralized in the latter group. It remains unclear whether this bias results from visuospatial, facial or emotional processing. Nonetheless, the results are consistent with some form of right hemisphere dysfunction.

Psychophysiological indices

Gruzelier & Venables (1974) found that skin conductance changes were less marked on the right in depressed patients and on the left in schizophrenics. Myslobodsky & Horesh (1978) found a similar pattern of results, consistent with right hemisphere overactivation in depression. However, other investigators have found no lateralized skin conductance responses when tested at rest (Storrie et al 1981). Myslobodsky & Horesh (1978) also examined the direction of the initial lateral eye-movement during auditory presentation of test questions, finding that depressed patients looked to the left more frequently, a result consistent with right hemisphere overactivity (Kinsbourne 1975), and again opposite to findings in schizophrenic patients (Schweitzer et al 1978). The problem of interpreting these findings is that they can equally well be explained by *underactivity*, of the contralateral hemisphere, if these functions are mediated by a balanced interaction between the hemispheres. Moreover, it appeared that the depressed patients (in contrast to controls) showed predominantly left eye-movements in response to spatial, emotional and neutral conditions as well, suggesting that the effects were psychologically non-specific.

In terms of EEG recording, using amplitude and variance of the waveform as indices of lateralized function, Perris and colleagues found a low left to right ratio in depressed (but not recovered depressed) patients, lower ratios corresponding to more severe depression and impaired verbal learning (d'Elia & Perris 1973, 1974, Perris, 1974). Flor-Henry (1976) also found predominantly right temporal lobe abnormalities in the manic phase of bipolar depression, and left temporal abnormalities in schizophrenics, when tested either at rest or in the performance of verbal or visuospatial tasks. At first sight, these results and others (see Silberman & Weingartner 1986) seem to support a right hemisphere overactivation hypothesis, but there are several problems of interpretation. For example, in the depressed phase of Flor-Henry's bipolar cases and in other depressed cases, there was abnormally high right parietal activity at rest, but also *left* temporal lobe activation during spatial tasks and *right* parietal activation during verbal tasks. This evidence is most consistent with a reversal of the normal pattern of dominance in depression, rather than specifically a right hemisphere dysfunction. Further studies by Perris's group reveal the possible complexity of linking depression specifically to right hemisphere dysfunction. For example, Perris et al 1978 and Perris & Monakhov (1979) have found that right frontal activity correlated with depressed *mood*, but left frontal activity with depressed *ideation*. These results confirm what one might expect; a complex affective and cognitive disturbance such as depression is unlikely to be linked in any simple way to lateralized hyper- or hypoactivity of the cerebral cortex.

Implications

The promise of this hypothesis has been that it has offered some way of countering Miller's (1975) suggestion that the neuropsychological pattern of performance in depression is not specific for this disorder and reflects merely general psychopathology. However, we are far from an integrated explanation of laterality effects in normals, let alone their relevance to mood disorders. For example, in depression, the psychophysiological evidence favours an overactivation of the right hemisphere, whereas neuropsychological results suggest deficits sometimes comparable with those following right-sided lesions. Nevertheless, it is difficult to predict the consequences for cognitive function of overactivation of the right hemisphere; would this be equivalent to underactivation, or would it lead to opposite dysfunctional effects? Furthermore, it should be realized that functionally lateralized changes could depend upon alterations in balance between the two hemispheres, rather than as a result of changes specific to the right hemisphere. For example, apparent right hemisphere dominance could result from underactivity of the left hemisphere or disturbed hemispheric communication via the corpus callosum. An additional possible complication is that the asymmetries result from changes in subcortical (e.g. monoaminergic) neurotransmitter systems. Either such change itself could be lateralized, or bilateral changes could amplify asymmetries in function at the cortical level. Neuroimaging studies could potentially rescue the laterality hypothesis from these tortured considerations, but the results so far have not been encouraging (see below).

DEPRESSION AS SUBCORTICAL DEMENTIA

The term 'subcortical dementia' refers to a clinical syndrome characterized by a slowing of cognition (often called 'bradyphrenia'), memory disturbances, difficulty with problem solving, visuospatial abnormalities and disturbances of mood and affect (Albert et al 1974, Cummings 1986). It is distinguished from 'cortical dementia' because of the absence of focal cortical signs such as aphasia and apraxia. Subcortical dementia implicates a dysfunction of the isodendritic core neurotransmitter systems and of such subcortical structures as the thalamus and striatum, along with their frontal cortex connections (Agid et al 1987). Thus, it has been usual to include basal ganglia diseases, particularly Parkinson's and Huntington's diseases, as well as progressive supranuclear palsy, as examples of subcortical dementia. However, the obvious question posed by the constellation of cognitive deficits comprising this syndrome is whether it is profitable to consider depression under the same heading. It is certainly true that these basal ganglia disorders are associated with forms of depression that are not simply related to the degree of motor impairment (e.g. Starkstein et al 1989, see Cummings 1986 for a review). Furthermore there is evidence, reviewed above, of memory disturbances in depression, and of deficits in 'effortful processing' similar to those seen in Parkinson's disease. Problem solving is also impaired in depression (Silberman et al 1983b) and there is some evidence of slowed thinking (Watts et al 1988).

A criticism sometimes levelled against the concept of bradyphrenia is that, because it is applicable to certain forms of cognitive task only, it may reflect alterations in speed/error trade-off functions rather than a generalized slowing of information processing. One approach aimed at answering this question utilizes the Sternberg short-term memory scanning paradigm. According to Sternberg (1969), several stages of information processing can be assessed independently by analysing the relation between task factors in their effect on reaction time. Thus, a linear relation holds between the time taken to compare a series of items with similar items in memory, and the number of items held in memory (as the memory load). In representing this relationship, the intercept is thought to measure the rate of perception and output factors, while the slope of the reaction-time/set-size function is a measure of the memory scanning process. The earlier studies came to much the same conclusion about short-term memory, that is, memory scanning is generally unimpaired in depressed patients (Hilbert et al 1976, Glass et al 1981, Koh & Wolpert 1983, Hart & Kwentus 1987). The study by Brand & Jolles (1987) however defined quite specific conditions under which a short-term memory processing deficit could be demonstrated in depression. They found that, in a group of subjects with unipolar depression, memory scanning was slower in three out of four tasks compared with controls, and in one case compared with a positive control group of anxious patients. However, there is considerable agreement (Koh & Wolpert 1983, being an exception) that depression is associated with slower responding in the *non-scanning* part of these tasks, as shown by higher values for the intercept in the reaction-time/set-size relationship.

Overall, the concept of depression as a 'subcortical' (or 'fronto-subcortical') dementia is worthy of further analysis. This will require detailed comparison of different patient groups with depression including Parkinson's or Huntington's diseases on the one hand, and dementia of the Alzheimer's type on the other along the lines begun by Wolfe et al (1987, see below).

COGNITIVE DEFICITS IN THE ELDERLY AND PSEUDODEMENTIA

Although it was realized as early as 1883 that severe affective disorder could lead to cognitive impairment (see Berrios 1985), the term pseudodementia was first used by Madden et al (1952) to describe cases in which the clinical presentation had led to a diagnosis of dementia subsequently to be changed because of remission of symptoms. Madden et al studied 300 patients over the age of 45 years and found that pseudodementia presented as disorientation, defects in recent memory, retention, calculation and judgment. This was particularly common in involutional psychoses and in psychoses associated with cerebrovascular disease and depression. Subsequently, pseudodementia has been associated with many additional psychiatric and medical conditions (Kiloh 1961, Marsden & Harrison 1972, Nott & Fleminger 1975, Wells 1979, Smith & Kiloh 1981).

McAllister (1983) reported that patients with depressive pseudodementia were significantly older than patients with other psychiatric illnesses. Thus, it is not surprising that the term pseudodementia is often used in clinical practice synonymously with depressive pseudodementia in the elderly, or that it poses severe problems of differential diagnosis with dementia. For example, a substantial proportion (8–10%) of patients initially diagnosed as demented were later considered to be suffering from affective disorder (Marsden & Harrison 1972, Ron et al 1979). Furthermore, in a recent study, the opposite form of misdiagnosis has been demonstrated. Sachdev et al (1990) reported a follow-up study of 19 patients with the diagnosis of pseudodementia made more than 10 years earlier (Smith & Kiloh 1981). Two cases were probably misdiagnosed, one of definite dementia and in the other dementia could not be excluded. The difficulty of differential diagnosis arises, in part, at clinical presentation due to the apparent similarity of the cognitive deficits. The true diagnosis only becomes evident during the course of the illness. At least until recently, dementia has been defined as an acquired, global condition of cognitive impairment which is progressive, irreversible, and occurs in the absence of clouding of consciousness (Trethowan 1979, Levy & Post 1982, Lishman 1987). In marked contrast, the hallmarks of pseudodementia are regarded as reversibility and lack of progression, since it is induced by a 'functional' illness and therefore symptomatology clears on recovery (Madden et al 1952, Kiloh 1961, Wells 1979).

Despite the lack of diagnostic specificity of the term pseudodementia, Sachdev et al (1990) have argued that, nevertheless, it has descriptive value for clinicians who find it useful to mean one or more of the following: 1) impairments in memory, learning, and related cognitive functions caused by psychiatric illness; 2) when the impairment is likely to be non-progressive and is potentially reversible if the primary illness is treated; and 3) either no neuropathological process can be identified, or if such a process exists, it is minor and insufficient to explain the severity of cognitive deficits. Although these criteria seem clear, two main questions remain to be answered: 1) Does normalization of cognitive function on recovery from depression occur? 2) Is the cognitive dysfunction associated with depression actually distinguishable from that of the dementias, either cortical or subcortical? As pointed out by Abas et al (1990) in answer to the first question, recovery from the cognitive deficits is frequently incomplete and dependent upon the precise functions tested (Whitehead 1973, Savard et al 1980, Jacoby et al 1981, Rabins et al 1984, Joyce & Levy 1988). Moreover, the residual deficits in these 'recovered' patients can be related to indicators of structural brain abnormalities (Abas et al 1990), thus rendering the term pseudodementia both unclear and misleading.

The question then remains as to the similarity of patterns of cognitive impairment between elderly patients with depression and patients early in the course of dementia of the Alzheimer type (DAT). Madden et al (1952) found that aphasia was not seen in their cases of pseudodementia, although language impairment is a frequent concomitant of DAT (Miller, 1989). In addition, apraxia and agnosia have not been widely reported to occur in pseudodementia and so these focal cortical signs may distinguish DAT from pseudodementia. However, the first and most prominent symptom to occur in DAT, as in pseudodementia, is usually deterioration in memory and learning (Corkin et al 1984, McKhann et al 1984, Sahakian et al 1988). Therefore, studies comparing the performance of depressed and DAT patients on tests of memory and learning should provide crucial information. In general, these comparisons have revealed quantitative differences in performance on particular tests, differences in the breadth of impairment and qualitative differences in the form of deficit.

Cross-study comparisons by Weingartner and colleagues (1981b, 1983, Cohen et al 1982) suggested that, unlike depressed patients, DAT patients have additional deficits in semantic encoding and retrieval, as well as in 'automatic' processing (see above). La Rue et al (1986) directly compared moderate/severe DAT patients with depressed patients and normal controls on the Inglis verbal paired associate learning test, the Benton test of ability to draw designs from memory and the Fuld test of recall of objects presented visually and tactually. They found the latter to be the most accurate diagnostic discriminator, with depressed patients having adequate storage but impaired retrieval relative to controls, while demented patients exhibited both storage and retrieval deficits. However, they were unable to confirm these results in a later study which also included comparisons with a heterogeneous group of 'subcortical conditions and multi-infarct states' (La Rue 1989).

Along similar lines, Hart et al (1987) compared patients with mild DAT and depressed patients with normal controls on the ability to learn and remember line drawings of common objects. Both depressed and DAT patients were impaired in acquisition compared with normal control subjects. In order to equate acquisition levels, and thus allow comparison of the three groups on retention ability, the exposure time of the line drawings was extended for the two patient groups.

Only the DAT patients showed faster forgetting over the first 10 minutes when compared with the other two groups.

Abas et al (1990) studied visual attention, memory and learning in groups of depressed, mild DAT and normal subjects. Depressed patients showed equivalent delay-dependent deficits in visual matching to sample performance, but less impairment in visuospatial paired associate learning compared with DAT patients. Qualitative differences were also found between the two patient groups with depressed subjects showing a different pattern of errors and a consistently prolonged latency of response which was independent of delay in a delayed matching to sample test. Therefore, the pattern of mnemonic performance in depression has some similarities, but also some differences, compared with DAT.

Rather than resembling cortical dementia, it has been suggested that the cognitive impairment of patients with pseudodementia may be more akin to that of subcortical dementia (Caine 1981, Cummings & Benson 1983, Cummings 1986, Hart & Kwentus 1987, but see Sahakian et al 1990). Neuropsychological deficits seen in subcortical dementia are described above and therefore will not be elaborated here, except to emphasize that psychomotor slowing appears to be the key feature linking subcortical and pseudodementia (Caine 1981, Cummings & Benson 1983, Hart & Kwentus 1987, but see Levy & Sahakian 1987). However, the pattern of deficits shown in Parkinson's disease and other basal ganglia disorders often considered to be examples of 'subcortical dementia' sometimes appears different from that seen in the elderly depressed. For example, delayed matching to sample performance appears to be qualitatively different in patients with Parkinson's disease and depression (Sahakian et al 1988, Abas et al 1990). In addition, performance on the Wisconsin Card Sorting Test, a test of frontal lobe function, may be impaired more drastically in Parkinson's disease and progressive supranuclear palsy than in the elderly depressed (Pillon et al 1986, Hart et al 1987).

In conclusion, it is an oversimplification to suggest that cognitive impairment in depression is akin either to that of 'cortical' or 'subcortical' dementia. Rather, it shares some features in common with both forms of dementia as well as showing some marked differences, thus retaining its own distinct cognitive profile. However, comparisons between depression and various dementing conditions are generally confounded by differences in the course and severity of the disorders and further studies are required.

COMPARISONS BETWEEN UNIPOLAR AND BIPOLAR DISORDERS

The distinction between unipolar and bipolar categories is likely to be of importance in the characterization of cognitive deficits in affective disorders. The two major issues are whether first, the manic and depressed phases in bipolar depression and, second, the depressed phases in unipolar and bipolar depression, produce qualitatively different forms of cognitive deficit, or whether both comparisons are confounded by the overall degree of disability.

Manic patients have proved to be difficult to assess with standard psychological procedures, although it has long been realized that this condition is associated with changes in cognitive as well as affective processes (Kraepelin 1921, Bunney & Hartmann 1965). Henry et al (1971) provided some evidence that serial word-list learning was impaired during the manic phase in patients with bipolar disorder. The learning impairments were accompanied by intrusions from idiosyncratic word associations formed by the patients to a much higher degree than observed in other studies of psychotic depression and schizophrenia. Another possibly characteristic feature of cognition in mania is the presence of more liberal response bias in recognition memory, contrasting with the generally conservative bias seen in depression (Corwin et al 1990b). The cognitive dysfunction in mania is often indistinguishable from that seen in schizophrenia, for example in tests of selective attention (Oltmanns 1978) or perceptual span (Strauss et al 1984), and so may therefore reflect changes associated with psychosis that are characterized by distractibility and thought disorder, rather than a trait specific to bipolar depression. However, in terms of localising features, there is some evidence of differences between mania and schizophrenia, with manic patients more likely to exhibit bifrontal and right hemispheric patterns of dysfunction than schizophrenics (see also above and review by Taylor et al 1979).

Several studies have shown that the degree of cognitive deficit is proportional to the severity of manic symptoms (Henry et al 1971); is reversible when the patient improves (Henry et al 1971, Savard et al 1980); and may normalize in remission (Kerry et al 1983), although the deficits in older bipolar patients can persist beyond the disappearance of affective signs (Savard et al 1980).

Comparisons between cognitive performance in the unipolar and bipolar depressed states are often confounded by the severity of depression and related factors that are difficult to control. Savard et al (1980) used the Halstead-Reitan Category test, which requires abstraction, rule-learning and concept formation, to compare groups of unipolar and bipolar depressed patients in the acutely depressed state with approximately the same level of rated depression on the day of testing, when not receiving medication. The bipolar depressed group were slightly older than the unipolar group, but made significantly more errors than either their age-matched control group of spouses or the unipolar group, who barely differed from the controls. Wolfe et al (1987) similarly found that bipolar patients performed worse than a unipolar group matched for age, years of education and severity of rated depression (but not in number of hospital admissions) in tests of both recall and recognition memory (modified Rey auditory verbal learning test) and verbal fluency (which was unimpaired in the unipolar group). In fact, the bipolar group was most similar in *level* of performance to a group of patients with Huntington's disease, although in *qualitative* terms the latter patients' performance most resembled that of the more mildly affected unipolar depressed patients, both groups showing more liberal response biases. The possible similarity of cognitive deficits in unipolar (but not bipolar) depression to those seen in basal ganglia disorder is relevant to the relationship of depression with 'subcortical dementia', but obviously requires more extensive analysis. Despite the methodological difficulties it now seems likely that bipolar depression may be associated with distinct cognitive deficits, as well as greater deficits than those seen in the unipolar condition.

BRAIN IMAGING AND AFFECTIVE DISORDERS

Structural imaging

Taking impetus from findings of enlarged ventricles in schizophrenia (e.g. Johnstone et al 1976), several studies have looked for this abnormality in affective disorders using computed tomography (CT) or magnetic resonance imaging (MRI). The majority have indeed found evidence of ventricular enlargement (Table 18.1). Whether this is accompanied by cortical shrinkage is controversial (Nasrallah et al 1982b, Dolan et al 1986, Dewan et al 1988a, b). CT brain density measures have not resolved these discrepant findings, there being evidence of both increased and decreased

regional density (Jacoby et al 1983, Schlegel & Kretzschmar 1987b, Schlegel 1988, Dewan et al 1988 a, b).

Table 18.1 CT studies of ventricular size in affective disorders. Unless specified, all measures refer to lateral ventricular to brain ratios (VBR). 'Mixed' refers to groups of subjects with unipolar, bipolar and other forms of depressive illness. All comparisons are with groups of normal controls

Normal ventricular size	
Jacoby & Levy 1980	mixed, elderly
Weinberger et al 1982	mixed
Iacono et al 1988	mixed
Johnstone et al 1989	bipolar, temporal horn
Increased ventricular size	
Nasrallah et al 1982a	manic, young
Standish-Barry et al 1982	mixed, elderly
Tananka et al 1982	mixed, elderly, frontal and temporal horns
Targum et al 1983	mixed, young
Luchins et al 1984	mixed
Dolan et al 1985	mixed, elderly
Schlegel & Kretzchmar 1987a	mixed, frontal horns, third ventricle
Abas et al 1990	mixed, elderly
Pearlson & Veroff 1981	psychotic, young
Scott et al 1983	psychotic, young
Dewan et al 1988a, b	bipolar, third ventricle
Andreasen et al 1990	mixed, young, bipolar males only

In general, no relationships have been found between ventricular enlargement and age, sex, age of onset, duration of illness or positive family history (Pearlson & Veroff 1981, Pearlson et al 1984a, b, 1985, Nasrallah et al 1984, Dolan et al 1985). However, several studies have related ventricular size to cognition. Kellner et al (1983) found a positive relationship between ventricular brain ratio (VBR) and performance on the Halstead-Reitan category test in a group of unipolar and bipolar depressives. Dewan et al (1988a, b) found a significant correlation between the impairment index from the Halstead-Reitan battery and VBR in bipolar patients. In the same vein, Coffman et al (1990) found global cognitive impairment in young bipolar patients which related to MRI indices of brain shrinkage.

Recent studies with MRI suggest that there may be a relationship between the presence of subcortical white matter changes (leucoencephalopathy) and mood disorder (Summergrad 1985, Coffey et al 1987, 1988, 1990, Joyce & Levy 1988, Krishnan et al 1988, Venna et al 1988). However, the majority of patients in these studies were elderly and had cardiovascular risk factors. These subcortical abnormalities would appear to represent cases of subcortical arteriosclerotic encephalopathy, the neuropathology of which was first described by Binswanger (see Biemond 1970 and Caplan & Schoene 1978). In contrast, *young* patients with bipolar depression may have an increased incidence of white matter changes unrelated to any organic condition (Dupont et al 1987, 1990). Furthermore, Dupont et al (1990) found that it was those subjects with lesions that had difficulty with tests of verbal fluency and memory.

Cerebral blood flow and metabolism in affective disorders

The advent of imaging modalities which allow visualization and measurement of brain function potentially revolutionizes our capacity to understand the neurobiological basis of affective disorders. Studies performed over the past decade have been limited largely to two techniques. One is xenon[133] cerebral blood flow (CBF), measured either by a fixed array of scintillation counters which detect cortical flow or by single photon emission computed tomography (SPECT), which also captures subcortical blood flow. The other method utilizes [18F]fluoro-2-deoxyglucose in conjunction with positron emission tomography ([18F]DG PET) to map the cerebral metabolic rate of glucose (CMRglu). Other metabolic tracers labelled with [15O] and [11C] have not been used with any regularity in studies of affective disorder (see Devous 1989, Holcomb et al 1989 for detailed accounts of SPECT and PET techniques). The two radiotracers (^{133}Xe, ([18F]DG) are limited in their capacity to elucidate such complex questions as the relationship between mood and cognition because they are unable to identify the contributions of the subcortical neurotransmitter systems which are so heavily implicated in affective disorders. The future availability of specific neurochemical radioligands will therefore add another crucially important dimension to functional imaging. Other technical factors exist which make those studies which have been performed difficult to compare (see Sackeim et al 1990 for a critique) and sources of variability with respect to subject populations (e.g. age, medication status, category of depression) further compound the problem of comparison.

Table 18.2 Global cerebral blood flow and metabolism in depression. 'Mixed' refers to groups containing subjects with unipolar, bipolar and other forms of depressive illness. All comparisons are with groups of normal controls

No difference		
Mixed	Gustafson et al 1981a, b	CBF
	Goldstein et al 1985	CBF
	Guenther et al 1986	CBF SPECT
	Reischies et al 1989	CBF SPECT
	Silfverskiold & Risberg 1989	CBF
Unipolar	Gur et al 1984	CBF
	Baxter et al 1985	[18F]DG PET
	Kuhl et al 1985	[18F]DG PET
	Kling et al 1986	[18F]DG PET
Bipolar	Rush et al 1982	CBF SPECT
Decreased		
Mixed	Mathew et al 1980a, b	CBF
	Warren et al 1984	CBF
	Raichle et al 1985	[15O] PET
	Sackeim et al 1990	CBF
Unipolar	Rush et al 1982	CBF SPECT
	Sackeim et al 1987	CBF
	Kishimoto et al 1987	[11C]glucose PET
Bipolar	Baxter et al 1985	[18F] DG PET
Increased		
Mixed	Silfverskiold et al 1986	CBF
	Rosenberg et al 1988	CBF SPECT

Most studies have examined cortical or hemispheric CBF and CMRglu in the resting state but no consensus has emerged for these global measures (see Table 18.2). As we shall see, more discrete regional analysis has proved to be more promising, although there are still many difficulties of interpretation. The limited progress may have resulted from the apparently pragmatic strategy of measuring solely the resting state. A more ambitious approach is to compare regional activity between the resting and activated state in the same patients. By activation, we refer to the use of defined test conditions for amplifying potential differences in regional cerebral activity. These may vary from the requirement for simple movements to the imposition of sensory stimulation and the performance of specific cognitive tasks (e.g. Buchsbaum et al 1984b, Gur et al 1984, Reischies et al 1989). While the use of such activation procedures has frequently been successful in demonstrating regional changes that reflect the neurobiological correlates of depression, they have not generally been designed explicitly to test psychological theories of the cognitive deficits. Nevertheless, such studies are sometimes relevant to these theories. For example, Warren et al (1984) compared a heterogeneous group of depressed patients with normals, both at rest and during the performance of mental arithmetic, a classical Working Memory task (Baddeley 1986), under different incentive conditions. Although the results were not especially clear-cut, this type of experimental design warrants further attention, particularly if placed in the theoretical context of Working Memory.

Comparisons between depression, euthymia and hypomania

In order to address the question of whether CBF or CMR changes reflect a pervasive abnormality or a trait marker, several studies have examined patients in different mood states. Although some studies have failed to find any global differences between various groups of depressed, manic, recovered and normal subjects (Gustafson et al 1981a, b, Silfverskiold and Risberg 1989), others have demonstrated changes which indicate that depression is related to decreased, and mania to increased, cortical or hemispheric activity (Rush et al 1982, Kishimoto et al 1987, Sackeim et al 1987). Baxter et al (1985) found that groups of bipolar-depressed and mixed affective state (i.e. hyperactivity with an irritable or depressed mood), but not unipolar-depressed patients, had decreased hemispheric CMRglu. Hypomanic patients were no different from controls as a group, but for individual patients with rapid cycling bipolar illness, there was increased CMRglu in the manic as compared to the depressed phase. In the same study they scanned five bipolar patients, both when depressed and when either euthymic or hypomanic; CMRglu always increased along with mood.

To support the conclusion that CBF or CMR changes are state-dependent, studies comparing either the same patients or separate groups of patients with affective disorder, when euthymic and when either depressed or manic, in general indicate that recovery is accompanied by normalization of brain activity (Rush et al 1982, Baxter et al 1985, 1989, Kishimoto et al 1987). In the same vein, Phelps et al (1983, 1984) describe an experiment in which 15 mg of the indirect catecholamine agonist methylphenidate was administered orally to a group of patients with major depression and focal metabolic asymmetries. These asymmetries worsened in the patients who became dysphoric under the drug and improved in those whose mood improved.

Lateralized changes

Functional imaging techniques would seem ideally suited to investigate whether there is right hemisphere dysfunction in affective disorders. However, studies addressing this question are contradictory. The majority report no difference in hemispheric symmetry between depressed and normal subjects (Buchsbaum et al 1984b, 1986, Gur et al 1984, Raichle et al 1985, Sackeim et al 1987, 1990, Silfverskiold & Risberg 1989), but some studies report lower right/left ratios in depressed subjects (Uytdenhoeff et al 1983, Baxter et al 1985, Devous 1989, Rush et al 1982).

Gur et al (1984) have examined CBF in depressed patients both at rest and during the performance of cognitive tasks designed to 'challenge' one hemisphere or the other. These were all medicated patients with unipolar depression who were asked to perform a verbal analogies test (left hemisphere) and a line orientation test (right hemisphere) on two separate occasions. At rest, there were generally no differences between depressed patients and controls in CBF. For both groups, cognitive activation produced increased CBF, more marked in the left hemisphere for the verbal task and in the right hemisphere for the spatial task. There were sex differences found in the pattern of CBF at rest and under cognitive challenge. Female depressed patients showed the same pattern as female normals but had higher CBF under all conditions. Male depressives had lower resting CBF than normal males. Under activation their CBF increased to that of normal males except over the right anterior probes. The authors suggest that this is consistent with right hemisphere dysfunction in depressed men. These results contrast with findings by the same group with medicated schizophrenics who showed higher left compared to right hemisphere CBF during both the verbal and spatial tasks (Gur et al 1983). In contrast to the less clear results for depressed patients, this indicates left hemisphere overactivation in schizophrenia.

Fronto-subcortical abnormalities

CBF studies of anterior–posterior gradients in normal subjects have repeatedly demonstrated relative hyper-frontality (but see Mathew 1989 for a critique). Several groups have also reported the normal pattern of CBF hyperfrontality in depressed patients (Warren et al 1984, Gur et al 1984, Goldstein et al 1985, Silfverskiold & Risberg 1989). On the other hand, Sackeim et al (1990) found a bilaterally reduced frontal to posterior CBF ratio and Buchsbaum et al (1984a, b) also found indices of reduced frontal activity using PET in depressives. In order to increase metabolism in the frontal lobes, Buchsbaum and colleagues examined the effect of delivering painful electric shock to one forearm during [^{18}F]DG uptake in a group of largely bipolar, medication-withdrawn depressed patients and controls. When comparing the ratio of anterior to posterior CMRglu they found that both groups had relative hyperfrontality but this was less apparent in the depressed group. In the same studies, schizophrenics exhibited similar effects and they have interpreted these findings as demonstrating hypofrontality in both schizophrenia and depression. However, in a later study, while replicating the finding of hypofrontality in schizophrenics and bipolar depression, they found higher than normal CMRglu in the frontal lobe in a small group of four patients with unipolar depression (Buchsbaum et al 1986).

Using more discrete regional measures in unipolar depressives, Uytdenhoeff et al (1983) found increased left frontal and decreased right posterior CBF expressed as a ratio to whole brain CBF, in a group with unipolar depression. Reischies et al (1989) confirmed the relative increase in left frontal flow in predominantly unipolar depressed patients with CBF SPECT. However, most regional studies point to decreased frontal function in depression. Baxter et al (1985) identified a subgroup of unipolar depressed patients with decreased left frontal CMRglu and, more recently, they showed that both unipolar and bipolar depressed patients have evidence of bilaterally reduced frontal CMRglu (Baxter et al 1989). Cohen et al (1989) found changes common to both schizophrenics and depressed subjects during performance of an auditory discrimination task. There was a relative reduction of CMRglu in frontal cortex and a relative increase in superior parietal cortex in both groups, although there were reductions in the temporal lobes specific to depression (see also Post et al 1987). Within the depressed patient group there were no differences between unipolar and bipolar cases.

Using sophisticated and rigorous statistical techniques, Sackeim et al (1990) examined a large group (41) of well-defined elderly patients with unipolar and bipolar depression who were withdrawn from medication. They found that the depressed group were distinguished by relatively lower flows in three frontal, one superior temporal and one anterior parietal region. They interpret the abnormal regional reductions uncovered by their statistical methodology as representing an abnormal neuronal network comprising areas of association cortex of the temporoparietal and frontal regions which are functionally interlinked to subserve arousal, attentional and motivational functions, as well as higher-order cognitive activity.

Reduced frontal metabolism, at least on the left side, appears to be independent of whether depression is primary or secondary to another disorder. Baxter et al (1989) included obsessive-compulsive disorder (OCD) patients both with and without secondary depression. Those with depression had lower frontal ratios than the euthymic OCD subjects, but only on the left side. Mayberg et al (1990) found that patients with depression associated with Parkinson's disease had relatively decreased orbitofrontal CMRglu, averaged across both sides, compared to a matched group of euthymic Parkinson's disease patients and healthy controls. In both of these studies, frontal CMRglu correlated inversely with the severity of depression as measured by the Hamilton Depression Scale.

Only three studies have examined subcortical regions in depressed subjects (Baxter et al 1985, Buchsbaum et al 1986, Cohen et al 1989), each suggesting that CMRglu is reduced in the caudate nucleus of depressed subjects, although Baxter et al found this only for unipolar, and not bipolar, depressives.

Implications and future directions

The utility of neuroimaging can be gauged from its capacity to illuminate neuropsychological theories of depression. Thus the evidence for fronto-subcortical changes in cerebral blood flow and metabolism in depression is consistent with the findings from structural imaging and generally seems more compelling than for lateralized changes. This knowledge must influence our further evaluation of these hypotheses.

The evidence of fronto-subcortical changes is, in fact, also relevant to several of the neuropsychological positions defined above, especially because of their sometimes overlapping relationships. For example, the cognitive deficits in depression can be viewed as resulting from deficiences in the allocation of attentional resources, whether manifested as 'effortful' processing or as the functioning of the Central Executive. Although these psychological concepts should not necessarily be mapped on to specific brain structures, the frontal lobes have been seen as contributing to those supervisory and coordinating functions characteristic of the Central Executive (Baddeley 1986). Brain imaging studies, as perhaps especially exemplified by the approach of Sackeim et al (1990), seem ideally suited to the measurement of such concepts as coordinated activity in different cortico – cortical, as well as cortical – subcortical domains, using sophisticated correlational techniques.

The realization that 'subcortical' dementia may result from dysfunctioning of the fronto-striatal axis further underlines the possibility of a synthesis that may be accelerated by the advent of functional imaging studies designed expressly to address these issues. These will also have to take into account the evidence of functionally segregated parallel fronto-striatal 'loops' (see Alexander et al 1986) and the likelihood of heterogeneity of function both within and between the frontal lobes.

If the fronto-subcortical hypothesis continues to be viable, it must address the very important issue of differentiating affective disorders from other conditions also associated with similar neuroanatomical structures, including basal ganglia disorders and schizophrenia. Furthermore, it must begin to explore the role of these structures in mood states. Again, selective functional imaging techniques may eventually lead to greater discriminatory power.

ACKNOWLEDGMENTS

We thank the Wellcome Trust for support of our experimental work. BJS thanks the Eleanor Peel Foundation for support.

REFERENCES

Abas M A, Sahakian B J, Levy R 1990 Neuropsychological deficits and CT scan changes in elderly depressives. Psychological Medicine 20: 507–520

Abrams R, Taylor M A 1987 Cognitive dysfunction in melancholia. Psychological Medicine 17: 359–362

Agid Y, Ruberg M, Dubois B, Pillon B 1987 Anatomoclinical and biochemical concepts of subcortical dementia. In: Stahl S M, Iversen S D, Goodman E C (eds) Cognitive neurochemistry, Oxford University Press, Oxford, p 248–271

Albert M L, Feldman R G, Willis A L 1974 The 'subcortical dementia' of progressive supranuclear palsy. Journal of Neurology, Neurosurgery and Psychiatry 37: 121–130

Alexander G E, De Long M R, Strick P L 1986 Parallel organization of functionally segregated circuits linking basal ganglia and cortex. Annual Review of Neuroscience 9: 357–381

Andreasen N C, Swayze V, Flaum M, Alliger R, Cohen G 1990 Ventricular abnormalities in affective disorder: clinical and demographic correlates. American Journal of Psychiatry 147: 893–900

Atkinson R C, Shiffrin R M 1968 Human memory: a proposed system and its control processes. In: Spence K W (ed) The psychology of learning and motivation, vol. 2. Academic Press, New York, p 89–195

Baddeley A 1986 Working memory. Clarendon Press, Oxford

Barnard P J, Teasdale J D 1991 Interactive cognitive subsystems: a systemic approach to cognitive-affective interaction and change. Cognition and Emotion, 5: 1–39

Baxter L, Phelps M, Mazziotta J, Schwartz J, Gerner R, Selin C, Sumida R 1985 Cerebral metabolic rates for glucose in mood disorders. Archives of General Psychiatry 42: 411–447

Baxter L R, Schwartz J M, Phelps M E, Mazziotta J C, Guze B H, Selin C E, Gerner R H, Sumida R M 1989 Reduction of prefrontal cortex glucose metabolism common to three types of depression. Archives of General Psychiatry 46: 243–250

Beck A T 1967 Depression: clinical, experimental, and theoretical aspects. Hoeber, New York

Berger-Gross P, Bruder G E, Quitkin F, Goetz R 1985 Auditory laterality in depression: relation to circadian patterns and EEG sleep. Biological Psychiatry 20: 611–622

Berrios G E 1985 'Depressive pseudodementia' or 'melancholic dementia': a 19th century view. Journal of Neurology, Neurosurgery and Psychiatry 48: 393–400

Biemond A 1970 On Binswanger's subcortical arteriosclerotic encephalopathy and the possibility of its clinical recognition. Psychiatrica, Neurologia et Neurochirugia 73: 413–417

Bradley B, Mathews A 1983 Negative self-schemata in clinical depression. British Journal of Clinical Psychology 22 : 173–181

Brand N, Jolles J 1987 Information processing in depression and anxiety. Psychological Medicine 17: 145–153

Breslow R, Kocsis J, Belkin B 1981 Contributions of the depressive perspective to memory function in depression. American Journal of Psychiatry 138: 227–230

Bruder G E 1988 Dichotic listening in psychiatric patients. In: Hugdahl K (ed) Handbook of dichotic listening: theory, methods and research. John Wiley, Chicester, p 527–653

Bruder G E, Sutton S, Berger-Gross P, Quitkin F, Davies S 1981 Lateralized auditory processing in depression: dichotic click detection. Psychiatry Research 4: 253–266

Bruder G E, Quitkin F, Stewart J W, Martin C, Voglmaier, Harrison W M 1989 Cerebral laterality and depression: differences in perceptual asymmetry among diagnostic subtypes. Journal of Abnormal Psychology 98: 177–186

Buchsbaum M, Cappelletti J, Ball R, Hazlett E, King A, Johnson J, Wu J, DeLisi L 1984a Positron emission tomographic image measurement in schizophrenia and affective disorders. Annals of Neurology Supplement 15: s157–s165

Buchsbaum M, DeLisi L, Holcomb H, Cappelletti J, King A, Johnson J, Hazlett E, Dowling-Zimmerman S, Post R, Morihisa J, Carpenter W, Cohen R, Pickar D, Weinberger D, Margolin R, Kessler R 1984b Anteroposterior gradients in cerebral glucose use in schizophrenia and affective disorders. Archives of General Psychiatry 41: 1159–1166

Buchsbaum M, Wu J, DeLisi L, Holcomb H, Kessler R, Johnson J, King A C, Hazlett E, Langston K, Post R M 1986 Frontal cortex and basal ganglia metabolic rates assessed by positron emission tomography with [^{18}F]2-deoxyglucose in affective illness. Journal of Affective Disorders. 10: 137–152

Bunney W E Jr, Hartmann E L 1965 A study of a patient with 48-hour manic-depressive cycles, I. An analysis of behavioural factors. Archives of General Psychiatry 12: 611–618

Caine E D 1981 Pseudodementia: current concept and future directions. Archives of General Psychiatry 38: 1359–1364

Calev A, Korin Y, Shapira B, Kugelmass S, Lere B 1986 Verbal and non-verbal recall by depressed and euthymic affective patients. Psychological Medicine 16: 789–794

Calev A, Ben-Tzvi E, Shapira B, Drexler H, Carasso R, Lerer B 1989 Distinct memory impairments following electroconvulsive therapy and imipramine. Psychological Medicine 19: 111-119

Caplan L R, Schoene W C 1978 Clinical features of subcortical arteriosclerotic encephalopathy (Binswanger's disease). Neurology 28: 1206–1215

Clark D M, Teasdale J D 1982 Diurnal variation in clinical depression and accessibility of memories of positive and negative experiences. Journal of Abnormal Psychology 91: 87–95

Coffey C E, Hinkle P E, Weiner R D, Nemeroff C B, Krishnan R R, Varia I, Sullivan D C 1987 Electroconvulsive therapy of depression in patients with white matter hyperintensity. Biological Psychiatry 22: 629–636

Coffey C E, Figiel G S, Djang W T, Cress M, Saunders W B, Weiner R D 1988 Leukoencephalopathy in elderly depressed patients referred for ECT. Biological Psychiatry 24: 143–161

Coffey C E, Figiel G S, Djang W T, Weiner R D 1990 Subcortical hyperintensity on magnetic resonance imaging: a comparison of normal and depressed elderly subjects. American Journal of Psychiatry 147: 187–189

Coffman J A, Bornstein R A, Olson S C, Schwarzkopf S B, Nasrallah H A 1990 Cognitive impairment and cerebral structure by MRI in bipolar disorder. Biological Psychiatry 27: 1188–1196

Cohen R, Semple W, Gross M, Nordahl T, King A C, Pickar D, Post R 1989 Evidence for common alterations in cerebral glucose metabolism in major affective disorders and schizophrenia. Neuropsychopharmacology 2: 241–254

Cohen R M, Weingartner H, Smallberg S A, Pickar D, Murphy D L 1982 Effort and cognition in depression. Archives of General Psychiatry 39: 593–598

Corkin S, Growdon J H, Nissen M J, Huff F J, Freed D M, Sagar H J 1984 Recent advances in the neuropsychological study of Alzheimer's disease. In: Wurtman R J, Corkin S H, Growdon J H (eds) Alzheimer's disease: advances in basic research and therapies. Center for Brain Sciences and Metabolism Charitable Trust, Cambridge, MA, p 75–93

Corwin J, Peselow E, Fieve R, Rotrosen J 1990a Memory deficits in depression: a test of task difficulty, store and task type explanations. (unpublished manuscript)

Corwin J, Peselow E, Feenan K, Rotrosen J, Fieve R 1990b Disorders of decision in affective disease: an effect of β-adrenergic dysfunction? Biological Psychiatry 27: 813–833

Cronholm B, Ottosson J-O 1961 Memory functions in endogenous depression. Archives of General Psychiatry 5: 101–107

Cummings J L 1986 Subcortical dementia. Neuropsychology, neuropsychiatry and pathophysiology. British Journal of Psychiatry 149: 682–697

Cummings J L, Benson D F 1983 Dementia: a clinical approach. Butterworth, London

d'Elia G, Perris C 1973 Cerebral functional dominance and depression. Acta Psychiatrica Scandinavica 49: 191–197

d'Elia G, Perris C 1974 Cerebral functional dominance and memory functions: an analysis of EEG integrated amplitude in depressive psychotics. Acta Psychiatrica Scandinavica (suppl): 143–157

Devous M D 1989 Imaging brain function by single-photon emission computer tomography. In: Andreasen N C (ed) Brain imaging: applications in psychiatry. American Psychiatric Press, Washington, DC, p 147–234

Dewan M J, Haldipur C V, Lane E E, Ispahani A, Boucher M F, Major L F 1988a Bipolar affective disorder: I. Comprehensive quantitative computed tomography. Acta Psychiatrica Scandinavica 77: 670–676

Dewan M J, Haldipur C V, Boucher M F, Ramachandran T, Major L F 1988b Bipolar affective disorder II. EEG, neuropsychological, and clinical correlates of CT abnormality. Acta Psychiatrica Scandinavica 77: 677–682

Dolan R J, Calloway S P, Mann A H 1985 Cerebral ventricular size in depressed subjects. Psychological Medicine. 15: 873–878

Dolan R J, Calloway S P, Thacker P F, Mann A H 1986 The cerebral cortex appearance in depressed subjects. Psychological Medicine 16: 775–779

Dunbar G C, Lishman W A 1984 Depression, recognition-memory and hedonic tone: a signal detection analysis. British Journal of Psychiary 144: 376–382

Dupont R M, Jernigan T L, Gillin J C, Butters N, Delis, D C, Hesselink J R 1987 Presence of subcortical signal hyperintensities in bipolar patients detected by MRI. Psychiatry Research 21: 357–358

Dupont R M, Jernigan T L, Butters N, Delis D C, Hesselink J R, Heindel W, Gillin J C 1990. Subcortical abnormalities detected in bipolar affective disorder using magnetic resonance imaging: clinical and neuropsychological significance. Archives of General Psychiatry 47: 55–59

Flor-Henry P 1976 Lateralized temporal-limbic dysfunction and psychopathology. Annals of the New York Academy of Sciences 280: 777–797

Flor-Henry P 1983 Neuropsychological studies in patients with psychiatric disorders. In: Heilman K, Staz P (eds) Neuropsychology of human emotion. Guildford Press, New York, p 193–220

Friedman A S 1964 Minimal effects of severe depression on cognitive functioning. Journal of Abnormal and Social Psychology 69: 237–243

Gjerde P F 1983 Attention capacity dysfunction and arousal in schizophrenia. Psychological Bulletin 93: 57–72

Glass R M, Uhlenhuth E H, Hartel F W, Matuzas W, Fischman M W 1981 Cognitive dysfunction and imipramine in depressive outpatients. Archives of General psychiatry 38: 1048–1051

Goldstein S G, Filiskow, S, Weaver L A, Ives, J O 1977 Neuropsychological effects of electroconvulsive therapy. Journal of Clinical Psychology 33: 798–806

Goldstein P C, Brown G G, Welch K M A, Marcus A, Ewing J R, Rosenbaum G 1985 Age related decline of rCBF in schizophrenia and major affective disorder. Journal of Cerebral Blood Flow and Metabolism 5(suppl 1): S203–S204

Golinkoff M, Sweeney J A 1989 Cognitive impairments in depression. Journal of Affective Disorders 17: 105–112

Gotlib I H 1981 Self-reinforcement and recall: differential deficits in depressed and nondepressed patients. Journal of Abnormal Psychology 90: 521–530

Gruzelier J M, Venables P H 1974 Bimodality and laterality of skin conductance orienting activity in schizophrenics: replication and evidence of lateral asymmetry in patients with depression and disorders of personality. Biological Psychiatry 8: 55–73

Guenther W, Moser E, Mueller-Spahn F, von Oefele K, Buell U, Hippius H 1986 Pathological cerebral blood flow during motor function in schizophrenic and endogenous depressed patients. Biological Psychiatry 21: 889–899

Gur R E 1978 Left hemisphere dysfunction and left hemisphere overactivation in schizophrenia. Journal of Abnormal Psychology 87: 226–238

Gur R E, Skolnick B E, Gur R C, Caroff S, Rieger W, Obrist W D, Younkin D, Reivich M 1983 Brain function in psychiatric disorders: I. Regional cerebral blood flow in medicated schizophrenics. Archives of General Psychiatry 40: 1250–1254

Gur R E, Skolnick, B, Gur R C, Caroff S, Rieger W, Obrist W D, Younkin D, Reivich M 1984 Brain function in psychiatric disorders: II. Regional cerebral blood flow in medicated unipolar depressives. Archives of General Psychiatry 41: 695–699

Gustafson L, Risberg J, Silfverskiold P 1981a Cerebral blood flow in dementia and depression. Lancet 1: 275

Gustafson L, Risberg J, Silfverskiold P 1981b Regional cerebral blood flow in organic dementia and affective disorders. Advances in Biological Psychiatry 6: 109–116

Hart R P, Kwentus J A, Taylor J R, Harkins S W 1987 Rate of forgetting in dementia and depression. Journal of Consulting and Clinical Psychology 6: 101–105

Hart R P, Kwentus J A 1987 Psychomotor slowing and subcortical-type dysfunction in depression. Journal of Neurology, Neurosurgery and Psychiatry 50: 1263–1266

Hasher L, Zacks R T 1979 Automatic and effortful processes in memory. Journal of Experimental Psychology: General 108: 356–388

Henry G M, Weingartner H, Murphy D L 1971 Idiosyncratic patterns of learning and word association during mania. American Journal of Psychiatry 128: 56–66

Henry G M, Weingartner H, Murphy D L 1973 The influence of affective states and psychoactive drugs on verbal learning and memory. American Journal of Psychiatry 130: 966–971

Hilbert N M, Niederehe G, Kahn R L 1976 Accuracy and speed of memory in depressed and organic aged. Educational Gerontology 1: 131–146

Holcomb H H, Winks J, Smith C, Wong D 1989 Positron emission tomography: measuring the metabolic and neurochemical characteristics of the living human nervous system. In: Andreasen N C (ed) Brain imaging: applications in Psychiatry. American Psychiatric Press, Washington DC, p 235–371

Holmes D S 1970 Differential change in affective intensity and the forgetting of unpleasant personal experiences. Journal of Personal and Social Psychology 15: 234–239

Iacono W G, Smith G N, Moreau M, Beiser M, Fleming J A E, Lin T, Flak B 1988 Ventricular and sulcal size at the onset of psychosis. American Journal of Psychiatry 145: 820–824

Jacoby R J, Levy R 1980 Computed tomography in the elderly: 3. Affective disorder. British Journal of Psychiatry 136: 270–275

Jacoby R J, Levy R, Bird J M 1981 Computed tomography and the outcome of affective disorder: A follow-up study of elderly patients. British Journal of Psychiatry 139: 288–292

Jacoby R J, Dolan R J, Levy R, Baldy R 1983 Quantitative computed tomography in elderly depressed patients. British Journal of Psychiatry 143: 124–127

Jaeger J, Borod J C, Peselow E 1987 Depressed patients have atypical hemispace biases in the perception of emotional chimeric faces. Journal of Abnormal Psychology 96: 321–324

Johnson O, Crockett D 1982 Changes in perceptual asymmetries with clinical improvement of depression and schizophrenia. Journal of Abnormal Psychology 91: 49–54

Johnson M H, Magaro P A 1987 Effects of mood and severity on memory processes in depression and mania. Psychological Bulletin 101: 28–40

Johnstone E C, Crow T J, Frith C D et al 1976 Cerebral ventricular size and cognitive impairment in schizophrenia. Lancet 2: 924–926

Johnstone E C, Owens D G C, Crow T J, Frith C D, Alexandropolis K 1989 Temporal lobe structure as determined by nuclear magnetic resonance in schizophrenia and bipolar affective disorder. Journal of Neurology, Neurosurgery and Psychiatry 52: 736–741

Jorm A F 1986 Controlled and automatic processing in senile dementia: a review. Psychological Medicine 16: 77–88

Joyce E M, Levy R 1988 Treatment of mood disorder associated with Binswanger's disease: a case report. British Journal of Psychiatry 154: 259–261

Kellner C H, Rubinow D R, Post R M 1983 Cerebral

ventricular size and cognitive impairment in depression. Journal of Affective Disorders. 10: 215–219

Kerry R J, McDermott C M, Orme J E 1983 Affective disorders and cognitive performance. Journal of Affective Disorders 5: 349–352

Kiloh L G 1961 Pseudo-dementia. Acta Psychiatrica Scandinavica 37: 336–351

Kinsbourne M 1975 The mechanism of hemispheric control of the lateral gradient of attention. In: Rabbitt P, Dornic S (eds) Attention and performance. V. Academic Press, London

Kishimoto H, Takazu O, Ohno S, Yamaguchi T, Fujita H, Kuwahara H, Ishii T, Matsushita M, Yokoi S, Io M 1987 ^{11}C-Glucose metabolism in manic and depressed patients. Psychiatry Research 22: 81–88

Kling A, Metter E J, Riege W, Kuhl D 1986 Comparison of PET measurement of local brain glucose metabolism and CAT measurement of brain atrophy in schizophrenia and depression. American Journal of Psychiatry 14: 175–180

Koh S D, Wolpert E A 1983 Memory scanning and retrieval in affective disorders. Psychiatry Research 8: 289–297

Kraepelin E 1921 Manic-depressive insanity and paranoia. E & S Livingstone, Edinburgh

Krishnan K R R, Goli V, Ellinwood E H, France R D, Blazer D G, Nemeroff C B 1988. Leukoencephalopathy in patients diagnosed as major depressive. Biological Psychiatry 23: 519–522

Kuhl D E, Metter E J, Riege W H 1985 Patterns of cerebral glucose utilization in depression, multiple infarct dementia, and Alzheimer's disease In: Sokoloff L (ed) Brain imaging and brain function. Raven Press, New York, p 211- 226

La Rue A 1989 Patterns of performance on the Fuld object memory evaluation in elderly inpatients with depression or dementia. Journal of Clinical and Experimental Neuropsychology 11: 409–422

La Rue A, d'Elia L F, Clark E O, Spar J E, Jarvik L F 1986 Clinical tests of memory in dementia, depression, and healthy aging. Psychology and Aging 1: 69–77

Levy R, Post F 1982 The dementias of old age. In: The psychiatry of later life. Blackwell Scientific Publications, Oxford, p 163–175

Levy R, Sahakian B J 1987 Subcortical dementia. British Journal of Psychiatry 150: 559–560

Lishman W A 1987 Organic psychiatry. Blackwell Scientific Publications, Oxford

Lishman W A 1972a Selective factors in memory. Part 1: Age, sex and personality characteristics. Psychological Medicine 2: 248–253

Lishman W A 1972b Selective factors in memory. Part 2: Affective disorder. Psychological Medicine 2: 248–273

Lishman W A, Toone B K, Colbourn C K, McMeekan E R L, Mance R M 1978 Dichotic listening in psychotic patients. British Journal of Psychiatry 132: 333–341

Lloyd G G, Lishman W A 1975 Effect of depression on the speed of recall of pleasant and unpleasant experiences. Psychological Medicine 5: 173–180

Luchins D J, Lewine R R J, Meltzer H Y 1984 Lateral ventricular size, psychopathology and medication response in the psychoses. Biological Psychiatry 19: 29–44

McAllister T W 1983 Overview: pseudodementia. American Journal of Psychiatry 140: 528–533

McDowall J 1984 Recall of pleasant and unpleasant words in depressed subjects. Journal of Abnormal Psychology 93: 401–407

McKhann G, Drachman D, Folstein M, Katzman R, Price D, Stadlan E M 1984 Clinical diagnosis of Alzheimer's disease: report of the NINCDS-ADRDA Work Group under the auspices of Department of Health and Human Services Task Force on Alzheimer's Disease. Neurology 34: 939–944

Madden J J, Luhan J A, Kaplan L A, Manfredi H M 1952 Nondementing psychoses in older persons. Journal of the American Medical Association 150: 1567–1570

Marsden C D, Harrison M J G 1972 Outcome of investigation of patients with presenile dementia. British Medical Journal 2: 249–252

Mathew R J 1989 Hyperfrontality of regional cerebral blood flow distribution in normals during resting wakefulness: Fact or artifact? Biological Psychiatry 26: 717–724

Mathew R J, Meyer J S, Francis D J, Semchuk K M, Mortel K, Claghorn J L 1980a Cerebral blood flow in depression. American Journal of Psychiatry 137: 1449–1450

Mathew R J, Meyer J S, Semchuk K M, Francis D J, Mortel K, Claghorn J L 1980b Cerebral blood flow in depression. Lancet 1: 1308

Mayberg H S, Starkstein S E, Sadzot B, Preziosi T, Andrezejewski A, Dannals R F, Wagner H N, Robinson R G 1990 Selective hypometabolism in inferior frontal lobe in depressed patients with Parkinson's disease. Annals of Neurology 28: 57–64

Meltzer K 1930 The present status of experimental studies on the relationship of feeling to memory. Psychological Review 37: 124–139

Miller E 1989 Language impairment in Alzheimer type dementia. Clinical Psychology Review 9: 181–195

Miller E, Lewis P 1977 Recognition memory in elderly patients with depression and dementia: A signal detection analysis. Journal of Abnormal Psychology 86: 84–86

Miller W 1975 Psychological deficit in depression. Psychological Bulletin 82: 238–260

Moscovitch M, Strauss E, Olds J 1981 Handedness and dichotic listening performance in patients with unipolar endogenous depression who received ECT. American Journal of Psychiatry 138: 988–990

Murphy D L, Henry G M 1972 Catecholamines and memory: Enhanced verbal learning during L-DOPA administration. Psychopharmacologia 27: 319–326

Myslobodsky M S, Horesh N 1978 Bilateral electrodermal activity in depressive patients. Biological Psychiatry 6: 111–120

Nasrallah H A, McCalley-Whitters M, Jacoby C G 1982a Cerebral ventricular enlargement in young manic males: a controlled study. Journal of the Affective Disorders 4: 15–19

Nasrallah H A, McCalley-Whitters M, Jacoby C G 1982b Cortical atrophy in schizophrenia and mania: a comparative CT study. Journal of Clinical Psychiatry 43: 439–441

Nasrallah H A, McCalley-Whitters M, Pfohl B 1984 Clinical significance of large cerebral ventricles in manic males. Psychiatry Research 13: 151–156

Newman R P, Weingartner H, Smallberg S A 1984 Effortful

and automatic memory; effects of dopamine. Neurology 34: 805–807

Nott P N, Fleminger J J 1975 Presenile dementia: the difficulties of early diagnosis. Acta Psychiatrica Scandinavica 51: 210–217

Oltmanns T 1978 Selective attention in schizophrenia and manic psychosis: The effect of distraction on information processing. Journal of Abnormal Psychology 87: 212–225

Pearlson G D, Veroff A E 1981. Computerised tomographic scan changes in manic-depressive illness. Lancet 2: 470

Pearlson G D, Garbacz D J, Breakey W R, Ahn H S, DePaulo J R 1984a Lateral ventricular enlargement associated with persistent unemployment and negative symptoms in both schizophrenia and bipolar disorder. Psychiatry Research 12: 1–9

Pearlson G D, Gabacz D J, Tompkins R H, Ahn H S, Gutterman D F, Veroff A E, Depaulo J R 1984b Clinical correlates of lateral ventricular enlargement in bipolar affective disorder. American Journal of Psychiatry 141: 253–256

Pearlson G D, Garbacz D J, Moberg P J, Ahn H S, DePaulo J R 1985 Symptomatic, familial, perinatal, and social correlates of computerized axial tomograph (CAT) changes in schizophrenics and bipolars. Journal of Nervous and Mental Disease 173: 42–50

Perris C 1974 Average evoked responses (AER) in patients with affective disorders. Acta Psychiatrica Scandinavica (suppl) 225: 89–98

Perris C, Monakhov K, VonKnorring L, Botskarev V, Nikiforov A 1978 Systemic structural analysis of the electroencephalogram of depressed patients: General principles and preliminary results of an international collaborative study. Neuropsychobiology 4: 207–228

Perris C, Monakhov K 1979 Depressive symptomatology and systemic structural analysis of the EEG. In: Gruzelier J, Flor-Henry P (eds) Hemisphere asymmetries of function in psychopathology. Elsevier North-Holland, Amsterdam.

Phelps M, Mazziotta J, Gerner R, Baxter L, Kuhl D 1983 Human cerebral glucose metabolism in affective disorder: drug-free states and pharmacologic effects. Journal of Cerebral Blood Flow and Metabolism 3 (suppl 1): S7–S8

Phelps M, Mazziotta J, Baxter L, Gerner R 1984 Positron emission tomographic study of affective disorders: Problems and strategies. Annals of Neurology 15 (suppl) S149–S156

Pillon B, Dubois B, Lhermitte F, Agid Y 1986 Heterogeneity of cognitive impairment in progressive supranuclear palsy, Parkinson's disease, and Alzheimer's disease. Neurology 36: 1179–1185

Post R M, DeLisi L E, Holcomb H H, Uhde T W, Cohen R, Buchsbaum M S 1987 Glucose utilisation in the temporal cortex of affectively ill patients: positron emission tomography. Biological Psychiatry 22: 545–553

Rabins P V, Merchant A, Nestadt G 1984 Criteria for diagnosing reversible dementia caused by depression: validation by 2-year follow-up. British Journal of Psychiatry 144: 488–492

Raichle M E, Taylor J R, Herscovitch P, Guze S B 1985 Brain circulation and metabolism in depression. In: Greitz T et al (eds) The metabolism of the human brain studied with positron emission tomography. Raven Press, New York, p 453–456

Reischies F M, Hedde J P, Drochner R 1989 Clinical correlates of cerebral blood flow in depression. Psychiatry Research 29: 323–326

Reus V I, Silberman E K, Post R M, Weingartner H 1979 d-Amphetamine: effects on memory in a depressed population. Biological Psychiatry 14: 345–356

Richards P M, Ruff R M 1989 Motivational effects on neuropsychological functioning: comparison of depressed versus non-depressed individuals. Journal of Consulting and Clinical Psychology 57: 396–402

Robertson G, Taylor P J 1985 Some cognitive correlates of affective disorders. Psychological Medicine 15: 297–309

Ron M A, Toone B K, Garralda M E, Lishman W A 1979 Diagnostic accuracy in presenile dementia. British Journal of Psychiatry 134: 161–168

Rosenberg R, Vorstrup S, Andersen A, Bolwig T 1988 Effect of ECT on cerebral blood flow in melancholia assessed with SPECT. Convulsive Therapy 4: 62–73

Roy-Byrne P P, Weingartner H, Bierer L M, Thompson K, Post R M 1986 Effort and automatic cognitive processes in depression. Archives of General Psychiatry 33: 219–224

Rush A J, Schlesser M A, Stokely E, Bonte F R, Altshuller K Z 1982 Cerebral blood flow in depression and mania. Psychopharmacology Bulletin 18: 6–8

Sachdev P S, Smith J S, Angus-Lepan H, Rodriguez P 1990 Pseudodementia twelve years on. Journal of Neurology, Neurosurgery and Psychiatry 53: 254–259

Sackeim H A, Prohovnik I, Apter S, Lucas L, Decina P, Mukherjee S, Prudic J, Malitz S 1987 Regional cerebral blood flow in affective disorders: relations to phenomenology and effects of treatment. In: Takahashi R, Flor-Henry P, Gruzelier J, Niwa S (eds) Cerebral dynamics: laterality and psychopathology. Elsevier Science Publishers, Hollingshead, N J, p 477–492

Sackeim H A, Prohovnik I, Moeller J R, Brown R P, Apter S, Prudic J, Devanand D P, Mukherjee S 1990 Regional cerebral blood flow in mood disorders: I. Comparison of major depressives and normal controls at rest. Archives of General Psychiatry 47: 60–70

Sahakian B J, Morris R G, Evenden J L, Heald A, Levy R, Philpot M, Robbins T W 1988 A comparative study of visuospatial memory and learning in Alzheimer-type dementia and Parkinson's disease. Brain 111: 695–718

Sahakian B J, Downes J J, Eagger S, Evenden J L, Levy R, Philpot M P, Roberts A C, Robbins T W 1990 Sparing of attentional relative to mnemonic function in a subgroup of patients with dementia of the Alzheimer type. Neuropsychologia 28: 1197–1213

Savard R J, Rey A, Post R M 1980 Halstead-Reitan category test in bipolar and unipolar affective disorders: relationship to age and phase of illness. Journal of Nervous and Mental Disease 168: 297–304

Schlegel S 1988 Brain density in depression: methodological and psychopathological aspects. Acta Psychiatrica Scandinavica 78: 610–612

Schlegel S, Kretzschmar K 1987a Computed tomography in affective disorders. Part I. Ventrical and sulcal measurements. Biological Psychiatry 22: 4–14

Schlegel S, Kretzschmar K 1987b Computed tomography in affective disorders. Part II: Brain density. Biological Psychiatry 22: 15–23

Schwartz J, Baxter L R, Mazziota J C, Gerner R H,

Phelps M E 1987 The differential diagnosis of depression: relevance of positron emission tomography studies.of cerebral glucose metabolism to the bipolar-unipolar dichotomy. Journal of the American Medical Association 258: 1368–1374

Schweitzer L, Becker E, Welsh H 1978 Abnormalities of cerebral lateralization in schizophrenia patients. Archives of General Psychiatry 35: 982–985

Scott M L, Golden C J, Ruedrich S L, Bishop R J 1983 Ventricular enlargement in major depression. Psychiatry Research 8: 91–93

Shallice T 1982 Specific impairments of planning. Philosophical transactions of the Royal Society B298: 199–209

Silberman E K, Weingartner H 1986 Hemispheric lateralization of functions related to emotion. Brain and Cognition 5: 322–353

Silberman E K, Weingartner H, Lorcia, M, Byrnes S, Post R M 1983a Processing of emotional properties of stimuli by depressed and normal subjects. Journal of Nervous and Mental Disease 171: 10–14

Silberman E K, Weingartner H, Post R M 1983b Thinking disorder in depression. Archives of General Psychiatry 40: 775–780

Silfverskiold P, Risberg J 1989 Regional cerebral blood flow in depression and mania. Archives of General Psychiatry 46: 253–259

Silfverskiold P, Gustafson L, Risberg J, Rosen I 1986 Acute and late effects of electroconvulsive therapy: clinical outcome, regional cerebral blood flow, and electroencephalogram. Annals of the New York Academy of Sciences 462: 236–248

Smith J S, Kiloh L G 1981 The investigation of dementia: results in 200 consecutive admissions. Lancet 1: 824–827

Snodgrass J G, Corwin J 1988 Pragmatics of measuring recognition memory: Applications to dementia and amnesia. Journal of Experimental Psychology: General 117: 34–50

Squire L, Zouzounis J A 1988 Self-ratings of memory dysfunction: different findings in depression and amnesia. Journal of Clinical and Experimental Neuropsychology 10: 727–738

Standish-Barry H M A S, Bouras N, Bridges P K, Bartlett J R 1982 Pneumoencephalographic and computerized axial tomography scan changes in affective disorder. British Journal of Psychiatry 141: 614–617

Starkstein S E, Preziosi T, Berthier M, Bolduc P L, Mayberg H S, Robinson R G 1989 Depression and cognitive impairment in Parkinson's disease. Brain 112: 1141–1153

Sternberg S 1969 Memory scanning: mental processes revealed by reaction time experiments. American Scientist 57: 421–457

Sternberg D E, Jarvik M E 1976 Memory functions in depression. American Journal of Psychiatry 33: 219–224

Storrie M C, Doerr M O, Johnson M H 1981 Skin conductance characteristics of depressed subjects before and after therapeutic intervention. Journal of Nervous and Mental Disease 69: 176–179

Strauss M E, Bohannon W E, Stephens J H, Pauker N E 1984 Perceptual span in schizophrenia and affective disorders. Journal of Nervous and Mental Disease 172: 431–435

Strauss M E, Weingartner H, Thompson K 1985 Remembering words and how often they occurred in memory impaired patients. Memory and Cognition 13: 507–510

Strupp B J, Weingartner H, Kaye W, Gwirtsman H 1986 Cognitive processing in anorexia nervosa: a disturbance in automatic information processing. Neuropsychobiology 15: 89–94

Summergrad P 1985 Depression in Binswanger's encephalopathy responsive to tranylcypromine: case report. Journal of Clinical Psychiatry 46: 69–70

Tananka Y, Hazama H, Fukuhara T, Tsutsui T 1982 Computerized tomography of the brain in manic depressive patients-a controlled study. Folia Psychiatrica et Neurologica Japonica 36: 137–144

Targum S D, Rosen L N, DeLisi L E, Weinberger D R, Citrin C M 1983 Cerebral ventricular size in major depressive disorder: association with delusional symptoms. Biological Psychiatry 18: 329–336

Tariot P, Weingartner H 1986 A psychobiologic analysis of cognitive failures. Archives of General Psychiatry 43: 1183–1186

Taylor M A, Greenspan B, Abrams R 1979 Lateralized neuropsychological dysfunction in affective disorder and schizophrenia. American Journal of Psychiatry 136: 1031–1034

Teasdale J D, Fogarty S J 1979 Differential effects of induced mood on retrieval of pleasant and unpleasant events from episodic memory. Journal of Abnormal Psychology 88: 248–257

Trethowan W H 1979 Psychiatry. Bailliere Tindall, London

Uytdenhoeff P, Portelange P, Jacquy J, Charles G, Linkowski P, Mendlewicz J 1983 Regional cerebral blood flow and lateralized hemispheric dysfunction in depression. British Journal of Psychiatry 143: 128–132

Venna N, Mogosci S, Jay M, Phull B, Ahmed I 1988 Reversible depression in Binswanger's disease. Journal of Clinical Psychiatry 49: 23–26

Warren L, Butler R, Datholi C, McFarland C, Crews E, Halsey J 1984. Focal changes in cerebral blood flow produced by monetary incentive during a mental mathematics task in normal and depressed subjects. Brain and Cognition 3: 71–85

Watts F N, Cooper Z 1989 The effects of depression on structural aspects of the recall of prose. Journal of Abnormal Psychology 98: 150–153

Watts F N, Sharrock R 1987 Cued recall in depression. British Journal of Clinical Psychology 26: 149–150

Watts F N, MacLeod A K, Morris L 1988 Associations between phenomenal and objective aspects of concentration problems in depressed patients. British Journal of Psychology 79: 241–250

Watts F N, Morris L, MacLeod A K 1987 Recognition memory in depression. Journal of Abnormal Psychology 96: 273–275

Weinberger D R, DeLisi L E, Perman G P, Targum S, Wyatt R J 1982 Computed tomography in schizophreniform disorder and other acute psychiatric disorders. Archives of General Psychiatry 39: 778–783

Weingartner H, Silberman E K 1982 Models of cognitive

impairment: cognitive changes in depression. Psychopharmacology Bulletin 18: 27–42

Weingartner H, Cohen R M, Murphy D L, Martello J, Gerdt C 1981a Cognitive processes in depression. Archives of General Psychiatry 38: 42–47

Weingartner H, Kaye W, Smallberg S A, Ebert M H, Gillin J C, Sitaram N 1981b Memory failures in progressive idiopathic dementia. Journal of Abnormal Psychology 90: 187–196

Weingartner H, Grafman J, Boutelle W, Kaye W, Martin R P 1983 Forms of memory failure. Science 221: 380–382

Weingartner H, Burns S, Diebel, R, LeWitt, P A 1984 Cognitive impairments in Parkinson's disease: distinguishing between effort-demanding and automatic cognitive processes. Psychiatry Research 11: 223–235

Wells C E 1979 Pseudodementia. American Journal of Psychiatry 136: 895–900

Wexler B E 1980 Cerebral laterality and psychiatry: a review of the literature. American Journal of Psychiatry 137: 279–291

Whitehead A 1973 Verbal learning and memory in elderly depressives. British Journal of Psychiatry 123: 203–208

Williams J M G, Scott J 1988 Autobiographical memory in depression. Psychological Medicine 18: 689–695

Wolfe J, Granholm E, Butters N, Daunders E, Janowsky D 1987 Verbal memory deficits associated with major affective disorders: a comparison of unipolar and bipolar patients. Journal of Affective Disorders 13: 83–92

Zuroff D C, Colussy S A, Wielgus M S 1983 Selective memory and depression: a cautionary note concerning response bias. Cognitive Therapy and Research 7: 223–232

19. Sleep and affective disorders

David J. Kupfer   Charles F. Reynolds III

The importance of sleep disturbance as a core symptom of affective disorder was recently highlighted by the NIMH Epidemiologic Catchment Area study of sleep disturbances and psychiatric disorders (Ford & Kamerow 1989). The major finding in this study of 7954 respondents was that 40.4% of those with insomnia and 46.5% of those with hypersomnia had a psychiatric disorder, as compared to 16.4% of those with no sleep complaints. Ford and Kamerow also reported that the risk of developing a *new* major depressive episode was much higher in those who had insomnia at both interviews (baseline, 1-year follow-up) compared to those whose insomnia had resolved by the time of follow-up. These data suggested the possibility that sleep disturbance may be critical in the pathogenesis of sleep disorders, particularly depression and anxiety, and 'that early recognition and treatment of sleep disturbance may prevent future psychiatric disorders'.

The concept of sleep as a 'marker' of psychiatric disorder, particularly of depression, raises two issues: 1) whether sleep alterations are neurobiologically fundamental in the pathogenesis of psychiatric disorders, or are merely sequelae or epiphenomena; and 2) whether sleep correlates of psychiatric disorders are in any way specific, or are similar across disorders. In this review of sleep and affective disorders, we will argue that electroencephalographic (EEG) sleep correlates provide a useful and valid indicator of depression; that such alterations in sleep are critical in the pathogenesis of depression; that they are relatively specific to major depression; and that sleep dysregulation should be viewed as part of the biological rhythm alterations that may be present in the affective disorders.

METHODOLOGICAL ISSUES

Most of the evidence reviewed in this chapter is based on cross-sectional psychobiological studies. However,

in the last 5 years particularly, relevant data from epidemiological and genetic studies have also been published, and a shift to longitudinal research designs has become more common. Such designs are more informative with respect to the questions raised by the concept of biological correlates generally and depression-related sleep changes in particular. Finally, most of the studies available report sleep changes under basal resting, or unchallenged, conditions. However, it is now accepted that the use of probes or challenges, whether naturalistic (e.g. sleep deprivation) or pharmacological, is frequently more informative with respect to the response characteristics and regulatory integrity of the sleep system in depression. Hence, in this chapter, we will review evidence from each type of study. It is appropriate to highlight the methodological advances in the past decade (Table 19.1) and several new informative research strategies, such as the use of non-somatic therapies (e.g. interpersonal psychotherapy or cognitive behavioural psychotherapy) to investigate the psychobiology of recovery from depression. From the viewpoint of sleep research, the major advantage conferred by

Table 19.1 Methodological advances in psychiatric sleep research 1980–1990

1. Increasing use of epidemiological and genetic strategies to complement traditional psychobiological approaches

2. Shift to longitudinal research design

3. Increasing use of naturalistic perturbations (e.g. partial and total sleep deprivation)

4. Use of pharmacological probes (e.g. clomipramine)

5. Use of structured psychotherapies to facilitate longitudinal psychobiological studies

6. Use of complementary automated approaches (period and spectral analyses) to ascertain the 'microarchitectures' of sleep in depression

this strategy is to permit an examination of the stability of sleep variables before, during, and after depression, solely as a function of clinical change, without the confounding effects of a somatic intervention. Another recent development has been the use of high-risk paradigms which employ sleep as a predictor of such salient clinical outcomes as relapse, recurrence or mortality. Finally, increasing reliance on the computer for quantifying phasic phenomena, such as the temporal distribution and integrated amplitude of rapid-eye movement (REMs) and electroencephalographic (EEG) slow-wave activity, has led to much finer-grained descriptions of sleep pathophysiology and microarchitecture. Period analyses have been paralleled by the application of spectral power analytical procedures. This in turn has made possible more sophisticated hypothesis generation and testing concerning hierarchical regulation and dysregulation, as well as age—disease interactions.

CONCEPTUAL ADVANCES

The conceptual advances in psychiatric sleep research 1980–1990 have been:

1. EEG sleep is abnormal in those at risk for depression.
2. The regulation of mood in affective illness is related to the regulation of sleep.
3. Some EEG sleep changes in depression are probably specific to depression, as suggested by genetic studies and studies of prognosis and treatment response.
4. There may be two distinct mechanisms of REM latency reduction in depression, one slow-wave sleep (SWS-) related and the other REM sleep (REMS-) related.

EEG sleep is abnormal in those at risk for depression

Major depression is a syndromal diagnosis and several clinically distinct subtypes have been proposed within this diagnostic grouping, e.g. bipolar, delusional and endogenous-melancholic forms. However, it is also likely that further biological heterogeneity exists within clinically distinct subgroups, both at the level of pathophysiology and at the level of treatment response (e.g. Giles & Rush 1982). Until recently, studies of sleep alterations have usually focused on more severely ill samples with endogenous or melancholic depressions.

Fortunately, a number of investigators are turning their attention to the longitudinal study of depressed outpatients who can be followed more easily during phases of the episode into recovery.

Relative to theory development, most sleep research on affective illness, especially unipolar subtypes, has focused on the pathophysiology that is concurrent with, or underlying, acute clinical signs and symptoms. To build a comprehensive pathophysiological model, however, it is necessary to develop lines of evidence bearing more directly on factors assessing vulnerability to affective illness. Identification of sleep physiological abnormalities that precede clinical episodes of major depression, especially the first episode, enables stronger inferences with regard to the potential aetiological role of these abnormalities. In other words, identification of a sleep abnormality does not necessarily imply aetiopathogenetic significance. Conceivably, a given disturbance of sleep may be present only during the episode of depression (state marker), may antedate the clinical episode (trait marker) or may persist during clinical recovery (i.e. be a marker of a past episode, 'scar' or a trait marker).

Viewed from this perspective, one can formulate testable hypotheses about such sleep abnormalities in depression as shortened rapid eye movement (REM) sleep latency. For example, is it possible to use shortened REM sleep latency as an independent variable to predict the likelihood of either a past history of affective disorder or the future development of affective disorder? The hypothesis suggested by such a question is that it is possible to predict the past or future occurrence of depression in a high-risk group if one knows the REM latency. Research to test this hypothesis is currently being conducted by Giles and colleagues (1989).

The concurrent study of sleep and genetics in depression is at an early but promising stage of development. For example, Giles et al (1988) are using sleep physiological data to define the risk pool with greater precision. To date, Giles has shown that reduced REM sleep latency is associated with increased lifetime prevalence of depression and occurs more commonly in the relatives of reduced REM latency probands. Specifically, in a sample of 37 first-degree relatives of reduced REM latency probands, 'the relative risk for unipolar depression among relatives with reduced REM latency was almost three times greater than for relatives with non-reduced REM latency' (Giles et al 1988). Giles has also reported that, in families in which the proband experienced an early onset (less than 20 years) of depression, reduced REM latency contributed independently to the rate of depression in family members. Based on these findings, Giles is now testing the hypothesis that reduced REM latency in the absence of a personal history of depression may predict those who will eventually develop depression.

The regulation of mood in affective illness is related to the regulation of sleep

In a similar context, longitudinal evaluation of change in clinical and sleep data may shed light on neurobiological and psychobiological mechanisms of response to treatment. Most effective somatic treatments are known to produce alterations in REM sleep and, with respect to tricyclic antidepressant therapy, acute suppression of REM sleep measures is significantly correlated with both clinical response and plasma tricyclic levels (e.g. Kupfer et al 1976, Gillin et al 1978, Höchli et al 1986). Vogel et al (1980) have proposed that REM sleep suppression is the key mechanism underlying treatment response (i.e. antidepressants work precisely because they are REM sleep suppressants), a suggestion based not only on the REM sleep-suppressant effects of efficacious antidepressant drugs, but also on the antidepressive effectiveness of REM sleep deprivation itself in endogenously ill patients (REM sleep disinhibition paradigm). Vogel et al (1980) have also reported that the extent of late REM sleep rebound following REM sleep deprivation is significantly correlated with final clinical response.

A related question is whether sleep abnormalities in affective illness are primary or secondary changes. That is, do sleep changes represent epiphenomena, or do they reflect the basic biological changes associated with, and responsible for, the presence of an affective illness and its responsiveness to treatment? The fact that sleep deprivation and REM deprivation have well-known antidepressant effects suggests that there must be links between the regulation of sleep and the regulation of mood in affective illnesses. Similarly, the fact that each intervention has its own distinctive time course of antidepressive efficacy may suggest that each works through different neurobiological mechanisms or, alternatively, that one is more powerful than the other. Furthermore, sleep changes may affect other biological rhythms, leading to abnormalities in neuroendocrine secretory patterns. For example, since the sleep—wake cycle itself affects the turning off of cortisol and the turning on of prolactin secretion, as well as growth hormone, it would appear that sleep abnormalities may affect various neuroendocrine rhythms. Further, the apparent persistence of sleep abnormalities into remission and their correlation with treatment response suggest that these abnormalities are not epiphenomenal but have instead a direct relation to aetiopathogenesis and the neuropsychobiology of treatment response.

EEG sleep changes in depression may be specific to depression

Despite the proliferation of studies in this area, there is still controversy about the sensitivity and specificity of the REM and NREM sleep changes observed in the state of depression (Buysse & Kupfer 1990). It is still not understood why some patients do not display the 'classic' sleep stigmata during depression, or, conversely, why some patients with other psychiatric or medical disorders display some of the sleep features associated with depression (Reynolds & Kupfer 1987). For example, Zarcone et al (1987) and Hiatt et al (1985) have demonstrated that some patients with the diagnosis of schizophrenia display shortened REM latency. Similarly, Hudson et al (1988) have reported shortened REM sleep latency during the manic phase of bipolar illness, while Thase et al (1989) reported normal REM sleep latency during the depressive phase of bipolar illness.

As stated previously, but germane to the issues of specificity, the traditional approach has been to focus on sleep features observed *during* an affective episode rather than before the illness begins or during a remission period. However, we believe that shortened REM latency during an episode is difficult to interpret unless one knows the patient's familial risk for depression. For instance, Giles et al (1987b) have shown that first-degree relatives of depressed probands, who have not necessarily had a personal episode of depression, are concordant for REM latency (i.e. reduced, non-reduced). Recently, Cartwright and colleagues (1988) suggested that a greater frequency of family history for depression is associated with short REM latency among divorcees with depression. Thus, under these conditions, one might view reduced REM latency as a vulnerability marker specific to affective illness.

This approach has also been applied to the study of schizophrenic patients, who have been shown to display shortened REM latency in some studies (Zarcone et al 1987, Hiatt et al 1985, Ganguli et al 1987). In a recent pilot study, Keshavan et al (1990) reported a significant difference in REM latency between schizophrenics and controls (71.8 minutes versus 49.4 minutes; $p < 0.002$).

However, when they examined the family history of the 25 schizophrenics, those with an affective family history (n = 8) had a REM latency of 37.9 minutes, significantly shorter than in the other patients. In summary, family history represents an important new feature that needs to be included when examining the specificity of biological variables in affective disorders.

One set of data supporting the specificity of REM latency in depression has explored the relationships among REM latency, prognosis and treatment response in depressed patients. There are now several studies suggesting that pretreatment REM latency has predictive value in terms of clinical outcome. Giles et al (1987a) have demonstrated that those individuals with a shortened REM latency have a poorer prognosis in terms of rapidity of relapse following remission than those with a more normal REM latency. Similarly, in a group of 27 geriatric depressives, Reynolds et al (1989) demonstrated that the four patients who suffered a recurrence within 18 months of treatment had a significantly shorter baseline REM latency than the 23 patients who did not. In other studies of the predictive utility of EEG sleep alterations in late-life mental disorders, Buysse et al (1988) found that pseudodemented depressed elderly had an antidepressant response to one night of sleep deprivation and a more robust REM sleep rebound than did patients with primary dementia and secondary depression. In the same group of patients with mixed depression and cognitive impairment, Hoch et al (1989) found significantly increased mortality at 2-year follow-up to be associated with baseline findings of apnoea-hypopnoea index greater than 3 and REM sleep latency longer than 40 minutes. Finally, our data from a population of recurrent depressives indicate that specific sleep features, including REM latency, are significantly associated with earlier time to recurrence (Kupfer & Frank 1989). Another body of data, using sleep measurements early in the course of tricyclic antidepressant treatment, has also indicated that REM sleep measures, particularly REM latency, may be useful in predicting clinical response (Kupfer et al 1976, 1980, 1981, 1983, Gillin et al 1978, Höchli et al 1986).

Synthesis: two distinct mechanisms for REM latency reduction in depression

We, as well as other investigators, have suggested that the weakening of the NREM system may actually contribute to the shortening of REM latency (Kupfer 1983, Feinberg et al 1988). The onset of the first REM period of the night may occur not only because of the emergence of REM sleep but perhaps because separate mechanisms have caused the first NREM period to terminate. Two possible roads to shortened REM latency may be present. In one path, REM sleep occurs earlier because NREM sleep, particularly slow-wave sleep (SWS), is reduced in length following sleep onset (Kupfer 1983). In the other path, discussed by Vogel et al (1980), REM sleep occurs earlier in the night because of so-called increased REM activity and 'pressure'. This distinction is important, since it suggests that two separate mechanisms may be responsible for the phenomenon of short REM latency, one SWS-related and the other REM sleep-related. These two possible paths for the shortening of REM latency have been labelled as type 1 and type 2 (Table 19.2).

Table 19.2   Two types of REM latency mechanisms

	Type 1	Type 2
Genetic familial transmission	+++	+
Slow-wave sleep	+++	+
REM sleep dysregulation	+	+++
Episode	±	+++
Aging-related	+++	+
Stress- and severity-related	+	+++
Antidepressant effects	+	+++
Neuroendocrine relationship	GRF	CRF (HPA Axis)

  +   moderate level of possible relationship
  ±   equivocal relationship
+++   strong relationship

The type 1 path represents a weakened SWS process that is manifested especially during the first NREM period of the night, or at least in the first 100 minutes of sleep. This type 1 effect on REM latency appears to be significantly altered by the impact of developmental factors on SWS. The aging process significantly and specifically reduces the amount and intensity of SWS (Smith et al 1977, Ehlers & Kupfer 1989), particularly during the first NREM period, as described by Feinberg (1974). With advancing age (above the age of 50 years), however, REM latency reflects the duration of SWS and eventually becomes significantly shorter (Ehlers & Kupfer 1989, Ulrich et al 1980, Gillin et al 1981). However, reduction in REM latency over the aging cycle is most probably associated with the factors regulating slow-wave activity, not REM sleep, since it has been amply demonstrated that the reduction in REM latency is positively correlated with changes in NREM period 1 rather than REM activity *per se* (Kupfer et al 1984, 1981). This is exactly what we observed in a recent study of 98 healthy, nondepressed elderly volunteers (aged 60–89) (Reynolds et al in press). Women had longer REM sleep latencies than men, a finding associated with higher rates of delta wave production in the first NREM sleep period of women than in men, but not with gender effects on tonic or phasic REM sleep measures.

Several studies of young, depressed subjects have demonstrated that, in non-suicidal adolescents, SWS markers may more clearly distinguish affectively ill subjects from age-matched controls (Hawkins et al 1985, Kupfer et al 1989a). Thus, changes in SWS, which can in turn modify REM latency, may precede actual changes in REM sleep in young, affectively ill individuals. Subjects with a family history of depression and older subjects might have a type 1 REM latency deficit, and this type of REM latency alteration may be associated with the other SWS abnormalities but not REM sleep alterations. The fact that aging and family history may produce some similar effects on SWS and REM latency is not surprising, since depression has in the past been suggested to produce a 'premature aging of sleep' (Ulrich et al 1980).

The type 2 REM latency path is envisioned to be more closely related to changes in arousal and REM sleep physiology itself. From available data, it appears to be episode-related and may also be associated with the severity of the depression or acute stresses that the patient is experiencing. The reduced REM latency seen in patients with other psychiatric and/or medical diseases that are devoid of family loading are also envisioned to be related to the type 2 path. This may also explain why decrease in REM latency is more prevalent in inpatients and during the acute phase of the illness, since it is thought to be sensitive to stress-related mechanisms. Type 2 REM deficits may produce sleep-onset REM periods. These ultra-early REM onsets appear to be found almost exclusively in inpatients and may therefore represent a correlate of various indices of severity of illness (e.g. lack of adequate response in an outpatient treatment regimen, presence of suicide risk or psychotic features) (Annseau et al 1984). These REM sleep alterations are usually, but not always, associated with sleep continuity disturbances and SWS changes.

CURRENT FINDINGS 1980–1990

The major current findings from EEG studies of depression 1980–1990 are:

1. Decreased sleep continuity in most unipolar depressives; increased sleep continuity in most non-psychotic bipolar depressives.

2. Diminished delta wave production, particularly during the first NREM sleep period.

3. Age range of sample, presence/absence of psychosis, severity, and inpatient/outpatient status all affect distribution of REM latency values in depression.

4. Increased power in higher bandwidths (18.0–28.0 Hz) among delusional depressives compared to non-delusional depressives.

5. Temporal redistribution of REM sleep in acute depression: prolonged first REM sleep period with heightened rates of REM production.

Sleep propensity and continuity

Although we have been focusing on shortened REM latency for the purpose of highlighting conceptual advances, it is clear that a *constellation* of findings characterizes the EEG sleep of depressive patients during the acute stage of the illness. First, the majority of patients with major depressive illnesses demonstrate sleep continuity disturbance usually associated with increased wakefulness or difficulty maintaining sleep. While younger depressive patients often report difficulty falling asleep, middle-aged and older depressive patients are more likely to complain of difficulty maintaining sleep, including early morning awakening. This range of complaints related to sleep continuity thus demonstrates an age-dependent continuum which has been confirmed objectively in sleep laboratory studies of younger, middle-aged and elderly depressives. A minority of patients with major depressive episodes, perhaps 10–20%, will demonstrate very high sleep efficiencies and will report spending more time in bed. This clinical feature is often associated with complaints of anergia and psychomotor slowing. Some, though not all of these patients, appear to suffer from bipolar depression (Thase et al 1989). When examined for the actual presence of excessive daytime sleepiness, using the multiple sleep latency test, anergic bipolar depressed patients showed normal multiple sleep latency test (MSLT) profiles, without evidence of pathological daytime sleepiness (Nofzinger et al in press).

Slow wave sleep

While it has been appreciated for many years that depressed patients show a reduction in slow-wave sleep (manifested by a reduction in the minutes and percentage of states 3 and 4 sleep), the application of automated (period) techniques to slow-wave sleep analysis has not shed considerable light on the nature of slow-wave sleep abnormalities in depression. Thus in young adult and middle-aged depressives there appears to be a reduction in both the absolute number of EEG delta waves during NREM sleep and in the density of such delta activity, that is, a decrease in the number of slow waves per minute of NREM sleep. Although such reductions appear to characterize all NREM periods, they are most marked in the first NREM period. While non-depressed healthy controls show a linear decrease in the density of EEG delta activity (i.e. delta counts per minute) across consecutive NREM periods during the night, by contrast, an altered temporal distribution of slow-wave activity is evident in the NREM sleep of major depressives, who show a reduction in the delta activity, particularly during the first NREM period compared to the second (Kupfer et al 1984, Reynolds et al 1985a). Such an alteration in the number and density of EEG slow waves (with a shift of slow-wave activity from the first to the second NREM period) has also been demonstrated in elderly non-demented depressives (Reynolds et al 1985b). This finding of weakened slow-wave activity, particularly in the first NREM period, is extremely interesting, since it is the length of the first NREM period which also defines the shortened REM latency in the majority of depressive illnesses (especially the endogenous forms) (Rush et al 1982). Finally, in a recent study of 302 depressed outpatients aged 20 – 69, we demonstrated a significantly higher percentage of slow-wave sleep and greater delta-wave counts in women than in men (Reynolds et al 1990).

Distribution of REM latency values in depression

The abbreviation of the first NREM period in depressive illnesses (i.e. shortening of REM sleep latency) remains a robust and widely replicated finding. However, one of the controversies that has beset the sleep and depression literature is whether REM latency in depression has a bimodal or normal distribution (Ansseau et al 1984). We believe that this issue has been resolved in the last 6 years, as we shall review. Specifically, it has become increasingly clear that the distribution of REM latency is determined by several independent, but probably interacting factors, including the age range of the sample studied, the severity of depressive symptoms and finally the subtype of depressive illness. Thus, very abbreviated REM latencies (shorter than 20 minutes) have been found in association with delusional depression (Coble et al 1981, Thase et al 1986), but also in association with *elderly* non-delusional depressives (Reynolds et al 1985b). If one's sample is heavily loaded with delusional depressives or with elderly depressives, a relatively high proportion of the REM latency values will be shifted leftward in the overall distribution, while if one is studying a group of middle-aged depressives without delusional features the REM latency distribution will be normal, with a mean value some 30 or 40 minutes below that of age-matched healthy controls. In other words, when age and psychosis are controlled, the apparently bimodal distribution of REM latency in major depressive patients may be replaced by a more continuous unimodal distribution, ranging from 0 to approximately 65 or 70 minutes (Ansseau et al 1984).

Temporal redistribution of REM sleep in depression

Finally, another robust and relatively specific feature of the sleep of acutely ill major depressives is the shift of REM sleep into the first REM period (Vogel et al 1980). In both middle-aged and elderly depressive patients, it has been shown that the length of the first REM period is consistently longer than that of age-matched healthy control subjects. The same may also be true of younger adult depressed patients, but this leftward shift of REM sleep into the first REM period appears to reflect, at least in part, an age-mediated disinhibition of REM sleep in depressive illnesses. In other words, the earlier appearance of REM sleep in depression appears to characterize more predictably the sleep of middle-aged and older major depressives than it does that of younger adult depressives (Kupfer et al 1985). Thus, the density of rapid eye movements in the first REM period appears to be greater in middle-aged and elderly depressives than it is in young adult depressives, whether determined visually or by computer-aided techniques.

Sleep in delusional versus non-delusional depression: findings from spectral analysis

Our increasing emphasis on spectral analysis has led us

to adopt this strategy to examine questions relating to delusional depression and to the process of aging. The most recent examination of this issue (Thase et al 1986) had suggested that the sleep of psychotic depression was characterized by increased wakefulness, decreased REM sleep percentage and decreased REM activity, even after controlling for clinical differences in age, severity and agitation. The aim of a more recent study was to examine, in a group of older individuals matched for age and sex, the specific EEG sleep profiles of depressive subtypes (Kupfer et al 1989b). Although the total number of individuals across all groups totalled only 18, the use of visual and spectral analysis facilitated the differentiation between normal sleep and the sleep of delusional and non-delusionally depressed patients. The sleep maintenance of the control group was significantly better than for either of the two groups of depressed patients. With respect to sleep architecture, our findings support the previous study by Ganguli et al (1987), who also reported an increase in Stage 2 sleep in the delusionally depressed subjects. EEG spectral analysis demonstrated significant differences between the control and the two patient groups. Increases in power in the higher bandwidths (18.0–28.0 Hz) suggest the prevalence of 'micro-arousals' or sleep lightening in the two depressed groups, which were even more prominent in the delusionally depressed groups. Decreased power in frequency bands 7.25–9.0 Hz) other than those related to SWS were also found when depressed subjects were compared to normal controls in an earlier sample (Borbély et al 1984). The increased power in the higher bandwidths in the delusionally depressed patients cannot be attributed to actual waking time differences, since awake time was not significantly different among the three groups.

ACROSS THE LIFE SPAN

It is now clear that there are important and robust interactions between age and disease in determining the sleep characteristics of depression (Gillin et al 1981, Kupfer et al 1982). Specifically, the sleep changes which characterize depression also occur, though to a lesser extent, during the course of normal aging itself. It is particularly the age-dependent increase in wakefulness after sleep onset and the decrease in slow-wave sleep which characterize both normal aging and depressive illness. At the same time, however, it is not firmly established from published data whether REM sleep latency itself shortens during the course of normal aging

and, if it does, how robust a trend this may be. On the other hand, the tendency for REM sleep periods to become progressively longer during the night is also significantly less in middle-aged and older persons than in young adults. That is to say, the capacity to sustain REM sleep inhibition during the first half of the night appears to be diminished by advancing age and, to a much greater extent, by the presence of depressive illness. It is precisely the shortening of REM sleep latency and the altered intra-night temporal distribution of REM sleep (with greater amounts of early REM sleep) that most specifically characterize the sleep of patients with major depressive disorders.

During the past 5 years, additional data on the sleep of childhood and elderly depressives have been published, and these data lend further support to the concept of an interaction between aging and disease in determining the sleep abnormalities of depression. In a large study of prepubertal children with major depressive illness, Puig-Antich et al (1982) have reported few differences between the sleep of depressed children and healthy controls matched for age, sex and pubertal status. On the other hand, when the depressed children were studied during clinical remission, their REM latencies showed a shortening compared to the controls (Puig-Antich et al 1983). Lahmeyer et al (1983) have suggested that the EEG sleep of adolescents with major depression is characterized by a constellation of findings similar to that of adult major depressives, particularly shortening of REM latency or first NREM sleep period. Emslie and colleagues (1990) also reported reduced rapid eye movement sleep latencies in prepubertal children with major depression. Thus, the literature has shown mixed results with respect to REM latency in childhood depression. To clarify this issue, further research is necessary, incorporating attention to possible family-history effects on sleep early in the life cycle. Further research should also utilize automated REM and delta-wave counting techniques to examine more subtle differences between the sleep of normal and depressed children. However, a recent report by Dahl and colleagues (1990), using automated delta-counting techniques, failed to detect slow-wave sleep changes associated with childhood depression.

At the other end of the life cycle, it has been demonstrated that very short REM latencies, prolonged first REM periods and extreme sleep-maintenance difficulty reliably characterize the EEG sleep of elderly non-bipolar and non-delusional (but predominantly endogenous) elderly depressives (Reynolds et al 1983, Reynolds et al 1985b). One of the more interesting findings to emerge from these studies has been the high frequency of sleep-onset REM periods in elderly endogenous depressives, where approximately 45% of REM latency values are less than 10 minutes. This finding stands in contrast to rates of 1.4% in healthy controls and 17% in non-depressed Alzheimer patients. It was also shown that the sleep-maintenance difficulties of the elderly depressives correlated significantly with the severity of depression, as indicated by Hamilton ratings. A concomitant finding was that the extent of cognitive impairment in the elderly depressives, as measured by the Folstein Mini-Mental state, was significantly and positively correlated with the amount of stage 1 sleep, another measure of sleep fragmentation.

In order to clarify further the nature of age-dependent changes in the sleep of depressed patients, normative sleep data across the life cycle, analysed by computer-aided techniques, is necessary. The expansion of the normative database will permit one to delineate more carefully differences between depressives and controls, in rates of age-dependent 'decay' of sleep maintenance, slow-wave sleep and REM sleep redistribution. It seems likely, in other words, that differences between the sleep of depressives and controls will be significantly influenced by the age of the samples studied. Younger depressives differ from controls more in measures of sleep initiation difficulty, for example, while older depressives differ more from controls in measures of sleep maintenance difficulty. Similarly, differences in absolute amount of slow-wave sleep may become somewhat attenuated with advances in age, although differences in the intra-night temporal distribution of slow wave activity *per se* may prove to be relatively age-stable. In other words, it appears likely that the reduction in delta activity in the first NREM period will be a robust finding across all age groups of depressives. This is likely to be intensively examined during the next decade of psychiatric sleep research.

ACUTE VERSUS LONGITUDINAL CHANGES (HIGH-RISK PARADIGMS)

Another potential application of EEG sleep measures in depression, which has been little reported to date, lies in the assessment of courses of illness and treatment beyond the immediate response to treatment in the acute episode. Currently, there is considerable investigative interest in ascertaining the residual sleep abnormalities in depressed patients during remission,

although to date, and particularly during the past 5 years, few data in this area have been published. Recent observations from the sleep research laboratories in Pittsburgh (Kupfer et al 1988) and in Dallas (Rush et al 1986) suggest that remitted depressed patients (particularly endogenous depressives) continue to show residual abnormalities of sleep, particularly a shortened REM sleep latency. The hypothesis being tested is that those individuals who are at high risk for relapse or for the onset of a new episode will continue to demonstrate sleep abnormalities no different from the acute episode or somewhat between the abnormalities found in the acute episode and in the normal state. However, it is not yet possible to determine if such residual abnormalities in the sleep of apparently remitted depressed patients actually represent a true trait (or marker of vulnerability), as opposed to being simply longer-lasting central nervous system effects of an episode of affective illness (i.e. a marker of past episode). This question will remain unanswered because we do not know if such patients ever had normal EEG sleep. A definitive answer to the issue of the state- versus trait-like nature of sleep abnormalities in depression can only be provided by longitudinal studies of sleep in the first-degree relatives of depressed patients, where such relatives have no personal history of affective disorder but are at increased risk for depression by virtue of their positive family history. Thus, if one found that the first-degree relatives of depressive probands had an increased frequency of polysomnographic abnormalities (e.g. decreased REM latency), even in the absence of a personal history of depression, then such abnormalities might be hypothesized to be markers of vulnerability. Presumably, also, such abnormalities would be more directly related to the aetiopathogenesis of depression. In summary, these observations suggest that more longitudinal psychobiological studies of sleep in depression are needed, with a dual focus both on remitted depressives and on the first-degree relatives of depressives before the clinical onset of illness.

MODELS OF SLEEP AND DEPRESSION

Sleep EEG studies have become increasingly important in examination of clinical and theoretical aspects of the neurobiology of depression. For instance, sleep EEG measures at baseline and following the acute administration of tricyclic antidepressants may predict ultimate response to antidepressant medication treatment (Kupfer et al 1976, 1981, Höchli et al 1986, Rush et al 1985, Zammit et al 1988). In a similar way, pretreatment REM latency may identify patients at risk for earlier and more frequent recurrences following successful psychotherapeutic treatment (Giles et al 1987a). Sleep studies are also being used to examine familial and genetic aspects of depression. Recent studies suggest that the REM sleep abnormalities of depressed patients may be found in their biological relatives as well (Giles et al 1987b, 1988, Coble et al 1988).

Models of sleep and mood build on the long-recognized interactions between sleep and mood regulation: depressed patients complain of sleep disturbance, which usually improves when they are treated. Further, sleep deprivation often leads to *improved* mood in depressed patients, but not in healthy control subjects. This suggests that sleep and mood may not only be correlated but causally related, and that the relation between sleep and mood is different for depressed patients than healthy subjects.

Since the early reports of beneficial effects from sleep deprivation in depressed patients (Pflug & Tolle 1971), several investigators have confirmed these effects (e.g. Gerner et al 1979, Duncan et al 1980). Several types of partial sleep deprivation have also been examined, including deprivation for part of the night, or of specific sleep stages (see Gillin 1983 for review). The therapeutic effects of sleep deprivation tend to be short-lived, with recurrence of depressive symptoms often noted even after brief naps, particularly those which contain REM sleep (Wiegand et al 1987). Specific REM sleep deprivation, on the other hand, appears to lead to more sustained remission of depressive symptoms (Vogel et al 1980). Clinical and biological correlates of positive responses to sleep deprivation, including neuroendocrine and baseline sleep measures, have been described (Joffe & Brown 1984, Duncan et al 1980, Gerner et al 1979, Joffe et al 1984). In general, patients with 'melancholic' or 'endogenous' depression, short REM latency or dexamethasone nonsuppression are more likely to have a beneficial response to therapeutic sleep deprivation.

Sleep deprivation has also been used as a diagnostic 'probe'. For instance, while baseline sleep characteristics differentiate elderly patients with depression and dementia from control subjects (Reynolds et al 1985b, 1988), sleep deprivation responses help to further distinguish these groups (Reynolds et al 1987). Specifically, these groups show similar delta sleep rebound following sleep deprivation, but the depressives also demonstrate a more robust delayed REM rebound. Subgroups of patients with concurrent symptoms of depression and dementia can also be differentiated by these REM sleep responses to sleep deprivation (Buysse et al 1988).

Sleep deprivation has also been used as a therapeutic adjunct. Potentiation of the clinical response to tricyclic antidepressants and lithium has been achieved with single or intermittent total sleep deprivations (Elsenga & Van den Hoofdakker 1983, Baxter et al 1986). Phase advance of the sleep — wake schedule, which may include sleep deprivation, can also act as an antidepressant (Wehr et al 1979, Souetre et al 1987), and may potentiate tricyclic medication antidepressant effects (Sack et al 1985).

The mechanism for sleep/mood interactions in depression is not known. Sleep and mood may not actually be related directly, but may interact through alterations of cholinergic/aminergic systems, neuroendocrine systems or circadian rhythms of temperature, rest and activity. In any case, sleep deprivation studies again point toward the REM sleep system's importance in the neurobiology of depression. Baseline REM measures are predictors of a positive clinical response to sleep deprivation; selective deprivation of REM sleep is associated with an antidepressant response; and REM measures during recovery sleep discriminate depressed from non-depressed patients and predict response to antidepressant medications.

NEXT STEPS

Since the major biological change and the most frequently experienced symptom of depression is, in fact, alteration in sleep patterns, this set of measures has represented a major biological focus of our investigation. EEG sleep analyses offer a unique quantitative opportunity to uncover a CNS 'signature' of depressive disorders. In using a variety of techniques to study changes in EEG sleep of normal and depressed individuals, a database now exists which demonstrates changes in the sleep of patients receiving different tricyclic antidepressants, the relationship of such changes to clinical response and the characteristics of an 8-hour window of combined sleep/neuroendocrine observations. The continued development and application of automated period and spectral techniques for 'micro-analysis' of sleep variables, the availability of antidepressant plasma levels and accurate assays for selected neuroendocrine measures, recent advances in the neuropeptide field and the expanding capability of conducting both intensive investigations and field studies have made it possible to take the next logical steps of continuing enquiries into EEG sleep in relation to affective illness.

Our focus in recent years on the sleep abnormalities in unipolar depression has led to a number of important observations which drive the studies which are proposed here. These observations include the fact that at least some of the sleep abnormalities once thought to be 'markers' of the episode (e.g. shortened REM latency) appear to persist not just early in remission but long into recovery (Cartwright 1983, Giles et al 1987a, Riemann & Berger 1989, Rush et al 1986, Steiger et al 1989) and that some of the abnormalities seen in depressed patients are also found in their never-ill first-degree relatives (Giles et al 1989). These observations, in turn, point to new questions. With respect to the persistence of some EEG sleep abnormalities, it is imperative that we examine data *on the same patient* from the onset of the episode, through remission, throughout recovery and in recurrence. Such long-term longitudinal data can only be interpreted, however, against a background of similarly collected longitudinal data on normal controls. In addition, the findings demonstrating that never-ill first-degree relatives may have somewhat shortened REM latency calls into question the value of all normative data gathered to date. It is now clear that truly 'normal' EEG sleep data can be obtained with confidence only in a population screened for psychiatric disorder in first-degree relatives. Finally, the nature of the EEG sleep abnormalities observed in the relatives of depressed probands must be better understood.

A guiding factor is the hypothesis that the mechanisms which regulate REM and SWS are specifically modulated in depression by certain biological (probably genetic) variables which ultimately lead to disturbed sleep physiology such as reduced REM latency. This hypothesis represents one of several hypothesized models which could potentially explain the alterations in sleep physiology associated with depression. In our current working model, disturbances in the mechanisms which regulate SWS and REM sleep are postulated to act through at least two 'paths' to produce such symptoms as a shortening of REM latency in depressives (Kupfer & Ehlers 1989). In one path, REM latency is postulated to be reduced because of a 'weakening' of NREM sleep, particularly slow-wave sleep, which causes the first NREM period of the night to end more quickly. In the other path, REM sleep occurs earlier in the night because of so-called increased 'REM pressure', i.e. REM sleep emerges earlier in the night due to an 'active dominance' of REM-related mechanisms. This distinction is important since it suggests that *two separate factors may be responsible for the phenomenon of short REM latency, a slow-wave-sleep related phenomenon and a REM-sleep related phenomenon.*

We have suggested that the combination of a shortened first NREM period and a lengthened first REM period in depressed patients may contain one potential key to understanding the sleep abnormalities in depressive illness. Data are now emerging from computer-assisted quantification of the first NREM/REM cycle which strongly suggest both a *diminution in slow-wave activity* (rate of production) during the first NREM period and a concomitant *increase in the rate of production of REMs* during the first REM period in depressed subjects. We continue to believe that this constellation of changes is a major feature of the sleep of depression and will have to be accounted for by any model of sleep—wake dysregulation in depression. However, the intriguing problems that need to be addressed are the facts that the constellation of these changes does not always appear in the same manner and that the clinical state may affect the manifestation of the persistent or episode-related sleep disturbances. Indeed, *a patient may demonstrate both persistent and episode-related sleep abnormalities during the clinical episode of depression.*

Future developments

Sleep research in affective illness has produced exciting advances in the past decade. Progress in conceptual and methodological arenas has yielded new insights into the dysregulation of sleep (and other biological rhythms) in depression, new information about sleep as a marker of genetic vulnerability to depression and new data about some of the more specific chronophysiological disturbances of depression. The field remains conceptually robust, as evidenced by such contributions as hypotheses of phase advance, cholinergic/aminergic imbalance, deficiencies in the homeostatic regulation of sleep (i.e. the Borbély two-process model), and the social zeitgebers hypothesis. Of the major challenges for the next decade, one will be to integrate biological and psychological concepts of aetiology in depression. The social zeitgebers hypothesis may well provide the conceptual machinery necessary for this. A particularly informative paradigm for testing the social zeitgebers hypothesis would be provided by studying such major mood-disturbing events as spouse bereavement. Another major challenge of the next decade will be to advance understanding of the specific neural substrates of depression and antidepressant response. The application of brain-imaging techniques which permit precise quantification/localization of changes in brain metabolic status during illness and recovery (e.g. PET, ^{31}P NMR spectroscopy) will allow psychiatric sleep research to look more directly at the brain than has been previously possible. Such an integration of structural and functional studies may prove to be particularly fruitful if erected upon the robust experimental paradigms provided by investigations using sleep-deprivation and pharmacological probes.

ACKNOWLEDGMENT

This work was supported in part by National Institute of Mental Health grants MH-24652, MH-30915, MH-37869, MH-00295, as well as a grant from the John D. and Catherine T. MacArthur Research Network on the Psychobiology of Depression.

REFERENCES

Ansseau M. Kupfer D J, Reynolds C F, McEachran A B 1984 REM latency distribution in major depression: Clinical characteristics associated with sleep onset REM periods (SOREMPs). Biological Psychiatry 19: 1651–1666

Baxter L R, Liston E H, Schwartz J M et al 1986 Prolongation of antidepressant response to partial sleep deprivation by lithium. Psychiatry Research 19: 17–23

Borbély A A, Tobler I, Leopfe M et al 1984 All-night spectral analysis of the sleep EEG in untreated depressives and normal controls. Psychiatry Research 12: 27–33

Buysse D J, Kupfer D J 1990 Diagnostic and research applications of electroencephalographic sleep studies in depression: Conceptual and methodological issues. Journal of Nervous and Mental Disorders 178: 405–414

Buysse D J, Reynolds C F, Kupfer D J et al 1988 Electroencephalographic sleep in depressive pseudodementia. Archives of General Psychiatry 45: 568–575

Cartwright R D 1983 Rapid eye movement sleep characteristics during and after mood disturbing events. Archives of General Psychiatry 40: 197–201

Cartwright R D, Stephenson K, Kravitz H, Eastman C 1988 REM latency stability and family history of depression. Sleep Research 17: 119

Coble P A, Kupfer D J, Shaw D H 1981 Distribution of REM latency in depression. Biological Psychiatry 16: 453–466

Coble P A, Scher M S, Reynolds C F, Day N L, Kupfer D J 1988 Preliminary findings on the neonatal sleep of offspring of women with and without a prior history of affective disorder. Sleep Research 16: 120

Dahl R E, Neidig M H, Ryan N D, Puig-Antich J 1990 Automated delta counts in childhood depression. Sleep Research 19: 365

Duncan W C, Gillin J C, Post R M et al 1980 Relationship between EEG sleep patterns and clinical improvement in depressed patients treated with sleep deprivation. Biological Psychiatry 15: 879–889

Ehlers C L, Kupfer D J 1989 Effects of age on delta and REM sleep parameters. Electroencephalography and Clinical Neurophysiology 72: 118–125

Elsenga S, Van den Hoofdakker R H 1983 Clinical effects of sleep deprivation and clomipramine in endogenous depression. Journal of Psychiatric Research 17: 361–374

Emslie G J, Rush A J, Weinberg W A, Rintelmann J W, Roffwarg H P 1990 Children with major depression show reduced rapid eye movement latencies. Archives of General Psychiatry 47(2): 119–124

Feinberg I 1974 Changes in sleep cycle patterns with age. Journal of Psychiatric Research 10: 283–306

Feinberg I, Baker T, Leder R, March J D 1988 Response of delta (0–3 Hz) EEG and eye movement density to a night with 100 minutes of sleep. Sleep 11: 473–487

Ford D E, Kamerow D B 1989 Epidemiological studies of sleep disturbances and psychiatric disorders: an opportunity for prevention? Journal of the American Medical Association 262(11): 1479–1484

Ganguli R, Reynolds C F, Kupfer D J 1987 Electroencephalographic sleep in young, never-medicated, schizophrenics: a comparison with delusional and nondelusional depressives and with healthy controls. Archives of General Psychiatry 44: 36–44

Gerner R H, Post R M, Gillin J C et al 1979 Biological and behavioural effects of one night's sleep deprivation in depressed patients and normals. Journal of Psychiatric Research 15: 21–40

Giles D E, Rush A J 1982 Relationship of dysfunctional attitudes and dexamethasone response in endogenous and nonendogenous depression. Biological Psychiatry 17: 1303–1314

Giles D E, Biggs M M, Rush A J, Roffwarg H P 1988 Risk factors in families of unipolar depression, I: Psychiatric illness and reduced REM latency. Journal of Affective Disorders 14: 51–59

Giles D E, Jarrett R B, Roffwarg H P, Rush A J 1987a Reduced rapid eye movement latency: a predictor of recurrence in depression. Neuropsychopharmacology 1: 33–39

Giles D E, Roffwarg H P, Rush A J 1987b REM latency concordance in depressed family members. Biological Psychiatry 22: 910–924

Giles D E, Kupfer D J, Roffwarg H P, Rush A J, Biggs M M, Etzel B A 1989 Polysomnographic parameters in first-degree relatives of unipolar probands. Psychiatry Research 27: 127–136

Gillin J C 1983 The sleep therapies of depression. Progress in Neuropsychopharmacology and Biological Psychiatry 7(2/3): 351–364

Gillin J C, Wyatt R J, Fram D, Snyder F 1978 The relationship between changes in REM sleep and clinical improvement in depressed patients treated with amitriptyline. Psychopharmacology 59: 267–272

Gillin J C, Duncan W C, Murphy D L et al 1981 Age-related changes in sleep in depressed and normal subjects. Psychiatry Research 4: 73–78

Hawkins D R, Taub J M, Van de Castle R L 1985 Extended sleep (hypersomnia) in young depressed patients. American Journal of Psychiatry 142: 905–910

Hiatt J F, Floyd T C, Katz P H, Feinberg I 1985 Further evidence of abnormal non-rapid-eye-movement sleep in schizophrenia. Archives of General Psychiatry 42: 797–802

Hoch C C, Reynolds C F, Houck P R et al 1989 Predicting two-year mortality in mixed depressed-demented patients using REM latency and apnea-hypopnea index. Journal of Neuropsychiatry and Clinical Neuroscience 4: 366–371

Höchli D, Riemann D, Zulley J, Berger M 1986 Initial REM sleep suppression by clomipramine: a prognostic tool for treatment response in patients with a major depressive disorder. Biological Psychiatry 21: 1217–1220

Hudson J I, Lipinski J F, Frankenburg F R et al 1988 EEG sleep in mania. Archives of General Psychiatry 45: 267–273

Joffe R T, Brown P 1984 Clinical and biological correlates of sleep deprivation in depression. Canadian Journal of Psychiatry 29: 530–536

Joffe R, Brown P, Bienenstock A et al 1984 Neuroendocrine predictors of the antidepressant effect of partial sleep deprivation. Biological Psychiatry 19: 347–352

Keshavan M S, Reynolds C F, Ganguli R, Brar J S, Houck P R, Kupfer D J 1990 EEG sleep in familial subgroups of schizophrenia. Sleep Research 19: 330

Kupfer D J 1983 Recent applications of automated sleep analysis in affective states. In: Mendlewicz J (ed) Advances in biological psychiatry. S Karger, New York, p 182–191

Kupfer D J, Ehlers C L 1989 Two roads to rapid eye movement latency. Archives of General Psychiatry 46: 945–948

Kupfer D J, Frank E 1989 EEG sleep changes in recurrent depression. In: Lerer B, Gershon S (eds) New directions in affective disorders. Springer-Verlag, New York, p 225–228

Kupfer D J, Foster F G, Reich L, Thompson K S, Weiss B 1976 EEG sleep changes as predictors in depression. American Journal of Psychiatry 133: 622–626

Kupfer D J, Spiker D G, Coble P A, Neil J F, Ulrich R, Shaw D H 1980 Depression, EEG sleep and clinical response. Comprehensive Psychiatry 21: 212–220

Kupfer D J, Spiker D G, Coble P A, Neil J F, Ulrich R, Shaw D H 1981 Sleep and treatment prediction in endogenous depression. American Journal of Psychiatry 138: 429–434

Kupfer D J, Reynolds C F, Ulrich R F, Shaw D H, Coble P A 1982 EEG sleep, depression and aging. In: Bartus R T (ed) Neurobiology of aging: experimental and clinical research. ANKHO International, Fayetteville, NY

Kupfer D J, Spiker D G, Rossi A, Coble P A, Ulrich R F, Shaw D H 1983 Recent diagnostic and treatment advances in REM sleep and depression. In: Clayton P, Barrett J (eds) Treatment of depression: old controversies and new approaches. Raven Press, New York, p 31–52

Kupfer D J, Ulrich R F, Coble P A et al 1984 Application of automated REM and slow wave sleep analysis II. Testing the assumptions of the two-process model of sleep regulation in normal and depressed subjects. Psychiatry Research 13: 335–343

Kupfer D J, Ulrich R F, Coble P A et al 1985 Electroencephalographic sleep of younger depressives: Comparison with normals. Archives of General Psychiatry 42: 806–810

Kupfer D J, Frank E, Grochocinski V J, Gregor M, McEachran A B 1988 Electroencephalographic sleep profiles in recurrent depression: a longitudinal investigation. Archives of General Psychiatry 45: 678–681

Kupfer D J, Frank E, Ehlers C L 1989a EEG sleep in young depressives: first and second night effects. Biological Psychiatry 25: 87–97

Kupfer D J, Reynolds C F, Ehlers C L 1989b Comparison of EEG sleep measures among depressive subtypes and controls in older individuals. Psychiatry Research 27: 13–21

Lahmeyer H W, Poznanski E O, Bellur S N 1983 Sleep in depressed adolescents. American Journal of Psychiatry 140: 1150–1153

Nofzinger E A, Thase M E, Reynolds C F, Himmelhoch J M, Mallinger A, Houck P, Kupfer D J Hypersomnia in bipolar depression: Part 1. A comparison with narcolepsy using the multiple sleep latency test. American Journal of Psychiatry (in press)

Pflug B, Tolle R 1971 Disturbance of the 24-hour rhythm, endogenous depression, and the treatment of depression by sleep deprivation. International Pharmacopsychiatry 6: 187–196

Puig-Antich J, Goetz R, Hanlon C et al 1982 Sleep architecture and REM sleep measures in prepubertal children with major depression. Archives of General Psychiatry 39: 932–939

Puig-Antich J, Goetz R, Hanlon C, Tabrizi M A, Davies M, Weitzman E 1983 Sleep architecture and REM sleep measures in prepubertal major depressives. Archives of General Psychiatry 40: 187–192

Reynolds C F, Kupfer D J 1987 Sleep research in affective illness: state of the art circa 1987 (state-of-the-art review). Sleep 10: 199–215

Reynolds C F, Spiker D G, Hanin I, Kupfer D J 1983 Electroencephalographic sleep, aging and psychopathology: New data and state of the art. Biological Psychiatry 18: 139–155

Reynolds C F, Kupfer D J, Taska L S, Hoch C C, Sewitch D E, Grochocinski V J 1985a Slow wave sleep in elderly depressed, demented, and healthy subjects. Sleep 8(2): 155–159

Reynolds C F, Kupfer D J, Taska L S et al 1985b EEG sleep in healthy elderly, depressed, and demented subjects. Biological Psychiatry 20(4): 431–442

Reynolds C F, Kupfer D J, Hoch C C et al 1987 Sleep deprivation as a probe in the elderly. Archives of General Psychiatry 44: 982–990

Reynolds C F, Kupfer D J, Hock P R et al 1988 Reliable discrimination of elderly depressed and demented patients by electroencephalographic sleep data. Archives of General Psychiatry 45: 258–264

Reynolds C F, Perel J M, Frank E, Imber S, Kupfer DJ 1989 Open-trial maintenance nortriptyline in late-life depression: Survival analysis and preliminary data on the use of REM latency as a predictor of recurrence. Psychopharmacology Bulletin 25(1): 129–132

Reynolds C F, Kupfer D J, Thase M E, Frank E, Jarrett D B, Coble P A, Hoch C C, Buysse D J, Simons A D Houck P R 1990 Sleep, gender, and depression: an analysis of gender effects on the electroencephalographic sleep of 302 depressed outpatients. Biological Psychiatry 28: 673–684

Reynolds C F, Monk T H, Hoch C C et al 1990 electroencephalographic sleep in the healthy 'old old': A comparison with the 'young old' in visually scored and automated period measures. Journal of Gerontology (in press)

Riemann D, Berger M 1989 EEG sleep in depression and in remission and the REM sleep response to the cholinergic agonist RS 86. Neuropsychopharmacology 2: 145–152

Rush A J, Giles D E, Roffwarg H P, Parker R C 1982 Sleep EEG and dexamethasone suppression test findings in outpatients with unipolar and major depressive disorders. Biological Psychiatry 17: 327–341

Rush A J, Erman M K, Schlesser M A et al 1985 Alprazolam vs. amitriptyline in depressions with reduced REM latency. Archives of General Psychiatry 42: 1154–1159

Rush A J, Erman M K, Giles D E et al 1986 Polysomnographic findings in recently drug-free and clinically remitted depressed patients. Archives of General Psychiatry 43: 878–884

Sack D A, Nurnberger J, Rosenthal N E et al 1985 Potentiation of antidepressant medications by phase advance of the sleep-wake cycle. American Journal of Psychiatry 142: 606–608

Souetre E, Salvati E, Pringuey Y et al 1987 Antidepressant effects of the sleep/wake cycle phase advance: Preliminary report. Journal of Affective Disorders 12: 41–46

Smith J R, Karacan I, Yang M 1977 Ontogeny of delta activity during human sleep. Electroencephalography and Clinical Neurophysiology 43: 229–237

Steiger A, von Bardeleben U, Herth T, Holsboer F 1989 Sleep EEG and nocturnal secretion of cortisol and growth hormone in male patients with endogenous depression before treatment and after recovery. Journal of Affective Disorders. 16: 189–195

Thase M E, Kupfer D J, Ulrich R F 1986 Electroencephalographic sleep in psychotic depression: a valid subtype. Archives of General Psychiatry 43: 886–893

Thase M E, Himmelhoch J M, Mallinger A G, Jarrett D B, Kupfer D J 1989 Sleep EEG and DST findings in anergic bipolar depression. American Journal of Psychiatry 146(3): 329–333

Ulrich R, Shaw D H, Kupfer D J 1980 Effects of aging on EEG sleep in depression. Sleep 3: 31–40

Vogel G W, Vogel F, McAbee R S, Thurmond A J 1980 Improvement of depression by REM sleep deprivation. Archives of General Psychiatry 37: 247–253

Wehr T A, Wirz-Justice A, Goodwin F K et al 1979 Phase advance of the sleep wake cycle as an antidepressant. Science 206: 710–713

Wiegand M, Berger M, Zulley J et al 1987 The influence of daytime naps on the therapeutic effect of sleep deprivation. Biological Psychiatry 22: 386–389

Zammit G K, Rosenbaum A H, Stokes P et al 1988 Biological differences in endogenous depressive placebo responders versus nonresponders: Dexamethasone suppression test and sleep EEG data. Biological Psychiatry 24: 97–101

Zarcone V P, Benson K L, Berger P A 1987 Abnormal rapid eye movement latencies in schizophrenia. Archives of General Psychiatry 44: 36–45

PART 3

Medication and physical treatments

20. Tricyclic and newer antidepressants

Guy M. Goodwin

Antidepressant drugs are an increasingly heterogeneous group of chemicals. In attempting a classification, there has been an historical emphasis upon innovations in stucture, hence tricyclics, bicyclics, quadricyclics or tertiary and secondary amino derivatives. However, such an approach diverts attention from the pharmacological properties and it is with these that clinicians should be familiar. Accordingly, the emphasis in this chapter will be upon the pharmacology of the compounds that act primarily by inhibiting monoamine reuptake. It will be convenient to distinguish between the older tricyclics, a few drugs that are atypical (e.g. mianserin, iprindole and trazodone) and newer compounds that are in several senses more selective (primarily for the reuptake of 5-hydroxytryptamine (5-HT)). In addition several other drugs, without actions on monoamine reuptake but not covered elsewhere in this book, will be mentioned.

The prototype tricyclic chemical iminodibenzyl was synthesized in 1895. The discovery that chlorpromazine, itself a tricyclic structure, was an effective antipsychotic, prompted an examination of the psychotropic properties of other tricyclic compounds. Kuhn (1958) discovered the antidepressant action of imipramine and the tricyclic era dates from his accurate clinical observation. Indeed, it is sobering to realise how little subsequent, more systematic investigation, has added to his account, which is still worth reading.

The pharmacology of tricyclic antidepressants has provided a dual focus, on the one hand for the development of new drugs, on the other for the understanding of the neurochemical abnormalities underlying depression. A number of the newer drugs have, like the tricyclics, a highly heterogeneous pharmacology (e.g. mianserin, trazodone), but there is currently an increasing specificity in the purposeful design and understanding of the pharmacology of new drugs. The drugs currently available for prescription in the UK that will be reviewed here are shown in Table 20.1. The tricyclic drugs are all very similar chemically and, what is more important, pharmacologically, as will be illustrated below.

Table 20.1 Tricyclic and newer antidepressant drugs currently available for prescription in the UK

Tricyclic and/related	'Atypical'	Selective 5-HT/ reuptake inhibitors
Amitriptyline	Iprindole	Fluvoxamine
Butriptyline	Mianserin	Fluoxetine
Clomipramine	Trazodone	
Desipramine		
Dothiepin	**'Miscellaneous'**	
Doxepin	Tryptophan	
Imipramine	Flupenthixol	
Lofepramine		
Maprotiline		
Nortriptyline		
Protriptyline		
Trimipramine		
Viloxazine		

BASIC PHARMACOLOGY

Binding affinity for different neurotransmitter receptors

It is now assumed that all the relevant actions of antidepressants are mediated by their binding to receptors of some sort. Most authorities would further assume that the receptors central to the actions of antidepressants have already been identified but this may not, of course,

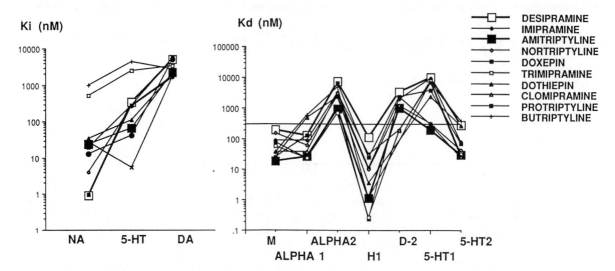

Fig. 20.1 The K_i (nM) for inhibition of monoamine uptake in vitro (left) and the K_d (nM) for binding to a range of receptors (right) of the classical tricyclic drugs. The affinity for the uptake site of noradrenaline (NA), 5-hydroxytryptamine (5-HT) and dopamine (DA) and for muscarinic (M), alpha₁-adrenoceptor (Alpha₁), alpha₂-adrenoceptor (Alpha₂), histamine-1 (H₁), dopamine D_2, 5-HT₁ and 5-HT₂ are shown. Data was obtained with human brain tissue in vitro. Original values are given for uptake sites in Richelson & Pfenning (1984), other receptors in Richelson & Nelson (1984) and Wander et al (1986).

The line indicating 200 nM affinity indicates the likely limit of drug action in vivo: K_d below this value indicates that a receptor may be a significant locus for drug action. Larger symbols have been used for the reference tricyclic, amitriptyline, and the most selective drug of this class, desipramine

prove to be correct. Drugs with a high affinity for a given receptor will occupy it at lower concentrations than drugs with low affinity. The K_d or equilibrium constant of binding is simply the concentration of a drug producing 50% occupancy of a given receptor; the lower the K_d, the higher the affinity and the greater the occupancy by drugs present at relevant concentrations (see below). The classical tricyclic drugs and their close chemical relatives are compared by means of their receptor affinities in Figure 20.1. These values are all taken from the most comprehensive existing summary which presented binding data for human tissue performed in a single laboratory.

The tricyclics have broadly similar properties and bind with high affinity to a range of receptor subtypes. The most important receptors are thought to be those mediating reuptake of the monoamines noradrenaline (NA), dopamine (DA) and 5-hydroxytryptamine (5-HT) (Fig. 20.1). The tricyclics have high affinities for NA and 5-HT transporters and, functionally, block transmitter reuptake. They do not have high affinity for DA reuptake. However, of the tricyclic group, both desipramine and clomipramine show important selectivity (for the NA and 5-HT transporter respectively).

In contrast, trimipramine has the lowest affinity for NA and 5-HT transporters.

Many of the older drugs also have important affinity for muscarinic, alpha₁-adrenergic and histamine-H₁-receptors (Fig. 20.1). They are not important dopamine receptor blockers with the exception of amoxapine, which is the only compound reported to cause extrapyramidal side-effects and to elevate prolactin. Since these motor and endocrine side-effects are quite specific to dopamine receptor blockade, they give a useful guide to the affinities that are relevant in vivo. Thus, clomipramine has a K_d for D_2 receptors of about 200 nM; the absence of extrapyramidal symptoms from its reported side-effects suggests that free drug levels of this magnitude are not achieved in clinical circumstances. Further, it suggests that the affinities shown for alpha₂-adrenoceptors and 5-HT₁-receptors are too low to implicate these receptors directly in the action of the classical antidepressants. Drug specificity can be seen to relate both to relative selectivity for one or other monoamine reuptake site and to affinity for other receptors. By both criteria, desipramine tends to be the most selective of the older drugs.

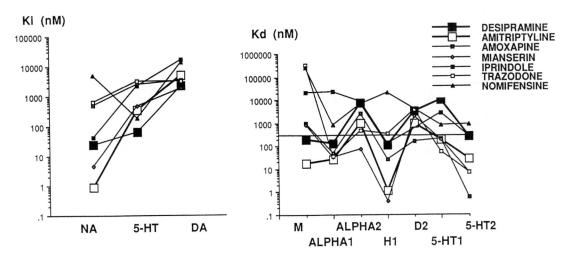

Fig. 20.2   The K_i (nM) for inhibition of monoamine uptake in vitro (left) and the K_d (nM) for binding to a range of receptors (right) of the atypical antidepressant drugs related to the tricyclic group. The affinity for the uptake site of noradrenaline (NA), 5-hydroxytryptamine (5-HT) and dopamine (DA) and for muscarinic (M), alpha$_1$-adrenoceptor (Alpha$_1$), alpha$_2$-adrenoceptor (Alpha$_2$), Histamine-1 (H$_1$), dopamine D$_2$, 5-HT$_1$ and 5-HT$_2$ are shown. Larger symbols have been used for the reference tricyclic, amitriptyline, and the most selective drug of this class, desipramine. Further details as in legend to Fig. 20.1.

The pharmacology of the atypical antidepressants such as mianserin, iprindole and trazodone has been held to be important in so far as it is different from the tricyclics. These drugs were identified in industrial screens by their tricyclic-like actions on brain function, manifest for example by electroencephalographic (EEG) changes rather than by their lower level pharmacology. In fact, only iprindole poses a particular puzzle because it has little affinity for any of the receptors illustrated (however, it may not be a very effective drug, see below). In contrast, mianserin and trazodone are more or less within the tricyclic profile but have lower affinity for muscarinic receptors and higher affinity for 5-HT$_2$-receptors (Fig. 20.2).

The pharmacology of all these drugs shows such a similar overall pattern, despite very major quantitative variation in affinities, that the likelihood of important differences in the mechanism of action between drugs, appears a priori improbable. Several of the older drugs not designed to show selectivity certainly have individual properties; e.g. mianserin has unusual affinity for alpha$_2$-adrenoceptors, trimipramine and doxepin have high affinity for histamine-H$_1$-receptors, amoxapine has apparently higher affinity for D$_2$ dopamine-receptors, and nomifensine blocks the dopamine transporter. However, it seems perverse to highlight these particular affinities in view of the overall similarity of action suggested by the properties that all

the older compounds share with the tricyclic group as a whole. We might, however, anticipate some minor differences in both efficacy and side-effects if this pharmacology is relevant.

The antidepressants that have been developed for their selectivity for either NA reuptake (maprotiline, oxaprotiline) or particularly 5-HT reuptake (zimeldine, fluvoxamine, paroxetine, fluoxetine sertraline and citalopram) are illustrated in Figure 20.3. It will be obvious that their profile is more selective than those of the tricyclics and they exhibit low affinity for muscarinic, adrenergic, histaminergic, dopaminergic and serotonergic receptors.

A final note of caution is necessary. The receptor affinities measured for a drug in vitro may be misleading if, after ingestion, it is metabolized to a pharmacologically active derivative. The information on the pharmacology of such compounds is often limited unless the active metabolite has itself been developed for use in man; desipramine, a derivative of imipramine and lofepramine, and nortriptyline, a derivative of amitriptyline, provide examples.

The mechanism of action of antidepressant reuptake blockers

The binding of antidepressant drugs to reuptake sites for NA, 5-HT and DA was established after the

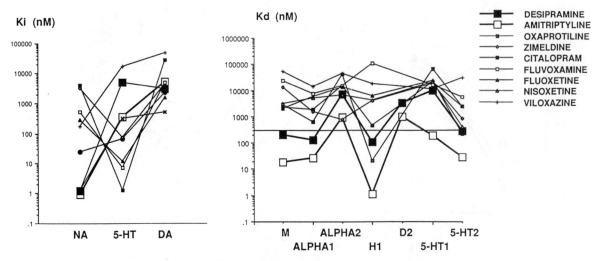

Fig. 20.3 The K_i (nM) for inhibition of monoamine uptake in vitro (left) and the K_d (nM) for binding to a range of receptors (right) of the newer more selective drugs. The affinity for the uptake site of noradrenaline (NA), 5-hydroxytryptamine (5-HT) and dopamine (DA) and for muscarinic (M), alpha$_1$-adrenoceptor (Alpha$_1$), alpha$_2$-adrenoceptor (Alpha$_2$), Histamine-1 (H$_1$), dopamine D$_2$, 5-HT$_1$ and 5-HT$_2$ are shown. Larger symbols have been used for the reference tricyclic, amitriptyline, and the most selective drug of this class, desipramine. Further details as on legend to Fig. 20.1

discovery of their antidepressant properties. Indeed, it was their efficacy that gave a massive stimulus to neuropharmacology in the 1960s and subsequently. The discovery of the mechanism of monoamine reuptake in animal studies was the first important fruit of this work, bringing the award of the Nobel Prize to Julius Axelrod for his part in it. Reuptake was immediately seen as an important basic mechanism by which neurotransmitter action could be regulated. Inhibition of reuptake would facilitate monoamine transmission and was seen as a sufficient model for antidepressant action. It also naturally suggested that depression might consist essentially of monoamine depletion. Exhaustive, if indirect, studies of neurotransmitter turnover have not demonstrated such depletion; however, some form of imbalance between the monoamines may still be claimed from such studies. Antidepressants certainly do modify the turnover of neurotransmitters in man and their effects tend to be both greater and more consistent than those associated with illness *per se*. Indeed, their prior use in drug-withdrawn patients is a major headache for biological investigations in this area. However, the central point is that the acute reversal of a transmitter deficit seems an unlikely explanation of how reuptake inhibitors work.

Apart from the failure to demonstrate transmitter depletion, doubts about the mechanism of action

arose from a comparison between the time course of effect of antidepressants upon depressive symptoms and upon indices of neuropharmacological effect. For example, Oswald et al (1972) drew attention to the apparent delay in action upon depressive symptoms both in published trials and in their own patients. This constrasted with the immediate effect that drugs must have on monoamine reuptake. At the time, it was not clear how evidence might best be obtained for effects of antidepressants with a slower onset than the primary inhibition of transmitter reuptake. Dunleavy et al (1972) drew attention to the adaptive changes in sleep architecture and the phenomenon of rebound increase in paradoxical sleep at the cessation of drug treatment. However, the more general point became how to move on from the acute effects of antidepressants to an understanding of their chronic effects.

Advances in neuropharmacology have provided an apparent solution. The function of any monoamine system can be analysed in terms of its three basic components:

1. **Presynaptic metabolism**. The rate of synthesis of transmitter or generation of metabolites can be estimated by the techniques of classical neurochemistry. In addition, release can be measured from brain

slices in vitro or from different brain regions in vivo using microdialysis.

2. **Receptor number** can be assayed by radioligand binding.

3. **Receptor function** can be assayed with appropriate agonist stimulation and functional response at any of several levels: membrane electrophysiology, biochemistry of second messengers or physiological/behavioural response.

In principle, chronic adaptive effects at any of these levels could be produced by drug administration (Sugrue 1981). Indeed, such changes have been reported for a wide variety of systems, although a review of them is beyond the scope of this chapter. There appear to be two classes of effect worth emphasising: those changes that occur in response to a whole range of different antidepressant treatments and those that are unique to particular treatments. Perhaps the best known example of the former is downregulation of beta-adrenoceptors and attenuation of their coupling to adenylate cyclase (Sugrue 1981). Another is the attenuation of the functional effects of the 5-HT_{1A} agonist 8-HO-DPAT at a presynaptic receptor mediating hypothermia in the rodent (Goodwin et al 1985). There is a poorly understood affinity between these systems, since beta-adrenoceptor stimulation facilitates the functional response mediated by 5-HT_{1A}-receptors. These effects are seen after chronic administration of tricyclic drugs, MAOIs and repeated electroconvulsive shock, all treatments derived independently of each other and more or less by serendipity. If these effects are, in fact, universal accompaniments of the best validated antidepressant treatments, what is their significance? The simplest view is that they are, in a fundamental sense, the core of antidepressant action; on this line of reasoning, any drug that produces these effects should be an antidepressant. Thus, 5-HT_{1A} partial agonists such as gepirone, or even GABA_B agonists like baclofen (Gray et al 1987), might turn out to be effective antidepressants. To refute the hypothesis we require at least one drug that produces the 5-HT effects but is not an antidepressant. Unfortunately the clinical data to show that drugs are not antidepressants are often little more than anecdotal.

The differences between the pharmacologies of different drug treatments are less interpretable than the similarities. For example, electroconvulsive shock (ECS) in animals enhances 5-HT_2 function while reuptake inhibitors and MAOIs reduce it (Goodwin et

al 1984). This differential effect, or the greater effect of ECS on dopamine function in animals might explain the greater efficacy of electroconvulsive therapy in more severe depressive states. Unfortunately, comparisons between basic pharmacology and clinical specificity are usually limited by our inability to subdivide depression reliably, and by uncertainty about the relative efficacy of different treatments. This approach is likely to remain attractive, nevertheless, because it has the virtue of simultaneously offering theoretical understanding (e.g. Deakin 1989) and practical insight into treatment.

Finally, irrespective of the endogenous pharmacology of depressive illness, better understanding of the pharmacology of treatments can guide strategies for augmentation of drug effects. Explicitly, let us assume that drug treatments facilitate recovery by enhancing the function of one or more neurotransmitters, usually but perhaps not necessarily monoamines. If animal studies suggest a synergistic interaction between two such treatments to boost neurotransmitter function, then the same combination may be more efficacious in treatment-resistant patients. This approach underlay the facilitation of MAOI action with tryptophan (Coppen et al 1963) and of tricyclic drugs with lithium (de Montigny et al 1983). It has also led to the attempt to augment antidepressant action with yohimbine (unsuccessfully, Charney et al 1986). In future one can envisage a range of potential augmentation strategies which are illustrated diagrammatically in Figure 20.4. The great advantage of this approach is that it equips clinicians with a strategy with which to treat refractory patients; the guidelines otherwise are anecdotal (Goodwin 1990).

CLINICAL PHARMACOLOGY

Pharmacokinetics

Most reuptake inhibitors are well absorbed after oral ingestion and show peak plasma levels at 2–4 hours. There is appreciable first-pass metabolism in the liver and this is an important determinant of bioavailability. The drugs are highly lipophilic and hence are strongly protein-bound. The small fraction of the drug that is free in plasma appears to be relatively fixed so that total plasma levels will be meaningfully related to free drug. The extensive apparent volume of distribution of these drugs means that, in overdose, there is no point in attempting haemodialysis.

They are metabolized by hydroxylation and N-

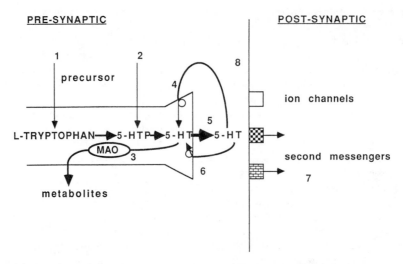

Fig. 20.4 The synaptic pharmacology of 5-HT is illustrated in diagrammatic form to illustrate the potential for the facilitation of neurotransmission by drugs

1) and 2) Primary or intermediate transmitter precursors can be used to increase transmitter synthesis; effects will be determined by enzyme kinetics so that appropriate compounds will either increase substrate supply or by-pass the rate limiting reaction. In the case of 5-HT, both tryptophan and 5-hydroxytryptophan have been employed. Enzyme cofactors such as pyridoxine or folate may also contribute to facilitate enzyme action in some circumstances

3) Transmitter metabolism can be inhibited. MAOIs do just this

4) Transmitter reuptake can be inhibited

5) Transmitter release may be facilitated by drugs like amphetamine or fenfluramine

6) Presynaptic autoreceptors can be blocked to prevent autoinhibitory effects of high transmitter levels

7) Postsynaptic actions on second messenger systems can be modulated (lithium provides an example)

8) Postsynaptic receptors can be selectively blocked or stimulated

There are many potential ways of augmenting function across a synapse of this sort by combining the effects of different treatments.
(Reproduced from Goodwin 1990, with permission)

oxidation in the liver and are conjugated with glucuronic acid. Irreversible demethylation of tertiary amino compounds to secondary amino derivatives also occurs to a variable, but sometimes considerable extent; amitriptyline, doxepin and imipramine yield nortriptyline, desmethyldoxepin and desipramine respectively. There are wide differences in the activities of the microsomal enzymes mediating drug metabolism. This is due to genetic polymorphism and can also be modulated by other drugs that either stimulate or inhibit enzyme activity (see below).

The clearance of all the tricyclic drugs and/or their active metabolites is relatively slow, with half-times of 12–48 hours (Amsterdam et al 1980). They can accordingly be prescribed on a once-daily basis. Steady-state levels are achieved within 7–21 days when fixed doses are employed.

Both first-pass metabolism and clearance may be less effective in the elderly, for whom lower doses of drug should generally be employed.

There is only limited information on the appearance of tricyclic drugs in breast milk. Amitriptyline and nortriptyline appear to be present at the same concentration as in plasma and hence can only be absorbed at negligible doses by a feeding infant (Bader & Newman 1980). On the other hand, clomipramine is said to be actively secreted in breast milk and should not be prescribed. There is little evidence bearing on the use of selective 5-HT reuptake inhibitors.

Drug interactions

Pharmacokinetic interactions occur with anticonvulsants and barbiturates which tend to increase the metabolism of tricyclics and lower plasma concentrations; conversely, fluoxetine, disulfiram, oral contraceptives and cimetidine have all been reported to increase tricyclic plasma levels.

Pharmacodynamic interactions occur because of a variety of synergistic effects. For example, increased antimuscarinic and histaminergic effects may result from joint prescribing with non-selective antihistamine and phenothiazine drugs; increased sedative effects occur with alcohol. Conversely, the actions of anticonvulsants, adrenergic neurone blockers (e.g. guanethidine) and clonidine may be decreased. Toxic interactions occur with the addition of 5-HT reuptake inhibitors to drug regimens including an MAOI. This has been established clinically for clomipramine and it may also be anticipated for the newer selective 5-HT reuptake inhibitors. The mechanism is increased release of 5-HT and the provocation of a 'serotonin syndrome' as it is called in animals (Marley & Wozniak 1983). Clinically, it consists of hyperarousal, anxiety, confusion, hyperthermia, hyperreflexia, tachycardia and hypotension. The endpoint can be coma and death. Particular care is also required on adding a potent 5-HT reuptake inhibitor after discontinuation of an MAOI. To add an MAOI to a non-selective tricyclic drug or to start both together is relatively safe (Pare 1985) although the combination is dangerous in overdose. Lithium promotes the serotonin syndrome in animals and may be expected to enhance the potential toxicity of tricyclic/MAOI and tricyclic/tryptophan combinations.

Dosage

The selection of dosage for tricyclic drugs remains an area of controversy. Recommended doses are in the region of 100–200 mg daily in the UK; doses recommended in the USA tend to be higher. (Data sheets should obviously be consulted for specific compounds.) However, it is widely believed that, in practice, the doses employed are often too low (Quitkin 1985). This is important because the response rates to conventional doses may only be 70% or so. For those tricyclic drugs that have been most intensively studied (imipramine, amitriptyline and desipramine) there is some evidence that doses up to 300 mg daily should be tried before the drug is said to have failed. Doses recommended in the USA tend to be in the higher ranges. Individuals vary greatly in the rate at which they metabolise the drugs and a single dose gives rise to a greater than tenfold range of plasma values (Åsberg 1976). Empirical investigation of the plasma levels associated with a favourable drug response suggests a range in the region of 100–200 ng/ml. Assuming plasma protein binding of 10–20% the free drug levels would be of the order of 10 ng/ml. A molecular weight of about 350 then gives a free drug activity of about 30 nmol/l in plasma.

The foregoing discussion implies that more is always best as long as side-effects are tolerated and the dose is safe. However, it was suggested by Åsberg et al (1971) that high plasma levels of drugs might be less effective because they would bind to receptors other than the reuptake sites. This would predict a bell-shaped plasma level/response relationship; i.e. poor responses should be associated with both too low and too high levels of drugs and good response with a therapeutic window. They actually reported this for nortriptyline (Åsberg et al 1971) and subsequently presented data to replicate the original finding (Kragh-Sørensen et al 1973) and to show that patients with high levels improved on *decreasing* the dose (Kragh-Sørensen et al 1976). A similar bell-shaped relationship has been described for amitriptyline (of which nortriptyline is the major metabolite) by Montgomery et al (1979a, b).

The identification of a reliable therapeutic window defined by plasma drug levels had obvious attractions. Unfortunately, the effect was not easily replicated (e.g. Coppen et al 1978, Hollister et al 1980) and, although this may have resulted from deficiencies in the later studies rather than necessarily in the originals, its validity has never gained general acceptance. There are, in fact, a number of purely practical problems that obscure the issue; these include the concomitant effects of other drugs upon plasma levels, inter-assay variability and reliability and timing of blood sample in relation to start of treatment. Thus, the precise numbers placed upon therapeutic windows are potentially misleading in any individual clinical situation.

However, uncertainty over what is or is not therapeutic should not obscure the value that levels do have in identifying extremes. It would be surprising if very low levels were not associated with treatment failure and many studies have confirmed that they are; they may also provide a valuable check on compliance. High values can arise in patients on average doses who are slow metabolizers of tricyclic drugs. While the probability of clinical response may or may not decrease in these patients, the risk of toxicity certainly increases.

This point is eloquently made in a review by Preskorn et al (1989) who suggest that CNS toxicity is increased appreciably with plasma levels about 450 ng/ml, and cardiotoxicity is a major risk with levels above 1000 ng/ml; about 7% of patients treated with 150 mg of amitriptyline daily will develop levels above 450 ng/ml. Provocatively, they also suggested that early toxicity produces symptoms such as impaired concentration that may be confused with worsening depressive symptoms and result in dangerous over-prescribing. The consequence of this line of reasoning would be to introduce another version of the therapeutic window, defined at its upper boundary by values associated with toxic side-effects rather than failure to improve. Thus, while routine measurement of drug levels is unlikely to be informative, there is good reason to measure levels where a treatment plan is not progressing well and uncertainty about compliance, side-effects or response is increasing.

In individual patients the dosage of amitriptyline, imipramine or desipramine should initially be raised to 150 mg and the patient should be examined carefully for clinical response. If there is little or no recovery within 2–3 weeks the dose should be increased towards 300 mg as far as side-effects permit. Doses beyond 300 mg are not commonly employed and an EEG should be done at this dose and for any increase beyond it. A strategy for the management of patients who do not respond to tricyclic drug treatment is given in chapter 26.

ADVERSE EFFECTS OF TRICYCLIC COMPOUNDS

The adverse effects of most of the typical and atypical antidepressants listed in Table 20.1 can be summarized together. Unusual risks associated with particular drugs will also be mentioned individually below. The Boston Collaborative Drug Surveillance Program (1972) reported that 15.4% of patients treated with tricyclic antidepressants experienced significant adverse effects ranging from drowsiness and mild symptoms of autonomic overactivity to severe reactions such as toxic confusional states. The major common risks are as follows.

Cardiovascular

The effects at therapeutic doses are reviewed by Glassman & Bigger (1981). Their main conclusion is that tricyclic drugs are safer than might be expected from their effects in overdose (see below). Relative tachycardia is a common accompaniment. Although this is usually attributed to antimuscarinic actions inhibiting vagal tone, it may be due to other effects on vasomotor integration. The increases in heart rate tend to be small. Large increases are unusual and should prompt investigation. Were large increases common the effects in patients with heart disease might be more important. By contrast, significant postural hypotension is common with tricyclic treatment. It occurs at relatively low doses of imipramine (75 mg daily) and is not made much worse by further increases in dose (Glassman et al 1979). It may be extremely inconvenient in younger patients but it is frankly dangerous in patients with heart disease and for the elderly, in whom it can produce falls. The most marked effects have been best documented for imipramine (Glassman et al 1979), but amitriptyline, doxepin, mianserin and trazodone have also been implicated (Warrington 1988). Glassman & Bigger (1981) argue strongly that postural hypotension is the most clinically important cardiovascular side effect of tricyclic treatment. Since it is so easy to measure it is curious that more information is not available. Nortriptyline appears to be the tricyclic least likely to cause the problem and may accordingly be the best choice among the older compounds in elderly patients.

Significant effects on myocardial conduction occur with therapeutic doses of tricyclics. They are usually attributed to quinidine-like or membrane-stabilizing properties of the drugs. Thus, prolongation of the P—R interval and QRS complex are easily demonstrated but these are not of clinical significance in healthy patients. They are, however, in patients with bundle branch block or other pre-existing conduction anomalies. For this reason, an ECG is a sensible precaution, particularly in patients over 50 or in anyone in whom cardiac problems may be suspected. Bundle branch block rather than a history of myocardial infarction *per se* is the main contraindication to the use of tricyclic drugs. An ECG should also be done if a tachycardia is pronounced or if unconventionally high doses of tricyclic drugs are contemplated.

The quinidine-like properties of tricyclics may actually be an advantage in the treatment of patients with extra beats of ventricular origin. Nevertheless, there are traditional concerns about tricyclics tending to impair cardiac output or as a cause of sudden death in patients. There is little definitive evidence favouring the view that tricyclic drugs have these effects at therapeutic doses (Glassman & Bigger 1981). The dangers in overdose, and perhaps less obviously in refractory patients receiving deliberately higher doses than usual, are increased and care must be exercised in both contexts.

It should be remembered that the risks of cardiac complications with treatment appear to be less than the risks of leaving depression without treatment (Avery & Winokur 1976).

Neurological

Sedation is a minor but unpleasant initial side-effect of most tricyclic drugs. It tends to be reduced by continuing drug administration, but a minor hangover effect in the morning often persists with the more sedative compounds. Patients should be cautioned not to drive or operate dangerous machinery while feeling sedated, and not to drink alcohol. The sedative effects are probably due to histaminergic, muscarinic and alpha$_1$-adrenoceptor affinity (Fig. 20.2).

Seizures are a particularly worrying but uncommon complication of tricyclic usage (Jabbari et al 1985). Limited evidence suggests that, at least in retrospect, a risk factor such as febrile convulsions, a family history of seizure disorder or possible brain injury is commonly identified. Maprotiline appears to be particularly proconvulsant while, until its withdrawal from use, nomifensine was regarded as particularly safe. The too sudden withdrawal of benzodiazepines may also contribute to the risk of a seizure and is an avoidable contributory factor. Finally, there may be some specific drug interactions that increase the risk of seizures: e.g. selective 5-HT reuptake inhibitors and lithium (Committee on Safety of Medicines 1989a). Unfortunately, following a seizure, even when an antidepressant can be reasonably said to have provoked it, patients should stop driving for one year and in the UK heavy goods or public service vehicle drivers are permanently disqualified.

Psychiatric

Tricyclic drugs are an important cause of confusional states. These are most common in the elderly or in patients with brain pathology (e.g. following stroke). The mechanism may be partly due to central antimuscarinic actions of the drugs, since this appears to be a cause of acute confusion in other circumstances (Tune et al 1981). It is also conventional to state that tricyclics can trigger manic states, although the status of such episodes is sometimes uncertain; patients with depres-

sion may develop mania because they have a bipolar illness, not simply as a side-effect of drug treatment. Antidepressants are certainly likely to make manic states worse and mis-diagnosis of sleep disturbance can result in their erroneous prescription.

Toxicity in overdose

The patient groups prescribed antidepressants, whether appropriately or inappropriately, are at risk of overdose and death. Tricyclic compounds, as already indicated, are both neuro- and cardiotoxic and they are a significant cause of death following deliberate overdose (or, indeed, accidental overdose in children). Nevertheless, tricyclic drugs only account for about 5% of deaths by poisoning in the UK (Henry & Cassidy 1986). In acute overdose, the ECG is probably the most useful predictor both of cardiac complications and of seizures (Boehnert & Lovejoy 1985); seizures were only seen with QRS lengthening over 0.1 s, and ventricular dysrhythmias with QRS over 0.16 s. How safe patients actually are when the QRS is below 0.1 is uncertain. Henry & Cassidy (1986) argue that it is the membrane-stabilizing actions of the tricyclics, and indeed of other drugs such as dextropropoxyphene and propranolol, rather than their primary pharmacology, that poses the major danger in overdose, although maprotiline appears to be particularly neurotoxic and outcome may not then be determined primarily by cardiac function. Otherwise, the cause of death is likely to depend on the availability of supportive medical care. In hospital, death is usually due to intractable arrhythmia, asystole or hypotension and therefore it is the support of cardiovascular function which is critical. Coma, seizures or respiratory depression may all contribute to death but are most dangerous in patients outside hospital. All the significant complications tend to occur within the 24 hours following ingestion of tablets. While a full account of the management of tricyclic poisoning is beyond the scope of the present chapter, it will be clear that it should normally be provided in a general hospital setting. Tricyclic overdose should be treated as would be a quinidine overdose, with bicarbonate or lactate infusion and cardiac pacing if necessary. Physostigmine can reverse coma but probably increases the risk of seizures and should not be used.

Different drugs appear to be associated with different risks of death (Table 20.2). Thus dothiepin (currently the most commonly prescribed tricyclic antidepressant in the UK) and amitriptyline show the highest mortality

Table 20.2 Fatal poisoning with antidepressant drugs 1975–1984 (England, Wales & Scotland) (data from Cassidy & Henry 1987).

Drug	Year introduced	Fatal poisonings		No of deaths per million prescriptions (95% confidence intervals)	
		No observed	No expected		
Desipramine	1963	13	5.7	80.2**	(36.6–123.8)
Dothiepin	1969	533	372	50.0***	(45.8–54.2)
Amitriptyline	1961	1181	886	46.5***	(43.9–49.1)
Nortriptyline	1963	57	51	39.2	(29.0–49.4)
Doxepin	1969	102	114	31.3	(25.2–37.4)
Imipramine	1959	278	342	28.4***	(25.1–31.7)
Trimipramine	1966	155	196	27.6**	(23.3–31.9)
Clomipramine	1970	51	160	11.1***	(8.1–14.1)
Protriptyline	1966	6	20	10.3**	(2.1–18.5)
Iprindole	1967	2	8.9	7.8**	(0–18.6)
Introduced 1974 and after					
Maprotiline	1974	83	77	37.6	(29.5–45.7)
Trazodone	1980	6	15	13.6*	(2.7–24.5)
Viloxazine	1974	2	7.4	9.4*	(0–22.4)
Butriptyline	1975	1	4.7	7.5	(0–22.2)
Mianserin	1976	30	187	5.6***	(3.6–7.6)
Nomifensine	1977	3	42	2.5***	(0–5.3)
Lofepramine	1983	0	3.7	3.7	
Monoamine oxidase inhibitors					
Tranylcypromine	1960	15	9.0	58.1*	(28.7–87.5)
Phenelzine	1959	24	36.7	22.8*	(13.7–31.9)
Isocarboxazid	1960	3	8.2	12.8	(0–27)
Tricyclic antidepressants 1970 and before		2384	61.9	38.5	(36.9–40.1)
Tricyclic and other anti-depressants 1974 and after		125	9.65	13.0	(10.7–15.4)
Monoamine oxidase inhibitors		42	1.57	26.7	(18.6–34.8)
All antidepressants		2551		34.9	(33.5–36.3)

p values: *<0.05 **<0.01, ***<0.001 for difference of a given drug from mean for all antidepressants

and, among the other commonly used drugs, mianserin and clomipramine show low rates. The interpretation of these relative risks is difficult. The low rates of death with clomipramine, for example, appear unlikely to be attributable to its pharmacology and it has been suggested that it may have a directly protective effect upon suicidal thoughts and compulsions (Montgomery et al 1988). However, there are other sources of uncertainty about the patient characteristics within the different drug groups and interactions with other drugs as the ultimate cause of death. It is their greater safety in overdose which is a particular apparent advantage of many newer compounds and, hopefully, the selective 5-HT reuptake inhibitors.

Hyperphagia and weight gain

While seldom emphasized this can in practice be a particularly inconvenient complication of long-term antidepressant treatment since it reduces patient compliance and self-esteem. It also tends to be fully developed only on prolonged treatment and can occur even on low doses of tricyclic drugs (Paykel et al 1973). The mechanism is poorly understood. Antagonism of 5-HT-receptors as by cyproheptadine is a possible explanation but most tricyclics have only modest affinity for $5-HT_1$- and $5-HT_2$-receptors, and drugs such as amitriptyline and mianserin have no worse a reputation for weight gain than those that do not block 5-HT-receptors (see Fig. 20.1). Since depressive illness is itself often associated with changes in appetite and weight the precise effect of drug treatment is sometimes difficult to isolate in the early stages of treatment.

Anticholinergic side-effects

The anticholinergic effects of tricyclics are manifest in a variety of actions on autonomic function. The dry mouth experienced almost universally by patients on tricyclic drugs is a subjective nuisance and contributes to dental problems on long-term administration. Excessive consumption of soft drinks may contribute to weight gain. More serious is the difficulty with micturition that can be provoked by tricyclics, especially in men with prostatic hypertrophy. There are also reports of sexual dysfunction in men on tricyclics, somewhat confused by the effects of depressive illness *per se*. Trazodone is unusual in having caused priapism. Effects on gut motility may be responsible for dyspepsia and constipation. Effects on the pupil and ciliary muscle of the eye produce troublesome blurring of vision and increase the risk of narrow-angle glaucoma.

Blood dyscrasias and other idiosyncractic reactions

As with many drugs, there are very occasional reports of agranulocytosis, aplastic anaemia or thrombocytopenia following the administration of antidepressants.

However, the only predictable risk is that mianserin can rarely cause a reversible neutropenia. Accordingly, regular full blood counts are recommended during continuing treatment with mianserin (Organon Laboratories revised Data Sheet 1986). There are also occasional hypersensitivity responses that may be linked to antidepressant drugs, including skin rashes, cholestatic jaundice and vasculitis.

ADVERSE EFFECTS OF SELECTIVE 5-HT REUPTAKE INHIBITORS, TRYPTOPHAN AND FLUPENTHIXOL

The newer 5-HT-selective drugs have different side-effect profiles from tricyclics. For example, fluoxetine produced subjective nausea in 25% of 1378 patients reviewed by Lader (1988). Nervousness or frank anxiety (in up to 30% of patients) and insomnia were also more often associated with fluoxetine than a tricyclic, as was headache. These side-effects are probably due to increased 5-HT neurotransmission. Important interactions also occur with tryptophan and probably also with lithium (Committee on Safety of Medicines 1989a). It must be appreciated that the frequency and importance of major adverse reactions have not been identified yet and it may well require longer and wider use of fluoxetine and other selective 5-HT reuptake inhibitors before they are. The drugs are free of many of the unwanted effects of tricyclics such as weight gain, cardiovascular effects and sedation. At low dose they show a very favourable side-effect profile but their efficacy may then be questionable, despite optimistic reports from preliminary fixed-dose studies (Hall 1988).

Tryptophan initially enjoyed a reputation for freedom from adverse effects matched only by its reputation for lack of efficacy in severe depression (see below). However, reports of a serious hypersensitivity syndrome tarnished its image as a simple foodstuff. This precipitated announcements that proprietary preparations of tryptophan had been withdrawn in a number of countries (Committee on Safety of Medicines 1989b). However, the adverse effects had resulted predominantly from over-the-counter health food supplements and the suspicion remains that a contaminant may have been responsible.

THE EFFICACY OF ANTIDEPRESSANT DRUGS

Antidepressant drugs have been subjected to evaluation of efficacy at a variety of different levels. Imipramine initially was accurately assessed to be an effective antidepressant by clinical observation without what would now be regarded as an adequate control treatment or subject randomization (Kuhn 1958). Such evidence depends crucially upon the experience and judgment of an individual clinician, and it is just such judgment that is traditionally the measure of the quality of an individual doctor. Controlled trials make a necessary sacrifice of this quality for the advantage of objectivity; they are now increasingly necessary to convince licensing bodies, and indeed scientifically-minded doctors, that treatments work. The methodology of such trials is clearly beyond the scope of this chapter but the ability to assess trials is an important part of a modern clinician's education. It will be worthwhile examining the most obvious pitfalls that apply generally to clinical trials before considering individual drug treatments.

Most trials compare the treatment of interest, A, with a placebo, P, or another standard treatment, X. Subjects should be randomized to the alternative treatments and assessed in double-blind fashion using an adequate instrument to estimate mood change. Outcome should then be expressed in binary terms (say 50% reduction in symptoms as a response) or as a change score. Problems tend to arise in the declaration and interpretation of the result. It is common to declare results in terms of statistical significance. Thus a comparison with placebo may show superiority of A at a $p < 0.05$ level, or a comparison with another active treatment may show no significant difference. Should we be confident in declaring that A is a better treatment than placebo or as good a treatment as the standard X? The answer depends on understanding that significance levels are crucially influenced by sample size. A highly statistically significant result in a very large trial may be entirely trivial; on the other hand, the failure to find a clinically significant difference between two active treatments may simply be due to small sample size. The confusion in part originates in the meaning of the term significant; indeed, statisticians often argue that discernible would be a better word (Wonnacott & Wonnacott 1977). However, more fundamental is the failure to think in terms of effect size and confidence intervals (Gardner & Altman 1990). The results of a trial are best expressed in terms of some convenient measure of effect size. For binary outcomes, the odds ratio has a number of advantages (Yusef et al 1985), among which is the easy calculation of a confidence interval. The most common situation in small trials is that effects are statistically significant but the con-

fidence interval is sufficiently wide to leave room for considerable and entirely legitimate uncertainty. The only solution to this dilemma is larger trials and the combination of trials of similar design for meta-analysis (Yusef et al 1985).

These considerations are of considerable importance both for clinical reasons, i.e. which is the best treatment?, and for theoretical reasons: does panic disorder have a differential treatment response to selective 5-HT reuptake inhibitors compared with selective NA uptake inhibitors?

Currently, there are other major problems that limit the applicability to general clinical experience of clinical trial data collected by companies testing new products. These include, on the one hand, the understandably self-defensive exclusion criteria that prevent many patients entering studies, on the other, the requirement to collate large amounts of information that discourages clincans from entering patients in studies. There is considerable need for simpler trials that will allow larger numbers of patients to be entered painlessly and which answer important clinical questions such as whether newer antidepressants are more effective than older ones and for whom and, more crucially, for how long treatments should continue.

Nevertheless, psychiatry has over the last 20 years subjected most of its traditional treatment methods to evaluation, in some cases with particularly severely disturbed patients. In addition, there is some practice that derives from uncontrolled clinical experience that understandably finds its way into current clinical recommendations.

Imipramine

As the first tricyclic to be available, imipramine has always been regarded as a reference compound for the evaluation of new antidepressants. It has been compared with placebo in nearly 50 individual studies (1334 patients). 30 of the studies presented data in a convenient form as binary outcome and can be combined to show 65% improvement on imipramine treatment compared with 30% on placebo. The doubling of the probability of response that this implies is an effect about which we can be extremely confident because of the large total number of patients (Davis & Glassman 1989). The corresponding p value, for what it is worth, is 10^{-31}. However, our certainty about the difference between imipramine and placebo does not much help the 30% or more patients who are not improved on active treatment. The disadvantages of imipramine are those typical of the tricyclic group as a class. It is a less sedating drug than amitriptyline, but can still be prescribed as a single dose at night.

Desipramine

Desipramine is relatively non-sedating and has the fewest anticholinergic side-effects of the older tricyclic group. This reflects its relative selectivity in vitro (Fig. 20.1).

Amitriptyline

Amitriptyline has been available since 1961. It has an active metabolite, nortriptyline, with a notably long half-life. Amitriptyline is the archetypical sedative tricyclic. Together with nortriptyline, it will tend to block reuptake of both 5-HT and NA. Its efficacy has been established both by placebo-controlled trials and by comparison of its efficacy with imipramine.

Nortriptyline

Nortriptyline appears to have an unusual dose/effect relationship which has been described in detail above. Its relative freedom from the side-effect of postural hypotension has made it a useful drug for the treatment of depression in the elderly.

Butriptyline, doxepin, dothiepin

These compounds have all been introduced as alternatives to amitriptyline and are very similar in their properties both to amitriptyline and each other. Dothiepin has been unusually successful in the UK, without any clear clinical evidence for particular advantages over the parent compound.

Protriptyline

Protriptyline is a less sedating compound than many other tricyclics especially amitriptyline, butriptyline, doxepin and dothiepin. It is recommended that single daily doses should not be taken within 6 hours of bedtime.

Amoxapine

Amoxapine is unusual in having pronounced affinity for D_2-receptors. It is the only tricyclic that has unequivo-

cally produced galactorrhoea, elevated prolactin secretion and extrapyramidal side effects. These effects may be attributable to additional action from a metabolite, 7-hydroxyamoxadine, which has even higher affinity for D_2-receptors. It appears to be quite a dangerous drug in overdose, in part because it tends to slow gastric emptying markedly.

Clomipramine

Of the older drugs, clomipramine shows the greatest affinity and selectivity for 5-HT transport in vitro. However, its metabolite desclomipramine is much less selective in this respect. Clomipramine is effective in depressive illness and is believed to have a wider spectrum of action than other tricyclics in relation to obsessive-compulsive and panic disorder. It should not be used in lactating mothers because it is said to be secreted in the breast milk. It is relatively non-sedating.

Lofepramine

Lofepramine is the most recent tricyclic to be introduced for clinical use in the UK. It is closely related to imipramine and is metabolized to desipramine. It is claimed that in vivo it remains a less active anticholinergic drug than its close chemical relatives and is less cardiotoxic. In part this may result from lower potency. However, desipramine is itself the most selective of the tricyclic drugs so the advantages of lofepramine may reside in part in its status as a pro-drug. There have been reports of abnormal liver function associated with lofepramine (Committee on Safety of Medicines 1988).

Iprindole

Iprindole has a low affinity for most receptor classes (Fig. 20.2). This 'atypical' profile was originally taken to be an important refutation of the idea that monoamine reuptake was the central action in the antidepressant mechanism of tricyclic drugs. However, a critical review of the efficacy of iprindole cast early doubt on its status as a first-line antidepressant (Zis & Goodwin 1979).

Mianserin

Like iprindole, mianserin was believed to be atypical at its introduction in the 1970s. It was introduced on the basis of its 'tricyclic-like' effect on the EEG rather than its effectiveness in animal screening tests. However, its binding profile is not markedly different from amitriptyline, albeit of lower potency for the monoamine transporters (Fig. 20.2). It certainly has a good reputation clinically for safety in overdose but there are doubts about its efficacy in severe depressive illness. The rare complication of neutropenia requires practical care in its use (see above).

Trazodone

Trazodone is a sedative antidepressant with, it is claimed, an important effect on anxiety symptoms. Its profile in vitro is unusual in exhibiting particularly low affinity for muscarinic receptors. It is apparently well-tolerated in the elderly. Its in vivo pharmacology is complicated by extensive metabolism to a non-selective 5-HT agonist, mCPP (m-chlorphenylpiperazine). The anti-anxiety effect may be, in part, due to the buspirone-like actions of mCPP.

Maprotiline

Maprotiline is quite selective for NA reuptake, but is otherwise similar in properties to the tricyclic group. It is particularly likely to provoke seizures, especially in overdose (Knudsen & Heath 1984).

Viloxazine

Viloxazine has side-effects of nausea, vomiting and headache that are similar to the selective 5-HT reuptake inhibitors. Like them, it is also non-sedative and has few anticholinergic side-effects. However, its in vitro pharmacology appears to show low affinity for the 5-HT reuptake mechanism, so the clinical profile is not easily explained.

Fluoxetine

Fluoxetine increases the plasma levels of tricyclic drugs, probably by impairing oxidative metabolism. This has practical implications for the process of switching between fluoxetine and many tricyclics, because it has a slow clearance (fluoxetine 2–3 days, desmethylfluoxetine 7–9 days). However, it is most clinically significant when a patient is switched from fluoxetine to an MAOI. For the reasons discussed earlier under Drug interactions the data sheet recommends a 5-week delay in starting an MAOI after fluoxetine.

Finally, there have been several case reports of fluoxetine producing significant extrapyramidal side-effects in patients who are taking or have taken neuroleptics. The mechanism is poorly understood (Ciraulo & Shader 1990).

Fluvoxamine

Fluvoxamine has similar in vitro selectivity for the 5-HT transporter to fluoxetine. Also similarly, it has been shown to be an effective antidepressant in placebo-controlled trials and has side-effects that include nausea and headache. It usually regarded as an alerting drug. There is little reason to anticipate major differences between the highly selective reuptake inhibitors and none have so far emerged.

Tryptophan

Tryptophan has been found to be effective in a study of depression in general practice patients (Thomson et al 1982). Otherwise, it can be used in combination with tricyclics or MAOIs (chapter 26). It is best prescribed at a dose of 3 g daily, since levels above this strongly induce liver enzymes that metabolize tryptophan. It had a good reputation for safety, unsurprising for a foodstuff, but this has been recently questioned (see above).

Flupenthixol

Flupenthixol, at a relatively low dose, may be an effective antidepressant. The major problem with its use is obviously the risk of both acute and chronic motor side-effects, as for other neuroleptic drugs. Its putative mode of action is inhibition of autoreceptors, which may be expected to increase dopamine release. It has never secured a clear indication in the management of depression.

THE USE OF ANTIDEPRESSANT DRUGS IN OTHER PSYCHIATRIC DISORDERS

There is a poorly explored but persistent idea in psychiatry that response to specific treatments might provide a defining classification of a particular illness category. It is therefore of considerable interest that conditions other than depression respond to treatment with antidepressant drugs.

Panic disorder

Imipramine was first suggested to be an effective drug in a range of patients with anxiety symptoms including what would now be called panic disorder (Klein & Fink 1962). Despite some initial scepticism (Marks et al 1983), reasonably directed to the possibility that imipramine might be relieving depressive symptoms, the efficacy of imipramine in panic-disorder patients without depression appears now to be widely accepted. Furthermore, clomipramine and the more selective 5-HT reuptake inhibitors also appear to be effective. Indeed, a selective inhibitor of 5-HT reuptake appeared to be more effective than a selective inhibitor of NA reuptake or a 5-HT$_2$-blocker (Westenberg & Den Boer 1989). The time course of the onset of positive effects was, however, rather prolonged. These most interesting findings point to the possibility of pharmacological dissection of a relatively homogeneous psychiatric disorder, something which has not yet proved feasible for depressive illness.

Obsessive-compulsive disorder (OCD)

Early claims for the efficacy of clomipramine have now been amplified with the apparent efficacy of more selective 5-HT reuptake inhibitors (fluvoxamine, Price et al 1987; fluoxetine, Levine et al 1989). The coexistence of depressive symptoms has made the claims for pharmacological efficacy the subject of some controversy, although the results of a number of small placebo-controlled trials have all been similar, assisted perhaps by the small size of placebo response. As for panic disorder, there is evidence for superior efficacy of a 5-HT reuptake inhibitor compared with an NA reuptake inhibitor (Goodman et al 1990). Nevertheless, the clinical impression is not one of particular efficacy; however statistically significant the improvement, the number of symptom-free OCD patients after treatment with clomipramine or a selective reuptake inhibitor may be rather few.

Bulimia nervosa

The response of some patients with bulimia nervosa to antidepressant treatments is of considerable interest. Again, the coexistence of depressive symptoms and the frequent family history of affective disorder complicates the interpretation, but more recent work appears to establish the efficacy of both 5-HT- and NA-selective drugs in the treatment of this sydrome without evidence for an antidepressant effect *per se* (Walsh 1988, Pope et al 1989).

Miscellaneous

The use of antidepressants in alcoholism, headache and other chronic pain syndromes is also of interest.

FUTURE PROSPECTS

There has been a lamentable tendency for new tricyclic drugs to be produced that are no improvement on the older ones. Since the most dangerous adverse effects in overdose are probably due to quinidine-like properties of the molecules, rather than their relevant pharmacology, newer drugs ought to be possible that have similar, relatively non-selective effects on monoamine function but are much safer in overdose.

It is not clear yet that selective inhibition of 5-HT reuptake represents an unequivocal therapeutic advance. This is most important in relation to efficacy (Danish University Antidepressant Group 1986, 1990). In addition, the side-effect profile at therapeutic doses, with nausea and headache prominent, may be different from tricyclics but is not necessarily better. Clinical definition of the relative efficacy of truly selective reuptake inhibitors is of great practical and theoretical importance.

The future development of antidepressant drugs requires advances in our understanding of how they work. Animal work shows that all the currently accepted antidepressant drugs appear to facilitate monoamine function. We are not certain that this is a necessary condition for effective action, but it remains the central working hypothesis that it is usually sufficient. Since there appear to be so many ingenious ways of producing increased monoamine function, new drugs are certain to appear. The monoamine theory of drug action therefore remains fruitful but it is less a testable hypothesis than a paradigm within which almost all new ideas currently have to develop. The essential parallel path is to seek greater understanding of the biological basis of depression and of treatment effects in man.

ACKNOWLEDGMENT

I wish to thank Norma Brearley for her careful preparation of the manuscript.

REFERENCES

Amsterdam J, Brunswick D, Mendels J 1980 The clinical application of tricyclic antidepressant pharmacokinetics and plasma levels. American Journal of Psychiatry 137: 653–662

Åsberg M 1976 Treatment of depression with tricyclic drugs – pharmacokinetic and pharmacodynamic aspects. Pharmacopsychiatry and Neuropsychopharmacology 9: 18–26

Åsberg M, Crönholm B, Sjöqvist F, Tuck D 1971 Relationship between plasma level and therapeutic effect of nortriptyline. British Medical Journal 3: 331–334

Avery D, Winokur G 1976 Mortality in depressed patients treated with electroconvulsive therapy and antidepressants. Archives of General Psychiatry 33: 1029–1034

Bader E F, Newman K 1980 Amitriptyline in human breast milk and the nursing infant's serum. American Journal of Psychiatry 137: 855–856

Boehnert M T, Lovejoy F H 1985 Value of QRS duration versus the serum drug level in predicting seizures and ventricular arrhythmias after an acute overdose of tricyclic antidepressants. New England Journal of Medicine 313: 474–476

Boston Collaborative Drug Surveillance Program 1972 Adverse reactions to the tricyclic-antidepressant drugs. Lancet 1: 529–531

Cassidy S, Henry J 1987 Fatal toxicity of antidepressant drugs in overdose. British Medical Journal 295: 1021–1024

Charney D S, Price L H, Heninger G R 1986 Desipramine-yohimbine combination treatment of refractory depression: implications for the β-adrenergic receptor hypothesis of antidepressant action. Archives of General Psychiatry 43: 1155–1161

Ciraulo D A, Shader R I 1990 Fluoxetine drug-drug interactions: 1. Antidepressants and antipsychotics. Journal of Clinical Psychopharmacology 10: 48–50

Committee on Safety of Medicines 1988 Lofepramine (Gamanil) and abnormal blood tests of liver function. Current Problems 23

Committee on Safety of Medicines 1989a Fluvoxamine and fluoxetine – interaction with monoamine oxidase inhibitors, lithium and tryptophan. Current Problems 26

Committee on Safety of Medicines 1989b L-tryptophan and eosinophilia-myalgia syndrome in the USA. Current Problems 27

Coppen A, Shaw D M, Farrell J P 1963 Potentiation of the antidepressive effect of a monoamine-oxidase inhibitor by tryptophan. Lancet 1: 79–81

Coppen A, Ghose K, Montgomery S, Rama Rao V A, Bailey J, Christiansen J, Mikkleson P L, van Praag H M, van de Poel F, Minsker E J, Kozulja V G, Matussek N, Kungkunz G, Jørgensen A 1978 Amitriptyline plasma-concentration and clinical effects. Lancet 1: 63–66

Danish University Antidepressant Group 1986 Citalopram: clinical effect profile in comparison with clomipramine. A controlled multicentre study. Psychopharmacology 90: 131–138

Danish University Antidepressant Group 1990 Paroxetine: a selective serotonin re-uptake inhibitor showing better tolerance, but weaker antidepressant effect than clomipramine in a controlled multicentre study. Journal of Affective Disorders 18: 289–299

Davis J M, Glassman A H 1989 Antidepressant drugs. In: Kaplan H I, Sadock B J (eds) Comprehensive textbook of psychiatry. Williams & Wilkins, Baltimore, p 1627–1655

de Montigny D, Cournoyer G, Morisette R, Langlois R, Caille G 1983 Lithium carbonate addition in tricyclic antidepressant-resistant unipolar depression. Archives of General Psychiatry 40: 1327–1334

Deakin J F W 1989 Role of 5HT receptor subtypes in depression. In: Archer T, Bevan P, Cools A (eds) Behavioural pharmacology of 5HT. Lawrence Erlbaum, New York, p 179–204

Dunleavy D L F, Brezinova V, Oswald I, MacLean A W, Tinker M 1972 Changes during weeks in effects of tricyclic drugs on the human sleeping brain. British Journal of Psychiatry 120: 663–672

Gardner M J, Altman D G 1990 Confidence – and clinical importance – in research findings. British Journal of Psychiatry 156: 472–474

Glassman A H, Bigger J T J 1981 Cardiovascular effects of therapeutic doses of tricyclic antidepressants. Archives of General Psychiatry 38: 815–820

Glassman A H, Bigger J T J, Giardina E V, Kantor S J, Perel J M, Davies M 1979 Clinical characteristics of imipramine-induced orthostatic hypotension. Lancet 1: 468–472

Goodman W K, Lawrence H P, Delgado P L, Palumbo J, Krystal J H, Nagy L M, Rasmussen S A, Heninger G R, Charney D S 1990 Specificity of serotonin reuptake inhibitors in the treatment of obsessive-compulsive disorder. Archives of General Psychiatry 47: 577–585

Goodwin G M 1990 Drug treatment of depression: what if tricyclics don't work? In: Hawton K, Cowen P J (eds) Dilemmas in the management of psychiatric patients. Oxford University Press, Oxford, p 1–15

Goodwin G M, Green A R, Johnson P 1984 5-HT$_2$ receptor characteristics in frontal cortex and 5-HT$_2$ receptor-mediated head-twitch behaviour following antidepressant treatment in mice. British Journal of Pharmacology 83: 235–242

Goodwin G M, De Souza R J, Green A R 1985 Presynaptic serotonin receptor-mediated response in mice attenuated by antidepressant drugs and electroconvulsive shock. Nature 317: 531–533

Gray J A, Goodwin G M, Heal D J, Green A R 1987 Hypothermia induced by baclofen, a possible index of GABA$_B$ receptor function in mice, is enhanced by antidepressant drugs and ECS. British Journal of Pharmacology 92: 863–870

Hall J 1988 Fluoxetine: efficacy against placebo and by dose – an overview. British Journal of Psychiatry 153: 59–63

Henry J A, Cassidy S L 1986 Membrane stabilising activity: a major cause of fatal poisoning. Lancet 1: 1414–1417

Hollister L E, Pfefferbaum A, Davis K L 1980 Monitoring nortriptyline plasma concentrations. American Journal of Psychiatry 137: 485–486

Jabbari B, Bryan G, Mars L E E, Gunderson C H 1985
Incidence of seizure with tricyclic and tetracyclic
antidepressants. Archives of Neurology 42: 480–481

Klein D F, Fink M 1962 Psychiatric reaction patterns of
imipramine. American Journal of Psychiatry 119: 432–438

Knudsen K, Heath A 1984 Effects of self poisoning with
maprotiline. British Medical Journal 288: 601–603

Kragh-Sørensen P, Åsberg M, Eggert-Hansen C 1973
Plasma-nortriptyline levels in endogenous depression.
Lancet 1: 113–115

Kragh-Sørensen P, Hansen C E, Baastrup P C, Hvidberg E F
1976 Self-inhibiting action of nortriptyline's antidepressive
effect at high plasma levels. Psychopharmacologia 45:
305–312

Kuhn R 1958 The treatment of depressive states with
G22355 (imipramine hydrochloride). American Journal of
Psychiatry 115: 459–464

Lader M 1988 Fluoxetine efficacy vs comparative drugs: an
overview. British Journal of Psychiatry 153 (suppl 3): 51–58

Levine R, Hoffman J S, Knepple E D, Kenin M 1989 Long-
term fluoxetine treatment of a large number of obsessive-
compulsive patients. Journal of Clinical
Psychopharmacology 9: 281–283

Marks I M, Gray S, Cohen D, Hill R, Mawson D, Ramm E,
Stern R S 1983 Imipramine and brief therapist-aided
exposure in agoraphobics having self-exposure homework.
Archives of General Psychiatry 40: 153–162

Marley E, Wozniak K M 1983 Clinical and experimental
aspects of interactions between amine oxidase inhibitors
and amine re-uptake inhibitors. Psychological Medicine 13:
735–749

Montgomery S A, Lambert M T, Lynch S P J 1988 The risk
of suicide with antidepressants. International Clinical
Psychopharmacology 3: 15–24

Montgomery S A, McAuley R, Rani S J, Montgomery D R
1979a Amitriptyline plasma concentrations and clinical
response. British Medical Journal 3: 1711

Montgomery S A, McAuley R, Rani S J, Montgomery D R
1979b Amitriptyline plasma concentrations and clinical
response. British Medical Journal 3: 230–231

Nelson J C, Jatlow P, Quinlan D M, Bowers M B 1982
Desipramine plasma concentration and antidepressant
response. Archives of General Psychiatry 39: 1419–1422

Oswald I, Brezinova V, Dunleavy D L F 1972 On the
slowness of action of tricyclic antidepressant drugs. British
Journal of Psychiatry 120: 673–677

Pare C M B 1985 The present status of monoamine oxidase
inhibitors. British Journal of Psychiatry 146: 576–584

Paykel E S, Mueller P S, De La Vesgne P M 1973
Amitriptyline, weight gain and carbohydrate craving: a side
effect. British Journal of Psychiatry 123: 501–507

Pope H G, Keck P E, McElroy S L, Hudson J I 1989 A
placebo-controlled study of trazodone in bulimia nervosa.
Journal of Clinical Psychopharmacology 9: 254–259

Preskorn S H, Jerkovich G S, Beber J H, Widener P 1989
Therapeutic drug monitoring of tricyclic antidepressants: a
standard of care issue. Psychopharmacology Bulletin 25:
281–284

Price L H, Goodman W, Charney D, Rasmussen S, Heninger
G 1987 Treatment of severe obsessive-compulsive disorder
with fluvoxamine. American Journal of Psychiatry 144:
1059–1061

Quitkin F M 1985 The importance of dosage prescribing
antidepressants. British Journal of Psychiatry 147:
593–597

Richelson E, Nelson A 1984 Antagonism by antidepressants
of neurotransmitter receptors of normal human brain in
vivo. Journal of Pharmacology and Experimental
Therapeutics 230: 94–192

Richelson E, Pfenning M 1984 Blockade by antidepressants
and related compounds of biogenic amine uptake into rat
brain synaptosomes: most antidepressants selectively block
norepinephrine uptake. European Journal of Pharmacology
104: 277–286

Sugrue M F 1981 Current concepts on the mechanisms of
action of antidepressant drugs. Pharmacology and
Therapeutics 13: 219–247

Thomson J, Rankin H, Ashcroft G W 1982 The treatment of
depression in general practice: a comparison of L-
tryptophan, amitriptyline, and a combination of L-
tryptophan and amitriptyline with placebo. Psychological
Medicine 12: 741–751

Tune L E, Damlouji N F, Holland A, Gardner T J, Folstein
M F, Coyle J T 1981 Association of postoperative delirium
with raised serum levels of anticholinergic drugs. Lancet 2:
651–653

Walsh B T 1988 Antidepressants and bulimia: where are we?
International Journal of Eating Disorders 7: 421–423

Wander T J, Nelson A, Okazaki H, Richelson E 1986
Antagonism by antidepressants of serotonin S_1 and S_2
receptors of normal human brain in vitro. European Journal
of Pharmacology 132: 115–121

Warrington S J 1988 The cardiovascular toxicity of
antidepressants. International Clinical Psychopharmacology
3: 63–70

Westenberg H G M, Den Boer J A 1989 Selective monoamine
uptake inhibitors and a serotonin antagonist in the
treatment of panic disorder. Psychopharmacology Bulletin
25: 119–123

Wonnacott T H, Wonnacott R J 1977 Introductory statistics.
John Wiley, New York, p 650

Yusuf S, Peto R, Lewis J, Collins R, Sleight P 1985 Beta-
blockade during and after myocardial infarction: an
overview of the randomized trials. Progress in
Cardiovascular Disease 27: 335–371

Zis A P, Goodwin F K 1979 Novel antidepressants and the
biogenic amine hypothesis of depression. Archives of
General Psychiatry 36: 1097–1107

21. Monoamine oxidase inhibitors

Jonathan R. T. Davidson

New treatments are sometimes discovered through serendipity: such was the case for monoamine oxidase inhibitors (MAOIs) when, in 1954, Bloch et al (1954) noted that tuberculous patients undergoing treatment with iproniazid became euphoric. The drug was known to inhibit MAO and, as a result of this observation, it was postulated that (1) MAOIs may have mood elevating properties and (2) mood elevation may be related to alteration of catechol or indole activity.

In short order, a flurry of publications attested to mood-enhancing effects of MAOIs in depression: over 1300 reports were published on this group of drugs between 1959 and 1962 (Laurence 1966).

During the 1960s, four critical developments threatened the existence of this group of drugs: 1) serious and life-threatening hypertensive reactions were reported in patients receiving MAOIs, when taken in conjunction with foods, beverages or medication (Blackwell et al 1967); 2) lethal interactions occurred between MAOIs, narcotics and hypoglycaemic drugs; 3) two major clinical trials (Greenblatt et al 1964, Medical Research Council 1965) concluded that MAOIs were no more effective than placebo in depression 4) other safer and more effective antidepressants became available. As a result of these events, the MAOIs came close to extinction, being reserved for use as drugs of last resort. They have since enjoyed a modest revival, yet still occupy only a small proportion of the market. In 1988, total USA dollar sales of MAOI drugs represented only 2.1% of all antidepressant sales.

Notwithstanding these observations, MAOIs have continued to attract a level of interest that goes far beyond their limited use. There are several reasons for this: 1) a number of depressed patients show preferential response to this class of drug; 2) MAOIs are effective in many other conditions besides depression; 3) there are good reasons for optimism that newer and safer MAOIs will become available.

TYPES OF MAO INHIBITOR

These drugs may be grouped according to chemical structure (i.e. hydrazine versus non-hydrazine), duration of action (reversible versus irreversible) or selectivity of enzyme action (selective for MAO-A or MAO-B versus non-selective) (see Table 21.1).

Hydrazine drugs are those which exhibit a N–N bond on the side chain (e.g. phenelzine, isocarboxazid, iproniazid). Non-hydrazine drugs (e.g. tranylcypromine, clorgyline, pargyline) do not exhibit this feature and are believed as a result to cause less hepatotoxicity. It is not clear, however, to what extent hepatotoxicity continues to be a problem with any concurrently marketed MAOI, except possibly for iproniazid.

Table 21.1 Classification of MAOI drugs by structure, selectivity and reversibility

Drug	Hydrazine	Selective	Reversible
Phenelzine	Yes	No	No
Isocarboxazid	Yes	No	No
Iproniazid	Yes	No	No
Nialamide	Yes	No	No
Tranylcypromine	No	No	No
Pargyline	No	Yes[1, 3]	No
Clorgyline	No	Yes[2]	No
Deprenyl	No	Yes[1, 3]	No
Moclobemide	No	Yes[2]	Yes
Brofaromine	No	Yes[2]	Yes
Amiflamine	No	Yes[2]	Yes

[1] Selective for MAO-B at lower doses

[2] Selective for MAO-A

[3] Become non-selective at higher doses

The standard MAOIs are irreversible, i.e. they form an irreversible, non-displaceable bond to the enzyme. As a result, upon discontinuation of a drug, new supplies of enzyme have to be synthesized by the body, a process which can take up to 2 weeks. The reversible drugs bind competitively to MAO and can be displaced by other substrates according to the law of mass action. The practical importance of this property is that tyramine-containing foods or sympathomimetic drugs are less hazardous and, in the case of some easily reversible inhibitors, may be safely taken with the drug.

The older MAOIs such as tranylcypromine, phenelzine, iproniazid and isocarboxazid are all non-selective inhibitors of both the A and B forms of MAO, whereas some newer drugs such as moclobemide and brofaramine are selective for MAO-A, while deprenyl is selective for MAO-B at lower doses. The importance of these properties is that an A-inhibitor will prevent the breakdown of noradrenaline (NA) and 5-hydroxytryptamine (5-HT), both of which are integral to depressive and anxiety states. B-inhibitors have less impact on these particular neurotransmitters, but affect dopamine (DA) to a greater extent and are less effective in depression (Lipper et al 1979).

The development of selective and reversible inhibitors such as moclobemide (Priest 1989) and brofaramine (Bieck et al 1983a) offer promise of safe and effective MAOI treatment.

INDICATIONS FOR MAOIs IN DEPRESSION

MAO inhibitors exert beneficial therapeutic effects across a wide range of both psychiatric and non-psychiatric disorders (Table 21.2). Some of these have been established through double-blind placebo-controlled trials, whereas others are based upon uncontrolled reports.

There is substantial evidence that phenelzine, isocarboxazid, iproniazid and tranylcypromine are effective in major depression or dysthymic disorder (Davidson et al 1988a, Razani et al 1983, Robinson et al 1973, Paykel et al 1982, Liebowitz et al 1984, Vallejo et al 1987, Kiloh et al 1959, Raft et al 1979). At higher doses, deprenyl also exerts antidepressant effects, although as a non-selective inhibitor (Mann et al 1989). Moclobemide is also more effective than placebo in depression (Versiani et al 1989).

Atypical depression

One sustaining factor behind the survival of MAO inhibitors has been the conviction that they are the preferred form of treatment for atypical depression (West & Dally 1959). Resolution of this issue depends partly upon the way in which atypicality is defined. It also depends upon the comparative treatment: i.e. it is quite possible that other non-tricyclic drugs besides an MAOI might benefit atypical depression.

Table 21.2 Clinical uses of MAOI drugs

Major depression	Double-blind placebo and active controls
Dysthymia	Double-blind placebo and active controls
Melancholia	Double-blind placebo-controlled and open trials
Panic disorder/agoraphobia	Double-blind placebo and active controls
Social phobia	Double-blind placebo and active controls
Post-traumatic stress disorder	Double-blind placebo and active controls
Obsessive-compulsive disorder	Open uncontrolled trial
Chronic pain/depression	Double-blind placebo and active controls
Parkinson's disease	Double-blind placebo control
Alzheimer's dementia	Double-blind placebo control
Neurodermatitis	Open uncontrolled trial
Rheumatoid arthritis	Open uncontrolled trial
Attention deficit disorder	Open uncontrolled trial
Herpes simplex	Open uncontrolled case report
Apthous ulcer	Open uncontrolled case report
Negative symptoms of schizophrenia	Open uncontrolled trial
Migraine	Open uncontrolled case reports

Atypical depression has been defined in different ways, most of which have either referred to depression with anxiety, chronic pain, reversed vegetative symptoms, rejection sensitivity or non-endogenous depression in general. The place of atypical depression in psychiatry, its definition, characteristics and diagnostic validity continue to be a matter of great interest and therefore invite further discussion in this chapter.

At this time, there is only a modest degree of validation for the concept. To some extent, this is accountable by the lack of a standard definition, but even when one definition is used (i.e. the Columbia group), validating data are still weak. The following approaches may be used in validating a disorder: longitudinal course, age at onset, treatment response, psychobiological markers, family history and symptomatology.

Age of onset and course

With respect to onset and longitudinal course, it is generally held that atypical depression begins in the teenage years of early adulthood, and that it follows a chronic or phasic course (Davidson et al 1982a).

Family studies

Rabkin et al (1990) report that in atypical depression, as defined by the Columbia criteria, there is increased prevalence of dysthymic disorder, alcoholism and atypical depression in relatives of atypical probands. They also noted a reduced prevalence of major depression.

Treatment response

With respect to treatment response, the Columbia group have found, in several studies, that so long as at least one of the following atypical features is present along with mood reactivity, then phenelzine is therapeutically superior to imipramine. These atypical features are: oversleeping, hyperphagia, weight gain, rejection sensitivity. The advantage for phenelzine is not based upon a heightened MAOI effect as much as it reflects a lack of imipramine effect. In patients who have only mood reactivity and none of the other atypical features, phenelzine and imipramine are therapeutically equivalent and are both superior to placebo (Rabkin et al 1990). Thus, one might conclude that, on the basis of current evidence, the Columbia criteria identify a type of depression which is somewhat unresponsive to imipramine, although the effects of imipramine would still appear to outweigh those of placebo.

Other investigators have reported somewhat different findings. Paykel and colleagues (1982) noted that phenelzine was superior to amitriptyline in atypical depression which was accompanied by an ICD-9 diagnosis of anxiety, but did not find that the Columbia criteria usefully predicted MAOI effects. They also found that phenelzine was less effective in the presence of 'characterological' depression, which might suggest that certain forms of personality disorder reduce the therapeutic effects of MAOIs more than they do for tricyclics.

In a recent multicentre study of isocarboxazid and placebo in atypical depression, Davidson et al (1988a) examined the independent contributions made to outcome by six different components of the 'atypical concept', as well as any possible specific interactive effects with the MAOI drug. The six elements were as follows: panic attacks, phobic avoidance, somatic anxiety, vegetative reversal, hostility and interpersonal sensitivity (IPS). IPS was found to account for the superior MAOI effect more than any other component, although the negative influence of phobic avoidance upon outcome was also reversed by the drug.

Psychobiological markers

The evidence from sleep studies (Rabkin et al 1990), tyramine excretion (Harrison et al 1984) and dichotic listening (Bruder et al 1990) shows that atypical depressives differ from melancholics, but not from normals. Atypical depressives are also more likely than melancholics to respond with dysphoria to intravenous amphetamine (Rabkin et al 1990).

Symptomatology

There have been few systematic clinical reports which have analysed the comparative symptomatology of atypical depressives and other relevant control groups. However, three classification studies have applied multivariate techniques to this question. Paykel et al (1983) found no cohesiveness to the three common definitions of atypicality (i.e. non-endogenicity, anxious depression, vegetative reversal).

Davidson et al (1988b) used Grade of Membership (GOM) analysis to derive subtypes of depression in a group of 190 depressed and anxious patients who had participated in clinical drug trials. The construct of atypicality was partially upheld, in that atypical vegetative symptoms were largely confined to two of the five groups, but the occurrence of panic attacks did not correspond to vegetative reversal. In a confirmatory GOM study (1989), Davidson et al again derived five subtypes which broadly corresponded to those obtained in the first study. Some support was provided for the concept of atypical depression, although in one of the emergent atypical subtypes MAOI response rates were low, indicating that a more severe end of the atypical spectrum may also exist and that not all atypicals can be expected to respond well to a traditional MAOI.

In summary, this author believes that a more solid foundation needs to be established before including atypical depression as a separate form of depression. Uniformity of construct needs to be developed, as better evidence for an unique neurobiological or familial pattern and stronger evidence for particular response to treatment.

Non-atypical depression

In addition to being effective in the treatment of atypical and (typical) major depression of non-melancholic type, it is likely that phenelzine, isocarboxazid and tranylcypromine are effective in melancholic depression (Davidson et al 1988a, c, McGrath el al 1986, 1987).

MAO inhibitors are less likely to benefit psychotic depression (Davidson et al 1977, 1978, 1982b, 1988c), but in combination with a neuroleptic they may be useful (Davidson et al 1982b).

Dose factors

Three different studies have shown that the therapeutic effect of an MAOI in non-endogenous depression is related to dose of drug and/or level of MAO inhibition which is achieved. 60 mg/day of phenelzine is more effective than 30 mg/day, which in turn was found to be no better than placebo in outpatients with non-endogenous depression (Ravaris et al 1976). Davidson et al (1984a) found that 50 mg/day isocarboxazid was more effective than 30 mg/day in non-endogenously depressed inpatients. In both studies, the higher MAOI doses produced greater platelet MAO inhibition which, in non-endogenous depression, appears to be proportionally related to the therapeutic effects of phenelzine (Ravaris et al 1976, Robinson et al 1978) and of isocarboxazid (Davidson et al 1986).

In a third study, Mann et al (1989) showed that deprenyl was more effective at higher doses (30 mg/day) than at lower doses, but time was a confounding factor in their report.

OTHER INDICATIONS FOR MAOIs

Panic disorder/agoraphobia

Double-blind studies by Tyrer et al (1973) and Sheehan et al (1980) have confirmed earlier suggestions (Kelly et al 1970) that phenelzine is effective in this disorder at doses of up to 60 mg/day. The study of Mountjoy et al (1977) is difficult to evaluate, since substantial amounts of benzodiazepine were also prescribed. Iproniazid is also effective in treatment of this disorder (Lipsedge et al 1973).

Kelly and Sheehan have expressed the opinion that phenelzine has a significant antiphobic action as well as being able to block panic attacks. Pretreatment with phenelzine can block lactate-induced panic (Kelly et al 1971).

Social phobia

Two placebo-controlled studies by Liebowitz et al (1988) and Versiani et al (1990) attest to an MAOI effect in social phobia. An open study with tranylcypromine has also demonstrated positive results (Versiani et al 1988). In the first study, phenelzine was shown to exceed placebo and atenolol in therapeutic efficacy, especially where avoidance was pervasive, while atenolol seemed effective in limited ('performance') social anxiety. In the second study, the new MAOI moclobemide was more effective than placebo in social phobia. The apparent benefit of an MAOI in this condition may suggest the relevance of rejection sensitivity or sensitivity to humiliation and criticism which characterize social phobia.

Generalized anxiety disorder (GAD)

Generalized anxiety disorder has been little studied as regards MAOI therapy. It is notable that Mountjoy et al (1977) found generalized tension to be associated with poor response to phenelzine.

Obsessive-compulsive disorder (OCD)

Despite clinical anecdotes favouring MAOIs in OCD, the one double-blind trial to compare an MAOI, clorgyline, to a tricyclic antidepressant (TCA), clomipramine, found the TCA to be more effective (Insel et al 1983). Nonetheless, it is likely that, in some cases, this often refractory disorder may respond to an MAOI.

Post-traumatic stress disorder (PTSD)

Early uncontrolled studies (Davidson et al 1987, Lerer et al 1987) suggested utility for phenelzine in PTSD. A short-term double-blind crossover trial of phenelzine and placebo found a time effect, but no treatment effect (Shestatsky et al 1988). An 8-week double-blind evaluation of phenelzine, imipramine and placebo reported good results with the MAOI in outpatients with minimal other comorbidity (Frank et al 1988).

Bulimia nervosa

Both isocarboxazid and phenelzine have been found, in double-blind placebo-controlled trials, to exert significant therapeutic effects upon symptoms of bulimia nervosa. Isocarboxazid up to 60 mg/day reduced binge eating and vomiting; the response was unrelated to other psychiatric comorbidity (Kennedy et al 1988). Walsh et al (1984), found that phenelzine also reduced bingeing in normal-weight bulimics, at doses of up to 90 mg/day.

Alzheimer's dementia

Tariot et al (1987) showed that deprenyl at a daily dose of 10 mg had positive effects on several symptom dimensions in Alzheimer's disease. A placebo control was less effective. Also, the authors observed that an increase in dose up to 40 mg/day did not produce further gains, which would indicate that the additional inhibition of MAO-A is unnecessary.

Parkinson's disease

The irreversible B-inhibitor L-deprenyl, in conjunction with L-DOPA/carbidopa, is effective in lessening the deterioration which can be seen during treatment with the L-DOPA/carbidopa combination. In particular, the addition of L-deprenyl may result in lowering the dose of L-DOPA/carbidopa, improvement of the 'on-off' phenomenon, akinesia, tremor and speech, and improved functional capacity (Golbe et al 1988).

Other indications

A number of disorders may respond to treatment with an MAOI, but at present no controlled data exist. Among these disorders are attention deficit disorder (Zametkin et al 1985), herpes simplex (Rosenthal & Fitch 1987), aphthous ulcers (Gelenberg 1988), rheumatoid arthritis (Lieb 1983), neurodermatitis (Friedman et al 1978) and the negative symptoms of schizophrenia (Bucci 1987). In two double-blind trials, chronic pain (Raft et al 1979) and atypical facial pain (Lascelles 1966) both improved more on phenelzine than on placebo in depressed patients.

ADVERSE EFFECTS OF MAOI DRUGS

A number of studies have reported the side-effect profiles of MAOI drugs. In general, while the dangers may have been exaggerated, it is probably accurate to say that even the 'run-of-the mill' side-effects of MAOI present more problems than do those of other antidepressants. In one multicentre trial, 6% of patients dropped out of treatment during a 6-week course of isocarboxazid because of side-effects (Zisook1984). It is useful to view MAOI side-effects as being either short-term or long-term, as there are some differences, and the late-emerging side-effects may undermine the therapeutic effects of an MAOI.

In general, the principle to follow calls for dosing up to a point where either therapeutic improvement sets in or there is some evidence of side-effects. Tranylcypromine is generally better tolerated than the hydrazine drugs and can be a useful alternative in patients who are unable to tolerate side-effects of these. Deprenyl is another useful drug in such a patient, although it is extremely expensive.

The most frequently occurring side-effects during short-term treatment with isocarboxazid are dizziness (32%), headache (14%), dry mouth (13%), insomnia (10%), constipation (8%), sedation (6%), blurred vision (6%), nausea (5%), peripheral oedema (5%), forgetfulness (3%), syncope (3%), tremor (3%), hesitancy of urination (3%), weakness (3%). The procedure used to establish these occurrences involved non-directively asking the patient at each visit whether he or she had noticed anything that had not been present at baseline, or which had worsened with treatment. All of the above events occurred more frequently on drug than on placebo (Zisook 1984).

Short-term effects of isocarboxazid upon blood pressure and pulse were noted to be maximal at weeks 3 and 4, possibly corresponding to the dose-increase schedule or to the effects of time. Mean drop in supine systolic blood pressure was 14 mmHg, and mean drop in supine pulse rate was 8 beats per minute.

It is likely that the cardiovascular effects of isocarboxazid are in some way connected with its antidepressant effects. Two lines of evidence can be cited in this regard: 1) the time course of therapeutic effect parallels the time course of vital sign changes described above; 2) recovery rates at 4 weeks are higher in depressed inpatients with a pretreatment systolic orthostatic change of ≥ 10 mmHg (Davidson & Turnbull 1986).

Hepatotoxicity was rare in the study of isocarboxazid. Five of 86 (5.8%) patients on isocarboxazid manifested transient mild elevation of SGOT or SGPT, and no patients showed elevations of bilirubin or alkaline phosphatase.

Intermediate and long-term side-effects

Studies by Evans et al (1982) and Rabkin et al (1984) have examined the incidence of side-effects with phenelzine and tranylcypromine. Over a 4–12-month interval, the problematic side-effects grow more apparent. During a 6-month maintenance placebo-controlled trial of phenelzine 45 or 60 mg/day, the following side-effects occurred: weight gain (43%), oedema (36%), muscle cramps (28%), carbohydrate craving (21%), sexual dysfunction (14%), pyridoxine deficiency (7%), hypocalcaemia with exacerbation of rickets (7%).

In a later report of side-effects of phenelzine, Rabkin et al (1984) noted sexual dysfunction or anorgasmia (22%), passing out/falling (11%), hypomania (8%), excessive weight gain (8%), hypertensive crisis (8%), disorientation (5%), urinary retention (5%).

Tranylcypromine was similar to phenelzine in respect of passing out/falling (17%) and hypomania (7%), but was less likely to produce disorientation, weight gain, oedema or sexual dysfunction. Although they observed fewer hypertensive crises with tranylcypromine, this appears unrepresentative of the drug, which in other series is associated with an 8% incidence (Blackwell 1963).

MAOI DRUGS, DIET AND THE TYRAMINE REACTION

Shortly after the MAOI drugs were introduced to psychiatry in the early 1960s, a number of reports described severe headaches in patients who were taking one of the drugs, in most cases tranylcypromine. The following vignette (Arora & Reed 1963) indicates how these reports were perceived at the time. The words are those of a patient writing to a physician, describing the effects of eating cheese: 'I get an attack similar to what I call "migraine" – heart thumping, head racked with pain and sickness within half an hour. Other patients

(taking the same MAOI) experienced this as well after cheese, but the doctors laughed at the idea . . .'

It was due to the efforts of Blackwell and colleagues (Blackwell 1963, Blackwell et al 1967) that the existence of this drug-food interaction was established, and its mechanism better understood (Blackwell & Marley 1966a, b). Their study also revealed that the risk was highest for tranylcypromine (8% of patients) and lower for phenelzine (1.5%), although it is likely that the dose of phenelzine was not comparable to that of tranylcypromine. Subsequent reports have also given an 8% incidence of hypertensive reaction with phenelzine (Wright 1978, Rabkin et al 1984). Hypertensive reactions have also been reported in 11% of patients who received tranylcypromine (Neil et al 1979), many of whom acknowledged non-compliance with treatment. One may conclude with dismay that the introduction of dietary advice has not in fact lowered the risk of hypertensive episodes, since in the three most recent studies all patients were given appropriate counselling. Two factors to consider are that phenelzine is now often used at higher doses and that, as treatment is continued for months or even years, the risk of dietary violation may increase (Neil et al 1979). These findings reinforce the need for careful selection of patients for MAOI therapy and for periodic reminders during treatment about dietary restrictions.

Recent surveys of MAOI diets have been made by Stewart (1976), Sullivan & Shulman (1984), Folks (1983) and McCabe & Tsuang (1982). These reviews concur that there are only a few foods and beverages which must be avoided.

In a review of 20 different recommended MAOI diets, Sullivan & Shulman found that the number of restricted substances ranged from eight to 32 categories, embracing 70 different items. All diets prohibited cheese, Chianti wine and pickled fish. Other items commonly, but not invariably, excluded were brewer's yeast extract, broad beans, beer and liver.

Folks (1983) has reviewed the foods and beverages which have reportedly been associated with a hypertensive reaction. There have been multiple cases where cheese, yeast extracts, smoked or pickled herring, broad bean pods, beer and Chianti wine were implicated. The following were mentioned in single reports: chicken liver (Hedberg et al 1966), beef liver (Boulton et al 1970), the peel of unripe bananas, avocado and guacamole (Generali et al 1981), non-alcoholic beer (Draper et al 1984), vermouth (Stewart 1976), New Zealand spinach (Comfort 1981) and the liqueurs Kahlua, Drambuie and Crème de Cacao (Neil et al

1979). It is hard to know what to make of a single case report, but it should not form the basis for an absolute proscription unless the link is entirely clear and has an understandable mechanism. Thus it is possible that the avocado was unfresh, and all unfresh or overripe food should be avoided because of bacterial decomposition, which can produce high tyramine levels. In the reported case involving beef liver, it was stated that the food was unfresh, yet it must be noted that the tyramine content of fresh liver is not insubstantial. The reaction with prickly spinach involved a large quantity of the vegetable. The skin of unripe bananas, which contains dopa, is rarely eaten in the United States, and hardly justifies the exclusion of banana. Broad bean (fava bean) pods are also rich in dopa.

McCabe & Tsuang (1982) make the point that tyramine content in an item of food may vary and cannot reliably be estimated without direct measurement. The tyramine content of a piece of cheese can vary from 0.002 mg/g to 2.1 mg/g (Sen 1969). Foodstuffs particularly high in tyramine are: pickled herring, with up to 3 mg/g; chicken liver, with 0.1 mg/g; Chianti wine, with 0.25 mg/ml; and beer, with 0.01 mg/ml. The tyramine content of various foods has been presented by Maxwell (1980), Sen (1969), Horwitz (1964) and Marley & Blackwell (1970). 6 mg of tyramine can induce a mild hypertensive reaction, 10 mg may induce a moderate reaction and 25 mg can lead to a severe hypertensive episode (Blackwell et al 1967, Sjoqvist 1965). Thus a significant reaction could follow 5 g cheese, 3 g pickled herring, 400 ml Chianti (i.e. 3–4 glasses). The fact that a patient may have violated his diet with impunity on one occasion in no way guarantees protection against further violation, because of the unpredictability of this reaction. Important considerations include the amount of tyramine in a particular food, rapidity of gastric emptying, duration of MAOI treatment, dose of drug and the time interval that has elapsed between dose and ingestion of food.

Suggested food and beverage restrictions

In light of the above, it does a disservice to patients and promotes non-compliance if they are taxed with unduly long lists of substances to avoid. The following foods and drinks should be avoided:

1) all cheese, except for cream, cottage and ricotta cheeses
2) red wine, sherry, beer and liqueurs
3) pickled or smoked fish
4) brewer's yeast products (e.g. Marmite, Bovril, some packet soups)
5) fava (broad) bean pods (i.e. Italian green beans)
6) beef or chicken liver
7) fermented sausage (bologna, pepperoni, salami, summer sausage)
8) any unfresh, overripe or aged food (especially pheasant, venison, spoiled fruit, unfresh meats, unfresh dairy products).

There are no good grounds for the exclusion of reasonable amounts of coffee, chocolate, colas or tea, any of which can produce untoward effects if taken in grossly excessive amounts, regardless of the MAOI drug. Yoghurt, fresh sour cream, soy sauce, tenderized meat, baker's yeast products (bread etc), avocados, bananas, sauerkraut, raisins and figs can also be safely consumed with an MAOI, on the basis of present evidence.

Alcoholic beverages not listed above can be consumed in moderation but are likely to be potentiated by the MAOI, so that as Sargant (1975) has pointed out, patients get intoxicated more easily. Comfort (1981) has also described a hazardous interaction between phenelzine and alcohol, and indeed other sedatives as well, in recovered patients, who develop toxic symptoms of disinhibited behaviour not unlike the effects of amphetamine. Because these unpredictable reactions may be socially embarrassing, Comfort recommends avoidance of all alcoholic drinks with MAOI drugs.

The hypertensive reaction

Presentation and diagnosis

All headaches are not hypertensive in origin, so that when a patient who is taking an MAOI reports this symptom it is important to be sure that other causes are not responsible. Some knowledge of the patient will help one to assess if it is a symptom of the underlying illness, a not uncommon finding in the MAOI patient who presents with various somatic complaints. The treatment of the patient is of course quite different in this case.

MAOI drugs can also produce a histamine headache, a distinct possibility when headache occurs in the absence of hypertension. Features which may be associated with a histamine reaction include hypotension, anginal pain, colic, diarrhoea, 'asthmatic' breathing, salivation and lacrimation. Some foods, including cheese and Marmite (Blackwell et al 1965) are rich in histamine, whose degradation is impaired by an MAO inhibitor. As suggested by Cooper (1967), an antihistamine would be the logical treatment for this condition.

The hypertensive reaction can occur with varying degrees of severity. It may present initially as a pounding occipital headache, which radiates frontally to become generalized. Patients will sometimes describe it as feeling as though their head was bursting. In some instances, the headache is preceded by sudden onset of palpitations, nausea or vomiting. In addition, there may be a feeling of apprehension, with complaints of chills, photophobia, sweating and restlessness. The physician or nurse may observe sweating, neck stiffness, chills, pallor, mild pyrexia, dilated pupils and motor agitation. A rise in systolic and diastolic blood pressure will be noticed. These reactions are characteristically of sudden onset, from within minutes up to $2\frac{1}{2}$ hours after ingestion of an incompatible food, drink or medication. Some authorities, however, say that hypertension can develop as long as 20 hours after ingestion of cheese (Klein et al 1981). The worst part of the headache will usually lift after an hour, but a dull ache may persist for some days (Dally & Connelly 1981).

The reaction may be severe, and can lead to more marked and/or persistent hypertension, alteration of consciousness, hyperpyrexia, convulsions and cerebral haemorrhage. The occurrence of fatalities led to the temporary removal of tranylcypromine from the market in the 1960s. We are unaware of any systematic study which examined the mortality rate from MAOI hypertensive reaction. From what we know, it is possible to make an educated guess, however. About 90% of deaths on tranylcypromine are due to hypertensive crisis (Freedman et al 1973); the death rate is 1 per 100 000 patients who receive the drug (Klein et al 1981). With a reported 8% incidence of hypertensive reaction on tranylcypromine (Neil et al 1979), one can assume that 8000 hypertensive reactions will occur in 100 000 patients. The fatality rate due to hypertensive crisis cannot then be higher than 1:8000 cases, i.e. 0.012%.

Treatment

The most frequently recommended treatment of a hypertensive reaction is to administer 5 mg phentolamine intravenously, which will produce a rapid response. Because it is often short-lived, the treatment may need to be repeated after a few hours. In addition, because of fluid retention associated with this treatment, administration of 40 mg frusemide may also be necessary (Davidson et al 1984b).

Alternative treatments include the infusion of diazoxide 300 mg, or of sodium nitroprusside 50–100 mg in 500 ml 5% dextrose in water (Davidson et al 1984b). These agents produce a longer-lasting response than phentolamine.

It has been recommended that patients carry around their personal supply of nifedipine to self-administer at the first sign of a hypertensive reaction. There is always the possibility of misdiagnosing the cause of headache, as well as the possibility of an overshoot leading to hypotension, if the recommendation is followed.

Incompatible combinations of MAOI and other medications include over-the-counter medications for coughs, colds, allergies, congestion, weight reduction and appetite suppression that contain indirectly-acting sympathomimetic agents which will, in combination with an MAOI, produce hypertension. The presentation and treatment of any ensuing reaction will resemble that caused by foodstuffs.

Pathophysiology of the tyramine interaction

A historical consideration will remind us that the amino acid tyrosine is named from the Greek word for cheese, *tyros*, which contains a plentiful supply of this substance. Under the influence of bacterial action, tyrosine can be decarboxylated to tyramine, a protein which has for a long time been known to exert pressor effects. Hare (1928) described tyramine oxidase as the enzyme responsible for tyramine degradation. Zeller (1938) proposed that it was a more general enzyme, which he named monoamine oxidase, which was present not only in liver but also in brain and was responsible for the breakdown of various monoamines, including catecholamines.

When iproniazid, a known inhibitor of MAO, was discovered to have antidepressant effects (Crane 1958), it is a remarkable oversight that, given the available knowledge at the time, the medical community failed to predict that hypertension would occur when a patient ingested tyramine-containing foods.

Why should such a reaction happen? Tyramine is an indirectly acting sympathomimetic, i.e. it is taken up in to the cell, where it releases stored catecholamine supplies into the free and active form. It thus leads to increased sympathetic function. This reaction would normally be self-limiting, because of the body's ability to degrade synaptic noradrenaline by catechol-o-methyl transferase (COMT), and to degrade intracellular noradrenaline via MAO, located in the mitrachondria. In a state of MAO inhibition, the major pathway of inactivation is blocked, so that the effects of noradrenaline will be intensified. This effect is further compounded by the fact that tyramine itself is inactivated by MAO, so there is even further magnification of response when MAO is inhibited.

There are rich supplies of MAO type A in the gut and the liver, so that any tyramine which is ingested by mouth will normally be in large part destroyed as it passes through these tissues. Faraj et al (1981) have shown that less than 1% of ingested tyramine passes unchanged into the systemic circulation. There is no question that there is considerable first-pass metabolism of tyramine (Simpson & White 1984).

Unavailability of MAO would certainly permit the access of substantially greater amounts of tyramine into the circulation. However, it appears unlikely that this adequately explains why hypertensive reactions take place. Indeed, the potentiation by an MAOI of tyramine effects may be unrelated to MAO inhibition.

Sandler (1981) studied the pig, an animal in which MAO-A is limited to the gut wall and which otherwise entirely possesses MAO-B. Administration of clorgyline did not protect the animal from a profound hypertensive reaction to intravenously administered tyramine, even though MAO was available to degrade both tyramine and clorgyline. On the other hand, deprenyl, which inhibited the pig's supply of MAO-B, failed to potentiate the hypertensive response.

One possible explanation is that the drug may facilitate the release of noradrenaline, as does tyramine, i.e. it has its own indirect sympathomimetic effect. This may explain why non-MAO inhibitors, such as isoniazid (Smith & Durack 1978) and indomethacin (Lee et al 1979), have resulted in hypertensive reactions. It might also explain why autotoxic reactions sometimes occur with an MAO inhibitor in the absence of any exogenous factor. This author has seen two such 'spontaneous' occurrences with phenelzine at 30 mg and isocarboxazid at 50 mg per day. In each case the patient was already in the hospital and other causes had been reasonably ruled out. There have been a number of reports in the literature where this has occurred with tranylcypromine (Cooper et al 1964, AMA Council on Drugs 1963, Nies 1984). Both phenelzine and tranylcypromine are known to have amphetamine-like noradrenaline-releasing effects from sympathetic nerve endings (Lee et al 1961), so that such spontaneous

reactions can be easily understood. We have seen one such case with isocarboxazid, although it has been stated that this is a 'pure' MAO inhibitor (Pare 1968). It is possible that this is merely a function of dose and that other properties of the drug become evident at higher doses.

Sandler (1981) also speculated that the amine-releasing property of MAOI drugs was a crucial part of their therapeutic effect. Deprenyl and pargyline have poor therapeutic effect, even when MAO-B has been extensively inhibited (Lipper et al 1979, Pare et al 1981), but it may be that MAO-A inhibition alone is sufficient for an antidepressant effect, since there will be substantial effects on noradrenaline and 5-HT.

Potentiating effects of MAOI drugs on tyramine have been studied by oral and intravenous administration of tyramine. Oral administration approximates most closely to the actual clinical situation, but such testing is more time-consuming and more hazardous. One has to contend with the possibility of delayed or variable absorption and prolonged response, so that increasing doses of tyramine can only be given at 30–60 minute intervals. Relatively few groups have used this strategy (Simpson & White 1984, Elsworth et al 1978, Lader et al 1970, Pare et al 1985).

Oral tyramine studies have shown that tranylcypromine results in a 10–20-fold potentiation of tyramine, i.e. approximately 15 mg tyramine is required to produce a 30 mmHg rise in blood pressure, compared to the 200–400 mg needed in unmedicated subjects (Bieck et al 1983b).

Pare et al (1982) reported that concurrent use of amitriptyline with an MAOI prevented the potentiation of intravenous tyramine, presumably by blocking uptake. However, with larger oral doses of tyramine this protection was not apparent (Pare et al 1985). Simpson & White (1984) have reported a hypertensive episode after oral tyramine in a patient who received combined tranylcypromine and amitriptyline. Deprenyl at low doses, which are selective for MAO-B, shows minimal potentiation of tyramine, but at the higher doses needed for antidepressant effect there is a greater potentiation (Simpson & White 1984).

PATIENT COUNSELLING

Many of the principles involved in counselling patients who are to receive MAOIs have been described by Walker et al (1984). Careful explanation is always owed to the patient about the nature of his or her illness, and about the treatment options that are available. This is especially important in the case of a person who is being considered for an MAOI. When other less toxic drugs are available, the physician should share his thinking with the patient as to why an MAOI is being recommended. This needs to be done with conviction and not in a half-hearted manner, since the patient will often have many doubts about embarking on a treatment which entails prohibitions and caveats. To keep a proper perspective, this author generally reminds the patient early on that *all* medicines are likely to have some unwanted effects, that they may impose certain restrictions and perhaps carry some slight risk, but that we consider these to be less than the risk of an untreated illness. It is emphasized early that, if the medicine brings about recovery of function and well-being, the disadvantages of the medicine may appear to be a price worth paying. In this context, the patient can be counselled as to dietary and medication restrictions which should be observed, as described earlier in the chapter.

A wallet-sized card is given to the patient, containing specific instructions. It may be pertinent to ask the patient to repeat these back to make certain that they are understood. The card also explains that the patient should not take any over-the-counter medicine without first obtaining clearance from a physician. It also instructs the patient, whenever they visit a doctor or dentist, to convey that they are taking the named drug. The physician can write his/her telephone number on the card, in the event that the patient needs to be in touch between visits or in an emergency.

With this approach, properly selected patients are usually quite willing to undertake a course of MAOI treatment, and initial preparation of this kind enables the patient to become more actively involved in the treatment process. Many of the MAOI responders have experienced chronic and previously treatment-resistant illness, and are more than willing to accept the risks entailed with MAOI drugs if they think that it will help them. Moreover, after having been somewhat disillusioned from failed treatment, and having perhaps sensed the frustrations of other therapists, they respond well to a new sense of optimism.

MECHANISMS OF ACTION

An initially appealing theory held that the antidepressant effects of an MAOI were directly related to the degree of peripheral MAO inhibition. In the case of phenelzine, this was shown by Robinson et al (1978) for outpatients and by Davidson et al for inpatients (Davidson et al 1978b). Unfortunately, these relationships have not been so clear-cut for other MAO inhibitors and they may also be subject to the clinical presentation of depression (Davidson & Pelton 1988, Davidson et al 1977).

Other properties of MAOI include the amphetamine-like release of stored amines (Tyrer 1982) referred to earlier. Its relevance to mechanism of action is unclear.

A second property, especially of tranylcypromine, is inhibition of reuptake. This may be of some importance, as demonstrated by Escobar et al (1974), who showed greater efficacy for the reuptake-inhibiting (-) isomer of tranylcypromine as compared to the MAO-inhibiting (+) isomer.

More recent work implicates central noradrenaline (NA) and 5-hydroxytryptamine (5-HT) systems. Hanger et al (1988) have shown a reduction in whole body NA turnover. This effect might result from increased adrenergic autoreceptor inhibition, with subsequent increased synaptic efficiency. Adaptive changes in second messenger systems and reduced alpha- and beta-adrenergic binding sites can result after chronic administration of clinically effective MAOI, but not after administration of clinically ineffective MAOI drugs such as pargyline and deprenyl (Murphy et al 1984).

There is also evidence from animal models to suggest that MAO inhibitors can produce long term changes within central 5-HT pathways. Clinically effective MAOI drugs, including the reversible MAO-A inhibitor amiflamine, result in enhanced 5-HT neurotransmission when 5-HT neurones discharge at their normal frequency in the presence of MAO-A inhibition. It is also of relevance that clorgyline induces an initial reduction of 5-HT firing, followed after 3 weeks by a return to normal, and that this return is paralleled by a threshold decrease in 5-HT autoreceptor sensitivity. This time course resembles the time taken for antidepressants to work in humans. Furthermore, these changes were not found after MAO-B inhibitor drug administration (Blier et al 1990).

The mechanisms of drug action in other states such as post-traumatic stress disorders and panic disorder, may be different from those of depression. In post-traumatic stress disorder and panic disorder it is likely that locus ceruleus downregulation may be of importance, along with the ability of an MAOI to reduce paroxysmal noradrenergic hyperactivity (Nutt & Glue 1989).

The effectiveness of phenelzine in social phobia has

speculatively been related by Liebowitz et al (1987) to its ability to increase the activity of dopamine, a neurotransmitter which may mediate social anxiety and interpersonal sensitivity.

WHERE DO MAOI DRUGS BELONG IN PSYCHIATRY?

Few people will choose to administer an MAOI as first-choice treatment, even through some studies have demonstrated excellent efficacy in atypical depression, social phobia and post-traumatic stress disorder, all of which are disorders for which there is no accepted standard treatment. They are generally suitable as second- or third-line treatments. As new antidepressants are developed, it may be expected that fewer patients will require the old hydrazine or non-hydrazine drugs. Of greater importance, however, is the development of safer selective and reversible MAO-A inhibitors such as moclobemide, which offer hope of equal efficacy compared with other antidepressants, without requiring dietary or medication restrictions or long washout periods. The therapeutic versatility of MAOI drugs is impressive, and a number of patients do exist for whom an MAOI remains the only effective agent.

REFERENCES

A M A Council on Drugs 1963 Paradoxical hypertension from tranylcypromine sulphate. Journal of the American Medical Association 254–294

Arora B, Reed A E 1963 Tranylcypromine and cheese. Lancet 2: 587

Bieck P, Antonin K H, Jedrychowski M 1983a Monoamine oxidase inhibition in healthy volunteers by CGP 11305 A, a new specific inhibitor of MAO-A. Modern Problems in Pharmacopsychiatry 19: 352–358

Bieck P R, Cremer G, Gleither C, Antonin K H 1983b Effect of the reversible MAO-inhibitor CGP-11305 A on blood pressure response after oral tyramine. Presented at the World Conference on Clinical Pharmacology and Therapeutics, Washington, DC

Blackwell B 1963 Hypertensive crisis due to monoamine oxidase inhibitors. Lancet 2: 849–851

Blackwell B, Marley E 1966a Interactions of cheese and of its constituents with monoamine oxidase inhibitors. British Journal of Pharmacology 26: 120–141

Blackwell B, Marley E 1966b Interaction of yeast extracts and their constituents with monoamine oxidase inhibitors. British Journal of Pharmacology 26: 120–142–161

Blackwell B, Marley E, Mabbitt I A 1965 Effects of yeast extract after monoamine oxidase inhibition. Lancet 1: 940–943

Blackwell B, Marley E, Price J, Taylor D 1967 Hypertensive interaction between MAOI and foodstuffs. British Journal of Psychiatry 113: 349–365

Blier P, De Montigny C, Chaput Y 1990 A role for the serotonergic system in the mechanism of action of antidepressant treatments: preclinical evidence. Journal of Clinical Psychiatry 51 (4): 14–20

Bloch R G, Dooneief A S, Buchberg A S, Spellman S 1954 The clinical effects of isoniazid and iproniazid in the treatment of pulmonary tuberculosis. Annals of Internal Medicine 40: 881–900

Boulton A A, Cookson B, Paulton R 1970 Hypertensive crises in a patient on MAOI antidepressants following a meal of beef liver. Canadian Medical Association Journal 102: 1394–1395

Bruder G, Quitkin F M, Stewart J M et al 1990 Cerebral laterality and depression: differences in perceptual asymmetry among diagnostic subtypes. Journal of Abnormal Psychiatry (in press)

Bucci L 1987 The negative symptoms of schizophrenia and the monoamine oxidase inhibitors. Psychopharmacology 91: 104–108

Comfort A 1981 Hypertensive reaction of New Zealand prickly spinach in a woman taking phenelzine. Lancet 2: 472

Comfort A 1982 Phenelzine therapy: the doctor, the patient and the wine and cheese party. Journal of Operational Psychiatry 13: 37–40

Cooper A J 1967 MAO inhibitors and headache. British Medical Journal 2: 426

Cooper A J, Magnus R V, Rose M J 1964 Hypertensive syndrome with tranylcypromine medication. Lancet 1: 527–529

Crane G 1958 Psychiatric side effects of iproniazid. American Journal of Psychiatry 112: 494

Dally P J, Connelly J 1981 An introduction to physical methods of treatment in psychiatry. Churchill Livingstone, New York, p 24

Davidson J R T, Pelton S 1988 A comparative evaluation of three discriminant scales for endogenous depression. Psychiatry Research 23: 193–200

Davidson J R T, Turnbull C D 1986 The effects of isocarboxazid on blood pressure and pulse. Journal of Clinical Psychopharmacology 6: 139–143

Davidson J R T, McLeod M N, White H L, Kurland A A 1977 A preliminary report on antidepressant drug therapy in psychotic depression. British Journal of Psychiatry 131: 493–496

Davidson J R T, McLeod M N, Lawyone B, Linnoila M 1978a A comparative study of phenelzine-amitriptyline and ECT in refractory depression. Archives of General Psychiatry 35: 639–644

Davidson J R T, McLeod M N, White H L 1978b Inhibition of platelet MAO activity in depressed subjects treated with phenelzine. American Journal of Psychiatry 135: 470–472

Davidson J R T, Miller R D, Turnbull C D, Sullivan J 1982a Atypical depression. Archives of General Psychiatry 45: 120–127

Davidson J R T, Turnbull C D, Miller R D, Dougherty G, Wingfield M 1982b Failure of isocarboxazid to alleviate delusional depression in a pilot study. Journal of Clinical Psychopharmacology 2: 408–411

Davidson J R T, Miller R D, Turnbull C D, Belyea M, Strickland R 1984a A two dose evaluation of isocarboxazid in depression. Journal of Affective Disorders 6: 201–207

Davidson J R T, Zung W W K, Walker J I 1984b Practical aspects of MAO inhibitor therapy. Journal of Clinical Psychiatry 45: 7(2): 81–84

Davidson J R T, Pelton S, Miller R D, Lipper S L 1986 Endogenous depression and the response to isocarboxazid. Clinical Neuropharmacology 9(4): 563–565

Davidson J R T, Walker J I, Kilts C D 1987 A pilot study of phenelzine in post traumatic stress disorder. British Journal of Psychiatry 150: 252–255

Davidson J R T, Giller E L Jr, Zisook S, Overall J E 1988a An efficacy study of isocarboxazid and placebo in depression, and its relationship to depressive nosology. Archives of General Psychiatry 45: 120–127

Davidson J R T, Woodbury M A, Pelton S, Krishnan K R R 1988b A study of depressive typologies using grade of membership analysis. Psychological Medicine 18: 179–189

Davidson J R T, Lipper S L, Pelton S et al 1988c The response of depressed inpatients to isocarboxazid. Journal of Clinical Psychopharmacology 8: 100–108

Davidson J R T, Woodbury M A, Zisook S, Giller E L Jr 1989 Classification of depression by grade of membership: a confirmation study. Psychological Medicine 19: 987–998

Draper R, Sandler M, Walker P L 1984 Clinical curio: Monoamine oxidase inhibitors and non-alcoholic beer. British Medical Journal 189: 308

Elsworth J D, Glover V, Reynolds G P et al 1978 Deprenyl administration in man: a selective monoamine oxidase inhibitor without the cheese effect? Psychopharmacology 57: 33–38

Escobar J I, Schiele B C, Zimmerman R 1974 The tranylcypromine isomers: a controlled clinical trial. American Journal of Psychiatry 131: 1025–1026

Evans D L, Davidson J R T, Raft D 1982 Early and late side-effects of phenelzine. Journal of Clinical Psychopharmacology 2: 208–210

Faraj B A, Carrana R A, Ali F M et al 1981 Studies of the effect of antidepressants on kinetics and metabolism of tyramine. Journal of Pharmacology Exceptional Therapy 218: 750–757

Folks D G 1983 Monoamine oxidase inhibitors: reappraisal of dietary considerations. Journal of Clinical Psychopharmacology 4: 249–253

Frank J B, Giller E L Jr, Kosten T, Dan E 1988 A randomized clinical trial of phenelzine and imipramine for post traumatic stress disorder. American Journal of Psychiatry 145: 1289–1291

Freedman D F, Kaplan H I, Sadock B J 1973 ECT mortality. In Comprehensive textbook of psychiatry, 2nd edn. Williams & Wilkins, Baltimore, MD

Friedman S, Kantor I, Sobel S, Miller R 1978 A follow-up study on the chemotherapy of neurodermatitis with a monoamine oxidase inhibitor. Journal of Nervous and Mental Disease 166: 349–357

Gelenberg A J 1988 Aphthous ulcers and antidepressants. Biological Therapies in Psychiatry 11: 37

Generali J A, Hogan L C, McFarlane M et al 1981 Hypertensive crisis resulting from avocado and a MAO inhibitor. Drug Intelligence and Clinical Pharmacology 15: 904–906

Golbe L I, Lieberman A N, Muenter M D et al 1988 Deprenyl in the treatment of symptom fluctuations in advanced Parkinson's disease. Clinical Neuropharmacology 111: 45–55

Greenblatt M, Grosser G H, Wechsler H 1964 Differential response of hospitalized depressed patients to somatic therapy. American Journal of Psychiatry 120: 935–943

Hanger R L, Scheinin M, Siever L J et al 1988 Dissociation of norepinephrine turnover from alpha$_2$ response after clorgyline. Clinical Pharmacology and Therapeutics 43: 32–38

Hare M 1928 Tyramine oxidase. I. A new enzyme system in the liver. Biochemistry Journal 22: 968–979

Harrison W, Cooper T B, Stewart J W et al 1984 The tyramine challenge test as a trait marker for melancholia. Archives of General Psychiatry 41: 681–685

Hedberg D L, Gordon M W, Glueck B C 1966 Six cases of hypertensive crisis in patients on tranylcypromine after eating chicken livers. American Journal of Psychiatry 122: 933–937

Horwitz D 1964 MAO inhibitors, tyramine and cheese. Journal of the American Medical Association 188: 1108–1110

Insel T R, Murphy D L, Cohen R M, Alterman I, Kilts C D, Linnoila M 1983 Obsessive-compulsive disorder: a double-blind trial of clomipramine and clorgyline. Archives of General Psychiatry 40: 605–612

Kelly D, Guirgius W, Frommer E, Michell-Heggs N, Sargant W 1970 Treatment of phobic states with antidepressants. British Journal of Psychiatry 116: 387–398

Kelly D, Mitchell-Heggs N, Sherman D 1971 Anxiety and the effects of sodium lactate assessed clinically and physiologically. British Journal of Psychiatry 119: 129–141

Kennedy S H, Warsh J J, Mainprize E et al 1988 A trial of isocarboxazid in the treatment of bulimia. Journal of Clinical Psychopharmacology 8: 391–396

Kiloh L G, Child J P, Latner G 1959 A controlled trial of iproniazid in the treatment of endogenous depression. Journal of Mental Science 106: 1139–1144

Klein D F, Gittleman R, Quitkin F, Rifkin A 1981 In diagnosis and drug treatment of psychiatric disorders. Williams & Wilkins. Baltimore, MD, p 464

Lader M H, Sakalis G, Tansella M 1970 Interactions between sympathomimetic amines and a new monoamine oxidase inhibitor. Psychopharmacology 18: 118–123

Lascelles R G 1966 Atypical facial pain and depression. British Journal of Psychiatry 112: 651–659

Laurence D R 1966 Clinical pharmacology. Churchill, London, p 309

Lee W C, Shin Y H, Shideman F E 1961 Cardiac effects of several monoamine oxidase inhibitors. Journal of Pharmacology and Experimental Therapeutics 133; 180–185

Lee K Y, Beilin J L, van Dongen R 1979 Severe hypertension after ingestion of an appetite suppressant (phenylopropanolamine) with indomethacin. Lancet 1: 1110–1111

Lerer B, Bleich A, Kotler M, Garb R, Herzberg M, Levin B 1987 Post traumatic stress disorder in Israeli combat veterans. Archives of General Psychiatry 44: 976–981

Lieb J 1983 Remission of rheumatoid arthritis and other disorders of immunity in patients taking monoamine oxidase inhibitors. International Journal of Immunopharmacology 5: 353–357

Liebowitz M R, Quitkin F M, Stewart J W et al 1984 Phenelzine v. imipramine in atypical depression. Archives of General Psychiatry 41: 669–677

Liebowitz M R, Campeas R, Hollander E 1987 MAOIs: impact on social behaviour. Psychiatry Research 22: 89–90

Liebowitz M R, Gorman J M, Fyer A J et al 1988 Pharmacotherapy of social phobia: an interim report of a placebo-controlled comparison of phenelzine and atenolol. Journal of Clinical Psychiatry 49: 252–257

Lipper S L, Murphy D L, Slater S, Buchsbaum M S 1979 Comparative behavioural effects of clorgyline and pargyline in man: a preliminary evaluation. Psychopharmacology 62: 123–128

Lipsedge M S, Hajioff J, Huggins P et al 1973 The management of severe agoraphobia: a comparison of iproniazid and systematic desensitization. Psychopharmacologia (Berlin) 32: 67–80

McCabe B, Tsuang M T 1982 Dietary consideration in MAO inhibitor regimens. Journal of Clinical Psychiatry 43: 181–184

McGrath P J, Stewart J W, Harrison W, Wager S, Quitkin F M 1986 Phenelzine treatment of melancholia. Journal of Clinical Psychiatry 47: 420–422

McGrath R J, Quitkin F M, Harrison W, Stewart J W 1987 Treatment of melancholia with tranylcypromine. American Journal of Psychiatry 141: 288–289

Mann J J, Aarons S F, Wilner P J et al 1989 Controlled study of antidepressant efficacy and side-effects of (−)-deprenyl: selective monoamine oxidase inhibitor 46: 45–50

Marley E, Blackwell B 1970 Interactions of monoamine oxidase inhibitors, amines and foodstuffs. In: Garattini S (ed) Advances in pharmacology and chemotherapy. Academic Press, New York, p 185–239

Maxwell M 1980 Reexamining the dietary restrictions with procrabazine (an MAOI). Cancer Nursing 12: 451–457

Medical Research Council 1965 Clinical trial of the treatment of depressive illness. British Medical Journal 1: 881–886

Mountjoy C Q, Roth M, Garside R F, Leitch I M 1977 A clinical trial of phenelzine in anxiety, depressive and phobic neuroses. British Journal of Psychiatry 131: 486–492

Murphy D L, Garrick N, Aulakh C S, Cohen R M 1984 New contributions from basic science to understanding the effects of monoamine oxidase inhibiting antidepressants. Journal of Clinical Psychiatry 45: 37–43

Neil J F, Licata S M, May S J, Himmelhoch J M 1979 Dietary noncompliance during treatment with tranylcypromine. Journal of Clinical Psychiatry 40: 33–37

Nies A 1984 Differential response patterns to MAO inhibitors and tricyclics. Journal of Clinical Psychiatry 7(sec 2): 70–77

Nutt D, Glue P 1989 Monoamine oxidase inhibitors: rehabilitation from recent research? British Journal of Psychiatry 154: 287–291

Pare C M B 1968 Recent advances in the treatment of depression. In: Coppen A, Walk A (eds) Recent developments in affective disorders. (Royal Medico-Psychological Association) Headley Brothers, Ashford, Kent, p 140–141

Pare C M B, Mendis N, Sandler M, Glover V, Stern G M 1981 Failure of the selective monoamine oxidase B. inhibitor, (−)-deprenyl to alleviate depression: relationship to tyramine insensitivity. In: Youdim M B H, Paykel E S (eds) Monoamine oxidase inhibitors – the state of the art. John Wiley, New York, p 171–176

Pare C M B, Kline N, Hallstrom C, Cooper T B 1982 Will amitriptyline prevent the 'cheese' reaction of monoamine oxidase inhibitors? Lancet 2: 183–186

Pare C M B, A L Mousaevi M, Sandler M, Glover V 1985 Attempts to attenuate the 'cheese' effect. Combined drug therapy in depressive illness. Journal of Affective Disorders 9: 137–141

Paykel E S, Rowan P R R, Parker R R, Bhat A V 1982 Response to phenelzine and amitriptyline in subtypes of outpatient depression. Archives of General Psychiatry 39: 1041–1049

Paykel E S, Rowan P R R, Rao B, Bhat A V 1983 Atypical depression: Nosology and response to antidepressants. In: Clayton P, Barrett J (eds) Treatment of depression: old controversies and new approaches. Raven Press, New York, p 237–251

Priest R G 1989 Editor's preface: antidepressants of the future. British Journal of Psychiatry 155 (6): 7–8

Rabkin J, Quitkin F M, Harrison W, Tricano E, McGrath R J 1984 Adverse reactions to monoamine oxidase inhibitors. Part 1: A comparative study. Journal of Clinical Psychopharmacology 4: 270–278

Rabkin J, Stewart J W, Quitkin F M, McGrath P J, Harrison W M, Klein D F 1990 Should atypical depression be included as a separate entity in DSM-IV? A review of the research evidence. Unpublished report

Raft D, Davidson J R T, Mattox A, Mueller R, Wasik J 1979 A double-blind evaluation of phenelzine, amitriptyline and placebo in depression associated with pain. In: Singer T, van Korff R, Murphy D L (eds) Monoamine oxidase: structure, function and altered functions. Academic Press, New York, p 507–516

Ravaris C L, Nies A, Robinson D S, Ives J O, Lamborn K R, Karson C 1976 A multiple-dose controlled study of phenelzine in depressive-anxiety states. Archives of General Psychiatry 33: 347–350

Razani J, White K, White J et al 1983 The safety and efficacy of combined amitriptyline and tranylcypromine treatment. Archives of General Psychiatry 40: 657–661

Robinson D S, Nies A, Ravaris C L, Lamborn K R 1973 The monoamine oxidase inhibitor, phenelzine, in the treatment of depressive-anxiety states. Archives of General Psychiatry 29: 407–413

Robinson D S, Nies A, Ravaris C L, Lamborn K R 1978 Clinical psychopharmacology of phenelzine: MAO activity and clinical response. In Lipton M A, DiMascio A, Killam K F (eds) Psychopharmacology: a generation of progress. Raven Press, New York

Rosenthal S H, Fitch W P 1987 The anti-herpetic effect of phenelzine. Journal of Clinical Psychopharmacology 7: 119

Sandler M 1981 Deprenyl, monoamine oxidase inhibition and the cheese effect: some outstanding problems. In: Youdim M G H, Paykel E S (eds) Monoamine oxidase inhibitors – the state of the art. John Wiley, New York, p 207–212

Sargant W W 1975 Interactions with monoamine oxidase inhibitors. British Medical Journal 2:

Sen N P 1969 Analysis and significance of tyramine in foods. Journal of Food and Science 34: 22

Sheehan D V, Ballenger J, Jacobsen G 1980 Treatment of endogenous anxiety with phobic, hysterical and hypochondriacal symptoms. Archives of General Psychiatry 37: 51–59

Shestatsky M, Greenberg D, Lerer B 1988 A controlled trial of phenelzine in post traumatic stress disorder. Psychiatry Research 24: 149–155

Simpson G, White K 1984 Tyramine studies and the safety of MAOI drugs. Journal of Clinical Psychiatry 7(2): 59–61

Sjoqvist F 1965 Psychotropic drugs. II. Interactions between monoamine oxidase (MAO) inhibitors and other substances. Proceedings of Royal Society of Medicine 58: 967–969

Smith C K, Durack D T 1978 Isoniazid and reaction to cheese. Annals of Internal Medicine 91: 793

Stewart M M 1976 MAOIs and food – fact and fiction. Adverse Drug Reaction Bulletin 58: 200–203

Sullivan E A, Shulman K I 1984 Diet and monoamine oxidase inhibitors: a reexamination. Canadian Journal of Psychiatry 29: 707–711

Tariot P N, Cohen R M, Sunderland T et al 1987 L-deprenyl in Alzheimer's disease. Archives of General Psychiatry 44: 427–433

Tyrer P J 1982 Monoamine oxidase inhibitors and amine precursors. In: Tyrer P J (ed) Drugs in psychiatric practice. Butterworths, London, p 249–279

Tyrer P J, Candy J, Kelly D 1973 A study of the clinical effects of phenelzine and placebo in the treatment of phobic anxiety. Psychopharmacologia 32: 237–254

Vallejo J, Casto C T, Catalan R, Salamero M 1987 Imipramine vs phenelzine in melancholias and dysthymic disorders. British Journal of Psychiatry 151: 639–642

Versiani M M F D, Nardi A E, Liebowitz M R 1988 Tranylcypromine in social phobia. Journal of Clinical Psychopharmacology 8: 279–283

Versiani M M F D, Oggero U, Alterwain P et al 1989 A double-blind comparative trial of moclobemide vs imipramine and placebo in major depressive episodes. British Journal of Psychiatry 155(6): 72–77

Versiani M M F D, Nardi A E, Mindim F D 1990 Pharmacotherapy of social phobia (unpublished)

Walker J I, Davidson J R T, Zung W W K 1984 Patient compliance with MAO inhibitor therapy. Journal of Clinical Psychiatry 45: 7(2): 78–80

Walsh J I, Stewart J W, Roose S P et al 1984 Treatment of bulimia with phenelzine: a double-blind placebo-controlled study. Archives of General Psychiatry 41: 1105–1109

West E D, Dally P J 1959 Effects of iproniazid on depressive syndromes. British Medical Journal 1: 1491–1494

Wright S P 1978 Hazards with monoamine oxidase inhibitors: a persistent problem. Lancet 1: 284–285

Zametkin A, Rapoport J L, Murphy D L et al 1985 Treatment of hyperactive children with monoamine oxidase inhibitors. Archives of General Psychiatry 42: 962–977

Zeller E A 1938 Uber den enzymatischen Abbau von Histamin und Diaminen. Helvetica Chimica Acta 21: 881–890

Zisook S 1984 Side effects of isocarboxazid. Journal Clinical Psychiatry 45(2): 53–58

22. Electroconvulsive therapy

Max Fink

We have witnessed a remarkable resurgence of interest in convulsive therapy in the past decade. The frequent failure of modern drug therapies, their neurotoxicity and cardiotoxicity, their intolerance by the elderly, and patient preference have led to its greater use, now well into the sixth decade since its discovery. Convulsive therapy was introduced in 1934 for the treatment of dementia praecox by the Hungarian neuropsychiatrist Ladislas Meduna (1935). The change from camphor and pentylenetetrazol to electrical inductions, demonstrated by Ugo Cerletti and his co-workers in Rome in 1938, made seizure induction relatively easy. The introduction of succinylcholine in 1953 encouraged the use of anaesthesia, enhancing the safety of the treatment. Continuous oxygenation, unilateral electrode placement and brief pulse currents, which reduced both the cognitive effects of the treatment and patients' fear, also encouraged greater use of electroconvulsive therapy (ECT).

Renewed interest in ECT has been accompanied by much social and political argument. The first convulsive treatments were done without anaesthesia, and for many patients they were experienced with fear and pain. Attitudes to consent in medical treatment were still primitive, and patients were often treated against their will and without their formal consent. In the United States, the war in Vietnam led to a backlash against authority and spawned an antipsychiatry movement. The re-introduction of ECT in the 1970s became a ready target, epitomized in the 1975 film *One Flew Over The Cuckoo's Nest*, in which a hapless patient is forcibly treated by threatening and unfeeling staff. In some venues, as in the State of California, legislative action prohibited the use of ECT, an action which was enjoined by the courts.

The anti-psychiatry movement forced the profession, notably the American Psychiatric Association (APA) and the National Institutes of Health (NIH) in the United States and the Royal College of Psychiatrists (RCPsych) in Great Britain, to undertake assessments of the treatment and to seek guidelines and standards for practitioners. Reports by the APA (1978, 1990), Royal College (Pippard & Ellam 1981, RCPsych 1989) and the NIH (Consensus Conference 1985) defined indications for the treatment, described practices which enhanced its safety and efficacy and established models for informed consent. The 1989 RCPsych and the 1990 APA reports were independently produced, yet they are almost identical in their concerns. These reports provide standards of care for ECT in these nations, and it is their main recommendations that are summarized in this review. To avoid an extensive citation list, specific references may be found in APA (1990), RCPsych (1989), Abrams (1988); for older citations, see APA (1978), Fink (1979), Pippard & Ellam (1981) and Kalinowsky et al (1982). For the treatment of high-risk patients the issue of *Convulsive Therapy* edited by Abrams (1989), and for theoretical discussions the issue of *Convulsive Therapy* edited by Sackeim (1989) are useful.

INDICATIONS FOR USE

Convulsive therapy is ordinarily reserved for patients so ill as to require hospitalization. The routine use of brief general anaesthesia makes ECT akin to surgery and thereby reserves it for those who require a major intervention. Present philosophy gives priority to trials with medications, despite indications of greater efficacy and safety for convulsive therapy for many conditions. The view that ECT is a 'last resort' therapy is encoded in many texts and in much clinical teaching. A feature of the 1990 APA report was the recommendation, more in keeping with British practice, that ECT may be considered a *primary treatment* for certain conditions:

Situations where ECT may be used prior to a trial of psychotropic agents include, but are not necessarily limited to, the following:

a) where a need for rapid, definitive response exists on either medical or psychiatric grounds; or
b) when the risks of other treatments outweigh the risks of ECT; or
c) when a history of poor drug response and/or good ECT response exists for previous episodes of the illness; or
d) patient preference. (APA 1990)

Examples of the primary use of ECT are where patients are so suicidal as to compel continuous observation; for patients in manic delirium, catatonic stupor or catatonic excitement, especially when these conditions are dangerous to the patient or to others and when they require continuous observation, restraints, isolation or parenteral feeding; where inanition is becoming so severe as to be life-threatening. Some psychiatrists prefer ECT as a primary treatment in patients with delusional or severely retarded depression, in first-episode acute schizophrenia in young adults, and in rapid-cycling manic patients in the awareness that psychoactive drugs are often less effective than ECT.

In the main, ECT is used in patients who have failed other treatments or in whom adverse effects preclude the continued use of standard drug treatments, especially for patients with depressive, manic, schizophrenic and schizoaffective disorders (APA 1978, 1990, Fink 1979, Pippard & Ellam 1981, RCPsych 1989).

Depressive disorders

Convulsive therapy is an effective antidepressant treatment, relieving the mood disorder of affectively ill patients, regardless of subtype. It is equally effective in those with unipolar or bipolar histories, especially when accompanied by psychosis. It is effective in patients with melancholia.

Some recent decriptions find ECT useful in the apparent dementias which may accompany severe cases of depressive illness, dementias which have been labelled 'pseudodementia' or 'reversible dementia' – the latter because of the response to effective treatment (Fink 1989a).

When depression is accompanied by psychosis, especially delusions of guilt, somatic concern or infidelity, it responds well to convulsive therapy. These signs are poor prognostic signs for treatment with antidepressant drugs. Depression with marked psychomotor retardation and depressive stupor also respond well.

Not all depressed patients are good candidates for ECT. Those with dysthymia (previously called neurotic depression) do not respond well; neither their depressive symptoms nor the accompanying symptoms of anxiety, hypochondria or hysteria improve. Much of the travail of electrotherapists and many of the ex-patients who are paraded by anti-psychiatrists as having been harmed by ECT are those whose conditions were mistakenly considered a primary depressive disorder but whose core illness was life-long dysthymia, persistent hypochondria, or somatization disorder (Fink 1979).

Patients with character disorders, or with drug dependence, in whom depressive symptoms may be situational and secondary to their social difficulties, are also poor candidates for convulsive therapy, often complaining more bitterly of their symptoms than before treatment.

Manic disorders

Patients with manic disorders respond well to ECT. In the anecdotal case material of the first few decades of its use, improvement among manic patients was consistently reported and often seen as dramatic and life-saving. With the introduction of lithium and antipsychotic drugs, such use was abandoned. In the past decade, however, descriptions of therapy-resistant manic patients, and of 'rapid-cyclers', have led to a re-assessment of ECT.

Schizophrenia

Convulsive therapy is effective in the treatment of acute schizophrenia, especially those conditions with acute onset and durations of less than 2 years. ECT is clearly effective in those with schizoaffective syndromes and those with catatonia. Combined with antipsychotic drugs, it is also effective in patients with positive symptoms who have failed drug therapies alone.

Other conditions

ECT is also effective in psychotic patients during pregnancy, with neuroleptic malignant syndrome, catatonia secondary to medical disorders, and Parkinson's disease (particularly those with the 'on-off' therapy phenomenon) (Fink 1988).

Among pregnant women with severe psychiatric illnesses, such as melancholia or mania, the risks of teratogenicity in the fetus preclude the general use of psychoactive drugs. This is especially true for the use of lithium and benzodiazepines, where the evidence of teratogenicity is considerable. The anaesthesia of the treatment is short and seems not to affect the developing fetus.

The neuroleptic malignant syndrome is a condition similar to 'malignant catatonia'. While withdrawal of neuroleptics and treatment with dantrolene and bromocriptine are most often recommended, ECT has been found to be effective. Similarly, the severe catatonia found among patients with lupus erythematosus and infectious diseases is responsive to courses of ECT (Fink 1990a).

Repeated seizures elicit a rise in seizure threshold, which may be useful in aborting status epilepticus. There is also a reduction in symptoms of Parkinson's disease, even among patients without clear evidence of severe depression.

CONTRAINDICATIONS

There are no 'absolute' physical or medical contraindications to the use of convulsive therapy in patients with conditions where there is a likelihood for clinical benefit. There are conditions of substantial risk, however, requiring special attention and skills (APA 1990). When treatment of a psychiatric condition is sufficiently compelling, as when patients are suicidal, debilitated or starving, contraindications may be set aside and convulsive therapy considered a prudent intervention. Such conditions include patients with recent myocardial infarction, cerebrovascular accident, cerebral vascular malformation or intracranial mass lesion, whose psychosis is so severe as to interfere with recovery from their medical illness. Patients with serious medical conditions are considered *high-risk* cases, requiring special expertise on the part of therapists. The prudent physician will not treat patients with these conditions with a therapy of any risk, unless the need is compelling. But when compelled, as when convulsive therapy is a safer alternative, treatments have been given. At such times, the skill of the psychiatrist and that of the anaesthetist determine the outcome (Abrams 1989, APA 1990).

RISKS

The main risks of convulsive therapy in its first decades were fracture, death, fear, tardive seizures and impairment of memory and cognition. Except for the effects on cognition, these concerns have been dissipated by barbiturate anaesthesia and suxamethonium relaxation, continuous oxygenation, changes in current type and dose and electrode placement and treatment by well-trained physicians (Fink 1979). Impairment of memory remains the main concern of patients and their families. Impairment is usually confined to the time of the illness and the events associated with the treatments, but there are some patients who describe a loss of memory of events earlier than the time of the illness.

Cognitive impairment results, in part, from the type and amount of electrical energy and the path of the electric currents used. Modern ECT devices with brief-pulse currents have lesser effects on cognition than the sinusoidal currents used in earlier decades. Seizures may be induced either through electrodes which are placed bilaterally (B/ECT) or on one side of the head (U/ECT). When electrodes are applied to the non-dominant hemisphere, the effects on cognition are less pronounced. But efficacy may be impaired. The 1989 RCPsych report argues: 'We believe that recent studies comparing B/ECT with U/ECT demonstrate that B/ECT is a more powerful antidepressant treatment, and that B/ECT shall be the treatment of choice... especially where speed of action is important.' The APA report remains ambivalent, and offers no specific guideline. My own preference is to follow the RCPsych suggestion, and to reserve the use of U/ECT for those patients in whom cognitive deficits are a concern in consent (Fink 1990b).

CONSENT

The stigma of 'shock therapy' is also a risk of treatment for patients, their families and their therapists. Convulsive therapy is controversial, and patients and their families may be confused as to why it is recommended (Consensus Conference 1985). Information about risks and the reasons for recommending ECT is central to a good outcome and good management. We no longer accept a patient's signature on a single-sentence consent to treatment as 'informed'. Both the APA and RCPsych guidelines encourage a full disclosure of risks and benefits before ECT. For those patients who are so ill as not to be able to make an intelligent judgment, consent from surrogates is generally provided in local law.

Our own practice is to give each patient and close family member a detailed explanation of the treatment

– what it entails, its risks and benefits and our understanding of its mechanism of action. This information is provided in a detailed consent form, which is discussed by a member of the treatment team (Fink 1979, APA 1978, 1990). This discussion is accompanied by the viewing of a videotape describing the benefits and risks of the treatment and demonstrations of actual treatments (Somatics 1986b). The videotape, produced in our own facility, has been very useful not only in assuring 'informed' consent, but in meeting institutional legal and ethical concerns.

MEDICAL EXAMINATIONS

When the decision to treat is made and consent is obtained, the medical history and physical examination are reviewed. Many patients referred for convulsive therapy need continuing treatment for hypertension, cardiac arrhythmia, diabetes, pulmonary disease and arthritis, conditions which increase anaesthetic risk. Therapies should be optimized and consultation with the patient's physician is useful.

There are no specific laboratory tests required before treatment. A pretreatment electrocardiogram is requested in patients with a history of cardiovascular disease or in those over the age of 40 years. Blood and urine tests are done to assure normal metabolic functions. Spine X-rays are no longer routinely obtained. In patients who have had prior courses of convulsive therapy, or in whom a disorder of the spine is suggested by the medical history, we obtain dorsal spine X-rays. (If they are done prior to treatment, we usually repeat X-rays after the course of therapy). Electroencephalogram, computed tomography scan and neuropsychological assessment are not routine examinations and serve no useful purpose in planning a course of convulsive therapy; these should be requested when the patient's history or examination raises questions for which the procedure may be helpful.

A dental examination is recommended, particularly in older patients, to determine the condition of the teeth or dentures. If the patient's psychiatric condition permits, repairs should be made and loose teeth should be secured before convulsive therapy is given.

The anaesthetist should meet the patient, review the medical record and discuss his procedures prior to the first treatment.

For a few years, there was a wave of enthusiasm that the dexamethasone suppression test would be a useful guide to treatment, but recent findings have not been reassuring. Interest in the test as applied to convulsive therapy has waned.

In some US institutions, medical 'clearance' for treatment is requested of external consultants. It is unclear what is expected. The decision to administer convulsive therapy is the responsibility of the attending psychiatrist, who must make the decision based on the severity of the patient's illness, treatment history, and risk—benefit analysis of the available psychiatric therapies. In requesting consultation we seek a better understanding and an optimization of the patient's medical condition, especially treatment for associated medical conditions. To ask for 'clearance for treatment', as if medical consultants have a special knowledge to judge the safety of a procedure as complex as convulsive therapy, is to ask for more than most consultants can answer. Such practice should not be condoned.

DRUG INTERACTIONS

Benzodiazepines or barbiturates given for night-time sedation raise seizure thresholds, making induction of seizures more difficult, especially in the elderly. The quality of the treatment may also be reduced, needlessly extending the course of therapy. Benzodiazepines should be discontinued before treatment.

Some antiarrhythmics, notably lidocaine, raise seizure thresholds and substitutes such as propranolol should be considered. Theophylline may increase the duration of seizures and lead to the development of prolonged seizures, especially when administered at high levels. Patients with glaucoma may continue their medications, unless they are receiving echothiopate, which should be discontinued. Diabetic patients should continue their medications, although dosages may be modified on treatment days. In patients with epilepsy, some authors decrease antiepileptic medications, especially phenytoin and phenobarbitone. This is not necessary, although the electrotherapist should be aware that seizure thresholds may be elevated and special manoeuvres may be necessary to ensure an adequate seizure.

It is difficult to decide whether or not to continue psychotropic drugs during ECT. For tricyclic antidepressant (TCA) drugs and monoamine oxidase inhibitors (MAOIs), there is little evidence of synergistic action with ECT. As cardiovascular risks may be increased by TCAs, especially in elderly patients, combined use is not usually recommended and TCAs are rapidly tapered off during treatment. Concerns have been expressed that a recent intake of MAOIs may increase the risks of hypertension during convulsive therapy, and some authors recommend that treatment be deferred until MAOI use has been suspended for 2 weeks. None of the recent reporters found evidence to support this practice, and such delay is not necessary.

Lithium administration may increase the risks of an organic mental syndrome and prolonged apnoea, and most therapists reduce dosages rapidly when convulsive therapy is being considered. The justification for such advice has been questioned, and combined therapy need not be fully proscribed.

There is some evidence of synergism in the combination of neuroleptic drugs with convulsive therapy, particularly in the treatment of manic and schizophrenic patients. These medications are usually continued during ECT. Reports of cardiovascular complications and death when reserpine was used with convulsive therapy suggest that such combined use is hazardous, but this injunction is limited to reserpine and is not generalized to other neuroleptic drugs. There is little information as to the safety of the concurrent use of anticholinergic drugs, so that most therapists use these substances only when clearly necessary.

TREATMENT PROCEDURES

Convulsive therapy is usually given with barbiturate-suxamethonium anaesthesia. An intravenous infusion line is established with dextrose in water or normal saline, and physiological monitors are put in place: blood pressure by cuff; ECG by three leads; frontal EEG; and oximetry (these procedures are not usually used outside the USA). For electric stimulation, the skin over the two stimulation sites is cleansed by a fat solvent and electrodes are applied using electrode-conducting jelly. The impedance of the circuit is checked and the contact of the electrodes is adjusted to an impedance within the specification of the instrument manufacturer.

For bilateral electrode placement, the electrodes are placed on both temples. For unilateral electrode placement, one electrode is placed on a temple, about midway between the outer canthus of the eye and the meatus of the ear. Many locations for the second electrode over the homolateral scalp have been proposed. As there is little therapeutic advantage for one locus over another, the second electrode is usually placed as far back on the scalp as is possible, near the middle (d'Elia location), as it induces a seizure with lower electrical dosage.

Some authors recommend the administration of intravenous atropine (0.6–1.2 mg) or glycopyrrolate (0.1–4 mg) to reduce the vagal effects of a seizure, especially in patients with cardiovascular disorders. Results in studies of such practice are ambiguous and their use is optional.

When an airway is assured, intravenous methohexitone (0.5–1.0 mg/kg) is given as a bolus. A blood pressure cuff on an extremity may be inflated to above the systolic pressure and intravenous suxamethonium (0.5–1.5 mg/kg) is given. The degree of motor paralysis is tested by the knee jerk, foot withdrawal to stroking the sole of the foot, or response to a nerve stimulator. Oxygenation is maintained throughout. When motor reactions are obtunded, a mouthguard is inserted and the treatment is given.

A concern in the treatment is the immediate effect of the seizure on blood pressure and heart rate. Both hypertension and hypotension occur, as do transient heart block and irregular heart rhythms. These effects ordinarily require no intervention, as they spontaneously normalize by the end of the seizure. For patients with established hypertension, however, intervention may be warranted. One may dissolve one or two nitroglycerine tablets (0.3–0.6 mg) under the tongue, 2–4 minutes prior to treatment. If hypertension is severe, or blood pressure control critical, the rapid-acting ganglionic blocking agent trimethaphan camsylate drip is used (Maneksha 1991).

For patients with a history of malignant hyperthermia, or those who develop fever with treatment, suxamethonium may be replaced by curare (3–6 mg/kg) or atracurium (0.5 mg/kg).

Seizure induction

A bilateral grand mal seizure with a minimum duration of 25 seconds in motor duration is the hallmark of an effective induction. Subconvulsive or sham treatments are less effective. While both sinusoidal and brief pulse currents were in use in the past decade, both the RCPsych and the APA now recommend the routine use of brief-pulse currents.

Present practice uses induction energies substantially above threshold, but not so high as to be associated with increased cognitive deficits or prolonged seizures. We use the cuff-monitored seizure duration as a guide. When seizure durations are between 25 and 30 seconds, we generally increase the dosage of the stimulation for the next treatment by 10%; when seizure duration is longer than 90 seconds, we reduce the dosage by about 10% for the next treatment.

Adequate treatment

An adequate treatment is conventionally defined as a convulsion with a duration greater than 25 seconds with cuff monitoring, with bilateral cerebral generalization as evinced by bilateral tonic and clonic components, and perhaps with a postseizure EEG electrical silence, usually defined by an abrupt EEG seizure termination. An adequate seizure results from the interaction of patient's age, degree of anaesthesia, type and dosage of electrical current and electrode placement (Fink 1989b).

The energy needed to induce a fit increases with age and is generally higher in men than in women. Thresholds are higher for bilateral electrode placements than for unilateral and they rise during the course of therapy. It is necessary, therefore, for the therapist to monitor seizure duration for adequacy. From time to time, seizure durations remain short and seizures are considered inadequate despite changes in electrical dosage and electrode placement. In such instances, therapists first check the placement of the electrodes, assuring an adequate contact (low impedance) between electrodes and the patient. Dosages of barbiturate anaesthetic may be reduced, or etomidate may be used instead of methohexitone. Benzodiazepine sedation should be stopped. If seizure durations remain short, augmentation by an analeptic agent may be tried. An intravenous bolus of caffeine sodium benzoate (500–750 mg), 5–10 minutes before seizure induction, may be successful. Oral theophylline the night before may lower seizure thresholds for an adequate seizure (Swartz & Lewis 1991). If seizures are prolonged, e.g. persisting for longer than 180 seconds, the seizure is interrupted by intravenous methohexitone (30–50 mg) or diazepam (2.5–5.0 mg).

Postseizure monitoring

The recovery period is a time of risk for the patient, and observation is continued by personnel able to manage an impaired airway or a change in cardiovascular status. Monitoring of vigilance, respiration, heart rate and, where used, ECG continue through the postseizure recovery period, until the patient is returned to his room. A simple scale of orientation and tests of aphasia are useful during recovery, to determine whether the mental changes are prolonged or aphasia persists. In such instances, a change in electrode placement or frequency of treatment is considered.

Number and frequency of seizures

Both the number of treatments and their frequency are defined by clinical progress. From seven to nine treatments for patients with severe affective disorders and from 12 to 20 for patients with mania and therapy-resistant psychosis are generally sufficient. The end-point of a course is defined by relief of the patient's symptoms.

It is conventional in the United States to treat patients three times a week, while in Great Britain and Ireland the pattern is twice weekly. Preliminary reports of an ongoing random assignment trial find that three times weekly ECT is associated with a more rapid improvement and shorter hospitalization, although the treatments are equally effective with the same cognitive effects at the end of the therapy (Lerer et al 1990).

Affectively ill patients show improvement, usually in the relief of vegetative symptoms and mood, within four to five treatments. When such changes are not observed, unilateral electrode placement should be changed. In severely ill patients, particularly those with manic delirium, daily treatments are useful. In patients with a severe manic disorder, schizophrenia or schizoaffective disorder, the number of treatments is generally greater, with initial courses of 12–20 treatments common. Some authors describe multiple treatments in one session – up to six seizures with one anaesthesia, known as 'multiple monitored ECT' – as being more effective and reducing the period of incapacity. The evidence that such modifications are more effective and as safe as conventional ECT is not compelling, and such courses are no longer recommended.

Continuation therapy

Convulsive therapy is an effective therapy, but the persistence of its effects is often short and continuation therapy is usually necessary. In psychoactive drug treatments, therapy is generally continued for months. Indeed, despite such continuation many affectively ill patients relapse. In convulsive therapy, continuation with antidepressant drugs or lithium reduces relapse rates when compared with no continuation or with sedative drugs. But for patients who have failed adequate drug treatment trials, continuation with the same medications may be of limited use. When drug therapies are used, treatment is usually maintained at half the clinical therapeutic dose, usually 150 mg daily for TCAs.

Continuation therapy with weekly or biweekly ECT was a regular feature of early practice. But such practice fell into disuse and the data are not available to provide adequate guidelines. In patients who rapidly relapse after a course of therapy, some practitioners induce seizures at weekly and biweekly intervals, proceeding to monthly intervals. Recent retrospective reports find continuation ECT useful, and such use was endorsed by the 1990 APA report.

FACILITIES

Psychiatrists administering convulsive therapy should be qualified, by preceptorship and experience, to assume responsibility for this complex treatment, since there is no longer any room for an attitude that accepts the least-qualified intern or junior as competent to manage these procedures. It is a reflection of the inherent safety of ECT and the tolerance of our patients for seizures that more reports of adverse effects do not fill the medical and legal literature. There is no accreditation procedure for practice, so it is the responsibility of each medical centre to establish guidelines for the proficiency of physicians responsible for these treatments (APA 1990). In addition to the psychiatrist, a trained nurse and nursing assistant with experience in intensive care and resuscitation are usually required. The role of the nurse has been described by the Royal College of Nursing (1987).

The administration of anaesthesia, even for a procedure as brief as convulsive therapy, requires skill in airway management and in resuscitation after cardiac or respiratory failure. Anaesthetists and nurse-anaesthetists are usually qualified in these practices and, in institutions equipped to treat high-risk cases, their skills should be part of the treatment team. In some countries this approach is used for all cases.

ECT is best given in a suite, consisting of a treatment room and a recovery area, on the psychiatric treatment unit. The use of operating rooms, their recovery areas or intensive care units invariably inhibits its proper use. It is neither required by the procedure nor does it facilitate the proper treatment of patients. Such usage usually reflects the dogmatism of the anaesthetist or the hostility of an administration to proper psychiatric practice.

ECT devices have undergone many modifications and there is little justification for using equipment designed or built prior to 1982. ECT is a repeated treatment, so that records are helpful in optimizing the treatment of individual patients. Records should include anaesthetic doses and adjuvant drugs; seizure induction parameters (instrument, dose, time, electrode placement); seizure duration measurements; blood pressures and/or heart rates; and notes as to any untoward events. A duplicate record kept in the treatment room is helpful, to assist in treating patients re-admitted after relapse.

Some educational materials are useful: the Consensus Development Conference Statement (1985); the experiences of a patient described in the autobiography by Norman Endler titled *Holiday of Darkness* (1982); and reports by the APA Task Force (1978, 1990) and the Royal College of Psychiatrists (Pippard & Ellam 1981; RCPsych 1989). Books by Fink (1979), Palmer (1981), Fraser (1982), Abrams & Essman (1982), Taylor et al (1985) and Abrams (1988) should be part of the library. Instruction manuals and videotapes describing treatment practice accompany many new instruments. An educational videotape for health professionals and students is available (Somatics 1986a). Videotapes made especially for patients and their families provide useful resources for consent (Somatics 1986b, Grunhaus 1989). The quarterly journal *Convulsive Therapy* (Raven Press, New York) is a source of case and research material, especially about high-risk cases. Subscribers and authors may also avail themselves of a citation service and 'hotline' for consultation.

MECHANISM OF ANTIDEPRESSANT ACTION

The repeated induction of bilateral grand mal seizures, two to five times weekly, for seven to 12 seizures remains essential for the antidepressant effect of convulsive therapy. We search for biochemical changes in the brain that follow repeated seizures for explanations, but seizures involve massive electrical and biochemical changes in brain tissues, stimulation of the autonomic nervous system, release of substances from endocrine glands and, unless there is neuromuscular blockade, severe tonic and clonic movements of body muscles. These activities elicit so many changes in the body that there is no dearth of demonstrable effects. We are unable to differentiate those changes which may be necessary for a therapeutic effect and those which may be clearly secondary (Fink 1979).

Additional difficulties that beset psychiatric research also affect convulsive therapy research: diagnostic and symptomatic variability of patients selected for study, difficulties in such procedures as cerebrospinal fluid examinations and the cost of procedures that delay treatment. These limitations compel studies in animals, but such studies have been of little help in our understanding of the convulsive therapy process. What progress has been made has come from human research, precisely because the conditions under study, the affective and psychotic disorders, have no duplicate in animal species.

Indeed, suggestions from animal studies have not been replicated in man. Cerebrospinal fluid studies do not find relations between catecholamine metabolites and seizures, and studies of naloxone fail to find connections between opioid receptors and convulsive therapy. Perhaps the single compelling observation from animal studies that has been replicated in humans is the increase in dopaminergic activity in centrencephalic regions, which suggested that parkinsonism might be helped by repeated seizures.

Many theories have been proposed to explain the clinical efficacy of convulsive therapy. These are summarized in the proceedings of the 1985 meeting at the New York Academy of Sciences (Malitz & Sackeim 1986), and in a special issue of *Convulsive Therapy* edited by Sackeim (1989). The main theories focus on the same neurohumoral mechanisms that are used to explain the action of antidepressant drugs. In a widely quoted formulation, the acute release of norepinephrine and dopamine and the increase in the turnover of norepinephrine in the brain that occur during cranial electroshock (ECS) are emphasized. Receptor sensitivity increase during ECS is also acknowledged. Sensitivity to agents mimicking the actions of brain monoamines is increased, such that postsynaptic responses mediated by 5-HT, dopamine and noradrenaline are enhanced. These biochemical changes are seen as reversing the pathophysiology of the depressive disorder and essentially follow formulations for the efficacy of TCAs and MAOIs.

Another view focuses on neuroendocrine dysregulation, which is prominent in patients with affective disorders, and which normalizes during the recovery process. Hypothalamic dysfunction (probably hypofunction) is postulated as central to endogenous depressive disorders. The antidepressant activity of convulsive therapy results from the stimulation of hypothalamic — pituitary centres, releasing natural substances, probably peptides, that modify mood, vegetative symptoms and behaviour associated with mood disturbances.

The theory considers that the grand mal seizure, with its centrencephalic features and release of brain substances, is essential to the treatment response. It claims nothing from the induction process or the peripheral manifestations. It recognizes that convulsive therapy is effective in relieving vegetative symptoms. It also takes advantage of observations that seizures release peptides from the central nervous system; that some peptides are behaviourally active; and that increased permeability of the blood—brain barrier is a regular feature of the convulsive therapy process.

Initially proposed by Fink & Ottosson (1980), this theory was restated by Fink & Nemeroff (1989) with resulting criticism (Cooper et al 1990) and by Fink (1990c) with debate (Sackeim & Devanand 1990, Post 1990, Nutt 1990, Fink 1990d).

REFERENCES

Abrams R 1988 Electroconvulsive therapy, Oxford University Press, New York, p 231

Abrams R (editor) 1989 ECT in the high-risk patient. Convulsive Therapy 6: 1–122

Abrams R, Essman W B 1982 Electroconvulsive therapy. Biological foundations and clinical applications. Spectrum, New York

American Psychiatric Association 1978 Electroconvulsive therapy. Task Force Report 14. American Psychiatric Association, Washington, DC

American Psychiatric Association 1990 The practice of electroconvulsive therapy: recommendations for treatment, training and privileging. APA Press, Washington, DC

Consensus Conference 1985 Electronconvulsive therapy. Journal of the American Medical Association 254: 103–108

Cooper S J, Scott A I F, Whalley L J 1990 A neuroendocrine view of ECT. British Journal of Psychiatry 157: 740–743

Endler N S 1982 Holiday of darkness John Wiley, New York

Fink M 1979 Convulsive therapy: theory and practice. Raven Press, New York

Fink M 1988 ECT for parkinson disease? Convulsive Therapy 4: 189–191

Fink M 1989a Reversible and irreversible dementia. Convulsive Therapy 5: 123–125

Fink M 1989b An adequate treatment? Convulsive Therapy 5: 311–313

Fink M 1990a Is catatonia a primary indication for ECT? Convulsive Therapy 6: 1–4

Fink M 1990b Electrode placement: a clinician's guide. Convulsive Therapy 6: 263–265

Fink M 1990c How does convulsive therapy work? Neuropsychopharmacology 3: 73–82

Fink M 1990d Response to critiques. Neuropsychopharmacology 3: 97–100

Fink M, Nemeroff C 1989 A neuroendocrine view of ECT. Convulsive Therapy 5: 296–304

Fink M, Ottosson J O 1980 A theory of convulsive therapy in endogenous depression: Significance of hypothalamic functions. Psychiatry Research 2: 49–61

Fink M, Shaw R, Gross G, Coleman F S 1958 Comparative study of chlorpromazine and insulin coma in the therapy of psychosis. Journal of the American Medical Association 166: 1846–1850

Fraser M 1982 ECT: a clinical guide. John Wiley, Chichester

Grunhaus L J, Barroso L W 1989 Electroconvulsive therapy: the treatment, the questions, the answers. MECTA Corporation, Lake Oswego, OR

Kalinowsky L B, Hippius H, Klein H E 1982 Biological treatments in psychiatry. Grune & Stratton, New York

Lerer B, Shapira B, Calev A, Kindler S, Lichtenberg P, Drexler H 1990 Optimizing ECT schedule: a double blind study. Presented at APA 143rd meeting, New York. Abstract NR453: 221

Malitz S, Sackeim H 1986 Electroconvulsive therapy: clinical and basic research issues. Annals of the New York Academy of Science 462: 1–424

Maneksha F 1991 Hypertension and tachycardia during electroconvulsive therapy: to treat or not to treat? Convulsive Therapy 7: 28–35

Meduna L 1935 Versuche über die biologische Beeinflussung des Ablaufes der Schizophrenie. I: Campher und Cardiozolkrämpfe. Zeitschrift für die gesamte Neurologie and Psychiatrie 152: 235–262

Meduna L 1937 Die Konvulsionstherapie der Schizophrenie. Carl Marhold, Halle

Nutt D 1990 (How does convulsive therapy work?) Not only but also. Neuropsychopharmacology 3: 93–96

Palmer R L 1981 Electroconvulsive therapy: An appraisal. Oxford University Press, New York

Pippard J, Ellam L 1981 Electroconvulsive treatment in Great Britain, 1980. Gaskell, London

Post R 1990 (How does electroconvulsive therapy work?) ECT: the anticonvulsant connection. Neuropsychopharmacology 3: 89–92

Royal College of Nursing 1987 RCN nursing guidelines for ECT. Convulsive Therapy 3 : 158–160

Royal College of Psychiatrists 1989 The practical administration of electroconvulsive therapy (ECT). Gaskell, London

Sackeim H A 1989 Mechanisms of action. Convulsive Therapy 6: 207–310

Sackeim H A, Devenand D 1990 (How does electroconvulsive therapy work?) Why we do not know how convulsive therapy works. Neuropsychopharmacology 3: 83–88

Somatics 1986a Informed ECT for health professionals. Videotape. Somatics, Inc., 910 Sherwood Drive, Lake Bluff, IL 60044

Somatics 1986b Informed ECT for patients and families. Videotape. Somatics, Inc., 910 Sherwood Drive, Lake Bluff, IL 60044

Swartz C M, Lewis R K 1991 Theophylline reversal of ECT seizure inhibition. Psychosomatics 32: 47–51

Taylor M, Sierles F S, Abrams R 1985 General hospital psychiatry. Free Press, New York

23. Lithium

Mohammed T. Abou-Saleh

The use of lithium in the management of affective disorders has proved to be one of the most rewarding therapeutic strategies in medical practice. In the management of bipolar disorders it has provided one of the most specific psychotropic drugs in psychiatry. Its unique chemical nature and neuropharmacology has extensively engaged neuroscientists and clinical scientists to investigate its mechanism of action and clinical effects in a variety of general medical and psychiatric conditions. The scope of this chapter is to review lithium therapy: historical origins; use and indications; efficacy and safety; optimal dosage and dosage regimen and important aspects of its routine use in psychiatric practice.

HISTORICAL ORIGINS

Lithium salts were used over 100 years ago in the management of various medical disorders such as gout, diabetes and epilepsy, antedating the discovery of its therapeutic effects in mania by Cade in 1949 (Amdisen 1987).

As early as 1845, lithium was used in the prophylactic treatment of gravel and gout. Garrod, in 1876, conceived that uric acid deposition in brain tissue caused mania and depression, which were incorporated into the group of gouty diseases, and recommended the use of lithium-containing mixtures of alkaline salts. Karl Lange, a Danish neurologist, added another 'gouty' condition which he named periodic depression and treated with prophylactic lithium. The Danish psychiatrist, H.G. Schou (father of Mogens Schou), recognized this recurrent, albeit mild and 'masked' periodic depression, but was against the use of lithium for its treatment. Lithium had also been used in antacid powders and was recommended as a diuretic drug until the 1960s.

Lithium was first entered into the British Pharmacopoeia in 1864 and by 1910 there were 25 preparations available for a variety of medical conditions. In the USA lithium was marketed in the late 1940s as a substitute for ordinary table salt for patients requiring salt-free diets. Its liberal use resulted in many deaths from lithium intoxication. This led the Food and Drug Administration to ban its use for about 20 years before it was released again in 1970 for use in mania and in 1974 as a maintenance treatment.

The psychiatric era of lithium started shortly after the Second World War, when John Cade discovered its therapeutic effects in mania, following observations of its calming effects in guinea pigs. These early observations provided the impetus for further studies by Schou, Gershon and Fieve. The discovery of the prophylactic effects of lithium is attributed to Hartigan (1963) in Canterbury, UK and Baastrup (1964) in Aarhus, Denmark, who independently reported on its prophylactic effects in recurrent affective disorders. The first systematic study was carried out by Baastrup & Schou (1967). The study showed a lower relapse rate during lithium treatment than the rate over a similar period before commencing lithium. This study was criticised by Blackwell & Shepherd (1968) on the grounds that the evaluation was not blind, that it depended on doubtful assumptions about the natural history of the illness and that improvement might have been not due to lithium but spontaneous. The demand for controlled studies led to a series of investigations with more stringent methodology of double-blind discontinuation and double-blind placebo-controlled prospective design.

INDICATIONS

Acute depression

The use of lithium in acute depression has been fraught with controversy. Prophylactic trials demonstrated

369

prophylactic antidepressant effects in both bipolar and unipolar illness. This, however, was not translated to recommendations for the treatment of acute depression, probably for two reasons: the availability of conventional antidepressants, which are less toxic than lithium, and the conception that lithium is less effective in unipolar than in bipolar depression. An early study by Stokes et al (1971), in which placebo was substituted for lithium in the acute phases of mania and depression, showed no benefit for lithium treatment in acute depression. The effects of lithium were assessed over 10 days, too short a time to expect a clinical effect. The second controlled placebo substitution study showed definite antidepressant effects of lithium (Mendels 1976). Further studies confirmed these antidepressant effects: 10 out of 13 studies showed lithium to be superior to placebo (seven out of nine studies), or as effective as tricylic antidepressants (Fieve & Peselow 1983). In these studies lithium was effective in 43% of unipolar patients, 60% of bipolar II patients and 76% of bipolar I patients. The study by Worrall and colleagues (1979) indicated that the clinical effects of lithium did not occur until the second or third weeks of treatment. There is a clear trend for bipolar depression to have a more favourable response than non-bipolar depression. In non-bipolar patients, those with an endogenous symptom profile, family history of mania, cyclothymic personality and postpartum onset respond more favourably.

Lithium can, therefore, be strongly recommended for the treatment of bipolar depression, rather than tricyclics which may provoke hypomanic episodes and increase the risk for the development of rapid-cycling illness. There is evidence that lithium alone is effective in depression that has failed to respond to tricyclic medication and in combination with other antidepressants in the management of resistant depression (see chapter 26).

Mania

Four placebo-controlled trials using the crossover design showed lithium to be superior to placebo in mania. These trials were, however, not comparable: diagnostic criteria and initial severity of illness varied; there were differences in treatment period and response criteria; and in only one study were plasma lithium levels used as a basis for adjusting dosage to a given range (Coxhead & Silverstone 1987). Double-blind comparative trials of lithium versus neuroleptics followed, with seven out of nine trials comparing lithium and chlorpromazine and two trials comparing lithium and haloperidol. Despite the variation in diagnostic criteria, severity of illness, dosage of both lithium and neuroleptics, the overall results showed comparable efficacy for lithium and neuroleptics in the majority of manic patients. The largest of these studies was the multicentre trial involving 255 patients (Prien et al 1972). This study showed chlorpromazine to be more effective than lithium in highly active manic patients with similar efficacy in the less active ones. Neuroleptics achieved their effects more rapidly than lithium, which took 2 weeks before its effects were noticed. Many patients who receive lithium, however, do not complain of the 'straightjacket' effect they experience with neuroleptics.

Lithium is the medication of choice in mania, except for highly active agitated or disturbed patients, who require neuroleptics for the rapid control of the condition, preferably in combination with lithium. Neuroleptics can then be withdrawn within 2–3 weeks, by which time lithium effects are established. This arrangement allows minimal exposure to neuroleptics and the use of lithium as continuation treatment for up to 3 months from the beginning of treatment, unless longer use of prophylactic lithium is indicated. Patients with affective disorders are highly vulnerable to develop tardive dyskinesia with brief intermittent exposure to neuroleptics (Mukherjee et al 1986). Neuroleptics can, however, be used alone in the management of mania in those patients who are intolerant of lithium and if there is any possibility of pregnancy. The elderly tolerate lithium well, but are highly susceptible to parkinsonian side-effects of neuroleptics. Lithium is less effective in manic patients with paranoid-destructive features than in those with grandiose-euphoric features (Murphy & Beigel 1974). Manic patients tolerate high doses of lithium due to increased influx into the intracellular space, but tolerance drops with improvement in association with increased plasma lithium levels. This necessitates frequent monitoring of lithium levels to prevent intoxication during recovery.

Schizophrenia

The use of lithium in the treatment of schizophrenia has not been satisfactorily established. The results of double-blind trials have been disappointing and neuroleptics are more effective than lithium. Lithium is effective in the affective component of schizoaffective disorder, particularly manic symptoms, while depressive symptoms are less responsive. There is little evidence that lithium has an antischizophrenic effect in patients with schizoaffective disorder who often require a combination of lithium and antipsychotic medication. Within schizophrenic disorders, lithium has been shown to be effective in schizophreniform, periodic types which may aetiologically be related to affective disorders. Studies have shown that patients with lithium-responsive schizophrenia have a higher familial incidence of affective disorders than those with lithium non-responsive schizophrenia (Sautter & Garver 1987).

Use in other psychiatric disorders

Lithium has also been recommended for affective disorders occurring in the setting of alcohol and drug misuse, premenstrual syndrome, eating disorders and personality disorders. Within personality disorders, those with cyclothymic, impulsive and aggressive traits benefit most from lithium. Lithium has been shown to have anti-aggressive effects in patients with personality disorders and mental handicap. Sheard & Marini (1976) found in a single-blind crossover study of prisoners, a significant reduction in violent incidents during lithium administration compared to the placebo period. Campbell & Small (1984), in a double-blind placebo controlled study of 66 prisoners, found a progressive reduction in violent episodes in the lithium-treated group with decreased ratings of hostility and excitement. There have been three double-blind placebo controlled studies of lithium in aggressive mentally handicapped patients, which found that 50–73% of patients showed improvement in aggressive behaviour on lithium, when compared with placebo (Worrall et al 1975, Tyrer et al 1984, Craft & Ismail 1987).

Lithium continuation therapy after ECT

Affective disorders are self-limiting and are by nature recurrent, and the necessity for continuation treatment following recovery from the acute episode has been well documented (Mindham et al 1973, Paykel et al 1975). An episode of depression or mania will often last between 3 and 6 months and may occasionally continue for more than a year before spontaneous remission. Five studies, of which four were prospective controlled investigations, examined continuation therapy with antidepressants or lithium to prevent early relapse after ECT (Abou-Saleh & Coppen 1988). Perry & Tsuang (1979) in a retrospective study found that lithium and

tricyclic antidepressants were equally effective in reducing relapses after a course of ECT. The usefulness of continuation treatment with lithium was evaluated in a double-blind placebo-controlled study for 1 year after recovery with ECT (Coppen et al 1981). Patients who received placebo spent an average of 7.8 weeks with an episode of depression, compared with 1.7 weeks for those who received lithium. Lithium continuation following recovery with ECT may have an advantage over tricyclic antidepressants in patients with a previous history of mania, elderly depressives and those with delusional depression (Abou-Sarleh & Coppen 1988).

There have, however, been anecdotal reports of the combination of ECT and lithium causing greater memory loss and confusion than ECT alone. Kukopulos and colleagues (1988) evaluated the efficacy and side-effects of ECT combined with lithium in 256 patients in comparison with 130 who received ECT only. They found no difference in response to ECT in these patients: 79% of those who received combined treatment had a good response to ECT compared to 75% who received ECT only. Among the 256 patients who had combined ECT with lithium, only three showed signs of acute brain syndrome in comparison with five of 130 patients who received ECT without lithium. Rudorfer and colleagues (1987), in a recent review, concluded that there were no demonstrable, pharmacokinetic or drug—drug interaction factors to preclude the combined use of lithium and ECT.

Prophylactic lithium

Affective disorders are recurrent illnesses and the discovery of the prophylactic effects of lithium opened a new era in their management. In a number of controlled investigations of varying stringency, lithium was shown to substantially reduce the long-term morbidity of both unipolar and bipolar disorders. An early study by Baastrup & Schou in 1967 showed that, in a group of 88 patients with affective disorders who had received lithium for periods of up to 5 years, affective morbidity was reduced to 2 weeks a year from an average of 13 weeks a year before lithium. These results were confirmed in studies of similar design (Angst et al 1970, Hullin et al 1972).

The second phase of evaluation was the discontinuation trial. Patients who were maintained on lithium for years were randomly switched to receive placebo or to continue with lithium. Discontinuation of lithium therapy for a period of 5 months was associated with relapse of 54% of patients compared with no relapse in patients who continued on lithium (Baastrup et al 1970).

Prospective trials were next. Coppen and his colleagues (1971) carried out the first placebo-controlled double-blind study of lithium over a period of 27 months. The results showed a very convincing advantage for the lithium-treated group. Patients who had received placebo and had *ad hoc* conventional treatment, including antidepressants, ECT or neuroleptics, spent 27% of their time as inpatients and a further 19% of their time with an outpatient episode. By contrast, patients treated with lithium spent only 5% of their time as inpatients and 7% of their time with an outpatient episode. The need for conventional treatment was also reduced greatly.

Two studies by Prien and colleagues (1973a, b) followed. The first was a placebo-controlled study for a period of 2 years; the second was a comparative study of placebo, lithium and imipramine. In unipolar depressives both lithium and imipramine had a prophylactic effect, but in bipolar patients lithium was significantly better than imipramine.

Further studies from Coppen and colleagues (Coppen & Abou-Saleh 1983) showed that lithium was superior to mianserin and maprotiline in the prophylaxis of unipolar illness. The Medical Research Council study in the UK showed lithium to be as effective as amitriptyline and both to be superior to placebo in the prophylaxis of unipolar depression (Glen et al 1981). The National Institute of Mental Health (NIMH) collaborative study, however, found that lithium was less effective than imipramine or their combination in the long-term management of severe unipolar illness, but found the three treatments equally effective in moderately ill patients (Prien et al 1984). The patients involved in the investigation, however, showed few clear-cut remission intervals, which may account for the different results found in this investigation.

Peselow et al (1990) evaluated the efficacy of lithium alone, antidepressants alone, lithium combined with antidepressants and placebo-no treatment in 222 unipolar patients over 4 years and found modestly but significantly lower relapse rates (40–50%) in patients receiving active medication, than those receiving placebo-no treatment (70%).

Overall, lithium is more effective in the prophylaxis of bipolar than unipolar illness. This appears to be related to the greater homogeneity of bipolar illness whilst unipolar illness remains the arena for the continuing controversy over its classification. The role of lithium in maintenance treatment is discussed further in chapter 25.

Who responds to prophylactic lithium

Among bipolar patients the group with rapid-cycling illness (those who suffer four episodes of illness per annum or more) have been shown repeatedly to be poor responders to lithium. Recent studies have examined the clinical and psychological characteristics of good and poor responders to lithium (Abou-Saleh & Coppen 1986, 1990). Among unipolar patients, those with endogenous illness and patients with pure familial depressive disease had comparatively better responses than those with non-endogenous, sporadic depressive and depression spectrum disease. In both bipolar and unipolar patients those with greater disturbance in their intermorbid personality responded less well than those with less personality disturbance. The most powerful predictor of long-term response, however, was an empirical one: the results of a trial of lithium for 6–12 months predicted response over many years. These results were confirmed in a recent study of lower doses/plasma level of lithium that also indicated that lithium is as effective in the elderly as in young and middle-aged patients (Coppen & Abou-Saleh 1988).

Aagaard & Vestergaard (1990), in a 2-year prospective study, showed that non-adherence to treatment was mainly predicted by substance abuse and many earlier admissions. Non-response in those who adhered to treatment was mainly predicted by female sex, younger age and a previous chronic course. A third of the population of patients studied, however, had a chronic illness and a half showed social deterioration prior to starting lithium.

Life events in the 12 months prior to starting lithium had no influence on outcome on lithium, confirming the findings of Hall et al (1977), who also found that those who relapsed had no more life events prior to their relapse than at other times. Priebe et al (1989), however, showed that patients living with high expressed emotion relatives had worse outcome.

SIDE-EFFECTS

Subjective side-effects

The occurrence of subjective side-effects during lithium therapy is well documented (Abou-Saleh & Coppen 1983a). Commonly reported side-effects in the early stage (within 6 weeks of starting lithium) include nausea, loose stools, fatigue, muscle weakness, polydipsia, polyuria and hand tremor. During maintenance weight gain, mild memory impairment and hand tremor are common complaints and polydipsia and polyuria may persist. The rate of occurrence of these side-effects and their severity are related to plasma lithium concentrations. Similar complaints, however, have been reported in patients who have received placebo, suggesting that these side-effects' are also symptoms of depression. Abou-Saleh & Coppen (1983a) investigated subjective side-effects in patients receiving lithium, drug-free depressed patients and normal control subjects. Side-effects reported showed a strong association with the presence of depression and personality disturbance in those patients. The reliability of side-effects as rated by clinicians and patients is moderate, with the clinicians rating side-effects less often and less severe than the patients themselves (Wancata et al 1988). Bech et al (1976) showed that patients who received antidepressants and neuroleptics complained of more side-effects than those on lithium alone or patients who discontinued their lithium. Lyskowski et al (1982) found that the presence of additional medication and mood disturbance contributed to the occurrence of side-effects.

Thyroid effects

In therapeutic plasma concentrations, lithium produces a transient decrease in thyroxine (T4) and triiodothyronine (T3) during the first 3 weeks or months of treatment. This leads to a compensatory increase in basal thyrotropin concentration, which restores plasma T4 and T3 concentrations to normal. Only a small percentage of patients develop hypothyroidism or clinical goitre. The frequency of hypothyroidism is around 5% and varies between studies in relation to sample size and criteria for diagnosing hypothyroidism. Thyrotropin concentrations are increased in 10–15% of patients. Women are more susceptible to developing hypothyroidism than men. This may be related to the increased disposition of women to develop autoimmune thyroid disease in middle age. Indeed preexisting thyroid disease is the major vulnerability factor for development of hypothyroidism during lithium therapy. Coppen & Abou-Saleh (1988) studied thyroid function in 125 patients receiving low-dose/plasma levels of lithium. Women had significantly higher levels of TSH than men, and all four patients with abnormally high TSH levels were unipolar women. Of the 11

patients who received replacement thyroxine, 10 were unipolar patients.

Thyroid dysfunction has been related to increased affective morbidity during prophylactic lithium and has been implicated in the development of rapid-cycling bipolar disorder.

Lithium and renal function

Hestbech and his associates (1977) presented alarming evidence of lithium nephropathy in postmortem and renal biopsy specimens from patients on long-term lithium therapy. Thirteen out of 14 patients investigated, five of whom had suffered one or more episodes of lithium intoxication, showed an increased proportion of sclerotic glomeruli, focal nephron atrophy and interstitial fibrosis. That report generated much concern and stimulated further research into renal function in patients on long-term lithium. Renal morphological abnormalities were demonstrated in a considerable proportion of patients on lithium. The results from five studies involving 124 patients showed a variable percentage of abnormal biopsies (range 16–100%). In studies where patients were selected on the basis of reduced kidney function, all biopsy specimens were abnormal, but a low rate of abnormality (16%) was found in studies where patients were selected on basis of time on lithium (Bendz 1983). Overall, 5–10% of patients on prophylactic lithium develop tubulointerstitial nephropathy complicated with glomerular pathology. There is no evidence that these changes are conducive to renal insufficiency. The rare incidents of renal failure on lithium were attributed to lithium intoxication or other causes. Glomerular filtration rate, as determined by 24-hour creatinine clearance, was shown to be abnormal (clearance below 70 ml/min) in 23% of cases (range 3–60%) in four studies involving 567 patients. Polyuria (24-hour urine volume greater than 3 litres) occurred in 29% of patients (mean of 10 studies involving 788 patients, range 1–57%). Renal concentrating ability was impaired in 33% of patients.

Coppen and his colleagues (1980), however, found little difference in kidney function between lithium-treated patients and patients with affective disorders who were never treated with lithium. The only difference shown was increased urinary volume in lithium treated patients.

These investigations suggest that there are potential hazards in the use of lithium that call for careful screening for evidence of renal disease before starting therapy. Patients with polyuria appear to be a high-risk group who need more regular monitoring of plasma lithium and kidney function.

Lithium intoxication

Prodromal symptoms and signs of lithium intoxication include nausea, vomiting, diarrhoea, coarse tremor, sluggishness and dysarthria, which occur if plasma lithium levels exceed 1.5 mmol/l. Plasma lithium levels exceeding 2.0 mmol/l are associated with moderate to severe intoxication with manifestation of clouded consciousness, muscular hypertonia, fasciculation, coarse tremor, hyper-reflexia, epileptiform seizures and, finally, a comatose state.

Management of lithium poisoning is primarily determined by the plasma level: patients with levels of 4.0 mmol/l and above, and levels between 2–4 mmol/l associated with kidney disease or renal failure, require peritoneal dialysis or haemodialysis.

Plasma lithium levels between 2–4 mmol/l in patients with normal renal function can be managed by: 1) close monitoring of plasma lithium and other electrolyte-concentrations, particularly sodium, while potassium concentration is best monitored on the ECG; 2) infusion of saline if the patient shows hyponatraemia (low plasma sodium causes a decrease in lithium clearance); 3) induction of diuresis using osmotic diuretics such as urea and mannitol, with alkalinization of urine; 4) general cardiopulmonary corrective measures and measurement of fluid input/output.

Lithium interactions

Lithium in therapeutic dosages shows several pharmacological interactions. The drug interacts synergistically with antithyroid medication used in the treatment of hyperthyroidism; with potassium chloride it may induce hypothyroidism.

The most alarming interaction is the observed neurotoxicity in patients receiving lithium combined with antipsychotic drugs, particularly haloperidol (Cohen & Cohen 1974). These patients, however, suffered from other pathology that could account for these findings. Whether this interaction is due to lithium, neuroleptics or their combination remains uncertain. Neurotoxicity reactions caused by lithium toxicity are similar to those reported on combined lithium and neuroleptics in their clinical features and prognosis. Moreover, these two syndromes are similar to neuroleptic malignant syndrome (NMS), except for the very high fever and high concentrations of creatinine phosphokinase in patients with NMS. Although these interactions are rare, it would be prudent to monitor patients for the possibility of their occurrence when combined lithium and neuroleptics are used, particularly in higher dosages. Neurotoxicity reactions have also been reported on lithium combined with carbamazepine. Lithium, however, may counteract the effect of carbamazepine to cause leukopenia, while carbamazepine may reduce lithium-induced polyurea.

Lithium may interact with beta-blockers, resulting in the slowing of heart rate and similar interactions have been noted when lithium is combined with digoxin, with reports of increased risk of sudden cardiovascular death on this combination in predisposed patients.

Thiazide diuretics reduce renal lithium clearance and increase plasma lithium levels by reducing plasma volume causing an increase in lithium and sodium reabsorption. This interaction is not observed with potassium-sparing diuretics and loop diuretics such as frusemide. Amiloride, however, has been used for treating lithium-induced polyuria and diabetes insipidus. Acetazolamide and osmotic diuretics increase renal lithium excretion and have been used to treat lithium toxicity.

Finally, the widely used non-steroidal anti-inflammatory drugs have been reported to reduce lithium clearance and increase plasma levels, except for aspirin and sulindac. Indomethacin, however, has been used to treat lithium-induced polyuria.

The young and the elderly

Bipolar affective disorder is rare in children, but less rare in adolescence, and the sole indication for the use of lithium is in the management of this disorder. Reports of the usefulness of lithium in hyperactivity are not convincing. Lithium, however, may be useful in the treatment of very aggressive children and is generally better tolerated than neuroleptics. Side-effects of lithium are minimal and youngsters who are starting lithium should be monitored closely, preferably with measurement of lithium in saliva in view of their aversion to venepuncture. Prophylactic lithium should only be considered for youngsters with frequent episodes of illness.

Lithium is an effective and safe treatment in affective disorders of old age (Himmelhoch et al 1980, Schulman & Post 1980). Abou-Saleh & Coppen (1983b) found no relationship between long-term efficacy and age of starting lithium. Moreover, low-doses/plasma levels (0.45–0.79 mmol/l) were as effective as high-doses/plasma levels (0.8–1.2 mmol/l) and were associated with fewer side-effects. The elderly, however, are more vulnerable to the adverse effects of lithium: Smith & Helms (1982) reported that 33% of the elderly experienced 'confusion' versus 12% of the younger group on plasma levels of 0.86–1.26 mmol/l. Lithium dose requirements show a decrease with increasing age, which is accounted for by decreased glomerular rate and lithium clearance (Vestergaard & Schou 1984).

Pregnancy

Animal studies using eight to nine times the mg/kg human dose suggested pathomorphic effects for lithium in mammals. An international register of lithium babies started in 1970 showed a high rate of congenital malformation (11%), mostly cardiovascular, in babies exposed to lithium during the first trimester of pregnancy compared to a rate of 3% in the general population. A Swedish study of a cohort of 287 cases showed that 7% of the cases involving lithium use during pregnancy resulted in a congenital heart defect compared to a rate of 1% in babies of manic-depressive women with no record of lithium use (Kallen & Tandberg 1983). Schou (1976) carried out a 5-year follow-up study of babies who had been exposed to lithium *in utero* and found no excess developmental abnormalities in these children compared with their non-lithium-exposed siblings. The study, however, was based on questionnaire data obtained from the doctors who had originally reported those babies to the Register and not on objectively assessed data. These findings suggest a considerable risk to a cardiovascular teratogenic effect for lithium and contraindicate its use in pregnancy during the first trimester. There is no evidence, however, that lithium is a behavioural teratogen.

Nursing mothers receiving lithium secrete it in considerable concentrations in their breast milk (30–100% of the mother's plasma concentrations). Breast feeding should, therefore, be discouraged. It has been suggested, however, that there is little likelihood that a few additional weeks of lithium exposure adds much in the way of developmental risk for an infant already exposed *in utero*.

Weinstein (1980) provided guidelines for the management of lithium therapy prior to and during pregnancy.

Women with childbearing potential should be informed of the teratogenic effects and therefore encouraged to avoid pregnancy or inform their doctors if they decided to become pregnant, and a pregnancy test is an essential screening test prior to starting lithium. Lithium should be stopped before conception and as soon as possible after an unplanned pregnancy is discovered.

The risk of relapse after lithium withdrawal appears lower in the earlier part of the pregnancy. If lithium is introduced after the first trimester of pregnancy, then plasma lithium levels should be monitored more frequently, particularly in the last few weeks of pregnancy, in view of its increased clearance and renal elimination. The lithium dose should be reduced to 50% in the last week of pregnancy and stopped at the onset of labour to prevent lithium intoxication. Lithium could then be reintroduced within the first week postpartum to avoid postpartum relapses.

Mortality on lithium

Affective disorders are associated with high mortality: studies have shown that 15% of depressed patients die by suicide and there is an additional increased risk for death by cardiovascular disease and secondary alcoholism. Treatment with lithium exerts a protective effect and lowers the rate of suicide and attempted suicide during prophylaxis (Causemann & Muller-Oerlinghausen 1988). Norton & Whalley (1984), in a naturalistic study of mortality in 791 subjects treated with lithium, observed a standardized mortality rate of 2.83 with excess mortality by suicide in the younger age-group (36 times) and cardiovascular disease in the older age-group (2.15 times), but no death from nephritis, cancer or leukaemia. It was worthy of note that all eight suicides had made previous suicide attempts and three of these eight suicides occurred within 3 months of starting lithium. Norton & Whalley also compared the 33 deaths with 33 matched patients selected from the 751 survivors and showed that patients who died on lithium had more severe psychiatric illness and showed more signs of physical disease than the controls: nine out of 14 patients who died of cardiovascular disease had clinical abnormalities attributable to disease of the cardiovascular system which were present before the introduction of lithium. The authors indicated the value of careful history-taking in the examination of the cardiovascular system, with measurement of blood pressure, recording of electrocardiogram and chest X-ray, before starting lithium and the close monitoring of lithium-treated patients with cardiovascular abnormalities. The findings by Norton & Whalley are in contrast to the results of a recent study by Coppen and colleagues (1990) of 104 patients attending a lithium clinic who were followed up for 10 years and who showed significantly lower mortality than would be expected from age/sex/year-specific rates for England and Wales. No patient died from suicide. These results suggest a protective effect for lithium.

The occurrence of sudden death in patients on lithium has been related to its effects on cardiac conduction mechanisms (Shopsin et al 1979).

CLINICAL USE

Plasma level and clinical response

The adequacy of a particular lithium dosage for the individual patient is best determined by the serum level achieved. The changes in plasma levels are determined by the size of the individual dose administered and the timing of subsequent doses. The previously accepted therapeutic range of plasma levels of 0.8–1.2 mmol/l 12 hours after the last dose was empirically determined from the earlier studies of the treatment of mania. Historically, the question has been more one of deciding on the non-toxic dosage and plasma levels than on establishing a therapeutic range, in view of the narrow therapeutic — toxic margin: while there is disagreement as to what is the minimum effective 12-hour serum plasma level, there is full agreement on the plasma toxic level (1.5 mmol/l).

Prien & Caffey (1976), in a restrospective study of a high risk group of 32 patients over 2 years, found that 55% of patients maintained on levels of 0.7 mmol/l or less had relapsed, compared with 14% of patients maintained on higher levels.

Jerram & McDonald (1978) carried out an open prospective study over 1 year in which they investigated the efficacy (relapse rates) in groups of bipolar and unipolar patients maintained at three different lithium levels: below 0.49, between 0.5 and 0.69, and above 0.7 mmol/l. Relapse rates in these groups were 18%, 13% and 20% respectively. To determine the minimum effective levels, Jerram & McDonald carried out a further study over 1 year and allocated patients to one of three groups with ranges of 0.25–0.39, 0.4–0.59 and 0.6–1.0 mmol/l. Relapse rates for the latter three groups were 62%, 15% and 18% respectively, showing a marked increase in the group maintained at the lowest levels, indicating that 0.4 mmol/l is probably the minimum effective lithium level. The study had the advantages of being prospective and including a repre-

sentative sample of the population of patients attending a lithium clinic. It was, however, an open study, in which evaluation of outcome did not consider sub-clinical morbidity in the form of lithium-modified episodes. 70% of the patients included in the study had a bipolar illness.

Three retrospective studies in bipolars (Sarantidis & Waters 1981) and unipolars (Decina & Fieve 1981, Sashidharan et al 1982) found better response rates in those maintained on serum lithium levels below 0.7 mmol/l. This association between poor clinical response and higher lithium levels may be related to the recognition by the treating physicians of high-risk patients and the prescription of high lithium doses in an attempt to prevent relapses.

Waters and colleagues (1982), in the first double-blind study, examined relapse rates of bipolar patients who were randomly assigned to lower levels (0.3–0.8 mmol/l) and higher levels (0.8–1.4 mmol/l) of lithium. Patients in each group were followed up for 6 months before being switched over to the other group for another 6 months. Waters et al found that significantly more of the relapses (83%) occurred during the low-level phase (mean 0.51 mmol/l), with only 17% occurring during the high-level phase (mean 0.99 mmol/l) of the trial.

A recent study from the USA suggested that bipolar patients require higher dosages to achieve plasma levels of 0.7 mmol/l (Gelenberg et al 1989). These workers have not, however, evaluated the efficacy of the middle range of levels between 0.6 and 0.8 mmol/l.

In our own study (Abou-Saleh & Coppen 1989a), we examined the morbidity and side-effects in 72 patients with recurrent affective disorders under double-blind conditions over a period of 1 year. The patients had been previously maintained on lithium dosages to give 12-hour plasma lithium levels of 0.8–1.2 mmol/l. The patients were randomly allocated either to remain on their previous dosage or to receive a 25% or 50% reduction in dose. No patient had a 12-hour serum lithium level of less than 0.45 mmol/l. Morbidity was assessed by a composite index which included measures of severity and duration of symptoms. We found that patients who were maintained at lower serum levels, below 0.79 mmol/l, had significant reduction in their morbidity (34%) while those who remained at levels of 0.8 mmol/l and above had a slight increase in morbidity. Similar results were found for both the unipolar and bipolar patients, except that in the former group those with non-endogenous illness had a more substantial reduction in morbidity (58%). These differences in morbidity were not related to differences in unwanted effects or the prescription of extra medication. The study, however, included patients who were not maintained solely on lithium. Patients who were maintained on plasma levels between 0.45 and 0.79 mmol/l following a 25–50% reduction of dosage experienced fewer side-effects, most notably in their complaints of tremor. Patients' weight was lower on lower levels of lithium. Measurements were also made of plasma thyrotropin (TSH) levels and 24-hour urinary volumes before and after starting the trial. It was found that patients who were maintained on lower plasma levels during the trial developed significant reductions in both measures, indicating a reduction in adverse effects on thyroid and renal functions.

Our findings are consistent with those of Schou & Vestergaard (1988) in their naturalistic prospective studies on a lithium cohort maintained on lower doses/serum levels (mean 0.68 mmol/l) over several years. They found no significant difference in urine volume, but significantly lower osmolality during lithium than before lithium was started. They compared these results with those obtained in a previous study, in which patients were maintained on higher doses/serum levels (mean 0.86 mmol/l) (Vestergaard & Amdisen 1981); lower serum levels of lithium were associated with lower urinary volume and higher osmolality. Vestergaard et al (1988) also studied the prevalence of side-effects such as tremor, thirst and excessive urination in their cohort: they found lower rates than in patients maintained on higher dosage. These observations, however, were made on naturalistically studied patients and comparisons were made between different populations.

The study by Milln & Patch (1988), using a similar design to the study by Coppen and colleagues (1983), failed to confirm these findings: patients who had 50% reduction in dosage (minimum plasma levels of 0.3 mmol/l) showed a significantly greater rate of relapse (58%) than those who had no reduction in dosage (17%).

The dosage regimen

Lithium, like most other psychotropic drugs, has tended to be prescribed routinely in a divided dosage regime of two to three doses per day. This regime has been advocated to avoid peak serum and tissue concentrations, assumed to be conducive to greater adverse effects, and to provide a reasonably uniform concentration, assumed to be necessary for a favourable clinical response. Slow or sustained-release preparations were introduced with the specific aim of meeting these two conditions. Lithium has a long elimination half-life (12–24 h) indicating that it need not be prescribed in more than one single dose per day. A few clinicians adopted this single daily dosage regimen from an early stage to encourage better compliance (Coppen et al 1971).

Single daily and divided daily dosage regimes produce quite different profiles of serum lithium levels over 24 hours. Lauritsen and colleagues (1981) showed that patients who were maintained on a single daily dosage regimen had early sharp peak lithium levels within 2–4 h of ingestion of the drug, but had lower levels in the second 12 hours of the day. Patients who had received a similar, but divided daily dosage regimen showed smaller peaks and had a relatively constant level throughout the 24 hours. The two groups had identical mean 12-hour and mean average levels over 24 hours. Other administration schedules will give different profiles. A 12-hour serum lithium level in a divided dosage regimen using a conventional preparation would be an underestimate of the amount of lithium to which the patient has been exposed, whilst a 12-hour serum lithium level in a single daily dosage regimen with a sustained release preparation would be an overestimate of such exposure.

Studies of the relationship between the dosage regimen and renal function followed. Plenge et al (1982) found that 24-hour urinary volume showed no association with maximum or 12-hour lithium levels, but was associated with minimal plasma levels: patients who had the greatest 24-hour urine volumes had the highest minimum plasma levels. They concluded that to avoid kidney damage during long-term lithium treatment it may be more important to have regular periods with low levels than it is to avoid peaks and they have accordingly strongly advocated a single daily dosage regimen.

These preliminary findings were confirmed in a study in which Plenge et al examined functional and structural changes in patients who had been given lithium in a single daily dosage regimen in comparison with patients who received it in divided doses. They found that the functional and structural changes were most pronounced in the group of patients who received their lithium in divided doses. They noted that the serum lithium profiles were markedly different between the two groups: those who had a single daily dosage regimen had the peak around 1.5 mmol/l within 4 h of ingestion, and 12-hour lithium levels around

1.0 mmol/l with a minimum level of 0.5 mmol/l before the next dose of lithium was given. For the group who had the divided dosage regimen, serum lithium levels never dropped below the 12-hour serum level of 0.7–1.0 mmol/l. A criticism that could be levelled at this study is that the group of patients who had the divided dosage regimen were patients who had been started on this regimen since the early 1970s or had come from other clinics and preferred to stay on it; treatment regimens were not, therefore, randomly allocated. Moreover, the two groups received different doses, with the group on the divided regimen receiving higher doses of lithium, which may have contributed to the greater functional and morphological changes in these patients.

Schou and colleagues (1982) instigated a similar study in collaboration with the Copenhagen group, to compare patients who had throughout received a slow-release preparation in a divided dosage regimen, with patients treated by the Copenhagen group with a conventional preparation in a single daily dosage regimen. It was noted that the Copenhagen group of patients were on average older, had been on lithium for longer and had slightly higher mean plasma concentrations. The results indicated that the dosage regimen had no effect on glomerular function (creatinine clearance) but did influence tubular function, as indexed by the 24-hour urinary volume, which was lower in the Copenhagen group. None of these studies, however, were carried out within the same clinic with random allocation of treatment regimen in conjunction with the assessment of clinical and unwanted effects.

These findings suggest that a dosage regimen with even longer intervals between doses, i.e. every second or third day, might be as effective as a daily regimen and less harmful to the kidney. Indeed, Jensen and colleagues (1990) evaluated the efficacy and side-effects of lithium given every other day in an open study of 10 patients with median duration of 13 months. There was no change in morbidity and side-effects were significantly reduced. Such a departure from a daily dosage regimen may lead to less compliance, unless, of course, dummy tablets were to be given on the non-dosage days.

Lithium preparations

Lithium preparations vary in their pharmacokinetic properties, which may influence the nature and severity of side-effects. The standard preparations are rapidly absorbed and show early peaks in plasma and shorter half-lives than slow or sustained-release preparations. Rapid absorption and early peaks in plasma lithium levels are associated with nausea and increased occurrence of tremor, while slow-release preparations are more often associated with complaints of diarrhoea and loose bowel motions. Slow-release preparations, with their slow absorption, may increase the chance of survival after an overdose but lead to more lithium accumulation, particularly in those with compromised renal function. Slow-release preparations are often given in a once-daily regimen, which encourages compliance and causes less renal toxicity (see above).

Earlier studies of the pharmacokinetic profiles of standard and slow-release preparations showed little difference between them (Tyrer et al 1976). More recent studies have found differences in pharmacokinetic characteristics and evidence for slow-release properties. These conflicting results may be related to methodological differences between studies, including frequency of blood sampling, whether the populations studied are patients or normal volunteers, patients' affective state and other variables altering the bioavailability, distribution and excretion of lithium, such as age, food, weight and extra medication. In a well-controlled study of four lithium preparations, slow-release characteristics were obtained at the expense of less bioavailability (Shelley & Silverstone 1987). Lower peak plasma levels obtained with a slow-release preparation may account for improved renal concentrating ability, suggesting that patients with symptomatic polyuria may benefit from a change to a slow release preparation from a standard one (Miller et al 1985).

THE ROUTINE OF LITHIUM THERAPY

The routine of lithium therapy as a long-term, if not a lifetime treatment, involves a number of important steps from the decision to refer patients for assessment by the general practitioner, assessment and screening procedures, indication for commencement of prophylactic therapy, monitoring progress, management of compliance, relapse and side-effects and finally the decision to terminate treatment.

Referral for assessment

Referrals for assessment for lithium therapy are often secondary and tertiary ones and very few general practitioners undertake such assessment and initiate treatment. Whilst bipolar patients are invariably referred to psychiatric clinics or, where available, the lithium clinic by their general practitioners, patients with unipolar illnesses are often treated by the general practitioner and the decision to refer them for prophylactic therapy is made following several episodes of illness with partial improvement. In the absence of a lithium clinic, psychiatrists often carry out the assessment and initiate lithium therapy and continue the long-term management in a hospital setting.

Assessment and indications

The assessment of patients involves general psychiatric assessment, with particular emphasis on age of onset, symptom pattern, frequency of episodes, the course of illness, family history and the physical condition. Patients with bipolar illness almost invariably receive prophylactic lithium, while patients with unipolar illness may also be considered for prophylactic antidepressant medication.

A crucial decision for the clinician is when to start prophylactic lithium. Angst (1981) analysed the course of illness in 159 unipolar, 95 bipolar and 150 schizoaffective patients over 27 years. He found that only 37% unipolars, 15% bipolar and 18% schizoaffective patients had suffered one episode of illness during that period. He decided it would be desirable to start prophylaxis if a patient was likely to suffer two further episodes in addition to the present one in the subsequent 5 years. He examined numerous criteria to see which identified those patients at risk. He found that the presence of two episodes in the previous 5 years in unipolars, in the previous 4 years in bipolars and in the previous 3 years in schizoaffectives provided satisfactory criteria for starting prophylactic lithium.

The World Health Organization has recently provided guidelines based on these findings: prophylactic treatment should be started in unipolar depression after three episodes, particularly if one discrete episode has occurred in the last 5 years, apart from the present episode. In bipolar illness, prophylactic treatment should be given after the second episode.

The list of routine investigations done prior to starting lithium and during treatment is shown in Table 23.1.

Monitoring progress

Once initiated, lithium should be estimated on a weekly basis, to adjust dosage to achieve therapeutic plasma levels of 0.6–1 mmol/l. This is particularly important if it is started during a manic episode, in view of the

Table 23.1 Routine assessments/investigations in lithium therapy

Prior to starting lithium

Physical examination

Haematology and clinical chemistry, including urea, creatinine electrolytes, thyroxine and TSH, urine test

Weight

Pregnancy test if necessary

ECG

During drug treatment

Investigation	Frequency
Physical examination, ECG, full blood count, 24 urine volume	once a year
Clinical chemistry, urea, creatinine T4, TSH and urine test	6-monthly
Weight and electrolytes	with each lithium estimation

fluctuations in plasma lithium levels with increased influx into the intracellular space, resulting in higher plasma levels, with the resolution of the illness. The occurrence of side-effects is monitored closely for the adjustment of dosage and the reassurance of patients. Once a reproducible plasma lithium level is obtained, patients are monitored less frequently at 6–8-weekly intervals. More careful and close monitoring is indicated in patients with thyroid, cardiovascular and renal disease.

Management of relapse

Up to 50% of patients will experience a recurrence of their illness over time. The main reason for failure of prophylaxis is poor compliance. Recurrences during lithium may be less frequent and modified to be less severe than before lithium was started, indicating partial improvement on lithium. A minority of patients experience as much morbidity after lithium as before its initiation, including the group with rapid-cycling illness. The management of the relapses depends on their causes, including poor compliance. Those who are true prophylaxis failures, but have nevertheless benefited from lithium therapy, can be treated with additional *ad hoc* antidepressant and antimanic medication. This extra medication can later be withdrawn on remission of the recurrence. Those who have shown no benefit from lithium should be considered for alternative medication: bipolar patients may benefit from anti-convulsants, such as carbamazepine, sodium valproate or clonazepam, whilst unipolar patients may require electroconvulsive therapy followed by prophylactic antidepressants, particularly selective 5-HT reuptake inhibitors such as fluoxetine.

The role of folate deficiency in the aetiopathogenesis of affective disorders, including relapses during lithium therapy, has been extensively investigated (Coppen & Abou-Saleh 1982, Abou-Saleh & Coppen 1985, 1989b) and therapeutic folate supplements have been shown to decrease the morbidity of patients receiving prophylactic lithium (Coppen et al 1986). Schou and colleagues (1986) reported low erythrocyte folate concentrations in affectively ill patients which were restored to normality after 12 months of lithium therapy. They suggested that folate supplements were not required during lithium therapy. The study, however provided no data on the morbidity of patients during lithium therapy and, while folate-deficiency may be corrected naturalistically, folate supplements may benefit patients who relapse during lithium therapy, who may require supratherapeutic levels of folate (Coppen et al 1986).

Termination of lithium therapy

There are no guidelines for the termination of lithium therapy and once started it could be continued indefinitely. The decision by the treating clinician to stop lithium is often related to the development of serious side-effects or adverse effects, such as renal toxicity, as well as situations when it is clearly of no benefit to the patient. Occasionally, patients instigate termination and more often they drop out from treatment for a variety of reasons. Patients who are likely to relapse are those who have not been well controlled on lithium, those who have discontinued its use whilst on extra medication and those with a history of many previous episodes of illness. Greil and colleagues (1981) found that patients who were maintained on antidepressants and neuroleptics in addition to lithium relapsed in 83% of cases, in contrast to 27% of those who were maintained on lithium alone.

The question of whether there is a lithium withdrawal syndrome has not been satisfactorily resolved. A few studies have reported the occurrence of anxiety, irritability, headache, insomnia, fatigue, nausea and diarrhoea and blurred vision within days of stopping lithium. Some of these patients progressed to experience a full-blown episode of illness, while others do not (Greil et al 1982). Whether these symptoms are related to anticipatory anxiety is uncertain. Sashidharan & McGuire (1983) argued against the notion of the lithium withdrawal syndrome on the basis of their findings in a discontinuation study: early relapses were part of the pattern of recurrences occurring over time, with no evidence of rebound episodes of illness. All lithium-related side-effects start to subside after stopping it, with renal concentrating ability and thyroid suppression showing a gradual recovery over a few weeks.

Management of compliance

Poor compliance with lithium is the main reason for prophylaxis failure. This occurs particularly in younger male patients with fewer episodes of illness. Reasons given by patients who stop lithium include side-effects, missing the 'highs', feeling less creative or productive, feeling well with no need to take lithium or being bothered by the idea that their moods are controlled by medication. Less frequently cited side-effects as reasons for discontinuing lithium are weight gain, increased thirst, tiredness, tremor, difficulties with memory, poor concentration and loss of enthusiasm (Jamison 1987a). Jamison (1987a) provided guidelines for maximizing lithium compliance which include monitoring of compliance with frequent enquiries, regular measurement of lithium levels and encouragement of patients to express their concerns about their treatment. Patients should be forewarned of side-effects, maintained on minimal effective levels and on a once-daily dosage regimen. Involving the family in therapy and the use of self-help groups may also be indicated. Cognitive psychotherapy was shown to improve compliance in patients. Jamison (1987b) advocated the use of psychotherapy with lithium in view of the serious personal, interpersonal and social consequences of severe and recurrent affective disorders. Psychotherapy for these patients requires considerable flexibility of style and technique, aiming to enhance the patient's sense of control over his illness, over and above the effects of lithium. Themes which often emerge in therapy include the loss of 'highs', productivity, creativity, decreased sexuality, fears of recurrence, denial of illness, effects of illness on family, the risk for children and the developmental difficulties in those with early-onset illnesses involving their individuation, development of intimate relationships and loss of career opportunities.

Numerous self-help groups and organisations

provide advice and support to patients and their families.

The lithium clinic

The complexities of the management of patients with affective disorders demands the expertise of a team that includes psychiatrists, nurses, social workers and laboratory technicians. These complexities are partly inherent in the nature of the illnesses and the nature of lithium therapy as the main long-term treatment.

The concept of the lithium clinic was pioneered by psychiatrists who carried out the earlier studies on its efficacy in the 1960s, and was part of the movement for the establishment of specialist clinics for patients with conditions such as diabetes, epilepsy and schizophrenia. Lithium-treated patients are also commonly treated in general psychiatric clinics. The proportion of the lithium-treated patients managed by their general practitioners is unknown, but presumably small.

Lithium clinics serve a number of functions. Primarily they provide expert assessment and treatment settings in which patients' treatment is supervised and their plasma lithium levels monitored on a regular basis with regular monitoring of thyroid and renal function. A few clinics provide education to patients and their families on the nature of their condition and the benefits/hazards of lithium therapy. They are often tertiary referral centres, receiving referrals from general psychiatrists, and are manned by psychiatrists, nurses, social workers and occasionally laboratory technicians. Some of these clinics have also provided a setting for research on lithium. It is estimated that there are at least 200 lithium clinics in the USA, with the large majority based in the University centres and commonly manned by specialist nurses under supervision from psychiatrists. In addition to all the aforementioned functions, these clinics provide psychotherapy services and support groups for patients and their relatives.

Studies in the USA have reported greater treatment compliance rates, lower rates of recurrence and fewer episodes of toxicity in patients attending these clinics compared to those attending general psychiatric clinics. Studies in the UK reported similar findings. A recent study, which compared a lithium clinic with psychiatric out-patient clinics and general practice supervision, found that the lithium clinic provided closest supervision and best control of plasma lithium at a lower mean level. Moreover, glomerular impairment occurred more often in general practice patients who were prescribed their lithium once daily (Masterson et al 1988).

The cost-effectiveness of the lithium clinic has been evaluated. Fieve & Peselow (1987) showed that the costs of managing patients in the lithium clinic were 2–5 times less than for those managed in other settings. We have recently evaluated the service requirements for a large cohort of patients attending the Lithium Clinic associated with the MRC Neuropsychiatry Laboratory in Epsom (Coppen & Abou-Saleh 1988). Of the 128 patients on lithium for the whole of 1983, 14% (four men and 14 women) received some treatment as inpatients for a relapse in their affective illness. These 18 patients required a total of 217 weeks of inpatient treatment, or an average for the whole clinic of 3.3% of the time. The average length of stay in the ward for those admitted was 12 weeks. In the control group of patients treated with placebo lithium, 76% of the group required admission to hospital. For affective disorder patients maintained on lithium therapy, approximately four inpatient beds are required per 100 patients. For patients not maintained on lithium, but receiving only *ad hoc* treatment, this figure rises to about 25 inpatient beds per 100 patients.

Lithium clinics are often held in the mornings, an ideal arrangement which allows measurement of plasma lithium levels 12 hours after the last dose. On arrival, patients have their blood taken for on-the-spot lithium estimation in the nearby laboratory. The patient then joins fellow patients in the waiting room, which provides informal contact and a 'therapeutic milieu': patients who are ill are reassured and encouraged by those who are well with access to the attending nurse and social worker as required. This time is also used for weighing and, if required, the completion of rating scales and a side-effects checklist. Once the plasma level is estimated, patients are seen by the clinician for an assessment of their physical and psychiatric status, including their experience of side-effects, adjustment of dosage, the prescription of extra medication if necessary and arrangement of routine laboratory investigations and supportive psychotherapy. In our own clinic we have used a chart (Fig. 23.1) to record all this information, which is also used to estimate the patient's affective morbidity over time by the calculation of an affective morbidity index (Coppen et al 1973). Patients are given free access to the clinic outside the regular appointments and those who fail to attend are called upon in case they experience a recurrence in their illness, for early intervention.

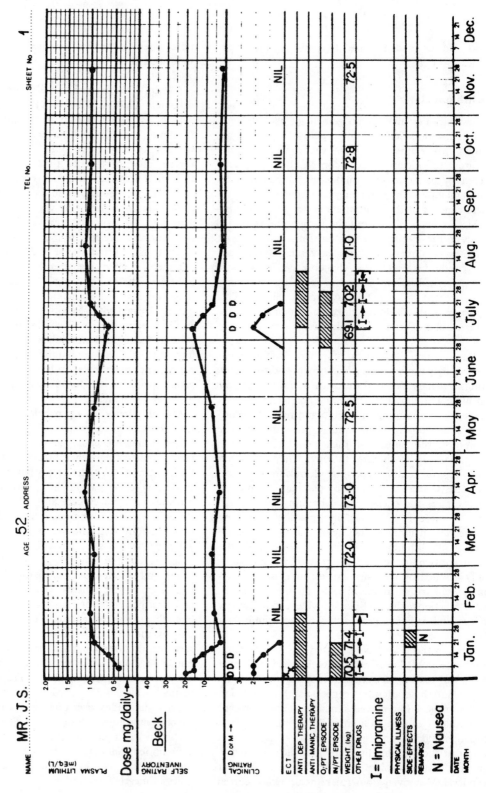

Fig. 23.1   A typical chart for a patient on lithium therapy

REFERENCES

Aagaard J, Vestergaard P 1990 Predictors of outcome in prophylactic lithium treatment: a 2-year prospective study. Journal of Affective Disorders 18: 259–266

Abou-Saleh M T, Coppen A 1983a Subjective side-effects of amitriptyline and lithium in affective disorders. British Journal of Psychiatry 142: 391–397

Abou-Saleh M T, Coppen A 1983b The prognosis of depression in old age: the case for lithium therapy. British Journal of Psychiatry 143: 527–528

Abou-Saleh M T, Coppen A 1985 The biology of folate in depression: implications for nutritional hypotheses for the psychoses. Journal of Psychiatric Research 20: 91–101

Abou-Saleh M T, Coppen A 1986 Who responds to prophylactic lithium? Journal of Affective Disorders 10: 115–125

Abou-Saleh M T, Coppen A 1988 Continuation therapy with antidepressants after electroconvulsive therapy. Convulsive Therapy 4 (4) 263–268

Abou-Saleh M T, Coppen A 1989a The efficacy of low-dose lithium: clinical, psychological and biological correlates. Journal of Psychiatric Research 23 (2) 157–162

Abou-Saleh M T, Coppen A 1989b Serum and red blood cell folate in depression. Acta Psychiatrica Scandinavica 80: 78–82

Abou-Saleh M T, Coppen A J 1990 Predictors of long-term outcome of mood disorder on prophylactic lithium. Lithium 1: 27–35

Amdisen A 1987 Historical origins. In: Johnson F N (ed) Depression and mania: modern lithium therapy. IRL Press, Oxford, p 24–28

Angst J 1981 Clinical indications for a prophylactic treatment of depression. Advances in Biological Psychiatry 7: 218–229

Angst J, Weis P, Grof P, Baastrup P C, Schou M 1970 Lithium prophylaxis in recurrent affective disorders. British Journal of Psychiatry 116: 604–614

Baastrup P C 1964 The use of lithium in manic-depressive psychosis. Comprehensive Psychiatry 5: 396

Baastrup P C, Schou M 1967 Lithium as a prophylactic agent against recurrent depression and manic-depressive psychosis. Archives of General Psychiatry 16: 162–172

Baastrup P C, Poulsen K S, Schou M et al 1970 Prophylactic lithium: double-blind discontinuation in manic-depressive and recurrent-depressive disorders. Lancet 2: 236–230

Bech P, Vendsborg P B, Rafaelsen O J 1976 Lithium maintenance treatment of manic-melancholic patients: its role in the daily routine. Acta Psychiatrica Scandinavica 53: 70–81

Bendz H 1983 Kidney function in lithium-treated patients: a literature survey. Acta Psychiatric Scandinavica 68: 303–324

Blackwell B, Shepherd M 1968 Prophylactic lithium: another therapeutic myth? An examination of the evidence to date. Lancet 1: 968

Campbell M, Small A M et al 1984 Behavioural efficacy of haloperidol and lithium. Archives of General Psychiatry 41: 650–656

Causemann B, Muller-Oerlinghausen B 1988 Does lithium prevent suicides and suicidal attempts? In: Birch N J (ed) Lithium: Organic, pharmacology and psychiatric use. IRL Press, Oxford, p 23–24

Cohen W J, Cohen N H 1974 Lithium carbonate, haloperidol, and irreversible brain damage. Journal of the American Medical Association 230: 1283–1287

Coppen A, Abou-Saleh M T 1982 Plasma folate and affective morbidity during long-term lithium therapy. British Journal of Psychiatry 141: 87–89

Coppen A, Abou-Saleh M T 1983 Lithium in prophylaxis of unipolar depression: a review. Journal of the Royal Society of Medicine 76: 297–301

Coppen A, Abou-Saleh M T 1988 Lithium therapy: from clinical trials to practical management. Acta Psychiatrica Scandinavica 78: 754–762

Coppen A, Noguera R, Bailey J et al 1971 Prophylactic lithium in affective disorders: controlled trial. Lancet 2: 275–279

Coppen A J, Peet M, Bailey J 1973 Double-blind and open prospective studies of lithium prophylaxis in affective disorders. Psychiatria Neurologia Neurochirurgia 76: 501–510

Coppen A, Bishop M, Bailey J, Cattell W, Price R 1980 Renal function in lithium and non-lithium treated patients with affective disorders. Acta Psychiatrica Scandinavica 62: 343–355

Coppen A, Abou-Saleh M T, Milln P 1981 Lithium continuation therapy following electroconvulsive therapy. British Journal of Psychiatry 139: 284–287

Coppen A, Abou-Saleh M T, Milln P, Bailey J, Wood K 1983 Decreasing lithium dosage reduces morbidity and side-effects during prophylaxis. Journal of Affective Disorders 5: 353–362

Coppen A, Chaudhry S, Swade C 1986 Folic acid enhances lithium prophylaxis. Journal of Affective Disorders 10 (1): 9–13

Coppen A, Standish-Barry H, Bailey J, Houston G, Silcocks P, Hermon C 1990 Long-term lithium and mortality. Lancet 335–1347

Coxhead N, Silverstone T 1987 The acute treatment of mania. In: Johnson F N (ed) Depression and mania: modern lithium therapy. IRL Press, Oxford p 31–35

Craft M, Ismail I A et al 1987 Lithium in the treatment of aggression in mentally handicapped patients. British Journal of Psychiatry 150: 685–689

Decina P, Fieve R R 1981 Prophylactic serum lithium levels in recurrent unipolar depression. Journal of clinical Psychopharmacology 1 (3): 150–152

Fieve R R, Peselow E D 1983 Lithium: clinical applications. In: Burrows G D, Norman T R, Davies B (eds) Antidepressants. Drugs in Psychiatry 1. Elsevier, Amsterdam, p 277–321

Fieve R R, Peselow E D 1987 The lithium clinic. In: Johnson F N (ed) Depression and mania: modern lithium therapy. IRL Press, Oxford, p 127–129

Gelenberg A J, Kane J M, Keller M B 1989 Comparison of standard and low serum levels of lithium for maintenance treatment of bipolar disorders. New England Journal of Medicine 321: 1489–1493

Glen A M I, Johnson A L, Shepherd M 1981 Continuation therapy with lithium and amitriptyline in unipolar depressive illness: a controlled clinical trial. Psychological Medicine 11: 409–416

Greil W, Broucek B, Klein H E, Engle-Sittenfeld P 1982 Discontinuation of lithium maintenance therapy: reversibility of clinical, psychological and neuroendocrinological changes. In: Emrich H M, Aldenhoff J B, Lux H D (eds) Basic mechanisms in the action of lithium. Excerpta Medica, Amsterdam, p 235–248

Greil W, Schmidt S 1987 Lithium withdrawal reaction. In: Birch N J (ed) Lithium: organic, pharmacology and psychiatric use. IRL Press, Oxford, p 149–153

Hall K S, Dunner D L, Zeller G et al 1977 Bipolar illness: a prospective study of life events. Comprehensive Psychiatry 18: 497–502

Hartigan G P 1963 The use of lithium salts in affective disorders. British Journal of Psychiatry 109: 810

Hestbech J, Hansen H E, Amdisen A et al 1977 Chronic renal lesions following long-term treatment with lithium. Kidney International 12: 205–213

Himmelhoch J M, Neil J F, May S J, Fuch C Z, Licata S M 1980 Age, dementia, dyskinesia and lithium response. American Journal of Psychiatry 137 (8): 941–945

Hullin R P, McDonald R, Allsopp M N 1972 Prophylactic lithium in recurrent affective disorders. Lancet 1: 1044–1046

Jamison K R 1987a Compliance with medication. In: Johnson F N (ed) Depression and mania: modern lithium therapy. IRL Press, Oxford, p 117–121

Jamison K R 1987b Psychological aspects of treatment. In: Johnson F N (ed) Depression and mania: modern lithium therapy. IRL Press, Oxford, p 121–124

Jensen H V, Olafsson K, Bille A, Andersen J, Mellerup E, Plenge P 1990 Lithium every second day: a new treatment regimen? Lithium 1: 55–58

Jerram T C, McDonald R 1978 Plasma lithium control, with particular reference to minimum effective levels. In: Johnson F N, Johnson S (eds) Lithium in medical practice. MTP Press, Lancaster, p 407–413

Källen B, Tandberg A 1983 Lithium and pregnancy: a cohort study of manic depressive women. Acta Psychiatrica Scandinavica 68: 134–139

Kukopulos A, Tondo A, Foggia D 1988 Electroconvulsive therapy. In: Johnson F N (ed) Depression and mania: modern lithium therapy. IRL Press, Oxford, p 177–179

Lauritsen B J, Mellerup E T, Plenge P, Rasmussen S, Vestergaard P, Schou M 1981 Serum lithium concentrations around the clock with different regimens and the diurnal variation of the renal lithium clearance. Acta Psychiatrica Scandinavica 64: 314–319

Lyskowski J, Nasrallah H A, Dunner F J, Bucher K 1982 A longitudinal survey of side effects in a lithium clinic. Journal of Clinical Psychiatry 43 (7): 284–286

Masterton G, Warner M, Roxburgh B 1988 Supervising lithium: a comparison of a lithium clinic, psychiatric out-patients clinics and general practice. British Journal of Psychiatry 152: 535–538

Mendels J 1976 Lithium in the treatment of depression. American Journal of Psychiatry 133: 373–377

Miller A L, Bowden C L, Plewes J 1985 Lithium and impairment of renal concentrating ability. Journal of Affective Disorders 9: 115–119

Milln P T S, Patch C 1988 Lithium dose reduction trial. In: Birch N J (Ed) Lithium: organic, pharmacology and psychiatric use. IRL Press, Oxford, p 33–34

Mindham R H, Howland C V, Shepherd M 1973 An evaluation of continuation therapy with tricyclic antidepressants in depressive illness. Psychological Medicine 6: 23–29

Mukherjee S, Rosen A M, Caracci G, Shukla S 1986 Persistent tardive dyskinesia in bipolar patients. Archives of General Psychiatry 43: 342–346

Murphy D L, Beigel A 1974 Depression, elation and lithium carbonate responses in manic patient sub-groups. Archives of General Psychiatry 31: 643–654

Norton B, Whalley L J 1984 Mortality of a lithium treated population. British Journal of Psychiatry 145: 277–282

Paykel E S, Dimascio A, Haskell D, Prusoff B A 1975 Effects of maintenance amitriptyline and psychotherapy on symptoms of depression. Psychological Medicine 5: 67

Perry A, Tsuang M T 1979 Treatment of unipolar depression following electroconvulsive therapy. Journal of Affective Disorders 1: 123–129

Peselow E D, Dunner D L, Fieve R R 1990 Psychopharmacology in clinical practice: the prophylaxis of unipolar depression. Lithium 1: 115–123

Plenge P, Mellerup E T, Bolwig T G, Brun C, Hetmar O, Ladefoged J, Larsen S, Rafaelsen O J 1982 Lithium treatment: does the kidney prefer one daily dose instead of two? Acta Psychiatrica Scandinavica 66: 121–128

Priebe S, Wildgrube C, Muller-Oerlinghausen B 1989 Lithium prophylaxis and expressed emotions. British Journal of Psychiatry 154: 396–399

Prien R F, Caffey E M 1976 Relationship between dosage and response to lithium prophylaxis in recurrent depression. American Journal of Psychiatry 133: 567–570

Prien R F, Caffey E M, Klett C J 1972 Comparison of lithium carbonate and chlorpromazine in the treatment of mania. Archives of General Psychiatry 26: 146–153

Prien R F, Caffey E M, Klett C J 1973a Prophylactic efficacy of lithium carbonate in manic-depressive illness. Archives of General Psychiatry 28: 337–341

Prien R F, Klett C J, Caffey E M 1973b Lithium carbonate and imipramine in prevention of affective episodes. A comparison in recurrent affective illness. Archives of General Psychiatry 29: 420–425

Prien R F, Kupfer D J, Mansky P A et al 1984 Drug therapy in the prevention of recurrences in unipolar and bipolar affective disorders. Archives of General Psychiatry 41: 1096–1104

Rudorfer M V, Linnoila M, Potter W Z 1987 Combined lithium and electroconvulsive therapy, pharmacokinetic and pharmacodynamic interactions. Convulsive Therapy 3: 40–45

Sarantidis D, Waters B 1981 Predictors of lithium prophylaxis effectiveness. Progress in Neuropsychopharmacology 5: 507–510

Sashidharan S P, McGuire R J 1983 Recurrence of affective illness after withdrawal of long-term lithium treatment. Acta Psychiatrica Scandinavica 68: 126–133

Sashidharan S P, McGuire R J, Glen A I M 1982 Plasma lithium levels and therapeutic outcome in the prophylaxis of affective disorders: a retrospective study. British Journal of Psychiatry 140: 619–622

Sautter F J, Garver D L 1987 Schizophrenia. In: Johnson F N (ed) Depression and mania: modern lithium therapy. IRL Press, Oxford, p 41–44

Schou M 1976 What happened to the lithium babies? A follow-up of children born without malformations. Acta Psychiatrica Scandinavica 54: 193–197

Schou M, Vestergaard P 1988 Prospective studies in a lithium cohort: renal function, water and electrolyte metabolism. Acta Psychiatrica Scandinavica 78: 427–433

Schou M, Amdisen A, Vestergaard P, Rafaelsen O J 1982 Lithium treatment regimen and renal water handling: the significance of dosage pattern and tablet type examined through comparison of results from two clinics with different treatment regimens. Psychopharmacology 77: 387–390

Schou M, Mortensen E, Vestergaurd P 1986 Erythrocyte folate before and during treatment with lithium. Human Psychopharmacology 1: 29–33

Sheard M H, Marini 1976 The effect of lithium on impulsive aggressive behaviour in man. American Journal of Psychiatry 133: 1409–1413

Shelley R, Silverstone T 1987 Lithium preparation. In: Johnson F N (ed) Depression and mania: modern lithium therapy. IRL Press, Oxford, p 94–98

Shopsin B, Temple H, Ingwer M, Kane S, Hirsch J 1979 Sudden death during lithium carbonate maintenance. In: Cooper T B, Gershon S, Kline N S, Schou M (eds) Lithium controversies and unresolved issues. Excerpta Medica, Amsterdam, p 527–551

Shulman K, Post F 1980 Bipolar affective disorder in old age. British Journal of Psychiatry 136: 26–32

Smith R E, Helms P M 1982 Adverse effects of lithium therapy in the acutely ill elderly patient. Journal of Clinical Psychiatry 43: 94–99

Stokes P E, Shamoian C A, Stoll P M et al 1971 Efficacy of lithium as acute treatment of manic-depressive illness. Lancet 1: 1319–1325

Tyrer S P, Hullin R P, Birch N J, Goodwin J C 1976 Absorption of lithium following administration of slow-release and conventional preparations. Psychological Medicine 6: 51–58

Tyrer S P, Walsh A, Edwards D E, Berney T P, Stephens D A 1984 Factors associated with a good response to lithium in aggressive mentally handicapped subjects. Progress in Neuropharmacology and Biological. Psychiatry 8: 751–755

Vestergaard P, Amdisen A 1981 Lithium treatment and kidney function: a follow up study of 237 patients in long-term treatment. Acta Psychiatrica Scandinavica 63: 333–345

Vestergaard P, Schou M 1984 The effects of age on lithium dosage requirements. Pharmacopsychiatry 17: 199–201

Vestergaard P, Poulstrup I, Schou M 1988 Prospective studies on a lithium cohort: tremor, weight gain, diarrhoea, psychological complaints. Acta Psychiatrica Scandinavica 78: 434–441

Wancata J, Simhandl C, Denk E, Lenz G et al 1988 Reliability of lithium related side-effects. In: Birch N J (ed) Lithium: organic, pharmacology and psychiatric use. IRL Press, Oxford, p 159–160

Waters B, Lapierre Y D, Gagnon A et al 1982 Determination of the optimal concentration of lithium for the prophylaxis of manic-depressive disorder. Biological Psychiatry 17: 1323–1329

Weinstein M R 1980 Lithium treatment of women during pregnancy and in the post-delivery period. In: Johnson F N (ed) Handbook of lithium therapy. MTP Press, Lancaster, p 421–429

Worrall E P, Moody J P, Naylor G J 1975 Lithium in non-manic depressives. British Journal of Psychiatry 126: 464–468

Worrall E P, Moody J P, Peet M 1979 Controlled studies of the acute antidepressant effects of lithium. British Journal of Psychiatry 135: 255–262

24. Anticonvulsants and novel drugs

Robert M. Post

Bipolar disorder presents unique difficulties in psychotherapeutic and pharmacological treatment. The illness is episodic, yet recurrent, with a tendency to faster if not more severe recurrences as a function of course of illness (Fig. 24.1). Thus, it behooves the physician and clinician to develop a systematic charting approach to mapping the course of illness, as this not only provides the best predictor of likely recurrences in the future, but is also of inestimable value in assessing the efficacy of prior treatment and thus in formulating novel treatment strategies for the future. A method for plotting the illness is illustrated in Figure 24.2 and

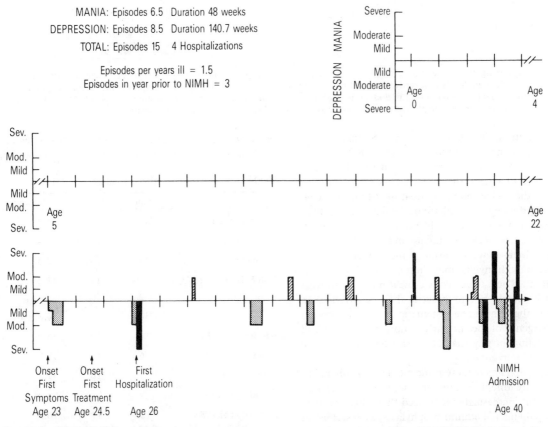

Fig. 24.1 Median course of affective illness in 82 bipolar manic-depressive patients admitted to NIMH. Note decreasing duration of well intervals between episodes (faster cycling) and increasing severity of illness

387

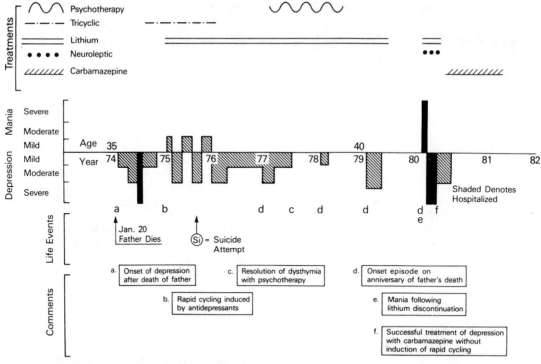

Fig. 24.2   Graphing the course of affective illness: prototype of a 'life chart'. Note how manic and depressive episodes can be plotted at three different levels of severity: mild = distinctly abnormal mood but no functional impairment; moderate = definite functional impairment in social or occupational roles; severe = functionally incapacitated or hospitalized (shaded). Medications and psychosocial stressors can be plotted concomitantly above and below the mood ratings respectively

described in more detail elsewhere (Squillace et al 1984, Roy-Byrne et al 1985, Post et al 1988a).

In addition to this recurrent and, at times, progressive course of illness, the impairments of the discrete episodes themselves often are treatment-limiting. That is, during the depressive phase of the illness the patient may be apathetic and guilt ridden and, therefore, unmotivated to seek treatment, and may be actively suicidal. In a converse fashion, the denial of illness associated with mania may impose equal treatment difficulties. Thus, it becomes critical not only to treat episodes acutely but to prevent their recurrence. In addition, there should be systematic contracting around the emergence of specific early symptoms that will lead to contacting the physician and institution of alternative treatment interventions.

Even with many of these principles closely adhered to in many treatment settings and sophisticated lithium clinics, it is increasingly recognized that a high proportion of patients fail lithium prophylaxis, as described in Table 24.1. Embedded in this overall non-response rate of some 40% is a variety of subtypes that are

peculiarly vulnerable to lithium non-responsiveness. As summarized in Table 24.2, the studies are consistent in

Table 24.1   Lithium prophylaxis failures: typical studies

	Failed	Total	% failures
Dunner et al 1976	44	96	46.0
Okuma et al 1973	8	18	44.4
Prien et al 1973	43	101	42.5
Itoh & Ishigane 1973	7	17	41.2
Page et al 1987	6	59	10.2 or
	30		50.8 (partial)
Kishimoto et al 1986	11	42	26.1
Prien et al 1988	6	16	37.5
Watkins et al 1987	5	16	31.2
Placidi et al 1986	7	14	50.0
Lusznat et al 1988	12	17	70.5
Totals	149	380	39.2

demonstrating the lack of acute and long-term responsivity in patients with dysphoric mania. In addition to these systematic studies, there is convergent data with the early observations of Baastrup & Schou (1967) that their patients with dysphoric mania were often non-responsive. As illustrated in Table 24.3, lithium non-response often occurs in patients with more rapid-cycling manic-depressive illness, although this is not invariable.

The sequential pattern of evolution of episodes is also a relative predictor of lithium non-response. Patients with the presentation of inital depressions followed by a swing into mania and then a well interval (D—M—I) are at a much higher risk of lithium non-response than those showing the converse pattern (M—D—I), i.e. mania, depression, well interval (Grof et al 1987, Haag et al 1987, Kukopulos et al 1980, Maj et al 1989b).

Table 24.2 Response to lithium in dysphoric mania

	Dysphoric manics	Non-dysphoric
Himmelhoch & Garfinkel 1986	11/26 (42%)	47/58 (81%)
Secunda et al 1987	2/7 (29%)	9/10 (90%)
Prien et al 1988		
Acute completers (not drop-out)	(39/99) (39%)	(59/101) (59%)
Prophylactic response	4/18 (22%)	16/17 (94%)
Totals	17/51 (33%)	72/85 (84%)

In addition, Kukopulos and associates (1983) and Altshuler et al (unpublished manuscript, 1990) have described patients with tricyclic-induced manias who appear to be at risk for the development of more rapid-

Table 24.3 Rapid cycling and response to lithium or carbamazepine

Good response	No prediction	Poor response
Lithium		
Schou 1973	Svestka & Nahunek 1975	Prien et al 1973, 1984
Page et al 1987	Dostal 1977	Dunner & Fieve 1974
	Itoh & Ishigane 1973	Misra & Burns 1977
	Kishimoto et al 1986 (but 10/42 cycling)	Kukopulos et al 1980, 1983
		Nolen 1983
		Hanus & Zapletalek 1984
		Abou-Saleh & Coppen 1986
		Goodnick et al 1987
Carbamazepine*		
Okuma et al 1973 (P)		
Post et al 1983b (P)		
Post et al 1987b (A)		
Post et al 1990b (P)		
Joffe et al 1990 (A,P) (unpublished manuscript)		
Joyce 1988 (P) (7/13 or 4/12)		
Nolen 1983 (P)		
Stromgren & Boller 1985 (P)		
Elphick 1985 (A,P)		
Post et al 1988a (P)		

*Studies were not necessarily predictive. (A) indicates acute study; (P) indicates prophylactic study.

cycling illness in spite of lithium prophylaxis. In the studies of Kukopulos et al (1980), patients with a continuous form of the illness also appear to be at high risk for lithium non-responsiveness.

Finally, there is some evidence that familial and, possibly, genetic factors are associated with lithium response and non-response. Studies are consistent in showing that a positive lithium response is highly associated with a family history of affective illness in first-degree relatives if not a history of lithium-responsive illness itself (Hanus & Zapletalek 1984, Mendelwicz et al 1973, Fieve et al 1976, Maj et al 1984).

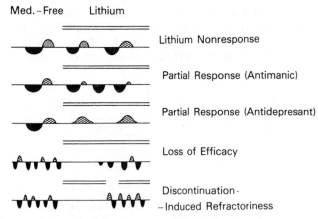

Fig. 24.3 Pattern of lithium non-responsiveness. Manic and depressive episodes are plotted above and below the line respectively. Lithium treatment is represented by double bar. Non-response and partial response are well recognized, but gradual loss of response in spite of continued treatment is a novel pattern suggested by a small minority of our NIMH patients and those of Maj et al 1989. The last pattern reflects the reappearance of episodes after lithium discontinuation; there is no longer a response to lithium when it is reinstituted

Thus, there is a panoply of presentations of the illness that are associated with non-response to traditional agents used in acute and prophylactic treatment. The patterns of non-response are illustrated in Figure 24.3, which highlights two processes for lithium non-responsiveness in addition to those traditionally recognized and described above. Loss of efficacy over time is not a widely appreciated clinical phenomenon and has not been systematically documented in the literature; it has not yet received the clinical investigative and theoretical attention that it deserves. The problem of loss of efficacy was recently reported by Maj et al (1989a), who followed a series of patients, all of whom showed an excellent and complete prophylactic

response to lithium for the first 2 years of treatment. However, upon follow-up at 5 years, they noted that 25 of 49 patients (51%) showed relapses. Four of these patients had three or more episodes in the last 2 years, suggesting clear loss of efficacy. These observations are consistent with our own unpublished data, indicating that a substantial subgroup (58%) of patients referred to the National Institute of Mental Health because of treatment refractoriness had shown an initial good response to lithium.

We have also recently observed several patients who demonstrated apparent lithium-induced discontinuation refractoriness; that is, patients who initially had a good response to lithium were withdrawn from the medication, experienced the onset of a new and severe episode, and then did not respond to the reinstitution of lithium (Altshuler & Post, unpublished observations, 1989). (One of these patients is illustrated in Figure 7 of Post 1990b.) While these observations have not been systematically documented in a large series of patients, they are not without precedent. Angst (personal communication, 1988) has found not only that 80% of his well-maintained patients show exacerbations on lithium discontinuation but that a substantial percentage appear to show this phenomenon of lack of renewal of clinical response to lithium once treatment is reinstituted. This raises the danger that not only may some patients show new episodes upon lithium discontinuation, and even show a withdrawal reaction (Mander & Loudon 1988), but the reappearance of episodes may engender a process of non-responsiveness. This may be the pharmacological equivalent of letting the manic-depressive horse out of the barn or the parallel of observations of refractoriness developing to primary treatments of tumours once they have metastasized. These data further emphasize the importance of maintenance of adequate prophylaxis, not only to prevent the occurrence of acute episodes but also to inhibit or forestall the potential sensitization phenomenon that comes with the occurrence of multiple episodes (Post et al 1984a, 1986b, 1988b).

We will review the emerging evidence for alternative treatments to lithium and the traditional unimodal antidepressants (heterocyclics and monoamine oxidase inhibitors [MAOIs]) and unimodal antimanics (neuroleptics and reserpine). The anticonvulsant drugs are best studied in this regard but other classes of compounds, such as the calcium channel blockers, appear to play an important role in treatment-refractory illness. In addition, we will mention several other groups of agents and pharmacological strategies that

Table 24.4 Controlled studies of carbamazepine (CBZ) and oxcarbazepine (OXCBZ)* in acute mania

Study	n	Diagnosis	Design	Dose of CBZ (mg/day) [blood level]	Other drugs	Duration	Results
Ballanger & Post 1978 Post et al 1984a; 1987b	19	M-D	D-bl, (B-A-B-A)	600–2000 [7–15.5 μg/ml]	None	11–56 days	12/19 improved – time course similar to neuroleptics; frequent relapses on placebo subsitution
Okuma et al 1979	32 CBZ 28 CPZ	M-D psychosis ICD-9	Bl. vs CPZ 150–450 mg	300–900 [2.7–11.7 μg/ml] [mean = 7.2 ± 3.4]	Bedtime hypnotics	3–5 weeks	21/23 improved on CBZ (marked to moderate) 15/28 improved on CPZ
Klein et al 1984	11	Manic	Blind vs placebo	600–1600 [6–18 μg/ml]	Halo, (15–45 mg/d) all patients	5 weeks	10/14 improved on CBZ + haloperidol
	3	Excited SA	addition to halo.				(7/13 improved on placebo + haloperidol)
Muller & Stoll 1984	6	M-D	Blind vs placebo	600–1200 mg	Halo. & hypnotics	3 weeks	7/6 p<0.01 better than placebo
Muller & Stoll 1984	10	M-D	Bld vs halo. (15–20 mg)	600–1200 mg OXCBZ	Halo. & hypnotics	2 weeks	7/10 OXCBZ = halo.
Grossi et al 1984	18 CBZ 19 CPZ	M-D	Blind vs CPZ randomized 200–500 mg CPZ	200–1200 mg 200–500 mg	?	21 days	10/15 improved on CBZ 13/17 improved on CPZ CBZ = fewer side-effects than CPZ
Emrich et al* 1985	7	Manic psychoses	D-Bl.(B-A-B)	1800–2100 OXCBZ	None	Variable	6/7 (>25% improved on IMPS)
Stoll et al 1986	14 CBZ 18 halo.	Manic	Randomized vs halo. 5–30mg/d	600–1200 mg	CPZ	3 weeks	12/14 improved on CBZ 12/18 improved on halo.
Lerer et al 1987	14 CBZ 14 Li	M-D	Bl. vs Li randomized	600–2600 mg (3.3–14 μg/ml)	Chloral hydrate Barbiturates H.S.	28 days	4/14 improved on CBZ 11/14 improved on Li CGI = p < 0.05 (Li) BPRS = n.s.
Lusznat et al 1988	22 CBZ	Manic	Bl. vs Li (0.6–1.4 mmol/l)	(0.6–1.2 mmol/l)	CPZ. Halo. Temazepam	6 weeks	No significant difference; CBZ required non-significantly more neuroleptics, however
Brown et al 1989	8 CBZ 9 Halo	Manic	Bl. vs halo. 20–80 mg/d	400–1600 mg	CPZ to 3 pts on CBZ to 7 pts on halo.	4 weeks	6/8 marked improvement CBZ 3/9 marked improvement halo. CBZ showed slower onset but higher completion rate (75% vs 22%) with fewer EPS & less procyclidine required

Table 24.4 Controlled studies of carbamazepine (CBZ) and oxcarbazepine (OXCBZ)* in acute mania — (contd)

Study	n	Diagnosis	Design	Dose of CBZ (mg/day) [blood level]	Other drugs	Duration	Results
Lenzi et al 1986	11 CBZ 11 Li	M-D & SA	Bl. vs Li	400–1600 mg (7–12 µg/ml) 900 mg (0.6–1.2 mEq/l)	CPZ all patients	19 days	Equal efficacy in CBZ & Li groups. Less CPZ required in CBZ group acutely. CBZ better on paranoia; less EPS
Desai et al 1987	5	Manic	Bl. vs placebo addition to Li	400 mb fixed dose	?	4 weeks	CBZ + Li ($p < 0.05$) better on BRMS scores than Li alone by 2nd week
Okuma et al 1988	50 CBZ 51 Li	M-D	Bl. vs Li	400–1200 mg	Neuroleptics	4 weeks	31/50 improved on CBZ 30/51 improved on Li onset earlier on CBZ
Okuma et al 1988	103 CBZ 98 plac.	SA; S; atypical P	Bl. vs placebo		Neuroleptics		50% improved on CBZ 30% improved on placebo
Small et al 1989	22 CBZ	M-D	Bl. vs Li		Hypnotics	6–8 weeks	No significant difference after 8 weeks. CBZ significantly better than Li in 2nd & 3rd weeks of treatment
Moller et al 1989	11 CBZ 9 plac.	Manic or SA	Bl vs placebo addition to halo.	600 mg	Halo. 24 mb/d all patients Levomepromazine	3 weeks	No significant difference. Less levomepromazine needed in CBZ group
Emrich 1990	17 OXCBZ 20 halo.	Acute mania	Bl vs halo. mean = 42 mg/d	2400 OXCBZ 600 CBZ	?	15 days	16/17 improved w/OXCBZ (excellent or good) 15/20 improved w/halo. (excellent or good)
Emrich 1990	29 OXCBZ 24 Li	Acute mania	Bl. vs Li	1400 OXCBZ 800 CBZ	?	15 days	27/29 improved w/OXCBZ (excellent or good) 22/24 improved w/halo. (excellent or good)
Total of all 19 studies	412 Patients on carbamazepine						155/221 (70%) improved w/CBZ.

Abbreviations: CBZ = carbamazepine; CPZ = chlorpromazine; Li = lithium; OXCBZ = Oxcarbazepine; IMPS = Inpatient Multidimension Rating Scale; BRMS = Bech-Raefelson Mania Scale; CGI = Clinical Global Impressions; BPRS = Brief Psychiatric Rating Scale; EPS = Extrapyramidal Side Effects.

are supported by some clinical or research evidence for their efficacy in acute or prophylactic treatment of bipolar illness.

CARBAMAZEPINE IN THE TREATMENT OF BIPOLAR ILLNESS

Acute mania

The studies documenting the acute antimanic efficacy of carbamazepine are summarized in Table 24.4. These include systematic comparisons with neuroleptics (six studies), lithium (six studies), placebo (five studies) or placebo crossover using an A-B-A design (two studies). Across the vast majority of these studies, acute antimanic efficacy of carbamazepine is documented. This tends to occur with a time course similar to that observed with neuroleptics, although several studies report slightly faster onsets of antimanic effects in the first several days of treatment (Cookson 1987, Post et al 1987b). However, by the end of the first week of treatment most studies show an approximately equal and parallel efficacy of these two treatment agents. Thus, the data suggest that antimanic onset with carbamazepine may be faster than that observed with lithium, based both on direct comparisons and also on the well-documented perspective that neuroleptics may show more rapid onset than lithium in the treatment of acute mania (Post et al 1980).

The clinical correlates of acute responsivity to carbamazepine in mania have not been systematically and extensively documented, although a preliminary clinical literature suggests that many of the patients with illness types described above, who are relatively non-responsive to lithium, may respond to carbamazepine acutely or prophylactically. Thus, in our series (Post et al 1987b), patients who showed excellent response to carbamazepine in acute mania were significantly more manic at the outset of treatment during the placebo period, showed a trend ($p < 0.10$) to be more dysphoric (i.e. to show prominent elements of anxiety and depression during their mania), and were significantly more rapid-cycling in the year prior to admission to the National Institute of Mental Health. In addition, they were characterized by a higher incidence of a negative family history of affective illness in first-degree relatives. These data are consistent with those of P. Grof (personal communication, 1983).

Our initial studies (Post et al 1983a) did not support a robust relationship between plasma levels of carbamazepine and degree of clinical response. Given the wide individual variation in the occurrence of side-effects and tolerance of carbamazepine (Tomson 1984), we would suggest slow initiation of treatment and upward titration of dose based on a side-effect profile. Typical side-effects likely to occur in the first several weeks of treatment include dizziness, ataxia, diplopia and sedation. As enzymes are induced within the first 2–3 weeks of treatment, doses that were not tolerated initially will often be well-accepted, so that slow upward titration to individual side-effect thresholds, rather than attempting to reach average doses of blood levels, appears to be the most expeditious treatment approach.

Acute depression

Acute antidepressant effects of carbamazepine are less well documented. In the only large systematic, double-blind study to date, we have observed good acute antidepressant responses to carbamazepine in approximately one-third of treatment-refractory depressed patients, as illustrated in Figure 24.4. It is of interest that those with a greater severity of initial depression, a history of more rapid cycling and of less chronic depression appear to be among those who responded best to carbamazepine (Post et al 1986c). Interestingly, non-

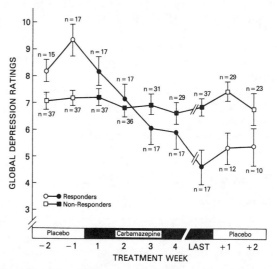

Fig. 24.4 Time-course of antidepressant response to the double-blind administration of carbamazepine. Note that significant improvement occurred in approximately one-third of our refractory patients following the second week and became clinically robust by the third, fourth and last weeks of treatment. Many patients did not relapse upon placebo substitution. Responders were chosen on the basis of two-point or greater weekly mean changes on Bunney—Hamburg depression scale (from placebo)

predictors appear to be minor EEG abnormalities, a history of robust psychosensory and psychomotor symptoms on systematic clinical interview and other measures that might reflect the possibility of a covert seizure disorder. While initial acute response to sleep deprivation appears to be associated with better acute antidepressant response to carbamazepine (Roy-Byrne et al 1984b), the addition of subsequent patients showed that this finding was no longer reliable. Paradoxically, we observed that those with the greatest decrements in thyroid indices showed greater degrees of antidepressant response (Roy-Byrne et al 1984a, Post et al 1987a).

Carbamazepine showed the usual lag in onset of antidepressant effectiveness in responsive patients, requiring some 3–4 weeks or longer to show maximum degrees of clinical efficacy. These data contrast with the more rapid onset of efficacy when lithium augmentation is utilized, where responses can often be observed in the first week of treatment. The degree of efficacy of carbamazepine as an augmentation strategy remains to be clearly delineated. However, in light of the data that traditional unimodal antidepressants such as the heterocyclics and MAOIs can be associated with a risk of manic induction, rapid cycling, or conversion of the bipolar patient to the continuous form of cycling, we would encourage the systematic clinical and research exploration of the use of carbamazepine as an alternative to the unimodal agents in the patient who is inadequately responsive to lithium alone.

An excellent and sustained antidepressant response, in a patient who required multiple courses of electroconvulsive therapy in order to treat her acute psychotic depression, is illustrated in Figure 24.5.

Prophylaxis

Clinical evidence

As summarized in Table 24.5, the data are not insubstantial for carbamazepine's effectiveness in long-term prophylaxis. Using a variety of designs, controlled clinical trials report a 71% marked or excellent response rate to carbamazepine. A substantially larger number of patients were studied in these partially controlled clinical trials, although systematic categorization of the response of individual patients was not always available. However, the response in these studies, approximately 71%, is even higher than that derived from the uncontrolled studies, where 288 of

449 patients (or 64%) have been reported to be responsive to institution of this treatment, usually as an adjunct to lithium and other previously ineffective treatment agents but, in some instances, to the use of carbamazepine alone. In our own study, we have observed sustained prophylactic response in some patients followed for more than 12 years (Post et al 1990a). However, as illustrated in Figure 24.6, a subgroup of patients show an initial good response to carbamazepine prophylaxis but then begin to show the emergence of episodes in the second, third or fourth year of treatment. Such a response is illustrated in an individual patient in Figure 24.7. This patient was a rapid and continuously cycling patient who was inadequately responsive to treatment with lithium and various antidepressants used either alone or adjunctively. She showed only an initial response to carbamazepine alone but, with the addition of lithium, demonstrated a complete remission of her ultrarapid cycling illness at the National Institute of Mental Health. She did well for approximately 4 years following discharge, with only minor episodes of dysphoria, but in the past year has begun to show the re-emergence of episodes in spite of good maintenance treatment with lithium and carbamazepine as well as adjunctive use of other treatments. We have discussed a variety of possible explanations for this loss of prophylactic efficacy (Post et al 1990a, Leverich et al 1990, Weiss & Post 1991a), but suggest that one possibility for this phenomenon is the development of tolerance to the psychotropic effects of carbamazepine similar to that reported previously for lithium (Maj et al 1989a).

Contingent tolerance as a mechanism for loss of efficacy

Weiss & Post (1991a) have documented an interesting preclinical model for the development of tolerance to the anticonvulsant effects of carbamazepine, which may be pertinent (on a very different time scale) to the emergence of tolerance to the psychotropic effects of carbamazepine in patients with manic-depressive illness. Remarkably, Weiss has shown that tolerance emerges only in animals repeatedly treated with carbamazepine prior to an amygdala-kindled seizure, but does not occur when the drug is administered after a seizure has occurred and then animals are switched to pretreatment. Moreover, once animals have become tolerant to the anticonvulsant effects of carbamazepine on amygdala-kindled seizures, this can be reversed by a period of administering kindled seizures without drug,

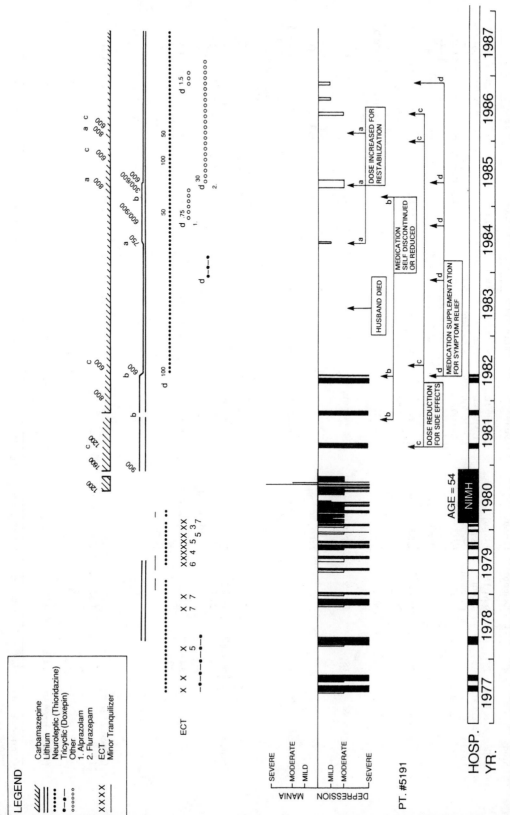

Fig. 24.5 Prophylaxis maintained with optimal management of dose titration (against side effects). Following a period of 11 hospitalizations and courses of ECT in spite of treatment with tricyclic antidepressants, lithium and neuroleptics, this patient was stabilized on the combination of carbamazepine and lithium. Breakthrough episodes occured in 1981–1982 because of reductions or discontinuations but, with careful dose titration and augmentation with neuroleptics or benzodiazepines, major episodes and the need for hospitalizations were aborted

Table 24.5 Controlled and quasi-controlled* studies of carbamazepine prophylaxis in manic-depressive illness

Study	n	Diagnosis	Design	Dose of carbamazepine mg/day	Other drugs	Duration	Results
Ballenger & Post 1978, Post et al 1983b	7	6 M-D 1 conf. psychosis	4 blind 3 open	800–2000 mg (11.3 µg/ml) (7.5–15.5 µg/ml)	None for 3 patients Li in 3 Neuroleptics in 1	6–51 months	6/7 improved, especially Li non-responsive cyclers
Okuma et al 1981	12 CBZ: 10 placebo	M-D	CBZ vs placebo Blind Randomized	400–600 mg (5.6 ± 2.0 µg/ml)	Acute treatments added during episode breakthroughs	12 months either R_x	6/10 improved on CBZ 2/9 improved on placebo ($p < 0.10$ diff.)
Placidi et al 1986	CBZ: 20 9 Li: 19 8	M-D SA M-D SA	CBZ vs lithium Blind Randomized	400–1600 mg (7–12 µg/ml)	Acute treatments added during episode breakthroughs	36 months	21/29 marked to moderate improvement on CBZ 20/27 on Li improved by relapse criteria
Kishimoto & Okuma 1985	18	BPI & II	Open crossover (A—B or B—A) vs Li (400–800 mg)	200–600 mg		> 1 year each $\bar{X}$ = 52.4 months CBZ $\bar{X}$ = 42.2 monghs Li	Significantly fewer hospitalization on CBZ; CBZ effective in Li non-responders
Watkins et al 1987	19 CBZ Li	7 UP 12 BP	CBZ vs Li D-blind Randomized	(5–12 µg/ml)	Antidepressants as needed		16/19 improved on CBZ 15/18 improved on Li $p<0.001$ increases in months of remission both drugs Li > CBZ
Bellaire et al 1988	50 CBZ	18 UP 24 UP	CBZ vs Li Open Randomized	600–800 mg (0.2–12.5 µg/ml)		24 months	Global efficacy and tolerance N.S. favour CBZ
Luznat et al 1988	20 CBZ 20 Li	M-D	CBZ vs Li Blind Randomized	(6–12 µg/ml)	Neuroleptics: antidepressants as needed	12 months	9/16 satisfactory on CBZ 5/19 satisfactory on Li CBZ nonsignificantly better than Li on readmission, depression, side-effects
Cabrera et al** 1986	4 CBZ 6 Li	3 BP 1 SA 5 BP 1 SA	BX vs Li Randomized	1050–1350 mg/d* (5.3–11.2 µg/ml)	Neuroleptic in 1 CBZ Neuroleptic in 2 Li	6–16 months	2/4 improved on CBZ 3/6 improved on Li
**Oxcarbazepine	4 CBZ	4 BP	Open	900–1200 mg/d (6.25–15.8 µg/ml)	Li in 1	16 months	2/4 improved on CBZ

Controlled studies = 60/85 (71%) response to carbamazepine. Uncontrolled studies = 288/449 (64%) response to carbamazepine. Total = 348/534 (65%) response.
*Blinded: crossover or randomized

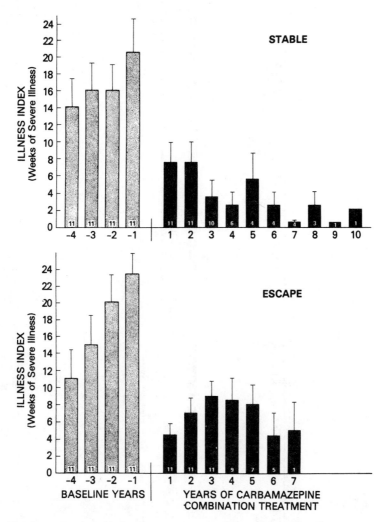

Fig. 24.6   Persistence of carbamazepine prophylaxis. One-half of our patients followed on carbamazepine show persistence of effective prophylaxis ('stable' group, top) while the other half show some loss of efficacy in the second, third or fourth years of treatment ('escape' group, bottom). During the baseline years of treatment before carbamazepine, the escape group showed a more rapid deterioration, as reflected in the illness index. The illness index is calculated on the basis of weeks ill/year times severity, with mild = 0.25; moderate = 0.5; severe = 1.0)

or giving the drug on a once-daily basis as before but immediately after a seizure has occurred. Tolerance does not dissipate with the mere passage of time, waiting either 11 days or 21 days. Tolerance also does not diminish if carbamazepine is administered without seizure induction. Thus, it would appear that the specific pairing of drug and seizure is required in order

to reverse the contingent tolerance phenomenon; i.e. a seizure is required to occur either without drug treatment or with carbamazepine treatment given after the seizure.

Interestingly, once animals demonstrated tolerance to the anticonvulsant effects of carbamazepine they showed responsivity to diazepam but not a drug (PK-

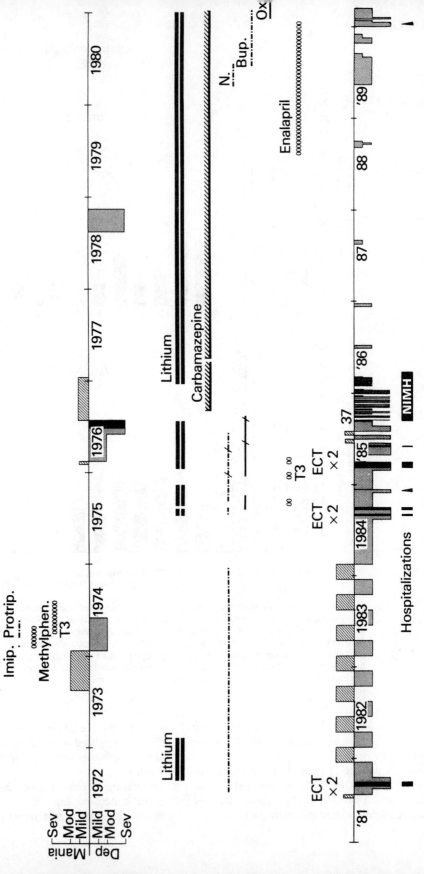

Fig. 24.7 Loss of prophylactic efficacy in a rapid-cycling bipolar II female patient. This patient illustrates progressive acceleration of the course of bipolar II illness with tricyclic-related continous cycling (1981–1983) and ultra-rapid cycling in 1985, in spite of lithium co-treatment. The patient showed a complete response to the combination of carbamazepine and lithium and maintained effective prophylaxis for 4 years. In 1989 she showed re-emergence of more protracted and severe episodes despite adjunctive treatment with nortriptyline (N), bupropion (Bup.) or oxazepam (Ox.), and required rehospitalization

11195) that acts as 'peripheral-type' benzodiazepine receptors, which are thought to be the locus of anticonvulsant action for carbamazepine (Weiss & Post 1991b). Thus, it would appear that there is crosstolerance to drugs acting through the same receptor mechanism but lack of cross-tolerance to drugs acting through different neuronal mechanisms (diazepam works through 'central' rather than 'peripheral-type' benzodiazepine receptors linked to the benzodiazepine GABA-chloride ionophore). Therefore, these preclinical data suggest the possible utility of switching patients who have become refractory to carbamazepine to other agents with different mechanisms of action or even, in the case of refractoriness of carbamazepine, the possible potential benefit of a period of medication-free evaluation with reinstitution of the drug at a later time. As in the contingent tolerance phenomenon observed clinically, it is possible that a period of time off medication, during which an affective episode has occurred, might be sufficient to renew psychotropic responsivity to a drug that had previously shown positive effects. Obviously, prospective clinical studies are required in order to document the validity of these two approaches to the treatment of patients in whom the drug has lost its efficacy.

In our preclinical model, merely treating the animals with an increased dose or raising the dose was insufficient to renew efficacy. It was of some interest that animals treated with higher doses of carbamazepine became tolerant at the same or an even faster rate than animals treated with a lower dose of drug (15 mg/kg i.p.). Thus, traditional responses of the clinician such as dose increases in the face of lost efficacy may or may not be adequate to renew responsivity if loss of efficacy is based on such a contingent tolerance phenomenon. We have observed at least one patient where renewed responsivity appeared to occur after a period of medication-free evaluation (Pazzaglia & Post 1991). Anecdotal evidence for renewed responsivity following a period off medication has also been reported by J. Fawcett (personal communication, 1988), B. Grosser (personal communication, 1988) and John Greden (personal communication 1988). Moreover, J. Engel (personal communication 1988) has reported that he has observed renewed responsivity to the anticonvulsant effects of carbamazepine following a period of medication-free evaluation, when patients experienced seizures during the evaluation for epilepsy surgery. In those patients who were not chosen for surgery and were replaced on medication, a period of at least transient increased

responsivity was observed, consistent with contingent tolerance.

Side-effect profile

The side-effects of carbamazepine in relationship to the pharmacotherapy of affective disorders are discussed in detail elsewhere (Uhde 1983, Joffe et al 1984, 1985, Post et al 1987a, Jefferson & Greist 1987, Pellock 1987, Post & Weiss 1989, Kramlinger & Post 1990, McElroy et al 1990). They are briefly summarized in Table 24.6, in comparison and contrast with those of lithium. Particularly noteworthy is the ability of lithium to reverse and override the benign white-count suppression of carbamazepine (Kramlinger & Post 1990). This appears to be occurring at the level of colony-stimulating factor, where carbamazepine consistently decreases these factors for platelets and megakaryocytes and lithium stimulates this effect at clinically therapeutic doses (Gallicchio & Hulette 1989). Thus adjunctive use of lithium in the face of benign white-count suppression may be attempted, but it is unlikely that lithium would be of utility in the more malignant or idiosyncratic cases of agranulocytosis and aplastic anaemia. This is all the more the case in the light of the evidence that lithium does not stimulate colony-stimulating factor for the erythropoietic series, which can also be involved in the process of carbamazepine-induced aplastic anaemia.

There is a wide variability in the recommendations for frequency of haematological monitoring during carbamazepine administration. Many authorities have conservatively suggested weekly monitoring in the first 4 months and monthly monitoring thereafter although, more recently, guidelines for monitoring have been made less specific in the *Physicians' Desk Reference*. Clearly, patients should be warned to consult their physician in the face of signs or symptoms that may be associated with agranulocytosis or aplastic anaemia. These would include the occurrence of rash, sore throat or other febrile illness, petechiae or other sign of bleeding disorder. These have been observed to occur, in some instances, in between regular monthly complete blood-count monitoring, further raising the question of the lack of clinical utility of even frequent monitoring in the face of rare but potentially serious and fatal idiosyncratic haematological complications. Obtaining a good informed consent and educating the patient regarding this potential problem are therefore of critical importance in the management of this infrequent drug side-effect.

Table 24.6   Comparative clinical and side-effect profiles of lithium and carbamazepine

	Lithium	Carbamazepine	Lithium carbamazepine combination
Clinical profile			
Mania	+ +	+ +	+ + +
Dysphoric	(+)	+	+ +
Rapid-cycling	+	+ +	+ + +
Continuous-cycling	(+)	+	+ +
Family history negative	+	+ +	+ + +
Depression	+	+	+ + +
Prophylaxis of mania and depression	+ +	+ +	+ + +
Epilepsy	0	+ +	?
Pain syndromes	0	+ +	?
Side effects			
White blood count	↑	↓	(↑),Li*
Diabetes insipidus	↑	↓	↑, Li*
Thyroid hormones T3, T4	↓	↓	↓↓
TSH	↑	--	↑,Li*
Serum calcium	↑	↓	?
Weight gain	↑	(--)	
Tremor	↑	--	
Memory disturbances	(↑)	?	
Diarrhoea	(↑)	--	
Teratogenesis	(↑)	(↑)	
Psoriasis	(↑)	--	
Pruritic rash (allergy)	--	↑	
Agranulocytosis	--	(↑)	
Hepatitis	--	(↑)	
Hyponatraemia, water intoxication	--	↑	
Dizziness, ataxia, diplopia	--	↑	
Hypercortisolism, escape from dexamethasone suppression	--	↑	

Clinical efficacy		**Side effects**	
0	none	↑	increase
+	effective	↓	decrease
+ +	very effective	( )	inconsistent or rare
+ + +	possible synergism	--	absent
( )	equivocal	↓↓	potentiation
		Li*	effect of lithium predominates

On the other end of the continuum is a side-effect that appears very common with the use of carbamazepine in psychiatric patients. We have observed a 12–14% incidence of rash following carbamazepine administration. This typically occurs between days 9 and 23 of treatment, although a late-appearing rash can also be experienced (Kramlinger et al, unpublished manuscript). The appearance of a macular rash and pruritus should lead to drug discontinuation, as reports have appeared of carbamazepine-induced rashes progressing to desquamation, exfoliation and the Stevens – Johnson syndrome. While some studies have suggested the possible rechallenge of patients with carbamazepine without reappearance of the rash, typically this is associated with earlier rash than on initial observation. If a patient appears to be a responder to carbamazepine and does not respond adequately or tolerate other agents, a retrial of carbamazepine can be initiated under the protection of glucocorticoid treatment. This has been reported in a series of three patients by Vick (1983) and has been widely practised by clinicians, with some success. However, when there is evidence of systemic allergy retrial of carbamazepine should not be attempted, as there are case reports that glucocorticoids are not helpful with cases where more generalized allergy appears to be occurring (Hampton et al 1985).

Carbamazepine and its congener oxcarbazepine have been associated with hyponatraemia and rare instances of water intoxication. Any patient presenting with signs or symptoms of confusion and possible water intoxication should be tested for hyponatraemia. There is some evidence that this may be more common in elderly patients and may be dose-related. Concurrent treatment with the antibiotic demeclomycin appears to be highly effective in reversing this potentially troublesome and/or serious side-effect. Vieweg et al (1987) have suggested the utility of lithium in reversing or preventing carbamazepine-induced hyponatraemia, although a systematic prospective study has not been conducted in order to test this hypothesis. However, in light of the divergent effects of carbamazepine and lithium on vasopressin function, one would surmise that this might be a clinically useful drug combination.

From the perspective of diabetes insipidus, the data suggest that carbamazepine is not able to overcome the effect of lithium in inducing diabetes insipidus. This occurs because carbamazepine appears to exert its action at or near the vasopressin receptor, while the effect of lithium occurs at the level of the second messenger or adenylate cyclase. Thus, even though carbamazepine is able to treat centrally-induced diabetes insipidus it is unable to reverse that caused by lithium.

VALPROATE

Clinical data

As reviewed in Table 24.7, substantial information is now available on the acute and prophylactic effects of valproate. While there are no double-blind studies of valproate prophylaxis, four studies exists for its efficacy in acute mania and each is positive. Two recent studies suggest the utility of valproate particularly in patients with dysphoric mania (Freeman et al 1990, McElroy et al 1990). These data, taken with the earlier observations of Emrich and associates (1980, 1984, 1985) and Brennan et al (1984) and a large series of uncontrolled observations, suggest the utility of this agent, particularly in rapidly cycling or dysphoric manic patients. The experience of Calabrese & Delucchi (1989) is of particular interest in this regard. They studied a series of patients who were unresponsive to lithium and, in many instances, to carbamazepine as well. They found a high incidence of acute antimanic responsivity in this patient population, as well as substantial evidence for long-term prophylaxis. These data, along with the different reports of carbamazepine's efficacy in rapid cyclers and dysphoric manic patients, suggest the utility of these two anticonvulsants in the treatment of lithium-refractory patients.

Differential response among anticonvulsants

In our case demonstration (Post et al 1984b) we observed some individual differences in anticonvulsant responsivity among the anticonvulsants. For example, one patient with malignant and continuous cycling between psychotic depression and psychotic mania showed an excellent response to carbamazepine, either alone or adjunctively with neuroleptics, but did not respond to valproate or phenytoin (Fig. 24.8).

In contrast, we have observed other patients who have not responded to carbamazepine and have responded to valproate (Fig. 24.9). The patient shown in Figure 24.9 is of particular interest since not only did she demonstrate non-responsivity to the combination of lithium and carbamazepine but attempts to treat residual depression with heterocyclic antidepressants and MAOIs appeared to incur a risk of the induction of cycling. This could not be controlled or ameliorated, in

Table 24.7   Studies of valproate response* in bipolar and schizoaffective illness

Study	Acute	Prophylaxis	Comment
Lambert 1984** Lambert et al 1975**		83/244 (34%)	Average dose 900 mg/d; M>D; Li plus valproic acid often required
Semadeni** 1976		23/32 (72%)	900–2400 mg/d for minimum of 2 years. Effective in some Li non-responders.
Emrich et al[B1] 1980, 1984, 1985	4/5 M (80%)	7/11 (64%)	Relapses on D/C in mania. 800–1800 mg/d; 48–102 µg/ml for prophylaxis; combination with Li may be required.
Puzynski & Klosiewicz** 1984		6/15 (40%)	Possible effects in BPII only; Poor effects on depression, 'fragmentations' (long episodes converted to shorter ones)
Vencovsky et al** 1984		?/38	Course similar to Li; fewer side effects (6–36 months)
Brennan et al 1984	6/8 M (75%)	4/4 (100%)	Relapse on D/C in 1/6 manics; Valproic acid increased GABA release, 900–3600 mg/day.
Prasad 1984	5/7 M (71%)		800–1500 mg/day
McElroy et al 1988b	33/56 (59%)		Initial relationship to EEG abnormality not sustained (750–3000 mg/d; 50–120 µg/ml. Two cases of abnormal liver function tests → D/C.
Post et al[B2] 1989, unpublished observations	4/6 M (67%) 1/5 D (20%)	6/9 M (67%) 2/11 D (18%)	2/4 M responders previously refractory to Li or CBZ Most prophylaxis patients were not studied in a blind fashion.
McElroy et al 1988a		6/6 (100%)	Six rapid cyclers resistant to Li, 5 resistant to CBZ
Brown 1989	BP 150/233 (64%) SA 38/66 (58%)		Community-based survey of clinicians; uncontrolled, global assessments, multiple medications
Hayes 1989b		30/35 (86%)	UP, BP, SA; Previous Li + CBZ non-responders; mean duration 1 year
Calabrese & Delucchi 1989, 1990	M 31/34 (91%) (9/10) Valp. alone D 16/34 (47%)	48/51 (94.1%) (19.20) Valp. alone 39/51 (76%)	Rapid cyclers; response in depression less than mania; acute and prophylaxis data are same patients 35/55 resistant to either lithium or carbamazepine 100% response in mixed mania
Sovner 1989		5/5 (100%)	Mentally retarded patients; two rapid cycling (1000–2000 mg/d; 61–80 µg/ml)
Freeman et al[B3] 1990	9/14 M (64%) Valp. (12/13 resp. in Li group)		Doses ranged from 1500 mg/d (week 1) to 3000 mg/d (week 3); particularly useful in dysphoric mania Rescue meds lorazepam and thiothixene
Huang et al 1990	14/15 (93%)		12 BP, 2 SA, 1 borderline personality disorder with manic symptoms; dose range: 500–2000 mg/d (25.6–96.1 µg/ml); good response in all but borderline; rapid response (< 7 days), relapse on D/C in 6/15; 3 patients became depressed
McElroy et al 1990[B4]	9/17 M (53%) Valp. Placebo 2/19		All Li-resistant. Placebo-controlled; rapid response (< 7 days); Rescue meds lorazepam to 4 mg in first 10 days, less lorazepam in valp. than placebo ($p<0.01$).
Totals Manic Depressed Overall	82/106 (77%) 17/39 (44%) 304/466 (65%)	220/461 (48%)	

B = blind; BP = bipolar disorder; CBZ = carbamazepine; D/C = discontinuation; Li = lithium; M = manic; SA = schizoaffective disorder; UP = unipolar. *Marked to moderate response; B1–4 = double-blind studies   ** = Dipropylacetamide

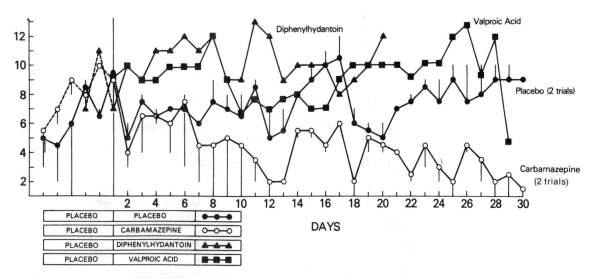

Fig. 24.8 Antimanic response to the anticonvulsant carbamazepine but not to diphenylhydantoin or valproic acid in a manic-depressive patient studied in a double-blind fashion. Note that mania ratings during treatment with phenytoin (at a dose of up to 600 mg/d, with blood levels reaching 19.8 ± 2.2 μg/ml) were substantially higher than those observed either during carbamazepine or placebo treatment. During treatment with valproic acid (up to 2500 mg/day, achieving blood levels of 88.8 ± 2.4 μg/ml), the patient showed little evidence of clinical response and again required seclusion for long periods of time. This patient therefore responded selectively to carbamazepine but not to valproate or phenytoin

spite of careful titration of dose, and the patient remained in a refractory condition in spite of the two mood-stabilizing agents (lithium and carbamazepine). She did not go into remission until valproate was substituted for lithium and carbamazepine and has subsequently done well over a period of several years.

These data agree with a recent report of good response to valproate in patients non-responsive to lithium and carbamazepine by McElroy and associates (1990). However, the study of Puzynski & Klosiewicz (1984) is less positive, indicating only partial antimanic responsivity and poor antidepressant responsivity in a group of refractory affectively ill patients.

Thus, the clinical and biological markers of who may respond to lithium versus the anticonvulsants, and to which of the anticonvulsants among the latter group, really remain to be delineated. Moreover, patients need to be followed up in the long term in order to assess the maintenance of degree of response. In this regard, we have observed that tolerance can occur, at least

partially, to the anticonvulsant effects of valproate on amygdala-kindled seizures (Weiss et al, unpublished data, 1990) and we have observed at least one patient where an initial response to valproate was subsequently lost (Post et al, unpublished observations). In this patient, the initial response to lithium and carbamazepine was also observed initially, with some loss of responsivity over time. Some patients may be uniquely predisposed to show loss of efficacy to a variety of psychotropic approaches to the long-term treatment of their illness.

Dose and side-effects

While the precise dose and blood level relationships to clinical response have not been clearly delineated, it is widely believed that blood levels between 50 and 100 μg/ml are useful in obtaining positive responses to valproate. This often is achieved with doses of drug between 750 and 2000 mg/day. Dose-related increases

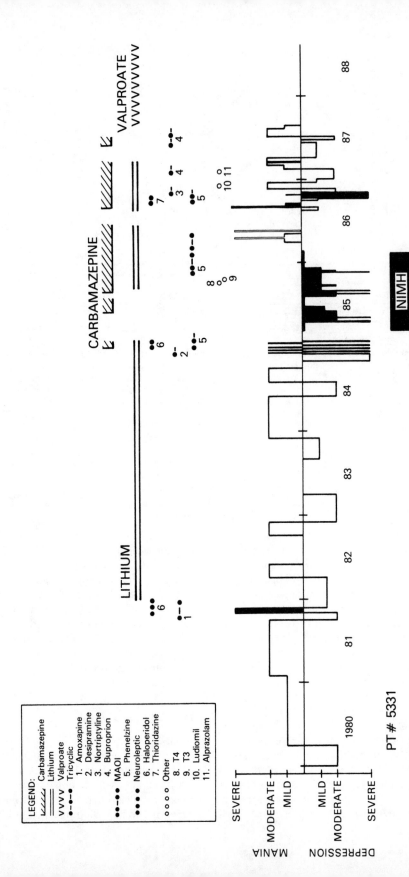

Fig. 24.9 Prophylactic response to valproate in a non-responder to lithium/carbamazepine. Non-response to lithium is documented in 1982–1984 with TCA and MAOI-induced rapid cycling in 1984. Carbamazepine appeared to be partially effective in ameliorating depressive symptoms but, in spite of lithium and thyroid potentiation, residual depression remained. Phenelzine augmentation was successful at NIMH in 1985, but the patient became irritable and angry, with other evidence of hypomania. A full-blown manic episode occurred shortly after discharge and adequate stabilization of mood was never achieved with various adjunctive treatments, in spite of combined use of two mood stabilizers (lithium and carbamazepine). Valproate made a dramatic impact on the illness, including a complete remission and clearing of the angry, irritable overlay which has previously been erroneously attributable to co-existing personality disorder

in tremor appear to be a relatively common side effect of valproate, as well as gastrointestinal distress, weight gain and, more rarely, alopecia.

It is recommended that baseline liver function tests be obtained and be monitored at regular intervals in light of the low but real risk of fulminant hepatitis which has been associated with mortality in children (Dreifuss & Langer 1987). The risk appears to be greater in children under the age of 10 and particularly under the age of 2, and in those treated with polypharmacy, but cases have also been reported in adults (Scheffner et al 1988). Conventional wisdom suggests that elevation of liver enzymes to two or three times normal can be watched cautiously, but higher values and those associated with symptoms should lead to drug discontinuation. Clearly, the patient should be warned that signs and symptoms of hepatic involvement should lead to physician consultation. These would include fever, chills, right upper quadrant pain, dark-coloured urine, malaise and jaundice. The liver toxicity on valproate appears to be of the toxic metabolic variety, as opposed to those with other anticonvulsants, which can be either toxic metabolic or allergic. Haematological problems, including granulocytopenia and thrombocytopenia, have also been reported on valproate but do not appear to be as common as those observed on carbamazepine.

CLONAZEPAM

A series of open clinical reports have suggested the utility of the treatment of acute mania with oral administration of high potency (anticonvulsant) benzodiazepines. These include clonazepam, clobazam and lorazepam. Orally-administered diazepam is not anticonvulsant and, while alprazolam is anticonvulsant, it appears to have unique properties based on its triazolo ring. Alprazolam, like antidepressants, has been reported to precipitate mania and thus should be used with caution in bipolar patients. The initial study of Chouinard et al (1983), reporting the efficacy of clonazepam compared with lithium on a double-blind basis, was really compromised by the use of neuroleptics in many of the patients studied, albeit in lower doses for those on clonazepam compared with lithium. Nonetheless, prospective double-blind and randomized clinical trials are required in order to establish the acute antimanic efficacy of the high-potency benzodiazepines. Until this is accomplished, we suggest the utility of using the high-potency benzodiazepines as adjunctive agents.

The sedating properties of clonazepam may be used in a positive fashion, particularly with bedtime dosing. In this fashion, one may interfere with initial evidence of mania breaking through and thus achieve rapid improvement of sleep in a patient with an incipient manic episode. Since Wehr (1989) has postulated that sleep loss can be not only a correlate of mania but a precipitant, one might in this fashion ameliorate the vicious circle effect of sleep deprivation in augmenting the manic process with high-potency benzodiazepines and thus avoid the use of neuroleptics.

While it has previously been thought that acute and intermittent dosing with neuroleptics might be sufficient to avoid the risk of tardive dyskinesia, a series of reports suggest that intermittent neuroleptics may pose equal or greater risks for tardive dyskinesia than chronic, continuous administration (Glenthoj et al 1988). Thus, neuroleptics should if possible be avoided in bipolar patients who appear to be at equal or greater risk of tardive dyskinesia than other psychiatric subtypes (Mukherjee et al 1986, Kane et al 1988, Waddington & Youssef 1988). In relation to this problem, sedating benzodiazepines may have a unique place.

The utility of high-potency benzodiazepines in the treatment of acute depression has not been systematically evaluated and reports from Japan suggest the possible development of tolerance to the therapeutic effects of clonazepam in prophylaxis of affective disorders in a high percentage of patients (Okuma & Kishimoto, personal communication, 1988). In addition, there are many reports of the rapid development of tolerance for the anticonvulsant effects of benzodiazepines in epileptic patients (Haigh et al 1988), suggesting that this therapy should be reserved for adjunctive use. Clearly, further systematic clinical trials of clonazepam and related agents are required to elucidate the clinical utility of these drugs in acute and prophylactic approaches to the illness. It is apparent that some patients may not be able to have clonazepam substituted for neuroleptics, as suggested in the study of Aronson and colleagues (1989), although these high-potency benzodiazepines would appear to play an important role as adjunctive treatment in patients with initial evidence of sleep loss.

OTHER ANTICONVULSANTS

Phenytoin

While initial reports concerning this anticonvulsant

were positive for the treatment of mania (Kalinowsky & Putnam 1943), subsequent open (Freyhan 1945, Kubanek & Rowell 1946) and double-blind studies (Post et al, unpublished observations) have not been equally positive. One well-documented case of a patient with schizoaffective illness exists in the literature (Freyhan 1945). This patient showed repeated therapeutic responses to the use of phenytoin with relapses upon drug discontinuation. Similar anecdotal cases are available in the literature and have recently been reported by Hayes (1989a). Thus, there would appear to be at least the occasional patient who might respond to this anticonvulsant, which might be considered in the absence of a response or in the case of intolerance to the other agents discussed above.

Pharmacotherapy as a function of stage of illness

From a theoretical perspective, the studies of Pinel (1983) are of considerable interest. He found that, while phenytoin was not highly effective in the initial phases of the epileptic kindling process, the drug was effective in the late phase of kindling characterized by spontaneous seizures. These data are consistent with observations that there are pharmacological dysjunctions in anticonvulsant responsiveness as a function of phase of kindling. For example, diazepam is highly effective in the initial phases of kindling development and completed kindled seizures, but is ineffective on the spontaneous variety. Carbamazepine blocks the completed amygdala-kindled seizure very effectively, but is without effect on the development of amygdala-kindled seizures (Weiss & Post 1987, Schmutz et al 1988). Conversely, carbamazepine is effective on the development of cocaine- and lidocaine-kindled seizures, but is without effect once these seizures have been completed or achieved with acute high doses. Given this differential anticonvulsant responsivity as a function of stage of kindling, we have asked whether similar dysjunctions are also observable in the course of treatment of affectively ill patients. In particular, we wonder whether some patients do not respond better to lithium in the early and mid phases of their illness but in the late phases, often characterized by rapid-cycling illness, require adjunctive treatments with anticonvulsants such as carbamazepine and valproate (Post et al 1986b). Whether phenytoin would play a role in some of these late phases of illness remains to be further systematically evaluated.

Acetazolamide

This carbonic anhydrase inhibitor is a clinically useful anticonvulsant. Inoue and associates (1984) reported that it was effective in some patients with atypical psychoses. Those patients with atypical confusional psychoses with dreamy states and also those with puerperal psychosis and menstrual psychoses appeared to be among the responders, suggesting the potential utility of this agent in patients with cyclic psychoses associated with endocrine alterations. We are not aware of further systematic clinical trials of this agent and look forward to their publication in the future.

Electroconvulsive therapy

Elsewhere we have discussed in detail the potent anticonvulsant properties of electroconvulsive therapy (ECT) (Post et al 1984c, 1986a). We would merely note in this regard that ECT is the one exception among the anticonvulsants that appears to be as effective or more effective in the treatment of acute depression than acute mania. However, evidence is sparse regarding its potential prophylactic efficacy (Thornton et al 1990, Grunhaus et al 1990, Fink 1984, Nakajima et al 1989) and the utility and practicality of prophylactic treatment in rapidly cycling bipolar patients is, at present, virtually undocumented and dubious. Systematic clinical trials are awaited. ECT may be used acutely in order to 'break' a refractory episode, but then the patient should be medicated with one of the other agents discussed in this chapter.

CALCIUM CHANNEL BLOCKERS

The calcium channel blockers are useful in the treatment of some seizure types but not others, and since their anticonvulsant effects are not generalized across the entire series of compounds they will not be considered under the category of anticonvulsants. However, it is noteworthy that nimodipine and flunarazine are highly potent anticonvulsants in some model systems and these agents at least deserve to be classified as anticonvulsants.

As illustrated in Table 24.8, considerable open and controlled clinical experience implicates the calcium channel blocker verapamil as an acute antimanic agent. However, studies are relatively lacking regarding its long-term efficacy in prophylaxis. Moreover, the study of Hoschl & Kozeny (1989) is particularly important in documenting not only the acute antimanic efficacy of

Table 24.8 Verapamil and other calcium channel blockers in affective illness

Study	Design	Response
Caillard & Masse 1982 (diltiazem)	Open	3/4 manic
Dubovsky et al 1982	Blind	1/1 manic
Dubovsky & Franks 1983	Blind	3/3 manic
Hoschl 1983	Blind	1/1 depressed
Giannini et al 1984, 1987	Blind vs Li	Equal effects in 10
Dubovsky et al 1985	Blind	1/1 blockade of phenelzine hypomania
Brotman et al 1986	Open	6/6 manic
Dose et al 1986	Blind	7/8 manic and SA
Dubovsky et al 1986	Blind	5/7 manic
Solomon & Williamson 1986	Open	2/2 bipolar (+ mania; − depression (trazadone required))
Barton & Gitlin 1987	Open	0/8 acute manic/hypomanic 2/4 prophylactic 2/2 drug-induced hypomanic (all patients resistant to conventional medications)
Patterson 1987	Open	1/1 manic

Hoschl & Kozeny 1989
86 depressed patients
  26 verapamil
  19 vs amitriptyline
  11 vs placebo
  30 vs eclectic
	Random
	Blind
		No difference between verapamil
		and placebo in depression.
		Amitriptyline and eclectic R_x
		superior to verapamil.

47 manic patients
  12 verapamil
  24 vs neuroleptics
  11 vs Li + neuroleptics
	Blind	Verapamil as effective as standard
		R_x in mania.

Brunet et al 1990 (nimodipine)	Open	6/6 manic; nimodipine (360 mg/d). significant improvement in most symptoms except sleep & psychosis.
Garza-Trevino 1990	Blind vs Li	17 manic; 43% reduction in Peterson Mania Scale score for verapamil; 40% reduction for Li

Total patients studied: 119   Moderate to marked responders: 40/54 (74%)

verapamil but the lack of acute antidepressant efficacy in comparison with amitriptyline or other antidepressant treatments. In this latter study of acutely depressed patients, verapamil was not more effective than placebo in acute depression.

Whether the other calcium channel blockers with a better anticonvulsant profile (nimodipine, flunarazine) have greater efficacy in acute depression or prophylaxis remains to be delineated. There is also some suggestion that this class of agents may act particularly in patients who are lithium-responsive, and the clinical and biological markers of response to the calcium channel blockers remain to be further studies. Given recent data

implicating calcium-active mechanisms in the anticonvulsant effects of carbamazepine and related agents (Post 1987, 1988, Post et al 1991a), the ultimate clinical utility of the calcium channel blockers remains an undocumented but theoretically intriguing proposition.

NEUROTRANSMITTER-TARGETED STRATEGIES

Alpha$_2$-agonist clonidine and alpha$_2$-antagonist iadozoxan

A series of studies has suggested the antimanic efficacy

of the alpha$_2$-agonist clonidine (Jouvent et al 1980, Maguire & Singh 1987, Hardy et al 1986). However, the most recent double-blind study of Janicak et al (1989) reports that clonidine is no more active than placebo in the treatment of acute mania. Thus further work is required in order to clarify the potential utility of this agent and describe the possible clinical and biological markers of responsivity. It is of some interest that, in our model of neuroleptic nonresponsivity on a preclinical level, we found that clonidine and clonazepam were effective in blocking both the development and the expression of context-dependent cocaine sensitization, whereas neuroleptics were active in blocking only the development but not the expression of this phenomenon (Weiss et al 1989). These data are of interest in relationship to the observations of Maguire & Singh (1987) reporting the potential utility of clonidine in neuroleptic-refractory manic patients. Thus this drug may deserve systematic clinical trials in patients unresponsive to other agents and, particularly, in the hypertensive manic patient.

Recent studies and reviews of Osman and associates (1990) and Montgomery (1989) have suggested the possible clinical utility of the alpha$_2$-antagonist idazoxan in the treatment of refractory bipolar patients. Interestingly, they did not report a high incidence of the induction of mania with this treatment, as might be theoretically predicted. Clearly, further systematic trials are necessary before the utility of this strategy can be adequately evaluated.

Beta-adrenergic active agents

It is of interest that several studies suggest the potential utility of beta-adrenergic agonists as antidepressants, although the degree of efficacy and sustained response remain to be adequately documented. Conversely, there is some evidence that high-dose beta-blocker treatment with propranolol may convey antimanic efficacy (Atsom et al 1971, von Zerssen 1976, Emrich et al 1979). However, in one study (Emrich et al 1979), equal antimanic efficacy was achieved with the d- and l-isomers. These observations, together with those that show that extremely high doses are required for the antimanic effect, suggest that non-beta-adrenergic receptor blockade properties of these drugs, potentially related to membrane stabilizing properties, may be involved in the antimanic effect with these compounds.

Dopamine-active compounds

Agonists: direct and indirect

Direct dopamine agonists such as bromocriptine (Colonna et al 1979, Nordin et al 1981, Waehrens & Gerlach 1981, Silverstone 1984) and piribedil (ET-495) (Shopsin & Gershon 1978, Post et al 1978) have been reported to have some success as antidepressant agents. These reports are of interest, in relation to recent evidence that amineptine is a highly effective antidepressant, and it is on the market in France (Kemali 1989, Mendis et al 1989, de Sousa and Tropa 1989). These data perhaps agree with recent data suggesting that bupropion increases dopamine release in the nucleus accumbens and striatum (Nomikos et al 1989), and this may account for its activity as a clinically useful antidepressant. Whether this agent will share the liabilities of other unimodal antidepressants in precipitating mania or increasing rapid cycling remains to be determined. However, preliminary reports by Shopsin (1983) and others (Wright et al 1985) are at least promising in relationship to the utility of bupropion in long-term prophylaxis.

Antagonists: neuroleptics

While the antipsychotic neuroleptics are of considerable use in the treatment of schizoaffective and psychotic manic and depressive patients, their long-term use is to be avoided because of the high risk of tardive dyskinesia in the patient population noted above. The recent availability of clozapine in the treatment of refractory schizophrenic patients and reports by Meltzer (1990) and others that schizoaffective patients appear highly responsive to this agent suggest the potential importance of systematic evaluation of clozapine in refractory affective disorders.

GABA-active treatments

The GABA-agonists progabide and fengabine have been reported in several studies (Morselli et al 1986, Weiss et al 1986, Perris et al 1986, Magni et al 1989) to have efficacy in the treatment of mild depression. These preliminary data are at least partially consistent with studies reporting deficits in plasma or cerebrospinal fluid GABA in affective illness (Emrich et al 1980, Berrettini & Post 1984). However, not all studies have been confirmed and the efficacy of these compounds in severe inpatient depressions remains to be documented. A recent outpatient placebo-controlled trial of fengabine was negative (Paykel et al, 1991).

While valproate has been reported in a series of studies (McElroy et al 1989, Post 1990a) to have acute and prophylactic antimanic effects, its efficacy in depressive phases of the illness are less well established. Nonetheless, compounds that indirectly increase $GABA_A$ function deserve further exploration.

We have explored the potential clinical efficacy of the $GABA_B$-agonist l-baclofen in manic and depressive illness based on several clinical and theoretical considerations. We wished to ascertain whether the antidepressant effects of carbamazepine might be mediated through a $GABA_B$ mechanism. This hypothesis was stimulated by the work of Terrence et al (1983), which indicated that not only was baclofen (like carbamazepine) effective in the treatment of trigeminal neuralgia, but the antinociceptive effects of both l-baclofen and carbamazepine could be reversed in an animal model using the inactive d-isomer of baclofen. These preclinical data, taken with the findings that virtually all antidepressant treatments upregulated $GABA_B$-receptors in the frontal cortex of rodents (Lloyd et al 1987), suggested that l-baclofen might possess antidepressant as well as antinociceptive properties.

In our initial clinical trial none of the first five patients studied responded to l-baclofen (Post et al 1991b). Three patients showed a pattern of increasing morbidity during double-blind treatment with l-baclofen in doses ranging from 10–55 mg/day and subsequent improvement during placebo substitution. One of these patients showed an exacerbation of his rapid cycling during baclofen treatment and attenuation of this pattern during placebo substitution. Taken together, these preliminary data suggest that not only is l-baclofen not effective in the treatment of depressed and bipolar patients but it may cause exacerbation of the illness. It is therefore possible that treatments aimed at reduction of $GABA_B$ tone may be worthy of further exploration. In this respect, use of a $GABA_B$-antagonist might be consistent with the data of Lloyd et al (1987); i.e. this type of compound that would presumably upregulate rather than downregulate $GABA_B$-receptors.

s-adenosyl-methionine

s-adenosyl-methionine is reported in controlled and uncontrolled studies to show a high incidence of antidepressant response and to be relatively devoid of side effects. Most noteworthy, however, is the high incidence of switches in bipolar patients (Carney et al 1988, 1989). Further studies of this compound may thus lead us to novel mechanisms of antidepressant action and help reveal target systems of antimanic action.

ADJUNCTS FOR PROPHYLAXIS

Thyroid augmentation

This strategy has had a long history since the early systematic observations of Gjessing (1975) on the use of suppressive doses of thyroid in the treatment of periodic catatonia. Stancer & Persad (1982) and Wehr and colleagues (1988) have also used this strategy in refractory bipolar patients. However, both of these groups observed loss of efficacy with continued administration and have observed a relatively high incidence of medical side-effects when this agent is used as the sole treatment. In contrast to attempts to use suppressive thyroid treatment as the sole active modality, Bauer & Whybrow (1988, 1990) recently reported success in a small series of patients using high-dose thyroid treatment in order to augment inadequate responses to lithium, carbamazepine and other primary treatment strategies. These investigators reported success with levothyroid in the dosage range of 0.15–0.4 mg/day in order to produce a 150% increase in the free thyroxin index adequate to suppress TSH. Severity of manic and depressive ratings was noted to decrease with this augmentation strategy, independent of initial thyroid status. However, relapses were observed in a number of patients, only some of whom re-responded to augmenting thyroid treatment. Thus long-term systematic observations of the utility of adjunctive treatment with this agent are required before definitive conclusions can be reached. However, as illustrated in Figure 24.10, we have observed the occasional patient who responds to thyroid augmentation of other partially effective treatment modalities. In this case, a patient with a history of refractory affective disorders and ultra-rapid cycling over a 30-year period was inadequately responsive to a combination of carbamazepine, lithium and valproate. However, when nonsuppressive doses of T3 were added to the regimen a remission was observed that lasted for a period of approximately nine months. Thus, although Bauer & Whybrow (1988, 1990) suggested that some patients may need suppressive doses of thyroid, the role of thyroid augmentation with T3 versus T4, as well as the need for suppressant doses, remains to be adequately delineated.

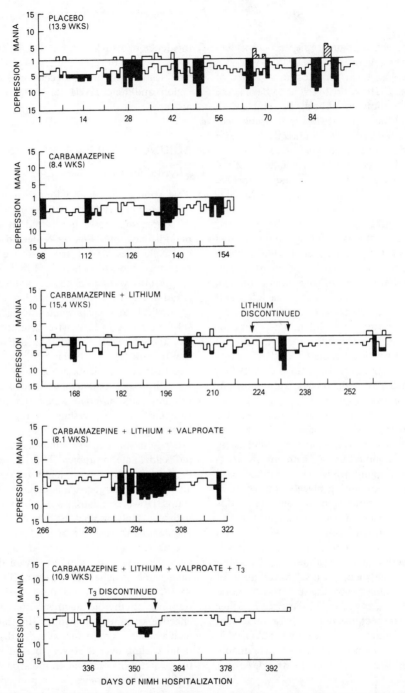

Fig. 24.10 Pharmacological response in an ultra-rapid cycling manic-depressive patient. This patient presented with an almost 30-year history of ultra-rapid cycling non-responsive to traditional psychotropic medication. Nurses rated the patient daily on the global Bunney—Hamburg Scale for Depression and Mania, blind to medication status. During placebo, her persistent ultra-rapid cycling (bipolar II) pattern was documented and confirmed. Moderate to severe depression rapidly attentuated with brief periods of mood elevation. During carbamezepine treatment (line 2), hyponamia was elimated but depression persisted. The additiona of lithium (line 3) may have further attenuated the depressions, while valpraote (line 4) appeared to slow the cycling at the cost of a longer period of depression. The addition of T_3 (last line) was associated with a persistent period of euthymia and the patient was able to be discharged

Other adjuncts for prophylaxis

Folic acid and ascorbic acid have both been reported to be useful as adjunctive treatments in acute or prophylactic treatment of refractory affective illness (Coppen et al 1986, Naylor & Smith 1981). In light of the benign nature of these treatments and the relative lack of side-effects, this would appear to be an ideal area for investigation and systematic trials, many of which could be conducted by clinicians in private practice, in order to delineate better evidence of the long-term efficacy of these treatment agents.

The use of methylene blue (based on theory that vanadium levels are increased in bipolar patients and that this agent catalyses the conversion to vanadyl, which is less metabolically active) has received preliminary support in a controlled trial. 17 patients completed a 2-year blind crossover trial (with lithium cotreatment). They were significantly less depressed during the year on methylene blue (300 mg/day) than during the year on inactive treatment (methylene blue 15 mg/day) (Naylor 1985, Naylor et al 1986). Interestingly, carbamazepine is reported to reverse vanadate-induced inhibition of Na-K ATPase (Naylor 1985).

Psychotherapy

While the use of psychotherapy in the treatment of recurrent unipolar and bipolar affective illness has been reviewed in detail elsewhere in this volume, it is worth re-emphasizing that a variety of techniques have been shown to be important in preventing relapse in unipolar, if not bipolar, affective disorder. We would support the systematic clinical application and evaluation of a variety of targeted psychotherapeutic techniques in maximizing treatment of the bipolar patient. Clearly, maximizing psychotherapeutic and pharmacotherapeutic intervention in this recurrent, potentially life-threatening, disorder is indicated in order to optimize treatment outcome. Interpersonal therapy, supportive techniques, cognitive and behavioural approaches would be particularly helpful as the patient enters relatively late and 'automatic' phases of the illness characterized by rapid and frequent cycling. A strong psychotherapeutic relationship may also assist in the maintenance of medication compliance and an appropriate appreciation of the need for vigilance in order to treat emergent symptoms as early as possible.

REFERENCES

Abou-Saleh M T, Coppen A 1986 Who responds to prophylactic lithium? Journal of Affective Disorders 10: 115–125

Altshuler L L, Post R M, Leverich G, Rosoff A 1990 Antidepressant-induced switches, rapid and continuous cycling. Unpublished manuscript

Aronson T A, Shukla S, Hirschowitz J 1989 Clonazepam treatment of five lithium-refractory patients with bipolar disorder. American Journal of Psychiatry 146: 77–80

Atsom A, Blum I, Wijsenbeek H, Maoz B, Steiner M, Ziegelman G 1971 The short term effects of adrenergic blocking agents in a small group of psychotic patients. Psychiatria, Neurologia and Neurochirurgia 74: 251–258

Baastrup P C, Schou M 1967 Lithium as a prophylactic agent: its effect against recurrent depressions and manic-depressive psychosis. Archives of General Psychiatry 16: 162–172

Ballenger J C, Post R M 1978 Therapeutic effects of carbamazepine in affective illness: a preliminary report. Communications in Psychopharmacology 2: 159–175

Barton B M, Gitlin M J 1987 Verapamil in treatment-resistant mania: an open trial. Journal of Clinical Psychopharmacology 7: 101–103

Bauer M S, Whybrow P C 1988 Thyroid hormones and the central nervous system in affective illness: interactions that may have clinical significance. Integrative Psychiatry 6: 75–85

Bauer M S, Whybrow P C 1990 Rapid cycling bipolar affective disorder. II. Treatment of refractory rapid cycling with high-dose levothyroxine: a preliminary study. Archives of General Psychiatry 47: 435–440

Bellaire W, Demish K, Stoll K-D 1988 Carbamazepine versus lithium in prophylaxis of recurrent affective disorders (abstract). Psychopharmacology (suppl) 96: 287

Berrettini W, Post R M 1984 GABA and affective illness. In: Post R M, Ballenger J C (eds) Neurobiology of mood disorders. Willims & Wilkins, Baltimore, p 673–685

Brennan M J W, Sandyk R, Borseek D 1984 Use of sodium-valproate in the management of affective disorders: basic and clinical aspects. In: Emrich H M, Okuma T, Muller A A (eds) Anticonvulsants in affective disorders. Excerpta Medica, Amsterdam, p 56–65

Brotman A W, Farhadi A M, Gelenberg A J 1986 Verapamil treatment of acute mania. Journal of Clinical Psychiatry 47: 136–138

Brown R 1989 US experience with valproate in manic depressive illness: a multicenter trial. Journal of Clinical Psychiatry 50: 13–16

Brown D, Silverstone T, Cookson J 1989 Carbamazepine compared to haloperidol in acute mania. International Clinical Psychopharmacology 4: 229–238

Brunet G, Cerlich B, Robert P, Dumas S, Souetre E, Darcourt G 1990 Open trial of a calcium antagonist, nimodipine in acute mania. Clinical Neuropharmacology 13: 224–228

Cabrera J F, Muhlbauer H D, Schley J, Stoll K D, Muller-Oerlinghausen B 1986 Long-term randomized clinical trial on oxcarbazepine vs lithium in bipolar and schizoaffective disorders: Preliminary results. Pharmacopsychiatry 19: 282–283

Caillard V, Masse G 1982 Traitement de la manie par un inhibiteur calcique. Etude preliminaire. Encephale 8: 587–594

Calabrese J R, Delucchi G A 1989 Phenomenology of rapid cycling manic depression and its treatment with valproate. Journal of Clinical Psychiatry 50: 30–34

Calabrese J R, Delucchi G A 1990 Spectrum of efficacy of valproate in 55 patients with rapid-cycling bipolar disorder. American Journal of Psychiatry 147: 431–434

Carney M W P, Chary T K N, Bottiglieri T, Reynolds E H 1988 Switch and s-adenosylmethionine. Alabama Journal of Medical Sciences 25: 316–319

Carney M W P, Chary T K N, Bottiglieri T, Reynolds E H 1989 The switch mechanism and the bipolar/unipolar dichotomy. British Journal of Psychiatry 154: 48–51

Chouinard G, Young S N, Annable L 1983 Antimanic effect of clonazepam. Biological Psychiatry 18: 451–466

Colonna L, Petit M, Lepine J P 1979 Bromocriptine in affective disorders. A pilot study. Journal of Affective Disorders 1: 173–177

Cookson J C 1987 Carbamazepine in acute mania: a practical review. International Clinical Psychopharmacology 2: 11–22

Coppen A, Chaudhry S, Swade C 1986 Folic acid enhances lithium prophylaxis. Journal of Affective Disorders 10: 9–13

Desai N G, Gangadhar B N, Channabasavanna S M, Shetty K T 1987 Carbamazepine hastens therapeutic action of lithium in mania. Abstract, Proceedings of the International Conference on New Directions in Affective Disorders, Jerusalem

de Sousa M P, Tropa J 1989 Evaluation of the efficacy of amineptine in a population of 1229 depressed patients: results of a multicenter study carried out by 135 general practitioners. Clinical Neuropharmacology 12 (suppl 2): S77–S86

Dose M, Emrich H M, Cording-Tommel C, von Zerssen D 1986 Use of calcium antagonists in mania. Psychoneuroendocrinology 11: 241–243

Dostal T 1977 Double-blind study of the therapeutic and prophylactic effect of lithium salts in psychiatry. In: Research Institute of Psychiatry—Candidate dissertation, Prague

Dreifuss F E, Langer D H 1987 Hepatic considerations in the use of antileptic drugs. Epilepsia 28: S23–S29

Dubovsky S L, Franks R D 1983 Intracellular calcium in affective disorders: a review and an hypothesis. Biological Psychiatry 18: 781–797

Dubovsky S L, Franks R D, Lifschitz M, Coen P 1982 Effectiveness of verapamil in the treatment of a manic patient. American Journal of Psychiatry. 139: 502–504

Dubovsky S, Franks R, Schrier D 1985 Phenelzine-induced hypomania: effect of verapamil. Biological Psychiatry 20: 1009–1014

Dubovsky S L, Franks R D, Allen S 1986 Calcium antagonists in mania: a double-blind study of verapamil. Psychiatry Research 18: 309–320

Dunner D L, Fieve R R 1974 Clinical factors in lithium carbonate prophylaxis failure. Archives of General Psychiatry 30: 229–233

Dunner D L, Fleiss J L, Fieve R R 1976 Lithium carbonate

prophylaxis failure. British Journal of Psychiatry 129: 40–44

Elphick M 1985 An open clinical trial of carbamazepine in treatment-resistant bipolar and schizo-affective psychotics. British Journal of Psychiatry 147: 198–200

Emrich H M 1990 Studies with oxcarbazepine (Trileptal) in acute mania. International Clinical Psychopharmacology 5 (suppl 1): 83–88

Emrich H M, von Zerssen D, Moller H J, Kissling W, Cording C, Schietsch H J, Riedel E 1979 Action of propranolol in mania: comparison of effects of the d- and the l-stereoisomer. Pharmakopsychiatrica 12: 295–304

Emrich H M, von Zerssen D, Kissling W, Moller H-J, Windorfer A 1980 Effect of sodium valproate in mania. The GABA hypothesis of affective disorders. Archiv für Psychiatrie und Nervenkrankheiten 229: 1–16

Emrich H M, Dose M, von Zerssen D 1984 Action of sodium-valproate and of oxcarbazepine in patients with affective disorders. In: Emrich H M, Okuma T, Muller A A (eds) Anticonvulsants in affective disorders. Excerpta Medica, Amsterdam, p 45–55

Emrich H M, Dose M, von Zerssen D 1985 The use of sodium valproate, carbamazepine and oxcarbazepine in patients with affective disorders. Journal of Affective Disorders 8: 243–250

Fieve R R, Kumbaraci T, Dunner D L 1976 Lithium prophylaxis of depression in bipolar I, bipolar II, and unipolar patients. Archives of General Psychiatry 133: 925–929

Fink M 1984 Theories of the antidepressant efficacy of convulsive therapy (ECT). In: Post R M, Ballenger J C (eds) Neurobiology of mood disorders. Williams & Wilkins, Baltimore, p 721–730

Freeman T W, Clothier J L, Pazzaglia P, Lesem M D, Swann A C, Roache A 1990 Valproate in mania: a double-blind study. Abstracts of the 143rd Annual Meeting of the American Psychiatric Association no. NR393, p 198

Freyhan F A 1945 Effectiveness of diphenylhydantoin in management of non-epileptic psychomotor excitement states. Archives of Neurology and Psychiatry 53: 370–374

Gallicchio V S, Hulette B C 1989 In vitro effect of lithium on carbamazepine-induced inhibition of murine and human bone marrow-derived granulocyte-macrophage, erythroid, and megakaryocyte progenitor stem cells. Proceedings of the Society for Experimental Biology and Medicine 190: 109–116

Garza-Trevino E S 1990 Verapamil versus lithium in acute mania. Abstracts of the 143rd Annual Meeting of the American Psychiatric Association no. 27, p 78

Giannini A J, House W L, Loiselle R H 1984 Antimanic effects of verapamil. American Journal of Psychiatry 141: 1602–1603

Giannini A J, Taraszewski R, Loiselle R H 1987 Verapamil and lithium in maintenance therapy of manic patients. Journal of Clinical Pharmacology 27: 980–982

Gjessing L R 1975 Academic address: a review of periodic catatonia. Biological Psychiatry 8: 23–45

Glenthoj B, Hemmingsen R, Bolwig T G 1988 Kindling: a model for the development of tardive dyskinesia. Behavioural Neurology 1: 29–41

Goodnick P J, Fieve R R, Schlegel A, Baxter N 1987 Predictors of interepisode symptoms and relapse in affective disorder patients treated with lithium carbonate. American Journal of Psychiatry 144: 367–369

Grof E, Haag M, Grof P, Haag H 1987 Lithium response and the sequence of episode polarities: preliminary report on a Hamilton sample. Progress in Neuropsychopharmacology and Biological Psychiatry 11: 199–203

Grossi E, Sacchetti E, Vita A et al 1984 Carbamazepine vs chlorpromazine in mania: a double-blind trial. In: Emrich H M, Okuma T, Muller A A (eds) Anticonvulsants in affective disorders. Excerpta Medica, Amsterdam, p 177–187

Grunhaus L, Pande A C, Haskett R F 1990 Full and abbreviated courses of maintenance electroconvulsive therapy. Convulsive Therapy 6: 130–138

Haag H, Heidorn A, Haag M, Greil W 1987 Sequence of affective polarity and lithium response: preliminary report on Munich sample. Progress in Neuropsychopharmacology and Biological Psychiatry 11: 205–208

Haigh J R, Gent J P, Garratt J C, Pullar T, Feely M 1988 Disappointing results of increasing benzodiazepine dose after the development of anticonvulsant tolerance (letter). Journal of Neurology, Neurosurgery and Psychiatry 51: 1008–1009

Hampton K K, Bramley P N, Feely M 1985 Failure of prednisolone to suppress carbamazepine hypersensitivity (letter). New England Journal of Medicine 313: 959–959

Hanus H, Zapletalek M 1984 The prophylactic lithium treatment in affective disorders and the possibilities of the outcome prediction. Sbornik Vedeckych Praci Lekarske Fakulty Karlovy Univerzity V Hradci Karlove 27: 5–75

Hardy M C, Lecrubier Y, Widlocher D 1986 Efficacy of clonidine in 24 patients with acute mania. American Journal of Psychiatry. 143: 1450–1453

Hayes S G 1989a Anticonvulsants in long-term psychiatric treatment. 142nd Annual Meeting of the American Psychiatric Association Symposium, May 6

Hayes S G 1989b Long-term use of valproate in primary psychiatric disorders. Journal of Clinical Psychiatry (suppl): 35–39

Himmelhoch J M, Garfinkel M E 1986 Sources of lithium resistance in mixed mania. Psychopharmacology Bulletin 22: 613–620

Hoschl C 1983 Verapamil for depression? (letter). American Journal of Psychiatry 140: 1100–1100

Hoschl C, Kozeny J 1989 Verapamil in affective disorders: a controlled, double-blind study. Biological Psychiatry 25: 128–140

Huang C C, Young L D, Harsch H H 1990 Clinical trials of sodium valproate on manic patients. Abstracts of the 143rd Annual Meeting of the American Psychiatric Association No. NR71, p 73

Inoue H, Hazama H, Hamazoe K 1984 Antipsychotic and prophylactic effects of acetazolamide (Diamox) on atypical psychosis. Folia Psychiatrica et Neurologica Japonica 38: 425–436

Itoh K, Ishigane M 1973 On the clinical effectiveness of lithium carbonate for manic-depressive reactions: therapeutic and prophylactic effects. Shinyaku-to-Rinsho 22: 1001–1015

Janicak P G, Sharma R P, Easton M, Comaty J E, Davis J M 1989 A double-blind, placebo controlled trial of clonidine

in the treatment of acute mania. Psychopharmacology Bulletin 25: 243–245

Jefferson J W, Greist J H 1987 Lithium carbonate and carbamazepine side effects. In: Hales R E, Frances A J (eds) American Psychiatric Association Annual Review 6. American Psychiatric Press, Washington D C, p 746–780

Joffe R T, Post R M, Eil C 1984 Carbamazepine does not interact with thyroid hormone receptors in human fibroblasts. Neuropharmacology 23: 1301–1303

Joffe R T, Post R M, Roy-Byrne P P, Uhde T W 1985 Hematological effects of carbamazepine in patients with affective illness. American Journal of Psychiatry 142: 1196–1199

Jouvent R, Lecrubier Y, Puech A J 1980 Antimanic effects of clonidine. American Journal of Psychiatry 137: 1275–1276

Joyce P R 1988 Carbamazepine in rapid cycling bipolar affective disorder. International Clinical Psychopharmacology 63: 123–129

Kalinowsky L, Putnam T 1943 Attempts at treatment of schizophrenia and other nonepileptic psychosis with dilantin. Archives of Neurology and Psychiatry 49: 414–423

Kane J M, Woerner M, Lieberman J 1988 Tardive dyskinesia: prevalence, incidence, and risk factors. Journal of Clinical Psychopharmacology 8: 52S–56S

Kemali D 1989 A multicenter Italian study of amineptine (survector 100). Clinical Neuropharmacology 12 (suppl 2): S41–S50

Kishimoto A, Okuma T 1985 Antimanic and prophylactic effects of carbamazepine in affective disorders. Abstracts of the 4th World Congress of Biological Psychiatry, September 8–13, no 506.4, p 363

Kishimoto A, Omura F, Inoue K, Okazaki T, Hazama H 1986 A comparative study of carbamazepine and lithium for prophylaxis of bipolar affective disorder. Yonago Acta Medica 29: 76–90

Klein E, Bental E, Lerer B, Belmaker R H 1984 Carbamazepine and haloperidol vs placebo and haloperidol in excited psychoses. Archives of General Psychiatry 41: 165–170

Kramlinger K G, Post R M 1990 Addition of lithium carbonate to carbamazepine: hematological and thyroid effects. American Journal of Psychiatry 147: 615–620

Kramlinger K G, Phillips K A, Post R M 1990 Skin rash complicating carbamazepine treatment. (Unpublished manuscript)

Kubanek J L, Rowell R C 1946 The use of dilantin in the treatment of psychotic patients unresponsive to other treatment. Disease of the Nervous System 7: 47–50

Kukopulos A, Reginaldi D, Laddomada P, Floris G, Serra G, Tondo L 1980 Course of the manic-depressive cycle and changes caused by treatment. Pharmakopsychiatrica 13: 156–167

Kukopulos A, Caliari B, Tundo A, Minnai G, Floris G, Reginaldi D, Tondo L 1983 Rapid cyclers, temperament, and antidepressants. Comprehensive Psychiatry 24: 249–258

Lambert P A 1984 Acute and prophylactic therapies of patients with affective disorders using valpromide (dipropylacetamide). In: Emrich H M, Okuma T, Muller A A (eds) Anticonvulsants in affective disorders. Excerpta Medica, Amsterdam, p 33–44

Lambert P A, Carraz G, Borselli S 1975 Le dipropylacetamide dans le traitement de la psychose maniaco-depressive. Encephale 1: 25–31

Lenzi A, Lazzerini F, Grossi E, Massimetti G, Placidi G F 1986 Use of carbamazepine in acute psychosis: a controlled study. Journal of International Medical Research 14: 78–84

Lerer B, Moore N, Meyendorff E, Cho S R, Gershon S 1987 Carbamazepine versus lithium in mania: a double-blind study. Journal of Clinical Psychiatry 48: 89–93

Leverich G S, Post R M, Rosoff A S 1990 Factors associated with relapse during maintenance treatment of affective disorders. International Clinical Psychopharmacology 5: 135–156

Lloyd K G, Morselli P L, Bartholini G 1987 GABA and affective disorders. Medical Biology 65: 159–165

Lusznat R M, Murphy D P, Nunn C M 1988 Carbamazepine vs lithium in the treatment and prophylaxis of mania. British Journal of Psychiatry 153: 198–204

McElroy S L, Keck P E Jr, Pope H G Jr, Hudson J I 1988a Valproate in the treatment of rapid-cycling bipolar disorder. Journal of Clinical Psychopharmacology 8: 275–279

McElroy S L, Pope H G Jr, Keck P E Jr 1988b Treatment of psychiatric disorders with valproate: a series of 73 cases. Psychiatrie et Psychobiologie 3: 81–85

McElroy S L, Keck P E Jr, Pope H G Jr, Hudson J I 1989 Valproate in psychiatric disorders: literature review and clinical guidelines. Journal of Clinical Psychiatry (suppl) 50: 23–29

McElroy S L, Pope H G Jr, Keck P E Jr, Hudson J I 1990 A placebo-controlled study of valproate in mania. Abstracts of the 143rd Annual Meeting of the American Psychiatric Association No NR312, p 167

Magni G, Garreau M, Orofiamma B, Palminteri R 1989 Fengabine, a new GABA-mimetic agent in the treatment of depressive disorders: an overview of six double-blind studies versus tricyclics. Neuropsychobiology 20: 126–131

Maguire J, Singh A N 1987 Clonidine. An effective anti-manic agent. British Journal of Psychiatry 150: 863–864

Maj M, Del Vecchio M, Starace F, Pirozzi R, Kemali D 1984 Prediction of affective psychoses response to lithium prophylaxis. Acta Psychiatrica Scandinavica 69: 37–44

Maj M, Pirozzi R, Kemali D 1989a Long-term outcome of lithium prophylaxis in patients initially classified as complete responders. Psychopharmacology (Berlin) 98: 535–538

Maj M, Pirozzi R, Starace F 1989b Previous pattern of course of the illness as a predictor of response to lithium prophylaxis in bipolar patients. Journal of Affective Disorders 17: 237–241

Mander A J, Loudon J B 1988 Rapid recurrence of mania following abrupt discontinuation of lithium. Lancet 2: 15–17

Meltzer H Y 1990 Clozapine treatment: long-term social outcome. Symposium: 143rd Annual Meeting of the American Psychiatric Association

Mendis N, Hanwella D R C, Weerasinghe C, Illesinghe D S, De Silva D 1989 A double-blind comparative study: amineptine (survector 100) versus imipramine. Clinical Neuropharmacology 12 (suppl 2): S58–S65

Mendlewicz J, Fieve R R, Stallone F 1973 Relationship between the effectiveness of lithium therapy and family history. American Journal of Psychiatry 130: 1011–1013

Misra P C, Burns B H 1977 'Lithium non-responders' in a lithium clinic. Acta Psychiatrica Scandinavica 55: 32–40

Moller H J, Kissling W, Riehl T, Bauml J, Binz U, Wendt G 1989 Double-blind evaluation of the antimanic properties of carbamazepine as a co-medication to haloperidol. Progress in Neuropsychopharmacology and Biological Psychiatry 13: 127–136

Montgomery S A 1989 Theoretical and practical implications of a controlled trial of an alpha-2-adrenoceptor antagonist in the treatment of depression. In: Dahl S G, Gram L F (eds) Clinical pharmacology in psychiatry. Psychopharmacology Series 7. Springer-Verlag, Berlin, p 105–108

Morselli P L, Fournier V, Macher J-P 1986 Therapeutic action of progabide in depressive illness: a controlled clinical trial. In: Bartholini G, Lloyd K G, Morselli P L (eds) GABA and mood disorders: experimental and clinical research. Laboratoires d'études et de recherches synthelabo (LERS) monograph series 4. Raven Press, New York, p 119–126

Mukherjee S, Rosen A M, Caracci G, Shukla S 1986 Persistent tardive dyskinesia in bipolar patients. Archives of General Psychiatry 43: 342–346

Muller A A, Stoll K-D 1984 Carbamazepine and oxcarbamazepine in the treatment of manic syndromes: studies in Germany. In: Emrich H M, Okuma T, Muller A A (eds) Anticonvulsants in affective disorders. Excerpta Medica, Amsterdam, p 139–147

Nakajima T, Daval J L, Gleiter C H, Deckert J, Post R M, Marangos P J 1989 C-fos mRNA expression following electrical-induced seizure and acute nociceptive stress in mouse brain. Epilepsy Research 4: 156–159

Naylor G 1985 Reversal of vanadate-induced inhibition of Na-K: a possible explanation of the therapeutic effect of carbamazepine in affective illness. Journal of Affective Disorders 8: 91–93

Naylor G J, Smith A H 1981 Vanadium: a possible aetiological factor in manic depressive illness. Psychological Medicine 11: 249–256

Naylor G J, Martin B, Hopwood S E, Watson Y 1986 A two-year double-blind crossover trial of the prophylactic effect of methylene blue in manic-depressive psychosis. Biological Psychiatry 21: 915–920

Nolen A W 1983 Carbamazepine, a possible adjunct to or alternative for lithium in bipolar disorder. Acta Psychiatrica Scandinavica 67: 218–225

Nomikos G G, Damsma G, Wekstern D, Fibiger H C 1989 Acute effects of bupropion on extracellular dopamine concentrations in rat striatum and nucleus accumbens studied by in vivo microdialysis. Neuropsychopharmacology 2: 273–279

Nordin C, Siwers B, Bertilsson L 1981 Bromocriptine treatment of depressive disorders. Clinical and biochemical effects. Acta Psychiatrica Scandinavica 64: 25–33

Okuma T, Kishimoto A, Inoue K et al 1973 Anti-manic and prophylactic effects of carbamazepine on manic-depressive psychosis. Folia Psychiatrica et Neurologica Japonica 27: 283–297

Okuma T, Inanaga K, Otsuki S, Sarai K 1979 Comparison of the antimanic efficacy of carbamazepine and chlorpromazine: a double-blind controlled study. Psychopharmacology 66: 211–217

Okuma T, Inanaga K, Otsuki S et al 1981 A preliminary double-blind study of the efficacy of carbamazepine in prophylaxis of manic-depressive illness. Psychopharmacology 73: 95–96

Okuma O T, Yamashita I, Takahashi R et al 1988 Double-blind controlled studies on the therapeutic efficacy of carbamazepine in affective and schizophrenic patients. Abstracts of XVI CINP Congress no. TH18.05. Psychopharmacology 96: 102

Osman O T, Rudorfer M V, Manji H K, Grossman F, Potter W Z 1990 Idazoxan in treatment-resistant bipolar depression. Abstracts of the 143rd Annual Meeting of the American Psychiatric Association no NR432

Page C, Benaim S, Lappin F 1987 A long-term retrospective follow-up study of patients treated with prophylactic lithium carbonate. British Journal of Psychiatry 150: 175–179

Patterson J F 1987 Carbamazepine for assaultive patients with organic brain disease. Psychosomatics 28: 579–581

Paykel E S, Van Woerkom E, Walters D E, White W, Mercer J 1991 Fengabine in depression: a placebo-controlled study of a GABA agonist. Human Psychopharmacology 6: 147–154

Pazzaglia P J, Post R M 1991 Contingent tolerance and re-response to carbamazepine: A case study in a patient with trigeminal neuralgia and bipolar disorder. Journal of Neuropsychiatry and Clinical Neurosciences (in press)

Pellock J M 1987 Carbamazepine side effects in children and adults. Epilepsia 28: S64–S70

Perris C, Tjallden G, Bossi L, Perris H 1986 Progabide versus nortriptyline in depression: a controlled trial. In: Bartholini G, Lloyd K G, Morselli P L (eds) GABA and mood disorders: experimental and clinical research. LERS monograph series 4. Raven Press, New York, 135–138

Pinel J P J 1983 Effects of diazepam and diphenylhydantoin on elicited and spontaneous seizures in kindled rats: a double dissociation. Pharmacology, Biochemistry and Behaviour 18: 61–63

Placidi G F, Lenzi A, Lazzerini F, Cassano G B, Akiskal H S 1986 The comparative efficacy and safety of carbamazepine versus lithium: a randomized, double-blind 3-year trial in 83 patients. Journal of Clinical Psychiatry 47: 490–494

Post R M 1987 Mechanisms of action of carbamazepine and related anticonvulsants in affective illness. In: Meltzer H, Bunney W E Jr (eds) Psychopharmacology: a generation of progress. Raven Press, New York, p 567–576

Post R M 1988 Time course of clinical effects of carbamazepine: implications for mechanisms of action. Journal of Clinical psychiatry 49: 35–46

Post R M 1990a Alternatives to lithium for bipolar affective illness. In: Tassman A, Kaufman C, Goldfinger S (eds) APA annual review 9. APA Press, Washington, D C, p 170–202

Post R M 1990b Prophylaxis of bipolar affective disorders. International Review of Psychiatry 2: 277–320

Post R M, Weiss S R B 1989 Kindling and manic-depressive illness. In: Trimble M, Bowling T G (eds) The clinical relevance of kindling. John Wiley, Chichester, p 209–230

Post R M, Gerner R H, Carman J S 1978 Effects of a dopamine agonist piribedil in depressed patients: relationship of pretreatment HVA to antidepressant response. Archives of General Psychiatry 35: 609–615

Post R M, Jimerson D C, Bunney W E Jr, Goodwin F K, Sharpley P H 1980 Dopamine and mania: behavioural and biochemical effects of the dopamine receptor blocker pimozide. Psychopharmacology 67: 297–305

Post R M, Uhde T W, Ballenger J C, Chatterji D C, Greene R F, Bunney W E Jr 1983a CSF carbamazepine and its -10,11-epoxide metabolite in manic-depressive patients: relationship to clinical response. Archives of General Psychiatry 40: 673–676

Post R M, Uhde T W, Ballenger J C, Squillace K M 1983b Prophylactic efficacy of carbamazepine in manic-depressive illness. American Journal of Psychiatry 140: 1602–1604

Post R M, Ballenger J C, Uhde T W, Bunney W E Jr 1984a Efficacy of carbamazepine in manic-depressive illness: implications for underlying mechanisms. In: Post R M, Ballenger J C (eds) Neurobiology of mood disorders. Williams & Wilkins, Baltimore, p 777–816

Post R M, Berrettini W H, Uhde T W, Kellner C H 1984b Selective response to the anticonvulsant carbamazepine in manic-depressive illness: a case study. Journal of Clinical Psychopharmacology 4: 178–185

Post R M, Putnam F W, Contel N R, Goldman B 1984c Electroconvulsive seizures inhibit amygdala kindling: implications for mechanisms of action in affective illness. Epilepsia 25: 234–239

Post R M, Putnam F, Uhde T W, Weiss S R B 1986a ECT as an anticonvulsant: implications for its mechanism of action in affective illness. In: Malitz S, Sackheim H A (eds) Electroconvulsive therapy: clinical and basic research issues. Annals of the New York Academy of Sciences 462: 376–388

Post R M, Rubinow D R, Ballenger J C 1986b Conditioning and sensitization in the longitudinal course of affective illness. British Journal of Psychiatry 149: 191–201

Post R M, Uhde T W, Roy-Byrne P P, Joffe R T 1986c Antidepressant effects of carbamazepine. American Journal of Psychiatry 143: 29–34

Post R M, Kramlinger K G, Joffe R T, Gold P W, Uhde T W 1987a Effects of carbamazepine on thyroid function. Scientific Proceedings of the American Psychiatric Association 140: 190, abstract no 104D

Post R M, Uhde T W, Roy-Byrne P P, Joffe R T 1987b Correlates of antimanic response to carbamazepine. Psychiatry Research 21: 71–83

Post R M, Roy-Byrne P P, Uhde T W 1988a Graphic representation of the life course of illness in patients with affective disorder. American Journal of Psychiatry 145: 844–848

Post R M, Weiss S R B, Rubinow D R 1988b Recurrent affective disorders: lessons from limbic kindling. In: Ganten D, Fuxe S (eds) Current topics in neuroendocrinology. Springer-Verlag, New York, p 91–115

Post R M, Leverich G, Rosoff A S, Altshuler L L 1990 Carbamazepine prophylaxis in refractory affective disorders. A focus on long-term followup. Journal of Clinical Psychopharmacology 10: 318–327

Post R M, Altshuler L L, Ketter T, Denicoff K, Weiss S R B 1991a Anticonvulsants in affective illness: clinical and theoretical implications. In: Smith D B, Treiman D M, Trimble M (eds) Proceedings of the International Symposium on Neurobehavioural Problems in Epilepsy:

Scientific Basis, Insights, and Hypotheses. Raven Press, New York, p 239–277

Post R M, Weiss S R B, Ketter T, Joffe R T, Kramlinger K L 1991b L-baclofen: Lack of relationship of GABA$_B$ agonism to antidepressant effects of carbamazepine. International Clinical Psychopharmacology (in press)

Prasad A J 1984 The role of sodium valproate as an anti-manic agent. Pharmatherapeutica 4: 6–8

Prien R F, Klett C J, Caffey E M Jr 1973 Lithium carbonate and imipramine in prevention of affective episodes. A comparison in recurrent affective illness. Archives of General Psychiatry 29: 420–425

Prien R F, Kupfer D J, Mansky P A, Small J G, Tuason V B, Voss C B, Johnson W E 1984 Drug therapy in the prevention of the recurrences in unipolar and bipolar affective disorders. Archives of General Psychiatry 41: 1096–1104

Prien R F, Himmelhoch J M, Kupfer D J 1988 Treatment of mixed mania. Journal of Affective Disorders 15: 9–15

Puzynski S, Klosiewicz L 1984 Valproic acid amide as a prophylactic agent in affective and schizoaffective disorders. In: Emrich H M, Okuma T, Muller A A (eds) Anticonvulsants in affective disorders. Excerpta Medica, Amsterdam, p 68–75

Roy-Byrne P P, Joffe R T, Uhde T W, Post R M 1984a Carbamazepine and thyroid function in affectively ill patients: clinical and theoretical implications. Archives of General Psychiatry 41: 1150–1153

Roy-Byrne P P, Uhde T W, Post R M, Joffe R T 1984b Relationship of response to sleep deprivation and carbamazepine in depressed patients. Acta Psychiatrica Scandinavica 69: 379–382

Roy-Byrne P P, Post R M, Uhde T W, Porcu T, Davis D D 1985 The longitudinal course of recurrent affective illness: life chart data from research patients at NIMH. Acta Psychiatrica Scandinavica (suppl) 71: 5–34

Scheffner D, Konig S, Rauterberg-Ruland I, Kochen W, Hofmann W J, Unkelbach S 1988 Fatal liver failure in 16 children with valproate therapy. Epilepsia 29: 530–542

Schmutz M, Klebs K, Baltzer V 1988 Inhibition or enhancement of kindling evolution by antiepileptics. Journal of Neural Transmission 72: 245–257

Schou M 1973 Prophylactic lithium maintenance treatment in recurrent endogenous affective disorders. In: Gershon S, Shopsin B (eds) Lithium: its role in psychiatric research and treatment. Plenum Press, New York, p 269–295

Secunda S K, Swann A, Katz M M, Koslow S H, Croughan J, Chang S 1987 Diagnosis and treatment of mixed mania. American Journal of Psychiatry 144: 96–98

Semadeni G W 1976 Etude clinique de l'effet normothymique du dipropylacetamide. Acta Psychiatrica Belgica 76: 458–466

Shopsin B 1983 Bupropion's prophylactic efficacy in bipolar affective illness. Journal of Clinical Psychiatry 44: 163–169

Shopsin B, Gershon S 1978 Dopamine receptor stimulation in the treatment of depression: piribedil (ET-495). Neuropsychobiology 4: 1–14

Silverstone T 1984 Response to bromocriptine distinguishes bipolar from unipolar depression (letter). Lancet 1: 903–904

Small J G, Milstein V, Klapper M H, Kellams J J,

Sharpley P H 1989 Carbamazepine compared with lithium in the treatment of mania. Biological Psychiatry 25: 137A, abstract no. 278

Solomon I, Williamson P 1986 Verapamil in bipolar illness. Canadian Journal of Psychiatry 31: 442–444

Sovner R 1989 The use of valproate in the treatment of mentally retarded persons with typical and atypical bipolar disorders. Journal of Clinical Psychiatry 50 (suppl): 40–43

Squillace K, Post R M, Savard R, Erwin M 1984 Life charting of the longitudinal course of recurrent affective illness. In: Post R M, Ballenger J C (eds) Neurobiology of mood disorders. Williams & Wilkins, Baltimore, p 38–59

Stancer H C, Persad E 1982 Treatment of intractable rapid-cycling manic-depressive disorder with levothyroxine. Archives of General Psychiatry 39: 311–312

Stoll K D, Bisson H E, Fischer E et al 1986 Carbamazepine versus haloperidol in manic syndromes – first report of a multicentric study in Germany. In: Shagass C (ed) Biological psychiatry 1985. Elsevier, Amsterdam, p 332–334

Stromgren L S, Boller S 1985 Carbamazepine in treatment and prophylaxis of manic-depressive disorder. Psychiatric Developments 3: 349–367

Svestka J, Nahunek K 1975 Proceedings: the result of lithium therapy in acute phases of affective psychoses and some other prognostical factors of lithium prophylaxis. Activitis Nervosa Superior (Praha) 17: 270–271

Terrence C F, Sax M, Fromm G H, Chang C H, Yoo C S 1983 Effect of baclofen enantiomorphs on the spinal trigeminal nucleus and steric similarities of carbamazepine. Pharmacology 27: 85–94

Thornton J E, Mulsant B H, Dealy R, Reynolds C F 1990 A retrospective study of maintenance electroconvulsive therapy in a university-based psychiatric practice. Convulsive Therapy 6: 121–129

Tomson T 1984 Interdosage fluctuations in plasma carbamazepine concentration determine intermittent side effects. Archives of Neurology 41: 830–834

Uhde T W 1983 Carbamazepine in affective illness: controlled studies of efficacy and side effects. Presentation at the Annual Meeting of the American College of Neuropsychopharmacology (ACNP), San Juan, Puerto Rico

Vencovsky E, Soucek K, Kabes J 1984 Prophylactic effect of dipropylacetamide in patients with bipolar affective disorder – short communication. In: Emrich H M, Okuma T, Muller A A (eds) Anticonvulsants in affective disorders. Excerpta Medica, Amsterdam, p 66–67

Vick N A 1983 Suppression of carbamazepine-induced skin rash with prednisone (letter). New England Journal of Medicine 309: 1193–1194

Vieweg V, Glick J L, Herring S 1987 Absence of carbamazepine-induced hyponatremia among patients also given lithium. American Journal of Psychiatry 144: 943–947

von Zerssen D 1976 Beta-adrenergic blocking agents in the treatment of psychosis. A report of 17 cases. In: Carlsson C (ed) Neuro-psychiatric effects of adrenergic beta receptor blocking agents. Urban Schwarzenberg, Munich, p 105–114

Waddington J L, Youssef H A 1988 Tardive dyskinesia in

bipolar affective disorder: aging, cognitive dysfunction, course of illness, and exposure to neuroleptics and lithium. American Journal of Psychiatry 145: 613–616

Waehrens J, Gerlach J 1981 Bromocriptine and imipramine in endogenous depression: a double-blind controlled trial in out-patients. Journal of Affective Disorders 3: 193–202

Watkins S E, Callender K, Thomas D R, Tidmarsh S F, Shaw D M 1987 The effect of carbamazepine and lithium on remission from affective illness. British Journal of Psychiatry 150: 180–182

Wehr T A 1989 Sleep loss: a preventable cause of mania and other excited states. Journal of Clinical Psychiatry 50: 8–16

Wehr T A, Sack D A, Rosenthal N E, Cowdry R W 1988 Rapid cycling affective disorder: contributing factors and treatment responses in 51 patients. American Journal of Psychiatry 145: 179–184

Weiss E, Brunner H, Clere G et al 1986 Multicenter double-blind study of progabide in depressed patients. In: Bartholini G, Lloyd K G, Morselli P L (eds) GABA and mood disorders: experimental and clinical research. LERS monograph series 4. Raven Press, New York, p 127–133

Weiss S R B, Post R M 1987 Carbamazepine and carbamazepine-10,11-epoxide inhibit amygdala kindled seizures in the rat but do not block their development. Clinical Neuropharmacology 10: 272–279

Weiss S R B, Post R M, Pert A, Woodward R, Murman D 1989 Context-dependent cocaine sensitization: Differential effect of haloperidol on development versus expression. Pharmacology, Biochemistry and Behaviour 34: 655–661

Weiss S R B, Post R M 1991a Development and reversal of conditioned inefficacy and tolerance to the anticonvulsant effects of carbamazepine. Epilepsia 32: 140–145

Weiss S R B, Post R M 1991b Contingent tolerance to the anticonvulsant effects of carbamazepine. In: Carbamazepine: a bridge between epilepsy and psychiatry. Proceedings of a Conference, Milan, Italy, 10 June 1989.

Wright G, Galloway L, Kim J, Dalton M, Miller L, Stern W 1985 Bupropion in the long-term treatment of cyclic mood disorders: Mood stabilizing effects. Journal of Clinical Psychiatry 46: 22–25

25. Maintenance treatment

Robert F. Prien

This chapter deals with research findings, issues and strategies relating to the maintenance treatment of both bipolar and unipolar affective disorders. Three types of maintenance treatments are discussed: continuation therapy, preventive therapy and treatment of subacute chronicity. For the purposes of this chapter, the term unipolar disorder refers to a depressive disorder with no history of a manic or unequivocal hypomanic episode. Bipolar disorder refers to an affective disorder with a history of at least one manic episode. This disorder is sometimes referred to as Bipolar I to distinguish it from Bipolar II, an affective disorder with at least one episode of major depression and a history of hypomania but not mania.

COURSE OF ILLNESS

It is necessary to consider the longitudinal nature of affective disorder in maintenance treatment planning and research. A significant proportion of individuals with affective disorder have a course of illness characterized by recurrences and/or chronicity that may benefit from treatment extending beyond the acute episode. It is estimated that over 50% of individuals who have an initial episode of major depression and at least 80% who have an initial episode of mania will have one or more recurrences, often with serious psychological, social and economic consequences (American Psychiatric Association 1987, Klein et al 1980, NIMH/NIH Consensus Development Conference Statement 1985). Approximately 15–30% of individuals with a major affective disorder do not recover fully from any given episode (Akiskal 1982, Cassano et al 1983, Keller & Sessa 1990, Weissman & Myers 1978).

The failure to treat the longitudinal course of recurrent affective disorder adequately can have devastating effects on life functioning. A study of bipolar disorder sponsored by the United States Public Health Service (Medical Practice Project 1979) indicates that, without adequate treatment, the average woman experiencing the onset of bipolar disorder at the age of 24 can expect to lose about 9 years of life, 12 years of normal health and 14 years of major life activity, e.g. work, school and child-raising. Recurrent major depression has a similar deteriorative effect on quality of life and productivity and represents an equally critical public health problem (Wells et al 1989).

PHASES OF MAINTENANCE TREATMENT

The maintenance treatment of affective disorders can be classified into three phases or purposes.

1. **Continuation therapy**: the continuation of treatment after the initial control of acute symptoms for the purpose of maintaining control over the episode.

2. **Preventive therapy**: long-term treatment for the purpose of preventing or attenuating new episodes.

3. **Treatment of chronicity**: the treatment of 'subacute' affective disorders such as dysthymia, cyclothymia and other chronic or frequently-cycling disorders that do not meet the prevailing criteria for major depression or mania.

The three phases may overlap or be blurred in clinical practice. Continuation therapy becomes preventive therapy once the episode ends. The differentiation between continuation therapy and preventive therapy becomes blurred when there is no discernible clinical or biological marker to indicate that the drug-treated episode is over. Also, preventive therapy may serve the dual purpose of preventing new episodes and managing inter-episode chronicity. Despite the potential for overlap, these categories are useful for discussing the purposes of maintenance treatment.

419

CONTINUATION THERAPY

The concept of continuation drug therapy in affective disorder was introduced shortly after the introduction of imipramine (Post 1959). Continuation therapy is based upon the assumption that antidepressant and antimanic drugs can suppress manifest symptoms of the episode without immediately correcting the postulated psychopathological process underlying the episode, which continues its natural course (Ayd 1983, Klein et al 1980, Prien & Kupfer 1986). As a result, there may be a gap of several weeks or months between the disappearance of symptoms and the end of the episode. During this period, continuation of medication is required to maintain control over the episode. Withdrawal of the drug before the episode is over can result in the rapid return of symptoms.

There are two critical questions that may be asked about continuation therapy:

1. After drug-induced remission of symptoms, is there truly a need for continuation therapy?
2. Assuming that continuation therapy is required, how long should it continue and at what dosage?

Need for continuation therapy

Numerous placebo-controlled studies demonstrate the need for continuation treatment (Bialos et al 1982, Coppen et al 1978b, Harrison et al 1986, Klerman et al 1974, Mindham et al 1973, Prien et al 1973b, Prien & Kupfer 1986, Seager & Bird 1962, Stein et al 1980). All of these studies used a similar discontinuation design. In each study, an antidepressant or lithium was used to control acute symptoms, after which half of the sample received a placebo and the other half continued to receive the drug. The drugs evaluated were amitriptyline (Bialos et al 1982, Coppen et al 1978b, Klerman et al 1974, Mindham et al 1973, Stein et al 1980), imipramine (Mindham et al 1973, Prien et al 1973b, Seager & Bird 1962), lithium (Prien et al 1973b), phenelzine (Harrison et al 1986) and the combination of lithium and imipramine (Prien & Kupfer 1986).

Discontinuation studies following electroconvulsive therapy (ECT) show a relapse rate similar to that occurring after withdrawal of antidepressants or lithium (Imlah et al 1965, Kay et al 1970, Sackeim et al 1990, Seager & Bird 1962), suggesting that the symptom suppression model postulated for continuation treatment also applies to non-pharmacological somatic treatments. This model is also reinforced by research with sleep deprivation. Patients experiencing an antide-

pressant response to sleep deprivation tend to relapse after one night of sleep (Wu & Bunney 1990). Short naps can also activate severe relapses.

Duration of continuation therapy

General problem

When continuation treatment is successful in suppressing symptoms, it may be difficult to determine when the episode is over and continuation therapy is no longer required. This decision is complicated by the fact that it is not known whether pharmacotherapy eventually corrects the postulated underlying disorder, thereby shortening the episode, or merely suppresses symptoms until the episode completes its natural course.

The duration of a drug-controlled episode is not a problem if the patient is to be continued on the same drug for preventive treatment. However, if the intention is to withdraw the drug after recovery from the episode, uncertainty as to when the episode is over may result either in premature withdrawal of treatment, leading to a relapse, or in unnecessary prolongation of treatment. Some clinicians would rather chance the unnecessary extension of treatment than risk a relapse and may maintain the patient on medication for a long period – e.g. 12 months or more – to make sure that the episode is over. This practice, however, is not innocuous, even at stable maintenance doses. Lithium may produce fine hand tremor, weight gain, hypothyroidism and renal complications and has teratogenic effects that necessitate caution in women of childbearing age. Tricyclic antidepressants (TCAs) may produce uncomfortable or potentially dangerous cardiovascular or anticholinergic reactions which may be particularly troublesome as the individual ages. Newer classes of antidepressants may introduce a new set of risks—tardive dyskinesia with amoxapine, priapism with trazodone, insomnia and agitation with fluoxetine and seizures with bupropion. With all drugs there is the omnipresent risk of accidental or intentional misuse.

A frequently employed practice is to continue medication for about 6 months following initial control of symptoms and then gradually to reduce dosage while carefully monitoring the patient for signs of an emerging relapse. A problem with this procedure is that signs of a manic or depressive syndrome may not be detected quickly enough to prevent a full-blown relapse, which can be seriously disruptive for both the patient and the therapeutic alliance. In some cases, a relapse may not occur until the patient has been free of medication for 2 months or more and has infrequent contact with the physician.

Literature guidelines

The literature is of limited help in determining the duration of continuation treatment. There is evidence from natural course of illness studies that the duration of episodes tends to remain constant or lengthen slightly with each recurrence (Angst et al 1973, Zis & Goodwin 1979). This finding suggests that the length of the prior episode can be used as the lower estimate of the duration of the current episode. The problem with this strategy is that effective treatment of the prior episode may have masked symptoms and made the episode appear shorter than it was.

During the past decade there have been increased efforts to identify a biological marker of recovery from an episode (a state-dependent marker). Research has focused on rapid eye movement (REM) latency, slow-wave sleep activity, dysregulation in the hypothalamic – pituitary – thyroid axis (often indexed by thyrotropin-stimulating hormone blunting following thyrotropin-releasing hormone administration), and dysregulation in the hypothalamic – pituitary – adrenal axis (typically demonstrated by hypercortisolaemia or dexamethasone non-suppression of cortisol production) (Arana et al 1985, Belsher & Costello 1988, Bowie & Beaini 1985, Carroll 1982, Giles et al 1987, Greden et al 1983, Joyce & Paykel 1989, Kirkegaard 1981, Loosen 1986, Targum 1984). A valid and easily measured state marker would not only aid in determining when continuation therapy can be safely withdrawn but might also be useful in detecting an emerging episode before appearance of overt symptoms. At present, however, none of the findings for potential biological markers are at a stage where they can be applied in clinical practice. This concurs with the conclusion from the European Consensus Conference on the Methodology of Clinical Trials of Antidepressants (Angst et al 1989). It was concluded that no single biological marker could be recommended either for determination of the duration of depressive syndromes or for the evaluation of treatment outcome.

Results from a multicentre study on maintenance drug therapy in recurrent affective disorder coordinated by the National Institute of Mental Health (NIMH) suggest that the duration of symptom suppression can be used as a guide for when to withdraw continuation therapy in patients with major depression (Prien &

Kupfer 1986). The study indicates that withdrawal of continuation treatment is safe only after the individual has been free of significant symptoms or has returned to his or her usual level of inter-episode functioning for at least 4 months. A patient was considered to be free of significant symptomatology if he or she manifested no more than minimal or transient symptoms as defined by the Global Adjustment Scale (Endicott et al 1976). The investigators caution that generalization of findings is limited by the study admission criteria, which entered only individuals with a history of good recovery between episodes. A more chronically ill sample may have yielded different findings. The 4-month period of continuation treatment has been used in two recent maintenance treatment studies in depression (Frank et al 1990, Georgotis et al 1988, Georgotis & McCue in press). Both report a low rate of clinical worsening during the 2 months following withdrawal of medication.

The significance of residual symptomatology during continuation treatment is highlighted by a multicentre study on continuation therapy coordinated by the Medical Research Council in the UK (Mindham et al 1973). Patients with residual symptoms at the time of withdrawal of antidepressant medication had a significantly higher relapse rate over a 6-month period than patients with no symptoms at withdrawal. Faravelli et al (1986) also found that patients with residual symptoms were more likely to relapse.

Research implications

The difficulty in detecting the end of an episode that has been effectively treated with medication has research as well as clinical implications. Most studies evaluating preventive therapy randomly assign patients to preventive treatments following drug-induced 'recovery' from an acute (index) episode. If symptoms of the episode have been effectively suppressed, it may be difficult to determine whether reappearance of symptoms within the first few months of preventive treatment represents a new episode or the re-emergence of the index episode. Montgomery et al (1988) emphasize that some studies that purport to be evaluating preventive therapy are, in effect, only examining the continuation phase of treatment. Klerman & Paykel (1970) recognized this problem over two decades ago when they stressed the importance of differentiating a 'relapse', defined as the worsening of an ongoing episode, from a 'recurrence', defined as the occurrence of a new episode. The differentiation between relapse and recurrence may be particularly critical for studies of preventive treatment using a placebo control, where heavy attrition due to relapse may leave too small a sample to evaluate prevention of recurrence adequately.

Continuation treatment following ECT

In the treatment of major depression with ECT, it is standard practice to initiate continuation treatment with a TCA following the ECT-induced remission of acute symptoms. This practice is based primarily on three studies conducted in the UK in the 1960s (Imlah et al 1965, Kay et al 1970, Seager & Bird 1962). Continuation treatment with TCAs reduced the relapse rate from approximately 50% to 20%. A recent study by Sackeim et al (1990) indicates that response to the post-ECT continuation drug treatment is related to the pre-ECT response to antidepressant drug treatment. Patients who failed to respond to adequate antidepressant medication trials prior to ECT had a higher rate of relapse than patients for whom medication resistance was not well established. The investigators contend that patients should not be expected to benefit from continuation treatments that were ineffective in treating the acute episode. They suggest that one alternative is to continue ECT on an intermittent basis following symptomatic response. Although the use of continuation ECT is not an uncommon practice (Kramer 1987, Mantzen et al 1988, Thienhaus et al 1990), it has not been evaluated in systematic studies. Another alternative that warrants consideration is the use of monoamine oxidase inhibitors (MAOIs) or new classes of antidepressants as post-ECT continuation treatments in TCA-refractory patients.

Dosage of continuation therapy

There are three basic dosage strategies for continuation treatment: 1) dosage is maintained at the level that effectively controlled acute symptoms; 2) dosage is reduced to a fixed level – e.g. to 50% of the acute therapeutic dose or to the equivalent of 150 mg/day of imipramine; and 3) dosage is reduced in graduated steps over a period of months, with a rapid build-up at the first sign of reappearance of symptoms. A key issue is whether patients require the full therapeutic dose to maintain control over the episode or can remain stable at lower maintenance levels. There are arguments for both strategies. Some clinicians contend that the reemerging depression resulting from a subtherapeutic dose can be controlled by rapid reinstitution of the therapeutic level (Hollister 1978). Others argue that there is no evidence for using low doses during continuation therapy and that the maintenance dose should be similar to that used during treatment of acute symptoms (Coppen & Peet 1979, Kupfer et al 1989). Efforts at achieving a consensus recommendation for a preferred dosage strategy have been unsuccessful (NIMH/NIH Consensus Development Conference Statement 1985). This is clearly an area in need of well designed research.

PREVENTIVE TREATMENT

Who to treat

The decision to initiate preventive treatment should be based on careful evaluation of several factors: 1) the likelihood of a recurrence in the near future; 2) the potential impact of a recurrence on the patient's career, family and interpersonal functioning; 3) the patient's response to prior treatment; 4) potential contraindications to treatment; and 5) the patient's willingness to commit him- or herself to the treatment programme. The patient and family should share in the decision-making process and understand the potential benefits and risks of the treatment programme as well as the consequences of receiving no treatment. The support of family members, their attitude toward the illness and their capacity to recognize and report signs of an emerging episode are critical contributions to the success of preventive treatment programmes.

Most clinicians who have published an opinion on the use of preventive drug treatment recommend that the patient should have two or three episodes before receiving preventive therapy. However, some opt for more stringent guidelines, such as two episodes in 2 years or three episodes in 5 years (Markar & Mander 1989). There is general agreement that patients who have only a single episode, mild episodes or a lengthy interval between episodes – e.g. 5 years or more – should probably not be started on preventive treatment. The exception is the patient for whom a second episode would be life-threatening or would have a highly disruptive effect on overall functioning.

There is support from the research literature for initiating preventive treatment after two or three episodes. Naturalistic course of illness studies indicate that patients with multiple episodes are at high risk for an early recurrence or a chronic unremitting course (Angst 1981, Fukuda et al 1983, Keller et al 1983, Perris 1968). Angst (1981), reporting on a 20-year study of

400 patients, indicates that patients who have two major episodes within 5 years have a 70% probability of having two or more episodes during the following 5 years. In an earlier report, Angst et al (1973) indicate that cycle length (the period between the onset of one episode and that of the next) tends to decrease with each successive episode, reaching a plateau after four or five episodes. The average cycle length drops from 3 years following the first episode to 18 months after the third episode. Lee & Murray (1988), in a follow-up of patients first interviewed in the 1960s, report that individuals with a history of two or more hospitalizations for depression have a 50% chance of readmission within 3 years. Keller et al (1982b), in a report from an NIMH collaborative study of the naturalistic course of affective disorders, indicate that patients with three or more episodes are at increased risk for relapse or an unremitting chronic course.

Choice of treatment: bipolar disorder

Lithium

Lithium clearly is the drug of choice for the preventive treatment of bipolar disorder. Numerous studies demonstrate that lithium is significantly more effective than placebo in preventing both manic and depressive episodes (Baastrup et al 1970, Coppen et al 1971, Fieve et al 1976, Prien et al 1973a, b). In the placebo-controlled trials, the average failure rate for lithium is 33% and for placebo 81%. There has been no placebo-controlled study of preventive therapy with lithium in bipolar disorder since the early 1970s.

The more recent studies of preventive treatment with lithium are less positive than the earlier placebo-controlled trials. The multicentre study on the maintenance treatment of recurrent affective disorder sponsored by the NIMH between 1978 and 1983 (Prien et al 1984) found that only 33% of the patients receiving lithium remained episode-free over an 18- to 24-month period. A multicentre study organized by the Medical Research Council in the UK provided similarly unimpressive results with lithium (Glen et al 1984).

One explanation for the relatively poor results with lithium in later trials is provided by the report from a recent workshop on bipolar disorder (Prien & Potter 1990). The report notes that many of the earlier studies were initiated when lithium was still an investigational drug and study centres were among the few places where lithium was available. These studies tended to include a high proportion of patients with classic bipolar disorder characterized by clear-cut onset and recovery of episodes and euthymia during inter-episode intervals. Nowadays, many of the classic cases are treated satisfactorily in the community and are not referred to the large university medical centres or receiving hospitals that conduct most of the preventive treatment studies. Thus, the patient sample participating in current trials may include a larger proportion of difficult-to-treat patients who have failed to respond to lithium or other traditional therapies. These patients may manifest a wide spectrum of complications, including non-compliance in taking medication, rapid cycling, substance abuse and other common disorders that can pose problems for patient management and retention in clinical trials. The report concludes that an accurate estimate of the effectiveness of lithium will require study of the broader population of patients being treated with lithium at all levels of mental health care.

Clinical predictors of lithium response

Overall, maintenance lithium treatment appears to be most effective with patients who have a history of good inter-episode functioning (Grof et al 1979), episodes uncomplicated by mixed manic and dysphoric features (Himmelhoch & Garfinkel 1986, Post et al 1989, Prien et al 1988) and a pattern of course of illness characterized by a cycle starting with mania, followed by depression and then by a free interval (Kukopulos & Reginaldi 1980, Maj et al 1989). Other positive predictors include a family history of bipolar illness (Maj et al 1984, Mendlewicz et al 1973, Prien 1980, Prien et al 1974, Svestlca & Nahumek 1975) and positive response of first degree relatives to lithium therapy (Coryell & Winokur 1980). A recent multicentre study reports that preventive lithium therapy may be most effective with patients who have had fewer than three prior episodes and are treated with dose levels between 0.8 and 1.0 mEq/l (Gelenberg et al 1989). Perhaps the most useful predictor of long-term outcome with preventive lithium therapy, however, is the response to lithium over the initial 6 months of treatment (Abou-Saleh & Coppen 1990).

Negative predictors of response to lithium preventive treatment include a recent history of dysphoric mania or rapid/continuous cycling (Dunner & Fieve 1974, Himmelhoch & Garfinkel 1986, Maj et al 1989, Misra & Burns 1977, Post et al 1989, Prien et al 1988), a history of alcohol or drug abuse not associated with mood change (Himmelhoch et al 1976, 1983) and failure to comply with previous maintenance treatment programmes (Dunner & Fieve 1974, Post & Uhde 1987).

Predictors of lithium response and strategies for optimizing lithium treatment outcome are discussed in detail in chapter 23.

Alternatives to lithium

There is a need for carefully evaluated alternatives to lithium for preventive treatment. Even in the more favourable early trials with lithium, one-third of the patients were classified as treatment failures, despite the fact that most of the trials excluded patients with rapid cycling and other negative predictors of lithium response.

Anticonvulsants. Carbamazepine has received critical attention as a promising treatment for patients who do not respond adequately to lithium or are unable to tolerate lithium's adverse reactions (Post & Uhde 1987, Prien & Gelenberg 1989, Sachs 1989). Three randomized double-blind studies comparing carbamazepine to lithium (Lusznat et al 1988, Placidi et al 1986, Watkins et al 1987) and one comparing carbamazepine to a placebo (Okuma et al 1981) suggest that the drug may be a useful adjunct or alternative to lithium for preventive treatment. However, the studies collectively evaluated carbamazepine in only 50 patients and have serious design flaws that limit generalization of findings (Prien & Gelenberg 1989, Prien & Potter 1990). The strongest evidence of the efficacy of carbamazepine as a long-term treatment comes from other designs.

1. Longitudinal trials in which carbamazepine is periodically replaced by placebo (Ballenger & Post 1980, Post et al 1983).
2. Long-term open trials evaluating carbamazepine in patients resistant to traditional treatments (Fawcett & Kravitz 1985, Gaspar & Kielholz 1984, Joyce 1988, Kishimoto et al 1983, Post & Uhde 1985, Stromgen & Boller 1985).
3. Mirror-image longitudinal trials in which the course of illness during treatment is compared to the course of illness during an equivalent period preceding the treatment (Shulka et al 1985).

Results from these studies are generally positive and suggest that carbamazepine may be effective in patients who are refractory to lithium. One problem in interpreting the results is that the majority of patients had carbamazepine added to lithium or other ineffective regimens. As a result, there are only limited data on the use of carbamazepine alone.

The long-term use of carbamazepine alone and in combination with lithium requires further research to define the drug's specific indications and range of clinical effects. There is also need for the establishment of accepted guidelines for haematological monitoring for the rare but potentially lethal side-effects of agranulocytosis or aplastic anaemia (Balon & Berchou 1986, Luchins 1984). Despite research spanning two decades, there is still no well-designed, controlled study with sufficient sample size to confirm the efficacy of carbamazepine as a preventive treatment. Nonetheless, carbamazepine is the most extensively studied alternative or adjunct to lithium for long-term preventive therapy and may be the best choice among available treatments for patients who are resistant to or cannot tolerate lithium. It may even become a treatment of first choice for certain subgroups of patients, such as those with rapid cycles (Post & Uhde 1987).

Another potentially useful anticonvulsant is valproate. Several open trials report moderately good findings with the combination of valproate and lithium or valproate alone (Calabrese & Delucchi 1990, McElroy et al 1989). However, valproate has not been directly compared to lithium, carbamazepine or other treatments for bipolar disorder and suffers from the absence of a definitive long-term trial. Carbamazepine and valproate are discussed further in chapter 24.

Neuroleptics. Neuroleptics are not a treatment of choice for maintenance therapy, despite their frequent use as an adjunct or alternative to lithium in the control of acute manic symptoms. The risk of tardive dyskinesia and other adverse reactions limit their use on an extended basis. However, as Klein et al (1980) point out, if there are repeated 'breakthrough' manias on maintenance lithium the option of using a neuroleptic should be given careful consideration. In such cases, the risks associated with neuroleptic treatment must be balanced against the severely disruptive and life-threatening effects of repeated manic attacks. There is need for precise definition of the patient population for whom this option is justifiable and determination of the minimal effective dose required to maintain stability.

Antidepressants. Two multicentre studies indicate that the TCA imipramine is significantly less effective than lithium in preventing recurrences of mania (Prien et al 1973a, 1984). Over 50% of the imipramine-treated patients in the two studies developed a manic recurrence over a 2-year period. Studies also show that the combination of lithium and imipramine provides no advantage over lithium alone in preventing either manic or depressive episodes (Prien et al 1984, Quitkin et al 1981).

Bupropion, a unicyclic compound, is the only other antidepressant that has been evaluated as a preventive treatment for bipolar disorder. There is evidence suggesting that bupropion may be a useful alternative to lithium (Gardner 1983, Shopsin 1983, Wright et al 1985). Some clinicians view it as the most promising of the newer antidepressants for bipolar disorder because of its purported efficacy in protecting against manic recurrences (Gardner 1983, Wright et al 1985). However, further study is necessary to establish the efficacy of bupropion compared to lithium and to determine whether there is any advantage in combining the two treatments.

Breakthrough depression during lithium maintenance treatment poses special therapeutic problems. In clinical practice, a breakthrough depression is usually treated by adding an antidepressant to the lithium regimen. This practice has not been well studied and has been criticized by some clinicians who claim that the use of antidepressants to treat depression during lithium maintenance may precipitate rapid or continuous cycling in susceptible patients (Goodwin & Jamison 1990, Kukapulos & Tondo 1980). There is a need to develop research-based treatment strategies for breakthrough depressions. The difficulty is that studies designed to identify and treat breakthrough episodes that occur during maintenance treatment require a large patient sample and considerable staff resources. Such studies are beyond the scope of most individual investigators or treatment centres.

Other somatic treatments. The Report from the NIMH Workshop on the Treatment of Bipolar Disorder (in press) identified a large number of somatic treatments that have been proposed for the long-term treatment of bipolar illness, including calcium channel blockers, beta blockers, clonazepam, L-thyroxine (T4), triiodothyronine (T3), L-tryptophan, tyrosine, methylene blue, clonidine, reserpine and psychosurgery. It was concluded that while these treatments may be of heuristic interest, they are either impractical, ineffective or inadequately studied.

ECT is a long-standing treatment for acute manic and depressive states that are life-threatening or refractory to drug treatment. If the advantages of acute ECT were to be demonstrated for maintenance ECT, it could benefit select patients who have repetitive major

episodes and do not respond to maintenance medication. Another non-pharmacological technique that warrants attention is sleep manipulation (Wehr et al 1987, Wehr 1989). The interest in sleep therapy as a preventive treatment is generated by evidence that disruption or loss of sleep may be a triggering mechanism for hypomanic or manic episodes in some patients with bipolar disorder (Wehr 1989). Finally, bright light therapy might serve as a preventive treatment for selected patients with seasonal affective disorder if initiated during the weeks preceding the usual appearance of the episode. However, none of these modalities have been systematically evaluated as preventive treatments and may be impractical for extended use.

Choice of treatment: bipolar II disorder

There has been surprisingly little research on the long-term treatment of bipolar II disorder. One reason may be that depressed patients with a history of hypomania have been grouped with unipolar patients in therapeutic trials and have not been the focus of independent analysis. Another reason is that hypomanic episodes are sometimes overlooked in the documentation of psychiatric history for patients selected for therapeutic trials. The American Psychiatric Association's *Diagnostic and Statistical Manual of Mental Disorders* did not have a category for bipolar II disorder until the 1987 revision, DSM-IIIR, where it is included under the category of 'bipolar disorder not otherwise specified' (American Psychiatric Association 1987).

The few long-term studies that have reported outcome for a bipolar II sample suggest that lithium is an effective treatment. However, results are far from conclusive. Kane et al (1982) reported that lithium was more effective than imipramine and placebo in preventing depressive recurrences in bipolar II patients. Dunner et al (1976) found lithium to be more effective than placebo in reducing the frequency of hypomanic episodes but no more effective than placebo in preventing episodes of major depression. Peselow et al (1982) reported that lithium was more effective with bipolar II patients than with unipolar patients, but found relatively high recurrence rates for both groups – 51% and 64% respectively. A third subgroup consisting of cyclothymic patients had a 69% rate of recurrence.

Although lithium must be regarded as the treatment of choice for bipolar II disorder, its effectiveness is not nearly as well established as in bipolar I disorder. There has been no systematic study of alternatives to lithium for this population. Some clinicians caution against the use of TCAs because of the possibility of precipitating mania or rapid cycling (Akiskal 1988, Goodwin & Jamison 1990). They claim that the biggest problem in erroneously diagnosing a bipolar II disorder as a unipolar disorder is the risk of the patient receiving a TCA or other antidepressant capable of inducing rapid cycling or mania in susceptible patients. Carbamazepine or valproate may prove to be useful alternatives to lithium for this population. However, the first priority should be to determine the long-term efficacy of lithium in a well-designed study of carefully diagnosed patients.

Choice of treatment: unipolar disorder

Placebo-controlled studies

Table 25.1 lists preventive treatment studies that used a placebo control and had a duration of at least 12 months. To reduce the risk of confusing a relapse of the admission episode with the occurrence of a new episode, most of the studies required that patients complete a defined symptom-free period before receiving preventive treatment. The length of the symptom-free period ranged from 6 weeks (Coppen et al 1978b) to 6 months (Kane et al 1982). The drugs reported to be more effective than placebo in at least one study are lithium (Coppen et al 1971, Kane et al 1982, Prien et al 1973a, imipramine (Frank et al, 1990, Prien et al 1973a, 1984, amitriptyline (Coppen et al 1978b), fluoxetine (Montgomery et al 1988), nomifensine (Lendresse et al 1985) and zimelidine (Bjork 1983). The latter two drugs have since been withdrawn from the market because of adverse reactions.

A number of the placebo-controlled studies have methodological limitations. The studies by Coppen et al (1971), Glen et al (1984) and Prien et al (1973b) had

Table 25.1 Preventive treatment studies for unipolar disorder

Study	Symptom-free interval	Length of study (years)	Treatment	Total N	Outcome*
Coppen et al 1971	Undefined**	2	Lithium Placebo	26	L > P
Prien et al 1973b	Undefined**	2	Lithium Imipramine Placebo	88	L > P I > P L = I
Coppen et al 1978b	6 weeks	1	Amitriptyline Placebo	29	A > P
Kane et al 1982	6 months	2	Lithium Imipramine Placebo	19	L > P L > I I = P
Bjork 1983	4 months	1	Zimelidine Placebo	38	Z > P
Glen et al 1984	Undefined	3	Lithium Amitriptyline Placebo	28	L = A = P
Prien et al 1984	2 months or more	2	Lithium Imipramine Placebo	110	I > P I > L L = P
Lendresse et al 1985	2 months	1	Nomifensine Placebo	303	N > P
Montgomery et al 1988	18 weeks	1	Fluoxetine Placebo	220	F > P
Frank et al 1990	17 weeks	3	Imipramine Placebo	51	I > P

*   Based on $p \leq 0.05$ level of significance
**   Preventive treatment initiated at discharge from hospital

no defined symptom-free period and, as a result, may have failed to differentiate continuation treatment effects from preventive treatment effects. The studies by Glen et al (1984) and Kane et al (1982) had a very small sample size, with only seven and six patients respectively receiving the antidepressant drug. In the latter study, the investigators acknowledged that with a larger sample, the antidepressant (imipramine) might have proved to be more effective than placebo. Finally, one may question whether a 1-year study is long enough to evaluate preventive treatment. Survival analyses from two studies indicate that patients who survive the first year of active preventive treatment without a recurrence tend to survive the second year as well (Frank et al 1990, Prien et al 1984). However, in both studies the patient sample was at very high risk for a recurrence within the first year. Studies with a less vulnerable population may require at least 2 years to ascertain the full preventive potential of an effective treatment.

Despite the design and methodological problems with the long-term trials, the finding of a significant difference between drug and placebo in the majority of studies provides strong evidence that antidepressants and lithium can reduce the occurrence of new episodes in unipolar disorder. The findings also suggest that no drug is a panacea for recurrent affective illness. Even the most favourable results indicate failure in at least a quarter of the patients (Frank et al 1990, Montgomery et al 1988).

Lithium versus antidepressants

The decision as to whether to use lithium or an antidepressant for preventive therapy is complicated by conflicting findings regarding the relative efficacy of the two treatments. There are six preventive treatment studies comparing lithium and an antidepressant. One group of studies shows lithium to be more effective than imipramine (Kane et al 1982), mianserin (Coppen et al 1978a) and maprotiline (Coppen et al 1976). Other studies report no difference between lithium and imipramine (Prien et al 1973b) and lithium and amitriptyline (Glen et al 1984). One study indicates that imipramine is superior to lithium (Prien et al 1984). A critical review of these studies suggests that the difference in findings may be attributed in large measure to differences in design and patient populations (Prien et al 1984).

Guidelines for the selection of lithium or an antidepressant for preventive treatment are provided by the report from the Consensus Development Conference on Mood Disorders: Pharmacologic Prevention of Recurrences convened by the National Institutes of Health in the United States (1985). The conference report concludes that both lithium and the TCAs are effective preventive treatments for unipolar recurrent depression, each with advantages for certain patients.

The advantage of lithium over the TCAs and other antidepressants stems from its potent antimanic properties. The TCAs are ineffective in preventing manic episodes (Prien et al 1973a, 1984, Quitkin et al 1981) and, according to some reports (Kukopulos & Tondo 1980, Wehr & Goodwin 1987), may even precipitate hypomania, mania or rapid cycling in susceptible patients. The conference report notes that 10–15% of patients with a diagnosis of unipolar disorder will subsequently develop a manic episode (NIMH/NIH Consensus Development Conference Statement 1985). Because of the serious consequences of an unexpected manic attack, lithium therapy may be the preferred treatment where there is suspicion of a latent or previously unrecognized bipolar disorder or a higher than usual risk of developing a manic episode. Factors increasing the risk of a manic episode are a personal history of hypomania, a family history of bipolar illness and young age at onset of depression (Akiskal & Haykal 1988, Goodwin & Jamison 1990, Prien et al 1984).

The TCAs have a logistical advantage over lithium. Because the TCAs are used far more frequently than lithium in treating acute unipolar depression, the clinician wishing to use lithium as a preventive treatment may have either to discontinue an effective antidepressant and substitute lithium or to add lithium to the antidepressant drug regimen. Both options have drawbacks. Taking away a drug that is producing a good response can create logistical, compliance and ethical problems. Also, there may be a loss of control over symptoms during and after the substitution, particularly if the episode has not run its course. The option of adding lithium to the antidepressant regimen presents all the problems associated with drug combinations – e.g. uncertain guidelines for effective dosage, increased problems with compliance, difficulty in determining which drug is exerting the preventive effect and the possibility of increased risk of adverse reactions. Also, there is no evidence that the combination of lithium and an antidepressant is more effective than an antidepressant alone (Prien et al 1984).

Other treatment options

The option of continuing the original antide-pressant drug for preventive therapy should be given serious consideration. The problem with this option is that not all antidepressants have been evaluated in controlled studies of preventive efficacy. Thus far, however, newer antidepressants evaluated in long-term maintenance studies have provided positive results. These data suggest that agents used effec-tively during acute and continuation phases of treatment have preventive potential. Unless the original drug presents special risks when used on a long-term basis or has not been adequately evaluated for safety for long-term use, the advantages of con-tinuing the drug would seem to outweigh the dis-advantages.

The side-effect profile of a drug and its anticipated effect on the patient's health, functioning and com-pliance is often the decisive factor in selecting one drug over another for long-term treatment. The most cautionary statement regarding long-term use is for amoxapine because of the risk of tardive dyski-nesia and extrapyramidal reactions. MAOIs pose dietary and medication restrictions that can limit their long-term use, although a recent study indicates that with careful monitoring phenelzine can be used safely for preventive therapy (Robinson 1990). The terato-genic effects of lithium may prohibit its use as a mainte-nance treatment with women at childbearing risk. Orthostatic hypotension and arrhythmogenic effects of some TCAs can pose problems for elderly patients. Peripheral anticholinergic effects (constipation, delayed urination) also become troublesome as the individual ages. Newly marketed drugs may have long-term adverse effects that were not detected in the carefully selected samples used in investigational drug efficacy and safety trials.

In the large majority of cases, however, adverse reactions with extended use of lithium and antide-pressants are more annoying than harmful. Nonetheless, they should not be ignored. Side-effects considered by the physician to be relatively mild may have a serious impact on patient compliance in taking medication. Examples include fine hand tremor, weight gain and polyuria with lithium and weight gain, dry mouth and impotence with antidepressants. Comprehensive reviews of the side effects of lithium and the various classes of antidepressants are provided in chapters 20, 21 and 23.

Effectiveness of preventive therapy in unipolar disorder

The large majority of the placebo-controlled studies evaluating preventive drug therapy in unipolar disorder report the superiority of the active medication over placebo. However, the success with a given drug may vary significantly from one study to another. The classic examples are imipramine and lithium. Imipramine has been evaluated in four studies and lithium in seven. The recurrence rates for imipramine were 21% (Frank et al, 1990), 46% (Prien et al 1984), 48% (Prien et al 1973b) and 83% (Kane et al 1982). Corresponding recurrence rates for placebo were 78%, 71%, 92% and 100%. Frank et al (1990) suggest that the low incidence of recurrences with imipramine in their trial (21%) may have been due, at least in part, to the use of a relatively high maintenance dose. The mean dose at the start of the preventive phase was 208 mg/day and the median dose 200 mg/day. By contrast, the mean maintenance dose in the other three studies ranged from 135–137 mg/day, with doses seldom exceeding 150 mg/day. The investigators report that the higher doses were reasonably tolerated. They conclude that there is a distinct advantage to maintaining patients at a dose 'in the range of 200 mg/day', if tolerated, they suggest that the traditional practice of tapering the dose following resolution of the acute episode warrants re-examination.

The seven placebo-controlled studies evaluating lithium as a preventive treatment report recurrence rates of 0% (Baastrup et al 1970), 9% (Coppen et al 1971), 27% (Kane et al 1982), 29% (Glen et al 1984), 48% (Prien et al 1973b), 57% (Fieve et al 1976) and 68% (Prien et al 1984). The corresponding rates for placebo were 53%, 80%, 100%, 89%, 92%, 64% and 71%. The study by Baastrup et al (1970), which reported no recurrences on lithium, was terminated after only 5 months, based on the results of a sequential analysis showing a statistically significant difference between lithium and placebo.

Combined results from the four studies of imipramine show that 42 of the 88 patients receiving imipramine (48%) had a recurrence compared to 69 of 89 patients on placebo (78%). The combined results for lithium were only slightly better: 49 of 119 lithium-treated patients (41%) had a recurrence as did 91 of 124 patients receiving placebo (73%). If the study by Baastrup et al is excluded, the recurrence rates for lithium and placebo are 48% and 79% respectively, almost identical to those from the imipramine trials.

The differences in results from studies evaluating the

same drug may be due to a number of factors, including the nature of the patient population, the duration of the trial, the length and operational definition of the symptom-free period preceding preventive treatment, the maintenance dose of active medication and the criteria for defining a recurrence or treatment failure. In designing future long-term studies, more attention should be focused on these critical methodological factors. Also, practitioners applying study results to clinical practice should carefully examine the description of the patient sample and the study methodology to determine how closely they correspond to the intended application of treatment. For example, in most preventive treatment studies patients are dropped from the trial after the first recurrence and are declared treatment failures, regardless of the length of time they remained episode-free. In clinical practice, however, success or failure often is weighed against the course of illness *before* treatment. Accordingly, the patient who suffers a moderately severe episode every 2–3 years may be considered a treatment success if he or she had more frequent or severe episodes prior to treatment. The effect of treatment on inter-episode psychopathology or impairment may also be a factor in judging the success of treatment.

It is important that physicians and patients have realistic expectations regarding the effectiveness of long-term preventive drug therapy. Despite differing opinions as to the relative efficacy of specific drugs, there is general agreement that only a minority of patients achieve normalization during treatment. Schou, for example, indicates that only about a fifth of the patients who are eligible candidates for lithium therapy can be expected to have no recurrences during long-term treatment (Schou 1980). The remaining four-fifths have varying frequencies and severities of recurrences ranging from rare and mild attacks to frequent and severe episodes. Only 10% of patients receiving adequate lithium therapy will continue to have the same or worse frequency and severity of attacks as before treatment. The latter patients are definite candidates for an alternative therapy. It is the sizeable group that continues to have recurrences at reduced frequency and/or severity that poses difficulties for determining future course of treatment. Unfortunately, prospective placebo-controlled studies of 1–2 years duration do not provide a sufficient longitudinal data base to aid significantly in this decision. Longer-term follow-up studies are needed to chart the course of an effectively treated disorder over an extended period.

Duration of treatment

There is no evidence that long-term therapy cures recurrent affective illness. However, recurrences may cease spontaneously after many years. Angst & Grof (1976) report that one of every eight bipolar patients and one of three unipolar patients over 65 years of age with a long duration of illness stop having recurrences. There are no valid predictors for identifying patients who no longer require preventive drug treatment. The only way to determine whether the patient still needs medication is to withdraw the drug gradually and follow the patient for signs of a recurrence. In general, if the patient has remained well on medication for 3–4 years, the clinician and patient should discuss the benefits and risks of discontinuing the drug, taking into account the course of illness before and during treatment and the presence of any long-term adverse reactions (Schou 1989). Special precautions should be taken with patients who have a history of episodes characterized by suicide attempts, need for hospitalization or severe disruption of career or family functioning, particularly if prior episodes had a rapid onset.

TREATMENT OF CHRONICITY

Chronic depression

Several studies suggest a role for antidepressant drugs in treating chronic depression (Akiskal et al 1988, Harrison et al 1986, Kocsis et al 1988, Murphy & Checkley 1988, Rounsaville et al 1980, Stewart et al 1988, Ward 1979). However, much work remains for developing effective treatment strategies. Most of the therapeutic studies in chronic depression are uncontrolled short-term trials that provide little information on the effectiveness of treatments in modifying the long-term course of the disorder. In addition, diagnostic criteria and definitions of chronicity vary considerably among studies, making it difficult to compare results, identify treatment-responsive subtypes, and establish guidelines for treatment.

One classification system that has generated recommendations for treatment is provided by Akiskal (1983, 1990), who subdivides chronic depression into four subtypes, two of which are reported to be responsive to pharmacological treatments. One of the suggested treatment-responsive subtypes is an early-onset 'subaffective dysthymia', characterized by frequent mini-episodes of depression. This subtype is described as a lifelong primary affective disorder that displays a predominantly unipolar course with subtle bipolar characteristics such as brief hypomanic switches to TCA challenge and a bipolar familial history. Preliminary evidence suggests that a trial of TCAs and/or lithium combined with 'practical' psychotherapeutic modalities such as social skills training is an effective treatment (Akiskal 1990, Weissman & Akiskal 1984).

The other treatment-responsive subtype is a late-onset chronic primary depression that typically occurs after the age of 40 in patients who fail to recover from major depressive episodes. The residual state may develop in the absence of a premorbid history of depressive manifestations and, in some patients, may represent an inadequately treated major depression. Akiskal (1990) recommends vigorous pharmacotherapy with one of the standard antidepressants combined with supportive psychotherapy and interpersonal therapy, followed by a dissimilar TCA or one of the new antidepressants if the patient remains unresponsive. ECT may also prove effective.

The subtype with the poorest response to treatment is an early onset characterological disorder labelled 'character spectrum disorder'. This disorder is a chronic dysphoria with prominent lifelong personality disturbances and an absence of validating criteria for an underlying affective biology – e.g. shortened REM latency. This subtype corresponds closely to Winokur's depressive spectrum disease (Winokur 1979) and a subtype with lifelong characterological instability proposed by Klein et al (1980).

The fourth subtype is a chronic primary depression secondary to a non-affective psychiatric disorder or medical condition. The treatment for this disorder is dictated by the nature of the affective symptoms and the non-affective disorder.

Although Akiskal's subtypes have promising potential for the development of effective treatment strategies for chronic depression, they require more precise operational definitions and validation. It is particularly important to validate the distinction between subaffective dysthymia and character spectrum disorder and between the early- and late-onset disorders.

The only published controlled therapeutic study to focus exclusively on chronic depression is a 6-week trial conducted by Kocsis et al (1988), comparing imipramine to placebo in 54 patients with DSM-III criteria for major depressive disorder. This phenomena of a major depression superimposed on a chronic dysthymia is referred to as double depression (Keller & Shapiro 1982). Patients with depressive disorders secondary to other major DSM-III Axis I or medical disorders were excluded from the sample. The dose of imipramine was increased rapidly during the first 10 days to a maximum of 300 mg/day or the highest tolerated dose. By the end of week 6, 35% of the imipramine-treated patients and 15% of the placebo-treated patients had a remission from both the acute symptoms of the major depression and the deficits of the dysthymic disorder. It was concluded that some patients with chronic depression can benefit substantially, at least in the short run, from aggressive treatment with a TCA.

A less positive course of double depression is reported by Keller et al (1982a, 1983), who found that only 29% achieved remission from the superimposed major depression and dysthymic disorder within 1 year. The investigators note that patients often received inadequate antidepressant drug treatment. Of the patients who were prescribed drugs for major depression, only 34% received TCAs for longer than 4 weeks and, of these, only 12% had a dose exceeding 150 mg/day. About one in five patients received only antianxiety drugs. Other reports also suggest that patients with chronic depression often receive substandard treatment or no treatment at all (Kotin et al 1973, Lehmann 1974, Schatzberg et al 1983, Scott 1988, Weissman & Klerman 1977). Although more systematic study is necessary to establish the relationship of adequacy of treatment to chronicity, available evidence suggests that inadequate treatment is a contributing factor in the development and prolongation of chronic states in some patients.

Some investigators suggest that the combination of an antidepressant and psychotherapy may be the most effective treatment for ameliorating both symptomatology and impaired functioning in some patients with chronic depression (Akiskal & Haykal 1988, Weissman & Akiskal 1984). However, there are no definitive data indicating what combination of treatments can be expected to work with what patients. Also, there are no well-controlled studies on the efficacy of psychotherapy alone.

Cyclothymia

Cyclothymia is a disorder characterized by both hypomanic and depressive periods that are not of sufficient severity or duration to satisfy the prevailing criteria for major depression or mania. There has been less research on the treatment of cyclothymia than on bipolar II disorder. Many patients with the disorder do not require pharmacological treatment because of the mildness of symptoms and the short duration of episodes. With others, the characterological pathology often associated with the disorder may cause researchers to place less emphasis on psychotropic drug therapy.

There is speculation that cyclothymia, bipolar II disorder and bipolar I disorder exist on a continuum of related disorders (Akiskal 1988). In that case, one would expect lithium to be an effective treatment for the disorder. Small-sample open trials and anecdotal reports suggest that lithium has a mood-stabilizing effect with some cyclothymic patients (Jefferson et al 1987). Peselow et al (1982), however, found that lithium was less effective in cyclothymia than in bipolar II disorder and unipolar disorder.

Until an assessable relationship is established between cyclothymia and bipolar I or II disorder, it is questionable whether any investigator will mount a large-scale long-term trial to determine if control of cyclothymia will prevent the development of a more severe disorder. Some investigators contend that a more relevant problem may be the tendency of clinicians to overlook the significance of cyclothymia in treating superimposed major depression (Akiskal 1988). They contend that overzealous use of a TCA can lead to rapid cycling and chronicity. Regardless of whether one agrees or disagrees with this position, it demonstrates a common theme that underlies both short-term and long-term treatment of affective disorder – namely, the need to consider the longitudinal course of the illness in treatment planning.

DIRECTIONS FOR FUTURE RESEARCH

Alternatives to lithium for bipolar disorder

Despite over three decades of research with lithium and other treatments for bipolar illness, there are still critical gaps in our knowledge of how to treat the disorder. There is a special need for well-designed controlled studies to evaluate the efficacy of alternatives for lithium preventive treatment. Carbamazepine, the best studied of the alternatives or adjuncts to lithium, still requires more definitive research to establish the drug's specific indications when used alone and in combination with lithium. Other promising treatments such as valproate also await systematic long-term controlled trials. In addition, there should be studies evaluating the role of neuroleptics for patients who have breakthrough manic episodes on lithium and development of research-based treatment strategies for breakthrough depressive episodes and rapid cycling.

Identification of state markers

There should be increased efforts at identifying biological or physiological markers of episode length. Such markers would be of significant help to clinicians in determining when medication can be safely withdrawn following remission of acute symptoms and when a partial remission requires more aggressive treatment. A valid site marker that precedes the appearance of overt symptoms would aid in the early identification of an emerging recurrence and, in selected cases, obviate the need for continuous preventive treatment.

Treatment of chronicity

There should be increased efforts at developing strategies for treating chronic depression. Well-designed controlled trials are required. To maximize the contribution from therapeutic studies, there is a need to develop and validate subtypes of the disorder that have relevance for predicting course of illness and long-term treatment outcome. Akiskal's classification system is promising but requires more research before it can be translated into viable treatment recommendations for clinical practice. Other systems of classification have not generated much therapeutic research. There is a need for studies of psychotherapy alone and in combination with antidepressants. Another research requirement is the development of an assessment battery sensitive to treatment-induced changes in low-grade depressive symptoms and social and interpersonal functioning. From a clinical standpoint, it is necessary to use antidepressants at an adequate dose. Failure to increase dosage to the maximum tolerated level in patients resistant to lower doses may lead to the erroneous judgment that the disorder is refractory to treatment.

Dosage during maintenance treatment

With the notable exception of lithium, systematic dose — response studies for long-term use of psychopharmacological agents are practically nonexistent. Most textbooks on psychotropic drugs recommend that the clinician use the 'lowest effective dose' for preventive treatment, without indicating how this can be accomplished without exposing the patient to a relapse or recurrence. Recent reports on the effective long-term use of antidepressant drug doses at or near the level that initially controlled acute symptoms underscores the need for well-designed dose—response studies for both continuation and preventive therapy.

REFERENCES

Abou-Saleh M T, Coppen A J 1990 Predictors of long-term outcome of mood disorder on prophylactic lithium. Lithium 1: 27–35

Akiskal H S 1982 Factors associated with incomplete recovery in primary depressive illness. Journal of Clinical Psychology 43: 266–271

Akiskal H S 1983 Dysthymic disorder: psychopathology of proposed chronic depressive subtypes. American Journal of Psychiatry 140: 11–20

Akiskal H S 1988 Cyclothymic and related disorders. In: Georgotis A, Cancro R (eds) Depression and mania: a comprehensive textbood. Elsevier, New York

Akiskal H S 1990 Toward a definition of dysthymia: boundaries with personality and mood disorders. In: Burton S W, Akiskal H S (eds) Dysthmic disorder. Gaskell, London

Akiskal H S, Haykal R F 1988 Dysthymic and chronic depressive conditions. In: Georgotis A, Cancro R (eds) Depression and mania: a comprehensive textbook. Elsevier, New York

American Psychiatric Association 1987 Diagnostic and statistical manual of mental disorders, 3rd edn – revised. American Psychiatric Press, Washington, DC

Angst J 1981 Clinical indications for a prophylactic treatment of depression. In: Mendlewicz J, Coppen A, van Praag H M (eds) Depressive illness – biological psychopharmacological issues. Advances in Biological Psychiatry 7. S Karger, Basel

Angst J, Grof P 1976 The course of monopolar depressions and bipolar psychosis. In: Villeneuve A (ed) Lithium in psychiatry: a synopsis. Presses de l'Université Laval, Quebec

Angst J, Baastrup P C, Grof P, Hippius H, Poeldinger W, Weiss P 1973 The course of monopolar depression and bipolar psychoses. Psychiatrie Neurologie et Neurochirugie (Amsterdam) 76: 489–500

Angst J, Bech P, Boyer P, Bruinvels R et al 1989 Consensus conference on the methodology of clinical trials of antidepressants, March 1988: Report of the consensus committee. Pharmacopsychiatry 22: 3–7

Arana G W, Baldessarini R J, Ornsteen M 1985 The dexamethasone suppression test for diagnosis and prognosis in psychiatry. Archives of General Psychiatry 42: 1193–1204

Ayd F J 1983 Continuation and maintenance antidepressant therapy. In: Ayd F J, Taylor I J, Taylor B T (eds) Affective disorders reassessed: 1983. Ayd Medical Communications, Baltimore

Baastrup P C, Poulson J C, Schou, M, Thomsen K, Amdisen A 1970 Prophylactic lithium: double-blind discontinuation in manic-depressive and recurrent disorders. Lancet 2: 782–790

Ballenger J C, Post R M 1980 Carbamazepine (Tegretol) in manic-depressive illness: a new treatment. American Journal of Psychiatry 137: 782–790

Balon R, Berchou R 1986 Hematologic side effects of psychotropic drugs. Psychosomatics 27: 119–120

Belsher G, Costello C G 1988 Relapse after recovery from unipolar depression: a critical review. Psychological Bulletin 104: 84–96

Bialos D, Giller E, Jatlow P, Docherty J, Harkness L 1982 Recurrence of depression after discontinuation of long-term amitriptyline treatment. American Journal of Psychiatry 139: 325–329

Bjork K 1983 The efficacy of zimeldine in preventing depressive episodes in recurrent major depressive disorders – a double blind placebo-controlled study. Acta Psychiatrica Scandinavica 68: 182–189

Bowie P C, Beaini A Y 1985 Normalisation of the dexamethasone suppression test: a correlate of clinical improvement in primary depressives. British Journal of Psychiatry 147: 30–35

Calabrese J R, Delucchi G A 1990 Spectrum of efficacy of valproate in 55 patients with rapid cycling bipolar disorder. American Journal of Psychiatry 147: 431–434

Carroll B J 1982 The dexamethasone suppression test: new applications. British Journal of Psychiatry 140: 292–304

Cassano G B, Maggini C, Akiskal H S 1983 Short-term, subchronic, and chronic sequelae of affective disorders. Psychiatric Clinics of North America 6: 55–67

Coppen A, Peet M 1979 The long-term management of patients with affective disorders. In: Paykel E S, Coppen A (eds) Psychopharmacology of affective disorders. Oxford University Press, New York

Coppen A, Noguera R, Bailey J et al 1971 Prophylactic lithium in affective disorders. Lancet 2: 275–279

Coppen A, Montgomery S, Gupta R K, Bailey J E 1976 A double-blind comparison of lithium carbonate and maprotiline in the prophylaxis of the affective disorders. British Journal of Psychiatry 118: 479–485

Coppen A, Chose K, Rao V 1978a Mianserin and lithium in the prophylaxis of depression. British Journal of Psychiatry 133: 206–210

Coppen A, Montgomery S A, Rao V, Bailey J E, Jorgensen A 1978b Continuation therapy with amitriptyline in depression. British Journal of Psychiatry 133: 28–33

Coryell W H, Winokur G 1980 Predicting lithium responders and nonresponders: familial indicators. In: Johnson F N (ed) Handbook of lithium therapy. MTP Press, Lancaster

Dunner D L, Fieve R R 1974 Clinical factors in lithium carbonate prophylaxis failute. Archives of General Psychiatry 30: 229–233

Dunner D L, Fleis J L, Fieve R R 1976 Lithium carbonate prophylaxis failure. British Journal of Psychiatry 129: 40–44

Endicott J, Spitzer R L, Fleiss J L 1976 The global assessment scale. A procedure for measuring overall severity of psychiatric disturbance. Archives of General Psychiatry 33: 766–771

Faravelli C, Ambonetti A, Pallanti S, Pazzagli A 1986 Depressive relapses and incomplete recovery from index episode. American Journal of Psychiatry 143: 888–891

Fawcett J, Kravitz H M 1985 The long term management of bipolar disorders with lithium, carbamazepine, and antidepressants. Journal of Clinical Psychiatry 46: 58–60

Fieve R R, Kumbarachi T, Dunner D L 1976 Lithium prophylaxis of depression in bipolar I, bipolar II, and unipolar patients. American Journal of Psychiatry 133: 925–929

Frank E, Kupfer D J, Perel J M, McEachran M S, Grochocinski V J 1990 Maintenance therapies on recurrent depression protocol; treatment outcome. Archives of General Psychiatry 47: 1093–1099

Fukuda K, Etoh T, Iwadate T, Ishii A 1983 The course and prognosis of manic-depressive psychosis: a quantitive analysis of episodes and intervals. Tohoku Journal of Experimental Medicine 139: 299–241

Gardner E A 1983 Long-term preventive care in depression: the use of bupropion in patients intolerant of other antidepressants. Journal of Clinical Psychiatry 44: 157–162

Gaspar M, Kielholz P 1984 Carbamazepine treatment in therapy-resistant patients with manic-depressive psychosis. In: Emrich H M, Okuma T, Muller A A (eds) Preliminary results with anitconvulsants in affective disorders. Elsevier, Amsterdam

Gelenberg A, Kane J, Keller M et al 1989 Comparison of standard and low serum levels of lithium for maintenance treatment of bipolar disorder. New England Journal of Medicine 321: 1489–1493

Georgotis A, McCue R E in press Relapse of depressed patients after effective continuation therapy. Journal of Affective Disorders (in press)

Georgotis A, McCue R E, Cooper T B, Nagachandra N, Chang I 1988 How effective and safe is continuation therapy in elderly depressed patients? Factors affecting relapse rate. Archives of General Psychiatry 45: 929–932

Giles D E, Jarrett R B, Roffwarg H P et al 1987 Reduced REM latency: a predictor of recurrence in depression. Neuropsychopharmacology 1: 33–39

Glen A I M, Johnson A L, Shepherd M 1984 Continuation therapy with lithium and amitriptyline in unipolar depressive illness: a randomized double-blind controlled trial. Psychological Medicine 14: 37–50

Goodwin F K, Jamison K 1990 Manic depressive illness. Oxford University Press, New York

Greden J F, Gardner R, King D, Grunhaus L, Carroll B J, Kronfol Z 1983 Dexamethasone suppression tests in antidepressant treatment of melancholia: the process of normalization and test-retest reproductibility. Archives of General Psychiatry 40: 493–500

Grof P, Lane J, MacCrimmon D 1979 Clinical and laboratory correlates of the responses to long-term lithium treatment. In: Schou M, Stromgren E (eds) Origin, prevention and treatment of affective disorders. Academic Press, London

Harrison W, Rabkin J, Stewart J W, McGrath P J, Tricamo E, Quitkin F 1986 Phenelzine for chronic depression: a study of continuation treatment. Journal of Clinical Psychiatry 47: 346–349

Himmelhoch J M, Garfinkel M E 1986 Sources of lithium resistance in mixed mania. Psychopharmacology Bulletin 22: 613–620

Himmelhoch J M, Mulla D, Neil J F et al 1976 Incidence and significance of mixed affective states in a bipolar population. Archives of General Psychiatry 33: 1062–1066

Himmelhoch J M, Hills S, Steinberg B, May S 1983 Lithium, alcoholism and psychiatric diagnosis. Journal of Psychiatric Treatment Evaluation 5: 83–88

Hollister L E 1978 Clinical pharmacology of psychotherapeutic drugs. Churchill Livingstone, New York

Imlah N W, Ryan E, Harrington J A 1965 The influence of antidepressant drugs on the response to electroconvulsive therapy and on subsequent relapse rates. In: Bente D, Bradley P (eds) Neuropsychopharmacology. Elsevier, Amsterdam

Jefferson J W, Greist J H, Ackerman D L, Carroll J A 1987 Lithium encyclopedia for clinical practice, 2nd edn. American Psychiatric Press, Washington DC

Joyce P R 1988 Carbamazepine in rapid cycling bipolar affective disorder. International Journal of Psychopharmacology 3: 123–129

Joyce P R, Paykel E S 1989 Predictors of drug response in depression. Archives of General Psychiatry 46: 89–99

Kane J M, Quitkin F M, Rifkin A, Ramos-Lorenzi J R, Nayak D P, Howard A 1982 Lithium carbonate and imipramine in the prophylaxis of unipolar and bipolar II illlness. Archives of General Psychiatry 39: 1065–1069

Kay D W K, Fahy T, Garside R F 1970 A seven-month double-blind trial of amitriptyline and diazepam in ECT-treated depressed patients. British Journal of Psychiatry 117: 667–671

Keller M B, Sessa F M 1990 Dysthymia: development and clinical course. In: Burton S W, Akiskal H S (eds) Dysthymia disorder. Saskell, London

Keller M B, Shapiro R W 1982 Double depression: superimposition of acute depressive episodes on chronic depressive disorders. American Journal of Psychiatry 139: 438–442

Keller M B, Klerman G L, Lavori P W, Fawcett J A, Coryell W, Endicott J 1982a Treatment received by depressed patients. Journal of the American Medical Association 248: 1848–1855

Keller M B, Shapiro R W, Lavori P W, Wolfe N 1982b Relapse in major affective disorders. Archive of General Psychiatry 39: 911–915

Keller M B, Shapiro R W, Lavori P W, Lewis C E, Klerman G L 1983 Double depression: two year follow-up. American Journal of Psychiatry 140: 689–694

Kirkegaard C 1981 The thyrotropin response to thyrotropin-releasing hormone in endogenous depression. Psychoneuroendocrinology 6: 189–212

Kishimoto A, Ogura C, Hazama H et al 1983 Long-term prophylactic effects of carbamazepine in affective disorder. British Journal of Psychiatry 143: 327–331

Klein D F, Gittelman R, Quitkin F, Rifkin A 1980 Diagnosis and Drug treatment of psychiatric disorders: adults and children. Williams & Wilkins, Baltimore

Klerman G L, Paykel E S 1970 Long-term drug therapy in affective disorders. International Pharmacopsychiatry 5: 80–99

Klerman G L, DiMascio A, Weissman M, Prusoff B, Paykel E S 1974 Treatment of depression by drugs and psychotherapy. American Journal of Psychiatry 131: 186–191

Kocsis J H, Francis A J, Voss C, Mann J J, Mason B J, Sweeny J 1988 Imipramine treatments for chronic depression. Archives of General Psychiatry 45: 253–257

Kotin J, Post R M, Goodwin F K 1973 Drug treatment of depressed patients referred for hospitalization. American Journal of Psychiatry 130: 1139–1141

Kramer B A 1987 Maintenance ECT: a survey of practice. Convulsive Therapy 3: 260–268

Kukopulos A, Reginaldi D 1980 Recurrences of manic-depressive episodes during lithium treatment. in: Johnson F N (ed) Handbook of lithium therapy. MTP Press, Lancaster

Kukopulos A, Tondo L 1980 Lithium nonresponders and

their treatment. In: Johnson F N (ed) Handbook of lithium therapy. MTP Press, Lancaster

Kupfer D J, Perel J M, Frank E L 1989 Adequate treatment with imipramine in continuation treatment. Journal of Clinical Psychiatry 50: 250–255

Lee A S, Murray R M 1988 The long-term outcome of Maudsley depressives 153: 741–751

Lehmann H E 1974 Therapy resistant depression: a clinical classification. Pharmacopsychiatrica 7: 156–163

Lendresse P H, Cren M C, LeMarie J C 1985 Traitment prolongé par nomifensine 75 mg dans les états depressifs nevrotiques et reactionnels. Psychiatrie francaise 16 (suppl): 156–158

Loosen P T 1986 Hormones of the hypothalamic-pituitary-thyroid axis: a psychoneuroendocrine perspective. Pharmacopsychiatry 19: 401–415

Luchins D J 1984 Fatal agranulocytosis in a chronic schizophrenic patient treated with carbamazepine. American Journal of Psychiatry 141: 687–688

Lusznat R M, Murphy D P, Nunn C M H 1988 Carbamazepine vs lithium in the treatment and prophylaxis of mania. British Journal of Psychiatry 153: 198–204

McElroy S L, Keck P E, Pope H G, Hudson J I 1989 Valproate in psychiatric disorders: literature review and clinical guidelines. Journal of Clinical Psychiatry 50 (suppl): 23–29

Maj M, Del Vecchio M, Starace F, Pirozzi R, Kemali D 1984 Prediction of affective psychoses response to lithium prophylaxis. Acta Psychiatrica Scandinavica 69: 37–44

Maj M, Pirozzi R, Starace F 1989 Previous pattern of course of the illness as a predictor of response to lithium prophylaxis in bipolar patients. Journal of Affective Disorders 17: 237–241

Mantzen T A, Martin R L, Watt T J et al 1988 The use of maintenance electroconvulsive therapy for relapsing depression. Jefferson Journal of Psychiatry 6: 52–58

Markar H R, Mander A J 1989 Efficacy of lithium in clinical practice. British Journal of Psychiatry 155: 496–500

Medical Practice Project 1979 A state-of-the-science report for the Office of the Assistant Secretary for the US Department of Health, Education, and Welfare. Policy Research, Baltimore

Mendlewicz J, Fieve R R, Stallone F 1973 Relationship between effectiveness of lithium therapy and family history. American Journal of Psychiatry 130: 1011–1013

Mindham R H, Howland C, Shepherd M 1973 An evaluation of continuation therapy with tricyclic antidepressants in depressive illness. Psychological Medicine 3: 5–17

Misra P C, Burns B H 1977 Lithium non-responders in a lithium clinic. Acta Psychiatrica Scandinavica 55: 32–40

Montgomery S A, Dufour H, Brion S et al 1988 The prophylactic efficacy of fluoxetine in unipolar depression. British Journal of Psychiatry 153 (suppl 3): 69–76

Murphy D, Checkley S A 1988 A prevalence study and treatment study of ritanserin in dysthymic disorder. Psychopharmacology 96: 109–113

NIMH-NIH Consensus Development Conference Statement 1985 Mood disorders: prevention of recurrences. American Journal of Psychiatry 142: 469–472

Okuma T, Inanaga K, Otsuki S, Sari K, Takahashi R, Hazama H, Mori A, Watanabe S 1981 A preliminary double-blind study on the efficacy of carbamazepine in prophylaxis of manic-depressive illness. Psychopharmacology 73: 95–96

Perris C 1968 The course of depressive psychoses. Acta Psychiatrica Scandinavica 44: 238–248

Peselow E D, Dunner D L, Fieve R R, Lautin A 1982 Lithium prophylaxis of depression in unipolar, bipolar II, and cyclothymic patients. American Journal of Psychiatry 139: 747–752

Placidi G F, Lenzi A, Lazzerini F, Cassano G B, Akiskal H S 1986 The comparative efficacy and safety of carbamazepine versus lithium: a randomized double-blind 3 year trial in 83 patients. Journal of Clinical Psychiatry 47: 490–494

Post R 1959 Imipramine in depression (letter). British Medical Journal 2: 1252

Post R M, Uhde T W 1985 Carbamazepine in bipolar illness. Psychopharmacology Bulletin 21: 10–17

Post R M, Uhde T W 1987 Clinical approaches to treatment-resistant bipolar illness. In: Hales R E, Frances A J (eds) American Psychiatric Association annual review 6. American Psychiatric Press, Washington, DC

Post R M, Uhde T W, Ballenger J C, Squillace 1983 Prophylactic efficacy of carbamazepine in manic-depressive illness. American Journal of Psychiatry 140: 1602–1604

Post R M, Rubinow T W, Uhde P P et al 1989 Dysphoric mania. Archives of General Psychiatry 46: 353–360

Prien R F 1980 Predicting lithium responders and nonresponders: illness indicators. In: Johnson F N (ed) Handbook of lithium therapy. MTP Press, Lancaster

Prien R F, Gelenberg A J 1989 Alternatives to lithium for the preventive treatment of bipolar disorder. American Journal of Psychiatry 146: 840–848

Prien R F, Kupfer D J 1986 Continuation drug therapy for major depressive episodes: how long should it be maintained? American Journal of Psychiatry 143: 18–23

Prien R F, Caffey E M, Klett C H 1973a Prophylactic efficacy of lithium carbonate in manic-depressive illness. Archives of General Psychiatry 28: 337–341

Prien R F, Klett C H, Caffey E M 1973b Lithium carbonate and imipramine in prevention of affective episodes. Archives of General Psychiatry 29: 420–425

Prien R F, Caffey E M, Klett C J 1974 Factors associated with treatment success in lithium carbonate prophylaxis. Archives of General Psychiatry 31: 189–192

Prien R F, Kupfer D J, Mansky P A et al 1984 Drug therapy in the prevention of recurrences in unipolar and bipolar affective disorders. Archives of General Psychiatry 41: 1096–1104

Prien R F, Himmelhoch J M, Kupfer D J 1988 Treatment of mixed mania. Journal of Affective Disorders 15: 9–15

Prien R F, Potter W Z 1990 Report on the treatment of bipolar disorder. Psychopharmacology Bulletin 26: 409–427

Quitkin F M, Kane J, Rifkin A, Ramos-Lorenzi J R, Saraf K, Howard A, Klein D F 1981 Prophylactic lithium with and without imipramine for bipolar I patients. Archives of General Psychiatry 38: 902–907

Robinson D 1990 Continuation and maintenance treatment of major depression with the monoamine oxidase inhibitor phenelzine: a double-blind, placebo-controlled discontinuation study. Presented at the 30th Annual Meeting of the New Clinical Drug Evaluation Unit (NCDEU) Program, Key Biscayne, Florida, May

Rounsaville B J, Sholomskas D, Prusoff B A 1980 Chronic mood disorders in depressed outpatients. Journal of Affective Disorders 2: 73–88

Sachs G S 1989 Adjuncts and alternatives to lithium therapy for bipolar affective disorder. Journal of Clinical Psychiatry 50 (suppl): 31–39

Sackeim H, Prudic J, Devanand D P, Decina P, Kerr B, Malitz S 1990 The impact of medication resistance and continuation pharmacotherapy on relapse following responses to electroconvulsive therapy in major depression. Journal of Clinical Psychopharmacology 10: 96–104

Schatzberg A F, Cole J O, Cohen B M, Altesman R I, Sniffen C M 1983 Survey of depressed patients who have failed to respond to treatment. In: David J M, Maas J W (eds) The affective disorders. American Psychiatric Press, Washington, DC

Schou M 1980 Lithium treatment of manic-depressive illness. S Karger, Basel

Schou M 1989 Lithium treatment of manic-depressive illness. A practical guide, 4th edn. S Karger, Basel

Scott J 1988 Chronic depression. British Journal of Psychiatry 153: 287–297

Seager C P, Bird R L 1962 Imipramine with electrical treatment in depression – a controlled trial. Journal of Mental Science 108: 704–707

Shopsin B 1983 Bupropion's prophylactic efficacy in bipolar affective illness. Journal of Clinical Psychiatry 44: 163–169

Shulkla S, Cook B L, Miller M G 1985 Lithium-carbamazepine versus lithium-neuroleptic prophylaxis in bipolar illness. Journal of Affective Disorders 9: 219–222

Stein M K, Rickels K, Weisse C C 1980 Maintenance therapy with amitriptyline: a controlled trial. American Journal of Psychiatry 137: 370–371

Stevenson G H, Geoghegan J J 1951 Prophylactic electroshock: a five year study. American Journal of Psychiatry 107: 743–748

Stewart J W, Quitkin F M, McGrath P J et al 1988 Social functioning in chronic depression: effects of 6 weeks of antidepressant treatment. Psychiatric Research 25: 213–222

Stromgen L S, Boller S 1985 Carbamazepine in treatment and prophylaxis of manic-depressive disorder. Psychiatric Developments 4: 349–367

Svestlca J, Nahumek K 1975 The results of lithium therapy in acute phases of affective psychoses and some other prognostic factors of lithium prophylaxis. Activ Nerv Sup 17: 270–272

Targum S D 1984 Persistent neuroendocrine dysregulation in major depressive disorder: a marker for early relapse. Biological Psychiatry 19: 305–317

Thienhaus O J, Margletta S, Bennett J A 1990 A study of the clinical efficacy of maintenance ECT. Journal of Clinical Psychiatry 51: 141–144

Ward N G 1979 The effectiveness of tricyclic antidepressants in chronic depression. Journal of Clinical Psychiatry 40: 49–52

Watkins S E, Callender K, Thomas D R, Tidmarsh S F, Shaw D M 1987 The effect of carbamazepine and lithium on remission from affective illness. British Journal of Psychiatry 150: 180–182

Wehr T A 1989 Sleep loss: a preventable cause of mania and other excited states. Journal of Clinical Psychiatry 50 (suppl): 8–16

Wehr T A, Goodwin F K 1987 Can antidepressants cause mania and worsen the course of affective illness? American Journal of Psychiatry 144: 1403–1411

Wehr T A, Sack D A, Rosenthal N E 1987 Sleep reduction as a final pathway in the genesis of mania. American Journal of Psychiatry 144: 201–203

Weissman M M, Akiskal H 1984 The role of psychotherapy in chronic depressions: a proposal. Comprehensive Psychiatry 25: 23–31

Weissman M M, Klerman G L 1977 The chronic depressive in the community: under-recognized and poorly treated. Comprehensive Psychiatry 18: 523–531

Weissman M N, Myers J K 1978 affective disorders in a US urban community: The use of research diagnostic criteria in an epidemiologic survey. Archives of General Psychiatry 35: 1304–1311

Wells K B, Steward A, Hayes R D et al 1989 The functioning and well-being of depressed patients: results from the Medical Outcomes Study. Journal of the American Medical Association 262: 914–919

Winokur G 1979 Unipolar depression – is it divisible into autonomous subtypes? Archives of General Psychiatry 36: 47–52

Wright G, Galloway L, Kim J et al 1985 Bupropion in the long-term treatment of cyclic mood disorders: mood stabilizing effects. Journal of Clinical Psychiatry 46: 22–25

Wu J C, Bunney W E 1990 The biological basis of an antidepressant response to sleep deprivation and relapse: review and hypothesis. American Journal of Psychiatry 147: 14–21

Zis A P, Goodwin F K 1979 Major affective disorder as a recurrent illness: a critical review. Archives of General Psychiatry 36: 835–839

26. Resistant depression and psychosurgery

Paul Bridges

TREATMENT OF RESISTANT DEPRESSION

General management

Unfortunately, to some clinicians the clearly effective physical treatments now available for potentially crippling psychiatric illnesses unreasonably remain associated with the limited effectiveness of obsolete physical therapies. Before the remarkable discoveries of potent psychotropic medication of various kinds in the 1950s, physical treatments were, at best, of only symptomatic value and, at worst, some were not only useless but could be actually harmful (e.g. deep insulin coma therapy). Amphetamines were often used symptomatically for depression, while anxiety symptoms were treated with barbiturates. Of course, these unsatisfactory drugs were both potentially addictive and dangerous in overdose.

Many psychiatrists seem to continue the same general strategy. They appear to believe that contemporary medication, despite its much more specific activity, must be used in small doses, while non-physical treatments are often given an unreasonable priority. That is, tablets are prescribed reluctantly and therefore usually inexpertly while the emphasis is on psychodynamic and behavioural therapies.

Our specialized unit for the treatment of affective disorders, which also has psychosurgery available if needed, offers a unique opportunity to assess the treatments used by clinicians throughout the UK, which they have considered to be ineffective before an assessment for psychosurgery was sought. Virtually every letter referring these patients includes a long list of the various drugs that have been tried and have failed, but without giving doses. This suggests an expectation that one particular antidepressant will be found which is effective in an individual case rather than the possibility that, with resistant illnesses, while the antidepressant prescribed has relevance the dose given is of greater importance.

In recent years there have been a number of reports stressing the existence of a tendency in a variety of countries for the use of inadequate doses of psychotropic drugs (Bridges 1983, Quitkin 1985). In the USA Keller et al (1982) reported that only 34% of 217 patients with major depressive disorders were treated with antidepressant medication and only 25% of patients with psychotic depression received antidepressants. In general, the treatment most widely used was psychotherapy, and antianxiety drugs were the most frequently prescribed. In addition, when antidepressants are ineffective, frequently because of low doses, the drug may nevertheless be continued for long periods, even up to a year or more (Bridges 1983).

A number of factors seem to combine to encourage ineffective low-dose prescribing. The pharmaceutical companies are understandably cautious when recommending dose ranges, which must be suitable for populations rather than individuals. For example, the manufacturers of trimipramine in the UK have never recommended more than 75 mg, to be taken at night, although the British National Formulary (1990) recommends for trimipramine a maximum of 300 mg daily. The manufacturers of clomipramine in 1982 recommended for 'more severe cases, 75 mg daily or more if necessary', although by 1990 the recommendation was up to 150 mg daily (Monthly Index of Medical Specialities, November 1982 and March 1990). The importance of high doses for refractory cases will be stressed further later. The doses to be advocated are considerably higher than those officially recommended and when very high doses are used it is necassary to bring this to the attention of the patient and to ensure acceptance and cooperation.

A persuasive advocate of higher doses for the more resistant illnesses is Quitkin (1985). From his review of the literature he concluded that patients should receive up to 300 mg daily of imipramine or an equivalent tricyclic, and a separate trial of up to 90 mg of phenelzine before the case is considered to be treatment-resistant. He also considered, as do many others, that the medication should be discontinued if there was no clear improvement after about 6 weeks.

Even when the use of high-dose medication is accepted, prescribing approaches are often undesirable in other ways. For example, when an antidepressant has been effective the dose may be prematurely reduced to an assumed 'maintenance' level, although it is rarely clear how this is determined. Relapse is invited in this way. Sometimes where medication is being given at a progressively increasing dose, the onset of perhaps troublesome but not intolerable side-effects leads to a dose reduction. In these circumstances the more important aim of relieving a painful illness gives way to what is usually the less important need meticulously to avoid side-effects. This is especially so as side-effects tend to become better tolerated with time. When an illness fails to respond to whatever dose of an antidepressant is the highest used, some clinicians take this to mean that medication is not appropriate and therefore psychotherapeutic techniques are likely to be, which is not necessarily valid.

Yet another reason for limiting the use of medication, the so-called 'therapeutic window for tricyclics', seems to be advocated less frequently now. The 'therapeutic window' implied that doses producing blood levels that were either lower *or* higher than the recommended levels were likely to be less effective than doses giving blood values within the recommended range. In fact this phenomenon was only shown with any degree of reliability for nortriptyline and not for other tricyclics (Montgomery 1980).

The safety of determined prescribing

The over-cautious use of antidepressants is associated with a not unfounded apprehension about adverse reactions. Tricyclics may cause cardiotoxic complications and hypotension which sometimes results in falls and fractures. The monoamine oxidase inhibitors are also associated with potentially serious problems. There are the multiple interactions with tyramine in some foods and with anaesthetics and opioid analgesics. Tranylcypromine can cause hypertension and even strokes. Nevertheless, Bass & Kerwin (1989) have expressed the opinion that 'the main fears about the

interaction of MAO inhibitors with tyramine in foodstuffs have been grossly exaggerated', quoting McGilchrist (1975). Two anaesthetists, Coe & Laurent (1989), although acknowledging that the MAO inhibitors 'enjoy an infamous reputation for interactions with anaesthesia' and that the standard practice is to stop the antidepressant 3 weeks before elective procedures, consider this to be overcautious 'since careful anaesthesia in the absence of drugs known to cause problems – for example, ephedrine, pethidine and ketamine – is reported to be safe'. Whether certain precautions are entirely necessary or not, it is obviously safest to implement all those advocated unless there are clear grounds for making exceptions. Such exceptions will occur with severe, chronic and intractable illnesses.

There has been some concern over tricyclic antidepressants with respect to the mortality rate when overdoses are taken, especially with the availabilities of newer and apparently safer antidepressants such as trazodone, fluvoxamine and fluoxetine. Tricyclics nonetheless continue to be used frequently, probably partly due to their cheapness compared with new drugs, particularly because prescribers are familiar with them and they are reliably potent. There is no evidence that any of the newer antidepressants are more effective than those previously available. Tricyclics in particular can be used in high doses for enhanced efficacy because the side-effects are now so well known, while this would not be appropriate for newly available compounds of which there has been less clinical experience.

It achieves nothing to seek to avoid suicidal behaviour by giving a weak antidepressant, or prescribing one in too low a dose, when suicidal drive may increase as a result of worsening of the illness. On the other hand, giving high doses, although the patient may have a large number of tablets available, tends to avoid suicidal behaviour because the depression is effectively treated. In any case, if there are significant doubts about the suicide risk, admission to hospital should be considered.

It should be remembered that the newer antidepressants are safer than the older ones. Fatal poisonings with tricyclics before 1970 amounted to 38.5 deaths per million prescriptions and for tricyclics and other antidepressants after 1974 there were 13 deaths per million. Among the top four most lethal tricyclics are amitriptyline (46.5) and dothiepin (50), the most commonly used (Cassidy & Henry 1987). Equally it should be remembered that poorly controlled depressive illnesses are associated with death by suicide in 15% (e.g. Guze

& Robbins 1970). In addition, persistent, incapacitating depression causes great distress to the patient, increases social disabilities and places a great strain on close relationships. For these important reasons, chronic depressive and related illnesses must be treated effectively and as expeditiously as possible. Some risks are inevitable when using high doses, but over-cautious prescribing may be associated with the onset of a disabled lifestyle associated with intractable illnesses, including failure of the marriage, sale of the family home and unemployment. Sometimes there may be prolonged admissions to hospital and increasing institutionalization.

Strategies with antidepressants

Experience with patients referred for psychosurgery shows that treatment resistance is only very rarely present from the onset of an affective illness. It is more usual for there to be a progressive failure in the effectiveness of various antidepressant treatments and of electroconvulsive therapy (ECT) over a period of years. The interesting question is: why do some patients suffering episodes of illness continue to respond to routine treatments, although perhaps variably, throughout their lives while with others the illness becomes increasingly refractory?

In the early stages of the development of resistance, the dose of a given tricyclic should be progressively increased, with increments about every 10–14 days, up to an equivalent dose for the standard drugs of about 200–250 mg/day. This dose should preferably continue for about 6 weeks and if there has been no decisive response then the situation should be reviewed. The patient's compliance may need to be checked by obtaining a blood level of the drug. The diagnosis might need to be reviewed as well at this point.

Most clinicians would consider that the treatment options at this stage include the use of either ECT or an MAO inhibitor. ECT is the first choice if there are depressive delusions or a high suicidal risk, and in both cases admission to hospital is necessary. MAO inhibitors should be used if anxiety or phobic symptoms are prominent, or when there are reversed vegetative symptoms including hypersomnia and overeating. Alternatively, some would add lithium to the ineffective tricyclic. However this means embarking on an inconvenient lithium regimen and it may not be appropriate to risk adverse effects on the thyroid at an early stage of the illness.

It is stressed that the sequence of medication being discussed is not intended to be given consecutively and continuously. Thus at one point a patient may respond to an MAO inhibitor, having failed to improve on a tricyclic given previously. There may later be a remission and at the next attack of illness the clinical circumstances may indicate that ECT should be used as the primary treatment, rather than medication. At a subsequent attack a combination of antidepressants may be appropriate.

Antidepressant combinations

The next group of treatments in the sequence of prescribing comprises the antidepressant combinations. These may be of high potency and the theoretical risks may be commensurately higher, especially with patients who are careless about taking medication and are unreliable with dietary precautions. Probably the most potent combination, although the least desirable because of potential side-effects, is the use of tranylcypromine with either amitriptyline or trimipramine. In combinations with MAO inhibitors, clomipramine should never be used because death can occur. The specific 5-HT reuptake inhibitors, such as fluoxetine and fluvoxamine, are also contraindicated. The more commonly used combination consists of phenelzine with either amitriptyline or trimipramine and this combination does not seem to produce troublesome side-effects in practice (Young et al 1979). It is preferable to start the tricyclic before the phenelzine or to begin both together at a low dose. Currently available MAO inhibitors inhibit the enzyme irreversibly. Therefore, when this medication is stopped its effects will continue for about 2 weeks until adequate monoamine oxidase is reformed.

Combinations with lithium

There remain two combinations which have received increasing attention in recent years for use especially with resistant anxiety and affective disorders. Barker et al (1987) have suggested that both combinations should be re-evaluated. They have reported on the effects of phenelzine and lithium while we have found high-dose clomipramine and lithium particularly successful in cases of chronic illness referred for psychosurgery (Hale et al 1987). L-tryptophan was included in both combinations originally and the paper by Hale et al (1987) offers anecdotal evidence that the L-tryptophan seemed to be an essential ingredient in at least one case. However, in 1989, L-trytophan was reported to be associated with cases of the eosinophilia-myalgia syndrome, which is potentially fatal. After this possibility was announced in the USA, 1400 cases were reported, mostly in women, and there were 19 deaths. L-tryptophan was then withdrawn both in the USA and in the UK. It was suggested that a contaminant could be the cause but this has come to appear less certain (Medsger 1990).

One of the conditions necessary when psychosurgery is being considered is that all other appropriate treatments should have been tried and found to be ineffective. What is meant by 'all other appropriate treatments'? Different clinicians will have various views about this. In relation to accepting patients for psychosurgery, in the 1970s the policy of our Geoffrey Knight Unit was to leave the decision largely, but not exclusively, with the referring psychiatrist. When the psychiatrist felt that he had used all reasonable treatments without success the patient was likely to be accepted if the other criteria were appropriate. However, the clinican was sometimes asked to try one more course of ECT, for example, or to try lithium if that had not been used. Neglecting the use of lithium was frequent in the 1970s but has been almost unknown in recent years. Also, during the 1970s, about one-third of the patients referred had never had a tricyclic in a dose above 100 mg daily and few had been on a tricyclic at a dose above 150 mg daily. As time went on it was felt that the issue of 'adequate treatment' should be clarified and the Unit's policy was then to begin to admit some patients referred for possible psychosurgery, in order to try various antidepressant regimens.

In this way it became clear that high-dose tricyclic, lithium and, hitherto, L-tryptophan is a combination which does not often produce severe side-effects and is successful with many patients who would otherwise have had psychosurgery. Clinical experience has suggested that clomipramine is the most effective tricyclic, although dothiepin and amitriptyline are also often used successfully. Whichever tricyclic is chosen, it is essential that the dose should be progressively increased to about 300–400 mg/day. If the side-effects preclude doses at these levels, then another tricyclic is tried. Lithium is given such that the blood level is within the higher part of the usual range, say 0.8–1.0 mmol/l.

The Unit's successful experience of this combination gives rise to the suggestion that, with unipolar depression, failure to respond to two courses of ECT and to the high-dose tricyclic and lithium combination means that the case is resistant to all routine physical treatments and therefore the patient can reasonably be considered for possible psychosurgery.

Augmentors

These are drugs that potentiate the action of antidepressants although their properties in this role are not well understood. For example, while lithium has important antimanic and prophylactic properties, many would not regard it as an antidepressant when used alone. If this is accepted, then when given with tricyclics it would be regarded as an augmentor. Others consider that lithium has antidepressant activity alone. When given with a tricyclic it would then be regarded as falling within the concept of combined antidepressants: i.e. antidepressants with actions at different metabolic sites which increase their combined effectiveness.

Perhaps the most studied augmentation effects, after those of lithium, have been those of the thyroid hormones, when combined with tricyclic medication. Thyroxine or liothyronine may be used. It has been proposed that thyroid hormones enhance the activity of tricyclics by facilitating central nervous system beta-adrenergic receptor functioning (Whybrow et al 1972). It has also been suggested that they act by increasing thyroid function in those depressed patients who have some degree of hypothyroidism (Targum et al 1984), either as a contributory factor or as the primary cause of the depression (Gold et al 1981).

Some anticonvulsant medications are increasingly being used for affective disorders (see chapter 24). Carbamazepine is particularly useful for bipolar illnesses and some consider that its action is mood-stabilizing. Where lithium does not fully suppress bipolar symptoms, the addition of carbamazepine may improve the response. Similarly clonazepam and sodium valproate may be useful in bipolar illnesses.

Some neuroleptics have been reported to have antidepressant activity. Flupenthixol in small doses has been promoted as an antidepressant in the UK and both chlorpromazine and thioridazine have been reported to have antidepressant activity (Robertson & Trimble 1982). These two phenothiazines seem to enhance antidepressant activity, when combined with a tricyclic antidepressant. Considerable care is needed when using augmentors with tranylcypromine, because of its potency and direct stimulant actions.

PSYCHOSURGERY

Introduction

This treatment has a tradition of being seriously misunderstood and inappropriately condemned. Hence some basic principles need to be considered. Psychosurgery is not different in any way from some other forms of neurosurgery. Use of a separate word has led to the view that, while neurosurgery is simply a surgical specialty, psychosurgery is quite different and is unacceptable. It is justified if it is only used when there is severe distress and incapacity, and it can be dramatically effective in intractable illnesses that have been present for many years. It should not be regarded as a treatment for unusual psychiatric disorders, since it is most reliably effective with very typical affective disorders.

It is a treatment that is only used when all other routine treatments fail and, in the majority of cases, the illnesses appropriate for psychosurgery develop in a recognizable way. At first they respond to medication and ECT but over the years the symptoms become increasingly intractable and finally there is a total lack of response to routine therapies. It is essential to see psychosurgery as an end-point which follows the progressive failure of some severe psychiatric illnesses to respond to other treatments. In such dire circumstances, psychosurgery still allows the possibility of treating the patient successfully.

Thus, when psychosurgery is correctly indicated there will be no alternative treatment available, and the choice is relatively simple. When psychosurgery is offered, the only decision required is whether the patient wishes to take up this offer or not. The majority of patients understandably say that the prospect of a brain operation causes them anxiety but choose it because they cannot continue with their intolerable and untreatable symptoms. In these desperate situations, although rather higher chances of adverse side-effects would be acceptable, in practice the contemporary operations have usually proved to be remarkably safe.

Operative procedures

Early psychosurgery

It was probably inevitable that two intrepid clinicians in the past should have attempted cerebral surgery for psychiatric illnesses very prematurely, well before neurosurgical techniques had developed sufficiently for this to be reasonably tried. A Swiss psychiatrist, Burkhardt, and a Russian surgeon, Puusep, separately tried a few such operations in the late nineteenth century. The historical development of psychosurgery has been the subject of a number of publications (Bridges & Bartlett 1977, Valenstein 1980, Kiloh et al 1988).

Standard prefrontal lobotomy or leucotomy

Lobotomy (operation on a lobe) is the usual American term, while the British seem to prefer the term leucotomy (operation on white matter). It was the operation of standard prefrontal lobotomy that initiated the psychosurgery controversy, which has in the past been intense. However, this technique has been obsolete for nearly 40 years.

At the International Neurological Congress held in London in 1935, John Fulton, the American neurophysiologist, reported on the effects of removing the frontal association areas of two chimpanzees, the now famous Becky and Lucy. Situations were devised which, before the ablations, caused frustration, anger and fear. In these same situations afterwards, the animals remained calm and indifferent. Although some regarded the surgery as a relatively specific treatment for 'experimental neuroses', psychiatrists would now be more likely to view the animals as showing normal responses to various stresses and the ablations as producing non-specific emotional blunting.

Moniz, a Portuguese professor of neurology, was in the audience, and he asked whether the operation might be used as a treatment for disturbed psychiatric patients. With his neurosurgical colleague, Lima, he devised a surgical technique which was first carried out later in 1935. Moniz was involved in about 100 operations and then awaited assessments of outcome. He shared the Nobel Prize for Medicine in 1949 for this pioneering work.

Freeman and Watts, respectively neurologist and neurosurgeon in Washington, DC, first operated in 1936 and developed their own standard prefrontal lobotomy operation, which became very widely used in the Western world. Tooth & Newton (1961) reviewed the effects on over 10 000 patients who had this operation in the UK in the 10 years from the 1940s. About two-thirds of the patients were schizophrenic. Although 3% suffered personality destruction ('vegetable personality') and 4% died for surgical reasons, as many as 18% could be discharged from hospital. However, in the early 1950s chlorpromazine was introduced and proved to be a much more effective and considerably safer treatment for schizophrenia. Prefrontal lobotomy became obsolete, although a few operations have been carried out subsequently, and the diagnosis of uncomplicated schizophrenia ceased to be an indication for any kind of psychosurgery thereafter. Although a controversy developed subsequently as to whether prefrontal lobotomy should have been used, it should not be forgotten that no alternative effective treatment for schizophrenia was available at the time.

Refining the surgery

It was essential for the operations to be refined. It was never certain that the lesion of prefrontal lobotomy needed to be so large and, because a blunt knife (leucotome) was simply swept through the brain by hand, the size and site of the lesion varied a good deal. It was John Fulton (1951), the unintentional initiator of psychosurgery, who showed the way forward. He published a short book on psychosurgery, advocating that prefrontal lobotomy should be abandoned. He suggested that the lesion should be produced by electrocoagulation and that the sites should be the ventromedial quadrants of the frontal lobes or the cingulum. Although written at the end of the 1940s, Fulton's book quite accurately describes psychosurgical lesions used today. Perhaps understandably, Fulton was less clear about the appropriate psychiatric diagnoses.

Early modifications involved lesions 2 cm wide on each side of the midline, still using a freehand leucotome technique. Bimedial leucotomy (Greenblatt & Solomon 1952) had an entry from the vertex and the lesions extended vertically down into the ventromedial quadrants, anterior to the caudate nuclei. Scoville's orbital undercut (Scoville 1949) involved lesions on each side of the midline with an entry above the frontal sinuses extending forwards and downwards to end under the caudate nucleus. Thereafter the surgical techniques changed fundamentally and freehand lesion-making was completely superseded.

INTERNATIONAL EXPERIENCE

North America

Donnelly (1978) reviewed the use of psychosurgery in the USA and Canada for the years 1971–1973. He obtained information from a questionnaire sent to 1450 American and Canadian neurosurgeons, and 78% replied. He reported a total of 476 operations carried out for intractable pain, 1039 psychosurgical operations

and 162 operations that were for both intractable pain and psychiatric disorders. It is a curious observation that neurosurgical treatment for intractable pain in the UK is uncommon and is never associated with psychosurgical operations. Sweet et al (1977) describe the clinical concept behind this application. During 1971–1973 the annual number of operations in the USA was over 300, and in Canada the highest annual number was 27. These numbers have probably fallen considerably in recent years. The controversy concerning psychosurgery was intense in the USA (Breggin 1980).

A series of patients treated by means of a 'brain pacemaker' was reported by Heath (1977). This involved continuous electrical stimulation over many months using electrodes placed on the surface of the brain so that the brain was not entered. The wires were led out through the skull to the pacemaker. Previous studies with patients had suggested the sites appropriate for various emotional states. 'Psychotic behaviour' was associated with spike and slow waves in the septal region while 'intense emergency emotion' (rage, fear, violence, aggression) was associated with amplitude spindle activity in the hippocampus.

11 patients were treated because they had been pronounced incurable by two physicians (psychiatrists and/or neurologists). The follow-up period was 3–16 months, which the author accepted as short. Different diagnoses were deliberately included (violent behaviour, schizophrenia, neurotic behaviour). Among the 11 patients, 10 'responded positively', none were in hospital and one was on medication 'for behavioural symptoms' when reviewed. The remaining patient was not helped, it was suggested because of damage to the cerebellar cortex. Heath emphasised his aim as modifying behaviour, especially aggression, as opposed to treating illnesses. The modification of undesirable behaviour by surgery has been and remains highly controversial. Crow has in the past used chronically implanted electrodes, although not for stimulation (see United Kingdom, below). The general principle seems undesirable and is discussed later.

In recent years the most active neurosurgical department carrying out psychosurgery has been in Boston. Ballantine et al (1987) reviewed 198 stereotactic cingulotomy operations evaluated prospectively with a mean follow-up of 8.6 years. They observed that cases with affective disorders (61% of the sample) and those with anxiety states (7%) did best, while those with obsessional states (16%), schizophrenia (6%) and personality disorders (4%) 'improved less predictably'.

It is also reported that hemiplegias occurred in two cases. During the follow-up period as many as 9% of the patients had died by suicide. The authors regarded this as 'a major post-cingulotomy problem' and asked, 'Are these suicides a reflection of the personalities of the patients, of their psychiatric illnesses, or are they a side-effect of cingulotomy?' This problem suggests that the operation has serious limitations when used to treat depressive disorders. However, the operation seems to be fairly safe from immediate consequences, apart from the two hemiplegias reported in this series, in that with a larger series of 696 cases there were no postoperative deaths and the postoperative seizure rate was 1%. One table not often included in such reports shows that, in the 8 months before surgery, average medical expenses were $18 494 and in the 8 months postoperatively they were $588, of which $408 was for medication. The Boston group (Martuza et al 1990) have recently reviewed the use of stereotactic radiofrequency thermal cingulotomy for obsessive-compulsive disorders. Among 198 patients, 25% were functionally well and another 31% showed marked improvement. Comparisons with other results suggested that cases of anxiety did better with this operation than did obsessional-compulsive patients.

Holland

Van Manen & van Veelan (1988) report that in 1975 Belgian and Dutch neurosurgeons and neurologists formed a group to study the value of surgery in severe intractable psychiatric disorders and epilepsy. Subsequently 54 Dutch patients had psychosurgery for various indications. Compulsive neurosis was the commonest diagnosis (22 of 54). One diagnostic group included 'depression, anxiety, tension, automutilation', but outcome results were not separated between different diagnoses. Seven different operative techniques were used but the figures were presented in such a way that it is not possible to assess easily their separate efficacy (see Denmark, below).

Australia

Bailey et al (1973) reported on the clinical results from selective anterior cingulotomy (cingulo-tractotomy) carried out on 150 patients. Of the overall results, taking together 'well marked improvement', 'remission of all symptoms' and 'very marked improvement', there were 94.7% of the patients in these categories. This

finding suggests that different degrees of improvement may have been defined somewhat optimistically.

In a previous paper (Bailey et al 1971) the results after the first 50 operations were given. The authors observe that 'infection has been the most troublesome and alarming complication' and 'two of the early patients went into alarming status epilepticus'. The more recent paper records one death from a cerebral haemorrhage. The authors concluded that this operation was the treatment of choice for severe affective disorders and for obsessional disorders. More controversially, they suggested: 'It is probably the treatment of choice for psychosexual exhibitionism and compulsive antisocial behaviour, and it certainly offers a better chance for the offender than penal restriction.' This confusion about the place of treatment and punishment seems undesirable.

The operation was reported to be of no value for schizophrenia.

These papers no doubt contributed to the clinical interest leading to a symposium held in Sydney in 1974. The presentations were published in a book (Smith & Kiloh 1977) and the Introduction mentions that reports by Bailey et al (1973) and by Kiloh et al (1974) 'provoked considerable controversy'. The symposium led to widespread public concern. The late Dr H. Crow, a British representative at the meeting, described his controversial psychosurgical operation of multifocal leucocoagulation (see United Kingdom, below). Furthermore, the organisers gave considerable prominence to the psychosurgical treatment of 'anger', 'aggression' and 'rage', experiences which are not usually regarded as illnesses. As a result, psychosurgery was banned in the State of New South Wales and a Committee of Enquiry was set up which recommended Psychosurgery Review Boards for each state.

Denmark

A retrospective review was published from Copenhagen in 1982 (Hansen et al 1982). The study involved 65 patients operated on between 1965 and 1974 from 13 hospitals. Two patients had never been admitted to hospital. There were nine diagnostic groups and six operations. Unfortunately, nine patients had had previous psychosurgery. The diagnoses included 'character deviation, hysterical character neurosis, post-traumatic psychosis and presenile dementia'.

The results were not good. Overall the condition of only 25% was 'improved'. The diagnoses which did best were 'manic-depressive psychoses' (3 improved out of 10), 'borderline states' (2 of 6) and 'schizophrenia or infantile psychosis' (7 of 19). The authors pointed out that in some cases preoperative therapeutic possibilities had not been exhausted and they observed that many operations were carried out on the basis that the neurosurgeon accepted the recommendation of a single referring psychiatrist. During the follow-up periods of from 11 months to 12.5 years (median 5.5 years) there were eight deaths. Four (6%) were by suicide, one was due to a pulmonary embolism in a patient who became grossly overweight postoperatively, one was caused by status epilepticus and one was unconnected with the operation.

Sweden

Advanced technology has been a characteristic of Swedish psychosurgery. The operation has almost exclusively been capsulotomy and the results of 300 cases were reviewed by Mindus (1988). The operation was particularly used for 'anxiety disorders unresponsive to conventional therapy'. Even although DSM-III criteria for anxiety diagnoses were used, it may be that some of the cases suffered from mixed anxiety-depressions, since they were said to show a suicide rate similar to or even higher than primary depression. The capsulotomy was described as 'stereotactic bilateral anterior .capsulotomy', aiming 'to interrupt the frontolimbic connections which pass through the internal capsule'. The clinical results of operations performed during 1952–1957 had been reported previously (Herner 1961).

There are two surgical techniques in use at the Karolinska Hospital. Radiofrequency lesions are produced with local anaesthesia and the target area in the internal capsule is localized with stereotactic computed tomography. The size of the lesion is 8 mm by 8 mm (Herner 1961, Bingley et al 1977).

The other method is termed radiosurgical capsulotomy and may indicate the direction of further developments in psychosurgery as it is non-invasive. The lesions are produced by focusing 179 narrow beams of cobalt-60 radiation from a stereotactic gamma unit (Leksell & Backlund 1979, Leksell 1983). The results are equally good with both methods but the time courses are different (Rylander 1979, Mindus et al 1987).

The inclusion criteria involve DSM-III: phobic disorders (300.03), generalized anxiety disorder (300.20) or obsessive-compulsive disorder (300.30) and 5 years minimum duration of illness together with the usual

requirements for all other treatments to have failed and the patient giving informed consent. This contrasts with most other centres, in which depressions are the most common diagnoses. About ten operations are carried out each year.

There have been no deaths and so far no cases of postoperative epilepsy. Three cases of transient neurological complications are reported but all recovered without sequelae. In the earlier group, during 1952–1957, a postoperative frontal lobe syndrome occurred in two out of 18 patients. There have been no adverse personality changes with the more recent operations, using the Karolinska Scales of Personality and the Rorschach Test. The outcome for 300 patients published in a number of series is given, overall, as 'in 70% of the patients a statistically and clinically significant reduction of target symptoms was noted'.

United Kingdom

There has been much less controversy in the UK than in the USA. This may be related to the greater acceptance of physical treatment generally in psychiatry.

Barraclough et al (1978) carried out a survey of psychosurgery in Britain during the 3 years 1974–1976. All 44 neurosurgical units replied to a postal questionnaire. 13 (30%) had carried out no psychosurgery. At the remaining 31 units a total of 431 operations were performed. The Geoffrey Knight Unit at the Brook Hospital, London, undertook most of the operations (127, or 29%). This was followed by Atkinson Morley's Hospital, London, using limbic leucotomy (15%), then Birmingham (13%) and Bristol (9%). Snaith et al 1984 reported a survey of 144 general adult psychiatrists and psychogeriatricians. Of these, 112 (78%) had referred patients for psychosurgery or had not referred but considered that they might want to do so in the future. The remainder reported that they were either unlikely to, or never would, refer. Table 26.1 gives the numbers of operations in the UK at the beginning and the end of a 10-year period. This shows that the total annual referrals to the Brook Hospital Unit have not changed but the number of operations performed annually has fallen to between one-half and one-third over the 10-year period. This seems to have been due to the effectiveness of high-dose and combined medication, as described above.

Limbic leucotomy

Kelly et al (1966), a group keenly interested in

psychosurgery, wrote that they wanted 'to learn more about the proper and discriminative selection of suitable patients...'. To this end they reported on an objective method of assessing anxiety before and after psychosurgery, by the technique of forearm blood flow. Modified leukotomy operations were found to result in a decrease in forearm blood flow by 34% postoperatively. In a later paper, Kelly et al (1973) described how a probe was used at the beginning of the psychosurgical operation in order to produce local physiological stimulation and the site for the lesion was chosen when there was a marked increase in heart rate, forearm blood flow, sweat gland activity and respiration. The intention was to produce the smallest possible lesion and it was postulated that the lesion could be small because the site was very precisely located by the physiological responses observed.

Table 26.1 Psychosurgical operations 1979–1989 United Kingdom and the Republic of Ireland

	1979	1980	1988	1989
Brook Hospital				
Referrals	74	69	70	85
Operations	47	50	20	18
(as % of referrals)	64%	73%	29%	21%
Other Hospitals				
Operations	23	12	6	5

The operation of limbic leucotomy involves two or three lesions, sited by using this monitoring: in the lower medial quadrant of each frontal lobe and also in the cingulum bundle, bilaterally (Richardson 1973). Originally the lesions were produced by a cryogenic technique involving the production of a very low temperature at the tip of the probe, down to −70°C. Subsequently thermocoagulation was also used. Postoperative outome has been discussed by Mitchell-Heggs et al (1976) and by Kelly (1980). The latter publication gives the results for the largest group of patients, 148 at 20 months postoperatively. These authors used a 5-point scale, and they considered a good outcome in terms of categories I, II and III. Other reports using 5-point scales usually give good outcome in terms of categories I and II only (symptom-free and much improved).

Patients with obsessional neurosis ($n=49$) did best, with 61% (I and II) or 84% (I-III) who recovered or were much improved. In the case of chronic anxiety ($n=27$) the improvement rate was 30% (I and II) or 63% (I-III). With depression the figures were 39% (I and II) or 61% (I-III). The recovery rates are rather heavily dependent on the inclusion or otherwise of category III, which Kelly (1980) stresses means a 'definite improvement'. There were also 19 schizophrenic patients operated on, together with seven patients with personality disorders, five with anorexia nervosa and one each with depersonalisation, intractable pain, dementia (depression), paranoia and palilalia (parkinsonism). There were no deaths associated with the surgery but, by 20 months postoperatively, eight patients (5%) had died by suicide. In the previous paper (Mitchell-Heggs et al 1976) it is reported that no patient developed epilepsy after the operation but all patients were advised to take prophylactic phenytoin for 6 months following surgery. There have been a total of 16 limbic leucotomy operations carried out during the last 4 years (to 1989).

Multifocal leucocoagulation

This operation, reported by Crow (1973) is mentioned as a curiosity and the technique has also been noted above (see Australia). It is not easy to understand the theoretical basis. The surgical technique involved the implantation of a number of electrode sheaves, each consisting of 3–7 separate electrodes wound round each other. Several sheaves were implanted throughout the frontal lobes. In one paper there is mention of a patient having 45 electrodes implanted. The electrodes were connected to a plug on the outside of the head which remained for up to 7 months (Crow et al 1961). The lesions were built up using direct current to whichever group of electrodes was thought likely to be most effective, although how this was decided is not clear. The expansion of the lesion depended on reports from the patients of subjective changes experienced after the lesions were made and observations of behaviour.

The results of the treatment were reported for only 90 patients. This technique would have to be vastly more effective and safer than the other contemporary operations to justify the 6 months admission (stereotactic tractotomy requires 4 weeks), the potential dangers of chronically implanted electrodes and the seemingly random way that the lesions are made. Crow considered that the best results were with the 'syndrome of constitutional excessive fear', and 'complete' or 'very good' relief of symptoms were reported in 68% of 41 patients. During the last 10 years only one of these operations has been carried out, in 1981.

Knight's stereotactic subcaudate tractotomy

This British operation has been the most frequently used technique over the past 20 years; hence it is considered in some detail. Mr Geoffrey Knight established modern psychosurgery in a methodical way. He first decided which he considered to be the safest and the clinically most effective psychosurgical operation available at the time and he chose Scoville's orbital undercut technique (Scoville 1949). He then carried out over 300 of these operations, the results of which were subsequently assessed by a senior and independent psychiatrist (Sykes & Tredgold 1964). This was a freehand technique and the incidence of side-effects was high although they were generally not as serious as with standard prefrontal leucotomy. For example, one or more epileptic fits occurred with 32 patients and there were five deaths. However the clinical results were good.

Knight, in reconsidering the problem, fundamentally changed the technique and devised a modified operation. This operation is still in regular use at the Geoffrey Knight Unit in London. In the 25 years since the first operation was carried out, over 1200 have been performed and it is now well established, with considerable clinical experience of its safety, efficacy and side-effects.

The lesion is produced in a controlled way by means of beta-radiation produced by rods of yttrium-90, each rod being 7mm long and 1mm in diameter. The half-life is about 68 hours and yttrium-90 decays to zirconium-90, which is stable. Lethal radiation extends up to about 2 mm from the surface of the rods and the lesions in the cerebral white matter come to consist of a central necrotic zone with surrounding dense demyelination (Newcombe 1975). This method of lesion-making is obviously safer than the use of a leukotome and furthermore it allows of stereotactic placement of the yttrium rods which are therefore sited with considerable accuracy. The configuration of the rods is at present two rows of five bilaterally (Hale et al, submitted). The rods become inert and remain in place indefinitely without causing problems. This is a much more refined lesion when compared with the previously used orbital undercut, as has been demonstrated by Corsellis & Jack (1973).

Knight (1965, 1969) called this operation stereotactic subcaudate tractotomy (SST). The lesion, which is sited stereotactically, is partly beneath the head of the caudate nucleus. The term 'tractotomy' was intended to avoid the unhappy associations of the earlier 'leukotomy'.

Experience has shown the remarkable safety of this neurosurgical operation. There has been one death, due to a miscalculation when setting up the stereotactic calibrations, so that a rod was mis-sited (Knight 1973). There are two theoretically important hazards. One is operative or postoperative haemorrhage. In the series of 1200 patients, there was only one elderly patient with postoperative bleeding and this was corrected by a second, emergency operation with no sequelae. The other possibility is an infection, but this has not occurred so far.

Cerebral surgery is inevitably associated with an increased risk of epilepsy. We know that, among a series of 1000 patients, there were 16 who experienced one or more epileptic fits at some time after the operation, but several of these patients had suffered fits preoperatively. One fit usually does not need treatment, but a second requires anticonvulsant medication. Because of this possibility patients must not drive for 6 months after the operation. As far as is known, 1% of patients have died by suicide at some time since the operation.

The operation has been found to be well accepted. It is carried out with a general anaesthetic and the head is not shaved. It lasts about 90 minutes. It is carried out in a specialized and highly experienced unit, under the supervision of a neurosurgeon and a psychiatrist who have worked together for many years, and only after high-dose and combined antidepressants have clearly failed to work. There is also supervision by the Mental Health Act Commission.

Both Strom-Olsen & Carlisle (1971) and Goktepe et al (1975) reported 'minor or mild' personality changes following this operation. However, for some years now it has appeared that adverse personality changes do not occur, although the operative procedures have not changed. This was the opinion of the senior and independent psychiatrist who assessed the outcome of several hundred patients at 1 year, with interviews with relatives. In the earlier reports the relatives described irritability, outspokenness and volubility most commonly. It is possible that these characteristics are in fact related to recovery from a chronic illness and that the relatives described the return to the premorbid personality as undesirable changes. This tends to be confirmed by a report by Bouras et al (1986) which showed that some 50% of patients being assessed for psychosurgery or who have had this treatment have marriages which have either failed or are clearly failing.

Sometimes this is because spouses find it impossible to tolerate long episodes of a psychiatric disorder, but another important reason is that the spouse cannot adjust to the postoperative re-emergence of the patient's premorbid personality, after a long period of illness which is often associated with passivity, dependence and gratitude. The replacement of these by more positive attitudes on recovery may not be welcomed by the spouse.

The indications for SST have been discussed by Bartlett et al (1981). The commonest diagnosis is that of unipolar depression, but bipolar illnesses are now regularly accepted (Lovett & Shaw 1987, Poynton et al 1988a). There has been a traditional reluctance to use psychosurgery for bipolar affective disorders. This probably depended on the disinhibition that seems to have occurred with some of the older operations. Stereotactic tractotomy does not produce disinhibition and in fact it has been found to produce useful amelioration in many bipolar cases and dramatic recovery for some. Poynton et al (1988a) reviewed nine patients treated by SST. They reported a general tendency for mania to show a greater reduction in severity than depression but even in cases where there was limited improvement the amelioration of the swings appeared to be clinically worthwhile.

Other relevant diagnoses include anxiety states, chronic tension, phobic disorders and obsessional illnesses. With all diagnoses the more prominent the depressive symptoms the more likely it is that there will be a good outcome. Uncomplicated schizophrenia is not an indication but some schizoaffective illnesses with prominent affective symptoms may be appropriate.

The contraindications are not numerous. There is no upper or lower age limit. The youngest patient was 18 years old and suffered from a depressive disorder associated with multiple and dangerous suicidal behaviour; she recovered completely. With elderly patients there tends to be an increasing possibility of physical factors which preclude surgery. In general, the more there is evidence of any form of dementia the less chance there is of a good outcome. All patients have computed tomography scans in order to assist assessment of this aspect. Other cerebral abnormalities may also seem to be contraindications, but localization by scanning may permit psychosurgery. For example, a previous stroke does not necessarily preclude the use of SST as its site is likely to be distant from the stroke lesion.

Antisocial personality traits and, in particular, established addictions make the operation undesirable even when an appropriate diagnosis is present. However, personalities with inadequate or dependent traits are not a contraindication because it would be expected that the personality would function better without the burden of a major psychiatric illness. With the earlier operations a certain robustness of personality was required, presumably the better to adjust to possible disabling side-effects.

SST is indicated in the following circumstances:

1) an appropriate diagnosis is present
2) the illness is severe and recurrent or chronic. Some patients suffer from less severe but disabling and very chronic disorders, and psychosurgery might not be considered for such cases. Nonetheless a good deal of suffering may be experienced. Similarly, if the patient has a good personality, he or she may tolerate distress well and, as a result, the patient is sometimes expected to experience painful symptoms for too long before surgery is offered
3) absence or inadequacy of response to all other reasonable treatments, carried out in a determined way
4) absence of contraindications (see above)
5) the patient's consent and also the consent of the nearest relative, unless (for the second) there are reasons otherwise.

One of the most important characteristics of SST is that, while with a few patients there is a dramatic and early response to the operation, in the majority of cases recovery is gradual, often with fluctuating symptoms. It may take 3 months, 6 months and perhaps 12 months or more before the full advantages of the surgery are apparent. The reason for this delay is unknown and it can occur with patients who remain well-adjusted socially so that the delay does not depend only on the adequacy of the rehabilitation carried out. However, with most patients, active rehabilitation is important and involves encouraging and helping patients to overcome persisting illness behaviour and disabling lack of confidence due to long periods of a highly incapacitating illness.

When recovery after SST is established, a later relapse is rare. It used to be more common until the configuration of the yttrium rods was increased from two rows of three rods to two rows of five. This larger lesion cannot be further extended. This has apparently abolished late relapses with no increase in side-effects (Hale et al, submitted).

Psychosurgery is often regarded as the treatment of last resort. This is not strictly true. If psychosurgery does not help the patient, then medication and ECT may be repeated after the operation, and clinical experience is that these treatments are more likely to be effective postoperatively than they were previously.

The postoperative results have been reported by Strom-Olsen & Carlisle (1971), Goktepe et al (1975) and Poynton et al (1988b). The paper by Goktepe et al (1975) reported that, for depression, 68% showed considerable improvement or recovery at 1 year postoperatively (i.e. I 'recovered: no symptoms and no treatment' or II 'well: mild residual symptoms, little or no interference with daily life'). The comparable figures for anxiety in various forms was 63% (I and II) and for obsessional disorders 50% (I and II).

Mention has been made of the possibilities of placebo responses. However, in most cases the recovery is gradual and not often immediate, and among the patients who did well in the groups included above ($n=78$), 53% had been ill for over 10 years. Among these 78 patients who did well, 44 had had ECT in the 4 years or so before the operations, of whom four patients had one to three courses and four had four or more courses. During comparable periods for each patient after the operation, only six patients needed ECT (five had one course and one had two courses).

In the same group of 78 patients, 33 had made one or more suicide attempts in the review period before the operation. During comparable periods afterwards, only five did so. Postoperative suicide attempts and ECT were mainly in the first year, before recovery was established.

Longer-term reviews of SST show that death by suicide occurs at some time in 3% of those operated on. For the Boston operations the figure was 9% (see North America, above) and with limbic leucotomy it was 5%. This must be compared with the 15% rate found in representative long-term follow-ups including less chronic and intractable subjects (Guze & Robbins 1970).

Mental Health Act Commission

In the UK the Mental Health Act (1983) applies to England and Wales and separate legislation refers to Northern Ireland and to Scotland. A new Mental Health Act Commission was set up to ensure the effectiveness of the Act. The full Commission has a multi-professional membership which includes psychiatrists, psychologists, social workers, lawyers and lay-members.

It is Section 57 of the Act which is concerned with psychosurgery. The section applies to 'any surgical operation for destroying brain tissue or for destroying the functioning of brain tissues; and such other forms of treatment as may be specified for the purposes of this section by regulations made by the Secretary of State'.

The patient being considered for psychosurgery is required to be 'capable of understanding the nature, purpose and likely effects of the treatment in question and has consented to it'. Confirmation of this understanding and consent must be given by a registered medical practitioner (the Medical Commissioner), specifically appointed for the purposes of this part of the Act by the Secretary of State. The doctor cannot be the physician responsible for the patient's care and is accompanied by two other non-medical people, also specially appointed. The regulation of psychosurgery in some states in the USA has been discussed by Grimm (1980).

PROOF OF EFFECTIVENESS OF NEUROSURGERY

It is easy to attribute the effectiveness of psychosurgical operations to placebo activity because surgery in general is expected to produce decisive results. Certainly a convincing controlled trial has never been carried out in order to test this, an omission stressed by many writers (Robin & Macdonald 1975, O'Callaghan & Carroll 1982). Attempts have been made. Livingston (1953) carried out sham operations on four patients, making an incision and removing discs of skull only. These patients were with patients who underwent real cingulotomies and the ward staff did not know of the sham surgery. No improvement occurred in these four patients in 1–3 months, after which they had cingulotomies. Robin (1958) described an attempt at a controlled study.

The Royal College of Psychiatrists set up a Research Committee (1977) to devise a prospective controlled trial. It was soon realized that there was no treatment with which psychosurgery could reasonably be compared. Hence the plan decided on involved patients accepted for psychosurgery being randomized, with some having an operation soon after and others having the operation delayed for 1 year. The progress of both groups was to be carefully assessed at 6 months and 1 year after the selection into two groups. The acceptability of the design was seriously doubted by some, for various reasons. However, no funding could be obtained for the trial.

While a controlled trial of psychosurgery is particularly needed, the clinical requirements which are specifically associated with psychosurgery make this very difficult. That is, to be accepted for an operation the patient must have failed to respond to all other appropriate treatments, so no treatment is then available for purposes of comparison. The patients will necessarily be severely ill and considerably incapacitated, so unnecessary delay in carrying out the operation can be considered to be unethical. Very clear informed consent is essential in the case of psychosurgery and it would be a very rare distressed patient who would voluntarily agree to his or her operation being postponed or another treatment substituted.

Some predictions of response have been suggested by research. There seems promise in a biological marker, the tyramine load test (Hale et al 1989). Also, in the case of SST, it has been found for one group of patients that serial EEGs were normal one day before the operation and also 6 months later. However at 2 weeks postoperatively there were large frontal slow waves, which were characteristic. The amount and spread of these slow waves at 2 weeks showed a significant positive correlation with the clinical outcome at 1 year (Evans et al 1981). The more the EEG disturbance 2 weeks postoperatively, the better the outcome at 1 year, which suggested that the operation had a specific effect on the outcome.

REFERENCES

Bailey H R, Dowling J L, Swanton C H, Davies E 1971 Studies in depression: cingulotractotomy in the treatment of severe affective illness. Medical Journal of Australia 1: 8–12

Bailey H R, Dowling J L, Davies E 1973 Studies in Depression III. The control of affective illnesses by cingulotractotomy. Medical Journal of Australia 2: 366–371

Ballantine H T Jr, Bouckoms A J, Thomas E K, Giriunas I E, 1987 Treatment of psychiatric illness by stereotactic cingulotomy. Biological Psychiatry 22: 807–819

Barker W A, Scott J, Eccleston D 1987 The Newcastle chronic depression study. International Clinical Psychopharmacology 2: 261–272

Barraclough B M, Mitchell-Heggs N A 1978 Use of neurosurgery for psychological disorder in the British Isles during 1974–1976. British Medical Journal 2: 1591–1593

Bartlett J R, Bridges P K, Kelly D 1981 Contemporary indications for psychosurgery British Journal of Psychiatry 138: 507–511

Bass C, Kerwin R 1989 Rediscovering monoamine oxidase inhibitors. British Medical Journal 298: 345–346

Bingley T, Leksell L, Meyerson B A et al 1977 Long term results of stereotactic capsulotomy in chronic obsessive-compulsive neurosis. In: Sweet H, Obrador S, Martin-Rodriguez J A (eds) Neurosurgical treatment in psychiatry, pain and epilepsy. University Park Press, Baltimore, p 287–289

Bouras N, Vanger P, Bridges P K 1986 Marital problems in chronically depressed and physically ill patients and their spouses. Comprehensive Psychiatry 27: 127–130

Breggin P R 1980 Brain-disabling therapies. In: Valenstein E S (ed) The psychosurgery debate: scientific, legal and ethical perspectives. W H Freeman, San Francisco, p 467–492

Bridges P K 1983 '. . . and a small dose of an antidepresssant might help'. British Journal of Psychiatry 142: 626–628

Bridges P K, Bartlett J R 1977 Psychosurgery – yesterday and today. British Journal of Psychiatry 131: 249–260

British National Formulary 1990. British Medical Association and Royal Pharmaceutical Society of Great Britain, London, March

Cassidy A, Henry J 1987 Fatal toxicity of antidepressant drugs in overdose. British Medical Journal 295: 1021–1024

Coe A J, Laurent S 1989 Rediscovering monoamine oxidase inhibitors. British Medical Journal 298: 671

Corsellis J A N, Jack A B 1973 Neuropathological observations on yttrium implants and on undercutting in the orbito-frontal areas of the brain. In: Laitinen L, Livingston K E (eds) Surgical approaches in psychiatry. MTP Press, Lancaster

Crow H J 1973 Intracerebral polarisation and multifocal leucocoagulation in some psychiatric illnesses. Psychiatria Neurologia Neurochirurgia 76: 365–381

Crow H J, Cooper R, Phillips D G 1961 Controlled multifocal frontal leucotomy for psychiatric illness. Journal of Neurology, Neurosurgery and Psychiatry 24: 353–360

Donnelly J 1978 The incidence of psychosurgery in the United States, 1971–1973. American Journal of Psychiatry 135: 1476–1480

Evans B, Bridges P K, Bartlett J R 1981 Electroencephalographic changes as prognostic indicators after psychosurgery. Journal of Neurology, Neurosurgery and Psychiatry 44: 444–447

Fulton J F 1951 Frontal lobotomy and affective behaviour: a neurosurgical analysis. W W Norton, New York

Goktepe E O, Young L B, Bridges P K 1975 A further review of the results of stereotactic subcaudate tractotomy. British Journal of Psychiatry 126: 270–280

Gold M S, Pottash A L C, Extein I 1981 Hypothyroidism and depression: evidence from complete thyroid function evaluation. Journal of the American Medical Association 245: 1919–1922

Greenblatt M, Solomon H C 1952 Survey of nine years of lobotomy investigations. American Journal of Psychiatry 109: 262–265

Grimm R J 1980 Regulation of psychosurgery. In: Valenstein E S (ed) The psychosurgery debate. W W Freeman, San Francisco, p 421–438

Guze S B, Robbins E 1970 Suicide and primary affective disorders. British Journal of Psychiatry 117: 437–438

Hale A S, Procter A W, Bridges P K 1987 Clomipramine,

tryptophan and lithium in combination for resistant endogenous depression: seven case studies. British Journal of Psychiatry 151: 213–217

Hale A S, Sandler M, Hannah P, Bridges P K 1989 Tyramine conjugation test for prediction of treatment response in depressed patients. Lancet 1: 234–236

Hale A S, Bartlett J R, Bridges P K (submitted) Lesion size and outcome following the psychosurgical operation of stereotactic subcordate tractotomy.

Hansen H, Anderson R, Theilgaard A, Lunn V 1982 Stereotactic surgery. Acta Psychiatrica Scandinavica 66 (suppl 301)

Heath R G 1977 Modulation of emotion with a brain pacemaker: treatment for intractable psychiatric illness. Journal of Nervous and Mental Diseases 165: 300–317

Herner T 1961 Treatment of mental disorders with frontal stereotactic thermolesions. A follow up study of 116 cases. Acta Psychiatrica Scandinavica 36 (suppl 158)

Keller M G, Klerman G L, Lavori P W, Fawcett J A, Coryell W, Endicott J 1982 Treatment received by depressed patients. Journal of the American Medical Association 248: 1848–1855

Kelly D 1980 Anxiety and emotions. Charles C Thomas, Chicago, IL

Kelly D H W, Walter C J S, Sargant W 1966 Modified leucotomy assessed by forearm blood flow and other measurements. British Journal of Psychiatry 112: 871–881

Kelly D, Richardson A, Mitchell-Heggs N 1973 Neurophysiological aspects and operative technique. British Journal of Psychiatry 123: 133–140

Kiloh L G, Gye R S, Rushworth R G et al 1974 Stereotactic amygdaloidotomy for aggressive behaviour. Journal of Neurology, Neurosurgery and Psychiatry 37: 437–444

Kiloh L G, Smith J S, Johnson G F 1988 Physical treatments in psychiatry. Blackwell Scientific Publications, Oxford

Knight G 1965 Stereotactic tractotomy in the surgical treatment of mental illness. Journal of Neurology, Neurosurgery and Psychiatry 28: 304–310

Knight G 1969 Bifrontal stereotactic tractotomy. British Journal of Psychiatry 115: 257–266

Knight G 1973 Further observations from an experience of 660 cases of stereotactic tractotomy. Postgraduate Medical Journal 49: 845–854

Leksell L 1983 Stereotactic radiosurgery. Journal of Neurology, Neurosurgery and Psychiatry 46: 797–803

Leksell L, Backlund E O 1979 Stereotactic gammacapsulotomy. In: Hitchcock E R, Ballantine H T Jr, Meyerson B A (eds) Modern concepts in psychiatric surgery. Elsevier-North Holland, Amsterdam, p 213–216

Livingston K E 1953 Cingulate cortex isolation for the treatment of psychosis and psychoneuroses. Research Publications, Association for Research in Nervous and Mental Disease 31: 374–378

Lovett L M, Shaw D M 1987 Outcome in bipolar affective disorder after stereotactic tractotomy. British Journal of Psychiatry 151: 113–116

McGilchrist J M 1975 Interactions with monoamine oxidase inhibitors. British Medical Journal 271: 591–592

Martuza R L, Chiocca E A, Jenike M A, Giriunas I E, Ballantine H T 1990 Stereotactic radiofrequency thermal cingulotomy for obsessive compulsive disorder. Neuropsychiatric Practice and Opinion 2: 331–336

Medsger T A 1990 Tryptophan-induced eosinophilia-myalgia syndrome. New England Journal of Medicine 322: 869–881, 926–928

Mindus P 1988 Capsulotomy, a psychosurgical intervention considered in cases of anxiety disorders unresponsive to conventional therapy. National Board of Health and Welfare, Drug Information Committee, Sweden, p 151–167

Mindus P, Bergstrom K, Levander S E, Noren G, Hindmarsh T, Thuomas K A 1987 Magnetic resonance images related to clinical outcome after psychosurgical intervention in severe anxiety disorder. Journal of Neurology, Neurosurgery and Psychiatry 50: 1288–1297

Mitchell-Heggs N, Kelly D, Richardson A 1976 Stereotactic limbic leucotomy – a follow-up at 16 months. British Journal of Psychiatry 128: 226–240

Montgomery S A 1980 Measurements of serum drug levels in the assessment of antidepressants. British Journal of Clinical Pharmacology 10: 411–416

Monthly Index of Medical Specialities Medical Publications Ltd, London

Newcombe R 1975 The lesion in stereotactic subcaudate tractotomy. British Journal of Psychiatry 126: 478–481

O'Callaghan M A J, Carrol D 1982 Psychosurgery: a scientific analysis. MTP Press, Lancaster

Poynton A, Bridges P K, Bartlett J R 1988a Resistant bipolar affective disorder treated by stereotactic subcaudate tractotomy. British Journal of Psychiatry 152: 354–358

Poynton A, Bridges P K, Bartlett J R 1988b Psychosurgery in Britain now. British Journal of Neurosurgery 2: 297–306

Quitkin F M 1985 The importance of dose in prescribing antidepressants. British Journal of Psychiatry 147: 593–597

Research Committee (Royal College of Psychiatrists) 1977 Evaluation of the surgical treatment of functional mental illness: proposal for a prospective controlled trial. In: Sweet W H, Obrador S, Martin-Rodriguez J G (eds) Neurosurgical treatment in psychiatry, pain and epilepsy. University Park Press, Baltimore

Richardson A 1973 Stereotactic limbic leucotomy: surgical technique. Postgraduate Medical Journal 49: 860–864

Robertson M M, Trimble M R 1982 Major tranquillizers used as antidepressants: a review. Journal of Affective Disorders 4: 173–193

Robin A A 1958 A controlled study of the effects of leucotomy. Journal of Neurology, Neurosurgery and Psychiatry 21: 262–269

Robin A, Macdonald D 1975 Lessons of leucotomy. Henry Kimpton, London

Rylander G 1979 Stereotactic radiosurgery in anxiety and obsessive-compulsive states: psychiatric aspects. In: Hitchcock E R, Ballantine H T Jr, Meyerson B A (eds) Modern concepts in psychiatric surgery. Elsevier-North Holland, Amsterdam, p 235–240

Scoville W B 1949 Selective cortical undercutting as a means of modifying and studying frontal lobe function in man. Journal of Neurosurgery 6: 65–73

Smith J S, Kiloh L G 1977 Psychosurgery and society. Pergamon Press, Sydney

Snaith R P, Price D J E, Wright J F 1984 Psychiatrists' attitudes to psychosurgery: proposals for the organisation of a psychosurgical service in Yorkshire. British Journal of Psychiatry 144: 293–297

Strom-Olsen R, Carlisle S 1971 Bifrontal stereotactic tractotomy. British Journal of Psychiatry 118: 141–154

Sweet W H, Obrador S, Martin-Rodriguez J G (eds) 1977 Neurosurgical treatment in psychiatry, pain and epilepsy. Part IV. University Park Press, Baltimore

Sykes M A, Tredgold R F 1964 Restricted orbital undercutting: a study of its effects on 350 patients over the ten years 1951–1960. British Journal of Psychiatry 110: 609–640

Targum S D, Greenberg R D, Harmon R L et al 1984 Thyroid hormone and the TRH test in refractory depression. Journal of Clinical Psychiatry 45: 345–346

Tooth G C, Newton M P 1961 Leucotomy in England and Wales: reports on public health and medical subjects 104. HMSO, London

Valenstein E S 1980 The psychosurgery debate: scientific, legal and ethical perspectives. W H Freeman, San Francisco

van Manen J, van Veelen C W M 1988 Experiences in psycho-surgery in the Netherlands. Acta Neurochirurgia (suppl) 44: 167–169

Whybrow P C, Coppen A, Prange A J et al 1972 Thyroid function and the response to L-triiodothyronine in depression. Archives General Psychiatry 26: 242–245

Young J P R, Lader M H, Hughes W C 1979 Controlled trial of imipramine, monoamine oxidase inhibitors and combined treatment in depressed outpatients. British Medical Journal 2: 1315–1317

27. Prediction of treatment response

Peter R. Joyce

For each new patient with an affective disorder, the clinician must consider the likely natural history of the disorder and consider whether any available treatment could favourably alter this natural history. The process of diagnosis involves identifying those features which a patient has, which, based on previous research, will predict outcome. The validity of diagnosis in psychiatry is essentially dependent upon predictive ability; that is, how capable the diagnosis is of predicting outcome and treatment response (Kendell 1989). This chapter reviews current understanding about the prediction of outcome for patients with affective disorders and especially concentrates on the prediction of treatment response in patients with depressive disorders and bipolar disorder.

To understand how treatment affects outcome and to be able to predict treatment outcome requires a thorough understanding of the natural history of affective disorders (see chapter 7). This necessitates being aware of the possibility of spontaneous recovery, of recovery due to non-specific factors, and the tendency of affective disorders to relapse. The issues of what constitutes recovery and when after recovery do we talk about relapse have only occasionally been addressed. Furthermore, as the data are increasingly emerging that the long-term outcome for patients with affective disorders is seldom one of an uncomplicated recovery, but that degrees of chronicity and/or relapse occur in the majority of patients (Kiloh et al 1988, Lee & Murray 1988), the focus of treatment studies on short-term outcome (e.g. 4 or 6 weeks) appears of less importance than the more important question of long-term outcome. The issue as to the degree to which modern treatments can alter the generally poor long-term outcomes for patients with affective disorders has not been adequately studied.

These factors have made it difficult to study the prediction of treatment outcome and, although studies on bipolar patients using lithium have looked at long-term outcome, studies in depression have concentrated excessively on short-term outcome. Many studies on the prediction of treatment outcome only examine the response in a group of patients being given one treatment, although outcome is an amalgam of the natural history, non-specific and specific treatment factors. In these circumstances predictors of a better outcome could in fact be predictors of spontaneous recovery or of improvement due to non-specific factors, rather than improvement due to specific treatments. It is also likely that even some of the more specific treatments such as antidepressant drugs may be much less specific than has traditionally been believed, as evidence is increasing that these drugs are effective across a broad spectrum of depressive, anxiety and other disorders. Furthermore, with antidepressant drugs there may be general factors which predict outcome for a range of antidepressant drugs, as well as more specific factors which predict outcome for one class of antidepressant drug only (Joyce & Paykel 1989).

However, it can be argued that treatment non-response is of greatest clinical importance. The reason for this is that if an antidepressant drug is prescribed for a patient with a depressive disorder of at least moderate severity, then the important clinical issue is not why a patient improves, but whether improvement occurs. Thus it would be of benefit to clinicians if they could identify at an early stage those patients who were unlikely to improve with the given treatment.

PREDICTION OF TREATMENT RESPONSE IN DEPRESSION

Clinical predictors of antidepressant drug response

For antidepressant drugs to be effective they must be

453

prescribed and taken in an adequate dosage for an adequate length of time. Some authors suggest that an adequate antidepressant trial is a minimum dosage of 250 mg/day of imipramine or a related drug for a minimum of 6 weeks. However, this statement ignores the large individual differences in the pharmacokinetics of tricyclic antidepressants. For antidepressant drugs such as amitriptyline, nortriptyline, desipramine and imipramine, for which there is reasonable evidence for an established therapeutic blood level, an adequate trial should also be checked by ensuring that therapeutic levels of the drug have been achieved (Preskorn 1989).

Bipolar depressions

Although there now tends to be wide acceptance that bipolar and unipolar affective disorders should be considered separate disorders, there is still controversy about bipolar spectrum disorders (for instance bipolar II; see chapter 5) and some of the genetic evidence does not support the notion that bipolar and unipolar disorders are genetically totally distinct. However, there are an increasing number of findings which report on differences between bipolar and unipolar depressions including brain-imaging (Buchsbaum et al 1986). neuroendocrine (Joyce et al 1988, Rudorfer et al 1985), receptor (Kafka et al 1986) and cognitive deficit studies (Wolfe et al 1987). Clinically the distinction is important as the possibility that a patient may develop mania with antidepressant drugs is considerably higher in bipolar depressed patients, and this will influence pharmacological treatment. The acute treatment response in bipolar depression is probably comparable to that of major depression, but tends to be worse when there is mood cycling, mixed mood states (Keller et al 1986) and if the patient has a bipolar II disorder (Endicott et al 1985).

Although there is some evidence to suggest that bipolar depressions respond better to lithium than unipolar depressions (Goodwin et al 1972), and there are anecdotal case reports of favourable response to monoamine oxidase inhibitors (MAOIs; Quitkin et al 1981), treatment response in bipolar depression has received little attention. Most clinicians utilize cyclic antidepressants in bipolar depressions, although often in conjunction with lithium so as to prevent mania and/or cycling.

Major depression with psychotic features

In recent years there has been a growing literature which finds that depressed patients with delusions have a poorer response to both tricyclic and monoamine oxidase inhibitor antidepressant drug treatment than non-delusional patients (Spiker et al 1985, Janicak et al 1988). However, the placebo response rate in delusional depression is lower than in non-delusional depression, and may be very low (Spiker & Kupfer 1988). This means that the difference between placebo and an antidepressant drug in delusional depression (e.g. 0% versus 30%) may be as great as that in non-delusional depression (e.g. 30% versus 60%), but clinically the majority of delusional depressed patients will not respond to an antidepressant drug alone. However, the majority of delusionally depressed patients respond to combined antidepressant and antipsychotic drug, or with ECT.

Non-bipolar, non-psychotic major depression

Non-bipolar, non-psychotic major depression is almost certainly a heterogeneous diagnostic category, and the optimal approach to classifying these depressive disorders remains controversial. There is some consensus that there exists an endogenous or melancholic subgroup, with core symptoms being psychomotor retardation (possibly agitation), pervasive anhedonia, non-reactivity of mood, distinct quality of mood, diurnal variation, early morning awakening and guilt. However, different diagnostic criteria for melancholia do not consistently diagnose the same patients as having endogenous depression, although they overlap considerably (Davidson et al 1984, Copolov et al 1986).

While a number of studies have reported that endogenous depressions respond better to tricyclic antidepressants than non-endogenous depressions (Paykel 1972, Raskin & Crook 1976), there are dissenting findings (Simpson et al 1976, Maier et al 1989). These conflicting results could be explained by the findings of Abou-Saleh & Coppen (1983). They found a curvilinear relationship between Newcastle endogeneity scores and response to amitriptyline, such that patients with very low or very high endogeneity scores (possibly largely due to psychotic features) responded poorly to amitriptyline compared to patients with an intermediate endogeneity score. Of the individual symptoms studied there is evidence that the presence of psychomotor retardation is a predictor of a good therapeutic response to antidepressants (Paykel 1972, Raskin & Crook 1976). It has also been suggested that loss of interest and pleasure, non-reactivity of mood and diurnal variation may be favourable prognostic symptoms (Maier et al 1989). The symptoms of sleep and appetite disturbance have not been found to be predictive of response to antidepressants and, indeed, weight loss has been found to be a predictor of improvement in untreated non-endogenous depression (Parker et al 1985).

The severity of depressions may confuse the issue of the endogenous/non-endogenous dichotomy, because the more severe depressions tend to be the more endogenous. In part this reflects the instruments used to assess severity and endogenicity, as the Hamilton rating scale (frequently used as a measure of severity), and both the Newcastle (Carney et al 1965) and Michigan (Feinberg & Carroll 1982) endogenicity scales share common items such as guilt and psychomotor change. The National Institute of Mental Health Treatment of Depression Collaborative Program found comparable response to imipramine in the more and less severe depressions, but found a much lower response to placebo in the more severe; this suggests that the placebo–antidepressant difference may be greater in more severe depressions (Elkin et al 1989). Other studies also report that when the severity is below a minimal level (Hamilton score of less than 13 or 14) there may be no detectable difference between antidepressant and placebo treatment (Stewart et al 1983, Paykel et al 1988). Similarly, depressed patients with melancholic symptoms may have a lower response to psychosocial treatments or placebo than non-melancholic patients (Robbins et al 1989). Although the best response to tricyclic antidepressants is seen in patients whose severity and endogenicity are in the middle range, there is good evidence that these drugs are effective in a broad spectrum of depressed patients. It is also worth recalling that patients with mild depressions are more likely to drop out of antidepressant treatment than those with more severe depressions (Last et al 1985).

Atypical depression

The diagnostic category of atypical depression is not yet included in official diagnostic classification systems, but remains of interest to clinicians and researchers because of reports that these depressed patients may have a better response to monoamine oxidase inhibitor drugs than to tricyclic antidepressants. The term atypical depression has been used in a variety of ways (Paykel et al 1983, Davidson et al 1982), but in terms of monoamine oxidase inhibitor response it is largely used to describe those depressed patients who have marked interpersonal sensitivity, reversed vegetative symptoms (such as hypersomnia and hyperphagia), and/or who have associated anxiety or panic attacks.

In recent years there have been a number of antidepressant trials, usually of phenelzine against a tricyclic antidepressant or against placebo in varieties of depressed patients, some of whom were within the atypical depression spectrum (Ravaris et al 1980, Paykel et al 1982). The earlier studies suggested that the differential therapeutic effects between MAOIs and tricyclics were relatively small, but a number of recent studies support the notion that, in depressed patients with panic attacks and/or hypersomnia and hyperphagia, phenelzine may be superior to tricyclic antidepressants (Liebowitz et al 1984, 1988, Kayser et al 1985, 1988). Isocarboxazid may also be especially effective in atypical depressions (Davidson et al 1988). There is, however, little evidence for the effectiveness of tranylcypromine in such depressions (White & White 1986) and some clinicians find it effective in the more severe endogenous depressions.

Comorbidity and associated factors

Early studies on antidepressant response tended to find that those depressed patients with a gradual-onset depression of short duration and with no other psychopathology had the best response to treatment (Bielski & Friedel 1976). Although depressive episodes of short duration are generally more responsive to treatment than chronic depressions (Garvey et al 1989), not all studies find this (Croughan et al 1988). Furthermore, antidepressant drugs such as imipramine are clearly better than placebo in chronic depression (Kocsis et al 1989) and chronicity is itself associated with a lower response to placebo (Rabkin et al 1986). This raises the possibility that the placebo – antidepressant difference is the same in chronic and non-chronic depression although overall improvement is less in chronic illnesses.

In general, depressed patients with an associated personality disorder respond less well to antidepressants, and there appears to be a consensus that patients with neurotic, hypochondriacal or histrionic personality traits respond less well to tricyclic antidepressants (Bielski & Friedel 1976, Pfohl et al 1984, Hirschfield et al 1986). However, not all studies have found that the presence of a personality disorder is predictive of a poorer treatment response (Davidson et al 1985, Joffe & Regan 1989), although the latter of these studies noted that personality features such as assertiveness, independence and competitiveness distinguished responders from non-responders. With the increasing interest in the measurement and assessment of personality and personality disorder, it is expected that further light on this important question of how personality affects antidepressant response will be forthcoming in the near future. The hypothesis proposed by Cloninger (1986) which links personality traits to underlying neurotransmitter systems may provide an important framework within which to address these questions.

It has been suggested that concurrent sedative or alcohol abuse is associated with a poorer antidepressant response (Akiskal 1982), but in the most extensive study to date concurrent alcoholism did not adversely affect the outcome for depressed patients (Hirschfeld et al 1989). There are suggestions that secondary depressions have a poorer treatment response than primary depressions (Coryell et al 1985, Maier et al 1989). In recent years there has been considerable interest in the comorbidity of major depression and panic disorder, and it has been reported that depressed patients with comorbid panic disorder have a less favourable response to treatment with tricyclic antidepressants (Grunhaus et al 1988). This could be consistent with the observations that depressions accompanied by panic attacks may have a better response to monoamine oxidase inhibitors than tricyclic antidepressants.

While life events preceding the onset of depressions do not appear to influence treatment response, ongoing events during treatment may adversely affect treatment outcome (Reno & Halaris 1990). Similarly, a poor relationship with a spouse, or a spouse who is disabled may contribute to a less favourable outcome (Akiskal 1982, Hooley et al 1986). Poor nutrition and low food intake may also attenuate antidepressant response (Soubrie et al 1989).

Predictors of response to electroconvulsive therapy

Electroconvulsive therapy (ECT) remains an important treatment modality for some depressed patients, but in clinical practice it is now mainly used for those with very severe and delusional depressions and for those who have not responded to other treatments. Early studies on prediction of response to ECT suggested that sudden onset, short duration, delusions, guilt, retardation and weight loss were favourable predictors, while neuroticism, personality disorder and self-pity were unfavourable predictors of response (Hobson 1953, Carney et al 1965). More recent studies suggest that it is especially the presence of depressive delusions which predicts a favourable response to ECT (Crow et al 1984). Given that the presence of delusions also predicts no response to placebo and a low likelihood of response to tricyclic antidepressant drugs alone, this suggests that in delusional depression combinations of antidepressant with antipsychotic drugs or ECT are probably the treatments of choice. Non-response to previous adequate trials of medication is associated with a lower likelihood of response to ECT (Prudic et al 1990).

Predictors of response to psychotherapies

It is now well established that both cognitive and interpersonal psychotherapies are as effective as tricyclic antidepressant drugs in the treatment of outpatients with milder nonbipolar, nonpsychotic major depression (Dobson 1989). To date, however, there has been relatively little research looking at the issue of prediction of treatment response.

In the National Institute of Mental Health Treatment of Depression Collaborative Program, the general order of treatment effectiveness was imipramine + clinical management, interpersonal psychotherapy, cognitive therapy and placebo + clinical management. The antidepressant drug was superior to other treatments only in the initially severely depressed (Hamilton score ≥ 20) (Elkin et al 1989). Prusoff et al (1980) found that interpersonal psychotherapy, while generally effective, was not as effective as antidepressant drugs in those with an endogenous depression. Similarly, in hospitalized depressed adolescents, those with melancholia did not respond to psychosocial treatment (Robbins et al 1989). The presence of an abnormal biological marker such as dexamethasone non-suppression or a shortened REM latency may predict non-response to psychosocial and cognitive therapies (Rush 1983, Robbins et al 1989). These studies would thus suggest that, in the severely depressed, in those with melancholia or abnormal biological markers, psychotherapies alone may be less effective than antidepressant medications. Conversely, better general emotional health may be predictive of a better response to interpersonal psychotherapy (Rounsaville et al 1981).

There is no evidence for adverse interactions between antidepressant drugs and psychotherapy; indeed, some patients may do better with both treatments (Conte et al 1986). For instance, Miller et al (1990) have found that depressed patients with high levels of cognitive dysfunction do significantly better with combined antidepressant and cognitive-behavioural psychotherapy than with pharmacotherapy alone.

Biological markers and treatment response in depression

Over the past 25 years the amine hypothesis has guided neurobiological research on depression. One of the areas of enquiry has been whether levels of certain amines, their precursors, their metabolites or associated enzymes are able to predict response to antidepressant drugs; either any antidepressant or specific classes of antidepressants. Further, as brain amines regulate neuroendocrine secretion, sleep rhythms and other physiological functions, there has been interest in whether measurable changes in these other systems could predict antidepressant response, on the assumption that these parameters are indirect reflections of the underlying neurochemical changes associated with some depressions (Joyce & Paykel 1989, Balon 1989).

In the 1970s it was suggested that depressive disorders might be biochemically heterogeneous and that there were noradrenaline depletion depressions and serotonin depletion depressions. The noradrenaline depletion depressions were suggested to be characterized by low urinary 3-methoxy-4-hydroxyphenylglycol (MHPG), a mood brightening with amphetamine and clinical response to noradrenergic antidepressants such as imipramine, while serotonin depletion depressions were characterized by low cerebrospinal fluid 5-hydroxyindoleacetic acid (5-HIAA), high urinary MHPG, a dysphoric response to amphetamine and clinical response to serotonergic antidepressants such as amitriptyline (Maas 1978). There is little substantial evidence for the hypothesis of biochemically distinct subtypes of depression, and all antidepressants probably act via a final common pathway of beta-adrenoceptor downregulation; but an intact serotonergic system may be necessary for this downregulation to occur. Furthermore, while noradrenergic systems may have an important place in mood regulation, there is increasing evidence that serotonin is implicated in modulating a range of behavioural phenomena including impulse control, anxiety and mood.

This hypothesis of biochemical subtypes of depression has stimulated considerable research into the role of monoamine metabolites (especially urinary MHPG) and of the mood response to stimulant drugs as predictors of response to specific antidepressants. Over 20 studies have looked at the relationship between urinary MHPG levels and antidepressant response and, while low MHPG may have some predictive power as regards a likely beneficial response to imipramine, nortriptyline and maprotiline, a high MHPG does not appear to predict amitriptyline response (Kelwala et al 1983, Joyce & Paykel 1989, Balon 1989). However, it has recently been reported that it is not the levels of any monoamine metabolite in isolation, but the interactions between noradrenaline, dopamine and serotonin metabolites which may best distinguish antidepressant responders from non-responders (Hsiao et al 1987). This finding needs replication but is consistent with the ever increasing evidence for interactions between the neurotransmitter systems.

The stimulant challenge test has also been studied in regard to prediction of antidepressant response and, although there are some discrepant findings, a mood brightening with a stimulant drug may predict a more favourable response to a noradrenergic antidepressant drug such as imipramine or desipramine. Also of interest have been reports that a positive response to stimulant challenge may predict antidepressant response to lithium (Goff 1986).

The amino acids tryptophan and tyrosine are the precursors of serotonin and noradrenaline, and it has been suggested that the availability of these amino acids in relationship to competing large neutral amino acids (LNAA) in plasma provides an indicator of neurotransmitter turnover. One research group has reported that the tryptophan-to-LNAA ratio predicts response to amitriptyline while the tyrosine-to-LNAA ratio may predict response to nortriptyline and maprotiline (Moller et al 1986).

Many neuroendocrine abnormalities have been reported in depressive disorders, with cortisol hypersecretion the best documented abnormality, occurring in 25–50% of depressed patients (Joyce 1985). Cortisol hypersecretion is often assessed by means of the dexamethasone suppression test (DST). Of the variety of neuroendocrine abnormalities only the DST has been sufficiently studied in relationship to treatment response to comment upon at this time. If an initial DST is positive (i.e. the patient shows cortisol non-suppression after dexamethasone), then the test usually normalizes with antidepressant treatment and failure to normalize, even if there has been clinical improvement, is associated with a high likelihood of early relapse (Arana et al 1985, Targum 1984). It has been suggested that DST non-suppressors do both better and worse than suppressors with treatment, but it seems likely that there is no significant difference in response between those with or without an abnormal DST (Arana 1985). However, it is becoming increasingly clear that those depressed patients with a positive DST are unlikely to respond either to placebo or to psychotherapies (Rush 1983, Peselow et al 1989). This suggests that the presence of an abnormal DST indicates the need for a biological treatment; it also suggests that the difference between antidepressant and placebo response rates is greater in DST non-suppressors than in suppressors, despite the observations that the likelihood of response is similar in those with and without abnormal DSTs.

Like the DST, the presence of a shortened REM latency may predict a poor response to placebo or psychosocial treatments, but a high likelihood of response to tricyclic antidepressants (Coble et al 1979, Rush et al 1989). The degree of REM sleep suppression after an antidepressant may also predict antidepressant response (Hochli et al 1986).

A low urinary tyramine sulphate excretion after an oral tyramine load has been suggested to be a trait marker for affective disorder (Harrison et al 1984). Two studies have found that low tyramine excretion may predict antidepressant response, although a placebo-controlled study is required (Stewart et al 1988, Hale et al 1989).

Preliminary studies have suggested that behavioural observations such as speech pauses, head aversions, assertive behaviours and psychophysiological measures such as facial EMG may predict antidepressant response (Greden et al 1984, Troisi et al 1989).

Although there are a number of interesting findings to date, none are sufficiently established and practicable for routine clinical practice. There also needs to be greater attention to the interrelationships between the various biological markers, so that it becomes clear which markers assess aspects of a common underlying pathophysiology and which detect the undoubted heterogeneity of depression.

PREDICTION OF TREATMENT RESPONSE IN BIPOLAR DISORDER

Whereas in major depression the majority of treatment studies have concentrated on short-term antidepressant response, in bipolar disorder there are relatively few studies addressing the prediction of the short-term response to treatment for mania and even fewer for bipolar depression. However, given that bipolar disorder has a high rate of recurrence it is appropriate

that the majority of studies have focused on the prediction of prophylactic response to lithium. Only recently has interest started to focus on the prediction of treatment response to the increasing range of alternative pharmacological approaches to lithium-resistant bipolar disorder (Post 1988).

Predictors of drug response in mania

In the short term the likelihood of a manic patient recovering from the current episode is over 80%, which is higher than the short-term recovery rate for depression (Keller et al 1986). There are few well-established predictors of acute treatment response in mania (Taylor & Abrams 1981), and what studies there are do not always explicitly clarify whether patients were treated with lithium alone, neuroleptic drugs or both. The best established predictor of a poor short-term response is the presence of a mixed mood state and/or mood cycling. This association has been repeatedly found as regards acute lithium response, but probably also applies when manic patients are being treated with neuroleptic drugs with or without lithium (Secunda et al 1985). Poor short-term outcome has also been associated with a long episode duration and with medical or psychiatric comorbidity (Black et al 1988). Some studies have suggested that the presence of psychosis predicts a poorer short-term outcome, but other studies have not found this to be of any predictive significance.

One of the few sustained research projects on biological predictors of short term lithium response has been carried out by Garver et al (1984), studying a cross-section of psychotic patients, many of whom did not have a diagnosed affective disorder. They have reported that a high growth hormone response to apomorphine and a high intracellular-to-extracellular erythrocyte ratio (Hirschowitz et al 1982) predict lithium response over 2 weeks in psychotic patients. However, further replication of these findings and extension to patients with diagnosed affective disorders is required.

Predictors of prophylactic response in bipolar affective disorder

Although it is now well-established that lithium is an effective prophylactic treatment for bipolar disorder, it needs to be emphasised that perhaps fewer than 50% of bipolar patients prescribed lithium, even under the optimal conditions of control and supervision in a drug trial, will have no further episodes of depression or mania. In ordinary clinical practice maintenance lithium therapy may be even less effective than this (Dickson & Kendell 1986).

Lithium prophylaxis is usually considered when patients have suffered from a minimum of two episodes of illness within a limited time span such as 2–3 years. As lithium prophylaxis is a long-term treatment, patients who do not adhere to the treatment regimen will not benefit from lithium treatment. However, adherence or compliance is not an all-or-none phenomenon, and with time, the experiencing of further episodes of illness and education patients may accept long-term lithium treatment. Thus before deciding that a patient has not responded to an earlier trial of lithium it is essential to clarify that the patient has really had an adequate trial in terms of dosage (Gelenberg et al 1989), duration and compliance. An adequate trial of prophylactic lithium probably requires 12 months and, although an early response is a favourable prognostic indicator, early non-response should not lead to discontinuation as some will ultimately benefit from lithium.

As with many psychotropic drugs, a past history or family history of lithium response is a favourable predictor of outcome. In addition, a family history of bipolar disorder is probably a favourable predictor of lithium response. Of clinical features, the best predictor of response is in fact a predictor of non-response; namely, those patients with rapid cycling and/or mixed mood states are likely to do poorly (Prien et al 1988). It is also becoming apparent that the nature of the index episode and the previous pattern of illness are important predictors, in that those recovering from a manic episode are more likley to do well than those recovering from a depressive episode (Shapiro et al 1989). Similarly, those whose pattern of illness is of mania followed by depression or an erratic course are more likely to do well with lithium than those whose course of illness tends to be depression followed by mania (Maj et al 1989).

It has also been found that a favourable lithium response is more likely in those with a good pre-morbid personality, low neuroticism (Abou-Saleh & Coppen 1986), good inter-episode functioning (Goodnick et al 1987, Grof et al 1983) and good social support.

At the present time there are no established biological predictors of lithium response which justify clinical usage. As mentioned above, Garver et al (1984) have found that the intracellular — extracellular lithium ratio and the growth hormone response to apomorphine may predict a favourable response to lithium in psychotic patients. It has also been reported by some workers, but not others, that the presence of the HLA-A$_3$ antigen or a positive M antigen predicts a better response to lithium. There are also suggestions that bipolar patients with subclinical hypothyroidism or low plasma folate are less likely to respond well to lithium.

CONCLUSIONS

Although the majority of depressed patients who are given adequate treatment will improve, degrees of chronicity and recurrence remain disturbingly high. Many depressed patients, especially non-bipolar, non-psychotic ambulatory outpatients, will respond well to interpersonal or cognitive psychotherapy. However, if the depression is severe or has a number of melancholic features, or if abnormal biological markers are present, then it is unlikely that psychotherapies alone will be sufficient and antidepressant drugs are likely to be necessary. Tricyclic and related antidepressants are broad-spectrum drugs that are of benefit across a range of depressive disorders. The depressed patient with a good premorbid personality, psychomotor retardation and an intermediate level of severity and endogeneity but without psychotic features may be the patient who responds best to these drugs. The presence of psychotic features suggests the need for the use of ECT or additional antipsychotic drugs. The presence of 'atypical' features such as panic attacks and reversed vegetative symptoms suggests that a better response may be obtained with monoamine oxidase inhibitors than tricyclic antidepressant drugs. A bipolar history suggests that lithium alone or in combination with another antidepressant may be necessary (Joyce & Paykel 1989, Paykel 1989). Although biological predictors are of theoretical, and may in the future be of clinical importance, none are sufficiently established to be of current clinical utility.

In bipolar disorder the short-term response to treatment for mania is generally favourable, and the only well-established predictor of likely poor response is the presence of cycling and/or a mixed mood state. A favourable prophylactic response to lithium is most likely in bipolar patients with a good premorbid personality, good social support and adequate inter-episode functioning. The presence of rapid cycling, mixed mood states and a pattern of depression followed by mania are predictive of a poorer response to lithium. In those who fail to benefit from lithium a variety of alternative treatments, such as the anticonvulsant drugs, may be beneficial.

REFERENCES

Abou-Saleh M T, Coppen A 1983 Classification of depression and response to antidepressive therapies. British Journal of Psychiatry 143: 601–603

Abou-Saleh M T, Coppen A 1986 Who responds to prophylactic lithium? Journal of Affective Disorders 10: 115–125

Akiskal H S 1982 Factors associated with incomplete recovery in primary depressive illness. Journal of Clinical Psychiatry 43: 266–271

Arana G W, Baldessarini R J, Ornsteen M 1985 The dexamethasone suppression test for diagnosis and prognosis in psychiatry: commentary and review. Archives of General Psychiatry 42: 1193–1204

Balon R 1989 Biological predictors of antidepressant treatment outcome. Clinical Neuropharmacology 12: 195–214

Bielski R J, Friedel R O 1976 Prediction of tricyclic antidepressant response. A critical review. Archives of General Psychiatry 33: 1479–1489

Black D W, Winokur G, Hulbert J, Nasrallah A 1988 Predictors of immediate response in the treatment of mania: the importance of comorbidity. Biological Psychiatry 24: 191–198

Buchsbaum M S, Wu J, DeLisi L E, Holcomb H, Kessler R, Johnson J, King A C, Hazlett E, Langston K, Post R M 1986 Frontal cortex and basal ganglia metabolic rates assessed by positron emission tomography with (^{18}F)2-deoxyglucose in affective illness. Journal of Affective Disorders 10: 137–152

Carney M W P, Roth M, Garside R F 1965 The diagnosis of depressive symptoms and the prediction of ECT response. British Journal of Psychiatry III: 659–674

Cloninger C R 1986 A unified biosocial theory of personality and its role in the development of anxiety states. Psychiatric Developments 3: 167–226

Coble P A, Kupfer D J, Spiker D G, Neil J F, McPartland R J 1979 EEG sleep in primary depression. A longitudinal placebo study. Journal of Affective Disorders 1: 131–138

Conte H R, Plutchilk R, Wild K V, Karasu T B 1986 Combined psychotherapy and pharmacotherapy for depression. A systematic analysis of the evidence. Archives of General Psychiatry 43: 471–479

Copolov D L, Rubin R T, Mander A J, Sashidharan S P, Whitehouse A M, Blackburn I M, Freeman C P, Blackwood D H R 1986 DSM-III melancholia: do the criteria accurately and reliably distinguish endogenous pattern depression? Journal of Affective Disorders 10: 191–202

Coryell W, Zimmerman M, Pfohl B 1985 Short-term prognosis in primary and secondary major depression. Journal of Affective Disorders 9: 265–270

Croughan J L, Secunda S K, Katz M M, Robins E, Mendels J, Swann A, Harris-Larkin B 1988 Sociodemographic and prior clinical course characteristics associated with treatment response in depressed patients. Journal of Psychiatric Research 22: 227–237

Crow T J, Deakin J F W, Johnstone E C, MacMillan J J, Owen D G C, Lawler P, Frith C D, Stevens M, McPherson K 1984 The Northwick Park ECT trial:

predictors of response to real and simulated ECT. British Journal of Psychiatry 144: 227–237

Davidson J, Miller R, Turnbull C, Sullivan J L 1982 Atypical depression. Archives of General Psychiatry 39: 527–534

Davidson J, Turnbull C, Strickland R, Belyea M 1984 Comparative diagnostic criteria for melancholia and endogenous depression. Archives of General Psychiatry 41: 506–511

Davidson J, Miller R, Strickland R 1985 Neuroticism and personality disorder in depression. Journal of Affective Disorders 8: 177–182

Davidson J R T, Giller E L, Zisook S, Overall J E 1988 An efficacy study of isocarboxazid and placebo in depression, and its relationship to depressive nosology. Archives of General Psychiatry 45: 120–127

Dickson W E, Kendell R E 1986 Does maintenance lithium therapy prevent recurrences of mania under ordinary clinical conditions. Psychological Medicine 16: 521–530

Dobson K S 1989 A meta-analysis of the efficacy of cognitive therapy for depression. Journal of Consulting and Clinical Psychology 57: 414–419

Elkin I, Shea M T, Watkins J T, Imber S D, Sotsky S M, Collins J F, Glass D R, Pilkonis P A, Leber W R, Docherty J P, Fiester S J, Parloff M B 1989 National Instiue of Mental Health Treatment of Depression collaborative research program. General effectiveness of treatments. Archives of General Psychiatry 46: 971–982

Endicott J, Nee J, Andreasen N C, Clayton P J, Keller M B, Coryell W 1985 Bipolar II: combine or keep separate? Journal of Affective Disorders 8: 17–28

Feinberg M, Carroll B J 1982 Separation of subtypes of depression using discriminant analysis. British Journal of Psychiatry 140: 384–391

Garver D L, Hirschowitz J, Fleishmann R, Djuric P E 1984 Lithium ratio in vitro: diagnosis and lithium carbonate response in psychotic patients. Archives of General Psychiatry 41: 497–505

Garvey M J, Cook B L, Tollefson G D, Schaffer C B 1989 Antidepressant response in chronic depression. Comprehensive Psychiatry 30: 214–217

Gelenberg A J, Kane J M, Keller M B, Lavori P, Rosenbaum J F Cole K, Lavelle J 1989 Comparison of standard and low serum levels of lithium for maintenance treatment of bipolar disorder. New England Journal of Medicine 321: 1489–1493

Goff D C 1986 The stimulant challenge test in depression. Journal of Clinical Psychiatry 47: 538–543

Goodnick P J, Fieve R R, Schlegel A, Kaufman K 1987 Inter-episode major and subclinical symptoms in affective disorder. Acta Psychiatrica Scandinavica 75: 597–600

Goodwin F K, Murphy D L, Dunner D L, Bunney W E 1972 Lithium response in unipolar versus bipolar depression. American Journal of Psychiatry 129: 44–47

Greden J F, Price L H, Genero N, Feinberg M, Levine S 1984 Facial EMG activity levels predict treatment outcome in depression. Psychiatry Research 13: 345–352

Grof P, Hux M, Grof E, Arato M 1983 Prediction of response to stablizing lithium treatment. Pharmacopsychiatry 16: 195–200

Grunhaus L, Harel Y, Krugler T, Pande A C, Haskett R F 1988 Major depressive disorder and panic disorder: effects of comorbidity on treatment outcome with antidepressant medications. Clinical Neuropharmacology 11: 454–461

Hale A S, Sandler M, Hannah P, Bridges P K 1989 Tyramine conjugation test for prediction of treatment response in depressed patients. Lancet, February 4: 234–236

Harrison W M, Cooper T B, Stewart J W, Quitkin F M, McGrath P J, Liebowitz M R, Rabkin J R, Markowitz J S, Klein D F 1984 The tyramine challenge test as a marker for melancholia. Archives of General Psychiatry 41: 681–685

Hirschfeld R M A, Klerman G L, Andreasen N C, Clayton P J, Keller M B 1986 Psycho-social predictors of chronicity in depressed patients. British Journal of Psychiatry 148: 648–654

Hirschfeld R M A, Kosier T, Keller M B, Lavori P W, Endicott J 1989 The influence of alcoholism on the course of depression. Journal of Affective Disorders 16: 151–158

Hirschowitz J, Zemlan F P, Garver D L 1982 Growth hormone levels and lithium ratios as predictors of success of lithium therapy in schizophrenia. American Journal of Psychiatry 139: 646–649

Hobson R F 1953 Prognostic factors in electric convulsive therapy. Journal of Neurology, Neurosurgery and Psychiatry 16: 275–281

Hochli D, Riemann D, Zulley J, Berger M 1986 Initial REM sleep suppression by clomipramine: a prognostic tool for treatment response in patients with a major depressive disorder. Biological Psychiatry 21: 1217–1220

Hooley J M, Orley J, Teasdale J D 1986 Levels of expressed emotion and relapse in depressed patients. British Journal of Psychiatry 148: 642–647

Hsiao J K, Agren H, Bartko J J, Rudorfer M V, Linnoila M, Potter W Z 1987 Monoamine neurotransmitter interactions and the prediction of antidepressant response. Archives of General Psychiatry 44: 1078–1083

Janicak P G, Pandey G N, Davis J M, Boshes R, Bresnahan D, Sharma R 1988 Response of psychotic and nonpsychotic depression to phenelzine. American Journal of Psychiatry 145: 93–95

Joffe R T, Regan J J 1989 Personality and response to tricyclic antidepressants in depressed patients. Journal of Nervous and Mental Disease 177: 745–749

Joyce P R 1985 Neuroendocrine changes in depression. Australian and New Zealand Journal of Psychiatry 19: 120–127

Joyce P R, Paykel E S 1989 Predictors of drug response in depression. Archives of General Psychiatry 46: 89–99

Joyce P R, Sellman J D, Donald R A, Livesey J H, Elder P A 1988 The unipolar-bipolar depressive dichotomy and the relationship between afternoon prolactin and cortisol levels. Journal of Affective Disorders 14: 189–193

Kafka M S, Nurnberger J I, Siever L, Targum S, Uhde T W, Gershon E S 1986 Alpha-2-adrenergic receptor function in patients with unipolar and bipolar affective disorders. Journal of Affective Disorders 10: 163–169

Kayser A, Robinson D S, Nies A, Howard D 1985 Response to phenelzine among depressed patients with features of hysteroid dysphoria. American Journal of Psychiatry 142: 486–488

Kayser A, Robinson D S, Yingling K, Howard D B, Corcella J, Laux D 1988 The influence of panic attacks on response to phenelzine and amitriptyline in depressed outpatients. Journal of Clinical Psychopharmacology 8: 246–253

Keller M B, Lavori P W, Coryell W, Andreasen N C, Endicott J, Clayton P J, Klerman G L, Hirschfeld R M A 1986 Differential outcome of pure manic, mixed/cycling, and pure depressive episodes in patients with bipolar illness. Journal of American Medical Association 255: 3138–3142

Kelwala S, Jones D, Sitaram N 1983 Monoamine metabolites as predictors of antidepressant response: a critique. Progress in Neuro-Psychopharmacology and Biological Psychiatry 7: 229–240

Kendell R E 1989 Clinical validity. Psychological Medicine 19: 45–55

Kiloh L G, Andrews G, Neilson M 1988 The long-term outcome of depressive illness. British Journal of Psychiatry 153: 752–757

Kocsis J H, Mason B J, Frances A J, Sweeney J, Mann J J, Marin D 1989 Prediction of response of chronic depression to imipramine. Journal of Affective Disorders 17: 255–260

Last C G, Thase M E, Hersen M, Bellack A S, Himmelhoch J M 1985 Patterns of attrition for psychosocial and pharmacologic treatments of depression. Journal of Clinical Psychiatry 46: 361–366

Lee A S, Murray R M 1988 The long-term outcome of Maudsley depressives. British Journal of Psychiatry 153: 741–751

Liebowitz M R, Quitkin F M, Stewart J W, McGrath P J, Harrison W, Rabkin J, Tricamo E, Markowitz J S, Klein D F 1984 Phenelzine vs imipramine in atypical depression. Archives of General Psychiatry 41: 669–677

Liebowitz M R, Quitkin F M, Stewart J W, McGrath P J, Harrison M W, Markowitz J S, Rabkin J G, Tricamo E, Goetz D M, Klein D F 1988 Antidepressant specificity in atypical depression. Archives of General Psychiatry 45: 129–137

Maas J W 1978 Clinical and biochemical heterogeneity of depressive disorders. Annals of Internal Medicine 88: 556–563

Maier W, Philipp M, Schlegel S, Heuser I, Wiedmann K, Benkert O 1988 Diagnostic determinants of response to treatment with tricyclic antidepressants: a polydiagnostic approach. Psychiatry Research 30: 83–93

Maj M, Pirozzi R, Starace F 1989 Previous pattern of course of the illness as a predictor of response to lithium prophylaxis in bipolar patients. Journal of Affective Disorders 17: 237–241

Miller I W, Norman W H, Keitner G I 1990 Treatment response of high cognitive dysfunction depressed inpatients. Comprehensive Psychiatry 30: 62–71

Moller S E, de Beurs P, Timmerman L, Tan B K, Leijnse-Ybema H J, Cohen Stuart M H, Hopfner Peterson H E 1986 Plasma tryptophan and tyrosine ratios to competing amino acids in relation to antidepressant response to citalopram and maprotiline. Psychopharmacology 88: 96–110

Parker G, Tennant C, Blignault I 1985 Predicting improvement in patients with non-endogenous depression. British Journal of Psychiatry 146: 132–139

Paykel E S 1972 Depressive typologies and response to amitriptyline. British Journal of Psychiatry 120: 147–156

Paykel E S 1989 Treatment of depression. The relevance of

research for clinical practice. British Journal of Psychiatry 155: 754–763

Paykel E S, Rowan P R, Parker P R, Bhat A V 1982 Response to phenelzine and amitriptyline in subtypes of outpatient depression. Archives of General Psychiatry 39: 1041–1049

Paykel E S, Parker P R, Rowan P R, Rao B M, Taylor C N 1983 The nosology of atypical depression. Psychological Medicine 13: 131–139

Paykel E S, Hollyman J A, Freeling P, Sedgwick P 1988 Predictors of therapeutic benefit from amitriptyline in mild depression: a general practice placebo-controlled trial. Journal of Affective Disorders 14: 83–95

Post R M 1988 Approaches to treatment-resistant bipolar affectively ill patients. Clinical Neuropharmacology 11: 93–104

Peselow E D, Stanley M, Filippi A M, Barouche F, Goodnick P, Fieve R P 1989 The predictive value of the dexamethasone suppression test. A placebo-controlled study. British Journal of Psychiatry 155: 667–672

Pfohl B, Stangl D, Zimmerman M 1984 The implications of DSM-III personality disorders for patients with major depression. Journal of Affective Disorders 7: 309–318

Prien R F, Himmelhoch J M, Kupfer D J 1988 Treatment of mixed mania. Journal of Affective Disorders 15: 9–15

Preskorn S H 1989 Tricyclic antidepressants: the whys and hows of therapeutic drug monitoring. Journal of Clinical Psychiatry 50 (7 suppl): 34–42

Prudic J, Sackeim H A, Devanand D P 1990 Medication resistance and clinical response to electroconvulsive therapy. Psychiatry Research 31: 287–296

Prusoff B A, Weissman M M, Klerman G L, Rounsaville B J 1980 Research diagnostic criteria subtypes of depression: their role as predictors of differential response to psychotherapy and drug treatment. Archives of General Psychiatry 37: 796–801

Quitkin F M, McGrath P, Liebowitz M R, Stewart J, Howard A 1981 Monoamine oxidase inhibitors in bipolar endogenous depressives. Journal of Clinical Psychopharmacology 1: 70–74

Rabkin J G, McGrath P, Stewart J W, Harrison W, Markowitz J S, Quitkin F 1986 Follow-up of patients who improved during placebo washout. Journal of Clinical Psychopharmacology 6: 274–278

Raskin A, Crook T A 1976 The endogenous-neurotic distinction as a predictor of response to antidepressant drugs. Psychological Medicine 6: 59–70

Ravaris C L, Robinson D S, Ives J O, Nies A, Bartlett D 1980 Phenelzine and amitriptyline in the treatment of depression: a comparison of present and past studies. Archives of General Psychiatry 37: 1075–1080

Reno R M, Halaris A E 1990 The relationship between life stress and depression in an endogenous sample. Comprehensive Psychiatry 31: 25–33

Robbins D R, Alessi N E, Colfer M V 1989 Treatment of adolescents with major depression: implications of the DST and the melancholic clinical subtype. Journal of Affective Disorders 17: 99–104

Rounsaville B J, Weissman M M, Prusoff B A 1981 Psychotherapy with depressed outpatients: patient and process variables as predictors of outcome. British Journal of Psychiatry 138: 67–74

Rudorfer M V, Ross R J, Linnoila M, Sherer M A, Potter W Z 1985 Exaggerated orthostatic responsivity of plasma norepinephrine in depression. Archives of General Psychiatry 42: 1186–1192

Rush A J 1983 Cognitive therapy of depression: rationale techniques and efficacy. Psychiatric Clinics of North America 6, 105–127

Rush A J, Giles D E, Jarrett R B, Feldman-Koffler F, Debus J R, Weissenburger J, Orsulak P J, Roffwarg H P 1989 Reduced REM latency predicts response to tricyclic medication in depressed outpatients. Biological Psychiatry 26: 61–72

Secunda S K, Katz M M, Swann A, Koslow S H, Maas J W, Chuang S, Croughan J 1985 Mania: diagnosis, state measurement and prediction of treatment response. Journal of Affective Disorders 8: 113–121

Shapiro D R, Quitkin F M, Fleiss J L 1989 Response to maintenance therapy in bipolar illness. Effect of index episode. Archives of General Psychiatry 46: 401–405

Simpson G M, Lee H L, Cuche Z, Kellner R 1976 Two doses of imipramine in hospitalized endogenous and neurotic depressions. Archives of General Psychiatry 33: 1093–1102

Soubrie P, Martin P, Massol J, Gaudel G 1989 Attenuation of response to antidepressants in animals induced by reduction in food intake. Psychiatry Research 27: 149–159

Spiker D G, Kupfer D J 1988 Placebo response rates in psychotic and nonpsychotic depression. Journal of Affective Disorders 14: 21–23

Spiker D G, Weiss J C, Dealy R S, Griffin S J, Hanin I, Neil J F, Perel J M, Rossi A J, Soloff P H 1985 The pharmacological treatment of delusional depression. American Journal of Psychiatry 142: 430–436

Stewart J W, Quitkin F M, Liebowitz M R, McGrath P J, Harrison W M, Klein D F 1983 Efficacy of desipramine in depressed outpatients. Response according to Research Diagnostic Criteria diagnoses and severity of illness. Archives of General Psychiatry 40: 202–207

Stewart J W, Harrison W, Cooper T B, Quitkin F M 1988 Tyramine sulphate excretion may be a better predictor of antidepressant response than monoamine oxidase activity. Psychiatry Research 25: 195–201

Targum S D 1984 Persistent neuroendocrine dysregulation in major depressive disorder a marker for early relapse. Biological Psychiatry 19: 305–318

Taylor M A, Abrams P 1981 Prediction of treatment response in mania. Archives of General Psychiatry 38: 800–803

Troisi A, Pasini A, Bersani G, Grispini A, Ciani N 1989 Ethological predictors of amitriptyline response in depressed outpatients. Journal of Affective Disorders 17: 129–136

White K, White J 1986 Tranylcypromine: patterns of predictors of response. Journal of Clinical Psychiatry 47: 380–382

Wolfe J, Granholm E, Butters N, Saunders E, Janowsky D 1987 Verbal memory deficits associated with major affective disorders: a comparison of unipolar and bipolar patients. Journal of Affective Disorders 13: 83–92

PART 4

Psychotherapeutic, cognitive and social treatments

28. Psychoanalytically orientated psychotherapy

Jules R. Bemporad

PSYCHOANALYTICAL THERAPY

The theory of psychoanalysis and its practical application as a therapeutic modality have gone through a series of constant revisions and modification since the pioneer publications of Breuer and Freud almost a century ago. Analysts who left the psychoanalytic movement have presented divergent approaches to psychopathology and, even within the more traditional camp, a steady development of theory and practice has continued to evolve. As a result, it is difficult to give a definition of psychoanalysis or psychoanalytic psychotherapy which would be accepted by most practitioners without reservation. Perhaps the closest approximation of the essentials of psychoanalytic therapy may be found in a passage from Freud's own *History of the Psychoanalytic Movement*, which appeared in 1914. In this work, Freud parsimoniously reduced the essence of psychoanalysis to two cardinal features, as follows:

> It may be said that the theory of psychoanalysis is an attempt to account for two striking and unexpected facts of observation which emerge whenever an attempt is made to trace the symptoms of a neurotic back to their sources in his past life: the facts of transference and of resistance. Any line of investigation which recognizes these two facts and takes them as the starting point of its work may call itself psychoanalysis, though it arrives at results other than my own. (Freud 1914, p 16)

Transference may be loosely defined as the unconscious distortions of current significant others in adult life to fit personality patterns and expectations of important individuals from the past. Resistance is the attempt to block memories and other aspects of one's inner world that cause psychic pain from reaching conscious awareness. Therefore, if a practitioner accepts transference and resistance as the cornerstones of therapy, he or she implicitly also accepts that the sources of psychopathology lie in the shaping of the patient's personality during childhood and that the result of this developmental shaping, while directing the patient's behaviour, thinking and emotional responses, lies outside of consciousness.

The therapeutic work involved in undoing resistances and interpreting transference aims at allowing the patient a greater conscious knowledge of his inner world as it was formed in his or her interchange with significant others during the formative years of childhood. This greater self-knowledge gained in the current interaction with the therapist (or gained in the interaction with others but scrutinized in the therapeutic process) allows for the replacement of atavistic childhood estimations of oneself and of others with more appropriate adult judgments. As Offenkrantz & Tobin (1974) comment, the two phases of the analytic task are: 1) to make the here and now experience between patient and analyst come alive with feeling in order to discover the manner in which the past is still active in the patient's current perceptions and behaviour; and 2) to help the patient grasp how his present adult situation is different from his past. Through the retrieval of memories, a more appropriate perception of one's past and those individuals who played an important role in that past, awareness of one's continuing to act in a manner more appropriate to the past rather than the present, and a novel experience of oneself in the therapeutic dyad, the patient learns to identify those outmoded needs, fears and evaluations that precipitated or perpetuated psychopathology. Karasu (1990a) highlighted this emphasis on self-awareness as curative by stating that psychoanalytic therapy is largely based on the maxim that the unexamined life repeats itself.

APPLICATIONS TO DEPRESSION

The increase in awareness through the analysis of transference and resistance comes only gradually with the expenditure of much time and effort. This form of therapy, therefore, is not designed to deal directly or rapidly with symptoms of an acute depressive episode. There may be an initial amelioration of symptoms as a result of the patient finding an empathic listener, believing his needs will be met by a new significant other who is endowed with magical powers or venting his anger or misery. However, the forming of a supportive interpersonal relationship between patient and therapist is part of most verbal therapies and does not capture the discriminant contribution of psychoanalytic therapy as stated above. Such improvement, if it occurs, is welcomed but is not seen as due to the analytic process.

The goals of psychoanalytic psychotherapy are to strengthen the individual's basic abilities to cope with the vicissitudes of life and to overcome remnants of the past that increase vulnerability to everyday stresses. By distorting the environment less and by realigning needs, expectations and fears to correspond to actual and consciously realized events, the individual will hopefully be less prone to illness in the future. However, this beneficial alteration in the personality takes a long time to exert its effect on depressive symptoms, so that other therapeutic approaches are warranted if the magnitude of illness is so great as to cause severe and unnecessary suffering, impede functioning or lead to destructive actions. There is no inherent contradiction in utilizing the benefits of pharmacotherapy in relieving the patient of the pain of an acute depressive episode or in decreasing those symptoms that would diminish the patient's accessibility to therapeutic work. Medication may be particularly useful in treating the vegetative signs that accompany some forms of depression and which have been shown to be less responsive to verbal therapies (Klerman & Schechter, 1982).

The realistic role of medication should be explained to the patient in order to avoid the attribution of personalized meanings to the dispensing of pharmacological agents. Karasu (1990b) cites Luborsky (1984) as indicating three potential problems in administering medication during psychoanalytic therapy. These include: 1) the patient considers taking medications a loss of self-control or autonomy; 2) the patient views the prescription for drugs as an indication that psychotherapy has failed; and 3) the patient ascribes magical qualities to the medication and to the therapist who has prescribed it. Karasu (1990b) mentions other difficulties, such as the therapist misinterpreting drug side-effects as psychological phenomena or the thera-

pist defensively resorting to drug administration during difficult points in therapy. These problems can be avoided by a reasoned and open discussion of what effects can and cannot be expected from pharmacological action in comparison with the results of exploratory psychotherapy. It is also advisable to institute pharmacotherapy from the outset, if it is indicated at that time, and not to rely on medication later if symptoms have not abated secondary to verbal therapy.

The process of psychoanalytical therapy is inherently laborious, lengthy and, at times, quite threatening to the patient, as unpleasant past or present truths about others and one's self are acknowledged. Therefore, this form of treatment is not applicable to every individual who has experienced depression. The very severely ill who have suffered a psychotic depression may not be able to withstand the dysphoria engendered by the analytical process. Similarly, individuals with bipolar illness, even when maintained on lithium, may be unable to tolerate the intense affects, both positive and negative, that are evoked during therapy. These individuals can still benefit from modified analytical therapy that is more supportive, less exploratory, does not seek to reproduce older relationships in the therapeutic setting and is more concerned with current, everyday problems that face the patient.

Psychoanalytic therapy may be equally inappropriate for the very healthy, not because these individuals cannot tolerate the rigors of this type of treatment but because it may well be unnecessary. All individuals, no matter how psychologically sound, suffer from depression following a significant loss or frustration. This painful reaction is embedded in our genetic response repertoire and is indicative of our ability to care greatly about some individual, personal ideal or individual goal. In fact, Gut (1989) has recently argued that the capacity to bear depression and to learn from this reaction are signs of maturity and psychological health.

An individual with a history of adequate personal functioning who responds appropriately to a major trauma may still be helped by briefer, less exploratory therapy. Quite often, because of their psychic stamina, such individuals go through a devastating reaction to a profound loss in isolation and are treated with medication only. A good deal of their suffering may be avoided by engaging in a therapeutic relationship that allows for a ventilation of affect, the placing of the trauma in context and a sharing of painful affects during the process of natural recovery. A not uncommon finding is that these individuals may make ill-advised decisions while in the grip of a depressive episode that are later regretted and could have been averted by being in a reality-based, therapeutic relationship. Therapy with these healthier individuals aims at easing the pain of depression and at 'holding together' the personality until the individual recovers on his or her own. Psychoanalytical therapy may later be initiated if the individual wishes to learn more about his or her inner world, but this extensive procedure is not particularly indicated for a naturally self-limited adjustment reaction.

Those mood disorders in which psychoanalytic therapy may have its greatest applicability include so called 'characterological' depression. In this condition, the individual's every day mode of thinking, feeling and interacting serves to perpetuate and reinforce a chronic state of depression, although the intensity of this state may vary in correspondence to life events. Individuals who manifest chronic characterological forms of depression do appear to carry into adult life pathological remnants of their childhood upbringing which interfere with contentment or adult modes of satisfaction.

Psychoanalytical therapy is also useful in cases where a precipitant has brought to light a whole system of pathological self-assessment, distortions of others and atavistic beliefs. As will be further discussed below, the actual event that sets off the depressive process gains its power as a precipitant as it reverberates with dreaded archaic fears and memories that were kept out of awareness and were in contrast to relatively mature functioning of the personality. The pathogenic potential of the external event really resides in the meaning ascribed to it by the individual in terms of reawakening older, painful situations from childhood. The degree of the clinical reaction, often prompted by objectively minimal events, is actually commensurate with past rather than current self-appraisals as these are automatically re-experienced by the patient. Similar to individuals with characterological depression, these depressives have developed maladaptive modes of psychological functioning to hide or minimize these painful schemas. The traumatic aspect of the precipitant resides in its ability to strip away these protective devices, leaving the individual face to face with exquisitely painful realizations about himself and significant others in his life.

Psychoanalytical therapy is directed toward these outmoded irrational beliefs that persist in both characterological and episodic forms of depression. Symptoms are generally considered as manifestations of

the living out or sudden awareness of these atavistic cognitive-affective schemas.

COURSE OF THERAPY

An exact description of the process of psychoanalytical therapy for depression (or any other psychiatric condition) is beyond possibility. Each individual is unique, with his or her own particular history, particular current life situation and a particular unpredictable future. The specific strengths and vulnerabilities of individuals vary markedly and are tailored to specific environmental threats. One middle-aged patient, discussed below, was able to withstand repeated spouse abuse, financial reversals and relative estrangement from her children without manifest symptoms, only to become severely depressed when publicly rebuked by her aging mother. Psychoanalytical therapy was not designed specifically for depressive conditions (in fact, it was applied to melancholia rather late in its development) but for any disorder that was thought to be caused, in great measure, by the perpetuation of childhood psychic contents, albeit unconscious, into adult life. Therefore the best opposition that may be offered is a general framework of the therapeutic process dealing with themes, conflicts and developmental deviations that are commonly found in most, but not all, individuals who experience depression of clinical proportions.

For the purposes of presentation, the course of therapy has been divided into three stages, a demarcation which is artificial at best. The three stages as described present the major tasks of therapy which are usually achieved consecutively, although there may be a great deal of overlap, so that when one has worked through one particular problem, new material is presented which reiterates the entire sequence based on a novel theme. Therefore, each stage should be accepted as a step in the overall therapeutic process which can occur during the entire course of therapy.

Depressed individuals seek out treatment after some event in their lives has precipitated an acute episode or after some self-realization that their lives are unsatisfactory. Not uncommonly, the individual is not quite sure of what has caused the depressive decompensation or, even if he or she is able to identify some environmental stressor, cannot see a direct relationship between the alleged precipitant and the ensuing illness. Freud (1917), mentions this lack of certainty in his differentiation between mourning and melancholia, commenting that in the former the role of an external loss is quite evident while in the latter it is not clear what exactly has been lost. More recent empirical studies have confirmed this lack of clarity regarding the role of a precipitant in depression. Leff et al (1970) found that the cause of a clinical episode was not always immediately apparent and the patient could identify the role of a stressor only after some time in exploratory psychotherapy. On the basis of a large empirical study, Brown & Harris (1978) conclude that depression does follow a significant loss but that this loss is of an important idea or ideal rather than simply an environmental deprivation. They cite the case of a woman who became depressed after she learned that her husband had been unfaithful some years earlier. Although nothing material was changed in her life, this new knowledge obviously affected this woman's idea of herself, her husband and her marriage. The depressed patient is not always certain how an external precipitant has brought about an alteration of his or her self appraisals, nor of how a precipitant may have brought to awareness painful experiences of the past, nor of his or her own attempts to suppress these memories.

A middle-aged woman who became profoundly depressed following a staff party illustrates some of these findings. This woman had previously been ill with pneumonia, requiring that she have bed rest for a protracted time. Her mother, who lived some distance from the patient, offered to come and take care of her. This gesture was out of character for the mother, who usually did not help the patient in any way and, indeed, took every opportunity to criticize her. When the mother arrived, it became clear that she had come in order to go shopping and she forced the patient out of bed to drive her to various stores and shops. During one outing the mother essentially let the patient know that she never cared for her and preferred the patient's two brothers. The patient was shaken by her mother's outspoken and vicious hatred toward her and her sense of anger over never being able to measure up to her mother's standards. The upshot of this argument was that the mother returned home earlier than planned and the patient continued her convalescence, during which she attempted to drive the episode of her argument from her thoughts.

Upon her return to work, she learned that her immediate boss, whom she idolized, had been stricken with terminal cancer. It was her sad duty to clear out his office and to answer numerous calls regarding his health. A short time after her return to work, she attended a prearranged seminar to stop smoking. This session lasted most of the day, with the speaker repeating sentences over and over again, an experience which the patient found similar to being hypnotized. The following day the patient attended a farewell lucheon for a staff worker where, after drinking a few glasses of wine, she began crying, and angrily denounced her fellow workers as ungrateful and cruel. She was taken home, where she fell asleep and upon awakening experienced severe dysphoria, exhaustion and inability to concentrate. The dysphoria intensified but, despite her melancholic state, she was unable to cry. She gradually lost her appetite, her prior desire to work or see friends and lapsed into a severe depressive episode.

When this patient presented for therapy she could not understand the reasons for her depression. She acknowledged her sadness over the eventual death of her boss, her feelings of exhaustion from her bout with pneumonia and her anger towards her mother but did not consider any of these unpleasant factors to be responsible for the illness. After some time in therapy, she began to remember the contents of the smoking cessation seminar she had attended. She recalled that the leader kept repeating that if anyone in the audience died, not five people in the world would care. This caused her to think to herself the following sequence: that no one in the world cared for anyone, that no one cared about her boss dying, that her mother did not care about her, that no matter what she did her mother would never love her, that her mother had never loved her, that she had been a loveless child, that she was evil and undeserving of love. She found this last conclusion so mentally painful and physically distressing that she forcibly put it out of her mind and riveted her attention on the seminar leader. Her sense of herself as unlovable and alone continued to intrude into consciousness for the next few hours and it was only with great effort that she was able to suppress this thought. The next day, at the luncheon, she was reminded of what the seminar leader had said when she experienced her co-workers enjoying themselves while her boss was terminally ill. She felt herself to be worthless since she, too, had attended the luncheon. She was overcome with a sense of anger, despair and self-hatred, culminating in her making a scene and having to be taken home.

This woman's depression was prompted by the emergence of a dreaded realization that her mother would never love her because she was an evil, worthless person. Reconstruction of childhood experiences later revealed how this belief was founded on actual occurrences which were disguised or repudiated by the mother and by the patient. The coincidence of events at the time of her pneumonia and subsequent to it proved to her the truth of this painful belief which she then tried to suppress once more. The relevant point for this discussion is how a precipitant may be an idea that events force into consciousness and that calls into question the individual's whole mode of evaluation of the self and others.

Another depressed patient presented with a provisional diagnosis of bipolar disorder or seasonal affective disorder, since her depressions usually occurred in the late autumn after a period of frenzied activity. It turned out that this woman believed that she could only be worthy of her parents' (and later significant others') love if she worked at her maximum capacity, excelling in her career. She would begin the academic year as a teacher with great hopes of surpassing her colleagues and of gaining special recognition, thus proving her worth and the degree of her efforts. As the school year progressed and her expected recognition failed to materialize, she pushed herself and her pupils harder, embarking on special projects or insisting her classes obtain the best test results in the school. When even these efforts did not result in rewards or accomplishments, she began to perceive her work as proof of her innate inferiority and of her inability to obtain the love she so desired. It became harder and harder for her to face her pupils and fellow teachers, upon whom she transferred the strict demands of her parents, until she became so depressed she had to withdraw from teaching for the year.

These examples are presented in order to demonstrate the hidden nature of the precipitant and its close relationship to the patient's self-esteem regulation. One of the first tasks of therapy is to work with the patient to discover what precipitated the depression and how this thought or realization indicates the particular deep vulnerability of each individual. This process begins the search for self-understanding and aids the patient in looking inward to his or her thoughts, dreams, fantasies and distortions which in the past may have been dismissed from consciousness. This active inquiry also serves to allow the patient to feel less helpless, demonstrating that the episode of depression has a meaning and is potentially under one's control. The themes that commonly emerge as the patient identifies his or her particular vulnerability revolve around the desperate need for love and approval from a few significant others that are representative of the powerful parent of the past. Usually, the depressive believes that such love is obtainable by working harder, inhibiting areas of pleasure or slavish devotion to pleasing authority figures.

The revelation of this mode of functioning may be presented in a dream, laying bare the patient's persistent childhood distortions. For example, a depressed woman in the initial stages of therapy reported a dream in which she was happily buying frilly and exotic clothes for herself. In the dream she looked across the store and unexpectedly saw her mother, after which she lost all interest in the clothes and felt guilty for wasting money on such trivial purchases. These dreams serve as stimuli in recalling childhood events that were repressed or rationalized and lead to an understanding of those important factors that shaped the personality.

A process that occurs simultaneously with the search for internal distortions and vulnerabilites is the formation of the therapeutic relationship. Quite often, the depressed patient will unconsciously reinstate with the therapist duplicates of the relationship with a significant adult in childhood. The patient will transfer attitudes, values and expectations from the parent to the therapist and then behave accordingly. In the case of the woman whose dream was reported, she came to sessions in drab clothing, without make-up, and made a point of demonstrating her frugality in her communications, anticipating that the therapist would disapprove of buying attractive clothing just as her mother had done. During the formation of these early transferential distortions, the nature of the therapeutic relationship as a curative, neutral partnership is explicitly stated in order to separate appropriate adult reactions from the inappropriate reliving of childhood experiences.

Jacobson (1971, 1975) has written extensively about the potential dangers of transferential distortions of depressed patients during the early stages of therapy. She describes how patients may focus their whole existence on the therapist, who assumes great stature in their eyes. Such patients may re-enact prior relationships in which they demonstrate obedience and devotion to an esteemed other and then react with hurt and anger when the expected protection and nurture is not returned by the therapist. These transferential reactions are best interpreted immediately, demonstrating to the patient how he or she had formed automatically a dependent mode of being, utilizing others to bestow a sense of worth, esteem or meaning. A therapeutic stance of warmth and encouragement is advocated but it should be clear from the outset that the burden of clinical improvement rests with the patient's ability to work through the inner problems rather than by winning the therapist's love or approval through alleged exemplary behaviour. Kolb (1956) recommends that the therapist of a depressed patient should take pains to be honest and forthright about his own limitations and those of the therapeutic process. This openness helps to develop a true therapeutic alliance and is in corrective contrast to many depressives' prior relationships, which were rife with deceit, secret obligations and manipulation. Ideally, therapy should engender complete honesty without fear of criticism, retaliation or abandonment.

The amelioration of manifest symptoms, the beginning of an inward search for atavistic remnants of childhood interactions which continue as vulnerabilities and distortions and the adjustment of the therapeutic relationship in a mutually helpful but reality-based endeavour roughly comprise the initial stage of therapy. The second stage involves the patient recognizing his or her characterological patterns of interaction, basic beliefs systems and particular defensive operations, and ultimately relinquishing these intrapsychic characteristics for more appropriate adult appraisals of self and others. The accomplishment of these goals represents the major portion of therapy as maladaptive behaviour is examined, traced to its origins, against resistance to remembering and to re-experiencing painful affects associated with these recollections, and, in the light of mature judgment, altered or minimized. Everyday experiences involving stresses, relationships to others and evaluations are analysed for traces of atavistic reactions as are dreams, fantasies and attitudes toward the therapist.

This process may be illustrated by an event reported by a depressed middle-aged businessman who sought therapy for chronic dissatisfaction with his existence and for the continuous unwelcomed intrusion of depression, anxiety or anger into his conscious life. This man reported that the previous day he had received a phone call about a business reversal due to some technical error. Although the mistake could be remedied, he was immediately filled with rage followed by a period of profound depression, remaining aware that both reactions were out of proportion to the situation. In discussing this event in therapy the following day, the patient associated to a recurrent dream he had had since childhood. This dream was that he is infuriated at someone and wants to attack this other person but he cannot move his arms and feels he will be beaten severely, whereupon he awakens in a state of fear and anxiety. As he recounted the dream, he recalled instances in which he had been beaten and berated by his father as a child. While the patient knew he had been abused as a child, he had never allowed himself to remember these past experiences in detail nor with any

accompanying affect. As vivid memories flooded him during the session, he re-experienced the anger and shame at his maltreatment but also, for the first time, recalled that his mother had been present during his punishment. At this recollection, he expressed, with great sadness, that she could not have loved him as she often professed if she allowed him to be beaten. In this manner, the patient was beginning to understand, on the basis of concrete, lived experience, his misinterpreting any obstacle to his ambitions as a re-enactment of the numerous attacks from his father and abandonment by his mother.

Bowlby (1980) has noted three major overriding themes in the history of depressed individuals: 1) the experience of never having attained a safe, satisfying relationship with one's parents despite numerous efforts; 2) the experience of having been told repeatedly how unlovable, inadequate or incompetent one is; or 3) the experience of deprivation following the loss of a parent. For Bowlby, these repetitive childhood situations create irrational belief systems which distort the way that experience is processed in adult life and ultimately result in depression. Arieti & Bemporad (1978) have found similar recollections and transferential re-enactments of childhood in the therapy of depressed patients. They stress the undue parental instilling of dependency in the future depressive, together with punishment by shaming, humiliation and inducing guilt. The depressive appears to grow up desperately needing love and approval from an esteemed (dominant) other and believing that his worth depends on the attainment of such love. The depressive may try to obtain this approval or redemption by hard work, slavish devotion or self-inhibition of gratification, thereby perverting his everyday relationships or behaviour. It is when the individual can no longer tolerate this characterological mode of being or when an event occurs which strips away defensive manoeuvres and confirms an existence devoid of love or worth that depression ensues.

This deviant mode of everyday life, as expressed in maladaptive and atavistic defensive manoeuvres is examined, interpreted, partially re-lived and, hopefully, modified during this stage of therapy. The process of change carries with it inherent discomforts and disillusionments which in turn provide the potential for greater freedom and contentment. The patient realizes that he or she may not have been the favoured child nor the cleverest, most able or most loving, but this realization often lifts the burden of an inauthentic life from the patient's shoulders.

A dream of a depressed woman during this phase of therapy may illustrate the sense of loss and of subsequent relief that typifies the therapeutic process. This woman had always inhibited expression of her true feelings or ideas in order to please the chronically disapproving mother who, despite the patient's best efforts, refused to bestow the praise or love that was so greatly desired. As this relationship was being discussed in therapy, she related a dream in which she was with her family at a formal dinner. In the dream, the patient was careful about what she said and ate and how she behaved in general. She began to experience a headache and stomach cramps, as well as anxiety (as she did in real life), because she was not sure if she had acted properly. After the meal, she was standing outside a building feeling sick and noticed her mother walking away. She cried out to her mother 'Now will you call me?' To this the mother turned to the patient, revealing an angry, critical expression, and answered a resounding 'no' and then resumed her walking away in a mist. The patient recounted that in remembering the dream she felt saddened by the mother's refusal to acknowledge her good behaviour but also that she now understood that, no matter what deprivation she imposed on herself, she would never obtain the approval she sought. At this thought she felt liberated, sensing herself free of the many irrational dictates of her childhood that she continued to carry within herself and which she projected on to others. This understanding, or insight, allowed her to begin to alter her relationship with significant people in her life, to dare to allow herself to pursue interests of which she had formerly been ashamed and to attempt to see herself in a new light without the distortions of the past. The new feeling of autonomy is reinforced in therapy as the patient slowly consolidates realistic modes of self-assessment, avenues of meaning and pleasure, and a lessened reliance on the reactions of others.

The recalling of past traumatic events, together with an appropriate emotional response and a putting of such memories in perspective, are not usually sufficient for a working through of atavistic psychic contents. The manner in which these prior contents continue to affect the individual should also be discovered, even after a bringing to consciousness of relevant memories. An abstract awareness of the past is incomplete and the patient should realize how he or she continues to live out childhood scenarios.

One depressed woman, for example, came to understand how she had always desired her father to value her as a person and to redeem her alleged sins by granting her his true attention and care. In therapy she came to appreciate that her father was a perfunctory parent who wished her to do well and then would send her off on her own. She had always felt that he wanted to get away from her and went through the motions of parenthood without true concern for her. At the end of a particularly revealing session, her therapist complimented her on coming to grips with her need of her father and tracing this need to its origins. Shortly following this session, the patient began experiencing marked anger at her therapist and despair over the possibility of cure. Reporting these feelings in the next session, she found that she had interpreted the therapist's complimentary remarks as his indication that he was now finished with her and that he intended to discontinue therapy. She appreciated that this form of behaviour was actually typical of her father, who would withdraw from her whenever she was not in dire need. She had confused the therapist's encouragement with her father's dismissing her, even though she had just completed discussing the latter in detail. Therefore, recollection and reconstruction do not always lead to transferential changes which continue despite awareness of the past. These are corrected as they occur and are related to significant experiences in the history of the individual.

The last stage of therapy deals with a consolidation of change and the implementation of this change into daily practice. The latter object is not an easy matter, since family, spouses, friends and colleagues have become accustomed to the patient's former mode of behaviour and may resent or discourage the transformations so laboriously achieved in therapy. This attitude is particularly true of spouses who, while not wishing the patient to experience episodes of clinical depression, may automatically reinforce those attitudes and behaviours that culminate in repeated decompensations. When this presents a major problem, the spouse of the patient may be referred for his or her own therapy, or couples therapy may be instituted. However, in most cases, repeated open and free discussions between patient and spouse (or other significant others) suffice to establish a relationship on a new equilibrium.

A second task of the terminal stages of therapy is to deal appropriately with the patient's newly revised perception of his or her past experiences and relationships. All too frequently, there is a progression from defensive idealization of others to disillusionment, ultimately arousing bitter resentment and anger. The pathogenic actions of parents and others were usually the result of their own distortions and limitations. The patient should not dwell on past injustices in order to excuse current inappropriate behaviour but should focus mainly on his own perpetuation of pathogenic attitudes, values and behaviours into adult life.

Manifestations of long-lasting improvement that are observed at the end of therapy revolve around the patient's ability to derive meaning and worth directly from his or her own activities. This fundamental change permeates the individual's manner of relating to others, of estimating his sense of worth and of generating spontaneity and creativity. These alterations are reflected in the therapeutic relationship, which becomes a communal endeavour for mutual knowledge and for sharing rather than a struggle for obtaining desired feedback from an artificially inflated transference figure. This new freedom is generalized from the therapeutic situation to other significant activities and relationships in everyday life.

RELATIONSHIP TO OTHER THERAPIES

Psychoanalytical therapy shares many of the features of cognitive therapy and interpersonal psychotherapy while also demonstrating marked differences in significant areas. As described by Beck and colleagues (1979), cognitive therapy also seeks out the erroneous belief systems that create irrational estimations and distorted perceptions of events and that underlie psychopathologic responses. Interpersonal psychotherapy, as described by Klerman and colleagues (1984) also traces the roots of depression to problems in relationships, social supports and personal effectiveness. However, both cognitive therapy and interpersonal psychotherapy focus on the current situation and do not attempt to trace present problems to childhood events that persist, although their remnants may be outside of awareness. Also, these forms of psychotherapy do not utilize interpretations of transference (or other manifestations of unconscious processes), although both advocate the beneficial effects of a therapeutic relationship. The unifying basis of these therapies with psychoanalytical psychotherapy is the belief that depression results from prior experiences that create vulnerabilities in the ability to tolerate stresses and that depression is treatable through increased self-awareness in the context of a supportive encounter with another human being.

Some other not insignificant differences are that interpersonal psychotherapy and cognitive therapy were developed specifically for the treatment of depression and that their advocates have been able to describe the therapeutic process in manuals that allow for replication, communication and evaluation by other therapists. Preliminary findings have shown that both cognitive and interpersonal forms of therapy are quite effective in the treatment of depression, particularly in the prevention of relapses following an episode of major depressive disorder (Frank et al 1989).

Psychoanalytical therapy of depression does not lend itself easily to large scale, controlled studies of efficacy. Most psychoanalysis practitioners believe that each patient who presents with depression or any other disorder is so unique as to defy generalization. The particular constellation of childhood experience, current life situation and innate abilities varies so greatly between individuals that comparisons would not be valid. The best that could be hoped for would be a loose presentation of basic therapeutic principles as these apply to depressive states. Another difficulty in performing efficacy studies is in regard to the criteria for improvement. The very goals of psychoanalytical therapy, such as freedom from neurotic inhibitions or greater self-contentment, seem difficult to gauge accurately by objective measures or ordinal rating scales. Finally, most psychoanalytical therapists can treat only a handful of patients at a time over the course of years, making the collection of data on a sufficiently large sample of patients usually beyond the experience of any one practitioner.

Despite these theoretical and practical problems, two psychoanalysts have reported on their experience with the psychoanalytical treatment of depressed patients. Arieti (1977) described 12 severely depressed patients (nine females and three males) whom he treated as outpatients. 3 or more years following termination of therapy, Arieti reports that seven showed complete recovery without relapse, four showed great improvement and one had relapsed into depression. Jacobson (1971) describes the post-treatment status of severely depressed patients treated by her over the course of decades, without mentioning sample size or exact post-therapy length of duration at time of follow-up. She found that many of her patients continued to do well for many years after psychoanalytical therapy. Some would again experience episodes of depression of lesser magnitude when faced with environmental stressors. Despite these episodes of dysphoria, Jacobson reports that these former patients manifested great improvement in establishing satisfying relationships and were capable of better parental, social and professional functioning. Some returned for additional therapy at crisis points in their lives, which is described as helpful. According to Jacobson, patients who reported suicidal ideation in childhood and those who experienced severe chronic rather than episodic depression did not respond as well to therapy. These two individual reports are neither sufficiently large nor sufficiently objective but do indicate a long-term effectiveness of psychoanalytical therapy. A larger-scale study, sampling the experience of many psychoanalysis practitioners, as performed in the investigation of other disorders (Bieber 1962), could provide valuable data on the inherent characteristics of psychoanalytical therapy with depressed patients as well as on its efficacy.

REFERENCES

Arieti S 1977 Psychotherapy of severe depression. American Journal of Psychiatry 134: 864–868

Arieti S, Bemporad J R 1978 Severe and mild depression: the psychotherapeutic approach. Basic Books, New York

Beck A T Rush A J Shaw B F Emery G 1979 Cognitive therapy of depression. Guilford Press, New York

Bieber I et al 1962 Homosexuality – a psychoanalytic study. Basic Books, New York

Bowlby J 1980 Loss. Basic Books, New York

Brown G, Harris T 1978 Social origins of depression. Tavistock Press, London

Frank E, Kupfer D J, Perel J M 1989 Early recurrence in unipolar depression. Archives of General Psychiatry 46: 397–400

Freud S 1914 The history of the psychoanalytic movement. Standard Edition, Vol 14 (1957). Hogarth Press, London, p 3–66

Freud S 1917 Mourning and melancholia. Standard Edition, Vol 14 (1957). Hogarth Press, London, p 243–258

Gut E 1989 Productive and unproductive depression. Basic Books, New York

Jacobson E 1971 Depression. International Universities Press, New York

Jacobson E 1975 The psychoanalytic treatment of depressed patients. In: Anthony E J, Benedek T (eds) Depression and human existence, Little, Brown, Boston

Karasu T B 1990a Toward a clinical model of psychotherapy for depression. I Systemic comparison of three psychotherapies. American Journal of Psychiatry 147: 133–147

Karasu T B 1990b Toward a clinical model of psychotherapy for depression. II: An integrative and selective treatment approach. American Journal of Psychiatry 147: 269–278

Klerman G L, Schechter G 1982 Drugs and psychotherapy. In: Paykel E S (ed) Handbook of affective disorders, 1st edn. Guilford Press, New York, p 329–337

Klerman G, Weissman M M, Rounsville B J, Chevron E S 1984 Interpersonal therapy of depression. Basic Books, New York

Kolb L C (1956) Psychotherapeutic evolution and its implications. Psychiatric Quarterly 30: 1–19

Leff M L, Roatch J F, Bunney W 1970 Environmental factors preceding the onset of severe depression. Psychiatry 33: 293–311

Luborsky L 1984 Principles of psychoanalytic psychotherapy. Basic Books, New York

Offenkrantz W, Tobin A 1974 Psychoanalytic psychotherapy. Archives of General Psychiatry 30: 593–606

29. Group therapy

Joan L. Luby   Irvin D. Yalom

Group psychotherapy is a treatment modality in widespread use for affectively disordered patients. A substantial proportion of depressed patients, particularly in the hospital setting, find their way into groups. In this chapter we will address the question of whether groups are therapeutic for these patients, and if so, how? We will examine specific group approaches used for this patient population, their comparative mechanisms and outcomes.

These questions are complicated by definitional problems. First, the term 'affective disorders' is vague and general. What are the contents and boundaries of this category? For the purpose of this chapter, we will narrow our definition to the major mood disturbances, major depressive and bipolar disorder, as well as their milder variants.

'Group psychotherapy' refers to a myriad of treatment approaches that share few common philosophical assumptions. There are, to name only a few, support groups, self-help groups, crisis groups, cognitive behavioural groups, interpersonal groups and analytically-oriented groups. The only common thread among this multitude of forms is the attempt to treat several patients simultaneously. Groups specifically for depressed patients range from behaviourally-based 'courses' with an emphasis on the educative and training aspects of treatment (Lewinsohn et al 1985) to small long-term interpersonal groups in which the analysis of 'here and now' experience is used as the therapeutic template.

In this chapter we will address the use of specific forms of group psychotherapy for the treatment of major depressive and bipolar disorder. Although there are few controlled research studies on group therapy for the affectively disordered patient, the literature contains several clinical accounts of homogeneous groups for depressed and bipolar patients. The treatment of this population in interpersonal therapy groups with mixed psychiatric patients has also been described.

Yalom (1985) has defined a set of therapeutic factors that characterize the healing process in group psychotherapy: 1) instillation of hope; 2) universality; 3) imparting of information; 4) altruism; 5) the corrective recapitulation of the primary family group; 6) development of socializing techniques; 7) imitative behaviour; 8) interpersonal learning; 9) group cohesiveness; 10) catharsis; and 11) existential factors. The role played by each of these factors in a given group depends upon the group's content, purpose and phase of treatment. Some of these factors are entirely specific to a group format while others, although present in individual therapy, operate more powerfully in groups.

Several of these therapeutic factors seem particularly important to the treatment of depressed patients. A few stand out as immediately relevant and activating for the depressed patient initially entering a therapy group. Consider the therapeutic impact of universality, the recognition that one's life experience is similar to that of other people. This knowledge has an early and meaningful impact on depressed patients, who typically enter a group feeling isolated and potentially stigmatized. The awareness that other patients experience similar conflict and despair is liberating, breaking down the entrenched sense of shame and hopelessness that often characterizes their state. Further, patients learn that the vulnerability to depressive illness is widespread. For those who blame themselves for becoming depressed, this insight may promote more realistic explanations about how and why depression occurs.

Altruism, the sense of fulfilment gained from the act of helping others, can be an immediate and powerful experience for the depressed patient entering the group. Because depressed individuals suffer from doubts about their self-worth and competence in the interpersonal realm, they often are reluctant to offer feedback to peers in the group. In fact, depressed patients may fear that their contributions will have a detrimental effect on others. By supporting these patients and encouraging them to reveal their thoughts, the leader can help them rediscover their ability to contribute to the lives of those around them. The conviction that one has something positive to offer others is an important building block in the re-establishment of self-esteem.

Another therapeutic factor, the instillation of hope, is similarly pertinent to depressed patients. Hopelessness is a disabling symptom of depression that can be difficult to approach therapeutically and is often resistant to treatment strategies. In a group setting, a patient has an opportunity to witness the progress of peers and the resultant diminution of their depressive symptoms. This experience emphasizes the plasticity of the depressive state and the fact that recovery is an attainable goal. An important turning point in the treatment of depression may occur with this experience.

Interpersonal learning, another important therapeutic factor for depressed patients, rests on the assumption that human relationships are essential to psychological well-being and fulfilment. An interpersonal emphasis in the group addresses the patient's maladaptive social behaviours. It aims to explore the underlying intrapsychic distortions and false assumptions that operate in an interactive context to cause relationship failures. Although interpersonal learning is the central principle of the interpersonal group approach, it is unavoidably a component of all group treatment modalities. This factor is, of course, also at play in the transference relationship of individual psychotherapy but it is stimulated and facilitated to a greater degree in the social climate of the group.

Virtually every psychiatric disorder affects a patient's interpersonal functioning. The depressive disorders, however, are thought by some to be particularly tied to interpersonal pathology: depressed patients are known to be withdrawn, isolated and avoidant of social contacts. Further, the important interpersonal relationships of these patients are often fraught with distortions and conflict. Bemporad (1977), for example, describes the characteristic need for an idealized, dominant other in the relationships of depressed individuals. The depressive has deeply ambivalent feelings toward this idealized other, a mixture of desperate need and bitter resentment about the dependency. Arieti (1978) has also discussed this key interpersonal component of depressive psychodynamics. He

stresses the importance of the 'dominant other' in the modulation of the depressed patient's self-esteem, '(this) dominant other has . . . provided the patient with the evidence, real or illusory, or at least the hope that acceptance, love, respect, and recognition of his human worth were acknowledged . . .' (Arieti 1978). Any threat to this relationship can precipitate an exacerbation of illness; loss may cause decompensation. Thus these interpersonal dynamics may be intimately connected to the course of the illness and, in some cases, to its origins.

Beck's extensive work on depression (Beck 1967) also touches on the disordered interpersonal experience of depressed patients. He points to the devaluation of intimacy and loss of emotional attachments that occur. Loss of pleasure and satisfaction in pursuing interpersonal relationships seems to follow from weakened attachments and may progress to an apathetic or indifferent attitude toward previous love objects. Paradoxically, the same patients often have heightened and unrealistic dependency needs. These symptoms, along with the depressed patient's characteristic negative expectations and cognitive distortions, profoundly affect his or her interpersonal life.

A group of investigators have developed a form of psychotherapy for depression, based solely on the interpersonal pathology of the disorder (Klerman et al 1984). Interpersonal psychotherapy of depression (IPT) is a short-term psychological treatment focusing on the role of dysfunctional interpersonal relationships in the onset and perpetuation of depression (see chapter 31). A recent collaborative study, sponsored by the National Institutes of Mental Health, compared multiple treatments for depression (Elkin et al 1989). This investigation found that IPT was effective for the reduction of depressive symptoms and perhaps more successful than cognitive therapy. This and other work strongly suggests that this treatment emphasis is efficacious for depressed patients.

Although group therapy seems uniquely suited to address the psychopathology of depression, there are several inherent problems in application. The group therapist encounters formidable difficulty even persuading these patients to enter a therapy group. Consider the fundamental characteristics of depression: pessimism, hopelessness, withdrawal and lack of motivation. With these qualities, the depressed patient is not prone to be self-directed and treatment-seeking and can remain unidentified by mental health professionals. Further, of patients who are seen, another fraction will resist the prescription of group treatment due to an expectation that they will be negatively evaluated and ultimately rejected by a group. If these initial impediments can be overcome, however, the group is the ideal therapeutic arena to address many of the problematic features of depression.

INPATIENT GROUP TREATMENT

Significant attention has been brought to bear on the group treatment of depressed inpatients while relatively little work has addressed the use of groups for patients with bipolar disorder. Inpatient groups are a standard component of the treatment plan of many hospitalized depressed patients. Even though a patient in the throes of a severe neurovegetative depression will not be accessible to interpersonal learning, he or she may profit from other therapeutic factors. The simple immersion of a depressive into a social environment has therapeutic impact: breaking the habitual isolative pattern. The patient grows more aware of the outside world and is, at least temporarily, diverted from ruminative self-preoccupations. In addition, the therapeutic factors of universality and instillation of hope can also be active in the beginning phases of the inpatient group treatment of depression. In general, these benefits warrant the inclusion of even severely ill patients in a group; later, as they improve, they will be able to make use of other therapeutic factors.

The inpatient setting itself presents unique challenges to the group psychotherapist. Many of the problems peculiar to the inpatient unit will affect the functioning of any group in this setting independent of diagnostic composition. A very basic and significant difficulty that the group faces is the challenge of co-existing with other, possibly competing treatment modalities on the unit. The success of the group rests on a strong commitment by group members and this, in turn, requires a milieu that is strongly supportive of group participation. If the group is not fully accepted and valued by the staff, patients will not engage in treatment in a serious way. Milieu support is established through the education of staff about the mechanisms and proven effectiveness of group treatment. Thus it is imperative that therapists work closely with inpatient staff to ensure unified staff support for the group.

The frequent discharges that are characteristic of current inpatient units pose another challenge to the group process. Groups are subjected to rapidly changing membership and must tolerate repeated additions and losses. This is a difficult situation for most patients but the depressive is particularly vulnerable. The adaptation to new members and, more significantly, the loss of existing relationships will be stressful for depressed patients. The experience may re-enact previous traumatic losses, heightening the affective responses from these patients. Although this can be a disturbing rather than soothing process, it stimulates important material for therapeutic work. The focus on processing actual group events in combination with reality testing from peers helps the patient to identify internally driven distortions in his or her current emotional reactions. The group format provides the patient with the opportunity to re-experience painful emotions of loss in a supportive therapeutic environment.

One might expect this rapid patient turnover to pose an obstacle to the development of the necessary degree of cohesion among inpatient group members. Cohesion is a therapeutic factor that has been repeatedly associated with positive treatment outcome (Bednar & Lawlis 1971). Maxmen (1973) has shown however, that members of a diagnostically mixed inpatient group experiencing such rapid turnover still rate cohesion as a highly valued therapeutic component. Although group composition may change daily, the fact that inpatients live together in a specialized treatment milieu may be ample compensation. As Betcher (1983) points out, extra group contacts on the unit occur in such an intense and personal context that they serve as a catalyst to relationship development. Thus, despite the fleeting nature of these relationships, the level of intimacy achieved may be profound.

Another challenge for the leaders of inpatient groups is that the severity of psychopathology in hospitalized patients is likely to be high. Depressed patients, in particular, may be some of the most despairing and hopeless group members. Their tendency towards rumination and negative self-absorption pose obvious impediments to participation in and acceptance by the group. The initial goal with these patients is to help them gain insight into the way in which their interactive style perpetuates the loneliness and isolation that they feel. Patients can be encouraged to examine how their behaviour alienates and repels those around them. They can learn from group feedback, for example, that ruminative preoccupation is interpreted by peers as a lack of interest. In this way, the interactive pathology of depression is identified and mobilized in group psychotherapy.

The inpatient therapist must take a very directive role, because of the severity of members' interpersonal impairment. Thus the therapist must actively facilitate and support patient participation and interaction. Group leaders must be attuned to the existing ego strengths of different members and encourage their application to group process. A severely depressed patient, for example, despite outward withdrawal and apathy, may have the capacity for important insights and empathetic listening in the group. Contributions of this nature may require delicate prompting by the leader but once elicited are often far more valuable than those offered by the therapist. The objective of the group therapist, more challenging in the inpatient setting, is to facilitate the members' ability to initiate and ultimately play a part in directing the group process.

Similarly, the creation of an atmosphere of mutual support and acceptance has been shown to be of partic- ular value in outcome studies of group therapy (Cabral et al 1975). Such an environment cannot be fostered when patients remain withdrawn or apathetic. Active participation must then be encouraged both for the unique value of its content and for the more subtle ways in which it becomes the framework for trust and accep- tance in the group. The therapeutic effectiveness of a group depends on actively contributing members who can learn both to process psychological material and to express support of and interest in peers. The creation and maintenence of this specialized environment, with severely impaired patients in a short time-frame, is the major challenge of the inpatient therapist.

Not uncommonly, group leaders will be frustrated with the slow progress of the inpatient group in general and particularly its depressed members. Group leaders can become overwhelmed by the excessive needs, demands and immobility of these patients, especially in the time-limited treatment setting, and themselves experience demoralization and hopelessness. There are several important measures that therapists can take, however, to enhance patients' motivation and progress and accordingly prevent their own discouragement. Appropriate goal setting is fundamental to the mainte- nance of patients' desire and commitment to work in the group. Goals beyond the capacity of the patient can be overwhelming and serve only to reinforce negative self-evaluations. Accordingly, assistance in setting more reasonable goals and acknowlegement of these smaller but progressive steps will aid in maintaining a patient's morale. This in turn can contribute to group morale and group integrity in general. For group leaders as well, this method provides markers of recovery in what may, at times, feel like a sea of pathology.

The 'agenda group', as described by Yalom (1983), provides a useful framework for circumventing some of the unique difficulties of inpatient groups. An agenda is required of each member at the outset of the daily group. This agenda is a short-term interactive treat- ment goal that is chosen by the patient: it is timely, circumscribed and thus realizable, affectively significant and pertinent to current group dynamics. The agenda is ideally based on the wish to change an interactive problem that is recognized by the patient and manifested in the group. Group leaders often assist in the formulation of an appropriate agenda, but the idea should arise out of a grain of motivation and self- awareness in the patient. This kind of agenda secures the patient's investment in and responsibility for treat- ment and change. It is a tool used to focus on a treat- ment objective that is achievable within the limited time period of a single group session.

The agenda is of particular relevance to depressed patients who require tangible goals to enter meaning- fully and participate in a group. Typically, they are not proactive patients and have trouble with social initiative secondary to a poor self-concept and ruminative pre- occupation. Slife et al (1989) suggest further that depressed patients have diminished cognitive processing abilities which may interfere with their spontaneous group participation. The agenda is a contract between the group and patient which encour- ages the depressed patient's active group involvement and earnest pursuit of a meaningful treatment goal. For example, a female depressed patient who is often cold and sharp in interactions with men finds herself unable to form desired relationships in this area. An appro- priate agenda for this patient might be to become aware of the impact of her approach on the men in the group. This could be achieved by her requesting that male patients give her direct feedback if they experience her as distant and off-putting. The stated agenda encour- ages the patient to seek and to consider valuable (although at times negative) feedback from others. Therapists and peers can refer to an agenda to remind a patient of his/her originally stated goals when behaviours, perhaps unconscious, seem to contradict these intentions. Patients can act to avoid facing their problems at times, despite a desire on another level to deal with them. The agenda also serves as a guide in pursuing a manageable treatment goal within a single group session. This is crucial in the inpatient setting where the length of an individual's involvement in the group is unclear at the outset and, unfortunately, often short.

OUTPATIENT GROUP TREATMENT

Cognitive group therapy

A widely used approach to the outpatient group treatment of depression is modelled on Beck's cognitive theory of depression. This theory is based on the notion that depression arises out of a series of negative self-image distortions that become self-perpetuating. In effect, the patient develops a negative self-concept and pessimistic world view based on past experiences. The disease evolves and escalates by a process of habitual negative misinterpretations of new life situations (see chapter 31). Effective therapy must interrupt the process of cognitive distortion and modify maladaptive belief systems. Beck's theory is easily adapted to a diagnostically homogeneous group format. Cognitive distortions are readily identified in groups, standing out because of their lack of external verification by others. For example, a patient who inaccurately experiences another as rejecting and aloof will find that his or her perceptions are not borne out by observers. In this way, dysfunctional beliefs and misperceptions are made more accessible to treatment. Further, the social dynamics of a group will stimulate a depressed patient's underlying negative self-comparisons and bring core esteem issues to the fore. The homogeneous quality of the group allows these common themes to be the central focus and principal group agenda.

The cognitive group approach lends itself easily to systematic study. Treatment goals are specific and symptom-based and protocols are replicable. Several outcome studies suggest that cognitive groups are superior to placebo or behavioural group formats. Shaw (1977) compared a cognitive group format (based on Beck's model) with the behavioural group approach as described by Lewinsohn and a waiting-list placebo group in a population of depressed college students. He found the cognitive group to be most effective in alleviating depressive symptoms, with the behavioural group superior to placebo. Further support for cognitive group treatment is offered by Gioe (1975). Investigating a population of depressed student volunteers, he reported that cognitive modification in combination with a positive group experience was more efficacious than either treatment alone or a waiting-list control condition. Studies that have attempted to compare psychodynamic and cognitive group approaches are problematic, because of the greater difficulty in assessing psychodynamic techniques and goals. These studies will be elaborated on in a later section.

Covi and Roth have examined cognitive groups composed of a homogeneous population of depressed patients in both open-ended (Roth & Covi 1984) and closed-ended (Covi et al 1982) formats. They believe that a homogeneous composition is therapeutically efficient as it allows the leader to draw on a repertoire of cognitive-behavioural strategies applicable to common psychopathology. In early group meetings, the focus is on behavioural directives to address basic problems of passivity and the inability of function. Covi et al (1982) explain that 'while these and other behavioural techniques directly provide a degree of symptomatic relief, they are also used as a springboard for cognitive change'. That is, the experience of increased competence in life activities can be used to begin to refute a patient's feelings of uselessness.

Roth & Covi (1984) point out that this approach utilizes interactive group techniques and the group process to facilitate cognitive treatment goals. A basic example is the importance of group feedback. Reality testing and, more specifically, the checking of one's self-perceptions and interpretations against the observations of a peer group is a primary step in the interruption of the depressive cognitive construct. Further, we know that the group, by its social and interactive nature, will cause a patient's underlying negative self-comparisons to surface and be available for therapeutic change. Altruism, in addition to its therapeutic function discussed earlier, might have another benefit in a cognitive group. Beyond the increase in self-esteem that is gained by making useful contributions to others, the depressed patient's role in correcting the cognitive distortions of a peer may facilitate the undoing of his own negative misperceptions. 'Thus, the members of the group reality-test assumptions, and in so doing, increase their skills in correcting their own maladaptive reactions' (Hollon & Shaw 1979).

The closed-ended group, the most common cognitive group design for depressed patients, requires that all members begin and end a time-limited, short-term group simultaneously. The treatment duration is fixed and equal for all members; therefore the departure or initiation of patients to the group is not an issue during the course of therapy. The format of such a group, as described by Covi, is highly structured, with therapists playing an active and directive role. In an effort to conserve group time, patients formulate personal agendas in individual meetings prior to the start of the group. The therapists attempt to address these agendas but this may be limited by the need to engage in prescribed therapeutic exercises and review homework assignments. During the course of the group, progress is systematically marked by the weekly reporting of Beck Depression Inventory scores. During each session, the therapists aim to distribute the time equally between patients in an effort to reach everyone within the brief treatment period.

Covi et al (1982) describe three important phases to the closed-ended cognitive group. The first is an educative one in which the theory and rationale of cognitive-behavioural therapy is explained and practised. 'Graded task assignments' are used in an effort to help patients recognize negative self-conceptualizations in daily life and modify behaviour accordingly. Therapeutic tasks are carried out in a formal way, usually with the use of specific written assignments. During the second phase, tools learned in the first phase are implemented within the interactive group context. Here one's negative self perceptions are checked against those of group peers. The third phase centres on an examination of termination issues and reframing of the concept of cure. The primary goal is to encourage acceptance of the idea that future treatment needs do not imply failure. Therapists emphasize the fact that recovery from depression may be a lifelong process likely to require periodic return to some form of treatment.

In summary, the cognitive group psychotherapy of depression has clearly delineated treatment methods and objectives. It offers a short-term, cost-effective treatment alternative to patients suffering from this disorder. Unlike psychodynamic, or more specifically interactive group approaches, it has an advantage of being readily testable in the experimental setting and several studies have supported its use for symptom reduction in major depressive disorders.

Interactional group treatment

In contrast to cognitive therapy groups, interactional group therapy for depression functions most effectively with a diagnostically heterogeneous composition (e.g. including one or two depressed individuals in a group of patients with a variety of other diagnoses). The need for heterogeneity stems from the fact that a group of depressed patients in a loosely structured setting is at risk for disabling inertia, a failure of spontaneous social interaction and the possible escalation of symptoms. A critical mass of interactive ability is necessary to overcome these pitfalls. Further, a diversity of perspectives and defensive styles is an essential ingredient in the open structure of this treatment method.

The interactive group is, by design, a relatively unstructured setting. Unlike the prescribed exercises used to facilitate cognitive groups, an open format is essential to facilitate the therapeutic process of the interactive group. The lack of an externally imposed structure allows the group to develop freely into a social microcosm. Over time, the members will constitute a unique social system encompassing complex relationships involving power, alliance, intimacy and animosity. Interactions in the group will tend to recapitulate external relationship patterns. The surfacing of these important patterns within the supportive and protected environment of the group enables the psychological growth of the patient.

As the social microcosm develops, the interactive group therapist seeks to foster and maintain a 'here and now' emphasis by focusing on intra-group dynamics and de-emphasizing historical or genetic material. Working in the 'here and now' enhances the experiential potency of the group through a utilization of material immediately at hand. A vital loop of experience and processing of experience within the group is established, creating the therapeutic matrix of the interactive technique. Maladaptive behaviours displayed within the group are interpreted as re-enactments of psychopathology in patients' outside relationships. Developing insight into these extra-group connections is stressed but only as an adjunct to the experiential treatment objectives.

Systematic studies of interactive and, in general, psychodynamic groups for depression are scarce and problematic. These types of group are less amenable to study than cognitive groups, for example, due to difficulties in the control and replication of the therapeutic techniques. Further, statistically meaningful results on outcome measures would require an examination of an enormous number of groups, a requirement beyond the capacity of most centres. A few studies have looked at the question of efficacy in depression specifically and report little or none when psychodynamic group therapy is applied to homogeneous depressed samples. Covi et al (1974) find it no more effective than biweekly brief supportive contact in chronically depressed neurotic women. Steuer et al (1984), in a study of elderly depressed patients, report that psychodynamic groups are inferior to cognitive—behavioural groups when comparing Beck Depression Inventory scores, but equal by several other measures. The use of the BDI in this investigation may bias the comparison of these two treatment forms, as it is specifically designed to assess those symptoms that the cognitive — behavioural approach emphasizes.

Further, the study looked at only four groups in total, limiting interpretation of the results.

Although there are certain common behavioural features of major depression, the expression of depressive symptoms will be determined by a patient's underlying individual character traits. Accordingly, the interpersonal styles of depressed patients depend largely on these more subtle and specific elements. A depressed patient's behaviour in groups will then be a function of a more complex equation. Bearing in mind important individual variations, there are, however, commonalities to the interpersonal habits of this population upon which specific therapeutic manoeuvres can be based.

The clinical symptoms of depression are often associated with an underlying experience of impoverishment. Social withdrawal and inertia, for example, can be maladaptive responses to internal emptiness. The socially isolated depressed patient who enters the therapy group often does so with significant reservations. This fearful attitude may become a self-fulfilling prophecy as patients consciously or unconsciously act in such a way as to bring about the rejection or lack of support they had feared. Rage may also be an overt or covert characteristic of depressed patients that significantly impairs their interactive success. The rageful depressed patient repels others but is typically perplexed as to why this occurs.

A depressed patient, even if motivated to be interpersonally connected, will usually become the quiet, neglected member of the group. Given the mixed composition, the more socially comfortable and extroverted members will tend to dominate. The depressive will passively allow the agendas of these members to supersede his or her own, thereby missing important therapeutic opportunities. In the group, this pattern should be identified and addressed. These patients may have some underlying awareness of, and dissatisfaction with, the deprivation they impose upon themselves. The therapist can focus on even subtle indications that this behaviour pattern is ego-dystonic as a way to motivate change. It is also important for group leaders to oppose depressed patients' passivity actively by drawing them in whenever possible.

In a 16-week outpatient group, a young woman suffering from a major depression avoided interpersonal exploration and change, despite the leaders' concerted efforts. She was a highly intelligent and professionally successful person whose depression was precipitated by a break-up with a boyfriend months prior to entering the group. Although she offered useful feedback to other group members, she kept her own intrapsychic conflicts well concealed.

To further complicate this situation, the patient quickly made a strong alliance with a forceful and attractive female member. This behaviour appeared consistent with the depressive's characteristic pursuit of the dominant, idealized other described by Arieti (1978) and Bemporad (1977). The patient participated when an issue involved this chosen 'partner' and she became her ally in all interpersonal conflicts. This was done at the expense of her own stated goals, and perhaps as a means of avoiding them. Additionally, the behaviour prevented her from establishing an independent identity within the group. As Arieti predicts, the 'dominant other' played the vital role of verifying the esteem and well-being of this depressed patient. Thus this patient was driven to protect and please her partner, even at great personal expense.

The pair became an accepted alliance, serving the depressed patient's dependency and her partner's grandiosity. As the group developed, the pair gained insight into the dynamics of their relationship. Peers also began to question and challenge the alliance. The depressed patient's commitment to the compromise was so powerful that she chose to defend and maintain it even in the face of her partner's willingness to give it up. Although our depressed woman was not yet able to change, she became aware of her problem and its maladaptive social solution. In the open structure of this group, the complex interactive pathology was manifest in a clear and workable way.

Depressed patients in interactive groups often thwart interpersonal engagement either with passivity or by alienating and repelling approaches. In these cases, the leader can encourage peer feedback in an attempt to heighten a patient's awareness of his or her social image. For patients with limited social contacts, this is likely to be a new and enlightening opportunity. A dysphoric, isolated patient, for example, was highly desirous of social engagement. Though he participated diligently in the group, he expressed himself in an overly detailed and monotonous fashion without sensitivity to listeners' responses. During the course of therapy, he learned that his interpersonal style bored and distanced group peers. Gradually, after many sessions and ample feedback, he came to understand his own active role in his social isolation.

Although examples of the interactive group treatment of major depression can be given, there is no formulaic approach. Individual differences in interactive pathology defy the use of a standardized method. Bear in mind that one does not treat depression itself in these groups, but its individual interpersonal manifestations. Further, these manifestations, rather than being mere concomitants of depression, may be vital to the inception and maintenance of the illness. The treatment of depression, from this perspective, intervenes in an individual's interpersonal world rather than in the symptom state.

The issue of medication will invariably come up in the group treatment of depressed patients. Those patients requiring medication as an adjunct to psychotherapy may request that physician group therapists administer this treatment. For several reasons, medication monitoring should be sought outside the group. First, the mental status examination necessary for psychopharmacological assessment and maintenance cannot be obtained during typical group sessions unless it is a specific goal of the group as a whole. Barring this, extra-group contacts between the therapist and patient would be required to perform the task competently. Extra-group contacts with selected patients will have a detrimental effect on group transference dynamics by introducing the appearance of favouritism. It is important to preserve the tangible equality of the treatment relationship for all group members. Additional issues arise simply from the act of giving medication: depressed patients who receive medication may tend to define their disease as primarily biochemical, taking less responsibility for the interpersonal elements of the illness. The task of encouraging a patient's awareness of the interpersonal components of his or her depression can be accomplished with greater ease when the group therapist is operationally removed from that biochemical definition.

GROUP TREATMENT FOR BIPOLAR DISORDER

The notion that bipolar patients are not suitable group candidates has become a well-accepted belief among group therapists. Yalom (1975) has previously stated that the inclusion of a patient who became manic in a heterogeneous outpatient group is 'one of the worst calamities that can befall a therapy group'. A manic or hypomanic episode is a highly disruptive and energy-depleting event in the group as the pressured and uncontrolled manic patient will be unable to adhere to basic group norms, thus impeding productive group process.

It is a widely accepted belief that bipolar patients are poor psychotherapeutic candidates in general, due to the difficult defensive styles that characterize this patient population. While bipolar disorder has strong biological correlates, psychoanalytical investigators (Cohen et al 1954, Fromm-Reichmann 1949 Jacobson 1956) have also observed characteristic personality traits: superficiality, narcissism, a strong tendency toward conformity and underlying fears of intimacy. These qualities pose obvious impediments to adequate group participation and predict that bipolar patients would be poorly integrated members of heterogeneous therapy groups. In addition, the bipolar's tendency to display behaviours that inhibit and alienate peers during exacerbations of the illness can result in social failure in the interpersonally challenging environment of the therapy group. Following this rationale, bipolar patients are rarely treated in group psychotherapy, narrowing treatment options down to support and medication.

Several investigators have explored alternative group approaches for the treatment of this population. Davenport et al (1977) have investigated the use of a couples group for married bipolar patients following discharge from the hospital. 12 patients receiving couples group therapy in conjunction with lithium were compared with 11 others undergoing medication maintenance alone and 42 receiving lithium in community aftercare centres. Those 12 receiving conjoint group therapy had significantly superior post-hospital courses as measured by lower rates of rehospitalization and marital failure. This study suggests that couples groups may be well suited to the ongoing needs of the married bipolar patient. The authors speculate that 'spouse involvement counteracts efforts to distort, deny, and flee' on the part of the patient (Davenport et al 1977). The homogeneous couples format is also well suited to address the family and genetic issues that are an important part of the treatment of this disorder.

The bipolar's characteristic conformity and conventionality are traits that can lend themselves to the success of a homogeneous group structure. Patients with these qualities will tend to bolster and adhere to group norms. If all members share them, the effect will be amplified. This will, in turn, facilitate cohesion and the commitment of members to the group. In the couples group for example, the authors report, 'we have been impressed that these couples remain in treatment and rarely miss a group meeting' (Davenport et al, 1977).

The couples format can positively influence medication compliance by directly involving partners in the job of medication maintenance. Homogeneous groups of individual bipolar patients can also address medication issues and effectively break through the denial that contributes to non-compliance (Shakir et al 1979). These preliminary studies suggest that groups may be a viable treatment for the prevention of relapse in bipolar disorder. These studies do not, however, address the question of whether interpersonal psychotherapy goals can be achieved with bipolar patients.

Volkmar et al (1981) reported on the results of a long-term, open-ended outpatient therapy group of bipolar patients where medication management was initially a primary goal. The group was based on an interpersonal 'here and now' format in which expression of affect and the processing of interpersonal pathology enacted within the group was emphasized. The leaders reported a slow start with initial erratic attendance, stabilizing after ten sessions. They found that the introduction of new members was particularly stressful, with the 'initial period of wariness more prolonged than that typically associated with a new member's joining' (Volkmar et al 1981). Once these resistances were overcome however, cohesion was strong and perhaps even fostered by the common involvement with lithium. The group was preoccupied in early sessions by a discussion of lithium and its difficulties. Gradually, however, patients shifted the focus to interpersonal problems: marital conflicts, family conflicts and the impact of the illness on relationships.

The experience of Volkmar et al raises the possibility that the characterological features of bipolar patients are treatable in a homogeneous long-term group setting, once cohesion is established and basic diagnostic and medication questions have been addressed. Stresses in the group, such as relapse or regression of group members, might predictably cause a reversion back to the medication focus. A shifting between these levels seems a reasonable group adaptation. These authors suggest that the homogeneous character of the group may have been a critical component of its success. The group was less disrupted by hypomanic or depressive episodes, perhaps because they were familiar events to all patients.

The observations of Volkmar et al have been corroborated by other authors. More ambitiously, Wulsin et al (1988) set out to form a therapy group composed of bipolar patients where interpersonal issues were the central theme and medications were prescribed by outside practitioners. This group contained patients with severe and long-standing disease for whom hospitalization was not an uncommon occurrence. The authors describe problems with attendance, tardiness and a relatively high drop-out rate (55%). Intense affect and conflict at times escalated to the point of discomfort; 'heightened affect, so inherent in the illness, proved the most consistent obstacle to negotiating conflict, even among euthymic patients' (Wulsin et al 1988).

Wulsin et al report that these obstacles were surmounted and ultimately the group evolved into a hard-working one in which members discussed several important issues: the difficulty in initiating and maintaining relationships, coping with multiple losses and the appropriate and safe expression of anger. Some information about the illness and its effects were addressed in the group, although this was minimized by establishing a separate forum for these questions. Wulsin et al offer a compelling account of a long-term psychotherapy group for bipolar patients. These experiences lend hope to the idea that a homogeneous group focusing on interpersonal issues can be successful for this population.

SUICIDALITY IN GROUP THERAPY

In working with affectively disturbed patients, suicidality will invariably surface, presenting a challenging issue for a therapy group. The suicidal patient absorbs significant amounts of energy from the group and requires that attention be shifted from other ongoing issues. When ideation or gestures occur, anxiety is aroused in group leaders and members alike. Peers may feel compelled to come to the aid of the distressed patient, in spite of being overwhelmed by this task and distracted from their own therapeutic issues. When not appropriately addressed, suicidality will be a prohibitive stress for the group. For this reason, many therapists may unnecessarily exclude suicidal patients from group treatment.

When an acute suicide risk or threat does arise during an ongoing group, it can be processed in a way that is meaningful for the group as a whole. The suicidal patient's problem must take precedence but, despite its obvious urgency, members may harbour feelings of resentment about the shift in focus. It is important, therefore, to go back and explore these feelings once the crisis is resolved. A determination of the seriousness of the risk by the leaders is, however, the first order of business and may warrant individual sessions with one or both of the therapists. If hospitalization is not indicated but additional measures are required, group members can be recruited to participate in a temporary support network of frequent extra-group checks with the patient in crisis. This can serve not only to aid a suicidal patient through difficult times, but also to increase dramatically the sense of cohesion and trust in the group.

The crisis can stimulate a myriad of important interpersonal issues that should be addressed once the immediate dangers are settled. For the non-suicidal group members, feelings of helplessness or betrayal may arise. Group members will be shocked by the intensity of a peer's distress if it was not previously evident. Reactions range from a loss of faith in group treatment to personal guilt about their inability to provide adequate support to the patient. Additionally, suicidal ideation may be interpreted by more intimate peers as a disavowal of the importance of the relationship; it is seen as a betrayal of commitment.

Other practitioners have specifically treated suicidality by forming a homogeneous group of suicidal patients. Such groups may offer advantages to suicidally preoccupied patients unavailable in heterogeneous groups. Frederick & Farberow (1970), in a widely cited paper, discuss this issue and elaborate on the unique focus and format of the suicidality group. These authors alter fundamental aspects of the group framework. For example, they encourage supportive extra-group contacts between members in contrast to the standard position taken by most heterogeneous group leaders. Additionally, fixed time limitations do not apply; the termination date of the group will be flexible depending upon the needs of the members. Other authors go further to suggest that regular attendance should not be a requirement of this type of group (Asimos 1979). The commitment to weekly group meetings is entirely voluntary. Patients are presented with the concept that they are 'welcome to attend'. The objective is to make the group a non-judgmental, open environment that is available, safe and appealing to the suicidal patient (Billings et al 1974).

The leaders of suicidality groups describe rapid cohesion and a marked absence of resistance: 'The person is exposed by the flagrancy of his symptom from the moment he enters such a group. The pathology of a suicide attempter... cannot be easily hidden by defensive measures' (Frederick & Farberow 1970). The authors conclude that patients in these circumstances have such exposed psychopathology that resistance is not an obstacle in the treatment process. Another important advantage to this format is that the suicidal act loses much of its interpersonal power in these settings. 'The experience is openly discussed and seen not as unique but as an area of common experience' (Asimos & Rosen 1978). Further, suicidal patients are expected to play an active, supportive role in steering peers away from suicidal solutions. This is therapeutic for both the patient in crisis and group members offering help.

The course and direction of this type of group is largely dependent upon whether patients are immersed in or past the acute crisis. Obviously, a strongly supportive and practical approach is taken during times of crisis. These episodes may demand the input of outside sources such as individual therapists, friends or family; involvement and availability of external resources is an important component of the crisis management. After the suicidal crisis resolves, more self-reflective and probing work will be encouraged. Some group therapists suggest that the short-term suicidality group should be used for patients in acute crisis and that long-term groups are indicated for stabilized patients wishing to pursue a more insight-oriented path (Comstock & McDermott 1975).

Frederick & Farberow (1970) describe a decrease in the intensity of therapist – patient transference as another appealing element of the homogeneous group for suicidal patients. They regard this as an advantage in the treatment process in that it 'reduces the projection of blame by widening the base of the transference phenomenon' (Frederick & Farberow 1970). The group situation, by its very nature, diffuses the intensity of the patient's expressed feelings toward the therapist. A patient's affects are shared and absorbed by the group as a whole rather than by the therapist alone. In this way, the group format is well suited to cope with the intense and difficult emotions, sometimes overwhelming to the individual therapist, that occur in suicidal patients.

Moving beyond suicidal ideation, what is the impact of a completed suicide on a therapy group? This is experienced as a trauma of no small magnitude to the group and its leaders, stimulating powerful and painful issues. There are few case reports in the literature depicting the impact of a suicide on a therapy group and clinical experience with the phenomenon may be sparse. Kibel (1973) shares his account of a patient's suicide during an ongoing group and its effect on group process and content. He describes several stages that the group collectively moved through in reaction to the trauma. Initially the response was one of shock and sadness; this was rapidly followed by attempts to deny the loss by diminishing the importance of the deceased patient to the group. Regression was evident: members showed increased dependence upon the leader and reverted back to previous problematic behaviours. Some members withdrew emotionally from the group and a few dropped out.

As the slow process of working through the trauma continued, Kibel observed that some members reacted with guilt that the group had been unable to detect the patient's level of distress. Underlying anger and blame of the therapist also surfaced. It is notable that several patients were highly motivated toward intrapsychic change after this event. They accepted confrontation with increased openness and seemed to have a new found fervour to participate in therapeutic work.

Group therapists who have lost a member through suicide experience many complex and painful emotions. Kibel (1973) writes, 'typically there is a tremendous loss of self-esteem. The suicide is seen as both a personal failure and a sign of professional inadequacy'. The therapist wonders, had he done enough? Kibel (1973) reminds us that compounding this burden, 'the therapist must cope with his own embarrassment in front of the other patients while at the same time engaging in the formidable task of trying to mitigate their reactions to the suicide'. The therapist

must cope with his own counter-transference reactions and his genuine despair and sorrow over the event and distinguish these feelings from the group's projections and distortions about his role or responsibility. Although this kind of trauma is a relatively rare event, the group therapist who undertakes the treatment of depressed and suicidal individuals must be prepared to deal with it.

Obviously, the use of a cotherapist is invaluable in such difficult circumstances. The task of supporting and comforting frightened or guilty patients and keeping the group essentially intact through the crisis period is a substantial one. Maintaining group norms of open and honest disclosure while respecting the privacy of the deceased patient is also a challenge. The cotherapy model is useful in this process as leaders will be struggling with their own strong reactions and may be compromised. Co-leaders not only share this burden but, more importantly, provide each other with an objective perspective when processing the powerful transference that arises in these circumstances. Sharing leadership responsibility will help to maintain perspective and to steer the course in a therapeutically effective way.

REFERENCES

Arieti S 1978 On schizophrenia, phobias, depression, psychotherapy, and the farther shores of psychiatry. Brunner/Mazel, New York

Asimos C T 1979 Dynamic problem-solving in a group for suicidal persons. International Journal of Group Psychotherapy 29: 109–114

Asimos C T, Rosen D H 1978 Group treatment of suicidal and depressed persons: indications for an open-ended group therapy program. Bulletin of the Menninger Clinic 42: 517

Beck A T 1967 Depression: causes and treatment. University of Pennsylvania Press, Philadelphia

Bednar R L, Lawlis G F 1971 Empirical research in group psychotherapy. In: Bergin A E, Garfield S L (eds) Handbook of psychotherapy and behaviour change: an empirical analysis. John Wiley, New York, p 822–823

Bemporad J R 1977 Resistances encountered in the psychotherapy of depressed individuals. American Journal of Psychoanalysis 37: 207–214

Betcher R W 1983 The treatment of depression in brief inpatient group psychotherapy. International Journal of Group Psychotherapy 33: 365–385

Billings J H, Rosen D H, Asimos C, Motto J A 1974 Observations on long term group therapy with suicidal and depressed persons. Life Threatening Behaviour 4: 160–170

Cabral R J, Best J, Paton A 1975 Patients' and observers' assessments of process and outcome in group therapy: a follow-up study. American Journal of Psychiatry 132: 1052–1054

Cohen M, Baker G, Cohen R, Fromm-Reichmann F, Weigert E 1954 An intensive study of twelve cases of manic-depressive psychosis. Psychiatry 7: 103–137

Comstock B S, McDermott M 1975 Group therapy for patients who attempt suicide. International Journal of Group Psychotherapy 25: 44–49

Covi L, Lipman F S, Derogatis L R, Smith III J E, Pattison J H 1974 Drugs and group psychotherapy in neurotic depression. American Journal of Psychiatry 131: 191–198

Covi L, Roth D, Lipman R S 1982 Cognitive group psychotherapy of depression: the close-ended group. American Journal of Psychotherapy 36: 459–460

Davenport Y B, Ebert M H, Adland M L, Goodwin F K 1977 Couples group therapy as an adjunct to lithium maintenance of the manic patient. American Journal of Orthopsychiatry 47: 495–502

Elkin I, Shea T, Watkins J T et al 1989 National Institute of Mental Health treatment of depression collaborative research program. Archives of General Psychiatry 46: 971–982

Frederick C J, Farberow N L 1970 Group psychotherapy with suicidal persons: a comparison with standard group methods. International Journal of Social Psychiatry Spring: 103–111

Fromm-Reichmann F 1949 Intensive psychotherapy of manic-depressives. Confinia Neurologica 9: 158–165

Gioe V J 1975 Cognitive modification and positive group experience as a treatment for depression. Doctoral Dissertation, Temple University. Dissertation Abstracts

International 36: 3039B–3040B (University Microfilms 75–28, 219)

Hollon S T, Shaw B F 1979 Group cognitive therapy for depressed patients. In: Beck A T, Rush A J, Shaw B F, Emery G (eds) Cognitive therapy of depression. Guilford Press, New York, p 335

Jacobson E 1956 Manic-depressive partners. In: Eisenstein V (ed) Neurotic interaction in marriage. Basic Books, New York

Kibel H D 1973 A group member's suicide: treating collective trauma. International Journal of Group Psychotherapy 23: 42–53

Klerman G L, Weissman M M, Rounsaville B J, Chevron E S 1984 Interpersonal Psychotherapy of Depression. Basic Books, New York

Lewinsohn P M, Steinmetz Breckenridge J, Antonuccio D O, Teri L 1985 A behavioural group therapy approach to the treatment of depression. In: Upper D, Ross S (eds) Handbook of behavioural group therapy. Plenum Press, New York, p 311–325

Maxmen J S 1973 Group therapy as viewed by hospitalized patients. Archives of General Psychiatry 28: 404–408

Roth D, Covi L 1984 Cognitive group psychotherapy of depression: the open-ended group. International Journal of Group Psychotherapy 34: 67–82

Shakir S A, Volkmar F R, Bacon S, Pfefferbaum A 1979 Group psychotherapy as an adjunct to lithium maintenance. American Journal of Psychiatry 136: 455–456

Shaw B F 1977 Comparison of cognitive therapy and behaviour therapy in the treatment of depression. Journal of Consulting and Clinical Psychology 45: 543–551

Slife B D, Sasscer-Burgos J, Froberg W, Ellington S 1989 Effect of depression on processing interactions in group psychotherapy. International Journal of Group Psychotherapy 39: 79–104

Steuer J L, Mintz J, Hammen C L et al 1984 Cognitive-behavioural and psychodynamic group psychotherapy in treatment of geriatric depression. Journal of Consulting and Clinical Psychology 52: 180–189

Volkmar F R, Bacon S, Shakir S A, Pfeferbaum A 1981 Group therapy in the management of manic-depressive illness. American Journal of Psychiatry 35: 226–234

Wulsin L, Bachop M Hoffman D 1988 Group therapy in manic-depressive illness. American Journal of Psychotherapy 42: 263–270

Yalom I D 1975 The theory and practice of group psychotherapy, 2nd edn. Basic Books, New York, p 393

Yalom I D 1983 Inpatient group psychotherapy. Basic Books, New York

Yalom I D 1985 The theory and practice of group psychotherapy, 3rd edn. Basic Books, New York

30. Family and marital therapy

John F. Clarkin   Gretchen L. Haas   Ira D. Glick

Current models of affective disorder (e.g. Billings & Moos 1985, Brown & Harris 1978, O'Connell & Mayo 1988) emphasize the many causal pathways to the symptoms of depression and mania. Genetic transmission of biological vulnerabilities which interact with psychosocial variables (such as social skills, social support and family/marital distress) all figure prominently in the construction of these models. It is likely that the relative salience and weight of these biological and psychosocial variables is different for the various affective disorder diagnostic entities and from case to case. A brief review of these variables will provide a theoretical backdrop for the indications and goals of family/marital intervention as part of the treatment for these disorders.

THE INTERPERSONAL CONTEXT AND AFFECTIVE DISORDERS

There is growing evidence of a reciprocal impact between the individual with affective disorder and that person's family and marital unit. This interaction has been investigated most extensively with individuals who are either in a depressive episode or have experienced one in the past. There is less research on bipolar disorder, probably related to the prominence accorded to biological factors. However, there is some growing research on the impact on the family of a member with bipolar disorder and the relationship of family adjustment to the subsequent course of the disorder.

Depression

The interactional behaviour of individuals with depression, especially those with mild to moderate depression, has received much recent attention. An extensive body of research indicates that depressives have inadequate social problem-solving skills (Dobson & Dobson 1981, Fisher-Beckfield & McFall 1982). Specific deficits such as social passivity, dysfunctional interpersonal cognitions and inadequate verbal and nonverbal communication skills have been noted (e.g. Hammen et al 1980, Sanchez & Lewinsohn 1980). Problem-solving skills, family support, marital and family functioning during and after depressive episodes and parenting skills have all received research attention.

Family support

The support of a marital relationship buffers individuals from depression, not unlike the classical finding of Brown & Harris (1978) that a close intimate relationship protects from depression. For example, in a community survey (Pearlin & Johnson 1977), married individuals reported less depression than did unmarried individuals, even after controlling for such variables as gender, age and ethnicity. Married individuals were less exposed to various life strains than the unmarried. When samples were equated for levels of life strain, married individuals were still less depressed than the unmarried.

Since family support is probably a potent factor in protecting from depression, it is important to differentiate the nature and kind of support. Adults residing in families low in cohesion and expressiveness and high in interpersonal conflict reported more depressive symptoms (Billings & Moos 1982). Compared with matched non-depressed controls, unipolar depressed patients have less supportive marital relationships and their family environments are characterized by less cohesion and interpersonal expressiveness and more conflict (Billings et al 1983). In fact, the level of family support has effectively discriminated between depressed and non-depressed women (Wetzel 1978, Wetzel & Redmond 1980).

Marital interaction

A recent thorough review (Barnett & Gotlib 1988) concluded that marital distress and low social integration are involved in the aetiology of the depressive episode, whereas introversion and interpersonal dependency are enduring abnormalities in the interpersonal functioning of individuals with remitted depression. Many studies indicate that marital conflict is highly correlated with depression and with the course of depression. In addition, studies of the interpersonal behaviour of depressed patients in communication with a non-depressed spouse have identified characteristic dysfunctional aspects.

Marital and family functioning during depressive episodes. There is a body of research suggesting that the interaction between a depressed and a non-depressed individual typically gives rise to anger in the non-depressed person. Coyne (1976) found that subjects who interacted in a 20-minute telephone conversation with a depressed outpatient unknown to them showed negative mood and reacted negatively to the depressed person on the telephone. This striking illustration of the immediate impact of a depressed person on others has been repeated in other studies (Gurtman 1986). It is not totally clear what the depressed individual is doing that makes for such an immediate negative reponse. In experimental situations, depressed persons when placed in a high-power role tended to be exploitative and uncooperative and to communicate more self-devaluation and helplessness (Hokanson et al 1980). When placed in a low-power role they tended to blame their partners. While individuals in the intimate relationship of marriage may be expected to be more sympathetic and understanding than strangers in a laboratory, it has become clear in interaction studies that hostility and rejection are often prominent.

In a prospective study by Monroe et al (1986) when both initial symptom level and marital conflict were statistically controlled, marital support was not a significant predictor of subsequent depression. When both initial symptoms and marital conflict were controlled for statistically, marital support was a significant predictor of subsequent depression. O'Hara (1986) assessed nondepressed women who became depressed postpartum. As compared with non-depressed controls, these patients reported significantly lower marital adjustment.

Not surprisingly, social dysfunction occurs during the acute phase of the depressive disorder. Depressed women have been found to be most impaired in their roles as wives and mothers (Weissman & Paykel 1974). Marriages were characterized by interpersonal friction, poor communication, dependency and diminished sexual satisfaction. Hostility was frequently overt and there was a lack of affection toward mates. Clinically recovered depressed women continued to experience problems functioning in their parental and spousal roles several months after recovery from the depressive symptoms. Interpersonal friction, inhibited communication and the expression of hostility continued over the course of 8 months despite symptom improvement (Paykel & Weissman 1973).

A characteristic lack of autonomy and a tendency to cling to partners have been noted among endogenous depressives (Akiskal et al 1978). Others have noted a characteristic wish by the depressed spouse for the partner to be strong and to control or to set limits. Unipolar endogenous depressed patients tend to have episodes during a relationship rather than after separation and break-up, with the latter pattern more characteristic of non-endogenous depressives (Akiskal et al 1983).

Rounsaville et al (1979) found that over half of their sample of depressed women reported difficulties. In addition, if the marital difficulties persisted as treatment progressed, they were associated with poorer improvement and a greater likelihood of relapse. Depressives show lower levels of social and marital-role functioning as compared with normal individuals. In fact, differential levels of depression are associated with good versus poor marital adjustment (Birtchnell & Kennard 1983).

Observational studies of interpersonal interaction. In many ways, investigations that involve the observation and recording of behavioural interaction between affectively disordered individuals and intimate others (e.g. spouses, parents, and/or children) are the most relevant studies for the family therapist who seeks to intervene in repetitive pathogenic interactional patterns. A behavioural record of interaction sequences provides information regarding the functional link or interface between the symptomatology of the patient and the interpersonal context, giving clues as to the sequences that trigger and/or help maintain the affective disorder. An examination of interpersonal interaction sequences transcends linear models of causality and provides an opportunity to observe how the behaviour of each partner correlates with depressive symptoms. Clinically, such observation can guide intervention schemes to eliminate maladaptive interactional sequences and introduce more helpful ones.

The growing body of research on the interaction between partners where one member is depressed suggests that these couples 1) exhibit conflicted interactions 2) characterized by hostility and low self-disclosure 3) with a lack of task orientation, and 4) these interactions are distinguishable from those of other conflicted couples without depression.

Depressed psychiatric inpatients verbalize personal subjective experiences more frequently than do control (medical) patients, who tend to be more task-oriented in their verbalizations. In addition, depressed couples experience more negative tension than do control couples (Hinchliffe et al 1975, Hooper et al 1977). Depressed married women display less problem-solving behaviour than do their spouses, and the spouses manifest less self-disclosure. These couples express less facilitative behaviour than do control couples and depression tends to reduce aversive behaviour in the spouse (Biglan et al 1985).

Hautzinger et al (1982) have studied couples seeking marital treatment, including a subset in which one spouse presented with unipolar depression. Couples with a depressed partner exhibited negative and asymmetrical communication, with expression of dysphoric and uncomfortable feelings. Depressed individuals spoke negatively about themselves and positively about their spouses. In contrast, the non-depressed spouses rarely spoke of themselves but evaluated their depressed partners negatively. Since all of the patients in this study had marital conflict, there was no representation of those without it. However, Kowalik & Gotlib (1987) compared the interactions of depressed and non-depressed outpatients with those of non-depressed non-psychiatric controls and their spouses in an interactional task. Depressed psychiatric outpatients showed negativity, which was not evident in the non-depressed control couples. Kahn et al (1985) found that couples with a depressed spouse experienced each other as more negative, hostile, mistrusting and detached, and as less agreeable, nurturant and affiliative, than did non-depressed couples.

Not all couples with a depressed member manifest negative interaction, however. Hooley (1986) has investigated the interaction between depressed individuals and their spouses who were classified as having high or low expressed emotion (EE) on the basis of the Camberwell Family Interview. In a 10-minute face-to-face interaction between the patients and their spouses, high EE spouses were more negative and less positive toward their depressed partners, in terms of both verbal and non-verbal behaviours. They made critical remarks, disagreed with their partners more frequently and were less likely to accept what their mate said to them. The depressed mates of high EE spouses exhibited low frequencies of self-disclosure and high levels of neutral non-verbal behaviour. Thus, a high level of negative affect and a relative lack of positive, supportive communications seem characteristic of high EE depressed couples.

Control and power issues also surface in the interactions. These may be related to, and/or causative of, the hostility mentioned previously. Contrary to the theoretical assumptions regarding passivity and dependency of the depressed spouse, Hooper et al (1977) reported that depressed patients in their sample produced substantial control-oriented communication with their spouses during the acute depressive episode – more than during the post-treatment follow-up period. Merikangas et al (1979) recorded and rated therapeutic interaction between depressed female inpatients and their spouses. During early sessions, the patient was strongly influenced by the behaviour of his or her spouse, but by the last session there was a more equal balance of power.

While most of the interactional studies have involved depressed women, Gotlib & Whiffen (1989) utilized couples where either a man or a woman was hospitalized with depression, and contrasted them with couples including a non-depressed medical inpatient, and non-depressed/non-patient controls. The depressed couples were clearly dysfunctional in interactional behaviour when contrasted with the community controls. The medical patients and spouses, like the depressed couples, exhibited some dysfunctional behaviour but the depressed couples were unique in their negative affect following the interactions and in their negative appraisals of spouses' behaviour. The results did not reveal any striking differences between depressed men and women, suggesting that the findings for depressed females and their spouses are not gender-specific.

Marital/family functioning following depressive episode. Not only do depressed individuals interact in a dysfunctional way with their partners, in most studies marital dysfunction is found to continue following the remission of the depressive episode. In one sample (Beach et al 1983), 84% of the depressed patients exhibited a negative course of marital change in the 4 years following hospitalization.

Beach et al (1983) followed unipolar and bipolar depressives and schizophrenics 3–4 years after an episode involving hospitalization. While all groups reported marital distress at discharge, at follow-up only the unipolar depressed group differed from normal controls with a higher frequency of poor marital course. A study by Gotlib (1986) suggests there may be sex differences in this phenomenon. Following recovery from a depressive episode, couples in which the wife was depressed reported continued marital difficulties, whereas couples in which the husband was the patient reported significant improvement in marital satisfaction.

The construct of expressed emotion may relate to a poor course in affective disorder, as it does in schizophrenia. Most recently, Hooley & Teasdale (1989) found high EE, marital distress and the patient's perception of criticism from the spouse as predictors of 9-month relapse rates in hospitalized unipolar depressives. The single best predictor was the patient's perception of a critical stance on the part of the spouse.

Depression is also associated with upset in the spouse and disruption of the marital relationship (Bloom et al 1978). Coyne et al (1987) found that among the spouses of depressed individuals, 40% were so distressed that they met a criterion for referral for psychotherapy. Depressed divorced persons are more likely than non-depressed divorced persons to have discovered adultery by their ex-spouses (Briscoe & Smith 1973). The divorce rate in depressed patients 2 years following discharge is nine times higher than the expected rate (Merikangas 1984).

Parenting

Depressed individuals have difficulties in interactions with their children (Coyne et al 1986). Relationships between depressed women and their children have been characterized by a lack of involvement and affection, impaired communication, friction, guilt and resentment (Weissman & Paykel 1974). Children of a depressed parent have been found to be at risk for psychological symptoms and behavioural problems. As many as 40–50% of children with a depressed parent have diagnosable psychiatric disorders (Cytryn et al 1982, Decina et al 1983). Biglan and colleagues (1985) studied the interactions of family members in the presence of a depressed mother. Children of mothers who were depressed displayed significantly more irritability than did controls. The fathers and children reduced their irritated and sarcastic behaviour immediately following the mother's displays of dysphoric affect. Such apparent adaptations to the dysphoric display suggest that they represent a reaction to depressive symptoms rather than a *stimulus* for dysphoric response.

Bipolar disorder

Janowsky and colleagues (1970) were among the first to describe the interpersonal and family behaviour related to bipolar disorder. They described five types of interpersonal activity related to mania, including the manipulation of the self-esteem of others, perceptiveness and exploitation of vulnerability in others, projection of responsibility, progressive limit-testing and distancing and alienation from other family members. These investigators noted that the family members perceive the spouse as ill in the depressive phase with little responsibility or control, while they perceive the patient as wilful and spiteful during the manic phase. Patients speak of divorce and sexual advances to others quite frequently and the spouses feel trapped in an impossible situation.

Hoover & Fitzgerald (1981) compared marital interactions between bipolar patients and their spouses with normal community couples on a self-report scale. The bipolar couples reported significantly higher levels of conflict. More specifically, conflict was highest with bipolar I spouses, next unipolar spouses and finally bipolar II. Targum and colleagues (1981) found the most troublesome family issues when one member has bipolar disorder were financial difficulty, unemployment, marital problems, symptom recurrence and hospitalization and social withdrawal and depression. On self-report measures of family functioning, families of bipolar patients reported less disturbance (along with families with a schizophrenic member) than families with a patient with major depression, alcoholism and adjustment disorders (Miller et al 1986). In fact, the families of bipolar patients as a group showed the least amount of self-rated family dysfunction. On the other hand, there were substantial numbers of bipolar families with significant dysfunction, especially when patient scores (which minimized family pathology) were excluded.

Family interaction concepts of affective style (AS) and expressed emotion, which have been successful in helping to predict relapse in schizophrenia, have recently been applied to bipolar disorder (Miklowitz et al 1988). A sample of 23 bipolar manic adult patients hospitalized for an acute disorder were studied, all but one of whom were living with one or both parents. The two measures of family functioning, EE and AS, were unrelated to each other and interactive predictors of patient outcome upon follow-up. If either index of family functioning was poor, relapse was highly likely (94%). Conversely, only those families rated low on both family factors had a low relapse rate (17%). Neither family EE nor AS were related to medication compliance, and medication compliance was not in itself related to relapse in this brief 9-month follow-up period. Social adjustment at all three follow-up points was found to be independent of symptomatic status, but it was related to social adjustment scores. Those families with a benign AS score showed improvement in social adjustment, whereas those from a negative AS family showed a decrement.

Hooley et al (1987) used attribution theory to further the understanding of family conflict when one member is seriously disturbed. The authors hypothesized that florid symptoms of the disorder would be attributed to illness and beyond the control of the ill spouse, and be more accepted by the mate than negative symptoms (e.g. behavioural deficits). Results were consistent with this hypothesis, as spouses of patients with negative symptoms and impulse-control deficits reported significantly lower levels of marital satisfaction than spouses of patients with positive symptoms. The issue of attribution – to what does the mate or family member attribute the undesired behaviours of the patient is a crucial one and may provide some insight into the productive but elusive concept of expressed emotion that has had so much attention in the family research in schizophrenia.

As with depressed patients, there is evidence that bipolar patients have difficulties in parenting. Davenport et al (1984) investigated the parenting attitudes and behaviours of a small number of married couples, each of which contained one spouse who had diagnosed bipolar disorder. The bipolar mothers, in comparison to controls, were less attentive to their children's needs, emphasized performance, were more overprotective, displayed more negative affect toward their children and were more tense, unhappy and ineffective.

Given the family problems presented by the illness, it is not surprising that the divorce rate is high. In one sample (Brodie & Leff 1971), the divorce rate was 57% for bipolars and 8% for unipolars. The divorces in the bipolar group always occurred after a manic attack. In another sample, Coryell and colleagues (1985) found a 33% divorce rate in bipolar IIs, 21% in the bipolar Is and 17% in the non-bipolar depression.

While lithium treatment is quite effective for many patients, it does have its own impact on patients' inter-personal and family adjustment. O'Connell & Mayo (1981) found that patients maintained on lithium increased the direct care of children by both spouses, reduced marital friction and was followed by an increase in cooperative communication and planning. Likewise, Holinger & Wolpert (1979) found significant improvement in family relationships in the majority of families but in 39% there was no change. Apparently lithium treatment also reduces sexual interest and responsiveness. In one sample (Winokur et al 1969) 63% of patients with mixed bipolar disorder experienced a decrease in sexual interest. Lithium can lead to a decrease in sexual interest and a decrease in frequency of intercourse, but does not interfere with sexual enjoyment itself (Lorimy et al 1977). These issues may be relevant for psychoeducation.

IMPLICATIONS FOR FURTHER RESEARCH

There are a number of research steps that must be taken in exploring the relationship between marital/family discord and affective disorders. A programmatic research plan would involve: 1) establishing the covariation between family functioning and affective symptoms; 2) establishing the boundaries of this relationship; 3) determining the direction of causality; 4) establishing the possibility of experimental control of the linkage; and 5) finally, refining the model through descriptive empirical studies of the mediating and moderating variables (Beach & Nelson in press, Greenberg 1990). The relationships in each of these steps may be different for the heterogeneous group of depressive disorders and the more homogeneous and biologically determined bipolar disorder.

As our review indicates, there is data on step 1 suggesting that depression and marital dysfunction are highly correlated, both prior to and following a depressive episode. There seems to be little doubt that bipolar disorder, while not caused by family disruption, can result in much family stress and call upon extraordinary coping efforts.

Step 2 concerning the boundaries of the relationship between affective disorders and family disruption has not been very well established. We know relatively little about the relationship between marital dysfunction and the severity of affective disorder or the subtypes of the disorder. Most studies have been done on mild to moderately depressed individuals. It is common in research studies to utilize an instrument such as the Beck Depression Inventory (BDI) and define as 'depressives' those individuals who score above a certain cut-off score. This may or may not be accompanied by a diagnosis and the diagnosis may be clinical or made with a semi-structured interview. It may be that the different diagnostic subcategories within affective disorders are most relevant to planning of treatment with medication. However, it is conceivable that various diagnostic subcategories will also influence psychosocial interactions and treatments. It may well be, for example, that endogenous depressives interact differently from non-endogenous depressives. Many of the studies do not clearly indicate the stage of the affective illness/episode during which the interaction samples are recorded. It is likely that the patient interacts in different ways depending upon the phase of the affective episode – whether during the prodromal phase, during an illness episode or during the recovery period.

There is even less information on the third step, that of establishing the direction of causality between family dysfunction and affective disorder. While poor social integration and lack of intimate relationships may be related to subsequent depressions of various degrees of severity, in bipolar disorder it is clear that marital and family difficulty tend to follow the episode and less is known about prior conditions.

The fourth step involving experimental designs can include treatment studies in which the researcher intervenes either on affective symptoms or family functioning and measures the effect on the other variables. Probably the best data to date in this regard is the subsequent family and marital functioning following relatively successful symptom treatment of bipolar disorder.

Questions about the relative role of other variables still remain. For example, there is a need for the systematic assessment and study of concurrent personality disorders and of how such chronic behaviour patterns influence interaction patterns of patient and spouse. Interpersonal behaviour is influenced by *both* the affective symptomatology and the personality styles of the participants. Recent data (Shea et al 1987, Pilkonis & Frank 1988) suggests that a substantial number of depressives do have personality disorders and disorder traits, especially of the fearful and anxious cluster.

INDICATIONS FOR MARITAL/FAMILY TREATMENTS

Under what conditions is a marital/family treatment indicated when the identified patient is suffering from an affective disorder? What are the mediating goals of treatment of an affective disorder that would call for a marital/family intervention? From a theoretical point of view, the following situations are relevant indications that might call for family treatments (often combined with medication) with various foci:

1) On clinical examination, it appears that marital/family stressors have elicited or precipitated the onset of affective symptoms in a biologically predisposed individual.
2) Family stress or the lack of an intimate relationship may potentiate the effects of other environmental stressors, leading to a depressive episode in a biologically vulnerable individual.
3) On clinical examination, it appears that affective symptoms in one family member have triggered negative responses from other family members, thus acting to elicit further marital/family conflict and depressive symptoms in the patient.
4) Subclinical affective-characterological traits and behaviour patterns in one or more family members seems to have potentiated family discord, which, in turn, has triggered the onset of an affective episode.

It is unfortunately clear that these are only hypothesized indications, and we have limited evidence for them at the present time. However, as the review of the research literature on the family context and affective disorder above indicated, there is some accumulation of data suggesting these linkages in some form are important and quite plausible.

On a more practical level the clinician must assess for common family problem areas regardless of whether they predate, are concomitant with or follow from the affective symptoms in the patient. It is often impossible to sort out clearly the time sequence and causal relations between symptoms and interpersonal interactions and stressors. As the review in this chapter would suggest, family and marital areas of prime relevance to intervention would include marital conflict, spouse anger and rejection of the patient, lack of marital intimacy, poor parenting behaviour, hostility and overinvolvement (high EE) with the patient, poor medication compliance and lack of family support for such compliance.

In addition to the focus on presence or absence of common problem areas when one family member is depressed or has bipolar disorder, a sequence of possible levels of family intervention is available. We are talking here about a possible progression of family intervention from psychoeducation to routine communication training and problem solving skills enhancement, to more involved systems and psychodynamic intervention. It would appear to us that in any family in which a member has an episode of major depression or bipolar disorder family psychoeducation is indicated. In families who have excellent premorbid communication and problem solving, psychoeducation may be sufficient. In the majority of families, however, the insult and stress of a major depressive or bipolar episode will call for at least a planned, relatively brief family/marital intervention, mainly cognitive and behavioural in strategy and focused on assisting the family in coping with the disorder. Finally, there are a subset of families in which premorbid marital conflict, interpersonal difficulties and poor problem solving are endemic. In these situations the patient often has concomitant Axis II pathology and the spouse may also have moderate to serious psychopathology. In these situations, a longer and more involved family intervention may be of assistance, although it is in these cases where small gains are long in coming.

Throughout all situations the commitment of the spouses to the marriage itself is an important variable. As noted earlier, the divorce rate with affective disorder is relatively high, and impending divorce related to affective episodes can be an issue in itself. Obviously, when divorce is in progress, marital intervention as a format may not be the most appropriate.

ASSESSMENT OF AFFECTIVE DISORDER AND THE INTERPERSONAL CONTEXT

Given the presence of an affective disorder in a family member, the clinician must assess the marital and/or family context in order to: 1) ascertain if the situation meets the indications for family/marital treatment; 2) focus the intervention in the marital/family format; and 3) provide a baseline measure for subsequent assessment of change. These issues have been addressed in several places (Haas et al 1985, Gotlib & Colby 1987, Clarkin & Haas 1988a).

The family evaluation must be done in such a way as to yield a symptom diagnosis (Axis I) and personality disorder diagnosis (Axis II) for the members of the family, not just the identified patient. In addition, interactional patterns suggestive for a toxic environment for the patient with affective disorder must be explicated.

In addition to the diagnosis, one must assess the important psychosocial variables that we have highlighted in this review. This would include the assessment of marital conflict and the presence of family EE. This would involve assessment of closeness

and emotional support in the family, including the knowledge and acceptance of the affective disorder by other members of the family. Medication compliance should be evaluated not only in terms of the patient but also in terms of family support for and involvement in such compliance. There are a number of self-report and interview techniques to evaluate these crucial areas.

INTERPERSONAL TREATMENTS

Differential treatment planning must involve decisions regarding five different factors: 1) treatment setting (outpatient, day hospital, hospitalization; 2) treatment format (individual, family/marital, group); 3) strategies and techniques (dynamic, cognitive – behavioural, systems); 4) medication; and 5) duration and frequency of treatment (planned brief treatment, long-term intervention) (Frances et al 1984). The focus of this chapter is on the use of family and marital treatment formats for the affective disorders. These family and marital treatments are typically utilized in an outpatient setting but are of potential usefulness during the acute phase of the disorder when the patient is in an inpatient treatment setting. Family/marital treatments are often combined with appropriate medication. While there were earlier concerns in the family literature that medicating one patient would prejudice if not vitiate a family systems approach, this is not an issue if handled appropriately (Glick & Clarkin 1981). In terms of treatment strategies and techniques, the majority of the research has been done with cognitive—behavioural strategies. It is our impression that the major focus of attention should be on the mediating goals of treatment as demanded by the affective disorders and the family context, and that treatment strategies (behavioural, cognitive, systems, strategic) should be selected not from adherence to a treatment philosophy but as a practical step in accomplishing the goals in the individual case.

Psychoeducation

Providing information about a psychiatric disorder (its symptoms, aetiology, prognosis, course and treatment for patient and family) has recently become a common procedure and focus of investigation when the patient is suffering from schizophrenia (Clarkin 1989). As the multiple aetiologies of the major psychiatric disorders are explicated, the use of psychoeducation for patients of other diagnostic categories and their families is utilized more frequently in order to inform the patient, establish a positive treatment alliance with the patient and family and convince patient and family to change aspects of their life style (such as family stress and conflict) which have a bearing on the course of the disorder.

It would seem that bipolar disorder and major depression, which, like schizophrenia, have a multiple causal pathway involving biological and social factors, are also disorders that call for psychoeducation with patient and family. There are signs that this is beginning to occur. Lewinsohn and colleagues (Lewinsohn & Brown 1979, Lewinsohn & Hoberman, 1982) have used a psychoeducational package involving 12 2-hour class sessions over 8 weeks with outpatients experiencing depression. Utilizing her experience with a psychoeducational approach with schizophrenic patients and their families, Anderson (Holder & Anderson 1990) has described a psychoeducational family intervention for seriously depressed patients and their families. Using group meetings and a workshop format, the programme is designed to connect with the family, provide information and coping skills and facilitate the application of this information to the practicalities of everyday life. Our group (Clarkin et al 1990a) has utilized printed psychoeducational material and group discussion to assist couples and families in coping with the affective disorders in a family member. While the psychoeducational material can be delivered by mental health professionals to each family or in family groups, written material can also be made available. There are a number of books and pamphlets that families can read which provide information on the aetiology, course and medication treatment of depression and mania (see Goodwin & Jamison 1990, p 744).

Marital Treatment

Probably the most investigated family approach for affective disorder is that of marital intervention when one spouse is depressed. The success of various treatments for depression delivered in the individual format, most prominently cognitive — behavioural treatments and interpersonal psychotherapy (Bellack 1985), has led to the utilization of these treatment strategies in a marital treatment format. This is a logical progression, given the marital difficulties that accompany affective disorders as described earlier. The relative absence of research on the use of other strategies and techniques such as systems-oriented and psychodynamic techniques is unfortunate, however. The reasons for this research imbalance are not totally clear, but one suspects that the codification of cognitive — behavioural

techniques in a manual is much easier to accomplish than that for systems and dynamic approaches. This imbalance in research effort leaves an unfortunate discrepancy between the available data on one hand and the preponderance of systems and dynamic treatments in general clinical practice on the other hand.

In one of the first controlled studies, Friedman (1975) utilized a random-assignment, placebo-controlled, 12-week clinical trial to assess the relative effectiveness of amitriptyline and marital therapy, administered separately and in combination. The patients had a primary diagnosis of depression (reactive depression, psychotic depression, manic-depressive psychosis or involutional psychotic reactions). Both drug and marital therapies had beneficial effects compared to their respective control treatments. There were also some signs of differential effects. While drug treatment was associated with significant early improvement in clinical symptoms, the marital therapy was associated with significant long-term changes in patient self-report measures of family role functioning and marital relations.

Cognitive—behavioural treatments

McLean et al (1973) used behavioural techniques to intervene in the verbal interchange between couples in which one was clinically depressed. Half of the sample was given feedback boxes designed to signal positive and negative feedback during the ongoing conversation. Couples in the feedback box group showed significantly reduced negative interchanges with a significant reduction of remarks considered negative. The total behavioural treatment package, including the feedback procedure, training in the use of behavioural contracting and social learning principles, produced significantly more improvement on target complaints than occurred in the non-treatment comparison group.

Building on the proven efficacy of behavioural/marital treatment for marital distress, and the known efficacy of cognitive and behavioural interventions for depression in the individual treatment format, Dobson et al (1988) have articulated a cognitive—behavioural marital treatment for spouses one of whom is depressed. There are four general areas in which cognitive distortions or negative thinking can arise with such couples: 1) problem definition; 2) expectancies for self and one's spouse; 3) beliefs about change; and 4) attributions for behaviour. The principal intervention strategies of this cognitive—behavioural marital treatment (Berley & Jacobson 1984) are: 1) challenging myths, expectations and beliefs; 2) relabelling; 3) behavioural enactment; 4) mood and affect modification; 5) strategic interventions; and 6) use of vignettes that present therapeutic principles and rules. Depressed women were randomly assigned to one of three conditions: a social learning marital therapy, an individual cognitive therapy or a combined treatment of individual cognitive therapy and conjoint marital therapy (Jacobson et al 1987). Preliminary results suggest that cognitive therapy, either by itself or in combination with marital therapy, is effective in alleviating depression when the couple does not report marital distress. In the presence of marital distress, however, the marital treatment is as effective as individual cognitive therapy in reducing depression. In addition, changes in the depression are correlated with improvement in the quality of the relationship (Jacobson et al 1989).

O'Leary & Beach (1990) randomly assigned depressed women and their spouses to marital treatment, individual cognitive treatment or waiting-list control. All of the women met DSM-III criteria for major depression or dysthymia and, concomitantly, had a BDI score of 14 or more. Both active treatments were effective in reducing depressive symptoms. In addition, the women who received marital treatment had significantly higher marital satisfaction scores after therapy than did the women in the other two groups.

Interpersonal psychotherapy (IPT)

Interpersonal psychotherapy for depression (Klerman et al 1984) has been shown to be effective in the individual treatment format for mild to moderate depressions. Although it is delivered as individual treatment, the focus of the intervention is on the interaction of the patient with significant others, especially family members. The success of this treatment, both in independent clinical trials and in the recent collaborative multi-site National Institute of Mental Health study (Elkin et al 1989) raises the interesting question of whether or not it would be more effective in a marital format. A direct approach to interpersonal issues in a marital format may be more effective and efficient either in the short run or in long-term follow-up than the individual treatment format. In a recent study (Foley et al 1987), IPT as a spouse-involved treatment was as effective as IPT in an individual format in reducing depression and was more effective at improving the quality of marital relationship. IPT is discussed further in chapter 31.

Other approaches

Gotlib & Colby (1987) have described a systems-oriented marital and family therapy for the depressed outpatient. In this context, depression is seen as a symptom pattern that has powerful intra- and interpersonal causes and repercussions. Treatment interventions following from this conceptualization and basic techniques include joining with the family, reframing the depression or problem areas, enacting problematic family interchanges, restructuring the family relationship and altering the boundaries between the various subsystems and alliances in the family. Throughout this effort, the strengths of the family are emphasized and utilized.

Waring et al (1988) compared doxepin with placebo and a marital therapy focused on enhancing intimacy for depressed married females. The women treated with medication and marital therapy showed significant improvement on all depression measures and on the intimacy scale (Waring & Reddon 1983). The authors note the presence of the supportive husband as a therapeutic element in itself.

Coyne (1988) has described a strategic therapy for couples when one is depressed. Three foci are the depressed person, the response of the spouse and the marriage. Strategic interventions, such as positive retraining, encouraging a moderate level of involvement by the non-depressed spouse and the use of extra session assignments, are routinely utilized.

Family treatment

When the individual with the affective disorder is a child, adolescent or young adult living with parents, the potential usefulness of family treatment should be considered. There is little research to guide the clinician in these situations, so one must use research in related areas and collective clinical experience. In the case of bipolar disorder in a late adolescent or young adult living with parents, the research on the effectiveness of family therapy in schizophrenia is a useful paradigm. The efficacy of family psychoeducation and cognitive — behavioural intervention focused on assisting the family to cope with the stress-responsive disorder (Falloon et al 1982, Hogarty et al 1986) suggests that such an approach would be useful for bipolar disorder. We anticipate relevant research in this area in the near future.

Depression in a child, adolescent or young adult living with parents could have many conceivable uses in the treatment of such an individual. As in the marital treatment when one spouse is depressed, family treatment in these situations may be of assistance in enhancing family support, reducing family conflict, increasing family communication skills and problem solving efficiency and supporting medication compliance.

Phases of the affective disorder and family treatments

One salient characteristic of the affective disorders is their phasic nature. It is important for treatment planning to recognize and utilize the characteristics of the disorder in its different phases to achieve maximum effectiveness. The acute phase of depression and mania calls for symptom containment and reduction and role-induction into possible maintenance treatment. The non-acute phase or maintenance phase calls for improving skills and behaviours that will reduce the likelihood of a future acute upset, improve everyday coping skills and prepare for coping with possible future episodes.

Acute phase

Our group (Clarkin et al 1990a, b) has investigated a brief family intervention during the hospitalization of a patient in the acute phase of an affective disorder. Inpatient family intervention (IFI) is a brief, focused intervention for patient and family that utilizes the occasion of the hospitalization of a family member to begin a treatment process that recognizes the affective disorder, the need for medication and possible psychosocial intervention and coping, and uses the crisis intervention to start the process. Both empirical data and anecdotal case histories (Clarkin et al 1988b) suggest that such a focused family intervention during the crisis of hospitalization can be helpful in assisting the family unit to cope with the disorder in one member.

The bipolar patients were predominantly white (81%) and female (67%), with a mean age of 32. Marital status was quite varied, with 52% single, 33% married and 14% divorced. 48% had no previous hospitalizations and 33% had no previous episodes of illness. There was a more seriously disturbed subgroup (14%) with three or more previous hospitalizations, and 19% with three or more previous bipolar episodes. The unipolar patients were predominantly white (62%), with almost equal distribution of males (45%) and

females (55%). The mean age was 38. 31% of the patients were single, 52% married, and 17% divorced or separated. 62% of the patients had no previous hospitalizations and 48% had no previous episodes. In contrast, 14% had experienced three or more previous hospitalizations and three or more previous episodes.

Female affective disorder patients with IFI were doing significantly better on a composite patient symptomatology/global outcome measure than those in the comparison group at discharge; on the other hand, affective disorder males were little affected. Family attitude toward treatment was significantly better in IFI females than in comparison females. Family attitude toward the patient, a self-report measure analogous to EE, was significantly better in males who received the *comparison* treatment than in males who received IFI.

At both 6- and 18-month follow-up points there were no main effects of treatment on either of the two patient measures, nor on the two family composite measures for the total affective group. There were, however, significant effects by subdiagnosis. At both follow-up points, bipolar patients showed better outcome with IFI while unipolar patients did better without it. On a composite measure of patient symptomatology/global functioning there was a treatment by subdiagnosis trend which became significant at 18 months. It was clear from inspection of composite means that the bipolars did better with IFI whereas unipolars did better with the comparison treatment. The bipolar treatment effect was due to female patients only, while the negative effect on unipolars appeared in both sexes. On a composite measure of patient functioning at both follow-up points, again the bipolar patients did better with IFI and the unipolar patients did better with the comparison treatment. On family attitude to patient/burden, there was a treatment by subdiagnosis interaction effect at 6-month follow-up, again favouring the IFI bipolar patients.

The results suggest that for bipolar patients a brief, family intervention that is psychoeducational in nature may be helpful in subsequent course. The prominent sex-by-treatment interaction favouring the positive responsiveness of female bipolar patients and their families to IFI was unanticipated. One can only speculate as to the reasons for this finding, and further research is needed. The data are less clear for unipolar depressive patients. The depressed group may be a more heterogeneous one and a straightforward psychoeducational approach may be less appropriate for at least some of these patients and families. Much more research is needed, of course, and unfortunately this is the only existing empirical investigation of family treatment and affective disorder during hospitalization.

Maintenance phase

When the depressed or manic patient is out of the acute phase of the disorder, longer-range interventions can be utilized. This could occur after the patient has been discharged from an inpatient service and is stabilized following an acute episode, or in the course of a disorder that is not so severe as to call for hospitalization. Treatment at this point can focus on marital and family stressors and conflicts that seem relevant to the precipitation or maintenance of the symptoms.

For example, we have articulated and are investigating an outpatient psychoeducational and cognitive — behavioural marital treatment for couples in which one spouse is diagnosed as bipolar. While the treatment may begin in the latter stages of an acute episode (and during hospitalization), the major portion of the treatment is best delivered in an outpatient setting while the patient is between episodes. The focus is on psychoeducation and the learning of communication and problem solving skills to enable the couple to cope adequately with the disorder and reduce ambient stress that might exacerbate the situation.

Treatment complications

In evaluating and treating patients with affective disorder and their families, there are related issues which are often present and need therapeutic attention. In reference to the affective disorders, this would include management and treatment of suicide, drug abuse and impending separation and divorce. It seems appropriate to comment on the use of family and marital treatment formats in the management and treatment of these difficulties.

Suicidal behaviour in the context of an affective disorder episode is probably most effectively treated by treating the affective disorder itself. The most effective somatic treatments will be crucial in this regard. Family and marital treatment may be used as an ancillary crisis intervention during a suicidal period. Family support, surveillance and protection of the patient can be crucial at such times.

Drug abuse in the context of affective symptoms should most probably receive an independent treatment (Goodwin & Jamison 1990). Family treatments are sometimes useful ancillary approaches to the treatment of drug and alcohol addictions, as these addic-tions have tremendous impact on the family unit and the patient needs the support of the family members.

We have noted previously in this chapter the association of affective disorder and marital disruption and divorce. It is not uncommon for the clinician to be faced with a family in the intense throes of considering divorce with concomitant exacerbation or onset of affective symptoms in the patient. It seems reasonable to establish a sequence for the intervention, with first attention to reducing affective symptoms and subsequent attention to the long-term viability of the marital relationship.

CONCLUSIONS

There is a growing body of empirical literature that implicates the interpersonal context in the precipitation and/or maintenance of affective symptoms in the individual. As an aggregate, however, the results of the studies to date are difficult to interpret. It is unclear, for example, if marital and family disputes are causative (or part of the cause) of the onset of depression or are a result of the depression. It is also not clear if the different levels of severity of depressive symptoms, or the different diagnostic entities, relate differentially to the associated involvement of family and marital conflict. For example, it may be that marital conflict is causative of mild to moderate depression, which will lift if the conflict is resolved in one way or another. It is equally conceivable that, in more severe depressions, marital conflict is a result of the individual pathology or the marital conflict is only one of many causative events. While marital and family conflict may trigger a bipolar episode, a more conservative approach is one that sees the biological variables as primary.

Thus issues of the causal pathway to affective symptoms cannot be the primary or only focus for determining the usefulness of family/marital interventions when a family member is so afflicted. Family conflict may be one variable that leads to an illness episode, it may follow from such an episode or it may contribute to recurrence of the disorder. From a more positive point of view, while family conflict may not contribute to affective episodes, the presence of family support may provide the context in which the future course of the illness is attenuated and improved.

We have focused, therefore, on the areas of family functioning that emerge from the research literature as the most important ones for family intervention when one family member is suffering from an affective disorder. In this regard, there is accumulating empirical evidence that marital intervention when one spouse is depressed not only reduces depression but also alleviates marital distress, a double effect that is not accomplished in comparable individual interventions. Research on family and marital intervention with bipolar disorder patients and families is in its infancy.

Since family EE affects the course of bipolar disorder as it does in schizophrenia, it is anticipated that family intervention of a psychoeducational and cognitive — behavioural nature will be as useful in bipolar patients/families as it has been found to be with schizophrenic patients and their families.

REFERENCES

Akiskal H S, Bitar A H, Puzantian V R, Rosenthal T L, Walker P W 1978 The nosological status of neurotic depressions: A prospective three- to four-year follow-up examination in the light of the primary-secondary and the unipolar-bipolar dichotomies. Archives of General Psychiatry 35: 756–766

Akiskal H S, Hirschfeld M A, Yerevanian B I 1983 The relationship of personality to affective disorders: a critical review. Archives of General Psychiatry 40: 801–810

Barnett P A, Gotlib I H 1988 Psychosocial functioning and depression: Distinguishing among antecedents, concomitants, and consequences. Psychological Bulletin 104: 97–126

Beach S R H, Winters K C, Weintraub S, Neale J M 1983 The link between marital distress and depression: a prospective study. Paper presented at the annual meeting of the Association of the Advancement of Behaviour Therapy, Washington DC

Beach S R H, Nelson G M in press Pursuing research on major psychopathology from a contextual perspective: The example of depression and marital discord. In: Brody G H, Sigel I E (eds) Methods of family research: biographies of research projects. II: Clinical populations. Lawrence Erlbaum, Hillsdale, NJ

Bellack A 1985 Psychotherapy research in depression: an overview. In: Beckham E, Leber W (eds) Handbook of depression: treatment, assessment and research Dorsey Press, Homewood, IL, p 204–219

Berley R A, Jacobson N S 1984 Causal attributions in intimate relationships: Toward a model of cognitive—behavioural marital therapy. In: Kendall P (ed) Advances in cognitive—behavioural research Academic Press, New York, p 168–209

Biglan A, Hops H, Sherman L, Friedman L S, Arthur J, Osteen V 1985 Problem-solving interactions of depressed women and their spouses. Behaviour Therapy 16: 431–451

Billings A G, Moos R H 1982 Social support and functioning among community and clinical groups: a panel model. Journal of Behavioural Medicine 5: 295–311

Billings A G, Moos R H 1985 Psychosocial stressors, coping, and depression. In: Beckham E E, Leber W R (eds) Handbook of depression: treatment, assessment and research. Dorsey Press, Homewood IL, p 940–974

Billings A G, Cronkite R C, Moos R H 1983 Social-environmental factors in unipolar depression: Comparisons of depressed patients and nondepressed controls. Journal of Abnormal Psychology 92: 119–133

Birtchnell J, Kennard J 1983 Does marital maladjustment lead to mental illness? Social Psychiatry 18: 79–88

Bloom B, Asher S, White S 1978 Marital disruption as a stressor: A review and analysis. Psychological Bulletin 85: 867–894

Briscoe C W, Smith J B 1973 Depression and marital turmoil. Archives of General Psychiatry 29: 811–817

Brodie H K H, Leff M J 1971 Bipolar depression – a comparative study of patient characteristics. American Journal of Psychiatry 127: 1086–1090

Brown G W, Harris T O 1978 Social origins of depression: a study of psychiatric disorder in women. Free Press, New York

Clarkin J F 1989 Family education. In: Bellack A (ed) A clinical guide for the treatment of schizophrenia. Plenum Press, New York, p 187-205

Clarkin J F, Haas G L 1988a Assessment of affective disorders and their interpersonal contexts. In: Clarkin J F, Haas G L, Glick I D (eds) Affective disorders and the family: assessment and treatment. Guilford Press, New York, p 29-50

Clarkin J F, Haas G L, Glick I D 1988b Inpatient family intervention. In: Clarkin J F, Haas G L, Glick I D (eds) Affective disorders and the family. Guilford Press, New York, p 134–153

Clarkin J F, Glick I D, Haas G L et al 1990a A randomized clinical trial of inpatient family intervention. V: Results for affective disorders. Journal of Affective Disorders 18: 17–28

Clarkin J F, Glick I D, Haas G L, Spencer J 1990b Inpatient family intervention for affective disorders. In: Keitner G (ed) Depression and families: impact and treatment. American Psychiatry Press, Washington, DC, p 121–136

Coryell W, Endicott J, Andreasen N, Keller M 1985 Bipolar I, bipolar II, and nonbipolar major depression among the relatives of affectively ill probands. American Journal of Psychiatry 142: 817–821

Coyne J C 1976 Depression and the response of others. Journal of Abnormal Psychology 2: 186–193

Coyne J C 1988 Strategic therapy. In: Clarkin J F, Haas G L, Glick I D (eds) Affective disorders and the family: Assessment and treatment. Guilford Press, New York, p 89–113

Coyne J C, Kahn J, Gotlib I H 1986 Depression. In: Jacob T (ed) Family interaction and psychotherapy. Plenum Press, New York, p 509–533

Coyne J C, Kessler R C, Tal M, Turnbull J, Wortman C B, Greden J F 1987 Living with a depressed person. Journal of Consulting and Clinical Psychology 55: 347–352

Cytryn L, McKnew D H, Bartko J J, Lamour M, Hamovitt J 1982 Offspring of patients with affective disorders: II. Journal of the American Academy of Child Psychiatry 21: 389–391

Davenport Y B, Zahn-Wexler C, Adland M L, Mayfield A 1984 Early child-rearing practices in families with a manic-depressive parent. American Journal of Psychiatry 141: 230–235

Decina P, Kestenbaum C J, Farber S, Kron L, Gargan M, Sackeim H A, Fieve R R 1983 Clinical and psychological assessment of children of bipolar probands. American Journal of Psychiatry 140: 548–553

Dobson D, Dobson K 1981 Problem-solving strategies in depressed and nondepressed college students. Cognitive Therapy and Research 5: 697–705

Dobson K S, Jacobson N S, Victor J 1988 Integration of cognitive therapy and behavioural marital therapy. In: Clarkin J F, Haas G L, Glick I D (eds) Affective disorders and the family: assessment and treatment. Guilford Press, New York, p 53–88

Elkin I, Shea M T, Watkins J T, Imber S D et al 1989 National Institute of Mental Health treatment of depression collaborative research program: general effectiveness of treatments. Archives of General Psychiatry 46: 971–982

Falloon I R, Boyd J L, McGill C W et al 1982 Family management in the prevention of exacerbations of schizophrenia. New England Journal of Medicine 306: 1437–1440

Fisher-Beckfield D, McFall R M 1982 Development of a competence inventory for college men and evaluation of relationships between competence and depression. Journal of Consulting and Clinical Psychology 50: 697–705

Foley S H, Rounsaville B J, Weissman M M, Sholomskas D, Chevron E 1987 May Individual vs conjoint interpersonal psychotherapy for depressed patients with marital disputes. Paper presented at the annual meeting of the American Psychiatric Association, Chicago

Frances A, Clarkin J F, Perry S 1984 Differential therapeutics: a guide to the art and science of treatment planning in psychiatry. Brunner/Mazel, New York

Friedman A S 1975 Interaction of drug therapy with marital therapy in depressive patients. Archives of General Psychiatry 32: 619–637

Glick I D, Clarkin J F 1981 Family therapy when an affective disorder is diagnosed. In: Gurman A S (ed) Questions and answers in the practice of family therapy. Brunner/Mazel, New York, p 250–253

Goodwin F K, Jamison K R 1990 Manic-depressive illness. Oxford University Press, New York

Gotlib I H 1986 Depression and marital interaction: a longitudinal perspective. Paper presented at the annual convention of the American Psychological Association, Washington, DC

Gotlib I H, Colby C A 1987 Treatment of depression: an interpersonal systems approach. Pergamon Press, New York

Gotlib I H, Whiffen V E 1989 Depression and marital functioning: an examination of specificity and gender differences. Journal of Abnormal Psychology 98: 23–30

Greenberg L 1990 June Presidential address given at the twenty-first annual meeting of the Society for Psychotherapy Research (SPR), Wintergreen VA

Gurtman M B 1986 Depression and the response of others: Re-evaluating the re-evaluation. Journal of Abnormal Psychology 95: 99–101

Haas G L, Clarkin J F, Glick I D 1985 Marital and family treatment of depression. In: Beckham E E, Leber W R (eds) Handbook of depression: treatment, assessment, and research. Dorsey Press, Homewood, IL, p 151–183

Hammen C L, Jacobs M, Mayol A, Cochran S D 1980 Dysfunctional cognitions and the effectiveness of skills and cognitive-behavioural training. Journal of Consulting and Clinical Psychology 48: 685–695

Hautzinger M, Linden M, Hoffman N 1982 Distressed couples with and without a depressed partner: an analysis of their verbal interaction. Journal of Behaviour Therapy and Experimental Psychiatry 13: 307–314

Hinchcliffe M, Hooper D, Roberts F J, Vaughan P W 1975 A study of the interaction between depressed patients and their spouses. British Journal of Psychiatry 126: 164–172

Hogarty G E, Anderson C M, Reiss D J et al 1986 Family psychoeducation, social skills training and maintenance chemotherapy in the aftercare treatment of schizophrenia. Archives of General Psychiatry 43: 633–642

Hokanson J E, Sacco W P, Blumberg S R et al 1980 Interpersonal behaviour of depressive individuals in a mixed-motive game. Journal of Abnormal Psychology 89: 320–332

Holder D, Anderson C 1990 Psychoeducational family intervention for depressed patients and their families. In: Keitner G I (ed) Depression and families: impact and treatment. American Psychiatric Press, Washington DC, p 159–184

Holinger P C, Wolpert E A 1979 A ten year follow-up of lithium use. IMJ 156: 99–104

Hooley J M 1986 Expressed emotion and depression: interactions between patients and high versus low EE spouses. Journal of Abnormal Psychology 95: 237–246

Hooley J M, Teasdale J D 1989 Predictors of relapse in unipolar depressives: Expressed emotion, marital distress, and perceived criticism. Journal of Abnormal Psychology 98(3): 229–235

Hooley J M, Richters J E, Weintraub S, Neale J M 1987 Psychopathology and marital distress: the positive side of positive symptoms. Journal of Abnormal Psychology 96(1): 27–33

Hooper D, Roberts F J, Hinchcliffe M K, Vaughan P W 1977 The melancholy marriage: an inquiry into the interaction of depression. I. Introduction. British Journal of Medical Psychology 50: 113–124

Hoover C F, Fitzgerald R G 1981 Marital conflict of manic-depressive patients. Archives of General Psychiatry 38: 65–67

Jacobson N S, Schmaling K B, Salusky S, Follette V, Dobson K 1987 November Marital therapy as an adjunct treatment for depression. Paper presented at the annual meeting of the Association for the Advancement of Behaviour Therapy, Boston, MA

Jacobson N S, Holtzworth-Munroe A, Schmaling K B 1989 Marital therapy and spouse involvement in the treatment of depression, agoraphobia, and alcoholism. Journal of Consulting and Clinical Psychology 57: 5–10

Janowsky D S, Leff M, Epstein R S 1970 Playing the manic game: interpersonal maneuvers of the acutely manic patient. Archives of General Psychiatry 22: 252–261

Kahn J, Coyne J C, Margolin G 1985 Depression and marital conflict: the social construction of despair. Journal of Social and Personal Relationships 2: 447–462

Klerman G, Weissman M M, Rounsaville B J, Chevron E S 1984 Interpersonal psychotherapy of depression. Basic Books, New York

Kowalik D, Gotlib I H 1987 Depression and marital interaction: concordance between intent and perception of communications. Journal of Abnormal Psychology 96: 127–134

Lewinsohn P M, Brown R A 1979 Learning how to control one's depression: an educational approach. Presented at a meeting of the American Psychological Association, New York

Lewinsohn P M, Hoberman H M 1982 Behavioural and cognitive approaches. In: Paykel E S (ed) Handbook of affective disorders. Guilford Press, New York, p 338–345

Lorimy F, Loo H, Deniker P 1977 Effets cliniques des traitements prolonges par les sels de lithium sur le sommeil, l'appetit et la sexualite. Encephale 3: 227–239

McLean P D, Ogston K, Grauer L 1973 Behavioural approach to the treatment of depression. Journal of Behaviour Therapy and Experimental Psychiatry 4: 323–330

Merikangas K R 1984 Divorce and assortative mating among depressed patients. American Journal of Psychiatry 141: 74–76

Merikangas K R, Ranelli C J, Kupfer D J 1979 Marital interaction in hospitalized depressed patients. Journal of Nervous and Mental Disease 167: 689–695

Miklowitz D J, Goldstein M J, Nuechterlein K H, Snyder K S, Mintz J 1988 Family factors and the course of bipolar affective disorder. Archives of General Psychiatry 45: 225–231

Miller I W, Kabacoff R I, Keitner G I, Epstein N B, Bishop D S 1986 Family functioning in the families of psychiatric patients. Comprehensive Psychiatry 27: 302–312

Monroe S M, Bromet E J, Connel M M, Steiner S C 1986 Social support, life events, and depressive symptoms: a one-year prospective study. Journal of Consulting and Clinical Psychology 54: 424–431

O'Connell R A, Mayo J A 1981 Lithium: a biopsychosocial perspective. Comprehensive Psychiatry 22: 87–93

O'Connell R A, Mayo J A 1988 The role of social factors in affective disorders: a review. Hospital and Community Psychiatry 39(8): 842–850

O'Hara M W 1986 Social support, life events, and depression during pregnancy and puerperium. Archives of General Psychiatry 43: 569–573

O'Leary K D, Beach S R H 1990 Marital therapy: a viable treatment for depression and marital discord. American Journal of Psychiatry 147(2): 183–186

Paykel E S, Weissman M M 1973 Social adjustment and depression. Archives of General Psychiatry 28: 659–663

Pearlin L I, Johnson J 1977 Marital status, life strains, and depression. American Sociological Review 42: 704–715

Pilkonis P A, Frank E 1988 Personality pathology in recurrent depression: Nature, prevalence, and relationship to treatment response. American Journal of Psychiatry 145(4): 435–441

Rounsaville B J, Weissman M W, Prusoff B A, Herceg-Baron R L 1979 Marital disputes and treatment outcome in depressed women. Comprehensive Psychiatry 20: 483–490

Sanchez V, Lewinsohn P M 1980 Assertive behaviour and depression. Journal of Consulting and Clinical Psychology 48: 119–120

Shea M T, Glass D R, Pilkonis P A, Watkins J, Docherty J P 1987 Frequency and implications of personality disorders in a sample of depressed outpatients. Journal of Personality Disorders 1(1): 27–42

Targum S D, Dibble E D, Davenport Y B, Gershon E S 1981 The Family Attitudes Questionnaire: patient's and spouses' views of bipolar illness. Archives of General Psychiatry 38: 562–568

Waring E M, Reddon J R 1983 The measurement of intimacy in marriage: the Waring Intimacy Questionnaire. Clinical Psychology 39(1): 53–57

Waring E W, Chamberlaine C H, McCrank E W, Stalker C A, Carver C, Fry R, Barnes S 1988 Dysthymia: a randomized study of cognitive marital therapy and antidepressants. Canadian Journal of Psychiatry 33: 96–99

Weissman M M, Paykel E S 1974 The depressed woman: a study of social relationships. University of Chicago Press, Chicago, IL

Wetzel J W 1978 The work environment and depression: implications for intervention. In Hawks J W (ed) Toward human dignity: social work in practice. NASW Professional Symposium Service, New York

Wetzel J W, Redmond F C 1980 A person – environment study of depression. Social Service Review 54: 363–375

Winokur G, Clayton P J, Reich T 1969 Manic depressive illness. C V Mosby, St Louis, M O

31. Interpersonal psychotherapy

Gerald L. Klerman   Myrna M. Weissman

For decades, there have been debates about the usefulness and efficacy of psychotherapy (Eysenck 1965). Despite the doubts and controversy, a wide variety of psychotherapies have developed and the practice of psychotherapy has flourished, particularly in North America. Parloff et al (1978) identified over 200 different types of psychotherapy used in clinical practice. In a review of the literature, Glass et al (1980) summarized over 400 controlled studies of different psychotherapies and concluded that there was evidence for their efficacy in many disorders (Klerman 1988, Glass et al 1980).

One of the notable developments over the past decade has been the increasing number of controlled clinical trials testing the efficacy of psychotherapy for specific disorders, using methods comparable to those used in the testing of pharmacotherapy (see Weissman et al 1987 for summary). To facilitate these studies, a catalogue of outcome measures has been developed. There has been delineation of therapist characteristics that influence outcome; improved patient specification, usually involving selection according to standardized diagnostic criteria, such as RDC or DSM-III; improved treatment specification through the use of treatment manuals, which standardize the treatment and facilitate the training of therapists; and lastly, improved techniques for training therapists for participation in clinical trials of psychotherapies (Chevron et al 1983). Many of these techniques evolved gradually during the 1960s and 1970s. Almost all have been incorporated in a recent multicentre clinical trial undertaken by the National Institute of Mental Health to test the efficacy of two psychotherapies: cognitive and interpersonal psychotherapy for ambulatory depressed patients (Elkin et al 1989, Beck et al 1979).

For depressive disorders, in particular, the evidence for the efficacy of psychotherapy based on controlled clinical trials has been growing, although the evidence is not as conclusive as that for drug therapy. A number of new psychotherapies specifically for the treatment of depression have been developed (see Weissman 1978, Weissman et al 1987 for reviews). Some studies have included comparisons with medication or the combination of medication and psychotherapy. For a number of treatments, particularly cognitive – behavioural therapy and interpersonal psychotherapy (IPT), manuals have been developed that describe the procedure of the therapy. These new psychotherapies have been the subject of extensive and critical review. See Lewinsohn (1980), Rush (1982), Strupp & Binder (1984), Hersen (1986), Shea et al (1988).

This chapter will review recent developments in interpersonal psychotherapy, which was developed initially for depressed adults. Results of efficacy studies and recent adaptations of IPT for conditions other than major depression, for special populations and presented in different formats will be summarized.

CHARACTERISTICS OF IPT

Development of IPT

IPT was developed initially as a brief (usually 12–16 week), weekly psychotherapeutic treatment for the ambulatory, non-bipolar, non-psychotic depressed patient. It focused on improving the quality of the depressed patient's current interpersonal functioning and identifying the problems associated with the onset of the depressive episode. As will be described, IPT has been adapted for treatment of a longer duration and with different patient populations. IPT can be administered after appropriate training by experienced psychiatrists, psychologists and social workers. It can be used alone or with medication.

IPT has evolved over 20 years of treatment and research experience with ambulatory depressed patients. It has been tested alone and in comparison and in combination with tricyclics in six clinical trials with depressed patients, three of acute treatment (Elkin et al 1989, Sloane et al 1985, Weissman et al 1979); three of maintenance treatment (Klerman et al 1974, Kupfer et al 1989, Reynold & Imber 1988). The Reynold & Imber study is still in progress.

Adaptation of IPT has been developed and tested in a conjoint format for depressed patients with marital disputes (Foley et al 1990); for patients in distress but not clinically depressed (interpersonal counselling, Klerman et al 1987); for long-term maintenance treatment of recurrent depression (Frank et al 1989, 1990b); for the elderly (Frank et al 1988, Reynold & Imber 1988); for opiate addicts (Rounsaville et al 1983); for cocaine abusers (Rounsaville et al 1985); and for bulimia (Fairburn 1988). IPT has been adapted for bipolar patients (Frank et al 1990a), for HIV positive patients with depression (Markowitz & Klerman 1990) and for depressed adolescents (Mufson et al 1990). Trials are being planned for these populations.

Six studies have included a drug comparison group (Elkin et al 1989, Klerman et al 1974, Kupfer et al 1989, Reynold & Imber 1988, Sloane et al 1985, Weissman et al 1979), and four have included a combination of IPT and drugs (Klerman et al 1974, Reynold & Imber 1988, Weissman et al 1979, Kupfer et al 1989).

To standardize the treatment so that clinical trials could be undertaken, the concepts, techniques and methods of IPT have been specified and operationally described in a manual. The manual, which has undergone a number of revisions, is now published in a book (Klerman et al 1984). A training program for experienced psychotherapists of different disciplines providing the treatment for these clinical trials has been developed (Weissman et al 1982). There is, to our knowledge, no ongoing training programme for practitioners, although workshops are available from time to time. The book can serve as a guide for the experienced clinician who wants to learn IPT.

THEORETICAL, EMPIRICAL AND CLINICAL BACKGROUND

IPT derives from a number of theoretical empirical and clinical sources. For a full discussion, see Klerman et al 1984.

Theoretical sources

The ideas of Adolf Meyer, whose psychobiological approach to understanding psychiatric disorders placed great emphasis on the patient's relation to his/her environment, comprise the most prominent theoretical sources for IPT (Meyer 1957). Meyer viewed psychiatric disorders as an expression of the patient's attempt to adapt to his or her environment. An individual's response to environmental change is determined by prior experiences, particularly early experiences in the family and the individual's affiliation with various social groups. Among Meyer's associates, Harry Stack Sullivan stands out for his general theory of interpersonal relationships and for his writings linking clinical psychiatry to the emerging social sciences (Sullivan 1953).

Empirical sources

The empirical basis from which understanding and treating depression with IPT is derived includes the following: studies associating stress and life events with the onset and clinical course of depression; longitudinal studies demonstrating the social impairment of depressed women during the acute depressive phase and the following symptomatic recovery; studies by Brown et al (1977) that demonstrate the role of intimacy and social supports as protection against depression in the face of adverse life stress; and studies by Pearlin & Lieberman (1979) that show the impact of chronic social and interpersonal stress, particularly marital stress, on the onset of depression. The works of Bowlby (1969) and Henderson et al (1978) emphasize the importance of attachment bonds and show that the loss of social attachments can be associated with the onset of depression. Epidemiological data show a strong association between marital disputes and major depression (Weissman 1987).

Depression as conceptualized in IPT

Clinical depression in IPT is seen as involving three component processes:

1. Symptom formation, involving the development of the depressive affect signs and symptoms, which may derive from psychobiological and/or psychodynamic mechanisms

2. Social functioning, involving social interactions with other persons, which derives from learning based on childhood experiences, concurrent social reinforcement, and/or current personal efforts at mastery and competence

3. Personality, involving more enduring traits and behaviours – the handling of anger and guilt and overall self-esteem – that constitute the person's unique reactions and patterns of functioning and which may also contribute to a predisposition to symptom episodes.

IPT, as it was originally developed, intervenes in the first two processes. Because of the brevity of the treatment, the low level of psychotherapeutic intensity and the focus on the current depressive episode, no claim is made that IPT will have an impact on the enduring aspects of personality, although personality functioning is assessed.

Goals of IPT for Depression

IPT develops directly from an interpersonal conceptualization of depression. IPT does not, however, assume that interpersonal problems 'cause' depression but rather, whatever that cause, the current depression occurs in an interpersonal context. The therapeutic strategies of IPT are to understand that context. IPT facilitates recovery from acute depression by relieving depressive symptoms and by helping the patient to become more effective in dealing with current interpersonal problems associated with the onset of symptoms. Symptom relief begins with helping the patient to understand that the vague and uncomfortable symptoms are part of a known syndrome, which responds to various treatments and has a good prognosis. Psychopharmacological approaches may be used in conjunction with IPT to alleviate symptoms more rapidly.

Treating the depressed patient's problems in interpersonal relations proceeds by exploring the four problem areas commonly associated with the onset of depression – grief, role disputes, role transition and interpersonal deficit. The middle phase of IPT then focuses on the particular interpersonal problem as it relates to the onset of depression (Klerman et al 1984).

IPT compared with other psychotherapies

The procedures and techniques of many psychotherapies have much in common. Many therapies emphasize helping the patient to develop a sense of mastery and combatting social isolation. The psychotherapies differ, however, as to whether the patient's problems lie in the far past, the immediate past or the present. IPT focuses primarily on the patient's present; it differs from other psychotherapies in its limited duration, its attention to current depressive symptoms and the current-depression-related interpersonal context. Given this frame of reference, IPT includes a systematic review of the patient's current relations with significant others.

IPT was originally developed as a brief treatment. However, as noted previously, an adaptation with long duration but non-intensive monthly sessions for maintenance treatment for severe recurrent depression has been developed (Frank et al 1989). Although long-term more intensive treatment may still be required for maladaptive interpersonal and cognitive patterns and for ameliorating dysfunctional social skills, evidence for the efficacy of long-term psychotherapy is limited. There are no published clinical trials indicating the efficacy of any psychotherapy for personality problems. Long-term intensive treatment may have the potential disadvantage of promoting dependence and reinforcing avoidance behaviour. Psychotherapies that are short-term with specific goals or long-term but not intensive may minimize these adverse effects for many depressed patients.

IPT is focused and not non-directive, focusing on one or two problem areas in the patient's current interpersonal functioning. The focus is agreed on by the patient and the psychotherapist after initial evaluation sessions. The topical content of sessions is, therefore, not open-ended.

IPT deals with current, not past, interpersonal relationships, focusing on the patient's immediate social context just before and as it has been since the onset of the current depressive episode. Past depressive episodes, early family relationships, previous significant relationships and friendship patterns are assessed however, in order to understand overall patterns in the patient's interpersonal relations. The psychotherapist does not frame the patient's current situation as a manifestation of internal conflict or as a recurrence of prior intrafamilial maladaptive patterns, but rather explores the patient's current disorder behaviour in terms of interpersonal relations.

EFFICACY OF IPT FOR DEPRESSION

Acute treatment

The New Haven—Boston acute treatment study

The first study of IPT for the treatment of acute depression was initiated in 1973. It was a 16-week treatment study of 81 ambulatory depressed patients, both men and women, using IPT and amitriptyline each alone and in combination against a nonscheduled psychotherapy treatment (DiMascio et al 1979, Weissman et al 1979). IPT was administered weekly by experienced psychiatrists. This study demonstrated that both active treatments, IPT and the tricyclic, were more effective than the control treatment and that combined treatment was superior to either treatment. In addition, a 1-year follow-up study provided evidence that the therapeutic benefit of IPT was sustained for many patients. Patients who had received IPT either alone or in combination with drugs were functioning better than patients who had received either drugs alone or the control treatment (Weissman et al 1981). There was no effect on symptom relapse or recurrence. A fraction of patients in all treatments relapsed and additional treatment was required.

National Institute of Mental Health (NIMH) study

For ambulatory depressed patients, a multicentre controlled clinical trial of drugs and two psychotherapies, cognitive – behavioural therapy and IPT, in the treatment of acute ambulatory depression was initiated by the NIMH (Elkin et al 1989). 250 outpatients were randomly assigned to four treatment conditions for 16 weeks: cognitive therapy, IPT, imipramine and a placebo – clinical-management combination. Extensive efforts were made in the selection and training of the psychotherapists. Of the 250 patients who entered treatment, 68% completed at least 15 weeks and 12 sessions of treatment. Overall, the findings showed that all active treatments were superior to placebo in the reduction of symptoms over a 16-week period (Elkin et al 1989). The overall degree of improvement for all patients, regardless of treatment, was highly significant clinically. Over half of the patients were symptom-free at the end of treatment.

More patients in the placebo – clinical-management combination dropped out or were withdrawn, twice as many as for IPT, which had the lowest attrition rate. At the end of 12 weeks of treatment, the two psychotherapies and imipramine were equivalent in the reduction of depressive symptoms on many measures. Imipramine had a more rapid initial onset of action and more consistent differences from placebo than either of the two psychotherapies. Although many of the patients who were less severely depressed at intake improved with all treatment conditions, including the placebo

group, more severely depressed patients in the placebo group did poorly. For the less severely depressed group, there were no differences among the treatments.

44% of the sample were moderately depressed at intake. For the more severe group (Hamilton Rating Scale for Depression score of 20 or more at intake), patients in the IPT and the imipramine groups had better outcome scores on the Hamilton Scale than the placebo group. Of the psychotherapies, only IPT was significantly superior to placebo for the severely depressed group. For the severely depressed patients IPT did as well as imipramine on some outcome measures. More information on this study is still forthcoming.

Acutely depressed elderly patients

Sloane et al (1985) completed a 6-week pilot trial of IPT versus nortriptyline in 30 elderly depressed patients. They found partial evidence for the efficacy of IPT over drug, primarily because many elderly could not tolerate the side effects of the medication and dropped out early.

Maintenance treatment

The New Haven—Boston maintenance treatment study

The first systematic study of IPT began in 1967 and was of maintenance treatment (Klerman et al 1974, Paykel et al 1976). By today's standards, this study would be considered a continuation study. In 1967, it was clear that the tricyclic antidepressants were efficacious in the treatment of acute depression. It was unclear how long treatment should continue and what the role of psychotherapy was in maintenance treatment. This first study of IPT was designed to answer those questions.

150 acutely depressed outpatients who had responded to amitriptyline with symptom reduction were studied. Each patient received 8 months of maintenance treatment with drugs alone, psychotherapy (IPT) alone or a combination of both. The major findings were that maintenance drug treatment prevented relapse and symptom worsening (Klerman et al 1974, Paykel et al 1975) and the effect of IPT was to enhance social functioning (Weissman et al 1974). Moreover, the effects of psychotherapy were not apparent for 6–8 months. Because of the differential effects of the treatments, the combination of drugs and psychotherapy was the most efficacious (Paykel et al

1976, Klerman et al 1974), and no negative interactions between drugs and psychotherapy were found.

Long-term maintenance treatment for recurrent depressions (IPT-M)

Frank et al (1989) have modified IPT in a maintenance form (IPT-M) to deal with patients who have serious recurrent depressions. They have recently completed a clinical trial of five treatments: IPT maintenance (IPT-M) offered alone; with active imipramine treatment; with placebo; a medication clinic visit with imipramine; and a medication clinic visit with a placebo administration. Initial findings over the first 18 months were published in 1989. The authors noted that interpersonal psychotherapy was significantly related to a longer survival time in treatment (Kupfer et al 1989).

The first results of the full study, which included 128 patients treated over 3 years, were reported at the end of 1990 (Frank et al 1990b). The results showed that imipramine at an average dose of 200 µg was associated with a mean survival time of almost $2\frac{1}{2}$ years and was significantly better than placebo. While IPT added to imipramine did not improve this outcome in patients who were receiving medication, IPT was associated with significantly longer mean survival time (74–82 weeks) than medication clinic visits (45 weeks) among patients assigned to placebo or no pill conditions. Of interest is the fact that the positive result of IPT was shown even with the low doses of only monthly contact. Further results of this important study, particularly the effects of treatment on social functioning, will be forthcoming.

ADAPTATIONS OF IPT

Thus far, this chapter has reviewed the development of IPT for depression and summarized the evidence from systematic controlled studies of its efficacy in the treatment of acute depressive episodes as well as in continuation and maintenance treatment for the prevention of relapse and recurrence. At the same time, a number of investigators have adapted IPT for use in other patient populations or in other formats. In this section we will review these adaptations.

Conjoint IPT for depressed patients with marital disputes (IPT-CM)

Although the direction of causality may be complex, clinical and epidemiological studies have shown that marital disputes, separation and divorce are strongly associated with the onset of depression (Rounsaville et al 1979, 1980). When psychotherapy is prescribed, it is unclear whether the patient, the couple or the entire family should be involved. Some evidence suggests that individual psychotherapy for depressed patients involved in marital disputes may promote premature separation or divorce (Gurman & Kniskern 1978, Locke & Wallace 1976). There have been no published clinical trials comparing the efficacy of individual versus conjoint psychotherapy for depressed patients with marital problems.

Individual IPT was adapted to the treatment of depression in the context of marital disputes by concentrating on the treatment of interpersonal marital disputes. A treatment manual and a training programme like those used in IPT were developed for IPT-CM in the initial phase of this study.

Only patients who identified marital disputes as the major problem associated with the onset or exacerbation of their major depression were admitted into a pilot study. 18 patients were randomly assigned to IPT or IPT-CM and received 16 weekly therapy sessions. In IPT-CM, the spouse was required to participate in all psychotherapy sessions, whereas in IPT the spouse did not meet with the therapist. At the end of treatment, patients in both groups expressed satisfaction with the treatment and exhibited a significant reduction in symptoms of depression and social impairment from intake to termination of therapy. There was no significant difference between treatment groups in the degree of improvement in depressive symptoms and social functioning by end-point (Foley et al 1990).

However, Locke – Wallace Marital Adjustment Test scores (Locke & Wallace 1976) at session 16 were significantly higher (indicative of better marital adjustment) for patients receiving IPT-CM than for patients receiving IPT. Scores on the Spanier Duadic Adjustment Scale (Spanier 1976) also indicated greater improvement in marital functioning for patients receiving IPT-CM than for patients receiving IPT. At session 16, patients receiving IPT-CM reported significantly higher levels in affectional expression (i.e. demonstrations of affection and sexual relations in the marriage) than patients receiving IPT.

The results need to be interpreted with caution due to the pilot nature of the study – the small size of the sample, the lack of a no-treatment control group and the absence of a pharmacotherapy or a combined pharmacotherapy – psychotherapy comparison group. If the study were repeated, we would recommend that medication be freely allowed or used as a comparison condition and that there be more effort to reduce the symptoms of depression before proceeding to undertake the marital issue. Perhaps a sequential design would be useful, with initial treatment of medication to produce symptom reduction and the psychotherapy coming into effect as symptom reduction was proved to be effective.

Interpersonal counselling for stress or distress in primary care (IPC)

Previous investigations have documented high frequencies of anxiety, depression and functional bodily complaints in patients in primary-care medical settings (Brodaty & Andrews 1983, Goldberg 1972). Although some of these patients have diagnosable psychiatric disorders, a large percentage have symptoms that do not meet established criteria for psychiatric disorders. A mental health research programme formed in a large health maintenance organization in the greater Boston area found that 'problems of living' and symptoms of anxiety and depression were among the main reasons for individual primary-care visits. These clinical problems contribute heavily to high utilization of ambulatory services.

A brief psychosocial intervention, interpersonal counselling (IPC), was modified from IPT to deal with patients' symptoms of distress and was administered by nurse practitioners working in a primary-care setting. IPC comprises a maximum of six half-hour counselling sessions in the primary-care office, which focus on the patient's current functioning (Weissman & Klerman 1988). Particular attention is given to recent changes in life events, sources of stress in the family, home, and workplace, friendship patterns and ongoing difficulties in interpersonal relations. IPC assumes that such events provide the interpersonal context in which bodily and emotional symptoms related to anxiety, depression and distress occur. The treatment manual includes session-by-session instructions as to the purpose and methods for IPC, including 'scripts' to ensure comparability of procedures among the nurse counsellors.

Patients with scores of 6 or higher on the Goldberg General Health Questionnaire (GHQ; Goldberg 1972) were selected for assignment to an experimental group that was offered IPC or to a comparison group that was followed naturalistically (Klerman et al 1987). 64 patients were compared with a subgroup of 64 sex-matched untreated subjects with similar elevations in GHQ scores. Compared with a group of untreated subjects with initial elevations in GHQ scores, patients receiving the IPC intervention showed greater reduction in symptom scores over an average interval of 3 months. Many IPC-treated patients reported relief of symptoms after only one or two sessions. This study provided preliminary evidence that early detection and outreach to distressed adults, followed by brief treatment with IPC, can, in the short term, reduce symptoms of distress as measured by the GHQ. The main effect seems to occur in symptoms related to mood, especially in those forms of mild and moderate depression that are commonly seen in medical patients. However, IPC did not result in reduction of utilization of health-care services. In fact, there was an increase in use of mental health services as patients began to clarify the psychological source of their symptoms. Definitive evaluation of IPC awaits further study.

Depressed adolescents (IPT-A)

Despite the high prevalence of depression in adolescents and the associated suicidal risk and social morbidity, evidence for the efficacy of treatment is nearly absent. The few clinical trials testing the efficacy of pharmacotherapy in this age group have not demonstrated their effectiveness. While psychotherapy is widely used for depressed adolescents, there is not one published clinical trial testing the efficacy of any psychotherapy in this population. In order to carry out a pilot controlled clinical trial of interpersonal psychotherapy, IPT has been modified by Mufson and colleagues (Mufson et al 1990) for this age group.

The goals and techniques of IPT-A, including methods for diagnosing and educating the patient about depression and the specific strategies for dealing with the four problem areas commonly associated with the onset of depression in adults, have been maintained. The manual has been modified for adolescents by adding a fifth problem area, the single parent family, because of this frequent occurrence of problematic nature in adolescents. The treatment has been adapted to address developmental issues most common in adolescents, which include separation from parents, exploration of authority in relationship to parents, development of heterosexual relationships, initial experience with death of relative or friend and peer pressures. A pilot clinical trial is planned.

Recurrent late-life depression (IPT-LLM)

The problem of administering medication in the

elderly, particularly the anticholinergic effects, has led to the interest in psychotherapy in this age-group. Sloane et al (1985), as noted before, completed a 6-week pilot trial of IPT compared with nortriptyline and placebo for acute treatment in depresssed elderly patients. The Sloane group did not specifically modify their manual for the elderly. A more comprehensive study following the design of the Kupfer and Frank maintenance trial is underway at the University of Pittsburgh for recurrent late-life depression (IPT LLM) (Reynold & Imber 1988). Moreover, IPT has been explicitly modified for this study to deal with the special issues of the elderly patient with recurrent depression (Frank et al 1988).

Depressed patients at risk for AIDS – HIV seropositive (IPT-HIV)

While considerable psychosocial stress is faced by patients who are seropositive for the human immunodeficiency virus (HIV), and many diverse interventions have been proposed (including cognitive – behavioural therapy, aerobic exercise, relaxation training), clinical trials of psychological treatments are largely absent.

Noting that individuals affected with HIV are at risk for depression, the investigators have argued that they may be candidates for IPT. They are developing a manual to deal with the special issues of these patients and have completed a pilot open trial with 21 depressed subjects at risk for AIDS by virtue of being HIV seropositive. The authors note that the discovery of HIV seropositivity is a calamitous life event with significant interpersonal and personal repercussions. The four problem areas identified in IPT for depressed patients, they note, can easily describe the problems faced by HIV patients. They felt that the 'here and now' framework of IPT helped maintain a hopeful focus in the face of lethal infection, implying to the patient that life was not over. They avoid encouraging depressive ruminations on the there-and-then, including self-blame for contracting HIV.

Based on an open trial with 21 HIV patients, all homosexual or bisexual, the investigators have described their experience in treating the patients in terms of the four problem areas of IPT (Markowitz & Klerman, submitted).

Bipolar patients (IPT-BP)

IPT has been adapted for use in a clinical trial with bipolar patients by Frank and associates (1990a) at the University of Pittsburgh. The goals of both IPT and IPT-BP are the management of affective symptoms and interpersonal difficulties facing the patient. However, in contrast to IPT, the bipolar adaptation places considerably more emphasis on the management of symptoms. This emphasis persists throughout the maintenance treatment phase that has been planned. IPT-BP addresses somewhat different aspects of role transitions and role disputes, and constantly explores the interaction between changes in the interpersonal realm and symptoms. Preventive strategies include exploration of sources of interpersonal distress: frequency and intensity of social interactions, and overstimulation, such as the timing and regularity of sleep, work and other social rhythms. The goal is to regulate social rhythms in order to keep the patient's social triggers for disruption under control. Other than these modifications, the goals and strategies of IPT, including the four problem areas, have been kept intact. The Frank group is planning a maintenance clinical trial for bipolar patients fashioned after their study of persons with recurrent unipolar depression.

Bulimia nervosa

Fairburn (1988), at Oxford University, has adapted IPT for patients with bulimia nervosa. The modifications for bulimia are only for the first phase of treatment. The first four sessions are devoted to analysis of the interpersonal context of the development and maintenance of bulimia (Fairburn 1988, Fairburn et al in press). A clinical trial comparing cognitive and behavioural treatments and IPT in 75 patients over an 18-week period was recently completed. Patients with bulimia in all treatments showed a decrease in the level of general psychopathology, frequency of overeating and number of bulimic episodes. Cognitive – behavioural therapy was more effective in reducing frequency of self-induced vomiting and extreme dieting and in modifying attitudes towards shape and weight. This study did not have a no-treatment control group because the authors argue that previous studies show that patients with bulimia do not improve on waiting lists. Additionally, the results reported above are based on a sample of completers, which could affect results. Data on a 1-year follow-up are forthcoming.

Methadone-maintained opiate addicts

Based on the observation that methadone maintenance

programmes with and without loosely-defined counselling services have shown a trend for counselling to be associated with better programme retention or completion, Rounsaville et al (1983, Rounsaville & Kleber 1985) developed a clinical trial to evaluate short-term interpersonal psychotherapy as treatment for psychiatric disorders in opiate addicts who were also participating in a full-service methadone hydrochloride maintenance programme. Patients were randomly assigned to treatment and were compared with low-contact monthly treatment. All patients continued in the usual methadone programme.

The IPT consisted of a weekly, individual, short-term treatment. The IPT manual for depression with minor modifications was used for the opiate addicts. 72 opiate addicts randomly assigned to one of the two groups participated in the study. However, recruitment was a serious problem, as only 5% of the eligible addicts agreed to participate and only around half of them completed the study treatment. The outcome was similar in the two groups. Both obtained significant clinical improvement. Only 38% of the patients completed IPT and 54% completed the low-contact condition. The authors concluded that weekly IPT added to the usual drug rehabilitation programme does not offer any further benefits to opiate addicts. The patients were already receiving relatively intensive treatment, at least one 90-minute group psychotherapy session per week, in addition to daily contacts for urine specimens and meeting with the programme counsellor as needed. Thus, the once-a-week individual treatment, in which talking was required, seems to offer very little over and above the already intensive treatment. The authors also note that IPT, which has a short-term focus on one or two limited problems, may be at variance with the framework of a methadone maintenance programme, which is seen as comparatively long-term treatment. Most of the clients continued to be involved in the methadone programme following termination of psychotherapy.

Cocaine addicts

Rounsaville et al (1985) have also revised IPT for application to cocaine abusers. The goals in the adaptation were reduction or cessation of cocaine use and development of more productive strategies for dealing with social and interpersonal problems associated with the onset and perpetuation of cocaine use. The therapist's stance and phases of treatment were not changed in the adaptation. The focus on depressive symptoms was changed to a focus on reducing cocaine use. 42 outpatients who met DMS-III criteria for cocaine abuse were randomly assigned to one of two forms of psychotherapy, either relapse prevention RPT (a structured behavioural approach) or IPT for 12 weeks. Overall, there were no significant differences between treatments on continuous weeks of abstinence or recovery (Carroll et al, submitted). The trend was for greater efficacy of the behavioural approach when patients were stratified by initial severity of substance use. Among the more severe users, patients who received RPT as compared with IPT were significantly more likely to achieve abstinence and to be classified as recovered. The authors conclude that psychotherapy may be effective for many ambulatory cocaine abusers, but that severe abusers may require greater structure and direction offered by a treatment emphasizing learning and rehearsal of specific strategies to interrupt and control cocaine abuse.

CONCLUSION

The best results and the most trials of IPT have been for the ambulatory depressed patient, either as acute as maintenance treatment. The findings for conjoint marital treatment, for patients in primary care in distress and for persons with bulimia are promising, but the results are still based on small samples. Adaptation and testing of IPT for geriatric patients with recurrent depression, adolescents, HIV-seropositive patients and bipolar patients are still in development. The findings on IPT as a treatment for drug abusers, either cocaine or opiate addicts, are negative.

Obviously, many treatments may be suitable for depression. The depressed patient's interests are best served by the availability and scientific testing of different psychological as well as pharmacological treatments to be used alone or in combination. Ultimately, clinical testing and experience will determine which is the best treatment for particular kinds of patient.

Although the positive findings of the clinical trials of IPT in the NIMH Collaborative Study and the other studies described are encouraging, we emphasize a number of limitations in the possible conclusion regarding the place of psychotherapy in the treatment of depression. All the studies, including those by our group and by the NIMH, were conducted on ambulatory depressed patients. Moreover, these results should not be interpreted as implying that all forms of psychotherapy are effective for depression or, alternatively, that only IPT is effective. One significant feature of recent advances in psychotherapy research is in the development of psychotherapies specifically designed for depression – time-limited and of brief duration. Just as there are specific forms of medication, there are specific forms of psychotherapy. It would be an error to conclude that all forms of medication are useful for all types of depression; so it would be an error to conclude that all forms of psychotherapy are efficacious for all forms of depression.

REFERENCES

Beck A T, Rush A J, Shaw B F, Emery G 1979 Cognitive theory of depression. Guilford Press, New York

Bowlby J 1969 Attachment and loss. Hogath Press, London, vol 1

Brodaty H, Andrews G 1983 Brief psychotherapy in family practice: a controlled perspective intervention trial. British Journal of Pyschiatry 143: 11–19

Brown G W, Harris T, Copeland J R 1977 Depression and loss. British Journal of Psychiatry 130: 1–18

Carroll K M, Rounsaville B J, Gawin F H (submitted) A comparative trial of psychotherapies for ambulatory cocaine abusers: relapse prevention and interpersonal psychotherapy.

Chevron E, Rounsaville B, Rothblum E D, Weissman M M 1983 Selecting psychotherapies to participate in psychotherapy outcome studies: relationship between psychotherapist characteristics and assessment of clinical skills. Journal of Nervous and Mental Disease 171: 348–353

DiMascio A, Weissman M M, Prusoff B A, New C, Zwilling M, Klerman G L 1979 Differential symptom reduction by drugs and psychotherapy in acute depression. Archives of General Psychiatry 36: 1450–1456

Elkin I, Shea M T, Watkins J T, Imber S D, Sotsky S M, Collins J F, Glass D R, Pilkonis P A, Leber W R, Docherty J P, Fiester S J, Parloff M B 1989 National Institute of Mental Health Treatment of Depression Collaborative Research Program: general effectiveness of treatment. Archives of General Psychiatry 46: 971–983

Eysenck J 1965 The effects of psychotherapy. International Journal of Psychiatry 1: 99

Fairburn C G 1988 The current status of the psychological treatments for bulimia nervosa. Journal of Psychosomatic Research 32 (6): 635–645

Fairburn C G, Jones R, Peveler R C, Carr S J, Solomon R A, O'Connor M E, Burton J, Hope R A (in press) Three psychological treatments for bulimia nervosa: a comparative trial. Archives of General Psychiatry

Foley S H, Rounsaville B J, Weissman M M et al 1990 Individual versus conjoint interpersonal psychotherapy for depressed patients with marital disputes. International Journal of Family Psychiatry 10: 1–2

Frank E, Frank N, Reynold C F 1988 Manual for the adaptation of interpersonal psychotherapy to maintenance treatment of recurrent depression in late life (IPT-LLM). University of Pittsburgh School of Medicine, Pittsburgh, PA

Frank E, Kupfer D J, Perel J M 1989 Early recurrence in unipolar depression. Archives of General Psychiatry 46: 397–400

Frank E, Kupfer D J, Cornes C, Carter S, Frankel D 1990a Manual for the adaptation of interpersonal psychotherapy to the treatment of bipolar disorder (IPT-BP). University of Pittsburgh School of Medicine, Pittsburgh, PA

Frank E, Kupfer D J, Perel J M, Cornes C, Jarrett D B, Mallinger A G, Thase M E, McEachran A B, Grochocinski V J 1990b Three-year outcomes for maintenance therapies in recurrent depression. Archives of General Psychiatry 47: 1093–1099

Glass G V, Smith M L, Miller N 1980 The benefits of psychotherapy. Johns Hopkins University Press, Baltimore, MD

Goldberg D P 1972 The detection of psychiatric illness by questionnaire. Institute of Psychiatry Maudsley Monographs 21. Oxford University Press, Oxford

Gurman A S, Kniskern D P 1978 Research on marital and family therapy. Progress, perspective and prospect. In: Garfield S B, Bergen A B (eds) Handbook of psychotherapy and behaviour change. John Wiley, New York, p 817–902

Henderson S, Byrne D G, Duncan-Jones P, Adcock S, Scott R, Steele G P 1978 Social bonds in the epidemiology of neurosis. British Journal of Psychiatry 132: 463–466

Hersen M 1986 Pharmacological and behavioural treatment: an integrative approach. John Wiley, New York

Klerman G L 1983 Psychotherapies and somatic therapies in affective disorders. In: Akiskal H (ed) Psychiatric clinics of North America 6. W B Saunders, Philadelphia, p 85–103

Klerman G L 1988 Drugs and psychotherapy. In: Garfield S B, Bergen A B (eds) Handbook of psychotherapy and behaviour change. John Wiley, New York, pp 773–814

Klerman G L DiMascio A, Weissman M M, Prusoff B, Paykel E S 1974 Treatment of depression by drugs and psychotherapy. Americal Journal of Psychiatry 131: 186–194

Klerman G L, Weissman M M, Rounsaville B J, Chevron E S 1984 Interpersonal psychotherapy for depression. Basic Books, New York

Klerman G L, Budman S, Berwick D, Weissman M M, Damico-White J, Demby A, Feldstein M 1987 Efficacy of a brief psychosocial intervention for symptoms of stress and distress among patients in primary care. Medical Care 25: 1078–1088

Kupfer D J, Frank E, Perel J M 1989 The advantage of early treatment intervention in recurrent depression. Archives of General Psychiatry 46: 771–775

Lewinsohn P M 1980 A behavioural approach to depression. In: Friedman R J, Katz M M (eds) The psychology of depression: contemporary theory and research. John Wiley, Washington, DC

Locke H J, Wallace K M 1976 Short-term marital adjustment and prediction tests: their reliability and validity. Marriage and Family Living 38: 15–25

Markovitz J C, Klerman G L (submitted) Interpersonal psychotherapy of depressed patients at risk for AIDS.

Meyer A 1957 Psychobiology: a science of man. C C Thomas, Springfield, IL

Mufson L, Moreau D, Weissman M M, Klerman G L 1990 Interpersonal psychotherapy for depressed adolescents (ITP-A). Unpublished document, College of Physicians and Surgeons, Columbia University and Cornell Medical School, New York

Parloff M B, Wolfe B E, Washkow I E, Hadley S 1978 Assessment of psychosocial treatment of mental disorders: current status and prospects. Institute of Medicine, Washington, DC

Paykel E S, DiMascio A, Haskell D, Prusoff B A 1975 Effects of maintenance amitriptyline and psychotherapy on symptoms of depression. Psychological Medicine 5: 67–77

Paykel E S, DiMascio A, Klerman G L, Prusoff B A, Weissman M M 1976 Maintenance therapy of depression. Pharmakopsychiatrie und Neuropsychopharmakologie 9: 127–136

Pearlin L I, Lieberman M A 1979 Social sources of emotional distress. In: Simmons R (ed) Research in community and mental health. JAI 1: 217–248

Reynold C, Imber S 1988 Protocol. University of Pittsburgh, Pittsburgh, PA

Rounsaville B J, Kleber H D 1985 Psychotherapy/counselling for opiate addicts: strategies for use in different treatment settings. International Journal of Addiction 20 (6&7): 868–896

Rounsaville B J, Weissman M M, Prusoff B A et al 1979 Marital disputes and treatment outcome in depressed women. Comprehensive Psychiatry 20: 483–490

Rounsaville B J, Prusoff B A, Weissman M M 1980 The course of marital disputes in depressed women: a 48 month follow-up study. Comprehensive Psychiatry 21: 111–118

Rounsaville B J, Glazer W, Wilber C H, Weissman M M, Kleber H D 1983 Short-term interpersonal psychotherapy in methadone-maintained opiate addicts. Archives of General Psychiatry 40: 629–636

Rounsaville B J, Gawin F, Kleber H 1985 Interpersonal psychotherapy adapted for ambulatory cocaine abusers. American Journal of Drug and Alcohol Abuse 11 (3&4): 171–191

Rush A J 1982 Short-term psychotherapies for depression. Guilford Press, New York

Shea M T, Elkin I, Hirschfeld R M A 1988 Psychotherapeutic treatment of depression. In: Frances A J, Hales R E (eds) American Psychiatric Association review of psychiatry.

American Psychiatric Press, Washington, DC, vol 7, p 235–255

Sloane R B, Stapes F R, Schneider L S 1985 Interpersonal therapy versus nortriptyline for depression in the elderly. In: Burrow G D, Norman T R, Dennerstein L (eds) Clinical and pharmacological studies in psychiatric disorders. John Libbey, London, p 344–346

Spanier G B 1976 Measuring dyadic adjustment: new scales for assessing the quality of marriage and similar dyads. Journal of Marriage and Family Living 38: 15–25

Strupp H H, Binder J L 1984 Psychotherapy in a new key. Basic Books, New York

Sullivan H S 1953 The interpersonal theory of psychiatry. W W Norton, New York

Weissman M M 1979 The psychological treatment of depression: research evidence for the efficacy of psychotherapy alone, in comparison, and in combination with pharmacotherapy. Archives of General Psychiatry 36: 1261–1269

Weissman M M 1987 Advances in psychiatric epidemiology: rates and risks for major depression. American Journal of Public Health 77: 445–451

Weissman M M, Klerman G L, Paykel E S, Prusoff B A, Hanson B 1974 Treatment effects on the social adjustment of depressed patients. Archives of General Psychiatry 30: 771–778

Weissman M M, Prusoff B A, DiMascio A et al 1979 The efficacy of drugs and psychotherapy in the treatment of acute depressive episodes. American Journal of Psychiatry 136: 555–558

Weissman M M, Klerman G L, Prusoff B A et al 1981 Depressed outpatients: results one year after treatment with drugs and/or interpersonal psychotherapy. Archives of General Psychiatry 38: 52–55

Weissman M M, Rounsaville B J, Chevron E S 1982 Training psychotherapists to participate in psychotherapy outcome studies: identifying and dealing with the research requirement. American Journal of Psychiatry 139: 1442–1446

Weissman M M, Jarrett R B, Rush J A 1987 Psychotherapy and its relevance to the pharmacotherapy of major depression: a decade later (1976–1985). In: DiMascio A, Killam K F (eds) Psychopharmacology: the third generation of progress. Raven Press, New York, p 1059–1069

32. Cognitive therapy

David A. F. Haaga   Aaron T. Beck

This chapter describes the outpatient treatment of unipolar major depression with cognitive therapy (CT; Beck 1964). We begin by reviewing the theory of depression on which CT is based and then describe the treatment itself and its empirical status, concluding with a discussion of extensions of CT to inpatient treatment and to bipolar disorder.

COGNITIVE THEORY OF DEPRESSION

Recent elaborations of cognitive theory of depression (Beck 1987) differ somewhat from earlier formulations, which has prompted some confusion in the literature. In this section, to create a context for our description of CT, we describe cognitive theory of depression, show how it has evolved from earlier versions and summarize its empirical status.

Description

The proposals of cognitive theory regarding *descriptive* aspects of depression must be distinguished from its claims about *causes* of depression.

Descriptive model

According to the theory, people experiencing a depressive episode show a cognitive triad: automatic thoughts reflecting themes of loss and revealing negative views of the *self*, the *world* and the *future*. 'Automatic' refers here to thoughts that are repetitive, unintended and not readily controllable. The cognitive triad is considered characteristic of all depressions, regardless of clinical subtype. Subtype distinctions are important for causal aspects of cognitive theory, but according to the theory once someone becomes depressed, for whatever reason, cognitive content is similar. Moreover, these negative automatic thoughts are believed to be sustained by information-processing biases such as selective memory for negative material, overgeneralization of the implications of negative events and dichotomous thinking (e.g. regarding experiences as either all good or all bad, rather than recognizing partial successes).

The negative automatic thoughts just described are sometimes referred to in cognitive theory as 'cognitions'. Thus, depressotypic 'cognitions' are viewed as a characteristic of depression, not as a cause of depression. In other words, 'It seems unwarranted to assert that "cognitions cause depression". Such statements would be akin to saying that "delusions cause psychosis"' (Beck 1987, p 10). This non-causal status of cognitions in cognitive theory is often misunderstood, possibly because there is not a consensus on usage of the term 'cognitions'.

Causal model

Cognitive theory contends that the negative cognitions apparent during depressive episodes are surface manifestations of depressive schemas (or 'basic beliefs') that have been activated by stress (Kovacs & Beck 1978). For example, a person holding the belief that 'If I am not perfectly successful, then I am a nobody' would be expected to show negative cognitions ('automatic thoughts') and depressed mood after a failure at work. Dysfunctional beliefs are thus hypothesized diatheses for depression (Riskind & Rholes 1984). They are expected to be latent (i.e. not directly influencing mood and not readily available to awareness) prior to activation as a result of stress.

The personality modes of *sociotropy* and *autonomy* (Beck 1983) specify the types of stressors predicted to activate dysfunctional beliefs in a given depression-prone person. Sociotropy is defined as placing a high value on 'positive interchange with others, focusing on acceptance, intimacy, support and guidance' (Beck et al

1983, p 3). Autonomy, on the other hand, is defined as placing a high value on 'independent functioning, mobility, choice, achievement, and integrity of one's domain' (Beck et al 1983, p 3). Stressors that are congruent with a highly-developed personality mode (e.g. personal rejection for someone high in sociotropy) are expected to activate dysfunctional beliefs about the meaning of the stressor and thus lead to negative cognitions and depression.

In short, cognitive theory hypothesizes that non-endogenous unipolar depressions result from the interaction of: 1) *dysfunctional beliefs* about the meaning of certain types of experiences; 2) *high subjective value* attached to the importance of these experiences (stemming from one's personality mode); and 3) *occurrence of apt stressors* (viewed as important by the patient and impinging on his or her cognitive vulnerabilities).

It is important to underscore the point that this causal analysis pertains specifically to *non-endogenous ('reactive') unipolar depression*, not necessarily all depressions. As noted by Beck (1987), 'the longitudinal cognitive model should probably be restricted to the so-called reactive depressions; that is, those that are brought about by socially relevant events. We would then postulate that although the *negative cognitive processing* is similar for all types of depression, the factors precipitating the various disorders vary widely' (p 24, emphasis in original).

Evolution from earlier presentations

In many ways, the theory just outlined is consistent with even the earliest formulations of cognitive theory (e.g. Beck 1963). The most important change is the postulate that sociotropy and autonomy create specific vulnerabilities to different types of stressors as precipitants of depressive episodes (Beck 1983, Beck et al 1983). This hypothesis was influenced by Bowlby's (1977) work on disruption of social bonds as a precipitant of depression. It was observed clinically that another subtype of depressed patient (i.e. the highly autonomous) did not seem to fit the picture painted by Bowlby's theory.

More generally, reviewers (e.g. Coyne & Gotlib 1983, Krantz 1985) had pointed out that earlier versions of cognitive theory appeared to pay insufficient attention to the nature of the stressful circumstances often faced by depressed people (e.g. marital distress, loss experiences). Current cognitive theory acknowledges the importance of environmental stressors while still emphasizing individual differences in dysfunctional

beliefs as a determinant of which people will attach depressive *meanings* to these stressors and thereby become hopeless, self-critical and depressed.

Empirical status

The empirical status of cognitive theory of depression is controversial. Research concerning the theory has been cited as yielding mainly negative conclusions about the validity of its causal hypotheses (as opposed to its descriptive claims about depressive thinking; Coyne & Gotlib 1983), as promising and mostly supportive (e.g. Segal & Shaw 1986) and as conceptually and methodologically flawed and therefore inconclusive (e.g. Abramson et al 1988).

Although it is beyond the scope of this chapter to review this research in detail, a sense of the empirical fate of the theory is relevant to understanding cognitive therapy. In general, the theory's descriptive account of depressive thinking seems accurate. For example, depressed people routinely report more negative cognitions than do non-depressed people (e.g. Crandell & Chambless 1986) and in particular hold a more negative view of themselves (e.g. Bradley & Mathews 1988), their future prospects (e.g. Hamilton & Abramson 1983) and their personal world (e.g. Blackburn et al 1986b) than do the nondepressed. Negative cognitions, as predicted, appear to be equivalent across clinical subtypes of depression (e.g. Hollon et al 1986) and discriminate depressed patients from anxiety disorder (e.g. Beck et al 1987) and heterogeneous psychiatric (e.g. Dobson & Shaw 1986) control groups.

On the other hand, the notion that dysfunctional beliefs are stable, pre-existing vulnerability factors in reactive depression has to date received little empirical support (Barnett & Gotlib 1988). For instance, measures of dysfunctional beliefs are typically at normal levels in completely remitted depressed patients (e.g. Peselow et al 1990) and thus appear to be state-dependent depression features. Longitudinal research on depression relapse has provided some support for specific interactional predictions about personality modes and matching type of stressful events, but results have been inconsistent with regard to which mode (sociotropy; Segal et al 1989: or autonomy; Hammen et al 1989) is useful in predicting relapse.

Most studies of causal aspects of cognitive theory, though, have failed to consider that dysfunctional beliefs are hypothesized to be latent, unless primed by an apt stressor, when a person is not in a depressive episode. As such, these studies may not have provided powerful tests of cognitive theory's predictions. Miranda & Persons (1988) found that induction of negative mood elevated scores on a measure of dysfunctional beliefs only among people with a history of depression. This result implies that enduring cognitive vulnerability to depression may exist but may only be detectable if subjects are exposed to a stress or priming manipulation.

In sum, empirical research has provided consistent support for the descriptive account of depressive thinking offered in cognitive theory. By contrast, the theory's causal formulations have not been strongly supported in research, though these hypotheses may fare better in research taking fully into account their methodological implications (e.g. the need to prime tacit cognitive vulnerabilities in a non-depressed period).

COGNITIVE THERAPY OF DEPRESSION

Description

CT for depression is a brief, structured, directive treatment designed to alter the dysfunctional beliefs and negative automatic thoughts typical of depression. CT is prototypically conducted with outpatients in about 20 sessions over the course of 12–16 weeks, but length of treatment can vary considerably, depending on patient and therapist styles.

The structure of CT sessions is distinctive in several ways. First, cognitive therapists regularly solicit feedback from the patient about the conclusions she or he has drawn from the discussion as well as any reactions to the therapy or therapist. This technique illustrates the emphasis in CT on collaboration between therapist and patient and models the habit of viewing one's inferences as hypotheses and seeking evidence to test them. That is, the therapist does not assume knowledge of the patient's reaction to sessions but rather enquires about it.

Second, CT sessions typically start with the establishment of an agenda of topics for the session. This procedure is used to demonstrate the value of focusing and setting priorities so as to use time efficiently in treatment. Agenda-setting can also provide a concrete framework in which to realize one of the overarching process goals of CT, a shift of responsibility for treatment from therapist to patient. In early sessions the therapist might list several points to be covered in the session and ask if the patient has anything to add. This

balance would switch gradually until the patient is largely responsible for the agenda. Calling attention periodically to such shifts in responsibility might facilitate the patient's making internal attributions for treatment-related improvements, which in turn seem to be associated with enhanced maintenance of therapeutic change (Brehm & Smith 1986).

In the early stages of CT it is important to teach a cognitive rationale for depression and its treatment. The patient's own thoughts can be used to illustrate the model. For example, if the patient felt disheartened before a session, one might ask what thoughts were associated with this feeling. Responses to this inquiry could help demonstrate the connection between thoughts and feelings, the negative thoughts typical of depression and the different feelings that might have emerged had the patient thought differently in the same circumstances. Therapy, in turn, can be presented as a relatively short-term experiment with a treatment that often but not always shows rapid benefits (Fennell & Teasdale 1987, Piasecki & Hollon 1987). This framing might be useful in conveying optimism without leading the patient to perceive a demand for long-term commitment.

Behavioural techniques

Behavioural techniques may be particularly important early in therapy in order to interrupt a self-maintaining depressive cycle of reduced activity, sense of personal incompetence, hopelessness, lack of positive reinforcement and low mood (Beck et al 1979). The implementation of behavioural techniques in CT differs in at least two ways, however, from orthodox behavioural therapies for depression (e.g. Lewinsohn 1974).

First, increased activity with potential for positive reinforcement is not considered an end in itself, but rather a means to cognitive change. The results of behavioural assignments are thus used primarily as evidence that an optimistic, non-depressive outlook on the patient's circumstances may be justifiable. Rather than taking for granted that cognitive changes will follow predictably from successful applications of behavioural techniques, however, CT therapists take pains to increase the probability of this outcome. For instance, patient's predictions of the outcomes of behavioural assignments should be written down before the assignments are carried out. This practice may lower the probability that the patient will discount the implications of a success experience by adjusting expectations (e.g. elevating in hindsight the standards for a success). Second, because behavioural assignments are intended in CT as data-gathering exercises, they should be devised specifically to yield data relevant to the patient's cognitions. This differs from, for instance, selecting assignments based on how pleasant the patient is likely to find them.

Examples of common behavioural procedures in CT follow.

Activity scheduling. This technique, particularly useful for very inactive patients, involves helping the patient specify a highly detailed plan of action, beginning with relatively easy tasks (e.g. read a magazine article, go for a short walk). Activity scheduling should be presented as a low-demand study of the relationship between activity and mood. If an increase in activities improves mood, that is important information. Even if it does not, however, this result offers useful feedback on the behaviours chosen. There might have been too few 'wants' and too many 'should' activities on the list (Marlatt 1985), for instance. Or perhaps the patient carried out activities normally considered pleasant but discounted them as unimportant. These interfering thoughts would be addressed by cognitive interventions in subsequent therapy sessions.

Mastery and pleasure tasks. As indicated, depressed patients can sometimes increase activity level in an apparently appropriate manner but nevertheless gain little sense of enjoyment or enhanced self-confidence in the process. For example, they might be ruminating on negative thoughts during activities ('I'm not doing as well as I should'). A recent experiment is consistent with this line of reasoning. Non-clinical subjects in whom a sad mood had been induced reported greater alleviation of sadness if assigned a more active task to perform, but the benefits of activity were far smaller among subjects led to ruminate about their bad feelings than among those whose assigned task provided distractions from sadness (Morrow & Nolen-Hoeksema 1990).

A second possible cause of deriving little satisfaction from activities is that some depressed patients might believe that they do not deserve to do things for the sake of their own enjoyment. Such self-critical patients often need assistance in seeing that this outlook is self-defeating, that pleasant events can enhance their capacity for all tasks, including those they deem especially important.

To help identify such potentially problematic reactions to behavioural assignments, CT patients are asked to self-monitor (e.g. on 0–5 scale) the degree of pleasure and sense of mastery or competence associated with each activity. Use of a continuous rating scale is hypothesized to foster the recognition of partial successes, an antidote to dichotomous thinking. Monitoring the results of mastery and pleasure tasks can also help to offset mood-congruent memory biases (Blaney 1986). If asked to summarize the events of several days since the previous therapy session, a depressed person might conclude that only setbacks and disappointments had occurred, while detailed records might indicate at least a few positive experiences. Piasecki & Hollon (1987) suggest emphasizing this point by giving patients self-monitoring assignments with the rationale that it is unwise to rely on memory, given that it can be affected by depression.

Graded task assignments. Goal-oriented assignments can seem to a depressed person impossible to execute if they are considered in large chunks (e.g. arrange adequate care for a frail elderly relative). As is recommended in problem-solving therapy (Nezu et al 1989), breaking down this goal into more manageable chunks and starting with relatively easy sub-tasks (e.g. make a list of options in the surrounding community) can render the challenge less overwhelming. If the patient completes such an asssignment, the therapist would want to call attention to this success and the role of the patient's skills and effort in bringing it about, in order to facilitate persistent effort in the future when difficulties arise (Forsterling 1985).

Cognitive techniques

Cognitive procedures in CT are used to identify maladaptive automatic thoughts, evaluate and (often) alter these cognitions, assess dysfunctional beliefs and modify beliefs.

Identifying negative automatic thoughts. Cognitions targeted in CT are 'ideation that interferes with the ability to cope with life experiences, unnecessarily disrupts internal harmony, and produces inappropriate or excessive emotional reactions that are painful' (Beck 1976, p 235). Psychometric methods can indicate the degree to which a patient endorses cognitions typical of depressed people (e.g. the Crandell Cognitions Inventory; Crandell & Chambless 1986, the Cognitions Checklist; Beck et al 1987). However, cognitive assessment in the clinical practice of CT often proceeds idiographically, permitting identification of idiosyncratic automatic thoughts.

The first goal in assessing maladaptive cognitions is to teach the patient to self-monitor negative automatic thoughts (ATs). These may be defined as thoughts or images that arise without intentional control and are associated with feeling upset. A pragmatic definition some patients find useful is that ATs are whatever they would say if asked, 'What is going through your mind right now?' when feeling bad. Piasecki & Hollon (1987) suggested additional ways to facilitate assessment of ATs, including: 1) Ask for them when the patient shows an abrupt mood shift during a therapy session; 2) Illustrate the meaning of ATs by thinking out loud oneself; and 3) Avoid insisting that an AT must have *preceded* the patient's awareness of an emotional reaction.

Once the patient understands dysfunctional ATs, he or she is asked to monitor on a Daily Record of Dysfunctional Thoughts (DRDT; Beck et al 1979) upsetting situations and accompanying emotions (rated on a 0–100 scale of intensity, again to instill the habit of using continuous rather than dichotomous thinking) and ATs, also rated 0–100% for degree of belief. Some patients have difficulty with this self-monitoring procedure because the distinction between thoughts and emotions can at times seem minute (e.g. 'I can't stand it' versus 'I'm so upset'). These must be distinguished, however, in order to proceed with evaluating ATs. Emotional reactions themselves are not questioned; they are assumed to be sensible in light of the patient's cognitions.

Evaluating and modifying automatic thoughts. Reviewing self-monitored ATs in subsequent sessions permits the therapist to teach several techniques for evaluating them and thereby uncovering and challenging cognitive biases. These may be summarized as a series of questions the patient learns to ask herself or himself about negative inferences, rather than automatically assuming them to be valid.

'*What's the evidence?*' The first question of interest concerns the nature of the evidence for and against the validity of a thought (or inference or interpretation). A balanced review of evidence pertaining to a negative AT might decrease the patient's belief in it. Nevertheless, it is also customary for a negative thought to enjoy substantial supporting evidence. Research on the social relationships of depressed people, for instance, confirms that their interactions are often conflictual and experienced as burdensome by their intimates, which may lead in turn to negative reactions to the patient (Coyne 1976, Coyne et al 1987, Krantz 1985). Moreover, if negative information is available, depressed patients may exaggerate its significance and future implications. As noted earlier, depression is associated with easier access to negative memories

(Blaney 1986, Clark & Teasdale 1982) and, unless special pains are taken to counteract this tendency, people typically form predictions on the basis of easily retrieved events rather than on a balanced consideration of all evidence (Kahneman et al 1982).

'*Is there any other way to look at it?*' Even if there is ample evidence consistent with a negative view of a depressed patient's situation, it is still possible to explore alternative conceptualizations of this evidence. In other words, there might be other interpretations of the same facts as plausible as, yet more hopeful than, the patient's. Reattribution techniques (Forsterling 1985) can be used in generating possible benign explanations for the event or situation. In particular, explanations that suggest that change is possible (i.e. *unstable* explanations for negative events) are likely to promote persistence and hopefulness (e.g. Wilson & Linville 1982).

'*How could that be tested?*' Verbal discussions of evidence regarding negative ATs and possible alternative conceptualizations often prove insufficient for enduring cognitive change (Hollon & Beck 1986). Therapist and patient therefore collaborate to devise tests (often behavioural assignments as described earlier) of depressive and more benign interpretations of a situation. This emphasis on *prospective empirical hypothesis testing* seems to be a distinguishing feature of CT (Piasecki & Hollon 1987).

'*What is the worst that could happen?*' As in rational-emotive therapy (Ellis 1962), CT encourages examining negative thoughts with respect to their ultimate implications. That is, supposing that the present situation is indeed as it seems and that the patient's most hopeless expectancies are fulfilled, what would this mean for the patient's life?

'*What can I do about it?*' Finally, the patient is encouraged to explore the possible utility of taking action to change upsetting situations. CT integrates cognitive and behavioural treatment strategies; in addition to the primary goal of changing information processing, there is a clear emphasis on making behaviour changes and thus creating new information for the patient to process. For example, consider a socially dependent patient reporting ATs such as 'No one cares for me'. If evidence indicated that this patient was indeed rejected by most people, and no unstable attribution for this circumstance seemed plausible, CT practitioners would employ behavioural skill training methods (cf Hersen et al 1984). The intended cognitive change here would not be negative perceptions of the patient's present social situation but rather the hopelessness ('I can never learn to get along with people better') that may have developed about it.

Conclusion. The aim of this process of questioning a dysfunctional AT is to derive a convincing (to the patient) 'rational response' to it. The response is itself rated for believability on a 0–100% scale, and the outcome of this entire exercise is recorded in yet a fifth column of the dysfunctional thought record, including the strength of the patient's residual belief in the AT and her or his rating of negative emotion. Outcome ratings help reveal the impact of the intervention. If the patient does not believe the rational response, believes the original negative AT as strongly as before and continues to feel terrible, this pattern would indicate that the rational response needs improvement.

Identifying tacit beliefs. Increases in behavioural activity and modification of specific negative cognitions do not guarantee lasting improvement, according to CT theory. It is also necessary to alter the dysfunctional beliefs underlying negative cognitions. Assessment of such beliefs in clinical work has mainly been an idiographic process relying on clinical inference (Safran et al 1986), though standardized measures of typical dysfunctional beliefs (e.g. the Dysfunctional Attitude Scale: DAS; Weissman & Beck 1978) have been developed.

Clinical assessment of dysfunctional beliefs can be facilitated through the use of such techniques as the following:

Tying automatic thoughts to underlying beliefs via the 'downward arrow' technique (Burns 1980). This technique involves asking recursively something like 'What would be upsetting to you about that?' with respect to each thought in turn until a seemingly basic belief has been revealed. In this fashion, CT takes an inductive approach to the question of what a given negative thought might mean to a patient. It is not assumed that the same thought reflects the same underlying meaning to all patients, nor that therapists can reliably deduce from theory what this meaning must be (cf Huber & Altmaier 1983).

Exploring the meaning of ATs associated with stressful, emotional situations. As noted earlier in our discussion of basic research on cognitive vulnerability to depression, it appears that access to enduring dysfunctional beliefs lessens once depressive symptoms remit. For the purpose of relapse prevention, therefore, it may be necessary near the end of treatment intentionally to induce an affective response in sessions in order to identify lingering cognitive vulnerabilities. Hollon & Garber (1990) suggest for this purpose imaginal cogni-

tive rehearsal of being confronted by whatever aversive situations the patient would be likely to find especially stressful.

Modifying dysfunctional beliefs. Once basic beliefs are identified, methods for evaluating and modifying them are often the same as those used with negative automatic thoughts (e.g. evaluating the evidence for and against a belief). Also, it is sometimes useful simply to trace the origins of dysfunctional beliefs (e.g. in early experiences, parental beliefs or peer values). This process can help patients understand and accept how they could have developed seemingly self-defeating beliefs, yet at the same time begin to distance themselves from them.

Conclusion

CT for depression is an optimistic treatment. The therapist strives to maintain a constructive, problem-solving outlook (these negative thoughts are probably somewhat biased and there may be another way to view the situation, or there may be a way to change the situation, or the interpretations may be accurate but less devastating than the patient assumes, or...), rather than joining the patient in hopelessness if treatment does not lead to immediate benefits. This style makes sense in view of CT's basis in a theory identifying negative views of the self and the future as problematic features of depression.

The metatheory of CT could thus be encapsulated as 'A positive is a positive; a negative is a chance to gather information and practise the techniques' (Haaga & Davison, 1991, p 268). In so far as this orientation can be absorbed by depressed patients, they should become relatively resilient people able to cope more effectively with future difficulties and setbacks.

EMPIRICAL STATUS OF COGNITIVE THERAPY

Acute response and maintenance of gains

CT has received substantial empirical support as an effective treatment for unipolar major depression. An initial study found CT to be significantly superior to imipramine in relieving depressive symptoms (Rush et al 1977), though subsequent studies have more typically revealed non-significant differences in acute response between CT and tricyclic pharmacotherapies (e.g. Murphy et al 1984). Hollon & Beck (1986) noted that the Rush et al (1977) study, in which pharmacotherapy patients were gradually withdrawn from imipramine, may have inadvertently underestimated the efficacy of imipramine because 'examination of the weekly depression scores . . . suggested that patients in the pharmacotherapy cell actually worsened as a group during the 2-week medication withdrawal period *prior* to the post-treatment evaluation' (p 449, emphasis in original). The National Institute of Mental Health Treatment of Depression Collaborative Research Program recently reported (Elkin et al 1989) general equivalence in the milder cases of depression of short-term symptom relief among CT, interpersonal therapy (Klerman et al 1984), and imipramine with clinical management. There were some differences among more severely ill patients, favouring imipramine in particular.

The most frequent conclusion from individual studies, then, is that acute response to CT does not differ significantly from response to other structured psychotherapies for depression or to tricyclic pharmacotherapy. However, treatment experiments usually possess inadequate statistical power for detecting as significant the fairly small differences associated with comparisons of active treatments for depression (Kazdin & Bass 1989). A thorough quantitative review of studies of CT for depression reported from 1976 through 1987 concluded that CT achieves greater self-reported short-term symptom relief than waiting-list controls, pharmacotherapies, behavioural treatments or a heterogeneous set of 'other psychotherapies' (Dobson 1989).

In absolute terms, the amount of relief afforded on average by brief courses of CT is fairly consistent across studies. Rush et al (1977) reported a pre–post decline in mean Beck Depression Inventory (BDI; Beck et al 1979) scores from 30 to 7 for the CT group; subsequent studies have reported comparable pre–post decreases (e.g. 31 to 9 in Beck et al 1985; 27 to 10 in Elkin et al 1989 for treatment completers). This average level of response is encouraging, given that: 1) it is reliably greater than what can be expected from passage of time alone (Dobson 1989); 2) Taylor & Klein (1989) found that 31 of 37 subjects scoring 10 or below on the BDI at a follow-up assessment were judged as 'recovered' from a depressive episode by interview-based criteria; and 3) an average post-treatment score of 9 or 10 reflects only about 1 standard deviation above the mean of non-distressed samples (Nietzel et al 1987). However, these results should not be taken as cause for complacency, for post-treatment averages remain higher than for non-depressed samples and those patients who remain mildly dysphoric may be the most likely to relapse (Simons et al 1986).

Perhaps the most encouraging finding from research on CT is an apparent prophylactic effect. That is, CT has in several studies resulted in significantly greater maintenance of improvement in the year or two after the end of treatment than did pharmacotherapy alone (Blackburn et al 1986a, Evans et al 1989, Simons et al 1986); a non-significant trend in this direction was noted in the follow-up to the Rush et al (1977) study (Kovacs et al 1981). To be sure, continuation of pharmacotherapy after acute response would be typical clinical practice and apparently achieves the same level of relapse prevention as having provided CT in the first place (Hollon & Najavits 1988). Nevertheless, differential relapse rates after complete discontinuation of treatment suggest that something is learned in CT that patients find helpful after the acute phase of treatment.

Prediction and explanation of the efficacy of CT

Research thus suggests that CT can have a powerful short-term impact on depression, and perhaps an especially good record in leading to maintenance of these improvements. It therefore becomes important to ask what aspects of CT are therapeutic, for which depressed patients it might be indicated or contraindicated and *how* it works when it works. As is generally true of intervention research (Davison 1968), empirical support for the efficacy of CT *per se* does not establish the validity of cognitive theory's claims about how CT works, let alone its hypotheses about the causes of the onset or maintenance of depression (Oei et al 1989).

Therapy and therapist characteristics

The efficacy of CT may be attenuated somewhat when it is adapted to a group therapy format (e.g. Rush & Watkins 1981). One study of group treatment, for instance, found depressed patients' BDI scores to decline only from an average of 27 to an average of 16, leaving a typical patient still moderately dysphoric (Zettle & Rains 1989). Quite similar results were obtained by Neimeyer & Feixas (1990). These modest findings might have resulted from the provision of a fixed dosage of 12 sessions in 12 weeks (Zettle & Rains 1989) or 10 sessions in 10 weeks (Neimeyer & Feixas in press), rather than the more flexible scheduling procedure used in most of the individual-therapy outcome studies.

It is not yet clear to what extent the basic techniques

of CT are its active ingredients, nor what specific thera-pist actions promote optimal efficacy. On one hand, there is reason to believe that the essential cognitive and behavioural techniques of CT are quite powerful. For instance, components analyses have suggested that both cognitive and behavioural procedures contribute to the effectiveness of CT (Taylor & Marshall 1977, Wilson et al 1983). Moreover, in-session change in dysfunctional thoughts predicts the extent to which patients make progress in resolving important problems by the next session (Safran et al 1987). Also consistent with the view that basic prescribed CT techniques are powerful is the finding that 'purity' of CT (i.e. the extent to which only theory-consistent therapist actions were performed) was positively correlated with outcome in CT for opiate addicts (Luborsky et al 1985). A recent report even suggested that computer-administered CT could be effective for mild-to-moderately depressed outpatients (Selmi et al 1990).

On the other hand, it would be premature to conclude that the effectiveness of CT rests on therapist adherence to specific, highly effective techniques which can be easily taught and disseminated. The effective-ness of CT for severely depressed patients, relative to comparison treatments, varied substantially across sites in the National Institute of Mental Health Program (Elkin et al 1989). It will be of great interest to deter-mine whether measures of the fidelity and quality with which CT was practised (Shaw 1984) can account for this variance in outcome.

A difficulty in conducting and interpreting research on the impact of therapist actions on the outcome of CT is that competency or purity may be confounded with patient variables that could be the root causes of any correlations between therapist behaviour and out-come (Beckham & Watkins 1989). For instance, pa-tients who are for one or another reason more difficult may derive less benefit from CT and simultaneously make it difficult for therapists to adhere to CT techni-ques and perform them in an apparently competent manner. Conversely, successful courses of treatment may make adherence possible, rather than the other way around; Luborsky et al (1985) concluded that their data relating purity to treatment success might only mean that 'the better the outcome, the more the thera-pists did what they were "supposed to do"' (p 608).

Pre-existing patient characteristics

Contrary to some speculation, endogenicity does not appear to predict poor response to CT (Hollon &

Najavits 1988), nor does being of only average intelli-gence (Haaga et al 1991). Although further research is needed, severe marital discord may contraindicate individual CT. Social-learning-based marital therapy might address the depression in one spouse as well as does individual CT, and the relationship problems better than does individual CT (O'Leary & Beach 1990).

Simons et al (1985) found that CT is especially beneficial, in contrast to pharmacotherapy, for patients who initially appeared to be high in learned resourceful-ness (Rosenbaum 1980). This result can be interpreted as an indication that agreeing with the rationale of CT (you can control your thinking and learn to help yourself) improves response to CT. Also consistent with this notion is a *post hoc* analysis by Fennell & Teasdale (1987). Approximately one-half of their CT subjects responded very quickly (within 2 weeks), apparently on the basis of being presented with the CT rationale for depression and agreeing that it fitted their circumstances. These subjects did not differ from less responsive ones in pretreatment severity of depression but did score especially high on 'depression about depression' (Teasdale 1985). That is, they reported especially negative reactions to aspects of the experi-ence of being depressed itself. Taken together, these two studies provide some basis for optimism that specific psychological indications for CT may be found, but further confirmation of the results is needed. One subsequent study, for instance, failed to replicate the finding that high pretreatment learned resourcefulness predicts favourable response to CT (Kavanagh & Wilson 1989).

Mediating mechanisms

Hollon et al (1988) have distinguished three cognitive models of how CT might exert its effects:

1) the *accommodation* model, which holds that CT modifies dysfunctional beliefs and/or the processes maintaining them
2) the *activation–deactivation* model, which proposes that CT does not change dysfunctional beliefs or cognitive processes but instead leads to the deactiva-tion of depressive processing and the activation of (already existing) nondepressive beliefs and processing styles
3) the *compensatory skills* model, which contends that patients learn some skills for halting the spiral of negative thinking after CT, though depressive

beliefs remain and therefore can potentially be activated.

Based on a review of the empirical literature, Barber & DeRubeis (1989) concluded that there is as yet little support for the accommodation model as an explanation of effects specific to CT. Most critically, change in depressive beliefs appears to be non-specific in that any successful treatment reduces such beliefs (e.g. Imber et al 1990, Simons et al 1984, Zettle & Rains 1989). Similarly, Barber & DeRubeis (1989) argued against the activation — deactivation model on the grounds that it does not offer a compelling explanation of *differential* relapse rates between CT and antidepressant medication. If depressive beliefs remain fundamentally intact but simply go underground, so to speak, the risk of relapse when negative events that can reactivate them occur should be quite high in CT as well.

Barber & DeRubeis (1989) concluded that the most promising, albeit still unproven, account of CT's effects is the compensatory skills model. They argue that deliberate use of coping skills (e.g. problem-solving, generating and testing alternative explanations for negative events) when negative thoughts arise could lessen depression about depression (Teasdale 1985) and thereby help patients ward off relapse even when stressful events occur after therapy has ended.

Considered as a whole, then, the current research literature offers promising leads but little conclusive guidance concerning which depressed people are especially likely to respond to CT, which therapist behaviours promote optimal results or which specific mechanisms mediate response to CT. Accordingly, a recent review of research on psychotherapy for depression concluded that 'we do not yet have an empirical basis by which to recommend matching treatment components to patient characteristics' (McLean & Carr 1989, p 459).

ADAPTATIONS

In this subsection we comment on extensions of the basic model of CT for unipolar outpatients, in particular research on the utility of CT for inpatients and patients with bipolar disorder.

Inpatients

CT has recently been experimentally evaluated as an addition to antidepressant medication and standard milieu treatment for depressed inpatients. Bowers (1990) assigned inpatients to receive 1) CT + nortriptyline, 2) relaxation training + nortriptyline, or 3) nortriptyline alone, with all subjects spending about 30 days in the normal hospital milieu. CT was conducted individually during the hospitalization period on a daily basis for 12 sessions. For the 10 completers in each treatment condition there were no significant group X-time interaction effects on either self-reported or interviewer-rated depressive symptoms; depression was substantially reduced over the time of treatment across groups.

Another comparison of CT and medication (amitriptyline or desipramine, somewhat flexibly administered), social skills training and medication or medication alone, with all treatments continuing for 20 weeks after discharge from the hospital, found no significant differences between CT and social skills training as supplementary treatments (Miller et al 1989). However, a significantly higher proportion of patients assigned to one of the combined treatment conditions (54% versus 18% for medication only) maintained complete remission throughout a 1-year follow-up. It should be noted that, in this as in most naturalistic follow-up studies, many patients (about three-quarters) continued to receive some form of outpatient treatment (outside the study protocol) after discontinuation of formal treatment in the study, complicating interpretation of the follow-up data.

This research suggests that CT can play a useful role as an addition to standard medication and milieu treatments for depressed inpatients, perhaps especially in facilitating maintenance of improvements. It is not clear, however, that this is a unique effect of CT as opposed to the general effect of adding a structured psychotherapy to the usual treatment modalities utilized on an inpatient ward.

Bipolar disorder

Although CT alone is not recommended as a sole treatment for bipolar disorder, it may be a helpful adjunctive treatment. A particularly useful role for CT in the clinical care of bipolar disorder was illustrated by Cochran's (1984) experiment. Adding a CT intervention directly relating to lithium compliance to routine clinical care reduced both non-compliance with lithium therapy and frequency of hospitalizations during a 6-month follow-up period.

CONCLUSION

In this chapter we have described the main features and empirical status of cognitive therapy for depression as well as the theory of the psychopathology of depression on which it is based. A parallel development is evident in the domains of psychopathology and psychotherapy. Concerning psychopathology, cognitive theory appears to have: 1) offered a compelling, empirically supported description of depressive thinking as it appears during depressive episodes; 2) provided a causal theory of the origins of depression that holds promise and has not been clearly refuted; yet 3) has not been clearly supported in longitudinal research. Similarly, cognitive therapy for depression (particularly unipolar outpatients): 1) has a substantial effect on depressive symptoms and on prevention of relapse in the first year or two after treatment; 2) offers a plausible theoretical account of the therapist behaviours needed to achieve this effect and the client processes through which it is mediated; yet 3) has to date failed to establish clearly the truth of this theoretical explanation. Beckham (1990) referred to this state of affairs as a failure thus far to confirm the 'primary premise' ('the hypothesis that change in the targeted aetiological or maintaining variable causes greater symptomatic improvement than would occur from the natural history of the disorder', p 223) of CT, a failure shared with other theories of psychotherapy for depression.

At least two potentially useful directions for future work on cognitive theory and therapy may be discerned. First, *more of the same* may be required, but with methodological refinements. That is, in the case of the psychopathology theory, future research using priming procedures to activate otherwise latent dysfunctional beliefs might corroborate Beck's diathesis-stress hypothesis about the onset of depression. Likewise, refinements in the analysis of causal mediational hypotheses about therapeutic change (Hollon et al 1987) might bolster the case that CT has specific, unique effects on depression best explained by cognitive theory.

Alternatively, *integration* with other theories of the aetiology and treatment of depression may prove necessary. Several theorists have argued, for instance, that CT would benefit from integration with interpersonal theories, leading to a greater emphasis on use of the psychotherapy relationship as a laboratory for analysing and modifying patients' tacit beliefs about relationships and interactions between themselves and other people (e.g. Jacobson 1989, Safran 1990a, b). At present, such recommendations are supported more by detailed logical analysis and clinical observation than by systematic empirical work.

By the end of the current decade we anticipate being in a better position to judge whether, and in what ways, these alternative strategies for enhancing the explanatory power of cognitive theory and the clinical utility of cognitive therapy have been fruitful.

REFERENCES

Abramson L Y, Alloy L B, Metalsky G I 1988 The cognitive diathesis-stress theories of depression: toward an adequate evaluation of the theories' validities. In Alloy L B (ed) Cognitive processes in depression. Guilford Press, New York, p 3–30

Barber J P, DeRubeis R J 1989 On second thought: where the action is in cognitive therapy for depression. Cognitive Therapy and Research 13: 441–457

Barnett P A, Gotlib I H 1988 Psychosocial functioning and depression: distinguishing among antecedents, concomitants, and consequences. Psychological Bulletin 104: 97–126

Beck A T 1963 Thinking and depression: I. Idiosyncratic content and cognitive distortions. Archives of General Psychiatry 9: 324–333

Beck A T 1964 Thinking and depression: II. Theory and therapy. Archives of General Psychiatry 10: 561–571

Beck A T 1976 Cognitive therapy and the emotional disorders. International Universities Press, New York

Beck A T 1983 Cognitive therapy of depression: new perspectives. In: Clayton P J, Barrett J E (eds) Treatment of depression: old controversies and new approaches. Raven Press, New York, p 265–284

Beck A T 1987 Cognitive models of depression. Journal of Cognitive Psychotherapy 1: 5–37

Beck A T, Rush A J, Shaw B F, Emery G 1979 Cognitive therapy of depression. Guilford Press, New York

Beck A T, Epstein N, Harrison R 1983 Cognitions, attitudes and personality dimensions in depression. British Journal of Cognitive Psychotherapy 1: 1–16

Beck A T, Hollon S D, Young J E, Bedrosian R C, Budenz D 1985 Treatment of depression with cognitive therapy and amitriptyline. Archives of General Psychiatry 42: 142–148

Beck A T, Brown G, Steer R A, Eidelson J I, Riskind J H 1987 Differentiating anxiety and depression: a test of the cognitive content-specificity hypothesis. Journal of Abnormal Psychology 96: 179–183

Beckham E E 1990 Psychotherapy of depression research at a crossroads: directions for the 1990s. Clinical Psychology Review 10: 207–228

Beckham E E, Watkins J T 1989 Process and outcome in cognitive therapy. In: Freeman A, Simon K M, Beutler L E, Arkowitz H (eds) Comprehensive handbook of cognitive therapy. Plenum Press, New York, p 61–81

Blackburn I M, Eunson K M, Bishop S 1986a A two-year naturalistic follow-up of depressed patients treated with cognitive therapy, pharmacotherapy and a combination of both. Journal of Affective Disorders 10: 67–75

Blackburn I M, Jones S, Lewin R J P 1986b Cognitive style in depression. British Journal of Clinical Psychology 25: 241–251

Blaney P H 1986 Affect and memory: a review. Psychological Bulletin 99: 229–246

Bowers W A 1990 Treatment of depressed in-patients: cognitive therapy plus medication, relaxation plus medication, and medication alone. British Journal of Psychiatry 156: 73–78

Bowlby J 1977 The making and breaking of affectional bonds. British Journal of Psychiatry 130: 201–210

Bradley B, Mathews A 1988 Memory bias in recovered clinical depressives. Cognition and Emotion 2: 235–245

Brehm S S, Smith T W 1986 Social psychological approaches to psychotherapy and behaviour change. In: Garfield S L, Bergin A E (eds) Handbook of psychotherapy and behaviour change, 3rd edn. John Wiley, New York, p 69–115

Burns D D 1980 Feeling good: the new mood therapy. William Morrow, New York

Clark D M, Teasdale J D 1982 Diurnal variation in clinical depression and accessibility of memories of positive and negative experiences. Journal of Abnormal Psychology 91: 87–95

Cochran S D 1984 Preventing medical noncompliance in the outpatient treatment of bipolar affective disorders. Journal of Consulting and Clinical Psychology 52: 873–878

Coyne J C 1976 Depression and the response of others. Journal of Abnormal Psychology 85: 186–193

Coyne J C, Gotlib I H 1983 The role of cognition in depression: a critical appraisal. Psychological Bulletin 94: 472–505

Coyne J C, Kessler R C, Tal M, Turnbull J, Wortman C B, Greden J F 1987 Living with a depressed person. Journal of Consulting and Clinical Psychology 55: 347–352

Crandell C J, Chambless D L 1986 The validation of an inventory for measuring depressive thoughts: the Crandell Cognitions Inventory. Behaviour Research and Therapy 24: 403–411

Davison G C 1968 Systematic desensitization as a counterconditioning process. Journal of Abnormal Psychology 73: 91–99

Dobson K S 1989 A meta-analysis of the efficacy of cognitive therapy for depression. Journal of Consulting and Clinical Psychology 57: 414–419

Dobson K S, Shaw B F 1986 Cognitive assessment with major depressive disorders. Cognitive Therapy and Research 10: 13–29

Elkin I, Shea M T, Watkins J T, et al 1989 National Institute of Mental Health Treatment of Depression Collaborative Research Program: general effectiveness of treatments. Archives of General Psychiatry 46: 971–982

Ellis A 1962 Reason and emotion in psychotherapy. Lyle Stuart, New York

Evans M D, Hollon S D, DeRubeis R J, et al 1989 Differential relapse following cognitive therapy, pharmacotherapy, and combined cognitive-pharmacotherapy for depression: II. A two-year follow-up of the CPT project. Manuscript submitted for publication

Fennell M J V, Teasdale J D 1987 Cognitive therapy for depression: individual differences and the process of change. Cognitive Therapy and Research 11: 253–271

Forsterling F 1985 Attributional retraining: a review. Psychological Bulletin 98: 495–512

Haaga D A F, Davison G C (1991) Cognitive change methods. In: Kanfer F H, Goldstein A P (eds) Helping people change: a textbook of methods, 4th edn. Pergamon Press, Elmsford, NY, p 248–304

Haaga D A F, DeRubeis R J, Stewart B L, Beck A T 1991 Relationship of intelligence with cognitive therapy outcome. Behaviour Research and Therapy 29: 277–281

Hamilton E W, Abramson L Y 1983 Cognitive patterns and major depressive disorder: a longitudinal study in a hospital setting. Journal of Abnormal Psychology 92: 173–184

Hammen C, Ellicott A, Gitlin M 1989 Vulnerability to specific life events and prediction of course of disorder in unipolar depressed patients. Canadian Journal of Behavioural Science 21: 377–388

Hersen M, Bellack A S, Himmelhoch J M, Thase M E 1984 Effects of social skill training, amitriptyline, and psychotherapy in unipolar depressed women. Behaviour Therapy 15: 21–40

Hollon S D, Beck A T 1986 Cognitive and cognitive—behavioural therapies. In: Garfield S L, Bergin A E (eds) Handbook of psychotherapy and behaviour change 3rd edn. John Wiley, New York, p 443–482

Hollon S D, Garber J 1990 Cognitive therapy for depression: a social cognitive perspective. Personality and Social Psychology Bulletin 16: 58–73

Hollon S D, Najavits L 1988 Review of empirical studies of cognitive therapy. In: Frances A J, Hales R E (eds) American Psychiatric Press review of psychiatry 7. American Psychiatric Press, Washington, DC, p 643–666

Hollon S D, Kendall P C, Lumry A 1986 Specificity of depressotypic cognitions in clinical depression. Journal of Abnormal Psychology 95: 52–59

Hollon S D, DeRubeis R J, Evans M D 1987 Causal mediation of change in treatment for depression: discriminating between nonspecificity and noncausality. Psychological Bulletin 102: 139–149

Hollon S D, Evans M D, DeRubeis R J 1988 Preventing relapse following treatment for depression: the Cognitive Pharmacotherapy Project. In: Field T, McCabe P, Schneiderman N (eds) Stress and coping across development. Lawrence Erlbaum, Hillsdale, NJ, p 227–243

Huber J W, Altmaier E M 1983 An investigation of the self-statements of phobic and nonphobic individuals. Cognitive Therapy and Research 7: 355–362

Imber S D, Pilkonis P A, Sotsky S M et al 1990 Mode-specific effects among three treatments for depression. Journal of Consulting and Clinical Psychology 58: 352–359

Jacobson N S 1989 The therapist-client relationship in cognitive behaviour therapy: Implications for treating depression. Journal of Cognitive Psychotherapy: An International Quarterly 3: 85–96

Kahneman D, Slovic P, Tversky A 1982 Judgment under uncertainty: Heuristics and biases. Cambridge University Press, Cambridge

Kavanagh D J, Wilson P H 1989 Prediction of outcome with group cognitive therapy for depression. Behaviour Research and Therapy 27: 333–343

Kazdin A E, Bass D 1989 Power to detect differences between alternative treatments in comparative psychotherapy outcome research. Journal of Consulting and Clinical Psychology 57: 138–147

Klerman G L, Weissman M M, Rounsaville B J, Chevron E S 1984 Interpersonal psychotherapy of depression. Basic Books, New York

Kovacs M, Beck A T 1978 Maladaptive cognitive structures in depression. American Journal of Psychiatry 135: 525–533

Kovacs M, Rush A J, Beck A T, Hollon S D 1981 Depressed outpatients treated with cognitive therapy or pharmacotherapy: a one-year follow-up. Archives of General Psychiatry 38: 33–39

Krantz S E 1985 When depressive cognitions reflect negative realities. Cognitive Therapy and Research 9: 595–610

Lewinsohn P M 1974 A behavioural approach to depression. In: Friedman R J, Katz M M (eds) The psychology of depression: contemporary theory and research. Winston–Wiley, New York, p 157–178

Luborsky L, McLellan A T, Woody G E, O'Brien C P, Auerbach A 1985 Therapist success and its determinants. Archives of General Psychiatry 42: 602–611

McLean P D, Carr S 1989 The psychological treatment of unipolar depression: Progress and limitations. Canadian Journal of Behavioural Science 21: 452–469

Marlatt G A 1985 Lifestyle modification. In: Marlatt G A, Gordon J R (eds) Relapse prevention: maintenance strategies in the treatment of addictive behaviours. Guilford Press, New York, p 280–348

Miller I W, Norman W H, Keitner G I 1989 Cognitive-behavioural treatment of depressed inpatients: six-and twelve-month follow-up. American Journal of Psychiatry 146: 1274–1279

Miranda J, Persons J B 1988 Dysfunctional attitudes are mood-state dependent. Journal of Abnormal Psychology 97: 76–79

Morrow J, Nolen-Hoeksema S 1990 Effects of responses to depression on the remediation of depressive affect. Journal of Personality and Social Psychology 58: 519–527

Murphy G E, Simons A D, Wetzel R D, Lustman P J 1984 Cognitive therapy and pharmacotherapy: singly and together in the treatment of depression. Archives of General Psychiatry 41: 33–41

Neimeyer R A, Feixas G (1990) The role of homework and skill acquisition in the outcome of group cognitive therapy for depression. Behaviour Therapy 21: 281–292

Nezu A M, Nezu C M, Perri M G 1989 Problem-solving therapy for depression: theory, research, and clinical guidelines. John Wiley, New York

Nietzel M T, Russell R L, Hemmings K A, Gretter M L 1987 Clinical significance of psychotherapy for unipolar depression: a meta-analytic approach to social comparison. Journal of Consulting and Clinical Psychology 55: 156–161

Oei T P S, Duckham S, Free M 1989 Does cognitive behaviour therapy support cognitive models of depression? Behaviour Change 6: 70–75

O'Leary K D, Beach S R H 1990 Marital therapy: a viable treatment for depression and marital discord. American Journal of Psychiatry 147: 183–186

Peselow E D, Robins C, Block P, Barouche F, Fieve R R 1990 Dysfunctional attitudes in depressed patients before and after clinical treatment and in normal control subjects. American Journal of Psychiatry 147: 439–444

Piasecki J, Hollon S D 1987 Cognitive therapy for depression: unexplicated schemata and scripts. In: Jacobson N S (ed) Psychotherapists in clinical practice: cognitive and behavioural perspectives. Guilford Press, New York, p 121–152

Riskind J H, Rholes W S 1984 Cognitive accessibility and the capacity of cognitions to predict future depression: a theoretical note. Cognitive Therapy and Research 8: 1–12

Rosenbaum M 1980 A schedule for assessing self-control behaviours: Preliminary findings. Behaviour Therapy 11: 109–121

Rush A J, Watkins J T 1981 Group versus individual cognitive therapy: a pilot study. Cognitive Therapy and Research 5: 95–103

Rush A J, Beck A T, Kovacs M, Hollon S D 1977 Comparative efficacy of cognitive therapy and pharmacotherapy in the treatment of depressed outpatients. Cognitive Therapy and Research 1: 17–37

Safran J D 1990a Towards a refinement of cognitive therapy in light of interpersonal theory: I. Theory. Clinical Psychology Review 10: 87–105

Safran J D 1990b Towards a refinement of cognitive therapy in light of interpersonal theory: II. Practice. Clinical Psychology Review 10: 107–121

Safran J D, Vallis T M, Segal Z V, Shaw B F 1986 Assessment of core cognitive processes in cognitive therapy. Cognitive Therapy and Research 10: 509–526

Safran J D, Vallis T M, Segal Z V, Shaw B F, Balog W, Epstein L 1987 Measuring session change in cognitive therapy. Journal of Cognitive Psychotherapy 1: 117–128

Segal Z V, Shaw B F 1986 Cognition in depression: a reappraisal of Coyne and Gotlib's critique. Cognitive Therapy and Research 10: 671–693

Segal Z V, Shaw B F, Vella D D 1989 Life stress and depression: a test of the congruency hypothesis for life event content and depressive subtype. Canadian Journal of Behavioural Science 21: 389–400

Selmi P M, Klein M H, Greist J H, Sorrell S P, Erdman H P 1990 Computer-administered cognitive-behavioural therapy for depression. American Journal of Psychiatry 147: 51–56

Shaw B F 1984 Specification of the training and evaluation of cognitive therapists for outcome studies. In: William J B W, Spitzer R L (eds) Psychotherapy research: where are we and where should we go? Guilford Press, New York, p 173–188

Simons A D, Garfield S L, Murphy G E 1984 The process of change in cognitive therapy and pharmacotherapy: changes in mood and cognition. Archives of General Psychiatry 41: 45–51

Simons A D, Lustman P J, Wetzel R D, Murphy G E 1985 Predicting response to cognitive therapy of depression: the role of learned resourcefulness. Cognitive Therapy and Research 9: 79–89

Simons A D, Murphy G E, Levine J E, Wetzel R D 1986 Cognitive therapy and pharmacotherapy for depression:

sustained improvement over one year. Archives of General Psychiatry 43: 43–48

Taylor E B, Klein D N 1989 Assessing recovery in depression: validity of symptom inventories. Cognitive Therapy and Research 13: 1–8

Taylor F G, Marshall W L 1977 Experimental analysis of a cognitive—behavioural therapy for depression. Cognitive Therapy and Research 1: 59–72

Teasdale J D 1985 Psychological treatments for depression: how do they work? Behaviour Research and Therapy 23: 157–165

Weissman A N, Beck A T 1978 Development and validation of the Dysfunctional Attitude Scale: a preliminary investigation. Paper presented at the annual meeting of the American Educational Research Association, Toronto

Wilson T D, Linville P W 1982 Improving the academic performance of college freshmen: attribution therapy revisited. Journal of Personality and Social Psychology 42: 367–376

Wilson P H, Goldin J C, Charbonneau-Powis M 1983 Comparative efficacy of behavioural and cognitive treatments for depression. Cognitive Therapy and Research 7: 111–124

Zettle R D, Rains J C 1989 Group cognitive and contextual therapies in treatment of depression. Journal of Clinical Psychology 45: 436–445

33. Social and community approaches

Janine Scott

Depression is often referred to as the 'common cold' of psychopathology (Gilbert 1984). However, there are some dangers in this analogy. While it is certainly a prevalent disorder, it is often severe and debilitating and does not always have the good prognosis we have been led to expect (Scott 1988a). Advances in pharmacological treatments have had a significant effect on the management of affective disorders, but it is apparent that this has not enhanced the outcome for all patients in this diagnostic subgroup (Bebbington & Kuipers 1983). Thus additional non-pharmacological treatment options have been developed (Bennett 1981). Although debates continue into 'biological' and 'social' models of aetiology, in clinical practice artificial dualistic separations are best avoided (Paykel 1989). Careful assessment and a multi-axial classification of the patients' problems should inform the development of systematic, flexible and integrated therapy programmes. The management of affective disorders incorporates psychological, biological and social approaches, although the relative emphasis on these different components will clearly vary according to the formulation of the case. Before reviewing specific aspects of treatment, this chapter will begin with a brief overview of the theoretical place of social factors in depression.

SOCIAL PSYCHIATRY AND DEPRESSION

In the last decade, increasing attention has been given to the role of psychosocial factors in the onset of affective disorders (Brown & Harris 1978, Brown et al 1987), and to the influence of the disorder on the sufferers, their lifestyles and their families (Wing 1971, Munroe 1988). The place of psychosocial factors in shaping the presentation or maintaining the illness is perhaps less contentious than their role in the onset.

There are several possible explanations for the controversy surrounding the aetiological role of psychosocial factors. Firstly, affective disorders span both the neuroses and the psychoses and models that might aid the understanding of the causation of the former may hold less credence when trying to explain the origins of the latter. Secondly, while progress in the understanding of the role of social processes in the onset and maintenance of depression have paralleled similar advances in the field of biological psychiatry, work on these specific theories seems to have been pursued in isolation (Munroe 1988). Ironically, this has led to competing rather than complementary aetiological models being promulgated and a lack of attention to the development of more convincing integrated theories (Scott 1988b). This is disappointing, as the evidence points towards a multifactorial causation of affective disorders (Akiskal & McKinney 1975).

Most studies on the social causation of depression arise from work on female samples. However, this research is broadly applicable to male populations (Brown 1989). 'Stress-buffering' models dominate, and the factors most clearly identified as having a role in social models of the causation of depression are gender, socioeconomic status, employment status, loss of parent, level of social support, expressed emotion and the occurrence of certain types of life event (the part played by expressed emotion and life events is detailed in chapter 10). While empirical evidence for these associations is strong, the information as to whether individual variables act only as modifiers or independently as stress factors is less convincing. There may be significant interaction or interference effects between factors.

One of the most robust findings in community and patient surveys is the higher morbidity rates for depression in females when compared to males (Robins et al 1984, Weissman & Klerman 1977). Social explanations focus on female roles and their status in society (Weissman & Klerman 1977). Further support for this theory is adduced from the finding that, with regard to depressive disorders, marriage is detrimental to women but protective for men (Der & Bebbington 1987). Many studies have suggested an inverse relationship between socioeconomic status and depression (Brown & Harris 1978, Goldberg & Huxley 1980). In one study (which controlled for other social variables), socioeconomic status was the strongest predictor of individual scores on a self-rated depression inventory (Hesbacher et al 1975).

Whilst unemployment is likely to lead to lower socioeconomic status, its association with depression may arise from other mechanisms. In particular, the role of work in maintaining self-esteem has been noted previously (Bolton & Oakley 1987, Scott 1988a). Other factors may also influence self-esteem. It is postulated that loss of a parent may operate as a vulnerability factor for future adult depression through its negative impact on self-esteem (Harris et al 1986). However, difficulties arise in assessing the role of self-esteem in depression. Studies suggesting that low self-esteem may interact with life events to produce depression (Brown et al 1987) must be considered in the light of other studies which suggest that low self-esteem is itself a consequence of repeated depressive episodes (Ingham et al 1987). It is often difficult to divorce the role of psychological variables such as self-esteem or premorbid personality from that of social variables. This is further demonstrated in a study by Fergusson & Horwood (1987), which suggested that 30% of the variance in life-event reporting was attributable to a combination of social disadvantage and premorbid neuroticism. As Munroe (1988) points out, it seems that much life stress is an outgrowth of social and personal forces.

Social support may buffer self-esteem or modify the impact of life stresses. Background adversity and variation in levels of support may predict illness (Bhugra 1988). However, too much social support (which reduces the sense of personal control) may be as damaging as too little (Krause 1987). In addition, many depressives show deficits in making and sustaining relationships premorbidly (Bhugra 1989). The role of social support in depression is further complicated by differing interpretations of this concept. Brown & Harris (1978) have investigated the importance of a specific form of social support, namely the presence or absence of a confidant, in reducing or increasing vulnerability to depression. Recent attempts to identify the role of social support in depression have used a wider definition but suggest that perceived numerical

and qualitative deficiencies in close personal relationships may predict onset and course of the illness (Bhugra 1988).

The work above has focused mainly on studies aimed at defining 'high risk' groups. Most models attempt to explain the differential response to provoking factors, i.e. why some people become depressed as a consequence of a significant loss while others do not show this reaction. The interaction between the individual and stress factors in the environment occurs at many conceptual levels (Jenkins 1979). Jenkins (1979) describes the different aspects of these adaptive capacities. Psychological capacities include resourcefulness, problem-solving abilities, ego strength, flexibility and social skills. Interpersonal capacities focus on primary relationships (including family) and the social support networks. Sociocultural adaptive capacities are seen in terms of values, norms and practices, 'therapeutic' social institutions and systems of knowledge and technology. The model emphasizes that those with a strong array of adaptive capacities are less likely to reach the pathological end-state of depression in response to stress.

Pearlin & Schooler (1978) investigated further the structure of coping. They argue that a coping repertoire consists not only of what an individual does but also of what resources are available. They describe social and general psychological resources as well as specific coping responses. General psychological and social resources are defined in terms of intrapersonal and interpersonal factors respectively, while specific coping responses refer to behaviours, cognitions and perceptions that modify the impact of problematic social experiences. Not only do individual coping repertoires vary significantly, but the coping mechanisms used by people vary in their efficacy in responding to different stresses (Pearlin & Schooler 1978). Also, strength in one area of the specific coping response may compensate for deficits in another: a small but interesting study demonstrated that those showing cognitive distortions were less likely to become depressed if they engaged in other 'coping' behaviours (Burns et al 1987). It can be seen that the models of individual coping put forward (Jenkins 1979 Pearlin & Schooler 1978) are similar in as much as both define coping in terms of an inward perspective (e.g. personality, self-image, biological predisposition) that is balanced by an outward perspective (interactions with other people and the environment). Future research on individual vulnerability will hopefully try to bring these two components together.

One particular form of coping response is help-seeking behaviour. It is well-recognized that a significant proportion of those suffering from depressive disorders in the community fail to seek any form of professional help. As described by Goldberg & Huxley (1980), there are a number of important stages between the onset of symptoms and the decision to seek treatment. Individuals vary in their attitude towards any symptoms they recognize in themselves. The personal interpretation of the meaning of the symptoms and why the individual thinks they are occurring represents a crucial first stage (Suchman 1965). Further validation of the meaning of these experiences is often sought from family and friends and the individual may now exhibit illness behaviour (Mechanic 1977). The adoption of illness behaviour is strongly influenced by socially learnt ideas about depression (Bennett 1981) as well as by the severity of symptoms, the level of distress and the degree of impairment of day-to-day functioning. The concurrence of life events is also likely to increase the chances of attending the general practitioner (Ingham & Miller 1976). Legitimisation of the sick role is brought about through consultation with a professional (Goldberg & Huxley 1980).

General practitioners' ability to recognize the functional nature of the disorder varies widely depending on their own attitudes towards psychological complaints and the patients' tendency to somatize their problems to a greater or lesser extent (Goldberg & Huxley 1980, Blacker & Clare 1987). Females are more likely than males to express emotional difficulties to friends and professionals (Briscoe 1982). However, in female depressives, referral on by a general practitioner to a psychiatrist is largely dependent on how the symptoms are expressed (Brown & Harris 1978). Those living alone are also over-represented among samples of depressives presenting in general practice, perhaps, as they have fewer 'significant others' to give provisional validation or support (Goldberg & Huxley 1980). While older males are significantly under-represented in those seeking help from general practitioners (Blacker & Clare 1987), they are over-represented amongst first admissions to hospital inpatient units (Cooper 1966). Delay in help-seeking behaviour may mean that the illness is more severe on presentation (Horowitz 1977). An alternative hypothesis suggests that women are less likely to be admitted because of the attitude of the psychiatrist (Goldberg & Huxley 1980).

Remaining in the community or returning there after inpatient treatment is not synonymous with recovery (Gillis & Keet 1965). Even with symptomatic improvement, social impairment may remain a major problem in 30% of depressives (Lehmann et al 1988). Although major decompensation in social adjustment might be expected during the acute stages of an illness episode, it seems that improvement in social functioning is often delayed and even on recovery, many depressives remain more impaired than their non-depressed counterparts (Tanner et al 1975, Cassano et al 1983). Depressed individuals may demonstrate social impairment in their interpersonal relationships (Bothwell & Weissmann 1977), in their marital relationships (Weissman & Paykel 1974) and in their work and leisure roles (Delisio et al 1986). Recent studies suggest that functioning in work and leisure areas is particularly disturbed in depressives (Cassano et al 1990). Interestingly, Cassano and colleagues (1990) have suggested that impaired functioning in leisure activities may be a premorbid trait in individuals vulnerable to depression, as little improvement was found even after extended follow-up. Social impairment has been under-investigated in affective disorders but the apparent levels of morbidity suggest that increasing attention is required in future.

Other chapters in this book give details of particular aspects of the psychosocial models of affective disorders and the specific physical and psychological therapies currently available. In order to avoid duplication, the following pages will focus on the principles behind social and community approaches to treatment. A fundamental concept in social and community psychiatry is a commitment to prevention. It is therefore convenient to divide the rest of this chapter into three sections, looking at primary, secondary and tertiary preventive strategies. Primary prevention aims to bring about a reduction in the incidence of a disorder by eliminating factors that cause it or contribute to its onset in high risk groups. Secondary prevention aims to decrease the duration of an episode of illness, attempting to reduce the likelihood of superadded problems by early detection and early intervention with treatment. Tertiary prevention focuses on measures to limit the disability and handicap that may occur as a consequence of the disorder.

PRIMARY PREVENTION

As yet, no aetiological model of affective disorders is robust enough to allow for the development of interventions that eliminate factors that cause or contribute to the onset of depression (Scott 1989). In order to evolve such strategies long-term large-scale prospective follow-up studies will be required to delineate vulnerable groups. Such studies will be expensive to fund and difficult to coordinate. Before dismissing the concept of primary prevention entirely, however, it is worth briefly reviewing research in the area of the neuroses which provides some hope for the future.

Early loss of parent has been postulated as a vulnerability factor for the future development of depression (Brown & Harris 1978). Several studies have investigated how the loss translates into adult vulnerability and have concluded that lack of adequate parental care in childhood may be an important intervening variable (Bifulco et al 1987, Harris et al 1986). Inadequate parental care of a child may be caused by many factors (Munroe 1988). For example, it is proposed that high levels of controlling behaviour combined with low levels of parental concern in childhood increase the risk in adulthood of neurosis in general and depression in particular (Parker et al 1987, Perris et al 1986) (see chapter 11). This 'affectionless overprotection' may reduce self-esteem and adversely affect the development of social competence (Henderson 1988). It follows that if parental care can be improved or the self-esteem of the individual at risk can be enhanced it may be possible to prevent the onset of affective episodes at some future point. Attempts at enhancing self-esteem in young people are limited, although Jorm (1987) describes a project focused on reducing neurotic traits in adolescents through the use of rational emotive therapy.

Attempts to enhance parental care (focused predominantly on females) have been tried in both England and Australia. In England, two befriending projects are described by Newton (1988). Homestart is a community-based support programme which has demonstrated enhanced child development and improved parental functioning in families identified as 'at risk' (Eyken 1982). The 'Newpin' project relates more closely to those at risk of depression (Pound et al 1985). Mothers who are vulnerable to depression according to the Brown & Harris model (1978), who are isolated or who show problems in parenting form a contract with a volunteer supporter from a similar social background. Preliminary evaluation of the project did not use any recognized depression rating scales. However, self-evaluation by the women suggested that self-esteem, self-confidence and interpersonal relationships had improved and that the mothers related better to their children (Newton 1988).

In New South Wales, Parker & Barnett (1987) assigned highly anxious primiparous women (who had been shown by previous research to be at greater risk of neurotic and depressive disorders) postnatally to either professional support, lay support or a control group with no additional help offered. The results on the specific role of this social support were difficult to interpret, but those who received professional help showed a significant reduction in postnatal anxiety levels compared to the other groups. Those receiving lay support showed a non-significant reduction in their anxiety levels. In theory, these interventions might be seen as secondary prevention in the mothers, reducing their depression and enhancing their parental coping skills (Barnett & Parker 1985) and possibly represent primary prevention for their infants.

An alternative approach to prevention is event-centred intervention. Parkes (1981) and Raphael (1977) have demonstrated the beneficial effects of support and counselling in reducing psychiatric morbidity in those at risk of abnormal grief reactions. Maguire et al (1980) offered counselling and practical advice to women exposed to a threatening life event, namely receiving surgical treatment for breast cancer. 152 women were randomly assigned to counselling or a non-counselled control group. The prevalence of anxiety and depression was similar in both groups, but episodes were of shorter duration in the couselled group and they showed better social and psychological adjustment at 18-month postoperative follow-up. Although offering some evidence of a possible primary preventive intervention, Maguire and colleagues (1983) were themselves critical of the project. They rightly point out that the reduced morbidity during episodes might have been a function of early recognition and prompt referral to additional specialist services by the counsellor (i.e. secondary prevention).

As can be seen, the above projects provide only tentative support for the possibility of primary prevention of affective disorders. The studies offer a useful starting point, but they lack methodological rigour and more systematic research will be required before resources can be committed to this area with confidence.

SECONDARY PREVENTION

Essentially, the secondary prevention of affective disorders encompasses early detection of the illness and early initiation of treatment.

Early detection

Early detection of affective disorders depends in part on

the behaviour of mental health professionals, but also upon the attitude of the individual towards any symptoms he or she develops. Recent studies suggest that fewer than 50% of those developing depressive disorders in the community seek professional help (Dew et al 1988, Lehmann et al 1988, Meller et al 1989). Patients with endogenous depression were more likely to seek help (Meller et al 1989). Other important variables in help seeking behaviour were limitation in the ability to work (Meller et al 1989), impaired functioning and lack of social support (Dew et al 1988).

Factors affecting the early recognition of affective disorders by general practitioners have been analysed by a number of researchers (Freeling et al 1985, see also chapter 41). Many strategies may be proposed to overcome this problem. Social and community psychiatry approaches focus on practices that may enhance access to mental health services. Two methods of achieving earlier intervention are available from this model. The first involves the deployment of mental health professionals in a liaison-consultation role with the primary care team. Alternatively, those seeking help might be offered direct access to mental health professionals by self-referral to a community mental health centre. Research on the general efficacy of these service models is available (Talbott et al 1987, Tyrer et al 1990), but the specific use of these approaches in affective illnesses is under-researched.

Social approaches to treatment

Although classified here under secondary prevention strategies, social approaches to treatment have a widespread influence. Strategies used in secondary prevention overlap to a certain extent with approaches used in tertiary prevention, and secondary prevention with a patient may offer effective primary prevention for a significant other. Social approaches can be divided into two categories (Henderson 1988). These are :

1) Environmental manipulation: this involves alteration of the individual's social environment, changing the behaviour of others and reducing the level of social stress.

2) Behavioural change: efforts are directed at improving the patient's coping repertoire and social skills. The aim is to teach problem-solving behaviours to apply to both current and anticipated difficulties.

Environmental manipulation

The most obvious immediate environmental change that can be made in the treatment of acute affective disorders is hospitalization. Longer term environmental change at an individual level will involve some form of 'lifestyle counselling'. Changing the behaviour of others will predominantly focus on interactions between the individual and the family, although some attention should also be given to the extended social network.

Treatment setting. The majority of patients with affective disorders are treated as outpatients. Craft's (1958) early study reporting no significant difference in the outcome of depressives treated in the day patient and inpatient setting has recently been confirmed by Creed et al (1990). However, inpatient care has a vital role to play in the treatment of affective disorders. Clearly it is indicated for the suicidal, for those with severe or non-responsive illnesses and for those without a social support network or whose network is under strain. Admission provides a safe, structured and supportive environment in which to implement a treatment programme. In addition, many clinicans comment on the improvement in mental state that may occur through the non-specific effect of hospitalization (Paykel 1989). The timing of hospitalization may be important in order not to damage further the fragile self-esteem of the individual nor to foster dependency. Some patients fear stigmatization, but this anxiety can be reduced by educating the patient about the potential benefits of being allowed space to improve current coping responses in a less stressful environment.

Life-style counselling. As pointed out by Birchwood et al (1988), many sources of stress lie beyond the individual's control. This would suggest that there is limited scope for change. However, the work of McGuffin and colleagues (1987) demonstrated that adversity may be familial. Difficult life circumstances might then be a consequence of long-standing maladaptive coping strategies. Changing such behaviours is not feasible for all patients and it may be necessary to attempt to reduce stress by reducing the density of life events and difficulties. Practical help in dealing with financial, housing and other areas may be required. A change to a less stressful employment may be one of the most significant interventions. However, as with schizophrenic patients, reducing stress for an individual should not condemn him or her to an unfulfilling life (Birchwood et al 1988).

Enhancing social support. The family and significant others have been implicated in the onset, maintenance and relapse of affective disorders. However, depressed patients may show deficits in their ability to mobilize social support prior to the onset of their illness (Bhugra 1989). The size and quality of the network may have important prognostic implications, particularly in neurotic depressions (Bhugra et al 1987). Expressed emotion, marital distress and patients' perceptions of criticism from the spouse are also significantly associated with outcome in unipolar depression at 9 months (Hooley & Teasdale 1989).

Corney (1987) describes the value of social work support to depressed females with marital problems. Bennett (1981) describes the use of 'network therapy' to engage all members of the patient's primary social group in taking responsibility in initiating change. This type of intervention is less popular than working directly with the patient and his or her immediate family. Family therapy and related interventions are dealt with in chapter 30. However, living with or near someone with an affective illness may have other profound effects on individual and family functioning (Keitner et al 1987, Scott 1988c). Fadden et al (1987) found that, although relatives were uncomplaining, they suffered a fall in income, endured marked restrictions in their social and leisure activities and marital relationships became strained. The burden on the family and their difficulties in coping with their own attitudes toward the illness cause considerable individual distress (Jacob et al 1987). This suggests an important role for family support and education.

Anderson and colleagues (1986) describe a comparative study of the impact of educational group work (providing information and discussing coping strategies) versus process group work (emphasizing support, destigmatization and self-help) on families of patients with affective disorders. There were few significant differences between the groups in terms of knowledge about the illness and adjustment to it, but both patients and relatives reported significantly greater satisfaction with the psychoeducational group.

As well as the beneficial effects of family meetings on family functioning, significant others have an important role in helping the patient come to terms with the illness. Davenport and colleagues (1977) reported that bipolar patients receiving lithium prophylaxis and couples group therapy were better adapted to their illnesses than those receiving medication alone. Lastly, the family meeting allows professional carers to make accurate assessments of family interactions (Bennett 1981) rather than drawing premature conclusions about the 'good or bad behaviour' of a family member

(Fadden et al 1987). The greater emphasis on community care for the mentally ill suggests an increasingly important role for a family support component in any treatment package (Tantum 1989). Such interventions should improve the quality of the domestic environment and reduce the level of maladaptive behaviours in the patient and relatives.

Behavioural change

Improving coping skills. If exposure to specific life events cannot be reduced, it may be possible to alleviate the stress experienced by changing the meaning of the event for the individual or changing the behavioural response. As described earlier, Pearlin & Schooler (1978) identified three aspects to an individual's coping repertoire: social resources, general psychological resources and specific coping responses. General psychological resources comprise self-esteem, self-denigration and a sense of mastery. These can be translated into positive self-regard, negative self-regard and perceived locus of control (Bennett 1981). Change in these components may best be effected through cognitive techniques. Specific coping responses were subdivided into those which control the meaning of the event, those that change the situation and those that control the stress. These responses were found to be effective differentially in social and work settings. This is important as, on symptomatic recovery, re-adapting to role in the family and social network does not automatically mean that the individual will make a successful transition back to his or her work role. As yet, clinical application of this knowledge is underresearched.

Specific approaches to improving psychological adaptation are described in this book in the chapters dealing with individual therapies. However, at a general level all patients will benefit from broad-based problem-solving training. Rehearsing how to act or cope with anticipated difficulties will lead to the development of protective behaviours. One important example that should not be overlooked is compliance with medication. In one study of outpatients over 50% of depressives were not taking their medication (Wilcox et al 1965). Cochran (1982) reviewed treatment compliance in patients who were prescribed lithium. Interestingly, their ambivalence and anxiety about receiving this treatment increased over time. A brief programme focused on exploring attitudes to treatment combined with behavioural strategies was effective in reducing non-compliance (Cochran 1984).

Social skills training. Youngren & Lewinsohn (1977) found depressed individuals had fewer social activities and coped less well in social interactions than non-depressed individuals: depressives were also more likely to have a negative impact on the people they met. Weissman & Paykel (1974) rated depressed females as less socially adjusted than their non-depressed counterparts. Although these ratings improved over time, the women still demonstrated social impairment after apparent recovery from the depressive episode. Given the social skills deficits of patients with depression, several studies of varying quality have tried to evaluate the efficacy of social skills training in this disorder. Early case studies (e.g. Hersen & Bellack 1976) were encouraging but the results on larger samples remain inconclusive. Wells et al (1977) reported subjective and objective improvements in assertiveness, eye contact and verbal responsiveness in a small group of depressives. However, Zeiss et al (1977) found that a social behaviour package incorporating interpersonal style modification and assertiveness training was no more effective than a self-monitoring control condition.

The approaches outlined should not be viewed in isolation. There are important areas of overlap that may have prognostic significance. For example, individuals with low self-esteem who lack supportive relationships are more likely to interpret an event as stressful and suffer a more prolonged mood shift than those with high self-esteem and social support (DeLongis et al 1988). Those with more personal and environmental resources are also more likely to engage in active coping behaviours rather than avoidance behaviours in the face of stress (Holahan & Moos 1987). On this basis the above interventions should theoretically be used in combination for maximum effect. Severe affective disorders may impede the patient's ability to engage in these approaches immediately. The introduction of social strategies may need to be delayed until symptomatic improvement with pharmacotherapy is underway (Scott et al 1990).

TERTIARY PREVENTION

The failure to investigate or attempt to eliminate the residual disabilities in patients with affective disorders contrasts sharply with the extensive literature on the rehabilitation of schizophrenics. This is partly explained by the fact that individuals with schizophrenia form the majority of the hospital long-stay population (McCreadie et al 1983). In addition, the disabilities seen in schizophrenia tend to be global and more progressive than those found in chronic affective disorders, perhaps leading to more intensive efforts at rehabilitation (Bennett 1982).

Chronicity in unipolar disorders usually presents as unremitting depression, while in bipolar disorders the most common form of chronicity is rapid cycling (Keller 1985). At least 10–15% of affective disorders show symptomatic chronicity (Scott 1988a), with a further 10–30% of patients showing evidence of moderate or severe social impairment (Lehmann et al 1988). The latter is usually a consequence of affective symptoms, even if these are relatively trivial in themselves (Weissman & Paykel 1974). In a smaller number of cases social impairment arises from a loss of confidence and motivation because of the recurrence of illness episodes which seem beyond the patient's control (Bennett 1982). It is now recognized that there is a role for rehabilitation in the management of these patients, but the currently available models may not be appropriate (Bennett 1982).

The first step in the development of a rehabilitation programme is a careful assessment. This is essential in guiding therapeutic efforts. The psychosocial assessment must address the complex interaction of pre-existing personal and social problems: the disruptive effects of chronic affective disorder upon self-esteem and social functioning, and the current affective psychopathology (Scott et al 1990). In chronic mood disorders it is rare for these problems to 'disappear as the illness fades' (Shaw 1977).

Few patients with chronic affective disorder show persistent psychotic symptoms or gross behavioural disturbance (Scott 1988a). For the small subgroup who do show extreme levels of impairment the rehabilitation interventions parallel those used for other chronic mentally ill patients (Paul 1969). This incorporates four priority areas focusing on social skills and self-care, maximizing role performance, reducing or eliminating inappropriate behaviours and engaging the help of one close contact (who might support the individual on return to the community). Like others with chronic, severe mental illnesses, patients with chronic affective disorders living in the community will benefit from the support of a case manager who coordinates an appropriate package of medical and social care (Intagliata 1982).

For the majority of patients with affective disorder the primary aim of rehabilitation is to enhance personal adaptation (Bennett 1981). Shaw & Koch (1982) suggest that cognitive therapy may be useful in rehabilitating these individuals. Scott (1988c) describes a combined programme of cognitive therapy and pharmacotherapy that may be of benefit in chronic depressions. The treatment was carried out on an inpatient basis with an extended emphasis on behavioural approaches in the early stages. The course of cognitive therapy was more prolonged than with episodic depressives (see chapter 32) and continued for many months post-discharge. Family sessions were held to look at the attitudes of significant others to the illness and also to renegotiate the role of the patient in the group. Intensive work was undertaken to enhance self-esteem and to combat the hopelessness of the chronically depressed individual. Patients were then helped to resume the demands of their social role in a graded and cautious way (Scott et al 1990). In an open study 16 of the 24 patients showed a significant improvement (greater than 50% reduction on pre-treatment Hamilton and Beck ratings) after 14 weeks of treatment (Scott 1988c). This type of approach shows some promise, but much more research is required to determine its efficacy.

Compared to its application for patients with schizophrenia, vocational rehabilitation of patients with affective disorders focuses less on work performance and more on the potential of work for restoring confidence and self-esteem and enhancing feelings of mastery (Bebbington & Kuipers 1983). Weissman & Paykel (1974) reported that women working outside of the home showed less impairment following depression than housebound housewives. Brown & Harris (1978) also saw work as having a protective function in women at risk of depression. Re-employment may also reduce depression in socially-isolated men who were made redundant (Bolton & Oakley 1987). Again, only broad guidelines on vocational training for patients with affective disorders are currently available (Bennett 1982, Shaw & Koch 1982).

Chronic neurotic disorders may cause significant limitations in social functioning (Henderson 1988). These individuals and their families may benefit from the support of a community psychiatric nurse rather than merely receiving intermittent outpatient appointments (Paykel et al 1982).

CONCLUSIONS

Researchers working in the field of the social psychiatry of the affective disorders are particularly interested in the role of demographic variables, childhood environment, life events, social support networks and family interactions in the onset and maintenance of the illness. Arguments rage about whether these factors (alone or in combination) represent necessary or sufficient causes of the disorder (Munroe 1988). It is hoped that in the future a more sophisticated integrated aetiological model will inform treatment decisions. In practice, the uncertainty as to whether psychosocial variables are antecedent, concomitant or consequential factors should not disarm the clinician. Affective disorders do not occur in a vacuum (Scott 1988b) and from the perspective of the therapist the treatment interventions used illustrate an important principle in psychiatry, namely the value of a multimodal approach (Paykel 1989). However, an eclectic approach must not be a euphemism for woolly or ill-devised management plans.

Social approaches to secondary prevention involve the development of individual coping skills, the modification of stressful environments and the enhancement of social support networks, particularly in relation to immediate family members. The principles behind these interventions are necessarily broad-based to take into account the spectrum of disorders subsumed under the rubric of affective disorders. However, similar approaches appear to be relevant to rehabilitation. Chronic affective disorders have only recently become the subject of systematic research. This is disappointing, given that they are a source of considerable morbidity in both the patients and their carers (Scott 1988a). Until further studies have been completed, it should be feasible to reduce the prevalence of this problem by more effective treatment of acute illness episodes and more aggressive follow-up of those at risk of chronicity.

At this stage we can only speculate on the future role and efficacy of social approaches to the primary prevention of affective disorders. This is likely to be beyond our grasp as we cannot clearly determine how to offer proactive outreach effectively. Theoretically, to protect children from the risk of adult disorders would require help to be offered to many couples to change their parental style or the means to offer specific individual help to the child. To protect at-risk adults (such as those groups defined by gender-based vulnerability factors or employment status) would be as likely to require major changes at a societal level (focusing on housing, unemployment, offering child care) as much as at an individual level. This is more clearly the domain of politics than psychiatry.

Social approaches to affective disorders have not

been subjected to the same level of scrutiny as the interventions used in the management of schizophrenia. This state of affairs needs to be rectified.

Social treatments of affective disorders are now at a critical stage. This chapter illustrates the contrast between innovative thinking in the development of interventions and the lack of outcome and process evaluation of a sufficient standard to allow dissemination and replication of this work. Comprehensive investigations are required to give such approaches credibility.

Future research should not only address whether treatment approaches are of benefit in isolation, but also how they act in combination with other therapies.

Psychosocial or pharmacological therapies may show differential effects on interpersonal adjustment and biological symptomatology respectively (DiMascio et al 1979). It would be valuable to discover whether the effects of combined treatments are independent or additive and if these combinations interact in a positive or negative way. Ultimately, we wish to know who responds best to which specific therapy or combinations of therapies. This research must be distanced to some extent from work on the aetiology of affective disorders. Assumptions about aetiology cannot be made on the basis of the treatment response. Reparative and causal pathways are not necessarily linked (Parker & Barnett 1987).

REFERENCES

Akiskal H S, McKinney W T 1975 Overview of recent research in depression. Integration of ten conceptual models into a comprehensive clinical frame. Archives of General Psychiatry 32: 285–305

Anderson C M, Griffin S, Rossi A, Pagonis I, Holder D, Treiber R 1986 A comparative study of the impact of education versus process groups for families of patients with affective disorders. Family Process 25: 185–205

Barnett B, Parker G 1985 Professional and non-professional intervention for highly anxious primaparous mothers. British Journal of Psychiatry 146: 287–293

Bebbington P, Kuipers L 1983 Social management of depression. Physician August: 176–179

Bennett D H 1981 Social and community approaches. In: Paykel E S (ed) Handbook of affective disorders. Churchill Livingstone, Edinburgh, p 346–357

Bennett D H 1982 Management and rehabilitation of affective psychoses. In: Wing J K, Wing L (eds) Handbook of Psychiatry, Vol 3: Psychoses of uncertain aetiology. Cambridge University Press, Cambridge, p 173–176

Bhugra T S 1988 Social support. Current Opinion in Psychiatry 1: 206–211

Bhugra T S 1989 Social support and social networks. Current Opinion in Psychiatry 2: 278–282

Bhugra T S, Bebbington P, McCarthy P, Sturt E, Wykes T 1987 Social networks, social support and the type of depressive illness. Acta Psychiatrica Scandinavica 76: 664–673

Bifulco A, Brown G W, Harris T O 1987 Childhood loss of parent, lack of adequate parental care and adult depression: a replication. Journal of Affective Disorders 12: 115–128

Birchwood M, Hallett S, Preston M 1988 Schizophrenia: an integrated approach to research and treatment. Longman, London, p 268–285

Blacker C, Clare A 1987 Depressive disorder in primary care. British Journal of Psychiatry 150: 737–751

Bolton W, Oakley K 1987 A longitudinal study of social support and depression in unemployed men. Psychological Medicine 17: 453–460

Bothwell S, Weissman M 1977 Social impairment four years after an acute depressive episode. American Journal of Orthopsychiatry 47: 231–237

Briscoe M 1982 Sex differences in psychological well-being. Psychological Medicine, Monograph Supplement 1: 1–46

Brown G W 1989 Depression: a radical social perspective. In: Herbst K, Paykel E S (eds). Depression: an integrative approach. Heinemann Medical Books, Oxford, p 21–44

Brown G W, Harris T O 1978 Social origins of depression: a study of psychiatric disorder in women. Tavistock Press, London

Brown G W, Bifulco A, Harris T O 1987 Life events, vulnerability and onset of depression – some refinements. British Journal of Psychiatry 150: 30–42

Burns D, Shaw B, Croker W 1987 Thinking styles and coping strategies of depressed women: an empirical investigation. Behaviour Research and Therapy 25: 223–225

Cassano G, Magini C, Akiskal H 1983 Short-term, subchronic and chronic sequelae of affective disorders. Psychiatric Clinics of North America 6: 55–68

Cassano G, Perugi G, Maremmani I, Akiskal H 1990 Social adjustment in dysthymia. In: Burton S, Akiskal H (eds) Dysthymic disorder. Gaskell, London, p 78–85

Cochran S D 1982 Strategies for preventing lithium non-compliance in bipolar affective illness. Doctoral dissertation, University of California, Los Angeles

Cochran S D 1984 Preventing medical non-compliance in the outpatient treatment of affective disorders. Journal of Consulting and Clinical Psychology 52: 54–60

Cooper B 1966 Psychiatric disorder in hospital and general practice. Social Psychiatry 1: 7–10

Corney R 1987 Marital problems and treatment outcome in depressed women. A clinical trial of social work intervention. British Journal of Psychiatry 151: 652–659

Craft M 1958 An evaluation of treatment of depressive illness in a day hospital. Lancet 2: 149–151

Creed F, Black D, Anthony P, Osborn M, Thomas P, Tomenson B 1990 Randomised controlled trial of day patient versus inpatient psychiatric treatment. British Medical Journal 300: 1033–1037

Davenport Y B, Ebert M H, Adland M L et al 1977 Couples group therapy as an adjunct to lithium maintenance of the manic patient. American Journal of Orthopsychiatry 47: 495–502

DeLongis A, Folkman S, Lazarus R S 1988 the impact of daily stress on health and mood: psychological and social resources as mediators. Journal of Personal and Social Psychology 54: 486–495

Der G, Bebbington P 1987 Depression in inner London: a register study. Social Psychiatry 22: 73–84

Delisio G, Maremmani I, Perugi G 1986 Impairment of work and leisure in depressed outpatients. Journal of Affective Disorders 10: 79–84

Dew M A, Dunn L O, Bromet E J, Schulberg H C 1988 Factors affecting help-seeking during depression in a community sample. Journal of Affective Disorders 14: 223–234

DiMascio A, Weissman M M, Prusoff B A et al 1979 Differential symptom reduction by drugs and psychotherapy in acute depression. Archives of General Psychiatry 36: 1450–1456

Eyken W van der 1982 Homestart: a four year evaluation. Homestart Consultancy, Leicester

Fadden G, Bebbington P, Kuipers L 1987 Caring and its burdens. A study of the spouses of depressed patients. British Journal of Psychiatry 151: 660–667

Fergusson D, Horwood L 1987 Vulnerability to life event exposure. Psychological Medicine 17: 739–749

Freeling P, Rao B M, Paykel E S, Sireling L I, Burton R H 1985 Unrecognised depression in general practice. British Medical Journal 290: 1880–1883

Gilbert P 1984 Depression: from psychology to brain state Lawrence Erlbaum, London, p 1–3

Gillis I S, Keet, M 1965 Factors underlying the retention in the community of chronic unhospitalised schizophrenics. British Journal of Psychiatry 111: 1057–1067

Golberg D, Huxley P 1980 Mental illness in the community. Tavistock Publications, London, p 47–122

Harris T O, Brown G W, Bifulco A 1986 Loss of parent in childhood and adult psychiatric disorder: the role of lack of adequate parental care. Psychological Medicine 16: 641–659

Henderson A S 1988 An introduction to social psychiatry. Oxford Medical Publications, Oxford, p 73–156

Herson M, Bellack A S 1976 Social skills training for chronic psychiatric patients: rationale, research findings and future directions. Comprehensive Psychiatry 17: 559–580

Hesbacher P, Rickels K, Goldberg D 1975 Social factors and neurotic symptoms in family practice. American Journal of Public Health 65: 148–155

Holahan C J, Moos R H 1987 Personal and contextual determinants of coping strategies. Journal of Personal and Social Psychology 52: 946–955

Hooley J M, Teasdale J D 1989 Predictors of relapse in unipolar depressives: expressed emotion, marital distress and perceived criticism. Journal of Abnormal Psychology 98: 229–235

Horowitz A 1977 The pathways into psychiatric treatment. Some differences between men and women. Journal of Health and Social Behaviour 18: 169–78

Ingham J, Miller P 1976 The determinants of illness declaration. Journal of Psychosomatic Research 20: 309–316

Ingham J, Kreitman N, Miller P, Sashidaran S, Surtees P 1987 Self-appraisal, anxiety and depression in women – a prospective study. British Journal of Psychiatry 151: 643–651

Intagliata J 1982 Improving the quality of community care for the chronically mentally disabled: the role of case management. Schizophrenia Bulletin 8: 655–674

Jacob M, Frank E, Kupfer D J, Carpenter L 1987 Recurrent depression: an assessment of family burden and family attitudes. Journal of Clinical Psychiatry 48: 395–400

Jenkins C 1979 Psychosocial modifiers of response to stress. In: Barrett J, Rose R R, Klerman G L, (eds) Stress and mental disorders. Raven Press, New York, p 265–278

Jorm A F 1987 Modifiability of a personality trait which is a risk factor for neurosis. Paper presented at the World Psychiatric Association Symposium on Epidemiology and the Prevention of Mental Disorders, Reykavik, 15–17 September

Keitner G I, Miller I W, Epstein N B, Bishop D S, Frazzetti A E 1987 Family functioning and the course of major depression. Comprehensive Psychiatry 28: 54–64

Keller M B 1985 Chronic and recurrent affective disorders: incidence, course and influencing factors. In: Kemali D, Racagni G (eds) Chronic treatments in neuropsychiatry. Raven Press, New York, p 111–120

Krause N 1987 Understanding the stress process: linking social support and locus of control beliefs. Journal of Gerontology 42: 589–593

Lehmann H E, Fenton F R, Deutsch M, Feldman S, Engelsmann F 1988 An 11-year follow-up study of 110 depressed patients. Acta Psychiatrica Scandinavica 78: 57–65

McCreadie R G, Wilson A O, Burton L 1983 The Scottish survey of 'new chronic' inpatients. British Journal of Psychiatry 143: 564–571

McGuffin P, Katz R, Bebbington P 1987 Hazard, heredity and depression. A family study. Journal of Psychiatric Research 21: 365–375

Maguire P, Tait A, Brooke M, Thomas C, Sellwood R 1980 The effect of counselling on the psychiatric morbidity associated with mastectomy. British Medical Journal 281: 1454–1456

Maguire P, Brooke M, Tait A, Thomas C, Sellwood R 1983 The effect of counselling on physical disability and social recovery after mastectomy. Clinical Oncology 9: 319–324

Mechanic D 1977 Illness behaviour, social adaptation and the management of illness. A comparison of educational and medical models. Journal of Nervous and Mental Disorder 165: 79–87

Meller I, Fichter M, Weyerer S, Witzke W 1989 The use of psychiatric facilities by depressives: results of the Upper Bavarian Study. Acta Psychiatrica Scandinavica 79: 27–31

Munroe S M 1988 Social factors in depression. Current Opinion in Psychiatry 1: 165–175

Newton J 1988 Preventing mental illness. Routledge, London, p 134–196

Parker G, Barnett B 1987 A test of the social support hypothesis. British Journal of Psychiatry 150: 72–77

Parker G, Kiloh L, Hayward L 1987 Parental representations of neurotic and endogenous depressives. Journal of Affective Disorders 13: 75–82

Parkes C M 1981 Evaluation of a bereavement service. Journal of Preventative Psychiatry 1: 179–188

Paul G L 1969 Chronic mental patients: current status – future directions. Psychological Bulletin 71: 81–94

Paykel E S 1989 Treatment of depression. The relevance of research to clinical practice. British Journal of Psychiatry 155: 754–763

Paykel E S, Mangen S P, Griffiths J H, Burns T 1982 Community psychiatric nursing for neurotic patients: a controlled trial. British Journal of Psychiatry 140: 573–581

Pearlin L I, Schooler C 1978 The structure of coping. Journal of Health and Social Behaviour 19: 2–21

Perris C, Arrindell W A, Perris H, Eiseman M, Van der Ende J, Von Knorring L, 1986 Perceived deprived parental rearing and depression. British Journal of Psychiatry 148: 170–175

Pound A, Mills M, Cox T 1985 A pilot evaluation of Newpin. A home-visiting and befriending scheme in south London. Newsletter of the Association of Child Psychology and Psychiatry October: 2–4

Raphael B 1977 Preventative intervention with the recently bereaved. Archives of General Psychiatry 34: 1450–1454

Robins L, Helzer J, Weisman M, Orvashcel H, Gruenberg E, Burke J, Reiger D 1984 Lifetime prevalence of specific psychiatric disorders in three sites. Archives of General Psychiatry 41: 949–958

Scott J 1988a Chronic depression. British Journal of Psychiatry 153: 287–297

Scott J 1988b Psychological models of depression. Current Opinion in Psychiatry 1: 719–724

Scott J 1988c Cognitive therapy with depressed inpatients. In: Trower P, Dryden W (eds) Developments in cognitive psychotherapy. Sage Publications, London, p 177–189

Scott J 1989 Can depression be prevented? Bulletin of the Royal College of Psychiatrists 13: 583

Scott J, Cole A, Eccleston D 1990 Dealing with persisting abnormalities of mood. International Review of Psychiatry: in press

Shaw D M 1977 The practical management of affective disorders. British Journal of Psychiatry 130: 432–451

Shaw D M, Koch H C 1982 Affective disorders. In:

McCreadie R G (ed) Rehabilitation in psychiatric practice. Pitman, London, p 7–27

Suchman E A 1965 Stages in illness and medical care. Journal of Health and Human Behaviour 6: 115

Talbott J A, Clark G H, Sharfstein S S, Klein J 1987 Issues in developing standards governing psychiatric practice in community mental health centres. Hospital and Community Psychiatry 38: 1198–1202

Tanner J, Weissman M, Prusoff B 1975 Social adjustment and clinical relapse in depressed outpatients. Comprehensive Psychiatry 16: 547–556

Tantum D 1989 Familial factors in psychiatric disorder. Current Opinion in Psychiatry 2: 296–301

Tyrer P, Ferguson B, Wadsworth J 1990 Liaison psychiatry in general practice: the comprehensive collaborative model. Acta Psychiatrica Scandinavica 81: 359–363

Weissman M, Klerman G 1977 Sex differences and the epidemiology of depression. Archives of General Psychiatry 34: 98–111

Weissman M, Paykel E S 1974 The depressed woman : a study of social relationships. University of Chicago, Chicago, p 154–170

Wells K, Hersen M, Bellack A S, Himmelhoch J 1977 Social skills training for unipolar depressive females. Paper presented at the Association for the Advancement of Behaviour Therapy, Atlanta, 12–15 December

Wilcox D R, Gilan R, Hare E H 1965 Do psychiatric outpatients take their drugs? British Medical Journal 2: 790–792

Wing J K 1971 Social psychiatry. British Journal of Hospital Medicine 5: 53–56

Youngren M A, Lewinsohn P M 1977 The functional relationship between depression and problematic interpersonal behaviour. University of Oregon, Oregon, p 15–25

Zeiss A, Lewinsohn P M, Munoz R F 1977 Nonspecific improvement effects in depression using interpersonal social skills training, pleasant activity schedules, or cognitive training. Journal of Consulting and Clinical Psychology 47: 427–439

PART 5

Special aspects

34. Transcultural aspects

Julian P. Leff

Diagnostic systems within psychiatry are currently in a state of flux. A few examples will suffice to illustrate the pendular movements that have occurred in recent decades. At the time of the US:UK Project (Cooper et al 1972) the diagnostic category of schizophrenia as employed by American psychiatrists was very broad relative to the British category. It encompassed almost all of what British psychiatrists called mania and a sizeable proportion of psychotic depression as diagnosed in Britain. The deep division in diagnostic practice revealed by the US:UK Project and confirmed by the International Pilot Study of Schizophrenia (IPSS) (World Health Organization 1973), in conjunction with a swing away from psychoanalysis to biological psychiatry, set the diagnostic pendulum in motion. The outcome is a relatively narrow American definition of schizophrenia, as set out in DSM-III (American Psychiatric Association 1980), and a broader category of affective disorder than currently in use in Britain.

An example, local to the author, is the shift away from anxiety neurosis and towards depression recorded at the Maudsley Hospital from 1955 onwards which Hare (1974) noted and ascribed to the introduction of specific antidepressant medication. Why are psychiatric diagnoses so fickle, blown hither and thither by the winds of fashion? The answer is surely that they are not anchored by any known pathology. While other branches of medicine also have their diagnostic rag-bags, such as 'irritable bowel disease', for which there is no demonstrable pathology, the major disease categories are firmly established, with clearly defined anatomical and/or physiological changes, even if the aetiology remains unclear. This is not the case in psychiatry, in which categorization rests solely on patterns of signs and symptoms, with occasionally a historical feature included, as in DSM-III schizophrenia. As signs and symptoms are constituted by the patient's behaviour and experience, and these are clearly shaped by culture, there is ample scope for cultural influences on diagnostic categories.

THE CULTURAL RELATIVITY OF PHENOMENA

Psychotic phenomena

If we consider the phenomena on which a broad diagnosis of psychosis is based, namely delusions and hallucinations, we find that cultural factors exert a major influence. In the case of delusions, cultural factors are an integral part of the definition. It is not possible to decide in the abstract whether a person's belief is delusional or not. For this judgment it is essential to know and understand the beliefs held by the people who make up the individual's cultural group. Such groups may represent the majority culture shared by millions of people or minority sects with only a handful of followers.

Furthermore, no absolute standard by which to judge the pathological nature of hallucinations can be established. Within mainstream British culture it has been found that half of all bereaved people experience hallucinations of the dead person for years after the loss (Rees 1971). In many traditional cultures spirits of ancestors are believed to be capable of communicating with the living, and individuals who see or hear such spirits are viewed as specially favoured (e.g. Cheetham & Cheetham 1976). In the same vein, some religious sects in Western countries encourage the belief that the holy spirit can descend into worshippers and be manifested in various ways, such as 'speaking in tongues'. Schwab (1977) conducted a population survey in Florida and found that hallucinations were reported more frequently by black Baptists, black Methodists and members of the Church of God

539

than by Lutherans, Presbyterians, white Methodists, Episcopalians and Jews. Hence the experiencing of hallucinations is subject to cultural influences and a judgment about their pathological nature has to take account of the cultural affiliation of the individual.

Neurotic phenomena

The influence that culture exerts looms even larger when we consider neurotic phenomena. An important fact to take account of is that 'psychotic' experiences are relatively rare in the general population whereas 'neurotic' experiences are extremely common. In Schwab's (1977) survey the proportion of respondents reporting hallucinations ranged from a high of 21% to a low of nil, while in Western countries virtually everyone will experience depression or anxiety at some time in their lives. The near universality of these experiences raises the question of how to establish a threshold for pathology. At what level, for example, does depression as a mood state become depression as a symptom? In clinical practice we rely on a number of attributes of the lowered mood to judge whether it can be considered pathological. We enquire about the duration of the mood, whether it can be relieved by company or by watching an amusing programme, and about the intensity of the feeling of depression. The latter can only be conveyed subjectively, but it is usual to ask whether the person has periods of crying and if so whether these occur when they are alone or in company. With respect to this, cultural norms for the expression of emotion need to be taken into account; for instance among British whites it is more acceptable for women to cry in public than for men.

Another judgment that often contributes to the decision as to the pathological nature of lowered mood is whether it stems from an understandable cause. The most obvious example is the response to bereavement. Loss of spouse is judged by the public to be the most stressful life event (Holmes & Rahe 1967, Ulrich 1987) and it would be strange indeed if someone experiencing such a loss did not become depressed for a time. But how long a time is acceptable before a diagnosis of 'prolonged bereavement reaction' is made? In many traditional cultures the period for grieving is stipulated, as well as the behaviour to be exhibited. For example, orthodox Jews observe three periods of graded mourning after the death of a close relative. For the first 7 days no work is done, the bereaved person sits on the floor and does not cut his/her hair and regular visits are paid by kin and friends. For the next 3 weeks there is a return to work but other restrictions are observed, while during the following 11 months life is carried on as usual except that a prayer for the dead is recited at the start of each day. At the end of a year a headstone is set up at the grave and the period of mourning is at an end. It is considered impious to prolong mourning beyond this time. In cultures which specify clear guidelines such as these, abnormal grieving is easy to identify. When traditions lose their grip on a populace and mourning becomes a matter of individual choice, it is still possible to identify a common sequence of psychological responses (Parkes 1972), but the decision as to when the reaction is pathologically prolonged is much more difficult.

Judgments about the pathological nature of neurotic experiences often rest on the patient's social performance. This is most evident with obsessional behaviour, for which the distinction between a trait and a symptom hinges on the extent to which the behaviour encroaches on daily life. To a lesser degree, this is true of anxiety, both free-floating and situational. A moderate amount of anxiety is a spur to action, but at higher levels performance increasingly begins to suffer, and a pathological state ensues. A different situation exists with regard to phobic anxiety, since even low levels are inhibiting rather than stimulating. However certain of this class of symptoms are so common, for instance spider phobia, that to label them pathological is to rob the word of its meaning. It is only when they reach such a pitch that the sufferer's daily life is affected that we consider them to be disease states. Since the adequate performance of social roles is moulded by cultural values and expectations, any judgment that takes into account the individual's social performance is inevitably influenced by cultural factors. This point is illustrated by Orley's experience in a Ugandan village (personal communication). He noted villagers whom he considered to be suffering from depression. They complained of lassitude and stopped working, but did not seek help for this, nor did other villagers comment on their dropping out of the work force. This was because the staple foods were grown with relatively little effort, and there was no desire to create a surplus. Consequently the loss of one pair of hands was not socially damaging. By contrast, in a competitive Western society if someone does not turn up for work it is a matter for serious concern, and an explanation is demanded. Waxler (1977) makes the same point about Sinhalese society: 'while social withdrawal, lack of energy and feelings of sadness are commonly labelled "depression" in Western societies, in Sri Lanka the same phenomena receive less attention . . . and very little treatment'.

CULTURE OR BIOLOGY?

The argument that cultural factors cannot be ignored in judging the pathological nature of behaviour and experience is widely accepted by psychiatrists. However, a more radical view of the influence of culture on psychiatry as a discipline has been expounded as part of the 'new cross-cultural psychiatry' (Kleinman 1977, Littlewood 1990). This approach, which has an epistemological basis, considers psychiatry as a product of Western culture. Its application to non-Western peoples is then of dubious validity. Disease categories developed from experience with the mental disturbances of Westerners may be imposed across cultural boundaries, but this activity is tantamount to cultural imperialism. Local patterns of morbidity are ignored if they do not fit into the Western grid, and local conditions are inappropriately viewed as variants of Western categories. This argument is hard to sustain with a condition such as manic-depressive psychosis, the characteristic symptoms of which are recognized by traditional healers in the third world. For example a Kenyan healer interviewed by Onyango (1976) described a condition which he ascribed to worms inside the patient's head.

> The worms have hairy bodies and these interfere with brain function. When the worms are awake in the head, the patient becomes very excited, talkative, his voice changes and the eyes become red. But when the worms are sleeping, the patient becomes too sad, never talks, refuses food and he may become very violent as he is constantly irritated in the brain by the hair of the worms.

When it comes to a behavioural disturbance such as anorexia nervosa which is virtually confined to Western cultures, the above argument has much greater force. Littlewood (1990) has proposed that psychiatric conditions can be sited at various points along a spectrum extending from a biomedical pole to a sociological pole. The symptomatic and functional psychoses occupy the biomedical end of the spectrum, while school refusal, eating disorders and shoplifting belong at the sociological end. The accumulating evidence for anatomical, physiological and biochemical abnormalities in schizophrenic and manic-depressive psychosis goes some way to establishing their position close to the biomedical pole. The neuroses occupy an uncomfortable position intermediate between the two poles. This resurrects the perennial question of whether depressive neurosis lies on a continuum with manic-depressive illness or whether there is a discontinuity between them (Kendell 1968). In this context, however, the question shifts from the extent to which these conditions share a reactivity to environmental stress, to the degree to which they are cultural constructions as opposed to biological entities. In principle, though, the question is essentially the same: does culture exert an incremental effect as we move from manic-depressive psychosis to depressive neurosis, or is the former a biological illness and the latter a cultural product? We will address this complex question in stages, beginning with cultural influences on manic-depressive psychosis.

CULTURE AND MANIC-DEPRESSIVE PSYCHOSIS

The earliest relevant observation was made by Kraepelin (1921) as a consequence of his visit to Java. He noted that cases of manic-depressive insanity, as he termed it, were as common in the psychiatric hospital he visited as in European asylums. However, the Javanese patients suffered 'almost exclusively states of excitement and often confusion'. He was unable to find 'well-marked states of depression lasting for some time, such as fill the observation wards at home'. Makanjuola (1982, 1985, 1989), in a series of studies of Nigerian patients, has demonstrated the same preponderance of manic states. In a consecutive series of admissions to two teaching hospital psychiatric units in Ife, he observed that recurrent manic disorder without depressive episodes was the rule rather than the exception (Makanjuola 1982, 1985). Out of a sample of 104 patients, 55 suffered from recurrent unipolar manic disorder. There was no difference in the duration of history between these patients and the bipolar groups, rendering unlikely the explanation that the apparent excess of unipolar manics was due to too brief a period of observation. However it remains possible that depressed patients may be much better tolerated in the community in a rural environment, as discussed above, leading to a selective referral to hospital of patients with mania. The population studies required to resolve this issue have not been conducted.

Makanjuola (1982) also investigated the possible influence of culture on the prevalence of characteristic symptoms in manic states. He examined each patient in his sample with the Present State Examination (PSE) (Wing et al 1974) and charted the frequency of individual symptoms among the 45 manic patients. His findings can be compared with two epidemiologically

542 HANDBOOK OF AFFECTIVE DISORDERS

based samples of first-admission manic patients from Aarhus, Denmark and London, together totalling 46 individuals (Leff et al 1976). For none of the symptoms commonly experienced in mania was there a significant difference between the Nigerian and European patients, with the exception of the area of hallucinations. These were experienced by 17 (38%) of the Nigerian sample compared with none of the European patients. Of the 17 Nigerian patients, 14 were rated as having verbal hallucinations based on elation. This striking difference might be accounted for on the basis that only the most severely ill manic patients were admitted to the relatively scarce facilities in Ife. However, this is implausible, since there was no difference between the European and Nigerian samples in the frequency of delusions. A more probable explanation is that the threshold for experiencing or reporting hallucinations is lower in Nigeria as a result of more tolerant public attitudes to these experiences, as discussed above. Further support for this explanation is provided by a study of the clients of a traditional healer in Kenya. Of the 13 clients interviewed with the PSE, seven were rated as experiencing olfactory hallucinations (Gatere 1980). This is an uncommon symptom among Western psychotic patients.

A comparison of symptoms assessed with the PSE was made in the context of the International Pilot Study of Schizophrenia (WHO 1973). Although the main focus of the study was schizophrenia, a sufficient number of manic-depressive patients was collected in Aarhus, Agra and Prague to render comparison of symptom frequency feasible. When the 20 manic patients from Aarhus were compared with the 20 manic patients from Agra, striking differences were found in only two areas: derealization was much commoner among the Danish patients and lack of insight among the Indian patients. Comparison of the 19 psychotically depressed patients from Aarhus with the same number from Prague also revealed two main areas of difference: the Danish patients had a higher prevalence of lack of insight and of derealization than the Czech patients. The only consistent finding from these comparisons is the relatively high frequency of derealization among the manic and depressed patients from Aarhus. This is more likely to be due to rater bias than to cultural effects.

Another aspect of the epidemiological study by Leff et al (1976) has some bearing on cultural influences on manic symptoms. They found that 45% of the sample collected in London were born outside the United Kingdom. When these patients were compared with the native British, it was found that a significantly higher proportion were rated as having delusions of special ability, grandiose identity and a special mission. Since they had been born in a variety of Western and non-Western countries, and furthermore the Nigerian patients in Makanjuola's (1982) study did not show a high prevalence of these delusions, this difference cannot be attributed to factors operating in a particular culture. Instead, it seems likely that it is due to immigrant status itself. Some support for this suggestion is provided by a study by Brody (1973) of psychiatric first admissions in Rio de Janeiro. He found that a much higher proportion of the recently migrant exhibited grandiose delusions than of settled people. These migrants originated from the countryside rather than from other countries. From a psychological viewpoint the migrant, disadvantaged in many respects compared to his/her settled neighbours, may compensate for this by developing grandiose delusions when mania supervenes.

In view of the interesting questions raised by transcultural comparisons of manic-depressive illnesses, it is surprising that so little research has been conducted in this area since Kraepelin's pioneering observations. Indeed a Medline search for 1983–1989 inclusive identified only the papers by Makanjuola as containing material relevant to this topic.

CULTURE AND DEPRESSIVE NEUROSIS

The decline of hysteria

In attempting to define the extent to which culture influences the neuroses, it is useful to adopt a historical perspective in addition to a transcultural one. It is evident from the professional literature of the late nineteenth and early twentieth centuries that hysteria was one of the commonest manifestations of neurosis in Western Europe at the time (e.g. Breuer & Freud 1956). Numerical estimates of its prevalence are difficult to obtain, however, until the First World War. Culpin (1920) reviewed 415 case records of neurosis from military hospitals, and assessed the primary diagnosis as being hysteria in 28%, while anxiety state comprised 49% of the sample. It is important to note that what would now be diagnosed as depressive neurosis was subsumed under the term anxiety state. A comparable study was conducted by Hadfield (1942) during the Second World War. He found that hysteria occupied a similar proportion of admissions of soldiers to a neuropathic hospital, namely 24%, while the prevalence of anxiety neurosis was somewhat higher than Culpin's figure, being 64%. At this period depression was still included under the rubric of anxiety. A study by Abse (1950) of admissions to a military hospital in Chester during 1943 produced a figure for hysteria of 24% and for anxiety states of 50%. Abse also studied admissions to a military hospital in Delhi during 1944 and found a remarkable reversal of these figures; 57% with hysteria and 12% with anxiety states.

The figures for British soldiers during the First and Second World Wars indicate that hysteria, while about half as common as anxiety states, remained at a steady level throughout that period of 30 years. However over the subsequent 30 years the admission rate of hysteria to psychiatric hospitals in England and Wales showed a rapid and regular decline, as charted in Figure 34.1.

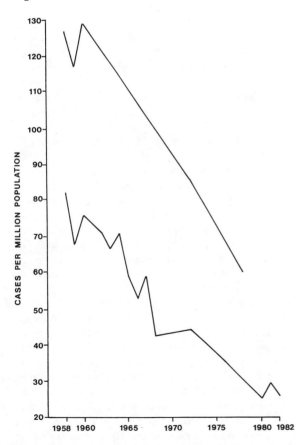

Fig. 34.1 Admissions, discharges and deaths with hysteria in NHS hospitals in England and Wales

The lower graph in the figure shows a similar reduc-

tion in discharges and deaths from hysteria in non-psychiatric hospitals (admission data are not available, but must be equivalent), indicating that there has not merely been a shift in the locus of care of hysteria from psychiatric to non-psychiatric hospitals. A comparable decline is not apparent in non-Western countries generally, although detailed figures are hard to obtain. However data are recorded in the Triennial Report of the Department of Psychiatry in Chandigarh, North India. Between 1975 and 1977 hysteria constituted 44% of the 126 admissions for neurosis and 23% of outpatient contacts for neurosis. In the University Psychiatric Clinic in Cairo in 1966 the proportion of neurotic outpatients with diagnoses of hysteria was 24% (Okasha et al 1968), while the comparable figure for Lebanon in 1964 was 22% (Katchadourian & Racy 1969). An impressionistic account of the clientele of a psychiatric clinic in Tonga is given by Murphy & Taumoepeau (1980): 'most cases have taken the form of a dissociative state or hysterical conversion syndrome. Paraesthesia, pseudo-paralysis, pseudo-epilepsy and hyperventilation are all to be encountered, just as if one were with Charcot a hundred years ago'.

There is at least one non-Western culture, Japan, in which, exceptionally, hysteria appears to be declining as in the West. Fukuda et al (1980) reviewed the records of the psychiatric departments of two general hospitals and calculated the rate over two decades (1952–1973) of all women attending with hysteria. Over this period hysteria in women as a proportion of new outpatients fell from 6% to 2%, despite a comparable attendance rate. This reduction of two-thirds is virtually identical to that affecting admissions for hysteria to psychiatric hospitals in England and Wales over the same period. Whatever cultural factors are responsible for the decline of hysteria in the West must also be present in the Japanese situation.

One can conclude that since the Second World War, hysteria in Western countries has been on the wane and has largely been replaced by anxiety and depressive neuroses, although for a time these were both grouped under the heading of anxiety. This raises the possibility that hysteria, anxiety and depression are various forms of an underlying dysphoric state, which we can refer to as distress. It has been suggested that patterns by which psychiatrists recognize these conditions may be better viewed as culturally determined idioms of distress, rather than disease entities (Nichter 1981) If this were the case, one would expect to find a considerable overlap between the symptom patterns during a process of transition from one idiom of distress to another.

Overlap between neurotic symptom patterns

Because of the period of time over which hysteria has been disappearing in the West, few studies of this condition employing standardized clinical instruments have been conducted. However, some clinicians have recorded their impressions of the coexistence of different symptom patterns. Head (1922) commented: 'In a large number of cases, especially in civil life, removal of hysterical symptoms is only a prelude to the discovery of an anxiety neurosis'. This observation suggests that the symptoms of anxiety (and depression, which were subsumed under anxiety at that time) were not apparent until the hysterical symptoms resolved. This is commensurate with the classical picture of hysteria, in which the patient exhibited a mood of *belle indifférence*. This was explained in psychodynamic terms as a consequence of denial of anxiety. However other studies have found symptoms of anxiety and depression to be present at the same time as conversion symptoms. Culpin (1920) advised that: 'Hysteria, anxiety state, psychasthenia and neurasthenia are not to be taken as the names of different entities...the different conditions must not be pictured as clearly separated from each other'. In a series of 438 cases admitted to a military hospital he found 29 with pure hysteria, 174 with an anxiety state and 67 with a combination of hysteria and an anxiety state.

More recently, Purtell et al (1951) examined 50 women admitted to a New England hospital with either hysterical conversion symptoms or a multiplicity of somatic complaints. They found that 74% complained of anxiety attacks and 58% of depression. Lader & Sartorius (1968) compared 10 patients with hysterical conversion symptoms with 71 patients suffering from anxiety states or phobias. The patients with hysteria were found to have higher self-ratings of anxiety than those with anxiety states. Meares & Horvath (1972) studied 17 patients with conversion hysteria, six of whom were in an acute state and remitted within a week, while the remaining 11 suffered from chronic symptoms. Both groups had neuroticism scores comparable with other neurotic patients and both were rated as having depressed mood, but depressive symptoms were much more severe in the chronic than in the acute group.

We have noted several times that depression has emerged relatively recently from the shadow of anxiety.

Consequently we would expect there still to be a considerable overlap in patients' experience of these sets of symptoms. Findings from a number of studies confirm this expectation. Snaith et al (1976) obtained self-reports from patients suffering from endogenous depression or anxiety neurosis. They completed a Leeds Self Assessment of Depression Specific Scale and an equivalent scale for anxiety. Of the patients diagnosed clinically as suffering from anxiety neurosis, only 24% had scores that did not overlap with those of the depressed patients. In a symmetrical fashion, only 26% of patients with endogenous depression had scores that did not overlap with those of anxious patients. Of the total group, 73% fell into the middle range of scores and were considered by Snaith et al to represent 'anxiety-depressions'.

In a more recent study of people aged 65 years and over in Southeast London, Lindesay et al (1989) interviewed 890 respondents using a structured schedule, which included depression scales and items covering the anxiety symptoms. They found that generalized anxiety and depression scores were significantly associated, with a correlation of 0.68, as were cases of those two disorders defined by threshold scores ($p < 0.001$).

We were interested in investigating the extent to which patients' concepts of anxiety and depression overlapped and to compare this with the concepts held by psychiatrists working in the same institution (Leff 1978). 20 patients suffering from neurosis and 10 experienced psychiatrists took part. Each subject was asked to rate feelings of depression, anxiety and irritability on 11 somatic and 11 psychological constructs. For instance, they were required to state whether when they felt depressed their heart beat fast (somatic construct) and whether they wanted to die (psychological construct). The patients were asked to rate their own unpleasant emotion, while the psychiatrists were requested to respond as they thought a typical neurotic patient would. The correlation coefficient between anxiety and depression on all 22 constructs was 0.62 for the patients, very similar to the correlation found by Lindesay et al (1989). However the psychiatrists' ratings produced a correlation of 0, indicating that they expected neurotic patients to make a perfect distinction between anxiety and depression. The important influence that psychiatrists' crystallized concepts of neurosis exert on the differentiation of these conditions by the public will be explored below.

The evidence reviewed so far indicates that hysteria, anxiety and depression often coexist in the same individual. Before exploring possible explanations for this phenomenon, we will take a broader look at the bodily symptoms that frequently accompany the neuroses.

The bodily expression of distress

We have already given some consideration to hysteria, which represents the transformation of distress into an extensive range of bodily symptoms mimicking, more or less convincingly, organic disease states. However another type of somatic experience is encountered much more commonly as a representation of distress, namely the autonomic accompaniments of emotional arousal.

Excitement and the pleasant states of arousal are universal, so everyone has experienced the effects of heightened autonomic activity; the pounding heart, the tight chest that results from rapid shallow breathing, the clammy hands, the sinking feeling in the stomach. The range of effects is very extensive, but these are among the commonest. In some patients in white British culture, and in the majority of patients in some other countries, these experiences dominate the complaints of distressed individuals. Are they merely a more intense form of everyday experiences or are they qualitatively different?

This important question has rarely been addressed, but there is one relevant study by Yanping et al (1986). They asked depressed Chinese patients to describe their experiences, and from the indigenous phrases or words used they constructed a Verbal Expression Style Investigation Schedule (VESIS). This was administered to samples of psychiatric patients with affective illness and to a control group of normal subjects. Depression was more frequently expressed somatically by depressed patients than by the controls, leading Yanping et al to conclude that patients who have experienced pathological depression place a greater emphasis on somatic symptoms than do normal subjects who have not been clinically depressed. This could result either from a heightened awareness of autonomic activity in those with affective disorders, or from actual quantitative or qualitative change in the autonomic accompaniments themselves. Whichever explanation proves to be correct, these somatic symptoms can constitute the presenting complaint of distressed individuals.

There are numerous reports from developing countries recording the observation that depressed patients manifest a much higher proportion of somatic complaints than in the West. German (1972) reports this for sub-Saharan Africa, Teja et al (1971) for Indians and Racy (1980) for Saudis, for example. The general assumption of these authors is that the patients in developing countries are suffering from an equivalent condition to depression in the West, but that they have somatized their complaints. This type of assumption has been criticized by Kleinman (1977) as representing a 'category fallacy'. He argues that there is no *a priori* reason to assume that categories of disease developed from experience with patients in the West can automatically be applied to patients in non-Western cultures. Thus the view that non-Western patients are presenting a debased or distorted version of depression reflects an ethnocentric Western stance.

A formulation that avoids this bias runs as follows: babies are born with a capacity to experience distress both somatically and psychologically. Recent research in neonatal psychology had demonstrated that very young babies are able to discriminate between smiles, frowns and expressions of surprise on adult faces (Field et al 1982). The culture into which the baby is born may choose to emphasize either the somatic or the psychological expression of emotion at the expense of the other. This does not necessarily mean that the individual fails to experience the full range of emotions. However, it does have an effect on the public expression of emotion, which includes consultations of patients with healers or doctors. We will consider these in detail below. An influence is also detectable on the language of emotion.

The language of emotion

It has been recognized for some time that it is difficult, if not impossible, to find equivalent terms for depression and anxiety in certain languages. The two phrases that were used for these terms in Yoruba were respectively back-translated as 'the heart is weak' and 'the heart is not at rest'. Marsella (1979) reviewed cross-cultural studies of depression and noted that research on indigenous categories of mental disorder in Malaysia, Borneo, Africa and among many American Indians revealed that there were no concepts that represented depression as either a disease, symptom or syndrome. It should be noted that this does not preclude the existence of words or phrases that convey sadness in everyday experience. The emphasis on the heart in the Yoruba vocabulary of emotion is repeated in other languages. Among Turkish-speaking peoples in Iran, emotional terms often contain a reference to the heart, for example *qualbim narahatdi* – 'my heart is upset, uncomfortable, distressed' (Good 1977). Among the Xhosa of South Africa, the word *mbilini* is used to indicate emotional instability, and refers to sensations of palpitation, throbbing, discomfort or pain in the epigastric region (Cheetham & Cheetham 1976). The Tswana use the phrase *pelo, pelo y tata* – 'heart, heart too much' – to express a variety of forms of distress (Ben-Tovim 1987).

In cultures in which the language of emotion refers directly to bodily experiences, there appears to be a wider range of somatic symptoms as expression of distress than in the West. For instance, Ebigbo (1982) recorded the somatic complaints of mentally ill patients in Nigeria, which included heat in the head, crawling sensation of worms and ants, a sensation of heaviness in the head and biting sensations all over the body. Verma & Wig (1976) constructed a questionnaire for eliciting the symptoms of neurosis in patients who spoke Hindi or Punjabi. Of the 50 items, 20 refer directly to somatic symptoms including: 'I often get watering of the eyes'; 'I belch a lot after eating'; 'I feel very thirsty'; 'I often have to go to the toilet straight after meals'; and 'I find difficulty in passing water'.

It appears that in cultures in which there is a greater emphasis on the somatic experiences of dysphoria than the psychological ones, this is reflected in a vocabulary of emotions which is firmly grounded in bodily sensations and the presentation of a wide diversity of somatic complaints by patients. However, we need to be aware that terms used in European language to convey the psychological experiences of emotional disturbance also derive their roots from bodily experiences. *Anxiety* derives from a Greek root which means to press tight or strangle, and is related to a number of Latin words, including *angina*, which all convey the notion of constriction and discomfort. In German the word *eng* means narrow, and its superlative form *engste* bears a close phonetic relationship to *Angst*, the word regularly used by Freud and translated as *anxiety*. The word *depression* is derived from the Latin root *depremere*, meaning to press down, and refers to the feelings of pressure in the head experienced by many depressed patients (Leff 1988).

Beeman (1985) raises the interesting possibility that all the words used in contemporary contexts for the psychological experiences of dysphoria are 'metaphorical extensions of what were originally thought of as somatic expressions'. He asserts that metaphor is the primary method of expressing emotion in all but the most clinical settings. This seems to be overstating the case, since in American and British cultures the term anxiety is used in common parlance for experiences which fall far short of clinical states, and yet its linguistic root in words denoting constriction in the chest is not at all apparent to the man in the street. On the other hand it is uncertain whether the Yoruba speaker using the local term for anxiety is referring to the heart metaphorically, as the English speaker would do when saying 'I am heart-broken', or whether the bodily experience is uppermost in his mind. It is not obvious how one would choose between these alternatives without requesting the Yoruba speaker to introspect about his associations to the phrase.

As we have seen, culture exerts a strong influence on the form in which patients present their distress. There are important clinical consequences stemming from the degree to which the doctor or healer is able to deal with the symptoms presented.

DOCTOR – CLIENT NEGOTIATION

Patients bring to the doctor a series of complaints which are in part moulded by the concepts of illness they hold, and in part by their expectations about what the doctor is prepared to deal with. The doctor translates the complaints into symptoms and then formulates a diagnosis on the basis of the symptoms. Doctors who are not alert to the fact that emotional distress may be presented as somatic complaints can easily make the wrong formulation and may then embark on an inappropriate series of investigations. Healers in developing countries appear to be well aware of the significance of somatic symptoms that signal distress. This may not be so easy for a doctor from another culture. Racy (1980) practised in Saudi Arabia and spoke Arabic fluently. Nevertheless he found that considerable effort was required to get beyond the somatic complaints of his patients to reach an understanding of their lives, concerns and troubles. When he was able to do so he found a series of common themes: 'neglect by the husband in favour of a younger and prettier wife, feelings of loneliness on separating from parents and siblings, lack of money or food, fatigue from prolonged child-rearing and conflicts with in-laws, since Arab homes tend to house several generations'.

The difficulty Racy encountered was probably due to his patients' reluctance to comment openly about their family relationships. In most of the developing world this is a delicate topic which can only be approached obliquely. Traditional healers are well aware of this, since they belong to the same culture as their clients, and are also in touch with the common conflicts in social relationships. Instead of speaking openly about such touchy matters, as a Kalanga diviner put it, 'we speak indirectly; we speak in allusions' (Werbner 1973). Often the healer translates the problems in human relationships to another, more acceptable, plane. In Ayurvedic medicine, the *pandit* discusses issues relating to family interrelationships and personal problems by referring to humoral imbalances (Nichter 1981). In Taiwan the *dang-ki* speaks of a devil, a ghost or a god, which can serve as a symbol of a significant person in the client's life. Thus the human difficulties can be referred to as ethereal spirit relationships (Tseng 1976). Similarly, in Tonga explanations about spirit interventions allow the expression of disharmony without open confrontation (Parsons 1984).

Although the healer's diagnosis is presented in displaced terms, his prescription usually involves a restoration of balance in the client's social relationships. However, this is also achieved by indirect means, since direct interventions are likely to fail, as recorded by Racy (1980): 'I have on occasion attempted to encourage Saudi women to assert and emancipate themselves. But I soon discovered that as a psychiatric consultant I could not be a social reformer. The patients belonged in their cultural set and distressing as it may be to them and to the observer, that reality could not be easily and safely altered.' Healers, however, are able to achieve social change without challenging the system. For instance they may prescribe an expensive ritual which requires the entire extended family to rally round the client in order to pay for it, and hence reinforces the social support that the client can draw on. A consideration of these healing practices raises the challenging question of whether they may be at least as effective in containing 'neurotic' morbidity as Western psychiatric treatments. We will discuss this question in the context of methods available to help individuals cope with loss in a variety of cultures.

LOSS AND THE 'WORK OF CULTURE'

The research of Brown & Harris (1978) has shown that events which cause significant loss to the individual, whether it is in terms of relationships, status or material objects, act to precipitate depression in vulnerable individuals. Loss events are a universal feature of human experience, but the way in which loss is coped with varies considerably between cultures. It is the process by which the individual is reconciled to loss that Obeyesekere (1985) calls 'the work of culture'. Three examples from the developing world will illustrate the variations in this process.

The Kaluli are a forest people of Papua New Guinea. Their society operates on a system of reciprocity. If a thief steals a pig, the deprived owner is allowed to steal a pig from the thief or to demand money in compensation. The same concepts are applied to other types of loss (Schieffelin 1985). The Kaluli have an extensive vocabulary for states of anger, which almost always contain the implication that the aggrieved person has suffered a loss of some kind, for which he expects to be compensated. The extent of a man's anger is proportional to the loss he has experienced. The response to a severe loss is public grieving, which is worked through in weeping and song and represents an appeal for retaliation and compensation. Although in reality the loss of a loved person can never be compensated for adequately, the public appeal evokes social support for the bereaved individual.

Iranian history is dominated by tragedy, injustice and martyrdom, which are central to the cultural ethos and are reflected in secular literature (Good et al 1985). The ability to express sadness appropriately and in a culturally approved manner is a component of social competence and is viewed as a mark of personal depth. Most children first learn to grieve in the context of religious ceremonies for Iranian martyrs. Thus grieving is not a solitary process but communal, and furthermore the loss experienced by the individual is dwarfed by the perspective of the historical tragedy of the Iranian people.

In Buddhism the lot of humanity is hopelessness, which can only be coped with by recognizing it as the reality and viewing the world of sense, pleasure and domesticity as illusory. In place of ennobling individual suffering, as does the Iranian culture, Buddhism aims to minimize the individual's sense of loss. The commonest form of meditation practised in Sri Lanka is probably that focused on revulsion (Obeyesekere 1985). The intention is to induce a sense of disgust for pleasures of the senses, which will emphasize the transitoriness of the body. The body is visualized as 'a clay pot, polished on the outside, but full of faeces'. This image is applied to people close to the meditator, such as parents, spouse and children, and is eventually extended to encompass the whole of humanity. In this way, the sense of loss is diminished by attenuating the emotional bonds of attachment.

These three examples of the 'work of culture' in helping individuals to cope with loss are set out in Table 34.1, where they are contrasted with the Western attitude, which Obeyesekere (1985) maintains is the medicalization of distress. In his view, Western biomedicine has invented a disease termed 'depression' to redefine painful emotions. This 'new definition of human suffering' leads to a different method of tackling the problems consequent on loss, namely the provision of a variety of treatments by a doctor. The psychosocial treatments, such as bereavement counselling and individual psychotherapy, bear some relation to the 'work of culture' in traditional societies. The physical treatments, such as antidepressant medication, do not.

Table 34.1 The 'work of culture' in dealing with loss

Culture or people	Coping mechanism
Kaluli	Compensation by society
Iran	Grief a communal act
Sri Lanka	Meditation on worthlessness
The West	Medicalization of distress

These comparisons raise complex questions, to which answers are not currently available. Are these cultural coping mechanisms effective in curtailing the emotional response to loss? If so, then is the prevalence of distress as it is presented to a healer less than that of depression in the West? How would one begin to answer this question given the uncertainty surrounding the equivalents in developing countries of Western depression? What would be the outcome if one treated indigenous categories of distress with Western remedies, such as antidepressants?

In fact an attempt to answer the last question has been made by Kleinman (1986). In China the term neurasthenia is in use for disorders that would mostly be diagnosed as one or other form of neurosis in the West. It corresponds with a number of conditions recognized by traditional Chinese practitioners, who categorize them according to the body organs believed to be affected by a decrease in vital energy or *qi*. Kleinman studied 100 patients attending a hospital in Hunan and given a local diagnosis of neurasthenia. He found that 87 of them satisfied the criteria for major depressive disorder, although 30% complained entirely of somatic symptoms and the remainder of a mixture of somatic and psychological symptoms with a strong emphasis on the former. He treated all 87 with a course of antidepressant medication. At a follow-up examination 6 weeks later, Kleinman found that 65% of patients reported that they were substantially improved. On the other hand 30% considered their social impairment to be worse and over one third sought further help from traditional Chinese practitioners. This indicates that although antidepressants removed the symptoms of the majority of patients with neurasthenia, there was a considerable proportion who remained dissatisfied. Kleinman concluded that 'medical treatment for chronic conditions without significant psychosocial intervention exerts only a limited effect on the overall illness'. This general statement is not confined to Chinese patients with neurasthenia, and would find strong support in the West with regard to patients suffering from depressive neurosis.

The question of the relative effectiveness of cultural resources in preventing a pathological outcome in response to loss could be tackled by taking bereavement as a starting point and comparing mourning practices across cultures. This field of study has recently been reviewed by Eisenbruch (1984), who raises the same question. However the problem of ensuring that one is measuring equivalent forms of pathological bereavement reactions remains a thorny issue.

DICHOTOMY OR CONTINUUM

Having reviewed the influence of culture on the manifestations of distress, we can return to the spectrum of psychiatric disorders extending from the biomedical to the sociological pole. We have adduced evidence for the proposition that disorders at the sociological end represent culturally determined modes of communicating distress which stems from psychosocial problems. How far along the spectrum can this view be said to predominate? Is there a distinct point at which biological factors become the overwhelming determinants of depression, or does one explanation merge imperceptibly with the other? The old issue of 'one depression or two' remains a vital one, for both theoretical and practical reasons. Cross-cultural studies are an important resource to the research worker seeking an answer.

REFERENCES

Abse D W 1950 The diagnosis of hysteria. John Wright, Bristol

American Psychiatric Association 1980 Diagnostic and statistical manual of mental disorders, 3rd edn. American Psychiatric Association, Washington DC

Beeman W O 1985 Dimensions of dysphoria: the view from linguistic anthropology. In: Kleinman A, Good B (eds) Cross-cultural psychiatry of affect and disorder. University of California Press, Berkeley, CA

Ben-Tovim D I 1987 Development psychiatry: mental health and primary health care in Botswana. Tavistock Publications, London

Breuer J, Freud S 1956 Studies on hysteria. Hogarth Press, London

Brody E B 1973 The lost ones. International Universities Press, New York

Brown G W, Harris T 1978 Social origins of depression: a study of psychiatric disorders in women. Tavistock Press, London

Cheetham W S, Cheetham R J 1976 Concepts of mental illness amongst the Xhosa people in South Africa. Australian and New Zealand Journal of Psychiatry 10: 39–45

Cooper J E, Kendell R E, Gurland B J, Sharpe L, Copeland J R M, Simon R 1972 Psychiatric diagnosis in New York and London. Maudsley Monograph 20. Oxford University Press, Oxford

Culpin M 1920 Psychoneuroses of war and peace. Cambridge University Press, Cambridge

Ebigbo P 1982 Development of a culture-specific scale for somatic complaints indicating psychiatric disturbance. Culture, Medicine and Psychiatry 6: 29–43

Eisenbruch M 1984 Cross-cultural aspects of bereavement: ethnic and cultural variations in the development of bereavement practices. Culture Medicine and Psychiatry 8: 315–347

Field T M, Woodson R, Greenberg R, Cohen D 1982 Discrimination and imitation of facial expression by neonates. Science 218: 179–181

Fukuda K, Moriyama M, Chibat T, Suzuki T 1980 Hysteria and urbanisation. British Journal of Psychiatry 137: 200–301

Gatere S 1980 Patterns of psychiatric morbidity in rural Kenya. Unpublished MPhil Thesis, University of London

German A 1972 Aspects of clinical psychiatry in sub-Saharan Africa. British Journal of Psychiatry 121: 461–479

Good B J 1977 The heart of what's the matter: the semantics of illness in Iran. Culture Medicine and Psychiatry 1: 25–58

Good B J, Good M, Moradi R 1985 The interpretation of human depressive illness and dysphoric affect. In: Kleinman A, Good B (eds) Studies in anthropology and cross-cultural psychiatry of affect and disorder. University of California Press, Berkeley, CA

Hadfield J A 1942 War neurosis. British Medical Journal 1: 281–285

Hare E H 1974 The changing content of psychiatric illness. Journal of Psychosomatic Research 18: 283–289

Head H 1922 The diagnosis of hysteria. British Medical Journal 1: 827–829

Holmes T H, Rahe R H 1967 The social readjustment rating scale. Journal of Psychosomatic Research 11: 213–218

Katchadourian H, Racy J 1969 The diagnostic distribution of treated psychiatric illness in Lebanon. British Journal of Psychiatry 115: 1309–1322

Kendell R E 1968 The classification of depressive illness. Maudsley Monograph 18. Oxford University Press, Oxford

Kleinman A 1977 Depression somatisation and the new cross-cultural psychiatry. Social Science and Medicine 11: 3–10

Kleinman A 1986 Social origins of distress and disease: depression neurasthenia and pain in modern China. Yale University Press, New Haven, CT

Kraepelin E 1921 Manic depressive insanity and paranoia, R M Barclay. E & S Livingstone, Edinburgh

Lader M, Sartorius N 1968 Anxiety in patients with hysterical conversion symptoms. Journal of Neurology Neurosurgery and Psychiatry 31: 490–495

Leff J P 1978 Psychiatrists' vs patients' concepts of unpleasant emotions. British Journal of Psychiatry 133: 306–313

Leff J P 1988 Psychiatry around the globe. Gaskell, London

Leff J P, Fischer M, Bertelsen A 1976 A cross-national epidemiological study of mania. British Journal of Psychiatry 129: 428–437

Lindesay J, Briggs K, Murphy E 1989 The Guy's age concern survey: prevalence rates of cognitive impairment depression and anxiety in an urban elderly community. British Journal of Psychiatry 155: 317–329

Littlewood R 1990 From categories to contexts: a decade of the 'new cross-cultural psychiatry'. British Journal of Psychiatry 156: 308–327

Makanjuola R O A 1982 Manic disorder in Nigerians. British Journal of Psychiatry 141: 459–463

Makanjuola R O A 1985 Recurrent unipolar manic disorder in the Yoruba Nigerian: further evidence. British Journal of Psychiatry 147: 434–437

Makanjuola R O A 1989 Socio-cultural parameters in Yoruba Nigerian patients with affective disorders. British Journal of Psychiatry 155: 337–340

Marsella A J 1979 Depressive experience and disorder across cultures. In: Triandis H, Draguns J (eds) Handbook of cross cultural psychology, vol 5, Allyn & Bacon, Boston, MA

Meares R, Horvath T 1972 'Acute' and 'chronic' hysteria. British Journal of Psychiatry 121: 653–657 1972

Murphy H B M, Taumoepeau B M 1980 Traditionalism and mental health in the South Pacific: a re-examination of an old hypothesis. Psychological Medicine 10: 471–482

Nichter M 1981 Negotiation of the illness experience: Ayurvedic therapy and the psychosocial dimension of illness. Culture Medicine and Psychiatry 5: 5–24

Obeyesekere G 1985 Depression Buddhism and the work of culture in Sri Lanka. In: Kleinman A. Good B (eds) Culture and depression: studies in anthropology and cross-cultural psychiatry of affect and disorder. University of California Press: Berkeley

Okasha A, Kamel M, Hassan A H 1968 Preliminary psychiatric observations in Egypt. British Journal of Psychiatry 114: 949–955

Onyango P P 1976 The views of African mental patients towards mental illness and its treatment. MA Thesis, University of Nairobi, Kenya

Parkes C M 1972 Bereavement: studies of grief in adult life. Tavistock Press, London

Parsons C D F 1984 Idioms of distress: kinship and sickness among the people of the kingdom of Tonga. Culture, Medicine and Psychiatry 8: 71–93

Purtell J J, Robins E, Cohen M E 1951 Observations on clinical aspects of hysteria. Journal of the American Medical Association 146: 902–909

Racy J 1980 Somatization in Saudi women: a therapeutic challenge. British Journal of Psychiatry 137: 212–216

Rees W D 1971 The hallucinations of widowhood. British Medical Journal 4: 37–41

Schieffelin E L 1985 The cultural analysis of depressive affect: an example from New Guinea. In: Kleinman A, Good B (eds) Culture and depression: studies in anthropology and cross-cultural psychiatry of affect and disorder. University of California Press, Berkeley

Schwab M E 1977 A study of reported hallucinations in a southeastern county. Mental Health and Society 4: 344–354

Snaith R P, Bridge G W K, Hamilton M 1976 The Leeds scale for self-assessment of anxiety and depression. British Journal of Psychiatry 128: 156–165

Teja J, Narang R, Aggarwal A 1971 Depression across cultures. British Journal of Psychiatry 119: 253–260

Tseng W S 1976 Folk psychotherapy in Taiwan. In: Lebra W P (ed) Culture-bound syndromes, ethnopsychiatry and alternate therapies. University Press of Hawaii, Honolulu

Ulrich H E 1987 A study of change and depression among Havik Brahmin women in a south Indian village. Culture, Medicine and Psychiatry 11: 261–287

Verma S K, Wig N N 1976 PGI Health Questionnaire N-2: construction and initial try outs. Indian Journal of Clinical Psychology 3: 135–142

Waxler N E 1977 Is mental illness cured in traditional societies? A theoretical analysis. Culture, Medicine and Psychiatry 1: 233–253

Werbner R P 1973 The superabundance of understanding: Kalanga rhetoric and domestic divination. American Anthropologist 75: 1414–1440

Wing J K, Cooper J E, Sartorius N 1974 Measurement and classification of psychiatric symptoms. Cambridge University Press, Cambridge

World Health Organization 1973 The international pilot study of schizophrenia, vol 1. WHO, Geneva

Yanping Z, Leyi X, Qijie S 1986 Styles of verbal expression of emotional and physical experiences: a study of depressed patients and normal controls in China. Culture, Medicine and Psychiatry 10: 231–243

35. Seasonal affective disorders

Dan A. Oren   Norman E. Rosenthal

Psychiatrists in the twentieth century have paid careful attention to social and psychological environmental factors that may modify affective states and illnesses. Disappointments, losses, rejections and stress are widely believed to influence the course of mood disorders. Recent decades have added genetic and biochemical perspectives to the understanding of depression and mania. Yet our physical environment has been neglected in the study of mood until the past decade, which has seen a burgeoning interest in the idea that seasonal variations can influence the course of some forms of affective disorder. Though this has been a highly controversial notion, the concept of seasonal mood disorders dates to the dawn of medicine (for review see Wehr & Rosenthal 1989a, b). Over the last decade, speculation and anecdotes have been bolstered by scientific inquiry. In this chapter we shall explore what today are known as the seasonal affective disorders.

HISTORICAL ASPECTS

Seasonal depressions were recorded circa 400 BC by physicians as ancient as Hippocrates (1931 edition). Eight centuries later Posidonius (Roccatagliata 1986) noted that 'melancholy occurs in Autumn, whereas mania in Summer'. The record of Greco-Roman physicians treating depression and lethargy with sunlight directed toward the eyes dates back to the second century (Adams 1856, Aurelianus 1950). Aristotle believed that changes in the temperature of bodily humours caused by changes in seasons could account for cheerfulness and despondency (Ross 1953).

Post-Enlightenment descriptions of seasonal depression appear in isolated reports over the psychiatric literature of the past two centuries (Wehr & Rosenthal 1989b). Cook's graphic descriptions (1894) are the earliest we have come across specifically linking seasonal loss of sunlight to a mood disorder. Accompanying Robert E. Peary on one of his early Arctic expeditions, Cook noted the profound influences of light on the voyagers and upon Eskimos. He depicted a syndrome, characterized by loss of sexual desire, fatigue, loss of energy and profoundly depressed mood, manifest not just in the observed Eskimos, but in the observers as well. Drawing on Cook's observations, Llewellyn (1932) suggested that visual pathways were linked to the powerful phenomenon of environmental light having an impact upon mood. The German psychiatrist Hellmut Marx (1946) described an engineer who had annual episodes of depression, fatigue and excessive appetite whose condition responded to sunlight or sunlamp treatments.

Surprisingly, in a century whose earliest decades saw humanity making great strides toward understanding the influence of environmental nutrients and pathogens on our health, there was little systematic interest in climatological influences upon mood disorders until the 1980s. Modern interest in patients with regularly recurring seasonal depressions was ushered in by the description of an engineer who had documented his own seasonal mood swings for 15 years and had hypothesized that changes in environmental light might have influenced their course (Lewy et al 1982, Rosenthal et al 1983). Thereafter, Rosenthal and colleagues (1984) recruited 29 further patients with regular winter seasonal depressions and described the syndrome of 'seasonal affective disorder' (SAD), based on clinical features, family history, course, laboratory studies and patients' preliminary response to light. Other groups (Boyce & Parker 1988, Garvey et al 1988, Hellekson 1989, Thompson & Isaacs 1988, Wirz-Justice et al 1986a) went on to confirm the existence of such patients whose clinical characteristics strongly resembled those originally described by Rosenthal and colleagues (1984). Wehr and colleagues

(1987a) have subsequently described a patient population with regular summer depressions. In the 1980s the study of seasonal affective disorders and the effects of light on humans became one of the most rapidly growing fields of biomedical research (Garfield 1988).

DIAGNOSTIC ASSESSMENT

The first set of diagnostic criteria for winter Seasonal Affective Disorder (Rosenthal et al 1984) used the seasons as their point of reference. In order to meet criteria for the condition, patients were required to have become depressed regularly during fall and winter and to have remitted regularly during spring and summer (see Table 35.1). In establishing a set of 'seasonal pattern' criteria, to be used as a modifier of any recurrent mood disorder, the creators of DSM-IIIR (American Psychiatric Association 1987) attempted to define more specific criteria. In a move away from the broader concept of seasons and toward specific dates, they specified that recurrent depressions had to start and end at dates within a 60-day window of one another. In addition, they required that the ratio of seasonal to non-seasonal episodes be at least 3:1. These latter criteria have been difficult to apply in the clinical situation and most clinicians and researchers in the field have remained with, or returned to, the original criteria of Rosenthal and colleagues (1984). Given the greater ease of administration of the original criteria and no evidence of any superiority of the DSM-IIIR revisions (Wirz-Justice, personal communication 1990), we and other researchers in the field suggest a return to the original criteria (Rosenthal et al 1984) for clinical and research purposes.

'Summer SAD' does not as yet have nearly the same status as its winter counterpart (Wehr et al 1987a). According to DSM-IIIR it is classified as 'seasonal pattern' according to criteria identical to those of the winter pattern SAD except opposite in the timing of onset and offset of depression. Although the far smaller amount of research on summer SAD has led some researchers to argue against assigning this condition to its own category at this time, others believe that it is distinct from winter SAD (G.L. Faedda et al, personal communication 1990) and should not be considered under the same descriptor. More research is required to evaluate whether this seasonal variant warrants a diagnostic category of its own.

Identification of a seasonal pattern can only be made if both patient and clinician actively look for it. If they fail to do so, many seasonal patients may be diagnosed as 'non-seasonals'. Although many winter SAD patients often meet criteria for 'atypical depression' (Liebowitz et al 1984) by virtue of their characteristic non-endogenous pattern of presentation, most 'atypicals' do not have strong seasonal histories, nor do they appear to respond to light therapy (Stewart et al 1990).

Clinical features

Characteristic symptoms of winter depression noted in SAD patients are dysphoria and decreased activity (see Table 35.2), usually accompanied by concentration difficulties, energy decreases, irritability, anxiety, decreased libido and social withdrawal. Unlike classi-

Table 35.1   Diagnosis of Seasonal Affective Disorder versus Major Depression, Seasonal Pattern

SAD criteria of Rosenthal et al (1984)	DSM-IIIR criteria (American Psychiatric Association 1987)
1) A history of major affective disorder, according to Research Diagnostic Criteria (Spitzer et al 1978)	1) A history of major affective disorder, according to DSM-IIIR Criteria
2) At least two consecutive previous years in which the depressions developed during fall or winter and remitted by the following spring or summer	2) At least three previous winter depressive episodes (two of which were consecutive)
3) Absence of any other Axis I DSM-III psychiatric disorder (American Psychiatric Association 1980)	3) Onset and full remission of each depressive episode which occur within specific 60-day periods of each year
4) Absence of any clear-cut seasonally changing psychosocial variables that would account for the seasonal variability in mood and behaviour	4) Seasonal episodes of mood disturbance outnumbered any non-seasonal episodes of mood disturbance that may have occurred by more than three to one
	5) Absence of any clear-cut seasonally changing psychosocial variables that would account for the seasonal variability in mood and behaviour

Table 35.2 Symptoms of depression in winter SAD around the world (*n* = number of patients surveyed – some individual questions had fewer respondents; % =percentage reporting symptom)

	London $n=51$ (Thompson & Isaacs 1988) %	Basel $n=81$ (Wirz-Justice 1990) %	Heidelberg $n=17$ (Kasper 1990) %	Tokyo $n=46$ (Takahashi 1990) %	Fairbanks, Alaska $n=17$ (Hellekson 1990) %	Bethesda $n=366$ %
Changes in affect:						
Sadness	96	95	77	80	94	96
Irritability	77	68	30	78	71	86
Anxiety	86	84	47	93	59	86
Decreased activity	100	80				95
Interpersonal difficulties	98	90	88	100	82	92
Changes in appetite:						
Increased	74	48	24	42	71	67
Decreased	16	26	47	23	6	16
Mixed or no change	10	26	24	28	24	17
Carbohydrate craving	82					71
Changes in weight:						
Increased	84	54	41	54	70	75
Decreased	6	20	24	7	6	9
Mixed or no change	10	25	30	39	24	17
Changes in sleep:						
Earlier onset			47		65	65
Increased duration	78	61	47	74	94	79
Changes in quality	71	79	77		65	75
Daytime drowsiness			83		35	81
Decreased Libido		38	59		65	65
Difficulties at work	100	96	100	100	76	86
Depression milder near equator			80		94	87
Menstrual exacerbation of symptoms			78		56	59

cally depressed patients, most SAD patients develop 'atypical' depressive symptoms of increased fatigue, increased sleep duration and increased appetite and weight. Not only do SAD patients crave carbohydrates in the winter (Rosenthal et al 1984, 1985a), but they actually report eating more carbohydrate-rich foods at these times (Kräuchi & Wirz-Justice 1988). Kasper's (personal communication, 1990) sample of SAD patients in Bonn complained predominantly of work and interpersonal difficulties and daytime drowsiness rather than changes in appetite and weight. Many patients are more disturbed by the lethargy and fatigue than by the mood changes themselves, especially in the early phases of their winter depression (Young et al 1990) and therefore often seek the help of a physician rather than a psychiatrist. An Alaskan sample of SAD patients, however, reported a lower incidence of daytime drowsiness than patients elsewhere, though this may be because more of them also slept longer during the depression than patients elsewhere (Hellekson, personal communication 1990). Depressions are usually mild to moderate, but 11% of our patients have needed hospitalization and 2% have been given electroconvulsive treatments (see Table 35.3).

SAD depressive episodes typically begin in

Table 35.3 Diagnostic and demographic features of winter SAD around the world (n = number of patients surveyed – some individual questions had fewer respondents; % = percentage reporting symptom)

	London $n=51$ (Thompson & Isaacs 1988) %	Basel $n=81$ (Wirz-Justice 1990) %	Heidelberg $n=17$ (Kasper 1990) %	Tokyo $n=46$ (Takahashi 1990) %	Fairbanks, Alaska $n=17$ (Hellekson 1990) %	Bethesda $n=366$ %
Sex ratio						
Female	90	80	86	59	94	78
Male	10	20	14	41	6	22
Mean age (years)	42	44	48	36	38	38
Mean age of onset (years)	24	32	32	26	25	23
Episode length (months)	4	5	4	4	6	5
Diagnosis						
Unipolar	29	94	71	63	82	33
Bipolar II	51	4	24	29	0	59
Bipolar I	20	1	5	17	18	8
Family history (at least one first degree relative affected)						
Major affective disorder	25	57	59	45	59	52
Alcohol abuse	8	25	24	13	41	37
Previous treatment						
None		23	20	33	41	23
Psychotherapy						73
Antidepressant drugs	49	45	80	63	35	43
Thyroid supplement			15		0	11
Hospitalization	18	12	35	22	6	11
Lithium	16	6	10	3	0	9
ECT	8		0	0	0	2

November for patients residing near the 38.9°N latitude of Washington, DC (Rosenthal et al 1984) when total hours of daylight in Washington drop below 10. Untreated, SAD depressive episodes generally resolve by springtime, although some individuals do not fully recover before the early summer. Many patients have reported that travel to latitudes nearer the equator resulted in remission or diminution of their symptoms (Rosenthal et al 1984). A history of briefly depressed moods recurring in spring or mid-summer if ambient light is reduced for any reason is common (Rosenthal et al 1984). SAD patients may experience a reversal of their winter symptoms in summer: mild hypomania with elation, increased libido, social activity and energy, and diminished sleep requirements, appetite and weight (Jacobsen & Rosenthal 1988).

Winter SAD is also seen in children, who present with fatigue, irritability, difficulty getting out of bed in the morning and school problems (Rosenthal et al 1986a). Anergia is often the central symptom (Sonis 1989). Rather than recognizing their symptoms as reflecting an internal change in mood, children with winter SAD tend to blame the external world (of parents and teachers) for treating them harshly.

The seasonal pattern of summer SAD is, by definition, opposite to that of winter SAD. In Washington, DC this variation corresponds to the period when the mean daily temperature is above 20°C. Patients with summer depression often report 'typical' endogenous vegetative depressive symptoms of insomnia and loss of appetite or weight (Boyce & Parker 1988, Wehr et al 1987a). Like most people, both summer SAD and winter SAD patients report that they sleep less and lose weight in summer and have the opposite pattern in winter (Terman 1988, Wehr & Rosenthal 1989b).

Epidemiology

Initial winter SAD studies indicated that most patients met criteria for bipolar II disorder (depressive and hypomanic episodes) (Spitzer et al 1978), while only a small proportion had bipolar I disorder (depressive and full manic episodes), or unipolar depression (Rosenthal et al 1985b, Thompson & Isaacs 1988). More recent work, however, has found the majority of patients to have unipolar depression, with a substantial minority of patients having bipolar II disorder and very few having bipolar I disorder (Sack et al 1990, Terman et al 1989a). Perhaps this discrepancy can be explained by the use of different sets of criteria. Thus more recent studies have used DSM-IIIR criteria, which are stricter than the RDC criteria used in earlier studies. While many SAD patients experience exuberance and extra energy in summer, this does not generally constitute a clinical problem. An alternative explanation for diagnostic differences across centres may be that they are due to different climatic conditions.

Familial factors may be involved in the disorder, given that over half the patients studied have reported a history of major affective disorder in at least one first-degree relative (Rosenthal et al 1984, Terman et al 1989a). Women are particularly vulnerable to SAD. The high proportion of women seen in research clinics may result from selection bias and may overstate the true relative prevalence of the disorder among women (Terman et al 1989a). In contrast to most research centres across the world, a relatively large proportion (41%) of Japanese SAD patients have been men (Takahashi, personal communication 1990). Patients often report disliking winter since their teenage years, though the problem generally becomes severe only in adulthood. The average onset of the disorder in our population has been at approximately age 23. These figures are nearly identical with those of Terman and colleagues (1989a) in New York. Patients seen in Germany and Switzerland, however, have reported a later age of onset, at about age 32 (Kasper, personal communication 1990, Wirz-Justice, personal communication 1990).

Though the geographical distribution of SAD has not been rigorously studied, some mail and newspaper surveys indicate that the prevalence of winter SAD increases with increasing latitude (Lingjærde et al 1986, Potkin et al 1986, Rosen et al 1990). Other studies, however, have not shown this pattern (Muscettola et al 1990, C.M. Shapiro et al, personal communication 1990). Clinical studies have documented the presence of the winter syndrome in North America, Europe, Africa, Asia, and Australia (Boyce & Parker 1988, Takahashi, personal communication 1990, Terman et al 1989a, Thompson 1986, Wirz-Justice et al 1989). Sub-clinical versions of the winter syndrome (S-SAD) (Kasper et al 1989a) also appear to increase in prevalence with increasing distance from the equator (Rosen et al 1990). One survey in the Washington area found approximately 4% of the population to have winter seasonal affective disorder and over 10% more to have sub-syndromal SAD (Kasper et al 1989b). Many more people among the general population may have mild seasonal symptoms as well (Kasper et al 1989b, Terman 1988). In one random survey, for example, 27% of respondents reported that changes with the seasons were a problem for them, 66% reported seasonal changes in energy level, 64% reported some seasonal changes in mood, and 49% reported seasonal changes in weight (Kasper et al 1989b).

TREATMENT

Light

Light has been the mainstay of treatments for winter depressions. The earliest recorded description of successful treatment of an apparent case of SAD was that by Esquirol (1838), who advised his patient to travel from Belgium to Italy during the winter. As noted earlier, Cook used bright artificial light on an Antarctic expedition in 1898 to combat the sadness and anergy of his crew (Cameron 1974). Hasselbalch (1905) reported that a 'light bath' including ultraviolet radiation produced feelings of increased energy, exhilaration and hypomania. Marx (1946) also noted that a recurrent winter depression responded to treatment with bright light. The first instance of phototherapy in modern times was the treatment of a single patient by extending the length of his day with bright artificial light (Lewy et al 1982). Thereafter, Rosenthal and colleagues (1984) treated a group of nine SAD patients in the first controlled study of light therapy, using a crossover design and blind raters.

The efficacy of light treatment has been demonstrated in over 20 placebo-controlled studies around the world (Rosenthal et al 1988b). Applying stringent criteria for remission of depression – drop in Hamilton Depression score (Williams 1988) by 50% or more to a level under eight – in a cross-centre analysis of data on 332 patients from 14 research centres, Terman and colleagues (1989c) demonstrated that phototherapy is capable of inducing remission in over half of SAD patients treated. Our clinical experience suggests that significant improvement in depressive symptoms occurs in at least three-quarters of SAD patients treated with light. SAD patients with suicidality or severe anhedonia, hypersomnia or carbohydrate craving as part of their symptom complex are particularly likely to benefit from phototherapy.

The placebo effect

It has been difficult to control for the placebo effect in phototherapy studies, especially since the patients often believe that light will be helpful and since the ideal standard of a double-blind design is not possible. Nonetheless, many attempts have been made to control for placebo effects of light by varying intensity, colour and timing of treatment, as well as directing the light to different parts of the body – the eyes or the skin. Raters have been kept blind and *a priori* expectations of the different treatments have been measured. Significant differences between active and control treatments have been found in many of these studies despite equivalent *a priori* expectations. Although the efficacy of light treatment for SAD has by now been widely accepted by clinicians (Rosenthal 1989), investigators continue to grapple with the problem of the placebo effect in treatment studies. Several parameters for optimal phototherapy of SAD have emerged from such trials.

Parameters for phototherapy

Brightness. Illuminance, measured in terms of quanta of light sensed over time by a certain surface area (Records 1979), was the first treatment variable studied systematically (Rosenthal et al 1988b). Critical to illuminance measurement is the distance of the subject from the light source. Initial researchers used a set of fluorescent light tubes in a metal fixture placed 90 cm from the subject to achieve an illuminance of 2500 lux (Rosenthal et al 1984). Light boxes delivering 100–850 lux were less effective than brighter units in a series of controlled cross-over studies (Rosenthal et al 1988b). Later studies indicated that an overall remission rate of 75% can be achieved using fluorescent light fixtures positioned to produce 10 000 lux at the level of the eye (Terman et al 1990a). The intensity-response curve for the antidepressant effects of light has not been

fully defined, however, and may be influenced by the nature of the light source. Thus, a recent study in which we used a head-mounted light visor suggested that lower illuminance values might be effective when the light source is within a few inches of the eye (Moul et al 1990).

Timing. Some researchers have found that morning is the most effective time for phototherapy, whereas others have found patients to respond well to light at other times of day (Blehar & Rosenthal 1989, Lewy et al 1985b). For example, several studies have found significant antidepressant effects following light exposure in the evening (James et al 1985, Wehr et al 1986, 1987b) or in the middle of the day (Jacobsen et al 1987). There is evidence of a carryover effect in the frequently performed crossover studies of phototherapy (Rosenthal et al 1988b). While in some instances such an effect might not have adversely affected the interpretation of a finding, there is recent evidence that, in studies of timing of light treatment, this effect might have had a major impact on such interpretation (Rafferty et al 1990). Since some studies have found morning light treatment to be superior to evening treatment, and no studies have found the reverse, if all other factors are equal, it is reasonable to start light treatment with morning exposure.

Duration. A few studies indicate that the greater the daily duration, the greater the antidepressant effect (Kripke 1981, Rosenthal et al 1988b, Terman et al 1988, 1989d, Wirz-Justice et al 1986b). There is little published evidence, however, that increased antidepressant effects may be achieved using greater than 2-hour light periods per day (Terman et al 1989d). Duration may be inversely related to intensity in determining efficacy of treatment. Consequently, treatment with 10 000 lux for 30 minutes in the morning appears to be as successful as 2500 lux for 120 minutes (Terman et al 1990b). This relationship may not be universally applicable, as evidenced by recent paradoxical findings with a portable, head-mounted light visor (Moul et al 1990).

Spectrum. The original studies of light therapy involved full-spectrum fluorescent lights, which largely reproduce the distribution and range of visible and ultraviolet sunlight. The results of more recent studies, however, differ in assessing the therapeutic effect of ultraviolet-free phototherapy (A. Frank et al, personal communication 1989, Lam et al 1989). Although there has been some discussion of the comparative merits of different brands of white fluorescent lamp emitting different amounts of ultraviolet radiation, we know of no study demonstrating the superiority of one form of white fluorescent lamp over another in winter SAD. There is some evidence that incandescent light sources may also be effective in the treatment of winter SAD (Moul et al 1990, Yerevanian et al 1986).

Apart from assisting in the development of optimal treatment sources, studies of the effects of different wavelengths may clarify the photoreceptors and pigments responsible for transducing the antidepressant effects of light. Inspired by this reasoning, we have found green to be superior to red light and others have found white to be superior to both red and blue (Brainard et al 1990). These findings are compatible with our understanding of the physiology of the retina, which absorbs light maximally in the green region of the spectrum (Dartnall et al 1983).

Route of delivery. Although one astonishing case report has documented the efficacy of phototherapy in a fully blind individual (Rosenthal et al 1989a), light appears to have its therapeutic effects through the eyes. In an experiment designed to tease out the antidepressant mechanism of light, Wehr and colleagues (Wehr et al 1987b) found that the eyes and not the skin appeared to mediate the effects of light treatment in SAD patients.

Light fixtures. Two types of 'light box' have been widely used in efficacy studies of light therapy for winter SAD. These boxes are essentially variations on common fluorescent ceiling fixtures. In one configuration, a rectangular box is placed horizontally on a table approximately 90 cm from the patient, so as to deliver 2500 lux to the eyes. In the second configuration, a square box is suspended diagonally above the patient, so as to deliver 10 000 lux to the eyes.

Two newer devices hold the promise of delivering light in a more convenient and less time-consuming fashion. A 'dawn-simulator' that mimics naturalistic springtime illumination patterns may offer patients the chance to receive effective phototherapy while they sleep (Terman et al 1989b). In an uncontrolled preliminary trial, seven of eight patients exposed to one 'dawn-simulator' had dramatic improvements after 2 weeks of phototherapy and relapsed when phototherapy was discontinued (Schlager et al 1989). A portable, head-mounted light visor has been considered as a plausible means of delivering light therapy in a multi-centre controlled trial (Moul et al 1990). The results of this study were surprising in that a dimmer visor (400 lux) proved more effective than a brighter (5000 lux) one. The chief advantage of this device over the light box is that it is easily portable. Further studies are needed to clarify the therapeutic efficacy and safety of these two newer fixtures.

Practical clinical guidelines

A reasonable initial light treatment approach would be to have the patient sit facing a 10 000 lux fixture for 30 minutes each morning. If this regimen fails to elicit an antidepressant response within the typical 2–5 day interval seen for SAD patients (Rosenthal et al 1985b), then extending the treatment time to an hour or dividing the treatments between morning and evening may be considered. (Most of the patients we have seen have required at least 45 minutes a day of phototherapy at the 10 000 lux illuminance). In previous years, we asked patients to glance briefly at the light units approximately once a minute: such direct glances may not be necessary as long as the patient is sure to face the lights directly. We have encouraged patients to engage in other activities while seated, as long as they continued to face the light (Jacobsen & Rosenthal 1988).

Our longitudinal experience suggests that the winter SAD patients who respond to phototherapy should be maintained on the treatment until they gain sufficient daily light exposure from other sources, typically from the sun in the spring. Over 90% of winter SAD patients will require phototherapy during January and February. Premature withdrawal from phototherapy usually results in a return of the depressive syndrome. Following the summer, it is often appropriate to resume phototherapy prophylactically near the calendar date when the patient's depressive episodes have begun historically.

Patients with winter SAD who are perennially light-deprived or live in a climate with extended spells of cloudy weather often find that phototherapy is helpful at any time of the year. In some cases where phototherapy brings about a partial but incomplete antidepressant response, our own group has found a combination of light treatment with standard antidepressant medications to be helpful, often resulting in remission at lower doses and with fewer side-effects. The advantages of such a combination must be weighed against the theoretical risks of combining phototherapy with a photosensitizing drug (Terman et al 1990).

Many social and personal factors can interfere with optimum light treatment. If the response to phototherapy is incomplete, one should always check on the patient's compliance with guidelines for distance, duration, and positioning. Lengthening the duration of light treatment, shifting the timing of treat-ment or replacing old light bulbs with new may all improve results. Increasing the patient's overall environmental lighting or setting a timer to turn on bedroom lights before wake-up time may also be helpful.

Adverse effects of phototherapy

Use of the bright white light treatment is generally a benign experience, with few side-effects (Rosenthal et al 1984). Some patients in our study, however, complain of eye strain, headaches, insomnia or hypomanic irritability. Eye strain, headaches and irritability often diminish after a few days of treatment, and they may be minimized by decreasing the duration of therapy or increasing distance from the light (Jacobsen & Rosenthal 1988, Rosenthal et al 1988b). Light adminis-tered too late in the evening sometimes results in difficulty falling asleep.

When properly administered, light treatment has no known irreversible side effects. Nevertheless, there is a theoretical possibility that overexposure to ultraviolet light might adversely affect the eyes or the skin (Oren et al 1990). Because fluorescent bulbs deliver small amounts of ultraviolet radiation, which may lead to the development of cortical cataracts after many years of excessive ultraviolet exposure (Taylor et al 1988), we recommend the use of ultraviolet-absorbing filters on fluorescent light fixtures. Two formal short-term studies (Gallin et al 1990, Rosenthal et al 1984) and several years of clinical experience with light treatment have not revealed any changes in eye function or anatomy with regular phototherapy, but a formal study of greater numbers of patients over time is still required (Remé et al 1990, M.Waxler, G.C. Brainard, personal communication 1990).

Patients should be discouraged from treating themselves by visiting tanning salons, which use light with a large amount of ultraviolet radiation directed at the skin.

Pharmacological approaches to winter SAD

Medications may also have a role in the treatment of SAD, but there are as yet no controlled studies of avail-able antidepressants for SAD. A promising treatment was studied by O'Rourke and colleagues (O'Rourke et al 1989) who found the serotonin-agonist d-fenfluramine to be a highly effective treatment for winter SAD. Our clinical experience suggests that

patients with SAD can be successfully treated with tricyclic and tetracyclic antidepressants, monoamine oxidase inhibitors or lithium. Recent use of the serotonin reuptake blocker fluoxetine in our clinic has also been helpful in several cases. Many SAD patients, however, turn to phototherapy to avoid the well-known side-effects of standard pharmaceutical agents.

Treatment of summer SAD

Although patients with summer depression appear to respond to traditional antidepressant medications, manipulations of the environmental stresses that prevail in summer, most notably heat and humidity, have not yet been demonstrated to be as convenient or as effec-tive as phototherapy for winter SAD. In a pilot trial, one patient was exposed to cold showers for 15 minutes several times a day and continuously isolated from heat in an air-conditioned house. Her depression responded dramatically on the fifth day of treatment, and returned 9 days after the treatment ended (Wehr et al 1987a). It is more difficult technically to perform controlled studies on the effects of environmental temperature as compared with light. A controlled study of six patients with summer SAD proved inconclusive in defining an effective treatment for the summer disorder (Wehr et al 1989).

PATHOPHYSIOLOGY OF WINTER SAD

We do not understand the aetiology of SAD. Nonetheless, two clinical observations that may help us understand the pathophysiology of the disorder are: 1) SAD is linked to a time of year when people are exposed to less sunlight than at other times; and 2) alteration of ambient light in winter can effectively treat the depression.

Several biological abnormalities have been found in winter SAD patients, including alterations in hormonal profiles, biochemical challenges, immune responses and visual evoked phenomena. Several biological parameters have been found to change following effec-tive light treatment, some of which form the basis of hypotheses about the mechanism of the antidepressant effects of light, which are discussed below.

The 'photon-counting' hypothesis

One possible explanation for the disorder is that the short days of winter deprive susceptible patients of sufficient quanta of light for some chemical process responsible for maintaining a euthymic state. By supplementing the deficient light of winter this 'photon' deficient' depression is treated. The initial report by Rosenthal and colleagues (1984) on SAD, documenting that bright light acted as an antidepressant whereas dim light did not, forms the cornerstone of this hypothesis. The failure of ordinary light to reverse winter depressions in this population indicated that delivering a large quantity of photons to patients was intrinsic to the antidepressant response. This hypothesis is supported by data indicating that there is a dose — response relationship for light as well as an inverse relationship between duration and intensity of light required for treatment of winter SAD (Terman et al 1989c, d). The great amount of light needed to reverse the symptoms of winter SAD in environments with low ambient light argues for the importance of light quantity as a treatment parameter. A limitation of this hypothesis is that it does not specify what intervening processes are influenced by these varying amounts of light, which in turn influence the outcome in winter SAD patients.

The 'melatonin' hypothesis

According to the 'melatonin hypothesis' the suppression of melatonin by light induces an antidepressant effect. No study has yet provided a definitive confirmation or disavowal of this theory (Oren 1991, Rosenthal et al 1985b). The potential importance of melatonin in SAD was suggested by the superior antidepressant effects of bright versus dim light, given the finding (Lewy et al 1980, 1982) that bright – but not dim – light suppresses melatonin blood levels in humans. The results of several studies argue against the validity of the melatonin hypothesis. First, the administration of melatonin to successfully treated SAD patients did not induce them to relapse significantly even though it exacerbated certain symptoms that are characteristic of SAD (Rosenthal et al 1986b). Second, depressed SAD patients have been treated with atenolol – a beta-adrenergic blocker that reduces night-time melatonin levels – and failed to improve (Rosenthal et al 1988a). Finally, Wehr and colleagues (1986) found no difference in antidepressant efficacy between pulses of light given early and late in the day so as to suppress melatonin and pulses given during the illuminated part of the day so as not to suppress melatonin. Besides arguing against the importance of melatonin suppression as a mediator of the antidepressant effects of light, this finding also suggested that these effects

were not photoperiodic, i.e. they did not require the day-length to be extended. At most, the suppression of pineal melatonin secretion may account for some symptoms that resolve during light therapy, but there is no convincing evidence yet that it is central to the disorder.

The 'phase-shift' hypothesis

Insofar as the melatonin hypothesis implied the need to expose winter SAD patients to bright light at certain times of day (the dark period), it was a circadian hypothesis. Another circadian hypothesis that has attracted considerable interest amongst researchers is the 'phase-shift' theory (Lewy & Sack 1986). This concept was built upon the capacity of bright light in the evening to delay the nocturnal rise of melatonin (Illnerová et al 1985) and of bright light in the morning to advance the rhythm (Lewy et al 1984, 1985a, b, 1987b). Two groups (Lewy et al 1987a, Terman et al 1987, 1988) have suggested that their patients had abnormally delayed melatonin rhythms, relative to sleep, that were advanced by bright light therapy in the morning. The association between the phase-advancing and antidepressant effects of light thus suggested a connection between delayed circadian rhythms and depression. Other groups have shown no systematic alterations in timing of melatonin secretion (Thompson et al 1988) or core body temperature rhythm (Rosenthal et al 1990b) before or after light treatment. In these studies, however, differences might have been masked by the way in which the rhythms were measured.

A few studies documenting the effectiveness of light treatment at different times of the day and evening do not support the phase-shift theory, since that theory postulates that time of day of phototherapy is critical to the antidepressant response (Isaacs et al 1988, Jacobsen et al 1987, James et al 1985, Wehr et al 1986). Indeed, it could be argued that evening light treatment should make patients worse whereas, in fact, it has been found to be antidepressant in some patients. Nevertheless, in a still-uncharacterized way, circadian rhythms may be linked to the response to phototherapy in winter SAD since the eye may be more sensitive to light in the early morning than at other times of day and a given number of photons might be more effective at one time of day than another (Bassi & Powers 1986, Knoerchen & Hildebrandt 1976, O'Keefe & Baker 1987). The still unanswered questions about this theory are: 1) Are rhythms really delayed in winter SAD? 2) If so, is this the central abnormality? 3) Is morning light more effective than evening light? 4) If so, are there mechanisms apart from advancing phase that might better explain this difference? and 5) How can the efficacy of evening light in some people be reconciled with the phase advance hypothesis? One point that is not in dispute, however, is the capacity of properly timed light and dark exposures to shift circadian rhythms (Czeisler et al 1989).

The 'amplitude' hypothesis

Depending upon the timing of light exposure, endogenous circadian amplitudes of variables such as temperature, melatonin and heart rate can be markedly suppressed or enhanced (Czeisler et al 1987). Kronauer has suggested that bright light exposure during the daytime in an individual entrained to a normal 24-hour day may have a significant amplitude enhancing effect (Kronauer 1987). On the basis of this model, still untested in SAD, Czeisler and Kronauer have suggested that an increased circadian amplitude induced by phototherapy may result in the antidepressant effect of light (Czeisler et al 1987, Kronauer 1987, Kronauer & Frangioni 1987).

Neurotransmitter-associated hypotheses

Two neurotransmitters have been postulated as playing central roles in the pathophysiology of winter SAD: dopamine and serotonin. Although cogent arguments have been made for the role of each of these, it seems likely that the two transmitters interact (Castrogiovanni et al 1989) and play important roles, perhaps in different areas or systems of the brain.

Dopamine

The 'behavioural facilitation system'. Depue and colleagues (1989b) initially proposed that dopamine might play a key role in SAD by modulating a 'behavioural facilitation system'. Two groups have found evidence of reduced prolactin secretion in SAD patients compared with normal volunteers in both winter and summer, suggesting that it might be a trait marker of the condition (Depue et al 1989a, Levendosky et al, personal communication 1990). Depue hypothesized that this finding might indicate a dopaminergic deficiency in SAD, since low basal prolactin secretion may result from compensatory up-regulation of D_2-receptors in the anterior pituitary

gland associated with low functional activity of dopamine (Jimerson & Post 1984). Depue'e group (1988, 1990) also found an increased frequency of eyeblinks in depressed patients with SAD. Because spontaneous eye-blink rates may reflect dopaminergic function in the nigrostriatal tract (Karson 1983), Depue suggested that a hypodopaminergic state in the nigrostriatal system may be associated with up regulation of dopamine receptors in the prefrontal cortex. His group also found that SAD patients had an abnormally inefficient heat loss response following exercise in winter that is normalized or exaggerated during light treatment and during summer. Since this response is partially dependent upon dopaminergic activity in the hypothalamic and nigrostriatal tracts, according to the dopamine hypothesis, the blunted thermoregulatory heat loss seen in SAD may represent another manifestation of a dopaminergic deficiency (Arbisi et al 1989). The above dopaminergic explanations are limited by the use of opposite mechanisms to explain different findings – downregulation in one case and upregulation in another. Despite this limitation, so many abnormalities in dopamine systems have been documented in SAD that it seems likely that these systems play some role in the pathophysiology of the condition.

Interactions with light and retinal melatonin. In animal models, bright light allows dopamine to be produced in the retina and suppresses the production of retinal melatonin. In the absence of bright light, a reduction in dopamine levels allows retinal melatonin to be produced. Oren (1991) has proposed that light may play its role in winter SAD by stimulating dopamine production in the eye. According to this putative 'retinal melatonin/dopamine hypothesis', sufficiently bright phototherapy may stimulate dopamine production and suppress melatonin in the retina, and thereby improve mood by mechanisms such as resetting a circadian ocular clock or triggering dopaminergic impulses affecting central neuronal structures. Patients with Parkinson's disease have been described as having delayed b-wave generation times after stimuli from a pattern electroretinogram and reduced electrooculogram Arden ratios (Bodis-Wollner & Onofrj 1987, Calzetti et al 1990, Economou & Stefanis 1978). Our group found that some patients with winter SAD have the former abnormality and another group (Lam et al 1990) has found that SAD patients have the latter. Both abnormalities imply that there may be a functional dopaminergic deficit in the retina of patients with winter SAD.

Serotonin

Several lines of research suggest that serotonin plays an important, if still somewhat uncharacterized, role in winter depressions. Coppen (1967) nominated this neurotransmitter as one whose functional deficiency might be responsible for depressive disorders in general. The therapeutic effects of some antidepressant drugs may be dependent on serotonin availability (Delgado et al 1990). Wurtman and colleagues (1981) have postulated that carbohydrate craving may reflect a functional serotonin deficiency, which would be consistent with the serotonin theory of SAD, given the prominence of carbohydrate craving in winter depressives (Jacobsen et al 1989, Rosenthal et al 1984). Rosenthal and colleagues (Rosenthal et al 1989b) have found that carbohydrate-rich meals activate patients with SAD and sedate normal controls. They have argued that this finding is consistent with a serotonergic abnormality in SAD. Additionally, winter reductions in serotonin concentrations have been observed in the human post-mortem hypothalamus (Carlsson et al 1980). Several studies from the NIMH group have shown abnormal behavioural and hormonal responses to infusions of the postsynaptic serotonin agonist m-CPP (Jacobsen et al, personal communication 1988, Joseph-Vanderpool et al, personal communication 1990). Recent reports that light exposure may alter serotonin receptor sensitivity in rat neurones (Cox et al 1986, Mason 1984) and in platelets of patients with winter SAD (Szádóczky et al 1989) are compatible with a serotonergic explanation of light therapy. The serotonergic agonist d-fenfluramine was found to be highly effective in reversing symptoms of the syndrome (O'Rourke et al 1989), which further supports the serotonin hypothesis. Therapeutic trials of medications that affect serotonergic systems, such as fluoxetine or trazodone, might be clinically useful and further our understanding of the roles of serotonin in SAD.

The role of the eye

Over four decades ago, Marx (1946) speculated that light exerts its antidepressant effects in winter depression through the eye and perhaps its connections with the hypothalamus. Several clinical trials support the hypothesis that the eye plays a special role in SAD, including the findings of abnormal electro-oculograms (Lam et al 1990) and electroretinograms (our own data, 1990) in SAD, as well as the phototherapy study suggesting that the antidepressant effects of light are mediated through the eyes not the skin (Wehr et al

1987b). Combined results from other controlled trials of light treatment suggest that green light is more effective as an antidepressant than either red or blue (Brainard GC et al, personal communication 1990, Oren et al, personal communication 1990). These findings are consistent with the maximal response to light for rod and cone photoreceptors at about 510 nm and 550 nm respectively (Bowmaker et al 1980, Fein & Szuts 1982, Records 1979). Our group has also observed that some depressed winter SAD patients are significantly more sensitive to dim light during a dark adaptation paradigm (Gunkel & Bornschein 1957) than matched normal controls (Oren et al, personal communication 1990). With so many studies implicating eye-related phenomena in SAD, it seems that the retina – the visual entrance to the central nervous system – might play a central role in SAD.

Hormones

Neuroendocrine measures classically undertaken in studying mood disorders have been applied to the research in SAD as well. Joseph-Vanderpool and colleagues (1990) have shown that depressed winter SAD patients have normal basal plasma cortisol and ACTH levels, but blunted ACTH responses to infusions of CRH, an abnormality that can largely be corrected with phototherapy. This blunted ACTH response may occur in hypercortisolaemic patients, such as melancholic depressives. Alternatively, it may reflect an underactive HPA axis associated with the lethargy, hypersomnia and hyperphagia typical of SAD as opposed to the agitation, insomnia and anorexia seen in melancholic depression. Though others have found thyroid abnormalities to be present in some forms of major depression, we have been unable to document any particular thyroid abnormality in seasonal affective disorder. Patients with winter SAD are not different from matched normal controls in free T4 or T3 levels or on hypothalamo – pituitary – thyroid challenge tests such as measuring TSH response to TRH infusion (Joseph-Vanderpool et al 1991, Rosenthal et al 1984). Table 35.4 summarizes current knowledge regarding the levels of various hormones that have been studied in winter SAD.

Miscellaneous biological findings in winter SAD

Temperature rhythms

Measurements of core body temperature may reveal certain elements of the pathophysiology of SAD in so far as they reflect circadian phase and amplitude and thermoregulation. Although we have found no difference in 24-hour core temperature measurements of SAD patients and normals either in winter (Rosenthal et al 1990b) or in summer (Levendosky et al, personal communication 1990), light treatment significantly enhanced the amplitude of the patients' circadian rhythms in winter. This finding supports the 'amplitude' hypothesis of phototherapy discussed above (Czeisler et al 1987, Kronauer 1987, Kronauer & Frangioni 1987).

Table 35.4   Hormonal profiles of SAD

	Substance	Change relative to normals
Plasma	Growth hormone	Delayed nocturnal peak*
	Cortisol	Unchanged*†
	Prolactin	Reduced* **
CSF	Homovanillic acid	Unchanged†
	MHPG	Unchanged†
	5-HIAA	Unchanged†
Challenges	m-CPP	Increased activation and euphoria in winter and increased cortisol and prolactin††
	DST	Unchanged***
	CRH	ACTH response blunted †††

    * Levendosky et al, personal communication 1990
    † Skwerer et al 1988
  ** Depue et al 1990
  †† Jacobsen et al, personal communication 1988, Joseph-Vanderpool et al, personal communication 1990
 *** James et al 1986
 ††† Joseph-Vanderpool et al, personal communication 1990

Sleep

Sleep studies reveal significant differences between SAD patients and normal controls. In consonance with patients' own reports, winter sleep in SAD patients is increased in length compared with summer. Although slow wave (delta) sleep is decreased in winter, SAD patients have more rapid eye movement (REM) and non-REM sleep. Light therapy partially corrects these abnormalities in sleep architecture (J.L. Anderson et al, personal communication 1990, Skwerer et al 1988).

Photoneuroimmunology

In contrast to those depressed patients who manifest decreased response of peripheral blood lymphocytes to mitogen stimulation (Kronfol et al 1983, Schleifer et al 1989), depressed SAD patients have been observed to have an abnormally increased response to the mitogens phytohaemaglutinin and concanavalin A (Skwerer et al 1988). Whereas eye exposure to bright white light enhanced lymphocyte blastogenesis in normals, in SAD patients the over-responsiveness was normalized (Skwerer et al 1988). Altered responses to mitogens could serve as a potential trait marker for SAD.

Sensory evoked potentials

In contrast to auditory P300s, C.C. Duncan and others (personal communication 1987) have shown that visual P300s are enhanced by light in SAD patients in direct proportion to its antidepressant effects. Such P300 measurements are a dynamic brain-event-related potential measuring the amount of brain attention or processing committed to a stimulus (Duncan-Johnson & Donchin 1982). The physiological meaning of this finding is not yet clear.

CRITICAL QUESTIONS: RESOLVED AND UNRESOLVED

Alternatives to light fixtures

As mentioned earlier, though SAD patients appear to be responsive to a variety of antidepressants, clinical trials of their efficacy in this condition have yet to be undertaken. A preliminary report suggests that regular early morning exposure to natural light may ameliorate winter SAD (Wirz-Justice et al 1990), but a controlled study of this treatment is necessary. The potential roles of diet and cognitive therapy in SAD are as yet unexplored.

Is light therapy just a placebo?

One controversy that attracts sceptics unfamiliar with the effects of phototherapy is the idea that phototherapy succeeds only as a placebo. While it is highly likely that there is a placebo component to the phototherapy response, several arguments suggest that placebo effects alone do not account for the efficacy of phototherapy. These arguments include the demonstration of the efficacy of light by several groups, the repeated responses within many individual patients over the course of years, the characteristic time course of response to treatment and relapse following treatment and withdrawal, the existence of a dose — response curve for light intensity and the evidence for a circadian rhythm of treatment sensitivity (Rosenthal et al 1988b). As new technologies allow the delivery of light through devices other than light boxes, more sophisticated placebo controls will probably confirm the clinical and research data that already suggest that light works by more than simply a placebo effect.

Light as a drug

If light is not merely a placebo, can it be considered as a drug? Parameters of drug delivery such as quantity, duration and timing are integral to light treatment. Preclinical studies of retinal physiology in frogs, rats, chickens and rabbits unequivocally demonstrate that light can stimulate or suppress the production of neurotransmitters and hormones as if it were a chemical compound. Students of chemistry are well aware that light may have profound reactions with molecules. This process, indeed, is the basis for vitamin D synthesis, vision and photosynthesis. As drugs often have effects beyond their traditional indications, a growing body of research suggests that there are specific syndromes beyond winter SAD in which light may play a therapeutic role. Among these are mild winter depression (sub-syndromal winter SAD) (Kasper et al 1989a, Rosenthal et al 1985a, Terman et al 1989d), non-seasonal depression (Kripke et al 1983), delayed sleep phase syndrome (Rosenthal et al 1990a) and shift work (Czeisler et al 1989).

Just as with a drug, toxic effects could result from too much light. In addition, light does have its therapeutic limitations. For example, two studies have failed to show any mood-altering effects in normal subjects (Kasper et al 1989a, Rosenthal et al 1987). Therefore light is not a universal euphoriant but appears to be rather a specific agent, helpful for specific conditions.

Past accomplishments and future directions

In the past decade, researchers have established a solid definition of the winter SAD syndrome and the efficacy of phototherapy for this syndrome. Summer SAD has been defined but has yet to be more thoroughly explored. Whether environmental manipulations are beneficial for this latter condition will require properly controlled therapeutic trials. The biological underpinnings of both winter and summer SAD syndromes might benefit from proper family studies exploring possible genetic or familial environmental factors that might contribute to these illnesses. Though some epidemiological studies of seasonal syndromes have been performed, future epidemiological surveys are needed to appreciate fully the incidence of these disorders and their impact on society. Forthcoming studies of seasonal affective disorders will need to address the question as to whether there are meaningful subtypes of winter SAD, perhaps based on typical versus atypical depressive symptoms, or phase-delayed versus phase-advanced circadian rhythms. A controversy exists as to whether phototherapy for winter SAD works better in the morning than other times of day. Though satisfactory methods of delivering light are available, better methods of light delivery are being developed. Phototherapy seems to have been quite safe to date, though formal studies of its safety, especially with long-term use, may be desirable. Finally, despite the development of several plausible theories of the aetiology and mechanisms of treatment of winter SAD, all these theories have limitations. Of course, researchers studying other forms of affective illness wrestle with the same uncertainty about the illnesses they study. The particular attraction of seasonal affective disorders to many researchers is that they are comparatively homogeneous, well-defined syndromes brought on and reversed by well-characterized stimuli. The responsiveness of a psychiatric disorder to relatively simple and measurable variations in the physical environment offers psychiatrists an outstanding model with which to understand these disorders and provides a neurochemical window into our understanding of brain function.

REFERENCES

Adams F 1856 The extant works of Aretaeus, the Cappadocian. Sydenham Society, London

American Psychiatric Association 1980 Diagnostic and Statistical Manual of Mental Disorders, 3rd edn. American Psychiatric Association, Washington, DC

American Psychiatric Association 1987 Diagnostic and Statistical Manual of Mental Disorders, 3rd edn – revised American Psychiatric Association, Washington, DC

Arbisi P A, Depue R A, Spoont M R, Leon A, Ainsworth B 1989 Thermoregulatory response to thermal challenge in seasonal affective disorder: a preliminary report. Psychiatry Research 28: 323–334

Aurelianus C 1950 On acute diseases and on chronic diseases. University of Chicago Press, Chicago

Bassi C J, Powers M K 1986 Daily fluctuations in the detectability of dim lights by humans. Physiology and Behaviour 38: 871–877

Blehar M C, Rosenthal N E 1989 Seasonal affective disorders and phototherapy. Archives of General Psychiatry 46: 469–474

Bodis-Wollner I, Onofrj M 1987 The visual system in Parkinson's disease. In: Yahr M D, Bergmann K J (eds) Advances in neurology. Raven Press, New York, p 323–328

Bowmaker J K, Dartnall H J A, Mollon J D 1980 Microspectrophotometric demonstration of four classes of photoreceptor in an old world primate, Macaca fascicularis. Journal of Physiology 298: 131–143

Boyce P, Parker G 1988 Seasonal affective disorder in the southern hemisphere. American Journal of Psychiatry 145: 96–99

Calzetti S, Franchi A, Taratufolo G, Groppi E 1990 Simultaneous VEP and PERG investigations in early Parkinson's disease. Journal of Neurology, Neurosurgery, and Psychiatry 53: 114–117

Cameron I 1974 Antarctica: the last continent. Cassell, London

Carlsson A, Svennerholm L, Winblad B 1980 Seasonal and circadian monoamine variations in human brains examined post-mortem. Acta Psychiatrica Scandinavica 61 (suppl 280): 75–85

Castrogiovanni P, Di Muro A, Maremmani I, Perossini M, Marazziti D 1989 Interaction between the serotonin and dopamine systems in humans: preliminary findings. Brain Research 504: 129–131

Cook F A 1894 Gynecology and obstetrics among the Eskimos. Brooklyn Medical Journal 8: 154–169

Coppen A 1967 The biochemistry of affective disorders. British Journal of Psychiatry 113: 1237–1264

Cox C M, Mason R, Meal A, Parker T L 1986 Altered 5-HT sensitivity and synaptic morphology in rat CNS induced by long-term exposure to continuous light. British Journal of Pharmacology 89: 528P

Czeisler C A, Kronauer R E, Mooney J J, Anderson J L, Allan J S 1987 Biologic rhythm disorders, depression, and phototherapy: a new hypothesis. Psychiatric Clinics of North America 10: 687–709

Czeisler C A, Kronauer R E, Allan J S et al 1989 Bright light induction of strong (type 0) resetting of the human circadian pacemaker. Science 244: 1328–1333

Dartnall H J A, Bowmaker J K, Mollon J D 1983 Human visual pigments: microspectrophotometric results from the eyes of seven persons. Proceedings of the Royal Society of London Series B 220: 115–130

Delgado P L, Charney D S, Price L H, Aghajanian G K, Landis H, Heninger G 1990 Serotonin function and the mechanism of antidepressant action. Archives of General Psychiatry 47: 411–418

Depue R A, Iacono W G, Muir R, Arbisi P 1988 Effects of phototherapy on spontaneous eye-blink rate in seasonal affective disorder. American Journal of Psychiatry 145: 1457–1459

Depue R A, Arbisi P, Spoont M R, Krauss S, Leon A, Ainsworth B 1989a Seasonal and mood independence of low basal prolactin secretion in premenopausal women with seasonal affective disorder. American Journal of Psychiatry 146: 989–995

Depue R A, Arbisi P, Spoont M R, Leon A, Ainsworth B 1989b Dopamine functioning in the behavioural facilitation system and seasonal variation in behaviour: normal population and clinical studies. In: Rosenthal N E, Blehar M C (eds) Seasonal affective disorders and phototherapy. Guilford Press, New York, p 230–259

Depue R A, Arbisi P, Krauss S et al 1990 Seasonal independence of low prolactin concentration and high spontaneous eye blink rates in unipolar and bipolar II seasonal affective disorder. Archives of General Psychiatry 47: 356–364

Duncan-Johnson C C, Donchin E 1982 The p300 component of the event-related potential as an index of information processing. Biological Psychiatry 14: 1–52

Economou S G, Stefanis C N 1978 Changes of electrooculogram (EOG) in Parkinson's disease. Acta Neurologica Scandinavica 58: 44–52

Esquirol E 1838 Des maladies mentales. J.-B. Baillière, Paris.

Fein A, Szuts E Z 1982 Photoreceptors: their role in vision. Cambridge University Press, Cambridge

Gallin P F, Rafferty B, Terman J S, Terman M, Remé C E 1990 Ophthalmological evaluation of SAD patients pre-and post-light therapy. In: Light treatment and biological rhythms. Society for Light Treatment and Biological Rhythms, New York, p 33

Garfield E 1988 Current research on seasonal affective disorder and phototherapy. Current Contents Life Sciences 31: 3–9

Garvey M J, Wesner R, Godes M 1988 Comparison of seasonal and non-seasonal affective disorders. American Journal of Psychiatry 145: 100–102

Gunkel R D, Bornschein H 1957 Automatic intensity control in testing dark adaptation. American Medical Association Archives of Ophthalmology 57: 681–686

Hasselbalch K A 1905 Die Wirkungen des chemischen Lichtbades auf Respiration und Blutruck. Skandinavisches Archiv für Physiologie 17: 431–472

Hellekson C 1989 Phenomenology of seasonal affective disorder: an Alaskan perspective. In: Rosenthal N E, Blehar M (eds) Seasonal affective disorders and phototherapy. Guilford Press, New York, p 33–45

Hippocrates 1931 Aphorisms. In: Hippocrates. Harvard University Press, Cambridge, MA p 128–129

Illnerová H, Zvolsky P, Vanecek J 1985 The circadian rhythm in plasma melatonin concentration of the urbanized man: the effect of summer and winter time. Brain Research 328: 186–189

Isaacs G, Stainer D S, Sensky T E, Moor S, Thompson C 1988 Phototherapy and its mechanisms of action in seasonal affective disorder. Journal of Affective Disorders 14: 13–19

Jacobsen F M, Rosenthal N E 1988 Seasonal affective disorder. In: Georgotas A, Cancro R (eds) Depression and mania: a comprehensive textbook. Elsevier Science, New York, p 104–116

Jacobsen F M, Wehr T A, Skwerer R A, Sack D A, Rosenthal N E 1987 Morning versus midday phototherapy of seasonal affective disorder. American Journal of Psychiatry 144: 1301–1305

Jacobsen F M, Murphy D L, Rosenthal N E 1989 The role of serotonin in seasonal affective disorder and the antidepressant response to phototherapy. In:

Rosenthal N E, Blehar M C (eds) Seasonal affective disorders and phototherapy. Guilford Press, New York, p 333–341

James S P, Wehr T A, Sack D A, Parry B L, Rosenthal N E 1985 Treatment of seasonal affective disorder with light in the evening. British Journal of Psychiatry 147: 424–428

James S P, Wehr T A, Sack D A, Parry B L, Rogers S, Rosenthal N E 1986 The dexamethasone suppression test in seasonal affective disorder. Comprehensive Psychiatry 27: 224–226

Jimerson D C, Post R M 1984 Psychomotor stimulants and dopamine agonists in depression. In: Post R M, Ballenger J C (eds) Neurobiology of mood disorders. Williams & Wilkins, Baltimore, p 619–628

Joseph-Vanderpool J R, Rosenthal N E, Chrousos G P et al 1991 Abnormal pituitary-adrenal responses to CRH in patients with seasonal affective disorder: clinical and pathophysiological implications. Journal of Clinical Endocrinology and Metabolism 72: 1382–1387

Karson C N 1983 Spontaneous eye-blink rates and dopaminergic systems. Brain 106: 643–653

Kasper S, Rogers S L B, Yancey A, Schulz P M, Skwerer R G, Rosenthal N E 1989a Phototherapy in individuals with and without subsyndromal seasonal affective disorder. Archives of General Psychiatry 46: 837–844

Kasper S, Wehr T A, Bartko J J, Gaist P A, Rosenthal N E 1989b Epidemiological findings of seasonal changes in mood and behaviour. Archives of General Psychiatry 46: 823–833

Knoerchen R, Hildebrandt G 1976 Tagesrhythmische Schwankungen der visuellen Lichtempfindlichkeit beim Menschen. Journal of Interdisciplinary Cycle Research 7: 51–69

Kräuchi K, Wirz-Justice A 1988 The four seasons: food intake frequency in seasonal affective disorder in the course of a year. Psychiatry Research 25: 323–338

Kripke D F 1981 Photoperiodic mechanisms for depression and its treatment. In: Perris C, Struwe G, Jansson B (eds) Biological psychiatry 1981. North Holland Biomedical Press, Amsterdam, pp 1249–1252

Kripke D F, Risch S C, Janowsky D 1983 Bright white light alleviates depression. Psychiatry Research 10: 105–112

Kronauer R E 1987 A model for the effect of light on the human 'deep' circadian pacemaker. Sleep Research 16: 621

Kronauer R E, Frangioni J V 1987 Modeling laboratory bright light protocols. Sleep Research 16: 622

Kronfol Z, Silva J, Greden J, Demginski S, Gardner R, Carroll B J 1983 Impaired lymphocyte function in depressive illness. Life Sciences 33: 241

Lam R W, Buchanan A, Clark C, Remick R A 1989 UV vs non-UV light therapy for SAD. In: First Annual Meeting of the Society for Light Treatment and Biological Rhythms. Society for Light Treatment and Biological Rhythms, Bethesda, MD, p 12

Lam R W, Beattie C, Buchanan A, Remick R A, Zis A P 1990 Retinal subsensitivity to light in seasonal affective disorder? In: Light Treatment and Biological Rhythms. Society for Light Treatment and Biological Rhythms, New York, p 34

Lewy A J, Sack R L 1986 Light therapy and psychiatry. Proceedings of the Society for Experimental Biology and Medicine 183: 11–18

Lewy A J, Wehr T A, Goodwin F K, Newsome D A, Markey S P 1980 Light suppresses melatonin secretion in humans. Science 210: 1267–1269

Lewy A J, Kern H A, Rosenthal N E, Wehr T A 1982 Bright artificial light treatment of a manic-depressive patient with a seasonal mood cycle. American Journal of Psychiatry 139: 1496–1498

Lewy A J, Sack R L, Singer C M 1984 Assessment and treatment of chronobiologic disorders using plasma melatonin levels and bright light exposure: the clock-gate model and the phase response curve. Psychopharmacology Bulletin 20: 561–565

Lewy A J, Sack R L, Singer C M 1985a Immediate and delayed effects of bright light on human melatonin production: shifting 'dawn' and 'dusk' shifts the dim light melatonin onset (DLMO). Annals of the New York Academy of Sciences 453: 253–259

Lewy A J, Sack R L, Singer C M 1985b Treating phase typed chronobiologic sleep and mood disorders using appropriately timed bright artificial light. Psychopharmacology Bulletin 21: 368–372

Lewy A J, Sack R L, Miller L S, Hoban T M 1987a Antidepressant and circadian phase-shifting effects of light. Science 235: 352–353

Lewy A J, Sack R L, Singer C M, White D M 1987b The phase shift hypothesis for bright light's therapeutic mechanism of action: theoretical considerations and experimental evidence. Psychopharmacology Bulletin 23: 349–353

Liebowitz M R, Quitkin F M, Stewart J W et al 1984 Phenelzine vs. imipramine in atypical depression. Archives of General Psychiatry 41: 669–677

Lingjærde O, Bratlin T, Hansen T, Gøtestam K G 1986 Seasonal affective disorder and midwinter insomnia in the far north: studies on two related chronobiological disorders in Norway. Clinical Neuropharmacology 9 (suppl 4): 187–189

Llewellyn L J 1932 Light and sexual periodicity. Nature 129: 868

Marx H 1946 'Hypophysäre insuffizienz', bei lichtmangel. Klinische Wochenschrift 24/25: 18–21

Mason R 1984 Effects of chronic constant illumination on the responsiveness of rat suprachiasmatic, lateral geniculate and hippocampal neurons to ionophoresed 5-HT. Journal of Physiology 357: 13P

Moul D E, Hellekson C J, Oren D A et al 1990 Treating sad with a light visor: a multicenter study. In: Second Annual Conference on Light Treatment and Biological Rhythms. Society for Light Treatment and Biological Rhythms, New York, p 15

Muscettola G, Barbato G, Beatrice M, Nelli A C 1990 Seasonality of mood in 'sunny' Italy. In: Second Annual Conference on Light Treatment and Biological Rhythms. Society for Light Treatment and Biological Rhythms, New York, p 9

O'Keefe L P, Baker H D 1987 Diurnal changes in human psychophysical luminance sensitivity. Physiology and Behaviour 41: 193–200

O'Rourke D, Wurtman J J, Wurtman R J, Chebli R, Gleason R 1989 Treatment of seasonal depression with d-fenfluramine. Journal of Clinical Psychiatry 50: 343–347

Oren D A 1991 Retinal melatonin and dopamine in seasonal

affective disorder. Journal of Neural Transmission 83: 85–95

Oren D A, Rosenthal F S, Rosenthal N E, Waxler M, Wehr T A 1990 Exposure to ultraviolet B radiation during phototherapy. American Journal of Psychiatry 147: 675–676

Potkin S, Zetin M, Stamenkovic V, Kripke D F, Bunney W E Jr. 1986 Seasonal affective disorder: prevalence varies with latitude and climate. Clinical Neuropharmacology 9 (suppl 4): 181–183

Rafferty B, Terman M, Terman J S, Remé C E 1990 Does morning light prevent evening light effect? A statistical model for morning/evening crossover studies. In: Second Annual Conference on Light Treatment and Biological Rhythms. Society for Light Treatment and Biological Rhythms, New York, p 18

Records R E 1979 Physiology of the human eye and visual system. Harper & Row, Hagerstown, M D

Remé C E, Rafferty B, Terman M, Terman J S, Gallin P F 1990 Ocular safety and potential hazards of light therapy. In: Second Annual Conference on Light Treatment and Biological Rhythms. Society for Light Treatment and Biological Rhythms, New York, p 26

Roccatagliata G 1986 A history of ancient psychiatry. Greenwood Press, Westport, C T

Rosen L N, Targum S D, Terman M et al 1990 Prevalence of seasonal affective disorder at four latitudes. Psychiatry Research 31: 131–144

Rosenthal N E 1989 Light therapy. In: Treatments of psychiatric disorders. American Psychiatric Association, Washington, p 1890–1896

Rosenthal N E, Lewy A J, Wehr T A, Kern H E, Goodwin F K 1983 Seasonal cycling in a bipolar patient. Psychiatry Research 8: 25–31

Rosenthal N E, Sack D A, Gillin J C et al 1984 Seasonal affective disorder: a description of the syndrome and preliminary findings with light therapy. Archives of General Psychiatry 41: 72–80

Rosenthal N E, Sack D A, Carpenter C J, Parry B L, Mendelson W B, Wehr T A 1985a Antidepressant effects of light in seasonal affective disorder. American Journal of Psychiatry 142: 163–170

Rosenthal N E, Sack D A, James S P et al 1985b Seasonal affective disorder and phototherapy. Annals of the New York Academy of Sciences 453: 260–269

Rosenthal N E, Carpenter C J, James S P, Parry B L, Rogers S L B, Wehr T A 1986a Seasonal affective disorder in children and adolescents. American Journal of Psychiatry 143: 356–358

Rosenthal N E, Sack D A, Jacobsen F M et al 1986b Melatonin in seasonal affective disorder and phototherapy. Journal of Neural Transmission 21 (suppl): 257–267

Rosenthal N E, Rotter A, Jacobsen F M, Skwerer R G 1987 No mood-altering effects found after treatment of normal subjects with bright light in the morning. Psychiatry Research 22: 1–9

Rosenthal N E, Jacobsen F M, Sack D A et al 1988a Atenolol in seasonal affective disorder: a test of the melatonin hypothesis. American Journal of Psychiatry 145: 52–56

Rosenthal N E, Sack D A, Skwerer R G, Jacobsen F M, Wehr T A 1988b Phototherapy for seasonal affective disorder. Journal of Biological Rhythms 3: 101–120

Rosenthal N E, DellaBella P, Hahn L, Skwerer R G 1989a Seasonal affective disorder and visual impairment: two case studies. Journal of Clinical Psychiatry 50: 469–472

Rosenthal N E, Genhart M J, Caballero B et al 1989b Psychobiological effects of carbohydrate- and protein-rich meals in patients with seasonal affective disorder and normal controls. Biological Psychiatry 25: 1029–1040

Rosenthal N E, Joseph-Vanderpool J R, Levendosky A A et al 1990a Phase-shifting effects of bright morning light as treatment for delayed sleep phase syndrome. Sleep 13: 354–361

Rosenthal N E, Levendosky A A, Skwerer R G et al 1990b Effects of light treatment on core body temperature in seasonal affective disorder. Biological Psychiatry 27: 39–50

Ross W D 1953 The works of Aristotle. Oxford University Press Oxford

Sack R L, Lewy A J, White D M, Singer C M, Fireman M J, Vandiver R 1990 Morning vs evening light treatment for winter depression. Archives of General Psychiatry 47: 343–351

Schlager D, Terman M, Rafferty B 1989 Dawn twilight therapy for winter depression. In: First Annual Meeting of the Society for Light Treatment and Biological Rhythms. Society for Light Treatment and Biological Rhythms, Bethesda, MD, p 25

Schleifer S J, Keller S E, Bond R N, Cohen J, Stein M 1989 Major depressive disorder and immunity. Archives of General Psychiatry 46: 81–87

Skwerer R G, Jacobsen F M, Duncan C C et al 1988 Neurobiology of seasonal affective disorder and phototherapy. Journal of Biological Rhythms 3: 135–154

Sonis W A 1989 Seasonal affective disorder of childhood and adolescence: a review. In: Rosenthal N E, Blehar M C (eds) Seasonal affective disorders and phototherapy. Guilford Press, New York, pp 46–54

Spitzer R L, Endicott J, Robins E 1978 Research diagnostic criteria: rationale and reliability. Archives of General Psychiatry 35: 773–782

Stewart J W, Quitkin F M, Terman M, Terman J S 1990 Is seasonal affective disorder a variant of atypical depression? Differential response to light therapy. Psychiatry Research 33: 121–128

Szádóczky E, Falus A, Arató M, Németh A, Teszéri G, Moussong-Kovács E 1989 Phototherapy increases platelet 3H-imipramine binding in patients with winter depression. Journal of Affective Disorders 16: 121–125

Taylor H R, West S K, Rosenthal F S et al 1988 Effect of ultraviolet radiation on cataract formation. The New England Journal of Medicine 319: 1429–1433

Terman J S, Terman M, Schlager D et al 1990 Efficacy of brief, intense light exposure for treatment of winter depression. Psychopharmacology Bulletin 26: 3–11

Terman M 1988 On the question of mechanism in phototherapy for seasonal affective disorder: considerations of clinical efficacy. Journal of Biological Rhythms 3: 155–172

Terman M, Terman J S, Stewart J W, McGrath P J 1987 The timing of phototherapy: effects on clinical response and the melatonin cycle. Psychopharmacology Bulletin 23: 354–357

Terman M, Terman J S, Quitkin F M et al 1988 Response of the melatonin cycle to phototherapy for seasonal affective disorder. Journal of Neural Transmission 72: 147–165

Terman M, Botticelli S R, Link B G et al 1989a Seasonal symptom patterns in New York: patients and population. In: Thompson C, Silverstone T (eds) Seasonal affective disorder. CNS (Clinical Neuroscience) Publishers, London, p 77–95

Terman M, Schlager D, Fairhurst S, Perlman B 1989b Dawn and dusk simulation as a therapeutic intervention. Biological Psychiatry 25: 966–970

Terman M, Terman J S, Quitkin F M, McGrath P J, Stewart J W, Rafferty B 1989c Light therapy for seasonal affective disorder: a review of efficacy. Neuropsychopharmacology 2: 1–22

Terman M, Terman J S, Quitkin F M et al 1989d Dosing dimensions of light therapy: duration and time of day. In: Thompson C, Silverstone T (eds) Seasonal affective disorder. CNS (Clinical Neuroscience) Publishers, London, p 187–204

Terman M, Remé C E, Rafferty B, Gallin P F, Terman J S 1990b Bright light therapy for winter depression: potential ocular effects and theoretical implications. Photochemistry and Photobiology 51: 781–792

Thompson C 1986 Seasonal affective disorder and phototherapy: experience in Britain. Clinical Neuropharmacology 9 (suppl 4): 190–192

Thompson C, Isaacs G 1988 Seasonal affective disorder-a British sample: symptomatology in relation to mode of referral and diagnostic subtype. Journal of Affective Disorders 14: 1–11

Thompson C, Franey C, Arendt J, Checkley S A 1988 A comparison of melatonin secretion in depressed patients and normal subjects. British Journal of Psychiatry 152: 260–265

Wehr T A, Rosenthal N E 1989a Light therapy and the seasonal affective disorder: in reply. Archives of General Psychiatry 46: 194–195

Wehr T A, Rosenthal N E 1989b Seasonality and affective illness. American Journal of Psychiatry 146: 829–839

Wehr T A, Jacobsen F M, Sack D A, Arendt J, Tamarkin L, Rosenthal N E 1986 Phototherapy of seasonal affective disorder: time of day and suppression of melatonin are not critical for antidepressant effects. Archives of General Psychiatry 43: 870–875

Wehr T A, Sack D A, Rosenthal N E 1987a Seasonal affective disorder with summer depression and winter hypomania. American Journal of Psychiatry 144: 1602–1603

Wehr T A, Skwerer R G, Jacobsen F M, Sack D A, Rosenthal N E 1987b Eye versus skin phototherapy of seasonal affective disorder. American Journal of Psychiatry 144: 753–757

Wehr T A, Giesen H, Schulz P M et al 1989 Summer depression: description of the syndrome and comparison with winter depression. In: Rosenthal N E, Blehar M C (eds) Seasonal affective disorders and phototherapy. Guilford Press, New York, p 55–63

Williams J B W 1988 A structured interview guide for the Hamilton depression rating scale. Archives of General Psychiatry 45: 742–747

Wirz-Justice A, Bucheli C, Graw P, Kielholz P, Fisch H-U, Woggon B 1986a Light treatment of seasonal affective disorder in Switzerland. Acta Psychiatrica Scandinavica 74: 193–204

Wirz-Justice A, Bucheli C, Schmid A C, Graw P 1986b A dose relationship in bright white light treatment of seasonal depression. American Journal of Psychiatry 143: 932–933

Wirz-Justice A, Graw P, Bucheli C et al 1989 Seasonal affective disorder in Switzerland: a clinical perspective. In: Thompson C, Silverstone T (eds) Seasonal affective disorder. CNS (Clinical Neuroscience) Publishers, London, p 69–76

Wirz-Justice A, Sand L, Graw P, Kräuchi K, Pöldinger W 1990 A short walk can do wonders: natural light therapy in seasonal affective disorder. In: Second Annual Conference on Light Treatment and Biological Rhythms. Society for Light Treatment and Biological Rhythms, New York, p 13

Wurtman J J, Wurtman R J, Growdon J H, Henry P, Lipscomb A, Zeisel S H 1981 Carbohydrate craving in obese people: suppression by treatments affecting serotonergic transmission. International Journal of Eating Disorders 1: 2–15

Yerevanian B I, Anderson J L, Grota L J, Bray M 1986 Effects of bright incandescent light on seasonal and nonseasonal major depressive disorder. Psychiatry Research 18: 355–364

Young M A, Watel L G, Lahmeyer H W, Eastman C I 1990 The temporal onset of symptoms in winter depression. In: Second Annual Conference on Light Treatment and Biological Rhythms. Society for Light Treatment and Biological Rhythms, New York, p 42

36. Depression after childbirth

John L. Cox

PSYCHOLOGICAL AND SOCIAL DIMENSIONS

Childbirth is undoubtedly a major and irreversible life event which is commonly portrayed in religious art and ritual. It is therefore not surprising that this event is so often associated with cosmic and meaningful affects of joy and anxiety, or of sadness following an actual, or threatened, loss of the baby or even loss of a 'cherished idea' (Brown et al 1987). Thus the baby can become a 'long-term difficulty' (Brown & Harris 1978) and paradoxically could therefore be rated as an 'entrance' event, or as an 'exit' (see chapter 10) from a valued life style which has exposed unresolved psychological problems for the parents such as their own maternal deprivation (see Cox et al 1989). Breen (1975) emphasized that childbirth is a complex biopsychosocial event which leads to the attainment of a new social status as a result of fundamental processes of development which permanently change the individual roles of parents as well as their relationship to each other.

Other psychoanalysts such as Deutsch (1947) describe the process of identification between the mother and her baby, and her own mother, which can cause difficulty with parenting, especially if this was a negative relationship or if there was earlier parental deprivation. Wolkind and colleagues (1976, 1980) found research evidence to support these psychodynamic theories and showed that those mothers who were themselves deprived of attention in childhood had greater difficulty in accepting their maternal role. Similarly, in a study by Frommer & O'Shea (1973), children whose mothers had themselves been separated from their mother were more likely to have sleeping difficulties and their mothers were more often depressed. Other support comes from the findings of Nilsson & Almgren (1970) that postpartum psychiatric disorders are more likely to occur to those women who had a poor relationship to their mother or were uncertain of their female identity.

Winnicott (1956, 1960) described the primary preoccupation of mother and baby as 'engrossment', but has emphasized that this mother who is vulnerable to the demands of her dependent baby needs only to be 'good enough'. Nevertheless the problems for some parents when confronted in their baby with their own infantile rage are usefully discussed by Joan Raphael-Leff (1986, 1989); she observed that this relationship can become 'out of step' and result in phobic withdrawal or a meticulous concern with orderliness. This obsessional 'regulator' mother requires the baby to fit into her own daily programme, in contrast to the 'facilitator' mother who is able to react more flexibly to the baby's changing demands. Raphael-Leff speculates that these adjustments to motherhood are accompanied by five fantasies; good mother/good baby, good mother/bad baby, bad mother/good baby, bad mother/bad baby and good-enough mother/good-enough baby. In the 'bad mother/good baby' fantasy a depressed mother regards herself as a bad mother in danger of affecting her good baby, which must therefore be protected from damage. For these women clinical depression could be even construed as a 'way out' of this real or fantasied partnership which has 'failed to thrive'.

Social anthropologists have also investigated child-rearing practices in different ethnic and racial groups, and it is within the parent – baby interaction that specific cultural variables are learnt and transmitted between generations (Lewis 1976). Those parents who are uncertain of their own cultural norms find this process of enculturation particularly difficult and their children have greater difficulty establishing their own cultural context. Aubrey Lewis (1965), in an introduction to a CIBA Symposium on Transcultural Psychiatry, emphasized the potential for a worthwhile research collaboration between psychiatrists and anthropologists, and studies of the relationship between maternal depression and child care is a particularly productive area for interdisciplinary research teams. Thus childbirth from an anthropological perspective is a Life Transition linked to the enactment of the 'rite de passage' (van Gennep 1960) in which there is a change in status from daughter to mother and wife to mother, or from husband to father. Most societies, therefore, attach much importance to this event because it procures the next generation which will assume authority (Mead & Newton 1967, McCormack 1982).

Many societies surround childbirth with rituals and taboos. In Europe these have included 'churching' the unclean mother (Valici-Bosio 1988) but more importance is attached in these days to ensuring the physical safety of the baby. However, in Chinese society this is less emphasized and more attention is still given to the role conflicts for the mother; in a statue in Singapore for example these dilemmas are publically portrayed – a mother must choose between feeding her starving baby with her older child dying, or sustaining her own frail mother. She chooses to offer the breast to her mother (Lau 1986). In China the status passage to motherhood is also more clearly demarcated than in the West; after childbirth for example a woman must 'do the month' when she must not leave home, nor eat chicken or be blown by the wind. She should not have intercourse with her husband, or cry. Pillsbury (1978) has speculated that these taboos might protect against postpartum affective disorder. Similarly, in India the 40 days post-partum are a time when much practical help is given to the mother, who sleeps in a separate house. In the Dominican Republic a chicken is killed on each of the 40 days post-partum, and the mother is also separated from her family (Garcia, personal communication).

These elaborate postpartum rituals and taboos contrast markedly with the present role ambiguity and lack of norms for new parents in the West, where a brief, 6-hour maternity-hospital admission is usually encouraged, rapid return to work and/or continuity of domestic responsibilities are expected and the postnatal examination, which symbolically is part of the 'rite of incorporation', marks the end of the 40-day period but is now less commonly held. Furthermore, childbearing is more often a result of a careful cost—benefit analysis and the evaluation of options. Oakley (1980) and Calvert (1985) regard the causes of postnatal depression as closely linked to the changing roles for women,

so that a complete understanding of this disorder may require recognition of feminist issues.

It is not surprising, because of the complexity of these psychosocial stresses, that childbirth is sometimes followed by severe emotional distress which may merge into a mental illness. The clinical problem for the psychiatrist is how to distinguish those mood disturbances which are morbid and require treatment from those which are self-limiting or associated with appropriate mourning. These problems of assessment are complicated further by the fact that some symptoms of a depressive illness, such as sleep disturbance and loss of libido, are not necessarily secondary to a low mood but result from the physical needs of the baby. Furthermore, as even moderate antenatal anxiety could influence the decision for obstetric intervention, active psychiatric management during pregnancy might be necessary.

On the title page of Vivien Welburn's book (1980) there is a quotation: 'You have to go around with that big smile on your face and people saying "aren't you lucky to have such a dear little baby" and you feel utter despair'. This underlines from a sufferer's perspective the need to consider the social and cultural contexts of childbirth if the nature of postnatal mental illness is to be fully grasped.

CLASSIFICATIONS: OFFICIAL AND FOLK

The present controversy about the optimum classification of postnatal mental illness is unresolved, and will persist. This is because the underlying assumptions of international classifications are largely based on a biomedical model of an illness which has distinctive symptoms and a biological cause, in contrast to the popular (folk) illness categories which are derived more directly from the experience of the sufferer. This unresolved controversy may have been anticipated by Hippocrates, who favoured an organic cause for postnatal depression as well as by Marcé (1858), who believed that postnatal psychosis was a distinctive syndrome. Although Marcé was later misquoted by Strecker & Ebaugh (1926) as believing that the puerperal psychoses had no specific features, Hamilton (1962) pointed out that Marcé *had* described a 'caractère speciale' that the postpartum period gave to symptomatology. It was the temporal and cotemporal variations of physiological and psychological states which led him to believe that there was a specific disorder. A temporal relationship does not, however, necessarily indicate a causal link; although this is the way in which the diagnoses of postnatal depression or puerperal psychosis are commonly understood.

Their exclusion from ICD-9 (World Health Organization 1978) and DSM-III (American Psychiatric Association 1980) has been a major disadvantage for aetiological, as well as service-orientated, research. Moreover, their continued exclusion as main diagnoses from DSM-IV and ICD-10 overlooks recent research findings which support the early observation of Marcé that confusion *is* particularly characteristic (Dean & Kendell 1981) and that puerperal, compared with non-puerperal, psychoses have more florid delusions and hallucinations and a better prognosis. In DSM-IV a postpartum onset will only be included as a modifier of major depression; it can be argued, therefore, that this classification commits the 'category fallacy' (Kleinman 1987) as it overlooks a 'popular' diagnosis. In ICD-10 puerperal psychoses are to be listed, but as a diagnoses only to be used if criteria for other psychiatric diagnoses are not fulfilled.

It is nevertheless unlikely that the diagnoses of 'postnatal depression' and 'puerperal psychosis' will not be used, even if official classifications do not include them, as popular usage and clinical observation both suggest that a major mental illness which occurs in a mother with a small baby is of particular importance, and could be hazardous. This fact was clearly grasped by William Wordsworth (1798) in his Lyrical Ballad *The Mad Mother.*

In some African countries the mental illnesses that follow childbirth are indeed given a distinctive name. The Baganda in Uganda, for example, believe that *amakiro* is caused by promiscuity of either parent during pregnancy and that its most frequent symptom is that a mother does not want to feed, or has a wish to eat, her baby (Orley 1970, Cox 1979a); similarly the terms puerperal psychosis and postnatal depression are embedded in much popular culture in the West and represent the 'common-sense' belief that this psychiatric disorder is distinctive in certain respects. The continued research interest in the causes and symptoms of postnatal mental illness in the UK and the US—although to a lesser extent in France (Gueli et al 1987) — may result from increasing concern about new patterns of parenting, a greater ambivalence about childbearing in general and the recognition that a search for a specific biomedical or psychosocial explanation could be rewarding. The Marcé Society, an international society of clinicians and researchers, has promoted the publication of three books on postnatal mental illness (Brockington &

Kumar 1982, Kumar & Brockington 1988, Oates 1990) that are evidence of this sustained clinical and research interest. Campbell & Winokur (1985) list several reasons why a postpartum illness should be identified as a separate diagnostic category: 1) research into these disorders will be encouraged; 2) a premature assumption that biological events of parturition are not causal or predisposing will not be made; and 3) these categories of postpartum illness help refine the understanding of all affective disorders and so reduce their heterogeneity.

Puerperal psychosis

Puerperal psychoses have been defined by Brockington & Cox-Roper (1988) according to the time interval between delivery and onset. This definition includes women who meet Research Diagnostic Criteria (RDC) for mania (Spitzer & Endicott 1978), schizoaffective mania, schizophrenia or undiagnosed functional psychosis within 2 weeks of childbirth irrespective of social circumstances. Patients who manifested similar symptoms during the ninth month of pregnancy are excluded, but those with depression or neurotic symptoms before delivery are included. A puerperal depressive 'psychosis' is defined thus:

1) Depression meeting RDC, or other widely used criteria, for major depression
2) Onset in the first 2 weeks after childbirth; if depression started later than that, 'probable' is added to the diagnosis
3) Presence of delusions, hallucinations or confusion

An optimum classification of puerperal psychosis will await results of further research about aetiology and natural history, yet such research will only be facilitated if women with a psychosis after delivery can readily be identified.

Postnatal depression

Postnatal depression is a diagnosis restricted to a non-psychotic depression (absent delusions or hallucinations), usually unipolar, which occurs later in the puerperium than puerperal psychosis. The disorder starts within 3 to 4 weeks but does not usually reach clinical levels of morbidity until the 4th to 5th month. Pitt (1968) described this depression as 'atypical' but later regretted using this term as the symptoms were similar to those found in a neurotic depression occurring at any other time, although the content (what the mother was depressed about) and the consequences of depression were considerably different.

Postpartum blues

The postpartum blues are not psychiatric disorders although, when severe, their differentiation from the early stages of mental illness can be difficult. They occur in up to three-quarters of women within 2 weeks of delivery (Robin 1962, Yalom et al 1965, Pitt 1973) and are characterized by marked contrasts of emotional state on successive days post-partum, including tearfulness, poor concentration and low spirits (Kennerley & Gath 1989). They tend to peak on the fourth to the sixth postpartum day (Kendell et al 1981). This emotionalism is restricted to women who have recently delivered, as the pattern of daily mood change is not found following elective gynaecological surgery (Isles et al 1989) but is reported following elective caesarian section (Kendell et al 1984). The interest of the postpartum blues for psychiatrists arises from the possibility that a greater understanding of their causation (which is likely to be neuroendocrine) may give clues to the aetiology of puerperal psychosis, which may also occur one week after delivery (Stein 1982).

There is conflicting evidence as to whether women with postpartum blues subsequently develop postnatal depression; several studies (Kendell et al 1981, Cox et al 1982, Hapgood et al 1988) have found such an association, and O'Hara et al (1991) regarded the blues as a variant of an affective disorder. Kennerley & Gath (1989), however, found no association between the blues and postnatal depression but, like Kendell et al (1981), reported that blues women were more likely to score highly on neuroticism. While it is possible that both neuroticism and the blues are related to changes in the level of circulating oestrogen and progesterone or changes in receptor sensitivity, it is more likely that a detailed examination of predisposing personality traits, especially vulnerability to the social, marital and intrapsychic stresses of childbirth, will yield important causal data. The development of a new self-report Blues Scale, which includes measures of depression (Isles et al 1989), will facilitate this research programme further.

PUERPERAL PSYCHOSES

Epidemiology

There is a dramatic rise in the admission rate of women to a psychiatric hospital in the first 3 months after child-

birth. Thus, in an important study carried out by Kendell et al (1987), using computer-linked data from obstetric and psychiatric case registers for a population of 470 000 in which there were 54 087 births over a 12-year period, 120 psychiatric admissions occurred within 90 days of parturition. They found that there was a substantial (sevenfold) increase in admission rates in the 30 days after childbirth, compared with the average monthly admission rate before pregnancy (68 versus 10), and that a higher admission rate was sustained, although to a lesser degree, for 2 years post-partum. This latter finding would suggest that the responsibilities of continuous childcare were important stressors, in addition to the specific and time-limited biological/psychological stress of the birth event itself.

The relative risk of admission associated with childbirth (calculated as the ratio of the rate of admissions immediately after childbirth to the average admission rate beforehand) varied, depending on the length of time after childbirth as well as on parity and diagnosis. When admission with a psychosis only was studied, these authors found 51 psychosis admissions in the first 30 days after parturition, more than in the whole of the previous 2 years. When the sample was reduced to women with no previous children who were admitted with a functional psychosis, then the relative risk was increased to a startling 35.

The RDC diagnoses of the 120 puerperal admissions illustrated the wide range of psychotic disorders; 46 out of 120 had major depressive disorder (28 definite, 18 probable), 22 were manic and only four had schizophrenia. 20 women had minor depressive disorder only – a finding of importance when considering whether an inpatient or day hospital unit is preferable. Their finding that in nine of the 120 women onset had occurred during pregnancy suggests that for a minority the birth event itself may have been coincidental. 13 women had 'unspecified functional psychosis', which could have included the discrete and specific puerperal psychosis. This study thus confirmed the earlier finding of Paffenbarger (1961) but failed to find an association with maternal age or obstetric complications. It also highlighted the need to consider psychosocial causes, such as marital disruption in the first-time mothers, as well as biological factors in women predisposed to manic-depressive psychosis.

However, as this research data was based on psychiatric admissions, it needed to be amplified further by community studies if an overall picture of postnatal mental illness, including non-psychotic postnatal depression, was to be achieved. Women with young children, for example, have low consultation rates; a disabling non-psychotic depressive illness, because it is 'understandable' and the mother may not appear distressed, is often overlooked (Cox et al 1982). Esquirol (1845), the teacher of Marcé, recognised specifically this possibility. 'There are', he said, 'a large number of mild to moderate cases of puerperal psychiatric illness cared for at home and never recorded' (quoted by Hamilton 1962). Jansson (1964) also concluded that 'preoccupation with psychosis has seriously distorted the understanding of psychic insufficiency states after partus'.

The fundamental nature of the puerperal psychoses, however, whether they are a specific discrete diagnosis or are related to manic-depressive illness which required admission to a psychiatric unit within 4 weeks of childbirth, has been considerably clarified in a study by Platz & Kendell (1988). These workers compared the frequency, nature and recurrence rate of 92 women with a puerperal psychosis to control women with a psychosis which had not occurred after childbirth. Both groups were followed up for a mean interval of 9 years, when adequate information was available for 72 of the 92 matched pairs. Their findings were clear-cut: women with puerperal psychosis were as likely to relapse with a non-puerperal depressive or manic psychosis as with a puerperal onset psychosis. The risk of psychiatric admission after a further pregnancy was the same in both groups – one in ten. However certain differences were found between index and control women; the puerperal women had fewer relapses, fewer committed suicide and the rate of psychiatric disorder in relatives (as reported in case notes) was lower. Their findings suggest that, although most puerperal psychoses were the same as affective illnesses occurring at other times, women with a puerperal episode might have lesser genetic predisposition.

The risk of relapse following a subsequent birth is very high (one in three or one in four) compared with the expected frequency for a first-time puerperal psychosis of one in 500, a finding which has important implications for prevention as well as aetiology. However, the failure to find differences in the levels of circulating steroid hormones in women with puerperal and non-puerperal psychoses (Deakin 1988) suggests that neuroendocrine factors are more likely to be related to changes in the sensitivity of steroid neuroreceptors than to absolute changes in their level. According to this hypothesis a psychosis occurs when neuroreceptor sensitivity is increased by a change in the balance of steroid hormones, or through some other

stress mechanism. Partial clinical confirmation for these biological models comes from studies which do not find a stressful life event to precede the early-onset postnatal psychoses (Dowlatashi & Paykel 1990, Martin et al 1989), as well as clinical evidence that for some women the onset is indeed sudden and 'out of the blue'.

Although it is likely that the higher rate of postnatal psychosis found in women than men is explained by these neuroendocrine factors—and in general men are at lesser risk of psychoses—the stresses of fatherhood are seriously underinvestigated at the present time. Although these stresses are sometimes different from those experienced by women, they may nevertheless be sufficient to precipitate a major paternal depressive illness. Harvey & McGrath (1988) have, for example, reported that a quarter of the fathers whose partners were admitted to hospital with a puerperal psychosis themselves had a psychiatric disorder, although Kendell et al (1976) found no increased rate of *admission* of fathers later in the puerperium.

Prevention

The identification of women at high risk for a puerperal psychosis can readily be carried out at an antenatal clinic; risk factors include a previous puerperal psychosis, family history of psychiatric disorder, previous psychiatric history, being a first-time mother and poor social support. Obstetricians and midwives can readily identify these risk factors and alert the liaison or general psychiatrist, the postnatal nurse, the health visitor or community nurse to those women at risk. Furthermore, as 15% of psychoses have an onset during pregnancy (Boyd 1942), active treatment of such antenatal mental illness should be undertaken. There is no absolute contraindication to electroconvulsive therapy or antidepressants being administered during the third trimester of pregnancy. Furthermore, Kumar & Robson (1984) have reported that 16% of married primigravidae have antenatal psychiatric morbidity, and similar rates were found in a controlled study by Cox (1983) and by Assael et al (1972) in Uganda.

Lithium prophylaxis is contraindicated during pregnancy because of the risk of congenital heart abnormalities and also because of difficulty in controlling the serum lithium levels at the time of delivery due to changes in renal function and other metabolic disturbances at that time. Lithium can be prescribed after childbirth, however, provided the mother does not breastfeed, although no controlled studies have as yet been carried out. The placebo effect of these clinical interventions is particularly substantial.

Support and specific counselling by a midwife, doctor or antenatal educator for women at high risk of developing a puerperal psychosis is helpful, as most such women and their partners are frightened of a relapse and readily recall their previous psychosis and the circumstances of the delivery. Some women experience features of the post-traumatic stress disorder (Bloor & Jones 1988) and recall with intense fear the abnormal or prolonged delivery and any inappropriate or insensitive advice received.

Wieck et al (1990), in a study which used growth hormone challenge by apomorphine and measures of prolactin secretion, found that hypersensitivity of the hypothalamic D_2-receptors was predictive of relapse of puerperal psychosis in a small sample of 'high-risk' women compared with controls; these dopamine receptors are known to be sensitive to reduction in oestrogen. This research will undoubtedly require to be replicated, as the sample size was small and women were assessed on the fourth day post-partum when the psychosis was already imminent. However, this important preliminary finding will encourage the identification of women at risk of relapse and the provision of assistance in the event of recurrence. Supportive psychotherapy and neuroleptic medication, such as thioridazine, has been found useful in a case report of a patient who had relapsed despite progesterone prophylaxis after an earlier pregnancy, but who avoided a subsequent psychosis after taking thioridazine (Murray 1990).

Treatment

Clinical experience and the reports of others (see Margison 1982) suggest that early diagnosis and active treatment of a puerperal psychosis reduces substantially the risk of suicide, non-accidental injury, bonding problems and marital breakdown. These treatments, however, are optimally carried out by a postnatal mental illness team led by a consultant psychiatrist but including a range of other mental-health professional workers. Margaret Oates (1988) in Nottingham has put forward plausible justification for each UK Health District to appoint a whole-time psychiatrist for women with a child under 1 year of age. She points out the specialist nature of this work and calculates that the workload is similar to a whole-time Sector Consultant in General Psychiatry. It is this author's experience that at least two sessions a week from a general or liaison psychiatrist is essential for the optimum care of more

recently delivered women (Appleby et al 1988). This consultant requires access to an inpatient mother and baby unit, although a purpose-built unit is not always essential provided an admission ward can be modified at short notice to care for a baby and there is adequate nursing staff available. These units must be safe from the intrusion of disturbed patients and preferably situated close to the paediatric and obstetric wards so that immediate advice and transfer of the mother and baby can be undertaken if necessary.

However some women with a postnatal mental illness do not regard themselves as 'mentally' ill or as similar to other psychiatric patients, and for these women additional community facilities with less psychiatric stigma are particularly desirable. For example, a day unit with a nursery, either as part of a general adult day hospital or as a full time specialist unit similar to the Parent and Baby Unit in Stoke on Trent, is justified in this writer's experience by the frequency of referrals (about 30 a month) and by the severity of the psychiatric disorders which present. Referred women tax to their full extent the training of the mental-health professionals on the team, including the consultant psychiatrists. A survey of clients' attitudes showed that a majority of subjects welcomed the key worker system and the non-institutional philosophy of the unit but wanted their partners to be more fully involved and for their older children to attend the nursery as well as their baby (Cox et al in preparation). Pregnant women at risk of puerperal psychosis and those experiencing a psychosis not requiring admission, as well as those recently discharged from an inpatient unit, are all optimally referred to the day unit, as well as those with new-onset postnatal depression. The other advantages of such day units include their educational and research potential and providing a focus for the Postnatal Mental Illness Service.

If a community crisis intervention team is established and includes a community nurse with special knowledge of postnatal mental illness, domiciliary management of psychotic women can be considered. The risk of infanticide is remote. Neonaticide is commonly linked with adverse social factors and an unwanted baby, but the killing of an older infant is commonly linked to mental illness (Resnick 1969, 1970, d'Orban 1979). This community service can only be successful if there are close links with an inpatient facility, and if mental-health professionals are readily available out of hours.

The treatment of puerperal psychosis is generally similar to a non-puerperal psychosis except that ECT is

DEPRESSION AFTER CHILDBIRTH 575

regarded as being particularly effective (Protheroe 1969, Deakin 1988), although no controlled studies of ECT in the treatment of puerperal psychosis have, as yet, been carried out. Constant attention also needs to be given to the safety of the baby and to its bonding with the mother. Support and explanation to the partner and to other family members is important, as such family members are often perplexed and angry that this illness has occurred at a time of expected happiness.

POSTNATAL DEPRESSION

The prevalence of postnatal depression varies according to the well-established high-risk factors for depression at other times, such as an increased frequency in working-class women with small children who are more likely to experience stressful life events unprotected by economic and family support. Such women may also have access to an inferior or less accessible obstetric care.

The finding of Brown & Harris (1978) that women with young children whose own mother is not available for support and those unable to work outside the home are vulnerable to depression is particularly relevant to understanding the causes of postnatal depression. Working-class women are less likely to identify with a middle-class institution such as the antenatal or postnatal clinic, or with some social support networks such as the National Childbirth Trust. Their finding that depressed women had twice the number of birth-related events than non-depressed women suggests that any complete explanation for the higher rates of depression in women than men must take into account child-bearing and child care. Bebbington et al (1991) have found that the rates of depression are higher in married parous women than in the non-parous, whose rates are similar to those of men. If these findings are replicated then, in addition to the small contribution to the prevalence of depression caused by puerperal psychosis, having small children may be directly associated with causing or maintaining depression. (Weissman et al 1972, Weissman & Paykel 1974, Weissman & Klerman 1985). Possible explanations for these findings include greater ambivalence towards parenting, and child-bearing being less welcomed than formerly as evidence of feminity or paternity, or as an event which 'creates the parents' (Lambo 1972). A small baby, therefore, with its continuous demands and initial dependence but subsequent emancipation, can become a 'long-term difficulty', be the 'event' which brings home the hopelessness of a mother's position (Brown & Harris 1978) or be a remainder of an unwanted partner.

There is, however, a tendency for researchers and clinicians to describe only negative sequelae of childbirth and to overlook the 90% of women in whom depression does not occur and for whom the maternal engrossment of the 'good-enough' mother, as well as paternal pride, may partially resolve neurotic conflict. It may therefore be necessary to devise more sensitive measures of the life events associated with childbirth and to develop further the innovative work of Barnett et al (1983).

Nevertheless, there remains the clinical need to help women who develop a non-psychotic postnatal depression, as several studies have found that at least 9-13% have a depressive disorder 3-6 months post-partum. (Paykel et al 1980, Cox et al 1982, Cox 1983, Kumar & Robson 1984, Watson et al 1984, Cooper et al 1988, O'Hara et al 1990). Nott et al (1982) found the highest frequency of new cases at 9 months post-partum and, like Kumar & Robson (1984) and Pitt (1968) found a strong tendency for these disorders to become chronic.

These studies have been fully summarized by O'Hara & Zekoski (1988) (Table 36.1), who point out that these rates are similar to those found in general population studies, an observation which has led some to question whether there is a need for a separate diagnosis of postnatal depression. Cooper et al (1988), for example, have drawn attention to the similarity of rates found in their prospective study with that found in a community study of depressed women in Edinburgh by Surtees et al (1986), although they found that new-onset depressions were more likely to occur within the first 3 months post-partum than later in the first postpartum year. The symptom profiles of depression in the puerperal women, however, showed greater depressed mood and loss of concentration and interest at 6 months, but not at 3 or 12 months, than the comparison group. In a US prospective controlled study O'Hara et al (1990) investigated the rates of depression in 182 postpartum women and a similar number of non-pregnant, non-puerperal acquaintance controls who were matched for age and marital status. Even allowing for methodological limitations of this study, which include the effect of serial measures, the selection criteria and timing of postnatal interviews, the findings of a non-significant increase of depression in index subjects compared with controls at 9 weeks post-partum, would suggest that the frequency of postnatal depression is much closer to that found in women with older children. This important finding, therefore,

Table 36.1 Incidence and prevalence of prenatal and postnatal depression: studies using conventionally defined diagnostic criteria (adapted from O'Hara & Zekoski 1988)

Study	Sample size and country of investigation	Prenatal incidence/ prevalence (%) (time of assessment)*	Postnatal incidence prevalence (%) (time of assessment)	Criteria	Comments
Pitt 1968	305 UK		—/10.8 (6–8 weeks)	Depressive symptoms that developed since delivery, lasting longer than 2 weeks, unusual in experience and to some degree disabling	2
Wolkind et al 1980	117 UK	—/16 (7th month)**	—/10 (4 months)** —/18 (14 months)**	Definite psychiatric disorder (mostly depression assessed in context of modified Present State Examination) (Rutter 1976)	3,6
Cox et al 1982	105 Scotland	—/4 (20 weeks)***	—/13 (4 months)	Pitt (1968) criteria assessed in context of Goldberg interview (Goldberg et al 1970)	2,6
Nott 1982	5200 UK	—/0.21 (entire pregnancy)	—/0.27 (9 months)	Depressive neurosis assessed in context of inpatient or outpatient psychiatric care	4,5
Cox 1983	183 Uganda	—	—/10 (3 months)	Depressive illness based on ICD-8 assessed in context of Goldberg interview	6
Cutrona 1983	85 USA	—/3.5 (3rd trimester)***	4.7/4.7 (2 weeks)*** 3.5/3.5 (8 weeks)*** 8.2/8.2 (combined)	DSM-III (American Psychiatric Association 1980); major depression	6,7
Kumar & Robson 1984	119 UK	12.0/13.4 (1st trimester) 2.5/7.6 (2nd trimester) 2.7/6.3 (3rd trimester)	14.0/14.9 (3 months)*** 4.5/11.2 (6 months)*** 4.6/6.5 (12 months)***	RDC major and minor depression in context of Goldberg interview	6
Nilsson & Almgren 1970	152 Sweden	27.6 moderate symptoms 17.1 pronounced symptoms (entire pregnancy)	26.3 moderate symptoms 19.1 symptoms (6 months)	Moderate symptoms affecting subject's wellbeing; pronounced psychiatric symptoms indicating clear mental disturbance	
O'Hara et al 1984	99 USA	—/9.0 (2nd trimester)	10/12.0 (9 weeks)	RDC major and minor depression, assessed in context of modified Schedule for Affective Disorders and Schizophrenia (Endicott & Spitzer 1978)	6,7
Paykel et al 1980	120 UK		20 (5–8 weeks)	Score greater than 6 on Raskin Three Area Depression Scale (Raskin et al 1970)	
Watson et al 1984	128 UK	—/9.4 (entire pregnancy)	7.8/12.0 (6 weeks) —/22.0 (entire postnatal year)	Neurotic depression as defined by ICD-9, assessed in context of Goldberg interview	6

* Period of coverage of assessment is entire pregnancy up to time of assessment or entire postpartum period up to time of assessment unless otherwise noted   ** Period of coverage is the previous 30 days   *** Period of coverage is the previous 7 days

Comments: 2 Validity of diagnostic criteria not established.   3 Anxiety disorders were included in addition to depression. 4 No control over method of diagnosis.   5 Case register study.   6 Structured interview.   7 Assessment of reliability of depression diagnoses.

required replication with larger samples and with a further consideration about the optimum choice of a control group and of measures of psychiatric morbidity. Cooper et al used the Present State Examination (Wing et al 1974), which is perhaps less sensitive to milder psychiatric morbidity, and O'Hara et al (1984) used the Beck Depression Inventory, although this scale is probably less discriminating for depression after childbirth than when administered at other times (Nott & Cutts 1982, O'Hara et al 1983).

However, the preliminary findings of the North Staffordshire Study of Postnatal Depression (Cox et al in preparation), which used 232 matched non-pregnant, non-puerperal controls obtained from general practitioner lists and measured prevalence and incidence of depression within 6 months of child-bearing, were like those of O'Hara. A non-significant increase in the rates of depression was found in the puerperal group as opposed to the controls. However, although the prevalence of depression was almost identical in the two groups, the proportion of new onset depressions was significantly greater within one month of childbirth than in the equivalent time period for controls. These results, therefore, suggest that the increased risk of a non-psychotic depression occurring after childbirth is not of the same order as the risk of developing a psychosis, and that the immediate impact of the birth event (psychological or physiological) is *far* less important in the aetiology of postnatal depression than was at one time believed. These findings lend some support to the hypothesis of a distinctive neuroendocrine aetiology of postnatal depression, in a small subgroup. A prospective study to elucidate any possible common neuroendocrine mechanisms for the pre-menstrual syndrome, the blues and postnatal depression is being undertaken to investigate further this biomedical hypothesis.

Aetiology

Contrary to much popular opinion there is no evidence for a causal association between postnatal depression and levels of circulating sex hormones, or with obstetric complications. There is, however, the probability of a small subgroup of women with postnatal depression having suppressed thyroid function, and Harris et al (1989a) suggest that this association could be causal for one in 100 women and not coincidental.

Several studies report that poor marital relationships are very commonly associated with postnatal depression (Nilsson & Almgren 1970, Braverman & Roux 1978, Paykel et al 1980, Cox et al 1982, Watson et al 1984 O'Hara 1986) and that stressful non-pregnancy-related life events also frequently occur. Thus in the study reported by Watson et al (1984) only three of the 30 women with postnatal depression had experienced no other stressful life event than childbirth. A past history or a family history of psychiatric disorder are also commonly found in women with postnatal depression (Kumar & Robson 1984, Paykel et al 1980); controlled follow-up studies of postnatal depression are therefore required to establish more clearly the relationship of postnatal depression to depression occurring at other times.

It is likely that a possible link between personality and the aetiology of postnatal depression will become more readily researched as more reliable measures of personality characteristics are developed. Pitt (1968) and Watson et al (1984) found an association with neuroticism and Cox et al (1982) with the woman's report that she was 'always a worrier'. However the use of new standardized personality questionnaires such as that developed by Tyrer et al (1989) may allow a more specific test of the hypothesis put forward by Tetlow (1955) that some women have a specific difficulty in mothering or with regard to their sexuality which predisposes them to develop postnatal psychiatric disorders – the 'Achilles heel' theory. Boyce et al (1991), for example, have found that high interpersonal sensitivity in the mother increased the risk of postpartum depression eightfold at 6 months postpartum.

Other causal theories using socioanthropological approaches to childbirth are also particularly plausible. Seel (1986) and Cox (1988a) have argued that the reason for the failure of childbirth to protect against depression is the present lack of postpartum ritual in Western society and especially of the 'rite of incorporation' into the new social role. If this was more reinforced by society through ceremony and sustained family support, it would assist the mother to achieve self-confidence in her new social role. Present-day ambivalance about motherhood can cause a lowering of self-esteem and, in some women, lead to clinical depression.

The several causal theories are illustrated in Figure 36.1. As with a depression that occurs at other times the causes are usually multifactorial, and the effective clinicians are those able to recognize the importance of several explanatory models (biomedical, sociocultural or psychological). In addition the woman's own explanation for her depression should always be listened to,

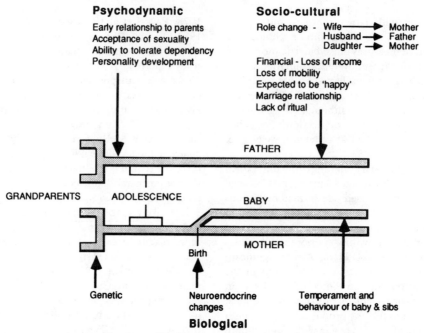

Fig. 36.1   Possible causes of postnatal depression

as failure to understand these explanations (such as hormonal deficiency or an unwanted pregnancy) may reduce compliance with important biological or social therapies.

Unlike the puerperal psychoses, however, in which a genetic predisposition and neuroendocrine abnormalities are important causes, personality traits (avoidant, histrionic and borderline), when linked to a specific difficulty with child care, are more likely to be vulnerability factors for postnatal depression.

Clinical features

In general the symptoms of postnatal depression are not substantially different from those found in depression at other times, although their impact on the family and on the baby in particular are distinctive. Anhedonia, for example, which is a common depressive symptom and regarded as central to the depressive syndrome (Snaith 1987), may be associated with loss of libido in excess of that expected in the puerperium and can further stress a marriage – especially if the partner is unprepared and already stressed by a diminution of sexual activity during pregnancy. Anger and irritability may then be directed outwards to the partner, who is himself seeking support, or to the baby, who is regarded as being a 'bad' baby.

The clinical presentation of postnatal depression has been summarized by Pitt (1968) on the basis of his research and clinical experience. Pitt correctly emphasized in this account the way in which depressive symptoms are coloured in their presentation by the mother's relationship to the baby, and by an understanding of additional stress caused by mothering difficulties:

It was after the return home that depression was always most evident, chiefly as tearfulness, despondency, feelings of inadequacy and inability to cope – particularly with the baby. ('Every other woman seems to be blooming.') Mood was often labile, and any diurnal variation took the form of greater distress in the evenings. Guilt was mainly confined to self-reproach over not loving or caring enough for the baby. Suicidal ideas were present only in the women admitted to psychiatric hospital, and feelings of actual hopelessness were not frequent. Yet many felt quite changed from their usual selves, and most had never been depressed like this before.

Depression was almost invariably accompanied, and sometimes overshadowed, by anxiety over the baby. Such anxiety was not justified by the babies' health; none was seriously ill, and most were thriving. Feeding worries were the commonest. Babies who would not sleep and kept crying were found hard to love, with consequent guilt and anxiety. Overt hostility to the child, though, was rare. Two mothers had great difficulty in accepting their babies as really theirs. A few, while able to satisfy their babies' physical needs, feared spoiling them. Multiparae tended to worry over the older children's jealousy of the new arrival.

Anxiety was also often manifest in hypochondriasis. Somatic symptoms abounded and formed the basis of fears of ill-health. One subject feared (falsely) that her ovaries had been removed in the course of Caesarian section, another feared tuberculosis, another regarded her thyroid as the root of her trouble, and another put her manifold disturbed sensations down to breast-feeding.

Unusual irritability was common, sometimes adding to feelings of guilt. A few patients complained of impaired concentration and memory. Undue fatigue and ready exhaustion were frequent, so that mothers could barely deal with their babies, let alone look after the rest of the family and cope with housework and shopping. Sometimes there was a loss of normal interests.

Anorexia, occasionally associated with nausea, was present with remarkable consistence. Sleep disturbance, over and above that inevitable with a new baby, was reported by a third of the patients, taking the form of difficulty in getting to sleep, and nightmares, more often than of early morning waking. Seventeen depressives, as compared with nine controls, lacked their normal sexual interest.

Such women may fail to attend a postnatal or child welfare clinic and disguise their depression, fearing that their baby would be taken away. They may report that it is the baby who is unwell or has difficulty feeding.

Prevention

Primary prevention

As with puerperal psychosis, women at risk of postnatal depression can readily be detected at the antenatal clinic. Such risk factors include a past history of psychiatric disorder, especially after childbirth, and marital difficulties. Leverton & Elliott (1989) have devised a screening questionnaire to detect those women vulnerable to postnatal depression and have research evidence that education and support given to first-time mothers during pregnancy may reduce the frequency of depression after delivery. Primary prevention of postnatal depression can also be facilitated by more widespread education of midwives (Ball 1987), obstetricians (Cox et al 1991, Elliott 1990), paediatricians (Zuckerman & Beardslee 1987), health visitors (Holden 1988, Taylor 1989) and maternal and child health nurses (Scott 1987).

Screening for depression at the postnatal clinic can readily be carried out by personal interview or by using a self-report questionnaire such as the Edinburgh Postnatal Depression Scale (EPDS) (Cox et al 1987) or the Depression subscale of the Symptom Check List 90-R (Derogatis 1983).

The main clinical use of the 10-item EPDS is to confirm or refute a health worker's belief that a mother may be depressed. As a research tool it can be used as a first-stage screening questionnaire in community studies, followed by a clinical interview of high scorers. The EPDS is sensitive to changes in depression over time and generally has satisfactory psychometric properties; it is also 'user-friendly' (Harris et al 1989b, Murray & Carothers 1990).

The scale was first validated on women at 3 months post-partum, when the depressive disorder was usually well established, but Carothers & Murray (1990) have now used the scale at 6 weeks on a larger community sample with only moderate reduction in sensitivity and specificity. The scale may also be administered during pregnancy or by computer (Glaze & Cox 1991) but is slightly less satisfactory than when used in the puerperium for detecting minor depression (Murray & Cox 1991). Antenatal psychiatric morbidity, especially depression, is particularly common (Nilsson & Almgren 1970, Kumar & Robson 1984, Assael et al 1972, Cox 1979b); to detect such major depression is therefore important. Antenatal depression requires active treatment and only rarely is a 'wait and see' policy justifiable. An untreated antenatal depression can merge into a prolonged and yet more disabling postpartum depression.

Secondary prevention

Secondary prevention is facilitated by early detection through using personal interview and self-report scales, as well as by making counselling skills available to health visitors and child welfare nurses. In a controlled study carried out by Holden et al (1987), for example, 8 weekly 30-minute sessions of non-directive counselling by a health visitor were beneficial for one-third of depressed women, although a further third did not improve with counselling alone. Indeed, it is for this latter group of women that a day hospital or other specialist community psychiatric team are important additional resources, since treatment of these more depressed women usually requires antidepressant medication as well as counselling from more specialist trained mental-health professionals, such as a community psychiatric nurse, psychiatrist or psychologist.

Group therapy (Morris 1987) and cognitive therapy (Elliott 1990) will also benefit selected patients. The scope for family assessments and for formal family therapy, which would include the assessment and treatment of younger children, is considerable and collaboration with child psychiatrists and child psychotherapists may be most helpful.

In Europe, Australia and North America the demand for improved postnatal mental illness services is consumer-led, as evidenced by the growth of such self-help groups as the Association of Postnatal Illness, the Meet-a-Mum Association in the UK, the Pacific Post Partum Support Group in Canada and the PANDA organization in Australia.

Tertiary prevention: impact of postnatal depression on the family

The close association between maternal depression and behavioural disturbance in older children is thoroughly documented by Cox (1988b) who observed that this association could readily be explained by the straight forward consequence of the child's exposure to depressive symptoms. Thus the immediate negative effect of postnatal depression on the baby is now well established (Murray & Stein 1989) and even possible long-term adverse sequelae on child development have been reported (Cogill et al 1986, Stein et al 1991, Wrate et al 1985). Furthermore, in addition to the distress of unexpected lack of libido and the mother's absent feeling for the baby, her partner may have difficulty himself adjusting to his partner's depression and may be experiencing marked psychiatric disorder. Indeed, the husband's personality and mental illness may have been the trigger for the mother's depressive disorder, which then leads to marital estrangement, separation or divorce. Clinical experience suggests that other unwanted sequelae of postpartum mental illness include the mother refusing a further pregnancy because of the memory of a previous psychosis, and admission to a psychiatric unit. Parents-in-law may believe that their daughter-in-law is unable to care for their grandchild, with a secondary increase in family tension. In addition an older sibling may make more demands on parents by clinging or antisocial behaviours. They may develop problems of attachment (Dunn 1985, Bowlby 1979), which prolong or initiate the threat to the mother's self-esteem, leading in turn to further clinical depression.

It is firmly established that a baby with a depressed mother who is withdrawn and less responsive protests by crying or turning away and will eventually become apathetic (Cohn & Tronick 1983, Murray 1988). Thus the mother/baby 'dance' becomes out of sequence, so that subsequent attachment difficulties occur and cognitive disabilities (object constancy) are reported at 9 months (Murray, personal communication). It is also possible that a maternal depression has been provoked by a temperamental difficulty in the infant (Cutrona & Troutman 1986). Furthermore, there is evidence that some cases of 'failure to thrive' of non-organic origin are caused by a mother's lack of interest in feeding or by neglect of child care associated with depression (O'Callaghan & Hull 1978). Other unwanted and serious sequalae of post partum depression, include infanticide which in 60% is associated with maternal suicide (d'Orban 1979) and rarely non-accidental injury (see Smith et al 1973). These findings suggest that paediatricians (Zuckerman et al 1987) and child psychiatrists, as well as obstetricians and psychiatrists, need to collaborate to establish a truly comprehensive clinical service for parents of young children.

REFERENCES

American Psychiatric Association 1980 Diagnostic and statistical manual of mental disorders, 3rd edn. American Psychiatric Association, Washington, DC

Appleby L, Fox H, Shaw M, Kumar R 1988 The psychiatrist in the obstetric unit: establishing a liaison service. British Journal of Psychiatry 154: 510–515

Assael M I, Namboze J M, German G A, Bennett F J 1972 Psychiatric disturbances during pregnancy in a rural group of African women. Social Science and Medicine 6: 387–395

Ball J A 1987 Reactions to motherhood. Cambridge University Press, Cambridge

Barnett B F W, Hanna B, Parker G 1983 Life event scales for obstetric groups. Journal of Psychosomatic Research 27: 313–330

Bebbington P E, Dean C, Der G, Hurry J, Tennant C 1991 Gender, parity and the prevalence of minor affective disorder. British Journal of Psychiatry 158: 40–45

Bloor R M, Jones R A 1988 Post traumatic stress disorders and sexual disfunction – a case report. British Journal of Sexual Medicine 15(5): 170–172

Bowlby J 1979 The making and breaking of affectional bonds. Tavistock Publications, London

Boyce P, Parker G, Barnett B, Cooney M, Smith F 1991 Personality as a vulnerability factor to depression. British Journal of Psychiatry 159: 106–114

Boyd D A 1942 Mental disorders associated with child bearing. American Journal of Obstetrics and Gynecology 43: 148–163

Braverman J, Roux J F 1978 Screening for the patient at risk for postpartum depression. Obstetrics and Gynaecology 52: 731–736

Breen D 1975 The birth of a first child. Tavistock Press, London

Brockington I F, Cox-Roper A 1988 The nosology of

puerperal mental illness. In: Kumar R, Brockington I F (eds) Motherhood and mental illness 2. John Wright, London

Brockington I F, Kumar R 1982 Motherhood and mental illness, Academic Press, London

Brown G W, Harris T 1978 Social origins of depression. Tavistock Publications, London

Brown G W, Bifulco A, Harris T O 1987 Life events, vulnerability and onset of the depression. British Journal of Psychiatry 150: 30–42

Calvert J 1985 Motherhood. In: Brook F, Davis A (eds) Women, the family and social work. Tavistock Publications, London

Campbell J L, Winokur G 1985 Postpartum affective disorders; selected biological aspects. In: Inwood D G (ed) Postpartum psychiatric disorders. APA Press, Washington, DC

Carothers A D, Murray L 1990 Estimating the prevalence of psychiatric morbidity: the use of logistic regression. Psychological Medicine 20: 695–702

Cogill S R, Caplan H L, Alexandra H, Robson K, Kumar R 1986 Impact of maternal postnatal depression on cognitive development of young children. British Medical Journal 292: 1165–1167

Cohn J F, Tronick E C 1983 Three month old infants' reaction to simulated maternal depression. Child Development 54: 185–193

Cooper P J, Campbell E A, Day A et al 1988 Non-psychotic psychiatric disorder after childbirth: a prospective study of prevalence, incidence, course and nature. British Journal of Psychiatry 152: 799–806

Cox J L 1979a Amakiro: a Ugandan puerperal psychosis? Social Psychiatry 14: 49–52

Cox J L 1979b Psychiatric morbidity and pregnancy: a controlled study of 263 semi-rural Ugandan women. British Journal of Psychiatry 134: 401–405

Cox J L 1983 Postnatal depression: a comparison of African and Scottish women. Social Psychiatry 18: 25–28

Cox J L 1986 Postnatal depression – a guide for health professionals. Churchill Livingstone, Edinburgh

Cox J L 1988a The life event of childbirth; sociocultural aspects of postnatal depression. In: Kumar R, Brockington I F (eds) Motherhood and mental illness 2. John Wright, London

Cox A 1988b Maternal depression and impact on children's development. Archives of Disease in Childhood 63: 90–95

Cox J L, Connor Y, Kendell R E 1982 Prospective study of the psychiatric disorders of childbirth. British Journal of Psychiatry 140: 11–17

Cox J L, Holden J M, Sagovsky R 1987 Detection of postnatal depression: development of the 10-item Edinburgh postnatal depression scale (EPDS). British Journal of Psychiatry 150: 782–786

Cox J L, Paykel E S, Page M L 1989 Childbirth as a life event. Duphar Medical Relations, Southampton

Cox J L, Murray D, Chapman G in preparation Controlled study of postnatal depression.

Cox J L, Cookson D, Jones J M (in preparation) establishing a day hospital and nursery in the potteries for women with postnatal depression; results of a Consumer Audit Health Trends

Cutrona C E 1983 Causal attributions and perinatal depression. Journal of Abnormal Psychiatry 92: 161–172

Cutrona C E, Troutman B R 1986 Social support, infant temperament and parenting self-efficiency; a mediational model of postpartum depression. Child Development 57: 1507–1578

Deakin J F W 1988 Relevance of hormone-CNS interactions to psychological changes in the puerperium. In: Kumar R, Brockington I F (eds) Motherhood and mental illness. John Wright, London

Dean C, Kendell R E 1981 The symptomatology of puerperal illnesses. British Journal of Psychiatry 139: 128

Derogatis L R 1983 SCL-90-R; administration, scoring and procedures manual. Clinical Psychosis Research, Baltimore

Deutsch H 1947 Psychology of women: Motherhood, vol 2. Research Book, London

d'Orban P T 1979 Women who kill their children. British Journal of Psychiatry 134: 560–571

Dowlatashi D, Paykel E S 1990 Life events and social stress in puerperal psychoses; absence of effect. Psychological Medicine 20: 655–662

Dunn J 1985 The arrival of a sibling. In: Nicol A (Ed) Longitudinal studies in child psychology and psychiatry. John Wiley, Chichester

Elliott S A 1990 Psychological strategies in the prevention and treatment of postnatal depression. In: Oates M R (ed) Psychological aspects of obstetrics and gynaecology. Baillière Tindall, London

Endicott J, Spitzer R L 1978 A diagnostic interview. The schedule for affective disorders and schizophrenia. Archives of general psychiatry 35: 837–844

Esquirol E 1845 Des maladies mentales. J Baillière, Paris

Frommer E A, O'Shea G 1973 Antenatal identification of mothers likely to have difficulty managing their infants. British Journal of Psychiatry 123: 149–156

Glaze R, Cox J L 1991 Validation of a computerised version of the 10-item (self-rating) Edinburgh Postnatal Depression Scale. Journal of Affective Disorders 22: 73–77

Goldberg D P, Connor B, Eastwood M R et al 1970 A standardised psychiatric interview for use in community surveys. British Journal of Preventive and Social Medicine 24: 18–23

Gueli J D, Boyer P, Consol S, Oliver-Martin R 1987 Psychiatrie. Presses Universitaires de France, Paris

Hamilton J A 1962 Postpartum psychiatric problems. C V Mosby, St Louis

Hapgood C C, Elkind A S, Wright J T 1988 Maternity blues: Phenomona and relationships to later post partum depression. Australian and New Zealand Journal of Psychiatry 22: 299–306

Harris B, Fung H, Johns S 1989a Transient post partum thyroid dysfunction and postnatal depression. Journal of Affective Disorders 17: 243–249

Harris B, Huckle P, Thomas R, Johns S, Fung H 1989b The using of rating scales to identify postnatal depression. British Journal of Psychiatry 154: 813–817

Harvey I, McGrath G 1988 Psychiatric morbidity in spouses of women admitted to a mother and baby unit. British Journal of Psychiatry 152: 506–570

Holden J M 1988 Detection and treatment of postnatal depression. A counselling manual for health visitors. (unpublished)

Holden J M, Sagovsky R, Cox J L 1987 Counselling in a general practice setting: a controlled study of health visitor intervention in the treatment of postnatal depression. British Medical Journal 298: 223–226

Isles S, Gath D, Kennerley H 1989 A comparison between post operative women and postnatal women. British Journal of Psychiatry 155: 363

Jansson B 1964 Psychic insufficiencies associated with childbearing. Acta Psychiatrica Scandanavica 39 (suppl 172)

Kendell R E, Wainwright, Hailey A, Shannon B 1976 The influence of childbirth on psychiatric morbidity. Psychological Medicine 6: 297–302

Kendell R E, McGuire R J, Connor Y, Cox J L 1981 Mood changes in the first three weeks after childbirth. Journal of Affective Disorders 3: 317–326

Kendell R E, MacKenzie W E, West C, McGuire R J, Cox J L 1984 Day to day mood changes after childbirth: further data. British Journal of Psychiatry 145: 620–625

Kendell R E, Chalmers L, Platz C 1987 The epidemiology of puerperal psychoses. British Journal of Psychiatry 150: 662–673

Kennerley H, Gath D 1989 Detection and measurement by questionnaire. British Journal of Psychiatry 155: 356

Kleinman A 1987 Anthropology and psychiatry: the role of culture in cross cultural research in illness. British Journal of Psychiatry 157: 447–454

Kumar R, Brockington I 1988 Motherhood and mental illness 2: causes and consequences. John Wright, London

Kumar R, Robson K M 1984 A prospective study of emotional disorders in childbearing women. British Journal of Psychiatry 144: 35–47

Lambo T A 1972 Characteristic features of the psychology of the African. Totus Homo 4: 8–17

Lau A 1986 Family therapy across cultures. In: Cox J L (ed) Transcultural psychiatry. Croom Helm, London

Leverton T J, Elliott S A 1989 Transitions to parenthood groups: a preventive intervention for postnatal depression. In: Van Hall E V, Everard W (eds) The free woman. Parthenon Publishing, Carnforth

Lewis A 1965 Chairman's introduction. In: De Reuck A V S, Porter R (eds) Transcultural Psychiatry. CIBA Symposium. Little, Brown, Boston

Lewis I M 1976 Social anthropology in perspective. Penguin Books, Harmondsworth

McCormack C P 1982 Ethnography of fertility and birth. Academic Press, London

Marcé L V 1858 Traité de la folie des femmes enceintes, des nouvelles accouchées et des nourrices. J. Bailliere, Paris

Margison F 1982 The pathology of the mother—child relationship. In: Brockington I F, Kumar R (eds) Motherhood and mental illness. Academic Press, London

Martin C J, Brown G W, Goldberg D P, Brockington I F 1989 Psycho-social stress and puerperal depression; Journal of Affective Disorders 16: 283–293

Mead M, Newton N 1967 Cultural patterning of perinatal behaviour. In: Richardson S A, Guttmacher A F (eds) Childbearing – its social and psychological aspects. Williams & Wilkins, Baltimore

Morris J B 1987 Group psychotherapy for prolonged postnatal depression. British Journal of Medical Psychology 60: 279–281

Murray L 1988 Effects of postnatal depression on infant development: Direct intervention. In: Kumar R, Brockington I F (eds) Motherhood and mental illness 2. John Wright, London

Murray D 1990 Recurrence of puerperal psychosis not prevented by prophylactic progesterone. Journal of Nervous and Mental Diseases 178: 537–538

Murray L, Carothers A D 1990 The validation of the Edinburgh Postnatal Depression Scale on a community sample. British Journal of Psychiatry 157: 288–290

Murray D, Cox J L 1990 Screening for depression during pregnancy with the Edinburgh Depression Scale (EPDS). Journal of Reproductive and Infant Psychology 8: 99–107

Murray L, Stein A 1989 The effects of postnatal depression on the Infant. In: Oates M R (ed) Psychological aspects of obstetrics and gynaecology. Baillière Tindall, London

Nilsson A, Almgren P E 1970 Parental emotional adjustment – a prospective investigation of 165 women. Acta Psychiatrica Scandinavica: suppl 220

Nott P N 1982 Psychiatric illness following childbirth in Southampton: a case register study. Psychological Medicine 12: 557–561

Nott P N, Cutts S 1982 Validation of the 30-item General Health Questionnaire in post partum women. Psychological Medicine 12: 409–413

Oakley A 1980 Women confined: towards a sociology of childbirth. Martin Robertson, Oxford

Oates M 1988 The development of an integrated community orientated service for severe postnatal mental illness. In: Kumar R, Brockington I F (eds) Motherhood and mental illness. John Wright, London

Oates M 1990 Clinical obstetrics and gynaecology: psychological aspects of obstetrics and gynaecology. Baillière Tindall, London

O'Callaghan M J, Hull D 1978 Failure to thrive or failure to rear? Archives of Disease in Childhood 3: 788–793

O'Hara M W 1986 Social support, life events, and depression during pregnancy and the puerperium. Archives of General Psychiatry 43: 569–573

O'Hara M W, Zekoski E M 1988 Postpartum depression: a comprehensive review. In: Kumar R, Brockington I F (eds) Motherhood and mental illness 2. John Wright, London

O'Hara M W, Rehm L P, Campbell S B 1983 Post partum depression: a role for social network and life stress variables. Journal of Nervous and Mental Disease 171: 336–341

O'Hara M W, Neunaber D J, Zekoski E M 1984 A prospective study of postpartum depression: prevalence cause and predictive factors. Journal of Abnormal Psychology 93: 158–171

O'Hara M W, Zekoski E M, Phillips L H, Wright E J 1990 Controlled prospective study of postpartum mood disorders: comparison of childbearing and non-childbearing women. Journal of Abnormal Psychology 99: 3–15

O'Hara M W, Schlecht E J A, Lewis D A, Wright E J 1991 Prospective study of postpartum blues: biological and psychosocial factors. Archives of general psychiatry 48: 801–806

Orley J H 1970 Culture and mental illness: a study from Uganda. Makerere Institute of Social Research. East African Publishing House, Nairobi

Paffenbarger R S 1961 The picture puzzle of the postpartum psychoses. Journal of Chronic Disorders 13: 161–173

Paykel E S, Emms E M, Fletcher J, Rassaby E S 1980 Life events and social support in puerperal depression. British Journal of Psychiatry 136: 339–346

Pillsbury B L K 1978 Doing the month; confinement and convalescence of Chinese women after childbirth. Social Science and Medicine 12: 11–22

Pitt B 1968 'Atypical' depression following childbirth. British Journal of Psychiatry 144: 1325–1335

Pitt B 1973 Maternity blues. British Journal of Psychiatry 122: 431–435

Platz C, Kendell R E 1988 Matched control follow-up and family study of puerperal psychoses. British Journal of Psychiatry 153: 90–94

Protheroe C 1969 Puerperal psychoses: a long term study 1927–1961. British Journal of Psychiatry 115: 9–30

Raphael-Leff J 1986 Facilitators and regulators: conscious and unconscious processes in pregnancy and early motherhood. British Journal of Medical Psychology 59: 43–55

Raphael-Leff J 1989 Orientation and adjustment to early motherhood. Midwife, Health Visitor and Community Nurse 25: 372

Raskin A, Schulterbrandt J, Reatig N, McKean J 1970 Differential response to chlorpromazine, imipramine, and placebo. Archives of General Psychiatry 23: 164–173

Resnick P J 1969 Child murder by parents: a psychiatric review of filicide. American Journal of Psychiatry 126: 325–334

Resnick P J 1970 Murder of the newborn: a psychiatric review of neonaticide. American Journal of Psychiatry 126: 1414–1420

Robin A A 1962 Psychological changes of normal parturition. Psychiatric Quarterly 36: 129–150

Rutter M 1976 Research report. Isle of Wight studies 1964–1974. Psychological Medicine 6: 313–332

Scott D 1987 Maternal and child health nurse: role in post-partum depression. Australian Journal of Advanced Nursing 5: 28–37

Seel R M 1986 Birth rite. Health Visitor 59: 182–184

Smith S M, Hanson R, Noble S 1973 Parents of battered babies: a controlled study. British Medical Journal 4: 388–391

Snaith R P 1987 The concept of mild depression. British Journal of Psychiatry 150: 387–393

Spitzer R L, Endicott J 1978 Research diagnostic criteria. Rationale and reliability. Archives of General Psychiatry 35: 773–782

Stein G 1982 The maternity blues. In: Brockington I F, Kumar R (eds) Motherhood and mental illness. Academic Press, London

Stein A, Gath D H, Bucher J, Bond A, Day A, Cooper P J 1991. The relationship between post-natal depression and mother–child interaction. British Journal of Psychiatry 158: 46–52

Strecker E A, Ebaugh F C 1926 Psychosis occurring during the puerperium. Archives of Neurology and Psychiatry 15: 239–252

Surtees P G, Sashidharan S P, Dean C 1986 Affective disorder amongst women in the general population: a longitudinal study. British Journal of Psychiatry 148: 176–186

Taylor E 1989 Postnatal depression: what can a health visitor do? Journal of Advanced Nursing 14: 877–886

Tetlow C 1955 Psychosis of childbearing. Journal of Mental Science 101: 624

Tyrer P, Alexander J, Ferguson B 1989 Personality disorders: diagnosis, management and treatment. John Wright, London

Valici-Bosio S 1988 La mère et l'enfant dans l'ancienne France. PV, Paris

Van Gennep A 1960 The rites of passage. Routledge & Kegan Paul, London

Watson J P, Elliot S A M, Rugg A J, Brough D I 1984 Psychiatric disorder in pregnancy and the first postnatal year. British Journal of Psychiatry 144: 453–462

Weissman M, Klerman G L 1985 Gender and depression. Trends in the Neurosciences 8: 416–420

Weissman M M, Paykel E S 1974 The Depressed Women: a study of social relationships. University of Chicago Press, Chicago

Weissman M M, Paykel E S, Klerman G L 1972 The Depressed Woman as a Mother. Social Psychiatry 7: 98–108

Welburn V 1980 Postnatal depression. Fontana, London

Wieck A et al 1990 Dopaminergic function, oestrogen withdrawal and bipolar relapse in recently delivered mothers. Paper presented at Marcé Meeting in York.

Wing J L, Cooper J E, Sartorius N 1974 Measurement and classification. Cambridge University Press, Cambridge

Winnicott D U 1956 Primary maternal preoccupations. In: Masud M, Khan R (eds) Through paediatrics to psychoanalysis. Hogarth Press, London

Winnicott D U 1960 The theory of the parent infant relationship. In: Sutherland J D (ed) The maturational process and the facilitating environment. Hogarth Press, London

Wolkind M, Keuk S, Chaves L P 1976 Childhood experiences and psychosocial status in primiparous women; preliminary findings. British Journal of Psychiatry 128: 391–396

Wolkind M, Zajicek E, Ghodsian M 1980 Continuities in maternal depression. International Journal of Family Psychiatry 1: 167–182

Wordsworth W 1798. The mad mother. In: Collected works. Collins, London

World Health Organization 1978 Mental disorders: glossary and guide to their classification in accordance with the ninth revision of the International Classification of Diseases. WHO, Geneva

Wrate R M, Rooney A C, Thomas P F, Cox J L 1985 Postnatal depression and child development: a 3 year follow up study. British Journal of Psychiatry 146: 622–627

Yalom I D, Lunke D T, Moos R H, Hamburg D A 1965 Postpartum blues syndrome. Archives of General Psychiatry 18: 16–27

Zuckerman B S, Beardslee W R 1987 Maternal depression: a concern for paediatricians. Paediatrics 79: 110–117

37. Depression in childhood and adolescence

Ian M. Goodyer

THE MEANING OF DEPRESSION

The child psychiatric literature has been confused by the variety of meanings attached to the word depression over the years (Angold 1988a). As a result, there have been wide differences in definition of caseness, method and design of studies, making comparison of research findings difficult. In recent years, however, distinctions have been usefully drawn between the symptoms of mood change and the presence of a syndrome. The application of standardized methods for collecting signs and symptoms of psychopathology from children and adolescents as well as their parents has considerably improved (Gutterman et al 1987). Both epidemiological and clinical studies confirm the presence of a depressive syndrome occurring in children at least as young as 3 (Rutter 1986, Emde et al 1986).

These studies indicate important developmental influences on the symptoms and syndromes of depression (Rutter 1986). Age effects in prevalence of disorder, course and relapse, continuities and discontinuities between child and adult disorders, as well as the age influences on the effects of psychiatric risk factors are important considerations in the developmental psychopathology of depression. The relevance of developmental issues is highlighted within each section of this chapter.

ASSESSMENT OF DEPRESSION

Since the mid 1970s diagnostic criteria have been more carefully specified and many workers have adopted unmodified adult criteria of DSM-III to determine both prevalence and characteristics of depression. A wide range of measures have now been developed for assessing the presence of a major depressive episode.

Self reports

A large number of self-report measures for children and adolescents are available for clinical and epidemiological purposes (Costello & Angold 1988, Kazdin 1989, 1990). Such reports may be particularly important in assessing key internalizing symptoms such as worthlessness and hopelessness. The Children's Depression Inventory (CDI; Kovacs 1981) and the Edinburgh Depression Inventory (Birleson 1981) represent two of the more commonly used measures. The Children's Depression Inventory, for example, contains 27 items reflecting affective, cognitive and behavioural signs and symptoms of depression. Children may read the items themselves or, in a 'semi-interview' format, have them read to them. The CDI has been shown to have high internal consistency (e.g. Cronbach's alpha > 0.8), to have acceptable test-retest reliability from one week to six months, to be able to distinguish clinical from non-clinical groups and to correlate in the expected direction with measures of self-esteem, perceived personal competence, negative cognitive attributions and hopelessness (Kovacs 1986). In addition, normative data are available to facilitate evaluation of the level of dysfunction of children relative to their same-age and -gender peers (Finch et al 1985).

Self-report scales have produced a great deal of research. They have highlighted, however, the importance of determining age-related cut-off scores for potential caseness and the variation of reliability and validity with age. Currently, self-reports look promising for epidemiological and clinical studies in children of 11 years and over. Further refinements to items and scale construction seem needed in 8–11-year-olds before acceptable psychometric properties are achieved. Under the age of 8 little is known about the reliability and validity of self-reports.

Interviews

A number of structured and semi-structured interviews are now available for research purposes (Gutterman et al 1987). The Diagnostic Interview Schedule for Children and Adolescents (DISC) is an example of a highly-structured interview with multiple symptoms, rated on a three-point scale to cover DSM-III diagnoses. The interview is for use by lay or clinical interviewers and specifically developed for epidemiological studies (Costello et al 1985).

The Schedule of Affective Disorders and Schizophrenia for School Age Children (K-SADS; Chambers et al 1985), by contrast, is a semi-structured interview for children with psychiatric disorders, in which general questions are asked about the child's symptoms, the reasons for clinic attendance and general functioning at home and school. Specific questions are then asked about symptoms and ratings are made by the clinician of the severity of each symptom. Clinicians also rate the severity of physical signs. Multiple diagnoses can be derived from items.

The Children's Depression Rating Scale is a specific interview for depression consisting of 16 items rated on a six-point scale for severity (Poznanski et al 1984). This interview is derived from the Hamilton Depression Scale for adults. A child's Hamilton scale, retaining the same scoring formats, has also been used (Foreman & Goodyer 1988).

The choice of interview depends on the population under investigation and the questions being asked. Several studies using these and other similar interviews have now been published, demonstrating that reliable diagnoses can be obtained. Both child and parent versions of interviews are generally used, although evidence is accumulating that internalizing emotional symptoms and syndromes in general, and depression in particular, are more reliably obtained by direct interview of the children (Kovacs 1986, Edelbrock et al 1986).

Peers, as well as parents, have been used to rate psychopathology in children, including depression. Self-reports by friends and classroom peers and measures of overt behaviour such as social interaction and activity have all been used to delineate altered mood and behaviour as perceived by others. Each programme has tended to develop its own methodology, making generalizations across studies difficult (Kazdin 1990). The findings do suggest that altered behaviours such as social withdrawal are consistent features of depression (Altmann & Gotlieb 1988). Whether behavioural characteristics of depression vary in prevalence and form with age and gender remains unclear.

The availability of reliable assessment methods from multiple informants has resulted in a marked increase in reports of the prevalence, nature and, to a lesser extent, outcome of depression.

Most studies report rather low agreements between alternative different sources such as child, parents and teachers (Achenbach et al 1987, Ivens & Rehn 1988, Fleming et al 1989). While correspondence may be low, there is evidence that different informants may provide valid information about different aspects of depression. For example, child self-report measures correlate with suicidal ideation and attempt, hopelessness and low self-esteem (Kazdin et al 1983, Haley et al 1985). Parental reports of depressed children correlate with diminished social interaction and loss of expressed affect (Kazdin et al 1985a).

The choice of respondent and instrument therefore depends in part on the question being asked. If the purpose is to determine the presence of a depressive disorder, children and adolescents are necessary and may be sufficient informants. If the social concomitants and consequences are required, parents or others should be used. The possibility that parents or other adults over-report depression in the child as a consequence of their own psychopathology may need to be taken into account. Recent evidence suggests, however, that such reporting distortions may be over-emphasized (Richters & Pellegrini 1989).

CHARACTERISTICS OF DEPRESSION

Classification

Over the past decade there has been a marked advancement in classifying depressive psychopathology in childhood and adolescence (Strober 1989, Kazdin 1990). Original attempts at defining child-specific criteria have proved to be unnecessary in 7–16-year-olds, who have been shown in a number of studies to meet adult-based criteria (Ryan et al 1987). Current emphasis has been on identifying subjects who met DSM-III or DSM-IIIR criteria in either clinical or community populations (Kovacs et al 1984, Ryan et al 1987, Fleming et al 1989). As a result, depressive diagnoses in children over 7, adolescents and adults are comparable, at least on the core set of signs and symptoms that are required for diagnoses. This does not mean that the manifestations of the disorder are identical at different ages. The configuration of symptoms accompanying social disabilities, course and outcome of disorder may vary with age or with other developmental factors such as puberty.

DSM-IIIR recognizes that there may be different features for varying ages and developmental levels. For example, irritability may be a core 'mood' as well as depressive affect. At this time, however, there are few studies of descriptive psychopathology at different ages and stages of development. Indeed, the current classification of depression is unable to take into account potential developmental influences on mood disorders. This is particularly true for infancy and early childhood (Emde et al 1986). Whilst there are many anecdotal reports of cases of depression in young children meeting adult criteria, we lack the reliable techniques that have become available in other age groups. Situation-specific behaviours, the unreliability of recall and the fluctuating nature of signs and symptoms in younger children all influence the form of psychopathology to a greater extent than at other age periods. Further research would be necessary to determine whether or not a greater proportion of children in this age group exhibiting emotional and behavioural syndromes which do not meet adult criteria are in fact depressed.

Direct observational studies have been conducted in an effort to delineate specific depressive behaviour in a social context. Studies of inpatient depressed children have shown that they engage in significantly less social behaviour and show less affect-related social expression than non-depressed children (Kazdin et al 1985a). Solitariness, poor engagement on on-task behaviours, disruptiveness and failure to complete tasks have all been noted (Kazdin et al 1985b, Altmann & Gotlieb 1988, Kazdin 1990). Despite idiosyncratic observational methods and varying populations, there is a consistency of findings for deficits in social behaviour during a depressive episode. Whether or not observational methods of assessment contribute important information for diagnostic purposes beyond interview techniques remains unclear.

The availability of different sources of information and different methods of collection does not indicate that there is a well-developed assessment strategy for diagnosing childhood depression. Several studies have shown that multiple measures focused on the same person (child, parent or others) correlate with each other (Rotundo & Hensley 1985, Ivens & Rehn 1988). By comparison, child and parent evaluations using the same or similar instruments often show low agreement or occasionally disagreement (Herjanic & Reich 1982, Achenbach et al 1987, Ivens & Rehm 1988, Fleming et

al 1989). Adolescents identify themselves as depressed between two and six times more often than their parents or other informants so identify them (Fleming et al 1989). Recent findings suggest that teacher-identified rates of depression in preadolescents agree as closely with the children as do those of their parents (Fleming et al 1989). Teachers have been underutilized as a source of diagnostic information in the past.

Despite low correspondence between sources, evidence points to the validity of information about the child from self and parent reports. For example, child self-report measures of depression correlate with suicidal attempt and ideation, and parental reports correlate with diminished social interaction and diminished facial expression (Kazdin et al 1983, 1985a). There is also some evidence that teacher and peer reports of depression correlate with their own evaluations of the child's academic performance and popularity respectively (Tesing et al 1980, Tesing & Lefkowitz 1982, Fleming et al 1989).

Ratings of children's depression from alternative sources, therefore, reflect potentially useful diagnostic information from different social, emotional and behavioural dimensions. Internalizing symptoms of mood and thoughts are most likely to be obtained from the child and indicate the central importance of direct interviewing. Externalizing symptoms such as social interaction and expression may be best obtained from parents, peers and teachers. As yet, the relative contribution of different sources of information to predict onset, course, treatment and outcome rather than diagnosis *per se* is not known.

In addition, evidence is beginning to accumulate concerning the nature, course and outcome of depression in young people (Angold 1988a, b, Kovacs et al 1988, 1989, McGee & Williams 1988). These factors, together with signs and symptoms at presentation, can be taken into account in the future classification of depression in young people.

Age and symptoms

A range of studies using parent reports and self-reports with widely differing subject selection has suggested that depressive symptoms and syndromes may be organized differently as a function of age and gender of the child (Angold 1988a).

In a recent study on the clinical characteristics of clinic attenders, Ryan and colleagues showed, using systematic interview techniques, that depressed children between 6 and 12 years were likely to look sad, report somatic features and be agitated, whereas between 12 and 16 years they were more likely to report depressive feelings, including hopelessness, demonstrate impaired concentration and make suicide attempts (Ryan et al 1987). Insomnia, appetite disturbance, loss of energy and lack of interest in normal activities were apparent to varying degrees across all ages. Children commonly reported feelings of guilt and thoughts that they would be better off dead but rarely made suicidal attempts.

These findings suggest two developmental influences on the patterning and presentation of depression. Firstly, cognitive development related to age and probably pubertal change increases the likelihood of cognition-related symptomatology. Secondly, the marked absence of suicide attempts in children suggests some potential form of protection against self-injuries and suicidal behaviour. These two factors may represent a 'cognitive continuum' but at present the matter is unclear. Suicides do occur rarely in children and anxious, somatic and cognitive features of depression are found across all ages. By contrast, a consistent finding has been the predominant reporting of physical symptoms together with loss of interest across the age range.

Similar studies on the developmental psychopathology of mood disorders in this age group are urgently needed to delineate further the characteristics of mood disorder in young persons.

Although major depressive disorder, dysthymia and adjustment disorder with depressed mood have all been described and investigated in childhood and adolescence, symptoms of depression occur in other psychiatric disorders of childhood such as anxiety and conduct disorders. Often in such cases depressive symptoms arise specifically in relation to one theme such as separation or school refusal and are not pervasive components of mental state. Within depressive conditions themselves anxious and behavioural symptoms are often present and it has become apparent from a number of studies that children may meet criteria for more than one syndrome. This phenomenon of comorbidity is common but its implications remain unclear. For example, as many as 40% of children presenting with major depression are comorbid for anxiety disorder (Kovacs et al 1989). Of these, separation anxiety disorder is the commonest and panic disorder the rarest. Even when criteria for anxiety syndromes are not met anxiety *symptoms* are commonly present (Hershberg et al 1982).

A further 15% of major depressive disorders are comorbid for conduct disorder (Kovacs et al 1988). Whether or not anxious and behavioural symptoms and syndromes precede depression is an important and unresolved issue and longitudinal studies are required to determine if an evolutionary relationship exists between different patterns of symptoms. At present, the developmental and gender influences on the form and patterning of disorder is unclear. Boys with a depressive syndrome do appear more likely than girls to present with behavioural symptoms and conduct disorder at all ages (Kovacs et al 1988, Kazdin 1990).

The severity and intensity of disorder may also vary as a function of development. The most striking finding to date has been that adolescents are significantly more likely than children to experience hypersomnia during a depressive episode (Mitchell et al 1988, Kovacs & Gatsonis 1989).

Suicidal behaviour and depression

The lifetime prevalence rate of suicide attempts in 14–20-year-olds has recently been estimated as 2% (Kienhorst et al 1990). Kienhorst and colleagues investigated the characteristics of suicide attempters in 9393 Dutch adolescents using self-report questionnaires. They found that psychological factors (depression and poor self-image) were more important in discriminating youngsters with suicidal behaviour than were sociodemographic factors. Suicidal tendencies have also been shown to persist in young people. Pfeffer and colleagues (Pfeffer et al 1988) conducted a 2-year follow-up of 75 out of 101 12-year-olds originally seen for suicidal tendencies. 67 (88%) reported at least one further episode of suicidal ideation or act. Associations were found with depression and aggression but not with social status, age, sex, hopelessness or parental depression. These findings agreed with a previous report that suicide attempters are more likely to be depressed and have poor self-esteem (Smith & Crawford 1986). In addition, differences in the rate of suicide attempts have been noted as dependent on mood state (Kienhorst et al 1990). Thus 3% of youngsters with depressed mood reported attempting suicide for the first time compared with no first-time attempters in the rest of the study population. By contrast, repeated attempters were equally common in the depressed and non-depressed groups.

Studies on hospital populations of adolescent suicide attempters have demonstrated that, although mood disturbance commonly accompanies the attempt, less than half of those with mood symptoms meet the criteria for major depressive disorder (Taylor & Stansfield 1984, Hawton et al 1982).

The presence of dysphoria may increase and maintain the risk for suicidal behaviour in the population at large. Both clinical and community studies indicate, however, that in adolescents major depression is not a prerequisite for suicidal behaviour. In addition, the association between thoughts and acts of suicide in this age group remains unclear.

By contrast, completed suicide appears to be commonly associated with features of major depression according to case-notes or interviews from surviving relatives (Hoberman & Garfinkel 1988, Shaffer 1982, 1986). Such cases appear likely to be comorbid for antisocial and interpersonal aggression.

Violent suicide and self-inflicted injury has increased significantly in recent years (Sellar et al 1990, McClure 1987). This may be accounted for by the increase in male suicides of all ages except under 15. Whether or not behaviour symptoms (in the presence of mood disorder) precede the onset of completed suicides is unclear.

Unlike adolescents, children rarely show suicidal behaviour or completed suicide (Kienhorst et al 1987, Shaffer 1986). Children do know how to kill themselves and by the age of 8 comprehend the permanence of death (Lansdowne & Benjamin 1985). In addition, the prevalence of suicidal ideation appears equally common in depressed children and adolescents (Ryan et al 1987).

The factors that protect children from suicidal behaviour and depression remain unclear. Perhaps greater daily contact with and supervision by parents results in the necessary conversation and support to prevent suicidal tendencies. Other factors, however, such as the stage of moral development of the child and, possibly, a different physiological responsiveness in prepuberty to social adversities, have yet to be investigated.

Prevalence

The epidemiology of depression has been investigated in both community and clinical populations. The prevalence of depressive *symptoms* in the community has ranged from 1% to 10% but few of these subjects meet diagnostic criteria for major depressive disorder (Schoenbach et al 1984, Lefkowitz & Tesing 1985). In normal adolescents there is a significant increase in self-reported depressive symptoms with age. In the Isle of Wight sample there was a fourfold increase in such

feelings between pre- and postpubertal children and a significant difference by gender. In prepubertal children the rates of depressive feelings were approximately equal for males and females, whereas in postpubertal cases rates for females were significantly greater than those for males (Rutter et al 1976a). The symptom characteristics showed that nearly 50% of 14-year-olds reported feelings of misery at direct interview, 20% acknowledged self-denigrating ideas and 7% suicidal ideation (Rutter et al 1976b).

These findings demonstrate the important influence of puberty on rates of depressive symptoms in the general population. The mechanism for this effect remains unclear however. Kandel & Davis (1982) investigated the predictive significance of current depressive symptoms in 8000 13–18-year-olds in upstate New York, using a self-report checklist previously validated on depressed patients of the same age. Nearly 20% of the sample had mean scores equal to or greater than the mean scale score obtained by the depressed group. As with the Isle of Wight study, females above 14 years showed significantly higher mean scale scores than males.

Population studies of depressive disorder in adolescents employing systematic interview procedures are few. Kashani reported a 2% prevalence rate of major depressive disorder in 7–12-year-olds using DSM-III criteria (Kashani & Symonds 1979, Kashani et al 1983). Interviews were carried out by a child psychiatrist with 103 children and their mothers. Half of the children were clinic attenders and the other half were selected from the community. Only two were depressed but a further 18% were sad and reported more somatic complaints, restlessness and low self-esteem. In the Isle of Wight Rutter et al (1976a) found a prevalence of only 0.14% in 10-year-old children.

Cohen et al (1985) carried out independent parent and child diagnostic interviews in 757 families randomly selected from two counties in New York State. Children were 9–18-years old at the time of interview. A diagnosis of depression was not made under the age of 13 in any females and the prevalence derived from both mothers' and children's reports was 1.7%. Prepubertal depression occurred predominantly in males. Age-specific rates of disorder increased steadily among females from 1% at the age of 13 to 7% at the age of 19. A high proportion of this depressed cohort displayed non-affective symptoms, including disturbed behaviour and anxiety.

Kashani and colleagues (Kashani et al 1987) estimated the prevalence of major depression among

150 adolescents, 14–16 years of age, representing 7% of all adolescents attending public schools in Columbia, Missouri. Again using DSM-III diagnoses derived from direct interviews with the child and independently with parents, with the additional judgment that symptoms were sufficiently handicapping to warrant treatment, 4.7% met criteria for current or past major depression and an additional 3.3% met criteria for dysthymic disorder. Ten of the 12 cases were female and, as in the cohort studied by Cohen et al (1985), anxious and behavioural symptoms were frequent concomitants of depression in this small sample. Perhaps the best published study is that of Fleming et al (1989) who, as part of the Ontario Child Health Study, reported on the prevalence of depression in 2852 children and adolescents aged 6–16. This study used a qualitative measure of caseness based on clinical characteristics found at interview; three levels suggest that in the population at large between 0.5% and 2% of children and 2–10% of adolescents suffer major depressive disorder. Sex differences, however, may be different from those of adults. Thus depressive symptoms are more common in adolescent females. However, when caseness is the criterion rather than presence of symptoms alone there are no sex differences in severe cases and in the prepubertal group there may be more males than females. The presence of behavioural and anxiety symptoms may obscure depressive symptoms, particularly in boys and in those children of both sexes where irritability and loss of interest are the predominant presenting mood disorders.

Clinical course and outcome

Recent longitudinal studies have shown that depression in young people may be limited to a single episode but for some, perhaps as many as 30%, the first episode is the beginning of a relapsing disorder present throughout adolescence and a risk factor for depression in adult life (Goodyer et al 1991). Kovacs and colleagues (1988) followed a sample of 104 depressed subjects aged 8–16 years, half of whom had a major depressive disorder at presentation with a mean duration of disorder of 32 weeks. A further 20% had depressive adjustment reactions of a few weeks' duration and the other 30% had a dysthymic condition with a mean duration of 3 years. The median time to recovery of dysthymia was 3–5 years and much the slowest. High rates of recovery were found for the other two diagnoses, with over 90% of major depressives recovered by 9.3 months. Adjustment depressives recovered the quickest (median = 6.2 months). Kovacs & Gatsonis (1989) also studied the likelihood of new episodes of illness in relation to four possible outcomes: 1) a new episode of major depression; 2) a first episode of bipolar disorder; 3) secondary anxiety disorder; and 4) secondary conduct disorder.

Children with major depression or dysthymia had a high probability of a new episode of major depression within 5 years of first presentation. Those with depressive adjustment reactions, on the other hand, showed no such probability. There was also a smaller but significant risk for bipolar disorder and anxiety and conduct disorders in the major depressive groups.

Finally, the influence of comorbidity at presentation was examined for 1) time to recovery and 2) risk of relapse. Comorbid anxiety disorders did not exert a significant influence either on time to recovery or risk of relapse for any depressive group. Comorbid conduct disorder, which was not differentially associated with any kind of depression, did not influence time to recovery but was associated with an increased rate of long-term difficulties. McGee & Williams (1988) followed up a community sample of 40 children depressed at 9 and studied again at the ages of 11 and 13. As well as high rates of depressive symptoms at follow-up when compared with controls, there was some evidence to suggest that boys were more at risk from persistent symptoms with an association between subsequent conduct disorder and original index depression.

These findings demonstrated that the diagnosis of depression showed strong temporal stability and that relapse rates are high, perhaps as much as one in three cases. The significance of comorbidity for risk of relapse clearly requires further investigation.

Bipolar disorder

The diagnosis of mania in children and adolescents extends back at least to Kraepelin, who recognized the condition in about 3% of his patients by the age of 15 (Kraepelin 1921). More recently the lifetime prevalence of mania in a non-referred sample of 14–16-year-olds varied from 0.06% to 13.3% depending on criteria (RDC in the former; DSM-IIIR in the latter) and whether or not severity and duration were included (yes in the former; no in the latter) (Carlson & Kashani 1988). Frank mania or hypomanic psychosis appears very rarely before puberty but it may be more difficult to draw clear distinctions between periods of persistent elated mood and less florid hypomanic states (Carlson 1990).

Recognition of mania in adolescents and older children has been hampered by the strongly held (but unsupported) view that schizophrenia is the more common psychosis in young people. Two large clinical studies, together with numerous case reports, have now confirmed Kraepelin's original observation that bipolar disorder frequently begins in adolescence and young adulthood and the clinical psychopathology is not 'schizophreniform' as often supposed but classically manic (Joyce 1984, Loranger & Levine 1987). It is commonly found that youngsters manifest thought disorder and irritability during a hypomanic episode, suggesting that young people may be particularly predisposed to such symptoms, and that such symptoms may be easily misinterpreted as schizophrenic (Carlson & Strober 1978, Hassanyeh & Davison 1980, Joyce 1984, Hsu & Storgynski 1986).

Coexisting or comorbid symptoms, as in depression, may obscure the diagnosis of hypomania. The most frequently quoted comorbidity is disruptive and/or overactive behaviour rather than anxiety as in depression. The relationships are, however, far from clear as criteria for behaviour disorders and hyperactivity syndromes have changed markedly over time. In a recent review of diagnostic considerations in early onset hypomania, Carlson (1990) concludes that, while a significant history of past behavioural difficulties is found in many cases, further work is required to be confident of coexisting concurrent disorders, particularly in irritable thought disordered cases.

Treatment of hypomania and mania in prepubertal and pubertal cases is similar to treatment in adults, with lithium and neuroleptics reported as beneficial in acute episodes (Varanka et al 1988, Tomasson & Kuperman 1990). Currently, little is known about the long-term outcome of this group of disorders arising in childhood and adolescence. Early onset does not appear however to worsen prognosis (McGlashan 1988).

In adolescents presenting initially with major depression a bipolar course was found to be more likely in those who had delusions and psychomotor retardation during their index depressive episodes (Strober & Carlson 1982, Akiskal et al 1983). Such subjects also had increased rates of bipolar disorder in their families. None of the children was reported as developing schizophrenia, suggesting that schizophrenic and manic-depressive outcomes from depressive episodes in adolescence can be differentiated by careful attention to patterns of premorbid adjustment, family history and social adjustment between episodes (Strober 1989).

Adult outcome

Clinical studies have suggested that depressive disorder in childhood and adolescence increases the risk for poor social adjustment in adult life. Adults with a history of depressive disorder in childhood and adolescence have high rates of marital discord, poor work records and frequent episodes of psychological difficulties (Eastgate & Gilmour 1985, Keller et al 1988). A recent controlled study followed up and compared 80 subjects (at a mean age of 31 years) with a history of a depressive syndrome who had attended a child psychiatry service, with 80 individually matched child patients with non-depressive disorders (Harrington et at 1990). The childhood depression group had a rate of major depressive disorder in adult life several times higher than the group with other psychiatric disorders.

In cases with comorbid conduct disorder the adult outcome showed that adult criminality was as common an outcome in these subjects as in those with conduct disorders alone (Rutter et al 1990). These findings cast doubt on the premise that conduct problems arise as secondary manifestations of depression. These studies also confirm a much worse prognosis for major depression occurring in young people than was previously considered. The evidence suggests that it is cases at risk for relapse during adolescence who may be most at risk for later disorder in adulthood, but this has yet to be systematically investigated.

Neither is it clear if there are clinical characteristics at first presentation which specifically predict further depression or, as appears likely in some cases, serve to increase the risk non-specifically for poor adult social adjustment.

AETIOLOGICAL FACTORS

Family – genetic models

The Yale Family Study of Affective Disorders recently demonstrated that an onset of major depressive disorder before the age of 20 years in probands was associated with a marked increase in familial loading, there being no such loading when the onset was after the age of 40 years (Weissman et al 1984, 1986, Price et al 1987). An eight-fold increase of early onset major depression was demonstrated in the relatives of probands who themselves had an early-onset major depression. The same group also interviewed children in a high-risk family study and showed that the onset of major depression in the offspring of probands with a lifetime history of depression was several years earlier than in the offspring of controls (12–13 years compared with 16–17 years) (Weissman et al 1987). The relative risk of depression arising at or before the age of 15 years was 14.2 in the children of probands with an onset under 20 years compared with controls (Weissman et al 1988).

Uncontrolled studies of the families of depressed children have suggested high rates of affective disorders in first-degree relatives (Livingston et al 1985, Dwyer & Delong 1987). Bipolar disorders have been noted in the offspring and siblings of adult bipolar patients (Akiskal et al 1985). Strober and colleagues (Strober 1989) found a high lifetime prevalence of affective disorder in the mothers of non-bipolar major depressives (25.7/100). In a further controlled study of 50 probands with bipolar/affective disorder, compared with 31 probands with schizophrenia, there was a nearly fourfold increase in the rate of affective disorder in the relatives of bipolar compared with schizophrenic cases. A significant aggregation of bipolar illness in relatives of adolescent manics has also been reported (Strober & Carlson 1982). Major depression and alcoholism have also been shown to be about twice as common in first-degree relatives of depressed children (Puig-Antich et al 1989). The lifetime prevalence of depression in first-degree relatives of adults depressed as children has also been reported as about three times higher than a matched control group (Rutter et al 1990).

Familial loading for major affective disorder appears to be greater in first-degree relatives when the probands have exhibited symptoms before the age of 12 years. In many cases these are not specifically depressive in nature but contain behavioural and hyperactivity symptoms (e.g. Strober et al 1988).

These important findings demonstrate familial associations for affective disorder and suggest greater genetic liability in the offspring of probands. While there are substantive findings showing an increased risk for depression, and other forms of psychopathology, in the children of depressed parents, these do not clearly separate genetic from environmental mediation and there is an urgent need to employ research strategies that do so.

Adverse life experiences

The concept of loss as a psychological cause of depression has been studied extensively in adults but, surprisingly, less often in children and adolescents. Sadness,

crying and irritability were reported by 70% of children (aged 2–17 years, mean 11 years) 1 month after bereavement, but by 13 months depressive symptoms were rare (Van Eerdewegh et al 1982). The proportion of children with subclinical depressive symptoms (14%) was significantly higher, however, than in matched controls (4%).

High levels of psychological symptoms have been found in children of divorced and divorcing parents (Hetherington 1989). Depressed mood and anxiety are commonly reported but so are a wide range of behavioural difficulties. It is not clear how many of these children are suffering from a depressive disorder as such. Furthermore, the degree of psychological difficulty depended on both the antecedent family relations and the postdivorce social and family environment as well as the divorce *per se* (Block et al 1988). This suggests that loss may not of itself be the only causation of disturbance.

Exit events occur more commonly in behavioural and mood disorders in child and adolescent psychiatric cases than in controls and may be more frequent in depressive conditions (Goodyer et al 1985). The association appears far from all-embracing and depressive cases within this age group also occur without such exits. The current position suggests that loss and separation events are associated with increases in anxious and depressive symptoms but that only some children develop major depressive disorders. Other social factors may ameliorate or amplify the effects of loss over the ensuing 12 months. It remains a matter for further research to determine which children are most at risk for major depression following divorce. Such losses and separations appear to exert latent effects for later adult depressive disorder through their impact on subsequent parental care (Bifulco et al 1987).

Some of the children may have been depressed, however, and contributed, through their psychiatric disorder, to consequent difficulties in subsequent interpersonal relations.

Cross-sectional case-control studies have established a potentially causal association between recent adverse life experiences rated for undesirability and the onset of anxious or depressive disorders in 8–16-year-olds (Goodyer et al 1985, 1988). Life events occurring prior to the onset of disorder and carrying a moderate to severe degree of undesirability occur in some 50% of major depressive disorders and carry a direct risk for the onset of depression even in the presence of other environmental risk factors. Recent life events combine in many cases with other more persistent family and social adversities, and it is the patterning and configuration of these factors that determine the magnitude of risk and mechanism of effects. For example, the combination of maternal distress, poor confiding relations in mother's own life and undesirable life events focused on the child increases the risk of affective disorder for children some one hundredfold. (Goodyer et al 1988).

Friendship difficulties in the 12 months prior to the onset of disorder are also associated with the onset of depression and anxiety (Goodyer et al 1989). Unlike undesirable life events and family adversities, friendship difficulties vary with pubertal status in their effect on the form of disorder. Thus in prepubertal children friendship difficulties are equally likely to be associated with anxiety and depression whereas, in postpubertal children, friendship difficulties are twice as likely to occur in anxiety than in depression. Perhaps adolescents are more resilient or participate more frequently in friendship change and are less prone to profound loss or disappointment from these relationships. The role of non-familial close relationships as a risk factor for affective disorder in young people requires further investigation.

Events, family adversities and friendship difficulties all exert direct provoking effects on the risk for depression and anxiety disorder. Unlike the findings of adult studies, there appear to be no specifically stress-buffering vulnerability factors within these recent social adversities. The absence of recent social achievements (such as no scholastic, social, community or sporting activities that have brought social recognition regardless of the level of success) within the same time frame as other life experiences, has been found to exert an increased risk for depression and anxiety in the presence of friendship difficulties but not in the presence of undesirable life events (Goodyer et al 1990). This indirect risk factor acts as a specific 'enhancer' to the likelihood of disorder but only within the social (non-familial) dimension of adverse life experiences. This preliminary evidence suggests relatively independent pathways of effect for adverse family and social experiences.

However, none of these social mechanisms specifically predicts major depressive disorder. Indeed, anxiety disorders appear equally likely and some 10% of both anxiety and depressive disorders occur with no recent social adversities in the year prior to the onset of disorder. The specificity between life adversities and comorbid psychopathology remains uncertain and the contribution of these social factors to the form of symptomatology requires clarification. Current evidence would suggest that recent life adversities are neither necessary nor sufficient to explain all forms of depressive disorder. They are likely, however, to occur in some 90% of cases. The role of personal dispositions such as pubertal development or temperament differences on the impact of adverse life experiences requires urgent investigation (Goodyer 1990). In addition, a greater use of life-history methods is needed to investigate the impact of life experiences at greater distances in time than the 12 months prior to onset.

Psychological factors

Classical psychoanalytical models of depression have undergone little modification in recent years and are similar in explanation for children, adolescents and adults. Central themes in theory are the child's identification with parents and their values and the development of adequate internalized objects. Depression may arise when parents fail to fulfil necessary psychological functions towards the child, resulting in disappointment and an internal conflict in the child between 'real' and 'ideal' parent figures (Mendelson 1982). The child may feel 'unacceptable' degrees of anger and hostility towards the parent, with resultant blaming of the self rather than the parent. Self-blame, guilt and criticism arise as a consequence. These dynamic factors may express themselves cognitively, such as in the ways children perceive and value themselves as persons (Harter 1986). Clinical depression may arise if repeated patterns of disappointment with parent figures occur in early life. An unmet need for affection may result in personally directed aggression and a persistent need for gratification and comfort.

There is clearly an important need to investigate the psychological components of the self-system which have significant implications for personality, socioemotional development and psychopathology (Harter 1983, 1986, Rutter 1987). Recent advances in the methodology for investigating the impact of maternal psychopathology on infant development may result in a clearer elucidation of some of the processes associated with early cognitive development and later self-esteem (Murray 1988). At present, the specific role of these psychoanalytical mechanisms for depression in school-age children is unclear.

Learning theory models derived from adult studies have also been proposed and have led to a cognitive behavioural model of depression in which symptoms are considered to result from deficits in interaction with the current environment and to determine the individual's negative appraisal and perception of himself in relation to others (Kendall & Bronswell 1984, Clorizio 1985). A number of theoretical models have been described, depending on the emphasis of the author. Social or life-skills deficits and family interaction deficits have been proposed as causal for depression through a loss of positive reinforcement and/or the presence of resentment or rejection by others (Mills et al 1985, Hops et al 1987). Systematic errors in thinking have been suggested which result in a misinterpretation of events and a predisposition to thoughts of helplessness or hopelessness, leading to depression (Teasdale & Dent 1987, Abramson et al 1989). Specific deficits in problem-solving skills, where individuals lack the ability to generate adaptive alternative solutions to here-and-now problems (Neyil & Ronan 1985) and may also lack self-regulatory control cognitions required to protect the self against unexpected and undesirable events such as may be seen in certain forms of denial at times of parental conflict (Smith & Rossman 1986), have also been suggested as aetiological models.

Currently, there is evidence to indicate that depressed children may show a negative bias in thinking and demonstrate aspects of learned helplessness and hopelessness and social skills deficits (Kazdin 1990). Whether such deficits are causes, concomitants or consequences of depression remains unclear. Overall the findings suggest that a specific association between any one cognitive–behavioural psychological mechanism and depression is unlikely. The indications are more encouraging, however, that a cognitive – behavioural approach in treatment may prove of value in some episodes of major depressive disorder in young people (Kendell & Bronswell 1984).

Biochemical factors

Abnormalities in hypothalamo—pituitary axis activity have been demonstrated in major depressive disorder in both children and adolescents (Foreman & Goodyer 1988, Puig-Antich et al 1989). Both resistance to the negative feedback effects of dexamethasone and increased episodes of cortisol hypersecretion during the circadian cycle have been documented. The dexamethasone suppression test shows similar abnormalities to adult studies, with some 45% of cases being non-suppressors (Doherty et al 1986, Foreman & Goodyer 1988, Pfeffer et al 1989). Non-suppression and hypersecretion do not always occur together, suggesting that they may represent different abnormalities of

the cortisol control system. In addition, a substantial proportion of major depressive disorders show no alteration in cortisol activity, particularly the prepubertal cases (Puig-Antich et al 1989, Dahl et al 1989).

Current evidence suggests that these cortisol changes recover with clinical recovery but may be associated with a risk of relapse (Puig-Antich et al 1989). The implications of dexamethasone non-suppression and circadian dysregulation for treatment and risk of relapse will not be clarified until longitudinal studies have been undertaken.

Recent advances in knowledge of the structure and function of steroid receptors will help clarify the mechanisms of cortisol activity in subgroups of depressive disorder (Gustaffson et al 1987). It has been established that glucocorticoids can downregulate receptor activity, though the mechanism is not fully understood. They may act directly on the expression of the receptor gene, although alterations in the receptor mRNA stability may also play a part (Gustaffson et al 1987). A recent important finding is that genetic mutants of glucocorticoid receptors have been described that bind steroid but activate suboptimally (Gustaffson et al 1987). These advances in molecular and cell biology of glucocorticoid activity suggest potential genomic differences in responsivity to circulating glucocorticoids.

Recent research in adults has focused on alterations in lymphocytic response to corticoids, demonstrating impairments of immune function that may accompany depression and whether or not these are a result of increased cortisol production or associated with dexamethasone nonsuppression (Murphy et al 1987, Lowy et al 1988, Cosyns et al 1989). Similar studies in young people are sparse, although preliminary evidence suggests that further research would be of interest, particularly if differences in lymphocyte responsivity were found between pre- and postpubertal depressives (Targum et al 1990). As yet no studies have reported as to whether or not genomic differences exist in the lymphocytes of children with or without cortisol hypersecretion during a depressive episode.

As in adult depressives, indirect studies of neurotransmitter function have been carried out. Puig-Antich and colleagues have documented blunting of growth hormone release in response to insulin induced hypoglycaemia in prepubertal children with major depressive disorder with endogenous symptoms, but no such response in depressed patients without endogenous symptoms (Puig-Antich et al 1981, 1984). These findings suggest that neurotransmitters responsible for growth hormone secretion are impaired during an episode of 'endogenous' depression.

Nocturnal secretion of growth hormone release has been studied in a few patients and the data remain sketchy (Puig-Antich 1986). Current evidence does not allow for any firm conclusions concerning the activity of growth hormone as a marker of neurotransmitter dysfunction either as a cause or a concomitant factor of depressive disorder.

Disturbances of cholinergic mechanisms have also been postulated to account for polysomnographic abnormalities found in adults who have recovered from a major depressive episode and were drug free at the time of investigation (Rush et al 1986). In many patients, however, abnormalities present during disorder normalize on recovery (Gillin et al 1984). In neither children nor adolescents have any abnormalities been found on sleep EEG recordings during an episode of depression (Puig-Antich et al 1982, Young et al 1982, Goetz et al 1986). It would appear that the characteristic alterations in polysomnographic measures found during depressive episodes in adults are absent in prepubertal and adolescent patients.

It has been suggested that it is with recurrent episodes of depression that individuals develop a propensity for biological dysregulation coupled with lower thresholds for the precipitation of new episodes (Post et al 1986). It may be that in childhood and adolescence the incidence of depression is higher than in adults and these 'first-episode' depressive disorders are less likely to contain altered biological responsivity compared to adult disorders which contain higher prevalence rates but may have lower incidence. Comparing the monoamine activity between new-onset and recurrent cases of depression at all ages and conducting longitudinal studies on early-onset depressive disorders incorporating serial measures of monoamine activity would considerably help to unravel the evolution of pathophysiology in affective disorders.

TREATMENT

Pharmacotherapy

There are no published reports of adequately controlled trials of antidepressants in childhood or adolescent depression. The studies to date have used small sample sizes and suffered from a range of methodological problems such as poor definition of cases, use of non-blind ratings and non-random assignment of children to groups. Recently two studies have been reported, one using imipramine and placebo and the other nortriptyline and placebo, with conflicting results. Preskorn and colleagues (Preskorn et al 1987) reported that 80% of prepubertal patients had symptomatic improvement at 3 weeks on imipramine compared with controls. They suggested a therapeutic window effect, with optimal response occurring with serum desipramine levels between 125 and 250 µg/ml. Below these levels there were no therapeutic effects whereas above them the response rate fell and signs of toxicity occurred. Being a dexamethasone non-suppressor also predicted response to antidepressants rather than placebo and (in the case of hospitalized adolescent patients) non-suppressors appeared to be more likely to respond to a combination of antidepressants and psychological treatment rather than psychosocial treatment alone (Robbins et al 1989). In the latter study melancholic subtype also predicted a better response to antidepressants, although a third of non-melancholic depressives were also rated as responders to pharmacotherapy. By contrast, Ryan et al (1986) showed no significant difference between imipramine and placebo in adolescents and Geller and colleagues (1989) reported similar negative findings for nortriptyline versus placebo.

Clinical reports have suggested that monoamine oxidase inhibitors may produce improvement in cases previously refractory to tricyclic antidepressants (Ryan et al 1986).

The contradictory findings concerning the efficacy of antidepressants in both children and adolescents may be clarified by subgrouping patients by cortisol activity and depressive symptoms rather than by symptoms alone. Other factors such as a family history of affective disorder may also be useful as potential predictors of response to pharmacotherapy in future research.

Psychological treatments

There are no adequately controlled studies of psychological treatment in young persons. A number of reports have been published which indicate that active brief treatments focusing on improving problem-solving, cognitive restructuring and social skills training significantly alleviate symptoms compared with no-treatment controls (Kazdin 1990). These studies have used a variety of methods and procedures, often with small numbers of subjects and varying methods of analysis. Overall they indicate the likelihood that brief focused psychological treatments are useful, but systematic evaluation is required. Recommendations for psychodynamic psychotherapy have also been made on theoretical and clinical descriptive grounds (e.g. Block-Lewis 1986). The current work (including selection of cases, randomized assignment and adequate measures of outcome) lags behind that of psychopharmacological studies.

CURRENT ISSUES AND FUTURE PROSPECTS

The psychopathology of childhood depression increasingly indicates the co-occurrence of another disorder in as many as 50% of cases (Anderson et al 1987, Fleming et al 1989), yet the meaning of this comorbidity is uncertain. Are anxiety disorders an evolutionary phase in a depressive condition? Is there a sub-group of depressed conduct disorders? The presence of comorbidity must be taken into account in future studies investigating cause, natural history and outcome of depressive disorders.

There is a dearth of information on treatment approaches to childhood depression. Pharmacotherapy studies need to consider patient selection on criteria other than descriptive psychopathology. The possibility that dexamethasone non-suppressors may be drug-responders requires further investigation. The absence of psychological treatment studies invites a wide-ranging series of approaches to this area. Such studies should include school-based treatments, already known to be effective for maladjusted and behaviourally disturbed children. Schools may be preferable environments for treatment: personal existing relationships with teachers can be utilized, as can school, health professionals and existing peer-group relations. An environmental 'status quo' for children can be maintained, avoiding the introduction of a novel environment such as a clinic.

Further research in causal theory is required. Recent social adversities are important but insufficient as an explanation of depression (Goodyer 1990). Early life experiences, such as the quality of attachment and relations with siblings, and personal qualities, such as temperamental attributes, need to be incorporated in future studies, which would also benefit from a longitudinal perspective. Family genetic studies, including twin and fostering and adoption designs, are required to investigate the genetic predisposition to these disorders (Rutter et al 1990). The possible implications of childhood depression for adult adjustment indicate the value of identifying a cohort for longitudinal study into adult life to elucidate the natural history of the disorder. No single study will encompass all aetiological questions, and a range of studies with differing methods and procedures is required to address the current outstanding questions.

REFERENCES

Abramson L Y, Metalsky G I, Alloy L B 1989 Hopelessness and depression: a theory based sub-type of depression. Psychological Review 96: 358–372

Achenbach T M, McConaughy S H, Howell C T 1987 Child/adolescent behavioural and emotional problems: implications of cross-informant correlations for situational specificity. Psychological Bulletin 101: 213–232

Akiskal H S, Walker P, Puyantian V R, King D, Rosenthal T L, Dranon M 1983 Bipolar outcome in the course of depressive illness: phenomenologic, familial and pharmacologic predictors. Journal of Affective Disorders 5: 115–128

Akiskal H S, Downs J, Jordan P, Watson S, Daugherty D, Pruitt D B 1985 Affective disorders in referred children and younger siblings of manic depressives: mode of onset and prospective course. Archives of General Psychiatry 42: 996–1003

Altmann E O, Gotlieb I H 1988 The social behaviour of depressed children: an observational study. Journal of Abnormal Child Psychology 16: 19–44

Anderson J C, Williams S, McGee R, Silva P A 1987. The prevalence of DSM-III disorders in pre-adolescent children: prevalence in a large sample from the general population. Archives of General Psychiatry 44: 69–76

Angold A 1988a Childhood and adolescent depression: 1. Epidemiological and aetiological aspects. British Journal of Psychiatry 152: 601–617

Angold A 1988b Childhood and adolescent depression: II. Research in clinical populations. British Journal of Psychiatry 153: 476–492

Bifulco A, Brown G W, Harris T 1987 Childhood loss of parent, lack of adequate parental care and adult depression: a replication. Journal of Affective Disorders 12: 115–118

Birleson P 1981 The validity of depressive disorder in childhood and the development of a self-rating scale: a research project. Journal of Child Psychology and Psychiatry 22: 73–88

Block J, Block H, Gherde P F 1988 Parental functioning and home environment in families of divorce: prospective and current analyses. Journal of the American Academy of Child and Adolescent Psychiatry 27: 207–213

Block-Lewis H 1986 The role of shame in depression. In: Rutter M, Izard C E, Read P B (eds) Depression in young people: developmental and clinical perspectives. Guilford Press, New York, p 325–339

Carlson G A 1990 Child and adolescent mania – diagnostic considerations. Journal of Child Psychology and Psychiatry 31: 331–341

Carlson G A, Kashani J H 1988 Manic symptoms in a non-referred adolescent population. Journal of Affective Disorders 15: 219–226

Carlson G A, Strober M 1978 Manic depressive illness in early adolescence: a study of the clinical and diagnostic characteristics in 6 cases. Journal of the American Academy of Child Psychiatry 17: 138–153

Chambers W, Puig-Antich J, Hirsch M et al 1985 The assessment of affective disorders in children and adolescents by semi-structured interview. Test-retest reliability of the K-SADS-P. Archives of General Psychiatry 24: 696–702

Clorizio H F 1985 Cognitive-behavioural treatment of childhood depression. Psychology in Schools 22: 308–322

Cohen P, Velez C N, Garcia M 1985 The epidemiology of childhood depression. Presented at the annual meeting of the American Academy of Child Psychiatry, San Antonio, TX

Costello E J, Angold A 1988 Scales to assess child and adolescent depression: checklists, screens and nets. Journal of the American Academy of Child and Adolescent Psychiatry 27: 726–738

Costello E J, Edelbrock C, Costello A J 1985 The validity of NIMH Diagnostic Interview Schedule for Children: a comparison between paediatric and psychiatric referrals. Journal of Abnormal Child Psychology 13: 579–593

Cosyns P, Maes M, Vandewoude M, Stevens W J, De Clerck L S, Schotte C 1989 Impaired mitogen-induced lymphocyte responses and the hypothalamic pituitary adrenal axis in depressive disorders. Journal of Affective Disorders 16: 41–48

Dahl R, Puig-Antich J, Ryan N et al 1989 Cortisol secretion in adolescents with major depressive disorders. Acta Psychiatrica Scandinavica 80: 18–26

Doherty M B, Madonsky D, Kraft J, Carter-Ake L L, Rosenthal P A, Coughlin B F 1986 Cortisol dynamics and test performance of the dexamethasone suppression test in 97 psychiatrically hospitalized children aged 3–16 years. Journal of the American Academy of Child Psychiatry 25: 400–408

Dwyer J T, Delong G R 1987 A family history study of 20 probands with childhood manic-depressive illness. Journal of the American Academy of Child and Adolescent Psychiatry 26: 176–180

Eastgate J, Gilmour L 1985 Long term outcome of depressed children: a follow up study. Developmental Medicine and Child Neurology 26: 68–72

Edelbrock C S, Costello A J, Dulcan M K, Conover N C, Kalas R 1986 Parent-child agreement on child psychiatric symptoms assessed via structured interview. Journal of Child Psychology and Psychiatry 27: 181–190

Emde R N, Harmon R J, Good W 1986 Depressive feelings in children: a transactional model for research. In: Rutter M, Izard C E, Read P B (eds) Depression in young people. Guilford Press, New York, p 135–162

Finch A J, Jn, Saylor C F, Edwards G L 1985 Children's Depression Inventory: sex and grade norms for normal children. Journal of Consulting and Clinical Psychology 53: 424–425

Fleming J E, Offord D R, Boyle M H 1989 Prevalence of childhood and adolescent depression in the community – Ontario Child Health Study. British Journal of Psychiatry 155: 647–654

Foreman D, Goodyer I M 1988 Cortisol hypersecretion in juvenile depression. Journal of Child Psychology and Psychiatry 29: 311–320

Geller B, Cooper J, McCombs H G, Graham D, Wells J 1989 Double-blind, placebo-controlled study of Nortriptyline in depressed children using a 'fixed plasma level' design. Psychopharmacology Bulletin 25: 101–108

Gillin J C, Sitoram N, Wehr, T et al 1984 Sleep and affective illness. In: Post R M, Ballenger J C (eds) Neurobiology of mood disorders. Williams & Wilkins, Baltimore, MD, p 157–189

Goetz R R, Puig-Antich J, Ryan N D et al 1986 Electroencephalographic sleep of adolescents with major depression and normal controls. Archives of General Psychiatry 44: 61–68

Goodyer I M 1990 Life experiences, development and childhood psychopathology. John Wiley, Chichester

Goodyer I M, Kolvin I, Gatzanis S 1985 Recent undesirable life events and psychiatric disorder in childhood and adolescence. British Journal of Psychiatry 147: 517–523

Goodyer I M, Wright C, Altham P M E 1988 Maternal adversity and recent stressful life events in anxious and depressed children. Journal of Child Psychology and Psychiatry 29: 651–667

Goodyer I M, Wright C, Altham P M E 1989 Recent friendships in anxious and depressed school-age children. Psychological Medicine 19: 165–174

Goodyer I M, Altham P M E, Wright C 1990 Recent adversities and achievements in anxious and depressed school-age children. Journal of Child Psychology and Psychiatry 31: 1063–1077

Goodyer I M, Germany E, Gowrusanker J, Altham P M E 1991 Social influences on the course of anxious and depressive disorders in school – age children. British Journal of Psychiatry 158: 676–684

Gustaffson J A, Carlstedt-Duke J, Poellinger L et al 1987 Biochemistry, molecular biology and physiology of the glucocorticoid receptor. Endocrine Reviews 8: 184–234

Gutterman E M, O'Brien J, Young D 1987 Structured diagnostic interviews for children and adolescents: current status and future directions. Journal of the American Academy of Child and Adolescent Psychiatry 26: 621–631

Haley G, Fine S, Marriage M, Moretti M, Freeman R 1985 Cognitive bias and depression in psychiatrically disturbed children and adolescents. Journal of Consulting and Clinical Psychology 53: 535–537

Harrington R C, Fudge H, Rutter M, Pickles A, Hill J 1990 Adult outcome of childhood and adolescent depression. I. Psychiatric status. Archives of General Psychiatry 47: 465–473

Harter S 1983 Developmental perspectives on the self system. In: Mussen P, Hetherington E M (eds) Handbook of child psychology, vol 4. Social and personality development. John Wiley, New York

Harter S 1986 Cognitive developmental processes in the integration of concepts about emotions and the self. Social Cognition 4: 119–151

Hassanyeh F, Davison K 1980 Bipolar affective psychosis with onset before age 16. Report of 10 cases. British Journal of Psychiatry 137: 530–539

Hawton K, O'Grady J, Osborn M 1982 Adolescents who take overdoses: their characteristics, problems and contacts with helping agencies. British Journal of Psychiatry 140: 118–123

Herjanic B, Reich W 1982 Development of a structured psychiatric interview for children: agreement between child and parent on individual symptoms. Journal of Abnormal Child Psychology 10: 307–324

Hershberg S G, Carlson G A, Cantwell D P, Strober M 1982 Anxiety and depressive disorders in psychiatrically disturbed children. Journal of Clinical Psychiatry 43: 358–361

Hetherington E M 1989 Coping with family transitions: winners, losers and survivors. Child Development 60: 1–14

Hoberman H, Garfinkel B 1988 Completed suicide in children and adolescents. Journal of the American Academy of Child and Adolescent Psychiatry 27: 689–695

Hops H, Biglan A, Sherman L, Arthur J, Friedman L, Osteen V 1987 Home observations of family interactions of depressed women. Journal of Consulting and Clinical Psychology 55: 341–346

Hsu L K G, Storgynski M S W 1986 Mania in adolescence. Journal of Clinical Psychiatry 47: 596–599

Ivens C, Rehn L P 1988 Assessment of childhood depression: correspondence between reports by child, mother and father. Journal of the American Academy of Child and Adolescent Psychiatry 27: 738–741

Joyce P R 1984 Age of onset of bi-polar affective disorder and misdiagnosis as schizophrenia. Psychological Medicine 14: 145–149

Kandel D B, Davis M 1982 The epidemiology of depressed mood in adolescents: An empirical study. Archives of General Psychiatry 39: 1205–1212

Kashani J H, Simonds J F 1979 The incidence of depression in children. American Journal of Psychiatry 136: 1203–1205

Kashani J H, McGee R O, Clarkson S E et al 1983 Depression in a sample of 9-year-old children. Archives of General Psychiatry 40: 1217–1223

Kashani J H, Carlson G A, Beck N C et al 1987. Psychiatric disorders in a community sample of adolescents. American Journal of Psychiatry 144: 584–589

Kazdin A E 1989 Identifying depression in children: a comparison of alternative selection criteria. Journal of Abnormal Child Psychology 17: 437–455

Kazdin A E 1990 Childhood depression. Journal of Child Psychology and Psychiatry 31: 121–160

Kazdin A E, French N H, Uris A S, Esveldt-Dawson K, Sherick R B 1983 Hopelessness, depression and suicidal intent among psychiatrically disturbed inpatient children. Journal of Consulting and Clinical Psychology 51: 504–510

Kazdin A E, Esveldt-Dawson K, Sherick R B, Colbus D 1985a Assessment of overt behaviour and childhood depression among psychiatrically disturbed children. Journal of Consulting and Clinical Psychology 53: 201–210

Kazdin A E, Sherick R B, Esveldt-Dawson K, Ranasello M D 1985b Non-verbal behaviour and childhood depression. Journal of the American Academy of Child Psychiatry 24: 303–309

Keller M, Beardslee W, Lavori P, Wunder J, Drs L D, Samuelson H 1988 Course of major depression in non-referred adolescents: a retrospective study. Journal of Affective Disorders 15: 235–243

Kendall P, Bronswell P 1984 Cognitive behavioural therapy of impulsive children. Guilford Press, New York.

Kienhorst C W M, Wolters W H G, Diekstra R F W, Otle E 1987 A study of the frequency of suicidal behaviour in children aged 5 to 14. Journal of Child Psychology and Psychiatry 28: 153–166

Kienhorst C W M, DeWilde E J, Van Den Bout J, Diekstra R F W, Wolters W H G 1990 Characteristics of suicide attempters in a population-based sample of Dutch adolescents. British Journal of Psychiatry 156: 243–248

Kovacs M 1981 Rating scales to assess depression in school age children. Acta Paedopsychiatrica 46: 305–315

Kovacs M 1986 A developmental perspective on methods and measures in the assessment of depressive disorders: The clinical interview. In: Rutter M, Izard C E, Read P B (eds) Depression in young people. Guilford Press, New York, p 435–465

Kovacs M, Gatsonis C 1989 Stability and change in childhood onset depressive disorders: longitudinal course as a diagnostic validator. In: Robbins L N, Barrett J E (eds) The validity of psychiatric diagnosis. Raven Press, New York, p 57–73

Kovacs M, Feinberg T L, Crouse-Novak M A, Paulauskas S L, Finkelstein R 1984 Depressive disorders in childhood: 1. A longitudinal prospective study of characteristics and recovery. Archives of General Psychiatry 41: 229–237

Kovacs M, Paulauskas S, Gatsonis C, Richards C 1988 Depressive disorders in childhood: III. A longitudinal study of comorbidity with and risk for conduct disorders. Journal of Affective Disorders 13: 205–217

Kovacs M, Gatsonis C, Paulauskas S, Richards C 1989 Depressive disorders in childhood: IV. A longitudinal study of comorbidity and risk for anxiety disorders. Archives of General Psychiatry 46: 776–782

Kraepelin E 1921 Manic depressive insanity and paranoia. E. & S. Livingstone Edinburgh

Lansdowne R, Benjamin G 1985 The development of the concept of death in children aged 5–90 years. Child Care, Health and Development 11: 13–20

Lefkowitz M M, Tesing E P 1985 Depression in children: prevalence and correlates. Journal of Consulting and Clinical Psychology 53: 647–656

Livingston R, Nugent H, Roder L, Smith G R 1985 Family histories of depressed and severely anxious children. American Journal of Psychiatry 142: 1497–1499

Loranger A P W, Levine P M 1978 Age of onset of bi-polar affective illness. Archives of General Psychiatry 35: 1345–1348

Lowy M, Reder A, Gormley G, Meltzer H 1988 Comparison of in vivo and in vitro glucocorticoid sensitivity in depression: relationship to the dexamethasone suppression test. Biological Psychiatry 24: 619–630

McClure G M G 1987 Suicide in England and Wales, 1975–1984. British Journal of Psychiatry 150: 309–314

McGee R, Williams S 1988 A longitudinal study of depression in 9 year old children. Journal of the American Academy of Child and Adolescent Psychiatry 3: 342–348

McGlashan T H 1988 Adolescent versus adult onset of mania. American Journal of Psychiatry 145: 221–224

Mendelson M 1982 Psychodynamics of depression. In: Paykel

E (ed) Handbook of affective disorders. Churchill Livingstone, Edinburgh

Mills M, Puckering C, Pound A, Cox A 1985 What is it about depressed mothers that influences their children's functioning. In: Stevenson J (ed) Recent advances in developmental psychopathology. Pergamon Press, Oxford

Mitchell J, McCauley E, Burke P M, Moss S J 1988 Phenomenology of depression in children and adolescents. Journal of the American Academy of Child and Adolescent Psychiatry 27: 342–348

Murphy D, Gardner R, Greden J F, Carroll B 1987 Lymphocyte numbers in endogenous depression. Psychological Medicine 17: 381–385

Murray L 1988 Effects of post-natal depression on infant development: direct studies of early mother-infant interactions. In Kumar R, Brockington I F (eds) Motherhood and mental illness. John Wright, London

Neyil A M, Ronan G F 1985 Life stress, current problems, problem solving and depressive symptoms: an integrative model. Journal of Consulting and Clinical Psychology 53: 693–697

Pfeffer C R, Lipkins R, Plutchik R, Mizruchi M 1988 Normal children at risk for suicidal behaviour: A 2-year follow-up study. Journal of the American Academy of Child & Adolescent Psychiatry 27: 34–41

Pfeffer C, Stokes P, Weiner A et al 1989 Psychopathology and plasma cortisol responses to dexamethasone in prepubertal psychiatric inpatients. Biological Psychiatry 26: 677–689

Post R M, Rulinow D R, Ballanger J C 1986 Conditioning and sensitization in the longitudinal course of affective illness. British Journal of Psychiatry 149: 191–201

Poznanski E O, Grossman J A, Buchsbaum Y, Boregas M, Freeman L, Gibbons R 1984 Preliminary studies of the reliability and validity of the Children's Depression Rating Scale. Journal of the American Academy of Child Psychiatry 23: 191–197

Preskorn S, Weller E B, Hughes C W, Weller R, Bolte K 1987 Depression in prepubertal children: dexamethasone non-suppression predicts differential response to imipramine vs placebo. Psychopharmacology Bulletin 23: 128–133

Price R A, Kidd K K, Weissman M M 1987 Early onset (under age 30 years) and panic disorder as markers for etiologic homogeneity in major depression. Archives of General Psychiatry 44: 434–440

Puig-Antich J 1986 Psychobiological markers: effect of age and puberty. In: Rutter M, Izard C E, Read P B (eds) Depression in young people: developmental and clinical perspectives. Guilford Press, New York, p 341–348

Puig-Antich J, Tabrizi M A, Davies M, Chambers W, Halpern F, Sachar E J 1981 Prepubertal endogenous major depressives hypersecrete growth hormone in response to insulin-induced hypoglycaemia. Biological Psychiatry 16: 801–818

Puig-Antich J, Goetz R, Hanlon C, Tabrizi M A, Davies M, Weitzman E D 1982 Sleep architecture and REM sleep measures in prepubertal major depressives during an episode. Archives of General Psychiatry 39: 932–939

Puig-Antich J, Davies M, Novacenko H et al 1984 Growth hormone secretion in prepubertal major depressive children III. Response to insulin induced hypoglycaemia in a drug-free, fully recovered clinical state. Archives of General Psychiatry 41: 471–475

Puig-Antich J, Goetz D, Davies M et al 1989 A controlled family history study of prepubertal major depressive disorder. Archives of General Psychiatry 46: 406–418

Richters J, Pellegrini D 1989 Depressed mothers' judgements about their children: an examination of the depression-distortion hypothesis. Child Development 60: 1068–1075

Robbins D R, Alessi N E, Colfer M V 1989 Treatment of adolescents with major depression: implications of the DST and the melancholic clinical sub-type. Journal of Affective Disorders 17: 99–104

Rotundo N, Hensley V R C 1985 The children's depression scale, a case study of its validity. Journal of Child Psychology and Psychiatry 26: 917–927

Rush A J, Erman M K, Giles D E et al 1986 Polysomnographic findings in recently drug free and clinically remitted depressed patients. Archives of General Psychiatry 43: 878–884

Rutter M 1986 The developmental psychopathology of depression: issues and perspectives. In: Rutter M, Izard C E, Read P B (eds) Depression in young people: developmental and clinical perspectives. Guilford Press, New York, p 3–30

Rutter M 1987 The role of cognition in child development and disorder. British Journal of Medical Psychology 60: 1–16

Rutter M, Tizard J, Yale W, Graham P, Whitmore K 1976a Isle of Wight Studies 1964–1974. Psychological Medicine 6: 313–332

Rutter M, Graham P, Chadwick O F D, Yule W 1976b Adolescent turmoil: fact or fiction. Journal of Child Psychology and Psychiatry 17: 35–56

Rutter M, Bolton P, Harrington R, Le Couteur H, Macdonald H, Simonoff E 1990 Genetic factors in child psychiatric disorders – II. Empirical findings. Journal of Child Psychology and Psychiatry 31: 39–84

Ryan N D, Puig-Antich J, Cooper T et al 1986 Imipramine in adolescent major depression: plasma level and clinical responses. Acta Psychiatrica Scandanavica 73: 273–288

Ryan N D, Puig-Antich J, Ambrosini P et al 1987 The clinical picture of major depression in children and adolescents. Archives of General Psychiatry 44: 854–861

Schoenbach V J, Garrison C Z, Kaplan B H 1984 Epidemiology of adolescent depression. Public Health Review 12: 159–189

Sellar C, Hawton K, Goldacre M 1990 Self-poisoning in adolescents: Hospital admissions and deaths in the Oxford Region 1980–1983. British Journal of Psychiatry 156: 866–870

Shaffer D 1982 Diagnostic issues in child and adolescent suicide. Journal of the American Academy of Child Psychiatry 21: 414–416

Shaffer D 1986 Developmental factors in adolescent suicide. In: Rutter M, Izard C, Read P B (eds) Depression in young people: developmental and clinical aspects. Guilford, New York, p 383–396

Smith K, Crawford S 1986 Suicidal behaviour among 'normal' high school students. Suicide and Life threatening Behaviour 16: 313–325

Smith W, Rossman R B 1986 Developmental changes in trait and situational denial under stress during childhood. Journal of Child Psychology and Psychiatry 27: 227–235

Strober M 1989 Affective disorders. In Hsu L K, Hersen M

(eds) Recent developments in adolescent psychiatry. John Wiley, New York, p 201–233

Strober M, Carlson G 1982 Bipolar illness in adolescents: clinical, genetic and pharmacologic predictors in a 3 to 4 year prospective follow-up. Archives of General Psychiatry 39: 549–555

Strober M, Morrell W, Burroughs J, Lampert C, Danforth H, Freeman R 1988 A family study of bipolar disorder in adolescence: early onset of symptoms linked to increased familial loading and lithium resistance. Journal of Affective Disorders 15: 255–268

Targum S D, Clarkson L L, Mague-Harris K, Marshall L E, Skwerer R G 1990 Measurement of cortisol and lymphocyte subpopulations in depressed and conduct disordered adolescents. Journal of Affective Disorders 18: 91–96

Taylor E A, Stansfield S A 1984 Children who poison themselves: 1. A clinical comparison with psychiatric controls. British Journal of Psychiatry 143: 127–135

Teasdale J, Dent J 1987 Cognitive vulnerability to depression: an investigation of two hypotheses. British Journal of Clinical Psychology 26: 113–126

Tesing E P, Lefkowitz M M 1982 Childhood depression: a 6 month follow up study. Journal of Consulting and Clinical Psychology 50: 778–780

Tesing E P, Lefkowitz M M, Gordon M H 1980 Childhood depression, locus of control and school achievement. Journal of Educational Psychology 72: 506–510

Tomasson K, Kuperman S 1990 Bipolar disorder in a prepubescent child. Journal of the American Academy of Child and Adolescent Psychiatry 29: 308–310

Van Eerdewegh J, Bieri M, Parilla R, Clayton P 1982 The bereaved child. British Journal of Psychiatry 140: 23–29

Varanka T M, Weller R A, Weller E B, Fristad M A 1988 Lithium treatment of manic episodes with psychotic features in prepubertal children. American Journal of Psychiatry 145: 1557–1559

Weissman M M, Leckman J F, Merikongas K R, Gammon D, Prusoff B A 1984 Depression and anxiety disorders in parents and children: results from the Yale Family Study. Archives of General Psychiatry 41: 845–852

Weissman M M, Merikanges K R, Wickmoratne P et al 1986 Understanding clinical heterogeneity of major depression using family data. Archives of General Psychiatry 43: 430–434

Weissman M M, Gammon G D, John K et al 1987 Children of depressed parents: increased psychopathology and early onset of major depression. Archives of General Psychiatry 44: 847–853

Weissman M M, Warner V, Wickramaratne P, Prusoff B A 1988 Onset of major depression in adolescence and early adulthood: findings from a family study of children. Journal of Affective Disorders 13: 269–277

Young W, Knowles J, MacClean A, Boag L, McCanville B J 1982 The sleep of childhood depressives: comparison with age and matched controls. Biological Psychiatry 17: 1163–1168

38. Affective disorders in old age

Elaine Murphy   Alastair Macdonald

Explorers of affective disorders in the elderly will find familiar country – the same signs, symptoms, treatment and responses as in younger patients, yet they will find differences, and this chapter attempts to chart these. Even so, it is an expedition rather than a survey; we map out a few areas of interest, and then withdraw, with no apology.

DEPRESSION

We know from surveys of mental disorder in a number of different communities that the great majority of elderly people do not feel depressed, unhappy or unfulfilled. Indeed, most old people feel that life has turned out better for them than they expected. Depression in old age has frequently been perceived as a predictable, understandable response to the losses and declines in the last season of life and the wintry themes of aging and sorrow have been closely linked in our minds. Professionals working with elderly people tend to meet those at greatest risk of feeling burdensome, unhappy, dependent and sad and we need to fight against the tendency to adopt the same stereotyped view of old age during the course of our daily work.

It is important not to exaggerate the extent of depression in the elderly population. Nevertheless, the minority of people who develop severe and significant depression generate a substantial demand for treatment and care.

In spite of the impact of depression on the sufferer and his family, the condition is easily overlooked or dismissed. The symptoms may be confused with organic physical disorder or regarded as an understandable and untreatable response to life stresses of later life. The importance of recognizing the symptoms of depression lies in the fact that the condition is treatable by a variety of medical and social measures and, in general, an isolated episode carries a favourable prognosis for recovery.

Classification

There are now few advocates of the notion that a diagnosis of depression connotes a homogeneous entity, or that mere severity of the condition accounts for all the apparent clinical sub-groups. There is as yet, however, no satisfactory scheme for the classification of depressive disorders at any age. This lack of an adequate nosology leads to even more confusion in depression in the elderly. We do not know whether to regard depressions occurring for the first time in 70- or 80-year-olds as similar or quite separate disorders from those in young or middle aged people. We are equally ignorant about what proportion of those who have a first episode in their teens or twenties will have subsequent depressions in later life.

Most classification systems aim to improve the distinction between subgroups in order better to indicate prognosis and choice of therapy. But the first question to be asked is how to define the distinction between depression as 'depressive illness' and depression as a normal, understandable response to unhappy circumstances. This question has bedevilled much epidemiological work, particularly in surveys of the elderly, in which those who have investigated the extent of simple depressed mood and other minor symptoms unaccompanied by biological changes find a very high prevalence in elderly people compared with younger counterparts. By contrast, where investigators have confined the concept of depression to a disorder lasting for at least some weeks, characterized by symptoms of mood disorder together with physiological and cognitive disturbances, far fewer elderly people are identified as cases in surveys and the difference in prevalence

601

between older and younger groups becomes much smaller.

Schedules designed specifically for use with the elderly population include the CARE (Comprehensive Assessment for Referral and Evaluation) schedule (Gurland et al 1983) and the GMS (Geriatric Mental State) schedule (Copeland et al 1976).

The issue of whether depression in old age represents a separate category of illness from that affecting younger people has led researchers to compare patients whose first illness began late in life with those with an earlier onset. Kay & Bergmann (1966) suggested that elderly patients with affective disorder fell into two groups. One consisted of patients who were retarded and showed depressive self-reproachful ideas or hypochondriacal and nihilistic delusions. This group appeared to correspond to the major 'endogenous' disorders of earlier life. Serious physical illness was relatively rare in this group. The second, 'late-onset', group was predominantly male; anxious, irritable, 'attention seeking', with many somatic complaints. Over half of this group had a serious physical illness and they often had a history of neurotic personality traits. However, the validity of separating the two groups has not been tested empirically and is not wholly supported by other research. Blazer and his colleagues (1987) found little to distinguish major depressive episodes in elderly people from those of young adults. The predominant view at present is that depression is depression at any age and that there is nothing which clearly distinguishes those whose first illness begins late in life from those whose first onset occurs in their younger days.

Other classifications of depression have been less useful in the elderly. Assignment to a class using the unipolar – bipolar distinction, for example, can only be made after several episodes of illness and then not with certainty – six episodes of depression in the 30s, 40s and 60s may be followed by one isolated episode of mania in the 70s. It is worth remembering, however, that both recurrent unipolar depressives and bipolar manic depressives grow old in time, carrying their psychiatric burden into old age. Episodes of illness sometimes become more frequent and more prolonged with age and it may be only in old age that these become frequent enough to persuade the patient and his family of the wisdom of taking prophylactic medication.

The classification of affective disorder in old age is unsatisfactory and confusing and likely to remain so until biochemical or genetic aetiological factors validate a classification system which can be confidently used to predict course, response to treatment and prognosis in individual cases. Shulman (1989) has challenged the notion that depression in old age is a primary mood disorder at all, postulating that depression is a final common pathway for central nervous system dysregulation. Only empirical studies will clarify whether depression in old age is different from that in younger people.

CHARACTERISTICS OF DEPRESSION IN OLD AGE

Clinically, depression in old age is generally the same as in younger people. However, there are sometimes misleading features, especially in those with concomitant physical illness. Depressed mood may be overshadowed by somatic complaints, delusional beliefs, bizarre behaviour disturbances or a picture resembling dementia.

Major depressive disorders in the elderly frequently present in florid form. Psychomotor agitation and retardation are common and often go together, seen as restless pacing, wringing of the hands and clinging, importunate begging for help which engenders a feeling of irritation in those around. At the same time the sufferer often feels slowed up, unable to think as fast as usual and answers questions in a retarded, monosyllabic and distracted fashion. Loss of concentration and muddled thinking, which are usual, can give the appearance of confusion. This, together with a lack of energy, prevents the sufferer from completing the simplest task effectively, which is often interpreted by the patient and sometimes by relatives or nursing staff as evidence of 'laziness' or as a sign of senility and dementia. Delusions of guilt, poverty and debt, severe illness – especially cancer, venereal disease – now including AIDS, punishment and impending death are often accompanied by somatic complaints of inability to swallow, blocked bowels and a feeling that the insides are rotting or diseased.

The classic presentation of an agitated depressive psychosis described here is characteristic of a severe illness seen in a cohort of elderly people born around the turn of the century. The psychopathology of future generations of elderly people may take a different form.

Depressive stupor

Retardation may be so severe that the patient appears stuporose, immobile and silent. This condition of akinetic mutism is rare but is easily confused with neurological stupor. A clue to the diagnosis is the determined rejection of food and drink, the alert, sometimes frightened, eyes and lack of neurological signs. The mortality rate of depressive stupor in old age is very high because of the rapid dehydration and risk of subsequent pneumonia. Rehydration and electroconvulsive therapy (ECT) may not only be life-saving but can be curative. However, the situation is made more complex by the fact that severe depressive stupor quite frequently occurs in the setting of cerebrovascular disease or other major physical illness.

Milder forms of depressive illness

Not all depressions are severe, and milder forms of major depressive disorders, presenting with querulous irritability, anxious clinging and apprehensive pessimism may be difficult to spot. Such elderly people are at risk of being labelled as having 'just personality problems' or 'getting crabby in old age'. Mistakes are easy to avoid if a good history is taken and a point in time of change from previously equable personality can be clearly established.

In hospital inpatients depression may present simply as withdrawal from the life of the ward, an overcomplaining attitude, a preoccupation with poor health out of keeping with the severity of the physical illness, profound pessimism about the future and so on. Since all these symptoms may, on the other hand, be appropriate to the person's real problems, careful interview and assessment of the overall situation are essential.

Depression may also present as acute phobic anxiety, usually an intense fear of being alone, complaints of despairing loneliness and fear. Someone who may have adjusted to years of widowhood and living alone will suddenly become determined to stay close to relatives or friends, needing constant reassurance and continuous company.

Distinguishing depression from dementia; 'pseudodementia'

Depressive and dementia syndromes (a preferred nomenclature: Mahendra 1983) can occur together for a number of reasons:

1) They can be coincidental.
2) Depression can complicate grief for one's former self, especially when insight is maintained, as in early multi-infarct dementia.

3) Depression can be caused by the structural changes causing the dementia syndrome ('organic depression').
4) Depression can perhaps cause structural changes that lead to dementia syndromes (Robinson et al 1986).
5) Severe depression can cause irreversible cognitive impairment, apathy and regression indistinguishable from a dementia syndrome ('depressive pseudodementia').
6) Depression can result from the systematic abuse-by-neglect that occurs in long-term residential settings for the demented.

The majority of elderly depressed patients show no evidence of impaired intellect or cognitive decline on specific tests. Depressed old people frequently complain of poor memory and fears of intellectual decline but on psychometric testing, performance on tests of immediate and delayed recall do not differ significantly from normal elderly people (Popkin et al 1982). The patient's perception is likely to be the direct consequence of concentration difficulties.

However, a small but important minority present a confused, withdrawn picture which is very difficult to distinguish from dementia. Psychological testing reveals numerous patchy gaps and lowered performance scores which are difficult to interpret. Computed axial tomography (CAT scan) may be equally unhelpful, a finding of mild cortical atrophy being of little significance. EEG may be helpful, although studies like those of Reynolds et al (1988) illustrate a problem in interpreting efforts to discriminate depression and dementia. The use of complex and powerful statistical methods allowed them to claim impressive accuracy using sleep EEG data – 78% correct classification: however, transposing this to clinical practice is problematic, since there seems no way of knowing whether the individual patient in front of the clinician would fall into the 22% or the 78%. Perhaps of more immediate relevance is the suggestion of Reynolds et al (1986) that early-morning wakening was more often associated with depression than dementia in a 2-year longitudinal study.

On balance, the syndrome of 'pseudodementia' is probably overdiagnosed. Previous history of depression, rapid onset and variable psychometric performance all point to a diagnosis of depression. It has been suggested that temporary impairment of cognitive functions may indicate some underlying unspecified cerebral organic disorder, consequent upon aging.

In clinical practice, if the physician finds it difficult to distinguish depression from dementia after lengthy interview, observation and a careful history from informants, then the issue will not be solved by psychological testing but by a therapeutic trial of antidepressant medication. The commonest reason for a puzzling mixed picture is that the patient has both depression and dementia occurring at the same time. Kral & Emery (1989) found that cognitive function returned to premorbid levels when depressive pseudodementia sufferers were vigorously treated for depression but that 89% of 44 subjects followed up for between 4 and 18 years had developed a dementia syndrome.

Hypochondriasis and pain

Hypochondriasis and somatic complaints in general are more commonly found in older than in younger patients (Gurland 1976, Zemore & Eames 1979). Pain of a persistent, unpleasant, unbearable quality which is difficult to pin down to a precise anatomical location is a common symptom of depression which carries a rather poor prognosis for treatment if it has been going on for many months or years. Physical facial pain is a variant which perhaps carries a better prognosis if vigorously treated (Feinmann et al 1964). Because physical disability and pain are legitimate triggers for sympathy and extra help from others in our society, anyone who is felt to be 'exaggerating', 'inventing' or 'imagining' illness is given short shrift by relatives and professionals alike and an overcomplaining depressed person often feels ostracized and neglected.

Depression presenting as behaviour disturbance

Behaviour problems of a wide variety are frequently symptoms of depression in elderly people who are heavily dependent on others for their day-to-day care. This happens, for example, in residential care, long-stay hospitals or where the elderly person is living with younger members of the family with whom they have a difficult relationship of long standing. Depressive behavioural problems often occur in the setting of mild intellectual impairment. Food refusal and wilful starvation, inappropriate urinary and faecal incontinence with faecal smearing of walls and furniture are reminiscent of the young child with a behaviour disorder. Persistent intermittent blood-curdling screaming, especially at night, frequently denied by the elderly person, seems usually to occur in response to anxious panic as a demand for instant help. In residential and nursing homes, the person who has recurrent, apparently wilful 'falls', throwing him- or herself on the floor in a theatrical fashion; the person who has recently 'fallen out' with all the other residents; the person who has begun to bite and scratch the caring staff, or become 'a management problem' should all be suspected of having a depressive disorder.

Depression, then, can be a rather chameleon-like disorder in elderly people, which is easily overlooked when the mood itself is not obviously sad or distressed. The key to diagnosis is a history of change in the person's mental state coming on over some days, weeks or a month or two rather than years.

EPIDEMIOLOGY OF DEPRESSION IN OLD AGE

A comprehensive and perhaps more optimistic picture is emerging from recent studies of the distribution of depression among the general population of elderly people. A clinician tends to see patients who are not only at the severest end of the spectrum of depressive disorders but also at the height of the disorder. It is difficult for a specialist to gain a broad perspective throughout the course of the illness.

The concept of a sub-clinical iceberg of unrecognized depression in elderly people in the community has been supported by a number of studies but the truth may be more complex. Recent studies have suggested that depression is generally recognized by family doctors but that very often no action is taken to investigate, treat or modify it with either a social or pharmacological approach (Macdonald 1986, Barsa et al 1986). This may be a consequence of the therapeutic nihilism which still bedevils the approach to treating all ailments in old age or may be a reflection of the family doctor's assessment that he has little to offer therapeutically to the mildly and understandably depressed person.

The major problem which has beset psychiatric epidemiologists has been the definition of what constitutes a 'case' of depression, Since depressed mood is an entirely appropriate response to unhappy circumstances and older people may carry a large burden of losses, social difficulties and health problems likely to cause sadness and unhappiness, studies in which a case has been identified merely by depressed mood may be expected to give a higher prevalence of the disorder among elderly people than younger people. This has indeed been the result of studies using these low threshold criteria, using self-rating scales or standard questionnaires (Zung 1967, Srole & Fischer 1980). Clinically this does not have much meaning, since the majority of dysphoric elderly people would not be considered appropriate for medical and/or social intervention. However society at large should perhaps be concerned that elderly people are often dissatisfied and unhappy.

Clinical epidemiologists wishing to seek out cases similar in severity to those seen in clinical practice have used different approaches to psychiatric case definition. This has given rise to problems in comparing results between studies. On the one hand, a quantitative symptom threshold assigns caseness on the basis of a predefined arbitrary cut-off level. Most community-based surveys of elderly populations have used global rating scales of psychiatric impairment (e.g. OARS community survey, Blazer 1978; US/UK community survey, Gurland et al 1983). The alternative approach is to have clearly defined operational criteria for specified case diagnosis. In this latter method, signs and symptoms are elicited by interviewers who are highly trained to rate reliably the answers to questions on a structured interview schedule. The ratings are then used to generate diagnoses for specific classification systems. For example the Diagnostic Interview Schedule (DSI) designed by Robins and colleagues (1981) has been extensively used in the United States in a number of studies sponsored by the National Institute for Mental Health, the Epidemiological Catchment Area (ECA) programme. It generates diagnoses using DSM-III criteria (American Psychiatric Association 1980). This is an attractive method but many clinicians question the usefulness of instruments developed to increase reliability of diagnosis in elderly people which were originally derived from symptomatology of younger adults. Elderly people seen in clinical practice do not always fit conveniently into existing classification schemes, as has been noted above.

The most surprising finding has been that the prevalence rates amongst elderly people for most non-organic mental disorders are in fact similar to or even slightly lower than at other stages of the life cycle (Myers et al 1984, Gurland 1976). Overall, women do not have an increased prevalence of depression in old age compared with younger ages; men show a small rise in prevalence through the 70s and 80s. The sex difference in prevalence between men and women is maintained throughout life, women having rates approximately 50% above that for men.

Depression in residential homes and hospitals

Only a small minority of elderly people are permanently resident in hospitals and homes, approximately 6% in the UK. Dementia is the major psychiatric problem found in elderly people in residential care and is the primary cause of admission in most cases. However, it is increasingly recognized that mentally alert residents and those with mild dementias have a markedly higher rate of depression compared with those living at home in the community. A survey of residents in old people's homes in one London borough found 38% had pervasive depression of a kind that was found in only 13% of the community-dwelling elderly in the same city (Mann et al 1984a). The rate in London homes was significantly higher than in similar institutions in New York and Mannheim, Germany but even in those cities the rate was higher than might be expected (Mann et al 1984b). It is possible that the drab quality of life provided in many residential homes is one reason for the high prevalence but it is also possible that chronically depressed elderly people are preferentially selected into residential care as a result of their dependence on others and failure to cope adequately alone at home.

PHYSICAL ILLNESS, DISABILITY AND DEPRESSION

Many authors have commented on the close association between physical ill health and depression in old age. However, since both occur commonly in old age, this is not surprising. The lack of clear evidence of an age-related increase in the prevalence of depressive illness lowers the probability that the observed relationship between these two types of morbidity occurs together more frequently than by chance alone. However, there is other evidence of more specific relationships in three areas: specific illnesses predisposing to a high rate of depression, the evidence that depression and bereavement may cause increased mortality and, last, the influence on course and outcome of depression by physical ill health.

Physical disease predisposing to depression

There are five possible reasons which could account for the association between depression and physical disorder:

1) Depression could be the consequence of treatment for physical illness.

2) Depression may be a direct consequence of the cerebral organic effects of certain specific physical disorders.

3) Depression may result from the psychological reaction to physical illness and the process of adapting to a future life of handicap and disability.

4) Depression may predispose to the onset of physical disease.

5) The behavioural consequences of depressed mood may cause physical ill health through starvation, self-neglect, self-harm and so on.

It is also possible that physical disorder and disability may increase the individual's vulnerability to other adverse life events which predispose to depression and may inhibit recovery from depression.

Treatment factors are important because they are a potentially avoidable cause of depression. Treatment for known conditions is often fatiguing or painful and a patient may not share the physician's understanding of the mechanisms of treatment or prognosis. But even treatments which in themselves are painless may contribute to depression. For example, more than 23 medications have been suggested to be depressogenic (Ouslander 1982).

We have already noted the association between stroke and depression. There is evidence that depression occurs more frequently in neurological disorders with specific reductions in neurotransmitters which have been linked to the monoamine theory of depression. For example, depression is common in Parkinson's disease and in Huntington's chorea, where one might postulate that a link between reductions in dopamine or GABA might predispose to imbalance of the neurotransmitter systems which maintain mood.

Many types of malignancy have been linked to severe depressions, especially carcinomas of the pancreas, stomach and bronchus. Other commonly described associations are between cardiovascular diseases and depression, and some metabolic and endocrine disorders (Ouslander 1982). The true incidence of depressive illness in the elderly following onset of physical disorder is not known. Biochemical explanations of depression in aging individuals are appealing in part because they suggest methods for intervention by biological treatments. However, physical disorder has a major impact on social well-being, dependence on others, the ability to maintain social activities and interpersonal relationships. Illness brings home to the individual the possible proximity of future mortality and in influencing the course of one's life, the meaning an illness has cannot be easily separated out from the biological components of causality.

Neuroradiological changes

The advent of computed axial tomography has brought a safe and non-invasive method of imaging the brain. There are changes in the brain with age in 15% of elderly people who have no evidence of psychiatric disorder, cortical atrophy and ventricular enlargement being the most common changes reported (Laffey et al 1984). A longitudinal study of the normal elderly population found that 16% had increased ventricular size at first assessment and a further 10% had enlarged ventricles at follow up at an average 2.5 years later. Ventricular enlargement was correlated with reduced scores on cognitive tests, as one might expect. There was also a higher than expected number of subjects with enlarged ventricles in the 9% of the total sample who developed depression during the follow-up study (Bird et al 1986). This contrasts with the earlier findings of Jacoby & Levy (1980) who found no difference in the proportion of depressed elderly patients with enlarged ventricles when compared with age matched controls. Interestingly, the nine out of 41 depressed elderly people who did have enlarged ventricles were described as clinically dissimilar from other depressed patients, being on the whole older and having more features of endogenous, retarded depression. At follow-up 2 years later, five of the nine with the enlarged ventricles were dead compared with only four of the 31 depressed with normal ventricles, suggesting that venticular enlargement may influence the course of depression.

The same investigators found that regional brain densities recorded on CAT scans of depressed elderly patients were intermediate between those of normals and those with dementia (Jacoby et al 1983), although at present the significance of this finding is unknown. It may be linked to the presence of cerebrovascular disease. The nature of the relationship between vascular disease generally and depression is unclear but many authors have suspected a close link. Kay (1962) found a higher than expected rate of cerebrovascular disease as attributed cause of death on death certificates in a mental hospital population diagnosed as having 'functional psychosis'. The evidence from studies of depression following stroke are far less clear. Robinson and his colleagues in Baltimore have claimed that up to 60% of patients may develop some form of depression following stroke (Robinson et al 1984a).

Further studies of stroke patients admitted to hospitals (Ebrahim et al 1987) have supported the very high rate of depression following stroke in this selected population. House, reporting from the Oxford Community Stroke Survey (House et al 1990) found that although there was the expected increase in depression 1 month after the stroke, by the end of a year stroke victims were not significantly more depressed than age-matched control subjects.

Physical illness caused by depression

Depression can be physically disabling. Fatigue, sleep disturbance and loss of appetite may be compounded by self-neglect, inactivity and reduction in the patient's motivation to take treatment for physical health problems. All this is fairly straightforward. But can depression and psychological adversity make people physically ill? The literature on this topic is vast and much research has been methodologically unsound. The best evidence is from Parkes's studies of recently bereaved people (Parkes 1964). He found an increased mortality from cardiovascular disease in 4500 widowers in the 6 months following death of the wife. The increased mortality was confined to men and limited to the first 6 months after the loss. However, these men would presumably already have had significant cardiovascular disease before the bereavement. The general public certainly believes that adverse life events can make people physically ill, particularly in the case of strokes and heart attacks, but the literature is unfortunately inconclusive on this point.

Influence on the course of depression

The course and outcome of depression does appear to be influenced by the presence of physical disorder. Murphy (1983) noted that physical illness during a 1-year follow-up period was significantly more common among depressed patients who had a poor psychiatric outcome compared with those who made a good recovery from depression. Shephard (1983) also showed that improved physical condition correlated with reduced psychological morbidity. These findings accord with clinical common sense and will surprise no-one.

PSYCHOSOCIAL FACTORS IN CAUSATION

Health, vigour and the well-being of the elderly have more to do with economics and social organization than with the biological inevitability of the laws of nature. Many of the problems of the elderly are susceptible to change by social evolution and political intervention. The exploration of how and to what degrees social factors are responsible for mental disorder in old age, especially depression, is therefore of great importance, since it has implications for prevention.

In Western societies, older people form a socially underprivileged group. They are in general poorer, more likely to live alone and to occupy the worst housing. They have more physical illness and are consequently less mobile, more likely to have poor sight and impaired hearing. Reduction of income, loss of status and sometimes of a useful role are commonplace events in old age. All this is not in doubt. But what empirical evidence is there that low social class, poverty, isolation or the loss events of old age really contribute to the onset of serious depressive illness?

Social class

The majority of studies, but not all, have demonstrated an inverse relationship between social class and the prevalence of depressive disorders at all ages but this is most marked in the milder forms of depression. There is less evidence for a social class effect in severe depressive psychoses. Probably of major importance in the elderly is the very wide variation in physical health status between the top and bottom ends of the social strata. There is also a difference in social isolation reported by elderly people in different classes.

Life events

There are two questions here. First, is there any causal link between events and the onset of a depressive illness? Second, do events act merely to trigger off an episode which would have occurred sooner or later anyway or can an event be the major formative factor, producing depression in someone who otherwise would have remained healthy?

The results of Murphy's 1982 study were very similar to the findings of Brown & Harris (1978) for younger subjects. 48% of depressed patients and 68% of depressed community subjects had experienced a severe life event in the year preceding onset, compared with only 23% of the normal group. The types of severe event which were commoner in depressed subjects were the death of a spouse or child, serious physical illness, life-threatening illness to someone close, severe financial loss and enforced change of residence as a result of a demolition programme. Major social difficulties, lasting 2 years or more, were also significantly associated with depression. The overall risk of developing an onset of depression in the year for the total general population sample was approximately 10%. The rate of preceding severe events did not distinguish the 'psychotic' group from the rest and the most severely ill were as likely to have predisposing social problems as the less severely ill.

Social circumstances and the events of a person's life do then seem to play an important role in depression. However, caution must be used in applying these research findings to individual clinical cases. Since in the above study almost a quarter of the normal elderly population experienced an event which did not lead to depression, in a given clinical case it is impossible to be sure whether a reported event is causal or not or whether it has occurred coincidentally.

Critics of life events research have pointed out that the magnitude of the effect of events on the causation of depression may be quite small and we must look for vulnerability factors which predispose individuals to depressive breakdown following life stress.

Social isolation

The question of how the quantity and quality of social relationships predisposes or protects from depression is a complex one in which research is fraught with methodological problems. Most authors are now agreed that simply living alone, or having relatively few daily contacts, are not especially disadvantageous for risk of developing depression. Furthermore, depressed people of all ages are more likely to report feeling lonely and unsupported but elderly people do not report more loneliness than younger age groups. The evidence overall is that the perceived quality of relationships and their perceived adequacy are the key factors emerging from most studies. It is likely that life-long personality adjustment and the capacity to form good social relationships are very important variables affecting vulnerability.

PROGNOSIS, COURSE AND OUTCOME

The introduction of ECT and specific antidepressant drugs have undoubtedly had a major impact on the short-term outcome of major depressive disorders in old age. In spite of the difficulties encountered in treatment, the majority of patients will respond well to treatment within a month (Jarvik et al 1982) although at least one-third will not respond very satisfactorily. However, the long-term course of depression in old age may be rather less optimistic than for younger people and there has been remarkably little improvement in long-term outcome over the past 15 years.

Mortality

The mortality of patients with depression has been consistently found to be higher than expected when compared with the general population. The increased mortality rate is particularly marked in males (Kay & Bergmann 1966). The straightforward explanation for this excess mortality is that elderly depressed patients have very poor physical health but this alone does not satisfactorily explain the excess mortality (Murphy et al 1988). However, this association between depression and excess mortality may not hold true for the milder degrees of depression found in community surveys.

Quality of long-term outcome

Post (1962) recorded a lasting complete recovery in 27% of inpatients admitted around 1950. In a later study (Post 1972) 26% of a series of patients admitted in 1966 and followed for 3 years were similarly described as well and lastingly recovered. This similarity in outcome between the two periods of study was interesting because of the introduction of antidepressant drugs between the two series. 14 years later, in Murphy's 1979–1980 series (Murphy 1983), 43% made a recovery at a 1-year follow-up and at 4 years this proportion had fallen to 25%, a figure very similar to Post's findings. Baldwin & Jolley (1986) reported a rather more optimistic outcome of 58% recovered at 1 year, but a similar result over the longer term.

The proportions who remain chronically unremittingly ill with depression also appear to have changed little over the years – 17% in 1950, 12% in 1966 and 14% in 1979–1980. Modern treatment does not seem to have reduced the hard core of persistently ill patients who make a very heavy demand on social and health services and pose a severe burden on the family.

There is a middle group, of between one-quarter and one-third of patients, who, while not remaining severely depressed, do not return to their former good mental health. While the biological symptoms remit, the person retains the cognitive and emotional changes of depressed mood. Post referred to this unsatisfactory outcome as 'residual depressive invalidism', a distressing, fluctuating condition which predisposes to further attacks of the full-blown disorder and which creates enormous social difficulties for the patient and family.

In conclusion, specific treatments appear to have shortened attacks of severe depression and far fewer patients remain in hospital in the long term than in earlier years of this century. However, a proportion remain severely depressed for many years, many more have residual problems and only one-third have the kind of good recovery which we would like all our patients to achieve.

We need to know more about prognosis from large, prospective series of a broader range of categories and severities of depressive illness. It is possible that the kind of depression treated in primary care settings has a more optimistic outlook.

NEUROCHEMISTRY AND THE SEARCH FOR BIOLOGICAL MARKERS FOR AFFECTIVE DISORDER IN THE ELDERLY

The relatively high prevalence of coexisting physical illnesses in the elderly, together with age-related changes in physiology and biochemistry, complicate the search for reliable biochemical markers for affective disorders in this age group. Increases in platelet monoamine oxidase activity over and above normal age-related increase have been reported in small studies (e.g. Schneider et al 1986a). There has been considerable interest in 3H-imipramine binding in the elderly as a means of distinguishing 'primary' depressive illness from depression secondary to physical illness (Schneider et al 1988a), a means of distinguishing depression from dementia (Nemeroff et al 1988, Galzin et al 1989), a prediction of response to antidepressant treatment (Georgotas et al 1987a) and a means of supporting distinctions between familial and non-familial depressions (Schneider et al 1986b). However, early promise of this test in younger patients has not borne the rich fruit that was originally hoped for, and the method has hitherto only been used to distinguish selected groups of elderly depressives; its performance in the hurly-burly of general psychogeriatric practice has yet to be evaluated. Furthermore, the small numbers used in initial evaluations of markers produce results that seem to be illusory; for instance, Houck et al (1988) found that the previously promising red blood cell/plasma choline ratio failed to distinguish elderly depressed and demented patients when larger numbers were tested.

A further example of the problems of defining a marker in depressive illness in the elderly is given by Greden et al (1986), who found that the effect of age was great enough to make the dexamethasone suppression test (DST) very difficult to interpret. This, coupled with the finding of abnormal DSTs in dementia (e.g. Gierl et al 1987), suggests that the DST is not a routinely useful clinical tool. Interest in rhythmic physiological changes continues, however: Teicher et al (1988) have reported changes in the timing and increased levels of activity of depressed elderly patients compared to controls and correlated phase delay with post-DST cortisol levels, but the sample was very small. The increase in circulating growth hormone provoked by desimipramine (Wilkins et al 1989) has yet to be shown in more realistic populations.

PHYSICAL TREATMENTS FOR DEPRESSION IN OLD AGE

There seems to be general consensus that the use of *specific* physical, as opposed to psychological, treatments for depression in the elderly has broadly the same indications as in younger age groups (Gerson et al 1988). While most authorities suggest lower doses of antidepressants in the elderly, clinical evidence suggests that, although a more gradual dose increase in older people is important, ultimate doses should be broadly comparable with those in younger patients if treatment is to be adequate. However, it could be that the dearth of specific non-medical treatment options in the elderly, probably related to the relatively low interest in this group by the disciplines of psychology and social work, may mean that physical treatments are being used inappropriately. Evidence for this is scant. Although Duncan & Campbell (1988) found 6% of a community sample of 761 70-year-olds and older taking long-term antidepressants, these were possibly unnecessary or apparently used as hypnotics in 17. The evidence for widespread use of benzodiazepines in the elderly, on the other hand, is overwhelming, although the point has been well made that most short-term use is related to physical illness and insomnia. A factor complicating research in this area is the methodology of drug histories in surveys: Jackson et al (1989) found discrepancies between histories given by the patient and drugs found in their homes in almost one-third of elderly outpatients, and depression was significantly correlated with this discrepancy. In that study, the number of 'extra' drugs was equal in the two assessments, but we (Macdonald 1986) found that, while the net tendency of GPs was to *add* to the prescriptions of elderly patients with high depression scores seen in their surgeries, follow-up at 9 months at home revealed that patients were taking fewer medications despite little change in depression scores, indicating an additional, perhaps fortunate self-regulating non-compliance.

Antidepressant treatment in the elderly

Various spectres haunt the feast of drug treatment in the elderly: pharmacokinetic and pharmacodynamic unpredictability, leading to sensitivity to unpleasant or dangerous adverse reactions; the increased suicide rate in the elderly in which powerful medications may play a part; and the dearth of alternative strategies leading to possible 'medicalization' of social or interpersonal problems. Until recently, there has been very little study of the relative efficacy and intolerance of antidepressants in the elderly (Gerson et al 1988), although the search by the pharmaceutical industry for replacements for traditional tricyclic antidepressants (TCAs) continues (e.g. Baldessarini 1987, Tempesta et al 1987, Wachtel et al 1988, Defrance et al 1988), based on a widespread perception of their toxicity in the elderly.

How justified is the trepidation with which TCAs for the elderly are viewed? Consideration of this topic cannot ignore a major problem in assessing the efficacy and relative safety of drug treatments: there is sometimes a wide discrepancy between the efficacy of medication in published trials and that perceived by clinicians in everyday practice. Reasons for this may include the absence of non-pharmaceutical funding for these trials, publication bias and subtle, perhaps as yet unrecognized methodological difficulties that may introduce inadvertent errors into the analysis. More alarming is the possibility that the same influences may lead to serious adverse reactions appearing more prominently in clinical practice than in published accounts. This discrepancy accounts for much of the reluctance by practitioners to try new medications, except *in extremis.*

Because of fears of irretrievable adverse reactions, there is much interest in possible predictors of response to TCAs in the depressed elderly. While Georgotas et al found that neither clinical features (1987c) nor DST response (1986a) predicted TCA response, Schneider et al (1986c) had already suggested that pre-existing postural hypotension was a predictor. The same author (Schneider et al 1987) suggested that a single dose of TCA (nortriptyline), followed by a blood level, was a useful predictor of ultimate TCA dose. However, this should be tested on larger samples.

Tricyclic antidepressants in the elderly

One of the principal sources of anxiety is the effect of TCAs on the cardiovascular system, especially cardiac conduction defects, cardiac output and postural hypotension. McCue et al (1989) found that ECG changes (P-R interval increase, QT_c interval and heart rate) with nortriptyline were unrelated to levels of nortriptyline and metabolites, unlike the report of Schneider et al (1988b) of elderly outpatients, four of whom developed conduction defects.

Kutcher et al (1986) found similar ECG abnormalities with desimipramine in elderly patients. Although Hartling et al (1987) found no effect of nortriptyline on left ventricular ejection fraction and left ventricular volumes, this was based on only eight patients. Postural hypotension is a common and potentially disastrous side-effect of TCAs in the elderly, but Schneider et al (1986c) seem to have confirmed a suggestion that *pretreatment* postural hypotension is a predictor of clinical response to TCAs in the elderly, thus raising an obvious and interesting paradox.

Urinary retention is a problem in elderly men with prostatism, but can also complicate treatment in women. It is sometimes possible to get away with tiny increments of TCAs, but the distress and pain of acute retention is very often a signal for a relapse of depression, and alternatives should be considered.

Generally speaking, the common forms of glaucoma in the elderly are not affected by TCAs – but 'closed-angle' glaucoma is almost always a contraindication.

Many elderly patients find constipation a severe problem with TCAs, for several reasons. Gut motility is reduced in old age; there may be a 'cohort' bowel fetish in the present elderly (and in future generations); constipation may be a feature of the depressive state; there is a high prevalence of lower intestinal pathology in the elderly; and dietary and exercise factors may also play a part.

In summary, although the few studies available suggest that TCAs have demonstrable effects on these functions, the *clinical* significance of these is unclear. Against the 50% chance of improvement suggested by Gerson et al (1988) from a meta-analysis are ranged largely theoretical objections, and a reasonably balanced view might be that TCAs are indicated when the diagnosis is clear or the patient's quality of life so poor, that dosage should be small to start with, gradually increasing over 3–4 weeks to levels that are similar to younger groups (e.g. 150 mg of dothiepin), limited only by the presence of symptomatic side-effects rather than, for instance, ECG abnormalities. If dose levels cannot be increased because of severe hypotension or dry mouth, a prolonged trial at the lower dose may be worthwhile (Lakshmanan et al 1986), rather than casting about for a new drug. Scathing comments on the low-dose treatment of depression (e.g. Bridges 1983) emanate from those unaware of referral bias; patients who do well on these regimes are not referred to specialists.

Newer antidepressants and the elderly patient

Lofepramine has been used extensively in younger patients in the UK. However, unless the patient is going to respond to low-dose antidepressant treatment (Lakshmanan et al 1986) it is necessary to use relatively high doses of lofepramine (e.g. 280 mg) in psychogeriatric practice to achieve the same results as older TCAs. At these levels, it appears that lofepramine is an expensive way of delivering desimipramine; effective, but with most of the side-effects of the older TCAs. It seems to have some alerting properties.

Mianserin. Widely marketed as a safer alternative to TCAs in the elderly, mianserin was widely prescribed for the elderly, particularly in primary care settings. Although apparently very safe in overdosage, there are considerable doubts about its efficacy, despite the results of several large-scale trials which have shown it to be as effective as TCAs (e.g. Altamura et al 1989).

Trazodone. Lader (1987) concluded from a review of studies of trazodone that it seemed to be an effective antidepressant but lacked the cardiotoxic properties of tricyclic antidepressants. Spar (1987) found no ECG effects whatsoever but also found, in a small series of elderly patients, that there appeared to be a therapeutic window in plasma concentrations. Side effects associated with trazodone include priapism, lethargy, dizziness, drowsiness and confusion; anticholinergic side effects seem minimal (Rakel 1987).

5-HT reuptake inhibitors: These new antidepressants have no anticholinergic activity, but are associated with mild tachycardia, sometimes very significant nausea and occasional hyponatraemia. Large-scale trials in the elderly appear not to have been carried out, so these drugs must suffer the fate of all new medication – to be used when other medication has failed.

Monoamine oxidase inhibitors (MAOIs)

There is a view that the dangers of these drugs were overestimated after the hypertensive crises reported in the 1960s, and they are sometimes advocated as being as effective as TCAs in the elderly (e.g. Georgotas et al 1986b). However, they may not be as effective as tricyclics in endogenous psychotic depression (Tyrer 1976). Furthermore, although anticholinergic effects are lesser, postural hypotension appears to be as frequent as with TCAs in the elderly (Georgotas et al 1987b), other side-effects lead to withdrawal from prolonged treatment (Georgotas et al 1988) and there remains the tyramine reaction as a major threat. MAOIs should perhaps be reserved as an adjunct in elderly patients in whom unusual admixtures of depressive symptoms and long-standing personality difficulties cannot be assisted by any other (particularly non-pharmacological) means.

Electroconvulsive therapy (ECT) in the elderly

The rarity of death associated with ECT in the elderly, compared with rates for TCA overdosage and the probability of other TCA-associated morbidity (e.g. fractures due to postural hypotension) is sometimes cited as evidence for the peculiar advantage that ECT holds over TCA treatment. However great the epidemiological fallacies revealed by such views, ECT is widely favoured, particularly in elderly patients with severe depression and delusions, in which it appears to be superior to combinations of TCAs and antipsychotic medication. Delusions of poverty, justified persecution, unworthiness, nihilism or fatal illness (particularly bowel disease) seem to be peculiarly susceptible; ECT can be a life-saving measure when refusal to drink would otherwise lead to dehydration and an untimely death. Pretreatment postural systolic hypotension appears to predict ECT response as well as TCA response (Stack et al 1988).

Kramer's retrospective review (1987) of brief pulse current ECT in 50 patients aged 61 to 88 revealed few serious complications and a 92% success rate. Burke et al (1987) found more complications in a larger sample, however: 35% of 40 patients over 60 had an 'untoward event'; deliria, falls and cardiac and respiratory problems accounted for most, although many in this sample clearly had pre-existing medical problems.

Memory impairment is a frequently encountered side-effect in elderly patients, and attempts have been made to reduce this by unilateral application, brief pulse currents and replacing atropine as premedication with glycopyrrolate (Sommer et al 1989). However, as with younger patients, it seems that unilateral or very brief pulse currents may be less effective than bilateral ECT which, provided it is administered no more often than twice a week, seems to produce few major, persisting memory deficits in those without pre-existing cognitive impairment. There have been no studies of persistent memory deficits following ECT in the elderly, since such a study would be complicated by the problem of dementia and depression which we have discussed.

ECT in dementia

Benbow (1987) has described the use of ECT in five patients with depression and dementia and avers that there is no need to withhold ECT in these patients. Yet many clinicians are aware of the profound decline in cognitive function that can occur with ECT in such patients and our impression is that this treatment should only be used in established dementia if depressive symptoms are very severely affecting the quality of life and cannot be dealt with any other way.

ECT in post-stroke depression

On the other hand, in depression following stroke, there appears to be no evidence that ECT has any sustained deleterious effects (Karliner 1978) and ECT should form part of the armamentarium that is deployed very actively in this distressing state.

Lithium in the elderly

Lithium is at least as useful in elderly patients as in younger ones for prophylaxis of unipolar or bipolar affective illness, for treatment of mania and as an adjunct to TCAs in resistant depression. Incipient or pre-existing renal impairment, thyroid deficiency and cardiac problems, as well as the consumption of drugs which will interfere with lithium treatment (thiazide diuretics and non-steroidal anti-inflammatory drugs in particular), are more common in the elderly, so careful physical examination and investigation are vital. Lithium can be used with caution in patients with mild renal or cardiac impairment; loop diuretics may be used and concurrent thyroxine treatment may be increased. Altered pharmacokinetics in the elderly (Hardy et al 1987) mean that dosage may be considerably less than in younger patients to achieve similar serum levels; also,

experience suggests that in patients over 70 lower serum levels (e.g. 0.4–1.0 mmol/l) may be adequate for prophylaxis, depending on the means of assay.

There is no evidence yet available on the use or utility of carbamazepine in affective disorders in the elderly, though there is no reason why it might not be as effective, especially if there are insuperable problems in maintaining lithium levels in the therapeutic range.

Maintenance treatment for depression in the elderly

The long-term nature of studies of maintenance antidepressant treatment, coupled with only recent interest in affective disorders in old age, means that there is very little evidence on which to answer several important questions (Reynolds et al 1989).

1) How long should antidepressant or ECT treatment continue in the elderly?
2) Is there a case for continued treatment (e.g. over a year)?
3) If maintenance therapy is indicated, should it be indefinite?
4) Are there serious consequences of prolonged antidepressant or lithium use in the elderly?

Such brief studies as are available suggest that initial TCA treatment in the elderly should be for at least 4 months (Georgotas & McCue 1989) and, while great caution should be taken before discontinuing long-term TCAs in patients from psychiatric settings (Cook et al 1986), a higher proportion of elderly starting long-term antidepressants in general practice can be discontinued, especially when the initial purpose of treatment was as a hypnotic or was unclear (Duncan & Campbell 1988).

There seems to be no evidence on which to answer other questions, though the very fact that the patients are elderly, with less life left to enjoy (or in which to recover from a relapse) might make one err on the side of caution when confronted by elderly patients on long-term treatment with a clear history of pervasive or severe disorder.

Resistant depression in the elderly

The principles of dealing with resistant depression are exactly the same as with younger patients, and the practice only differs in the speed with which high doses of combination medication are achieved. A careful review of the diagnosis is the first step, with special attention to social pressures and problems, some of which may have been produced by the depression. The possibility of an underlying dementing or other physical illness should be explored by physical reappraisal and re-investigation; even so, persistent depressive symptoms demand action on their own account, if only to clear the clinical picture. A review of past medication will reveal inadequate treatment approaches which can be pursued more vigorously – pharmacy staff may be able to provide an invaluable drug history from their records. Augmentation of TCA with lithium is a useful first step (Lafferman et al 1988) – patients in their 70s or 80s on combinations of a TCA at equivalent doses of 150 mg to 200 mg of TCAs, lithium and tryptophan (Hale et al 1987) are able to enjoy what would be denied them by a lily-livered approach to this most bleak condition. ECT may be considered, even when, perhaps through chronicity, the clinical picture may contain fewer biological symptoms. Apart from other pharmacological strategies like triiodothyronine and carbamazepine, combination antidepressants can also be used. Rarely, psychosurgery may be considered where there is persistent suffering without organic brain disease. In summary, old age, or even a certain degree of frailty should be no bar to any approach that might be considered for a younger patient; especially when the frailty can often be itself a consequence of protracted depression and its consequences.

Other physical treatments for depression in the elderly

Sleep deprivation

Cole & Muler (1976) have reported favourable results in an open trial of sleep deprivation in 15 elderly depressed patients. These patients were referred to the trial in an unspecified way – in particular, it is not clear whether or not they had a depression resistant to orthodox treatment – but the use of repeated (mean 3.6 treatments) 36-hour deprivation revealed two groups – those who responded after the first two treatments and those who did not respond at all. All patients appeared to be on 'thymoleptics' as well. There were no adverse affects other than the expected hypomanic swings.

Exercise

The effect of exercise on the mood of normal elderly people is still unclear (Hatfield et al 1987, Morin & Gramling 1989) Although it is recommended as part of treatment for psychological and physical illnesses

(Lampman 1987), the strong possibility that increased exercise levels (as opposed to activity levels (Teicher et al 1988)) are secondary to enhanced mood needs evaluation.

Stimulants

Amphetamine-related medication has been suggested as a treatment specifically for the elderly depressed, especially women in medical settings (Askinazi et al 1986). Accepting that the risk of dependence might be low, controlled trials seem to have indicated that these drugs are little better than placebo (Satel & Nelson 1989), and the social cost of a widespread reintroduction of legitimized psychostimulants would surely outweigh the relatively slender benefits.

DEPRESSION IN ELDERLY MEDICAL INPATIENTS

Management of depression in the elderly in medical settings poses significant problems, but also allows special opportunities. The problems include complications for diagnosis and management produced by often severe illnesses and their treatments, severely disrupted social roles and supports and the powerlessness and frustration felt when confronted by the occasional ignorant or uncaring staff member. The general level of understanding of affective states in staff in many medical settings is sometimes poor and, when the depression is associated with regression or other behavioural problems, the patient may become a focus for staff dispute which is seldom therapeutic. Opportunities include the possibility of regular, reliable information from nursing staff on key symptoms, constant surveillance, a consistent approach and rapid attention to complications of management. We shall now pick out problems specific to the elderly that require special mention, although they may equally well be encountered outside medical settings.

Depression after stroke

The diagnosis of depression after stroke in the elderly is complicated by 'normal' grief, fear, frustration, communication problems, transient cognitive impairments and, perhaps above all, pessimism in carers and victim alike, leading to a preference for the error of omission to that of commission. A perception of 'giving up', with decline in mobility, interaction and determination may be the first sign, but the diagnosis rests on exactly the same symptoms and signs as at any other age. Whatever the outcome of the discussion on the relationship between lesion and depression after stroke (Robinson et al 1984b, House 1987, Eastwood et al 1989), most authors agree that effective treatment can improve depressive symptoms, 'emotionalism' and cognitive impairment, and may even have an impact on underlying structural changes (Robinson et al 1986), and there is no reason to withhold physical means of treatment.

Depression in Parkinson's disease

The same case is even stronger for depression in Parkinson's disease (Taylor et al 1986), in which the 'organic depression' component may have an important relationship to the Parkinsonian symptoms themselves, and treatment of depression may have a beneficial effect on these.

Depression versus 'turning to the wall'?

One of the most difficult clinical and ethical decisions is the assessment of the physically ill elderly person who appears to have 'given up', lost interest in the world, relatives, eating, drinking or even movement. Enquiry about sleeping, weeping and eating are fruitless; nor is the patient apparently willing to say anything. The absence of any immediate physical cause for decline is often striking, although there is almost always a dependency-creating disorder such as severe arthritis, cardiovascular or respiratory disorder. The question is whether one treats the patient as suffering from a severe depressive disorder, using TCAs (if the patient will accept medication at all) or even ECT, and risk turning a dignified retreat towards death into a disastrously painful debacle, or whether one simply allows the patient to die, possibly missing a treatable illness and further life of whatever quality. Simon (1989) has called these patients 'silent suicides', and seems to indicate that the latter mistake (of 'omission') is more often made than the former (of 'commission'). If the state originated with clear depressive symptoms, then perhaps an aggressive approach is warranted, even if it eventually fails. The relatives' wishes must, of course, be considered, though the decision is the doctors – the survey by Wasserman (1989) of patients attempting suicide in more direct ways indicated that knowledge of the relationships between the patient and key relatives is important in assessing the relatives' attitudes, especially to elderly patients.

The problem posed by elderly patients with terminal cancer is, by contrast, a straightforward judgment of the relative influence of treatment or non-treatment on the quality of remaining life (Kinzel 1988), although the possibility of error by omission or commission must be acknowledged.

DEPRESSION IN ELDERLY PRIMARY CARE PATIENTS

The primary care physician is ideally placed to recognize and treat depression in elderly patients (Hedley et al 1986). However, whether general practitioners should be encouraged to screen for affective disorders is not established – Macdonald (1986) found that GPs had little difficulty identifying depressed and dysphoric elderly attenders, but preliminary results from a subsequent study (D. Jenkins, personal communication 1990) suggest that referral to specialist services is possibly helpful only for a minority, particularly elderly men.

Bereavement

Fasey (1990) has recently reviewed the surprisingly scanty literature on bereavement in the elderly and concludes that it seems to run much the same course, respond to the same interventions but, surprisingly, may produce fewer physical symptoms (as opposed to morbidity) than in younger age-groups. He concludes with a plea for further work in this obviously important area.

Depression in carers

A specific group (not necessarily elderly, but many are) at risk of depression are the carers of the demented elderly (Goldman & Luchins 1984), although this does not appear to be a simple matter. For instance, there seem to be complex interactions between gender and psychological distress (Moritz et al 1989), and levels of cognitive impairment in patients do not seem necessarily related to prevalence of depression in carers (Eagles et al 1987). The finding of Drinka et al (1987) that carer depression correlated better with levels of depression, rather than with dementia, in the sufferer, coupled with the increasing awareness of psychiatric and behavioural complications of the dementias, reinforces the clinical view that depression in carers should always be enquired about, especially when there are behavioural problems or depressive symptoms in the patient or when there are known, pre-existing relationship or personality problems in either. Depression in a carer requiring treatment will not respond to measures to reduce burden alone, and treatment of the carer can bring about definite reductions in the perceived behavioural problems of the dementia sufferer. It seems that emotional support for carers is of more use than information (Sutcliffe & Larner 1988) for carers in general, though of course the latter is very important.

OTHER AFFECTIVE DISORDERS IN THE ELDERLY

Mania

Studies of elderly people with bipolar affective disorder have suggested that few cases begin in old age; approximately 90% of patients have been identified as bipolar by the age of 50 years. However, this does not seem to be the case with mania alone where the number of first admissions remains steady or may be slightly higher in older people (Broadhead & Jacoby, 1990). A number of authors have pointed out the high association between mania in old age and organic physical disease, but there appears to be no association with dementia.

The symptoms of mania in old age are indistinguishable from those occurring in younger patients, and admixtures of depressive symptoms are common. In addition, Broadhead & Jacoby found the time course of the episode and the outcome very similar between younger and older manic patients.

Treatment of acute manic illness is similar in all ages, with the proviso that much smaller doses of neuroleptic medication may suffice to control symptoms in older patients and the extrapyramidal side effects of butyrophenones may be disabling and long-lived. For recurrent episodes, lithium is effective, but needs very careful monitoring, especially in those with concurrent heart, lung or kidney disease. Even mild dehydration as a result of an infection may give rise to lithium toxicity, and hypothyroidism is an almost universal consequence in elderly people.

Anxiety states in the elderly

Lindesay has surveyed the literature on anxiety states in the elderly and divides his analysis into studies before 1975, and thus before the development of standardized diagnostic criteria for phobic disorder, and those after. Rates for all forms of neurosis in the first group appear to be between 7.5% and 25% of community samples; in the latter group the prevalence of all phobic disorder (including agoraphobia and specific phobias) is between 2.2% and 11.7% (J. Lindesay; personal communication 1990). Anxiety disorders are thus frequent in the community elderly and appear to be rarely referred for specialist help, and there is extensive comorbidity with depressive states. In his population studies, Lindesay found that very few subjects were receiving appropriate psychological treatments. Generalized anxiety and agoraphobia were associated with decreased social functioning, and an important association between the development of late-onset agoraphobia and traumatic physical health event raised the possibility of preventive work by geriatric physicians and surgeons. There is no evidence for the widely-held view that anxiety disorders in the elderly are less susceptible to treatment than in earlier life.

REFERENCES

Altamura A C, Mauri M C, Rudas N et al 1989 Clinical activity and tolerability of trazodone, mianserin and amitriptyline in elderly subjects with major depression: a controlled multicenter trial. Clinical Neuropharmacology 12 (suppl 1): S25–S33; S34–S37

American Psychiatric Association 1980 Diagnostic and statistical manual of mental disorders, 3rd edn. American Psychiatric Association, Washington, DC

Askinazi C, Weintraub R J, Karamouz N 1986 Elderly depressed females as a possible subgroup of patients responsive to methylphenidate, Journal of Clinical Psychiatry 47: 467–469

Baldessarini R J 1987 Neuropharmacology of s-adenosyl-L-methionine, American Journal of Medicine 83: 95–103

Baldwin R C, Jolley D J 1986 The prognosis of depression in old age. British Journal of Psychiatry 149: 574–583

Barsa J, Jones J, Lantigua R, Gurland B 1986 Ability of internists to recognize and manage depression in the elderly. International Journal of Geriatric Psychiatry 1: 57–62

Benbow S M 1987 The use of electroconvulsive therapy in old age psychiatry. International Journal of Geriatric Psychiatry 2: 25–30

Bird J M, Levy R, Jacoby R J 1986 Computed tomography in the elderly: change over time in the normal population. British Journal of Psychiatry 148: 80–86

Blazer D G 1978 The OARS Durham surveys: description and application. In: Multidimensional functional assessment: the OARS methodology, 2nd edn. Centre for the Study of Ageing and Human Development, Duke University, Durham, NC

Blazer D, Bachar J R, Hughes D C 1987 Major depression with melancholia: a comparison of middle-aged and elderly adults. Journal of the American Geriatrics Society 35: 927–932

Bridges P K 1983 . . . and a small dose of an antidepressant might help. British Journal of Psychiatry 142: 626–628

Broadhead J, Jacoby R 1990 Mania in old age: a first prospective study. International Journal of Geriatric Psychiatry 5: 215–222

Brown G W, Harris T O 1978 Social origins of depression. Tavistock Press, London

Burke W J, Rubin E H, Zorumski C F, Wetzel R D 1987 The safety of ECT in geriatric psychiatry. Journal of the American Geriatrics Society 35: 516–512

Cole M, Muler H F 1976 Sleep deprivation in the treatment of elderly depressive patients. Journal of the American Geriatrics Society 42: 308–313

Cook B L, Helms P M, Smith R E, Tsai M 1986 Unipolar depression in the elderly. Reoccurrence on discontinuation of tricyclic antidepressants. Journal of Affective Disorders 10: 91–94

Copeland J R M, Kelleher M J, Kellett J M et al 1976 A semistructured clinical interview for the assessment of diagnosis and mental state in the elderly. The Geriatric Mental State Schedule: 1. Development and reliability. Psychological Medicine 6: 439–449

Defrance R, Marey C, Kamoun A 1988 Antidepressant and anxiolytic activities of tianeptine: an overview of clinical trials. Clinical Neuropharmacology 11 (suppl 2): S74–S82

Drinka T J, Smith J C, Drinka P J 1987 Correlates of depression and burden for informal caregivers of patients in a geriatrics referral clinic. Journal of the American Geriatrics Society 35: 522–555

Duncan A J, Campbell A J 1988 Antidepressant drugs in the elderly: are the indications as long term as the treatment? British Medical Journal 296: 1230–1232

Eagles J M, Beattie J A, Blackwood G W, Restall D B, Ashcroft G W 1987 The mental health of elderly couples: I. The effects of a cognitively impaired spouse. British Journal of Psychiatry 150: 299–303

Eastwood M R, Rifat S L, Nobbs H, Ruderman J 1989 Mood disorder following cerebrovascular accident. British Journal of Psychiatry 154: 195–200

Ebrahim S, Barer D, Nouri F 1987 Affective illness after stroke. British Journal of Psychiatry 151: 52–56

Fasey C 1990 Grief in old age: a review of the literature. International Journal of Geriatric Psychiatry 5: 67–75

Feinmann C, Harris M, Cawley R 1964 Psychogenic facial pain: presentation and treatment. British Medical Journal 288: 436–438

Galzin A M, Davous P, Roudier M, Lamour Y, Poirier M F, Langer S Z 1989 Platelet 3H-imipramine binding is not modified in Alzheimer's disease. Psychiatry Research 28: 289–294

Georgotas A, McCue R E 1989 Relapse of depressed patients after effective continuation therapy. Journal of Affective Disorders 17: 159–164

Georgotas A, Stokes P, McCue R E et al 1986a The usefuless of DST in predicting response to antidepressants: a placebo-controlled study. Journal of Affective Disorders 11: 21–28

Georgotas A, McCue R E, Hapworth W et al 1986b Comparative efficacy and safety of MAOIs versus TCAs in treating depression in the elderly. Biological Psychiatry 221: 1155–1166

Georgotas A, Schweitzer J, McCue R E, Armour M, Friedhoff A J 1987a Clinical and treatment effects on 3H-clonidine and 3H-imipramine binding in elderly depressed patients. Life Sciences, 40: 2137–2143

Georgotas A, McCue R E, Friedman E, Cooper T B 1987b A placebo-controlled comparison of the effect of nortriptyline and phenelzine on orthostatic hypotension in elderly depressed patients. Journal of Clinical Psychopharmacology 7: 413–416

Georgotas A, McCue R E, Cooper T B, Chang I, Mir P, Welkowitz J 1987c Clinical predictors of response to antidepressants in elderly patients. Biological Psychiatry 22: 733–740

Georgotas A, McCue R E, Cooper T B, Nagachandran N, Chang I 1988 How effective and safe is continuation therapy in elderly depressed patients? Factors affecting relapse rate. Archives of General Psychiatry 45: 929–932

Gerson S C, Plotkin D A, Jarvik L F 1988 Antidepressant drug studies, 1964 to 1986: empirical evidence for aging patients. Journal of Clinical Psychopharmacology 8: 311–322

Gierl B, Groves L, Lazarus L W 1987 Use of the dexamethasone suppression test with depressed and demented elderly. Journal of the American Geriatrics Society 35: 115–120

Goldman L S, Luchins D J 1984 Depression in the spouses of demented patients. American Journal of Psychiatry 141: 1467

Greden J F, Flegel P, Haskett R, Dilsaver S, Carroll B J, Grunhaus L, Genero N 1986 Age effects in serial hypothalamic – pituitary – adrenal monitoring. Psychoneuroendocrinology 11: 195–204

Gurland B 1976 The comparative frequency of depression in various adult age groups. Journal of Gerontology 31: 283–292

Gurland B, Copeland J, Kuriansky J, Kelleher M, Sharpe L, Dean L L 1983 The mind and mood of ageing. Haworth, New York

Hale A S, Procter A W, Bridges P K 1987 Clomipramine, tryptophan and lithium in combination for resistant depression: seven case studies. British Journal of Psychiatry 151: 213–217

Hardy B G, Shulman K I, Mackenzie S E, Kutcher S P, Silverberg J D 1987 Pharmacokinetics of lithium in the elderly. Journal of Clinical Psychopharmacology 7: 153–158

Hartling O J, Marving J, Knudsen P, Dahl A, Hoilund-Carlsen P F, Hartling L 1987 The effect of the tricyclic antidepressant drug nortriptyline on left ventricular ejection fraction and left ventricular volumes. Psychopharmacology (Berlin) 91: 381–383

Hatfield B D, Goldfarb A H, Sforzo G A, Flynn M G 1987 Serum beta-endorphin and affective responses to graded exercise in young and elderly men. Journal of Gerontology 42: 429–431

Hedley R, Ebrahim S, Sheldon M 1986 Opportunities for anticipatory care with the elderly. Journal of Family Practice 22 : 141–145

Hendrickson E, Levy R, Post F 1979 Average evoked responses in relation to cognitive and affective states in elderly psychiatric patients. British Journal of Psychiatry 134: 494–501

Houck P R, Reynolds C F, Kopp U, Hanin I (1988) Red blood cell/plasma choline ratio in elderly depressed and demented patients. Psychiatry Research 24: 109–116

House A 1987 Depression after stroke. British Medical Journal 294: 76–78

House A, Dennis M, Warlow C, Hawton K, Molyneux A 1990 Mood disorders after stroke and their relation to lesion location: a CT scan study. Brain 113: 1113–1130

Jackson J E, Ramsdell J W, Renvall M, Swart J, Ward H 1989 Reliability of drug histories in a specialized geriatric outpatient clinic. Journal of General Internal Medicine 4: 39–43

Jacoby R J, Levy R 1980 Computed tomography in the elderly: 3. Affective Disorder. British Journal of Psychiatry 136: 270–275

Jacoby R J, Dolan R, Levy R, Baldy R 1983 Quantitative computed tomography in elderly depressed patients. British Journal of Psychiatry 143: 124–127

Jarvik L F, Mintz J, Steuer J, Gerner R 1982 Treating geriatric depression: a 26 week interim analysis. Journal of the American Geriatrics Society 30: 713–717

Karliner W 1978 ECT for patients with CNS disease. Psychosomatics 19: 781–783

Kay D W K 1962 Outcome and cause of death in mental disorders of old age: a long term follow up of functional and organic psychoses. Acta Psychiatrica Scandinavica 38: 249–276

Kay D W K, Bergmann K 1966 Physical disability and mental health in old age. Journal of Psychosomatic Research 10: 3–12

Kinzel T 1988 Relief of emotional symptoms in elderly patients with terminal cancer. Geriatrics 43: 61–65; 68

Kral V A, Emery O B 1989 Long term follow up of depressive pseudo-dementia of the aged. Canadian Journal of Psychiatry 34: 445–446

Kramer B A 1987 Electroconvulsive therapy use in geriatric depression. Journal of Nervous and Mental Disease 175: 233–235

Kutcher S P, Reid K, Dubbin J D, Shulman K I 1986 Electrocardiogram changes and therapeutic desipramine and 2-hydroxy-desipramine concentrations in elderly depressives. British Journal of Psychiatry 148: 676–679

Lader M 1987 Recent experience with trazodone. Psychopathology 20 (suppl 1): 39–47

Lafferman J, Solomon K, Ruskin P 1988 Lithium augmentation for treatment-resistant depression in the elderly. Journal of Geriatric Psychiatry and Neurology 1: 49–52

Laffey P, Peyster R, Nathan R, Haskin M, McGinley J 1984 Computed tomography and ageing: results in a normal elderly population. Neuroradiology 26: 273–278

Lakshmanan M, Mion L C, Frengley J D 1986 Effective low dose tricyclic antidepressant treatment for depressed geriatric rehabilitation patients. A double-blind study. Journal of the American Geriatrics Society 34: 421–426

Lampman R M 1987 Evaluating and prescribing exercise for elderly patients. Geriatrics, 42: 63–65; 69–70; 73–76

McCue R E, Georgotas A, Nagachandran N et al 1989

Plasma levels of nortriptyline and 10-hydroxynortriptyline and treatment-related electrocardiographic changes in the elderly depressed. Journal of Psychiatric Research 23: 73–79

Macdonald A J D 1986 Do general practitioners 'miss' depression in elderly patients? British Medical Journal 292: 1365–1367

Mahendra B 1983 'Pseudodementia': a misleading and illogical concept. British Journal of Psychiatry 143: 202

Mann A H, Graham N, Ashby D 1984a Psychiatric illness in residential homes for the elderly: a survey in one London borough. Age and Ageing 13: 257–265

Mann A H, Wood K, Cross P, Gurland B, Schieber P, Hafner H 1984b Institutional care of the elderly: a comparison of the cities of New York, London and Mannheim. Social Psychiatry 19: 97–102

Morin C M, Gramling S E 1989 Sleep patterns and aging: a comparison of older adults with and without insomnia complaints. Psychology of Aging 4: 290–294

Moritz D J, Kasl S V, Berkman L F 1989 The health impact of living with a cognitively impaired elderly spouse: depressive symptoms and social functioning. Journal of Gerontology 44: S17–S27

Murphy E 1982 Social origins of depression in old age. British Journal of Psychiatry 141: 135–142

Murphy E 1983 The prognosis of depression in old age. British Journal of Psychiatry 142: 111–119

Murphy E, Smith R, Lindesay J, Slattery J 1988 Increased mortality rates in late life depression. British Journal of Psychiatry 152: 347–353

Myers J K, Weissman M M, Tischler G L et al 1984 Six month prevalence of psychiatric disorders in three communities. Archives of General Psychiatry 41: 959–967

Nemeroff C B, Knight D L, Krishnan R R, Slotkin T A, Bissette G, Melville M L, Blazer D G 1988 Marked reduction in the number of platelet-tritiated imipramine binding sites in geriatric depression. Archives of General Psychiatry 45: 919–923

Ouslander J G 1982 Physical illness and depression in the elderly. Journal of the American Geriatrics Society 30: 593–599

Parkes C M 1964 Recent bereavement as a cause of mental illness. British Journal of Psychiatry 110: 198–204

Popkin S J, Gallagher D, Thompson L, Moore M 1982 Memory complaint and performance in normal and depressed older adults. Experimental Ageing and Research 8: 141–145

Post F 1962 The significance of affective symptoms in old age. Maudsley Monographs 10. Oxford University Press, London

Post F 1972 The management and nature of depressive illness in late life: a follow through study. British Journal of Psychiatry 121: 393–404

Rakel R E 1987 The greater safety of trazodone over tricyclic antidepressant agents: 5 year experience in the United States. Psychopathology 20 (Suppl 1): 57–63

Raskind M, Peskind E, Rivard M, Veith R, Barnes R 1982 DST and cortisol circadian rhythm in primary degenerative dementia. American Journal of Psychiatry 179: 1468–1471

Reynolds C F, Kupfer D J, Hoch C C, Stack J A, Houck P R, Sewitch D E 1986 Two year follow up of elderly patients with mixed depression and dementia. Clinical and electroencephalographic sleep findings. Journal of the American Geriatrics Society, 34: 793–799

Reynolds C F, Kupfer D J, Houck P R, Hoch C C, Stack J A, Berman S R, Zimmer B 1988 Reliable discrimination of elderly depressed and demented patients by electroencephalographic sleep data. Archives of General Psychiatry 45: 258–264

Reynolds C F, Perel J M, Frank E et al 1989 Open, trial maintenance pharmacotherapy in late-life depression: survival analysis. Psychiatry Research 27: 225–231

Robins L N, Helzer J, Croughan J, Ratcliff K S 1981 National Institute of Mental Health Diagnostic Interview Schedule: its history, characteristics and validity. Archives of General Psychiatry 38: 381–389

Robinson R G, Starr L B, Price T R 1984a A two year longitudinal study of mood disorders following stroke: a six month follow-up. British Journal of Psychiatry 144: 256–262

Robinson R G, Kubos K L, Starr L B, Rao K, Price T R 1984b Mood disorders in stroke patients: importance of location of lesion. Brain 107: 81–93

Robinson R G, Bolla-Wilson K, Kaplan E, Lipsey J R, Price T R 1986 Depression influences intellectual impairment in stroke patients. British Journal of Psychiatry 148: 541–547

Satel S L, Nelson J C 1989 Stimulants in the treatment of depression: a critical overview. Journal of Clinical Psychiatry 50: 241–249

Schneider L S, Severson J A, Pollock V, Cowan R P, Sloane R B 1986a Platelet monoamine oxidase activity in elderly depressed outpatients. Biological Psychiatry 21: 1360–1364

Schneider L S, Fredrickson E R, Severson J A, Sloane R B 1986b 3H-imipramine binding in depressed elderly: relationship to family history and clinical response. Psychiatry Research 19: 257–266

Schneider L S, Sloane R B, Staples F R, Bender M 1986c Pretreatment orthostatic hypotension as a predictor of response to nortriptyline in geriatric depression. Journal of Clinical Psychopharmacology 6: 172–176

Schneider L S, Cooper T B, Staples F R, Sloane R B 1987 Prediction of individual dosage of nortriptyline in depressed elderly outpatients. Journal of Clinical Psychopharmacology 7: 311–314

Schneider L S, Severson J A, Sloane R B, Frederickson E R 1988a Decreased platelet 3H-imipramine binding in primary major depression compared with depression secondary to medical illness in elderly outpatients. Journal of Affective Disorders 15: 195–200

Schneider L S, Cooper T B, Severson J A, Zemplenyi T, Sloane R B 1988b Electrocardiographic changes with nortriptyline and 10-hydroxynortriptyline in elderly depressed outpatients. Journal of Clinical Psychopharmacology 8: 402–408

Shephard R J 1983 Physical activity and the healthy mind. Canadian Medical Association Journal 128: 525

Shulman K I 1989 Conceptual problems in the assessment of depression in old age. Psychiatric Journal of the University of Ottawa 14: 364–366

Simon R I 1989 Silent suicide in the elderly. Bulletin of the American Academy of Psychiatry and the Law 17: 83–95

Sommer B R, Satlin A, Friedman L, Cole J O 1989 Glycopyrrolate versus atropine in post-ECT amnesia in the elderly. Journal of Geriatric Psychiatry and Neurology 2: 18–21

Spar J E 1987 Plasma trazodone concentrations in elderly depressed inpatients: cardiac effects and short-term efficacy. Journal of Clinical Psychopharmacology 7: 406–409

Srole L, Fischer A K 1980 The midtown Manhattan longitudinal study versus the 'Paradise Lost' doctrine. Archives of General Psychiatry 37: 209–221

Stack J A, Reynolds C F, Perel J M, Houck P R, Hoch C C, Kupfer D J 1988 Pretreatment systolic orthostatic blood pressure (PSOP) and treatment response in elderly depressed inpatients. Journal of Clinical Psychopharmacology 8: 116–120

Sutcliffe C, Larner S 1988 Counselling carers of the elderly at home: a preliminary study. British Journal of Clinical Psychology 27: 177–178

Taylor A E, Saint-Cyr J A, Lang A E, Kenny F T 1986 Parkinson's disease and depression: a critical re-evaluation. Brain 109: 279–292

Teicher M H, Lawrence J M, Barber N I, Kinkelstein S P, Lieberman H R, Baldessarini R J 1988 Increased activity and phase delay in circadian motility rhythms in geriatric depression. Preliminary observations. Archives of General Psychiatry 45: 913–917

Tempesta E, Casella L, Pirrongelli C, Janiri L, Calvani M, Ancona L 1987 L-acetylcarnitine in depressed elderly subjects. A crossover study vs placebo. Drugs under Experimental and Clinical Research 13: 417–423

Tyrer P 1976 Towards rational therapy with monoamine oxidase inhibitors. British Journal of Psychiatry 128: 354–360

Wachtel H, Loschmann P A, Pietzuch P 1988 Absence of anticholinergic activity of rolipram, an antidepressant with a novel mechanism of action, in three different animal models in vivo. Pharmacopsychiatry 21: 218–221

Wasserman D 1989 Passive euthanasia in response to attempted suicide: one form of aggressiveness by relatives. Acta Psychiatrica Scandinavica 79: 460–467

Wilkins J N, Spar J E, Carlson H E 1989 Desipramine increases circulating growth hormone in elderly depressed patients: a pilot study. Psychoneuroendocrinology 14: 195–202

Zemore R, Eames N 1979 Psychic and somatic symptoms of depression among young adults, institutionalised aged and non-institutionalised aged. Journal of Gerontology 31: 283–292

Zung W W K 1967 Depression in the normal aged. Psychosomatics 8: 287–292

39. Bereavement

Warwick Middleton   Beverley Raphael

It is perhaps paradoxical that the very ubiquity of bereavement and its central place in so many theoretical structures has made it such a difficult area to study. Bereavement represents a meeting point for ethology, transcultural studies, life events research, psychoanalysis, behaviourism, sociology, psychosomatic medicine, personality theory and developmental psychiatry.

Faced with the complexities involved there has been a tendency to oversimplify the process or else to concentrate research on areas that seem to be more associated with 'pathology'. The difficulty in trying to establish parameters which separate 'normal' from 'pathological' forms of grief may be due to a preoccupation with the nature of the loss rather than with the powerful influences of pre-existing attachment and character of the bereaved.

Furthermore, the interrelationships between bereavement and depression have been confused. There is often an assumption that the phenomenology of grief is the same as that of depression, at least in overt affective parameters. Attempts to measure bereavement reactions have frequently involved the use of depression scales.

A common feature of the bereavement literature is the use of terms or concepts as if they had broad acceptance or there were widely agreed criteria that define them. Yet in this regard the bereavement literature lags behind that of many other research areas. Stroebe & Stroebe (1987) point out that the terms 'grief', 'mourning' and 'bereavement' are often used interchangeably. They attempt to differentiate between them by using 'bereavement' to refer to 'the objective situation of an individual who has recently experienced the loss of someone significant through that person's death' (p 7). They see bereavement as being the cause of both grief and mourning; where 'grief' is the individual's emotional response to loss, and includes a number of psychological and somatic reactions, and 'mourning' refers to expressive acts of grief that are influenced by the mourning practices of a particular society or culture.

It should be noted, however, that many writers use the term 'mourning' to describe intrapsychic processes occasioned by loss.

CONCEPTUAL PERSPECTIVES

Psychodynamic

Freud's father died in October 1886 and he wrote to Fliess describing the powerful effect which the loss had on him (Jones 1953, p 324). In 1917 Freud published *Mourning and Melancholia*, an attempt to compare grief and depression and to thus demonstrate that grief could be used as a model for clinical depression. In attempting to view both as reactions to loss, Freud had a difficulty in that with depressed subjects a loss could not always be identified, and he was left to suggest that the memory of such losses is sometimes repressed.

Freud's concept of mourning was based on his energy model and included in it was what he described as the 'work' of mourning, a process by which the mourner over time repeatedly examines aspects of the relationship with the lost person in such a way as to allow for the gradual relinquishment of libidinal bonds to that person. Freud (1977), however, stated: 'Why this process of carrying out the behest of reality bit by bit, which is in the nature of compromise, should be so extraordinarily painful is not at all easy to explain in terms of mental economics' (p 154).

Freud at this stage felt that healthy grief and depression could only be distinguished by the absence of guilt, self-reproach and lowered self-esteem in the former, and their presence in 'pathological' grief. Freud felt that the object of self-accusations for those with pathological grief was really the lost object and that the underlying reason for this happening was the existence of an ambivalent relationship with that person. As that person became introjected, the hostile side of the ambivalence which was focused on the lost individual thus became directed inwards against the bereaved's own ego, leading to depression.

Later, Freud (1923) modified his view that identification characterizes only pathological grief, concluding that libidinal withdrawal from any love object occurs through the ego identifying with that object.

In delineating the features of acute grief, Lindemann built upon Freud's model to produce the first detailed systematic description. While his choice of subjects was hardly typical of bereaved populations in general, his descriptions have endured. In 1944 he reported his observations on 101 bereaved subjects. In summary, the acute symptoms of normal grief included:

1) sensations of somatic distress, which included a feeling of tightness in the throat, choking with shortness of breath, need for sighing and an empty feeling in the abdomen, lack of muscular power and an intense subjective distress experienced as tension or mental pain
2) intense preoccupation with the image of the deceased
3) self-blame and strong feelings of guilt
4) a loss of warmth toward others, with a tendency to respond with irritability and anger
5) a loss of usual behaviour patterns, with aimless moving about and difficulty in initiating or sustaining organized activity.

To these Lindemann added a sixth characteristic, 'shown by patients who border on pathological reactions' and this was 'the appearance of traits of the deceased in the behaviour of the bereaved' (p 142). This identification with the deceased could be in the form of taking up activities previously associated with the lost person. The theme of decathexis was integral to Lindemann's description of grief work (Lindemann 1979).

> This grief work has to do with the effort of reliving and working through in small quantities events which involved the now-deceased person and the survivor; the things one did together, the roles one had vis-á-vis each other, which were complementary to each other and which one would pass through day by day in the day's routine. Each item of this shared role has to be thought through, pained through, if you want, and gradually the question is raised, How can I do that with somebody else? (p 234)

While suggesting that the normal grief process averaged about 4 months, Lindemann believed that the duration depended on the success of the bereaved person's 'grief work' or the 'emancipation from the bondage of the deceased, readjustment to the environment . . . and the formation of new relationships'.

Analytical works on bereavement include those by Deutsch (1937), Klein (1940), Anna Freud (1958) and Wolfenstien (1966). Pollock's (1961) model of mourning was of the initial stage of shock being followed by the grief reaction proper. This process is brought to conclusion by restructuring the representation of the lost object from one of reality to one of memory.

Engel (1961) took the somewhat extreme view of conceptualizing even 'uncomplicated adaptive grief' as a 'disease' in that it 'represents a manifest and gross departure from the dynamic state considered representative of health and well-being' (p 20). Anticipating later research, Engel suggested that biochemical or physiological processes associated with grief could allow for unfavourable somatic changes.

Attachment theory

It was the analyst John Bowlby (1971, 1975, 1981) who introduced a new dimension to views of bereavement by integrating analytical and ethological theories. Central to the theory is attachment, a behavioural system which, ethological studies suggested, was common to many species. Its function is to ensure personal and species preservation. Grief is thus seen as an extension of a general response to separation. It was on separation that Bowlby's earlier work concentrated (Robertson & Bowlby 1952, Bowlby 1960) in studying the responses of 2–3-year-old healthy children temporarily separated from their mothers in hospital or residential-care nurseries. These children responded to the initial separation by protesting tearfully and angrily. After several days hope for a quick reunion appeared to fade and the children appeared preoccupied and despairing. Hope and despair would often alternate until, after more prolonged separation they appeared detached and, if then reunited with their mothers, would be unresponsive for hours or even days. When this unresponsiveness subsided it was then replaced by manifestations of overanxious attachment, such as clinging behaviour or rage and anxiety at even the briefest separation. In Bowlby's model an attachment object, particularly a mother, provides a secure base from which the child can explore his/her environment.

Confronted with a threat the child retreats to the attachment object, but if that attachment object is missing the retreating child becomes terrified. Applying this principle, Bowlby accounts for why distress is so universal in response to separation from an attachment object.

While a restricted definition of attachment emphasizes the role of the adult in providing for and protecting the dependent child, the theory has been extended by many to include the maintenance of a mutually reinforcing relationship with a particular adult. Many of the key responses on the part of the bereaved reflect similar themes to the phenomena of separation. Central to Bowlby's theories in his thesis that: 'If . . . the urges to recover and scold are automatic responses built into the organism, it follows that they will come into action in response to any and every loss and without discriminating between those that are really retrievable and those, statistically rare, that are not' (Bowlby 1979, p 53).

Bowlby concluded that not only did mourning in mentally healthy adults last for longer than was often suggested, but several of the responses widely regarded as pathological were in fact common in healthy mourning. These included anger directed at third parties, the self and sometimes the lost person, disbelief that the loss had occurred and a tendency, often, though not always, unconscious, to search for the lost person in the hope of reunion (Bowlby 1982).

Thus Bowlby saw separation phenomena, particularly anxiety and anger, as part of the reaction to loss and when hope was given up for the return of the lost object sadness, depression and despair would supervene until acceptance and reorganization, with the formation of new attachments, was possible (Bowlby 1981). He put forward a phasic model which defined depressive phenomena as an inevitable part of the process of adjusting to the loss of an attachment figure.

In Bowlby's opinion manifestations of pathological grief could be linked to childhood experiences and the pattern of parental attachment behaviour. Bowlby believed that 'pathogenic parenting' had a marked detrimental impact and made vulnerable those individuals who experienced it, e.g. those adults whose childhoods were characterized by anxious attachment to parents would be likely to have insecure attachments to marital partners and be overly dependent and more vulnerable to developing chronic grief.

Another pattern of disordered attachment was compulsive self-reliance, in which the individual is reluctant to accept care and insists on doing everything by themselves. Such a person may deny loss or be vulnerable to delayed onset of grief.

Parkes (1972, 1985) has further delineated the attachment model of bereavement. He has highlighted particularly the 'searching behaviours' of the bereaved which include yearning and pining for the lost person and a perceptual set for that person reflecting the attachment to them.

It is interesting to note how powerful the influence attachment theory has been on senior researchers, clinicians and theoreticians in the field of bereavement. A survey (Raphael & Middleton 1989) showed that 75% of the group surveyed ($n = 60$) utilized attachment theory as a principal theoretical framework.

Cultural issues

Viewed from an ethological viewpoint it would be predicted that, while external manifestations may be modified by cultural practices, core elements of grief would be universal for members of the human species. From the admittedly incomplete evidence it would seem that grief is universally felt, though its manifestations in different cultures are extremely varied.

Attention has focused on how these core responses of grief have become integrated into diverse mourning practices and on whether particular practices mean that the members of certain cultures have advantages or disadvantages to their coping. One hypothesis is that those cultures that encourage the expression of grief may be more adaptive. For example, Miller & Schoenfeld (1973) describe the Navajo Indians as limiting their mourning to only 4 days, with excessive emotion even during this period being discouraged. They argue that this prohibition of mourning is linked to pathological grief, which principally takes the form of depression.

Crying and some form of emotional upset seem to be universal features of grief. Supporting this is the finding by Izard (1977) that the interpretation of facial expressions showing basic emotions is stable across cultures, supporting Charles Darwin's original observation that 'the power to bring the grief-muscles freely into play appears to be hereditary' (Darwin 1965, p 182). Across cultures the trend is for women to cry as frequently or more frequently than men following a loss (Rosenblatt et al 1976).

There is marked diversity in mourning rituals. The Kota Indians of Southern India have two funerals; the first, the Green Funeral, takes place shortly after the death and is attended by close relatives and friends of the deceased. Intense grief is expressed and, following cremation, a piece of skull bone is recovered and reverently stored until the Dry Funeral, which occurs yearly for all the deaths in the community and lasts 11 days. For the first 2 days of the Dry Funeral bereaved women wail while male counterparts weep. Strict mourning taboos apply and for the first week the dead are memorialized individually while the non-bereaved dance to distract the mourners. Finally, the bones and personal ornaments are placed on a pyre. Following the cremation the new dawn heralds an abrupt change of mood, with dancing and feasting continuing until nightfall when a pot is smashed, symbolizing the departure of the dead. Widows and widowers have sexual relations with the siblings of their dead spouses and festivities continue for 5 more days (Goldberg 1982).

Mourning customs such as these can serve the function of reinforcing the religious and social structure of the group as well as allowing emotional expression for the bereaved (Averill 1968). What is sanctioned or prohibited in one society may differ diametrically from what is or is not permitted in another.

Kleinman et al (1989) make the salient point that 'the contemporary Western practice of systematically looking for the health consequences of bereavement is so unusual in cross-cultural perspective that it can be regarded a result of Westernization' (p 205). In considering the features of complicated grief and its relationship to depression we need, for example, to keep in mind that three-quarters of the world's societies express depression with somatic rather than mental symptoms (Kleinman, quoted by Eisenbruch 1984).

Animal models

Animal studies formed an essential cornerstone of attachment theory.

Humans are a social species and, like many other primates, live in groups (Averill 1979). The acute responses of infants to separation are quite similar across species, including guinea pig, dog, human (Hirsch et al 1984).

The similarities in the response of human children and infant monkeys to separation has stimulated a body of research into behavioural, immunological, endocrine and other physiological parameters.

It was with Rhesus monkeys that Harlow and colleagues (Harlow & Mears 1979) carried out their observations on 6-month-old monkeys separated from their mothers for a 3-week period by a Plexiglas partition which allowed them to see each other. After extreme protest and attempts at breaking through, the infants over a few days became lethargic and withdrawn.

How much these models of animal separation-induced depression can be equated with the bereavement process is conjectural. Research in the area has demonstrated, for example, immunological changes in infant monkeys that parallel those seen in bereaved adult humans (Laudenslager, 1988). However there are basic physiological differences between Rhesus and squirrel monkeys in response to separation. For example, the squirrel monkey has a more labile endocrine response in terms of elevations in blood cortisol levels than does the Rhesus monkey or human. While demonstrating physical changes, such findings highlight the difficulties of interpretation.

PSYCHOSOMATIC ISSUES

Psychiatry has struggled with the best conceptualization of the influence of bereavement on biological and psychological parameters. Theories range from altered health behaviours to models such as Hofer's (1984), postulating relationships as psychobiological regulators which are disrupted by loss.

Stroebe & Stroebe (1987) feel that the most convincing evidence of a relationship between bereavement and health comes from mortality studies, although there are plausible alternative explanations for increased mortality findings, such as assortive mating or joint shared unfavourable environments.

Widowers have been identified as the bereaved group at greatest risk of increased mortality. Hypotheses for increased mortality have focused on a number of factors, cardiovascular disease being the most prominent. Suicide (Klerman & Izen 1977) may be more common than official statistics indicate.

While loss is a significant focus of psychosomatic medicine, it has proved to be difficult to establish whether health deterioration, when it occurs, is caused by loss accelerating or aggravating existing illnesses or whether loss can in fact cause new disease.

In their Harvard Study Glick and co-workers (1974) reported that four times as many bereaved as non-bereaved were hospitalized during the year following their bereavement. However, in statistically controlling for the possible effect of depression influencing health measures, Stroebe et al (1985) found no significant differences in self-reported physical health between married and widowed groups.

Other possible mechanisms for increased disease or

elevated death ratios include changes to the immune or endocrine systems, alteration in health-related behaviour such as increased smoking, dieting changes, increased alcohol and drug intake, or failure to identify or care for illness (Raphael & Middleton 1987).

The excess mortality seems to relate principally to cardiovascular events (Reich et al 1981), in accordance with the model of sudden and rapid death during psychological stress as described by Engel (1971). Parkes and co-workers (1969) reported heart and circulatory diseases as accounting for two-thirds of the increase in mortality during the first 6 months after bereavement.

Bartrop and colleagues (1977) produced the first demonstration of a relationship between bereavement and alterations in immune function when they monitored several aspects of the immunity of 26 surviving spouses of patients who had died following fatal injury and prolonged illness. Measured at 2 and 6 weeks, they found suppression of lymphocyte mitogenic stimulation in response to two particular mitogens (phytohemaglutinin and conA), but no other significant differences.

The essential findings were replicated (Schleifer et al 1983), while in a more recent study (Kiecolt-Glaser & Glaser 1986) the blood of 15 men whose wives had advanced cancer was collected before and after the death of their spouses. Their lymphocytes showed a poorer proliferative response after their wives' deaths than before.

Endocrine studies have failed to show a simple relationship between grief and adrenocortical activity and there is no evidence to date that endocrine parameters predict either medical or psychiatric illness in the bereaved (Jacobs 1987). Dexamethasone suppression tests have failed to demonstrate significant levels of non-suppression amongst the bereaved (Schuchter et al 1986).

RELATIONSHIP WITH DEPRESSION

While the key distinction that Freud (1917) made between grief and depression was that the former was not acompanied by lowered self-esteem, Stroebe et al (1985) demonstrated that young widows and widowers who were not clinically depressed nevertheless experienced lowered self-esteem when matched with married controls.

In Freud's conceptualization an ambivalent relationship with the person who was lost allowed the hate to be internalized and directed towards the self, e.g. turning murderous impulses into suicidal thoughts and behaviour. Raphael (1978) showed that there were increased levels of depression, and depression of greater intensity, among widows who had had ambivalent relationships with their deceased husbands and who had not had support to deal with these ambivalent aspects in their grieving. Bowlby (1981), however, noted that the loss of an ambivalently loved person was in many cases consistent with healthy mourning.

Adding to the complexity is the propensity for bereaved to become clinically depressed. Clayton & Darvish (1979), in prospective studies of widows and widowers, found that 42% at 1 month and 15% at 1 year had symptom constellations of sufficient severity to meet Feighner criteria for the diagnosis of depression.

Whether using clinical criteria or rating scales, the vast majority of studies have found the bereaved to have a heightened risk of depression. However, given the differing criteria and the high refusal rates inherent in many longer-term studies, caution is required in interpreting figures. Typifying the trend in the longer term, Zisook and colleagues (1987) observed depression to be present in around 32% of surviving spouses at 1 month and to steadily decline to a prevalence of under 10% 4 years later.

As Stroebe & Stroebe (1987) point out, 'the absence of a clear boundary separating normal grief from clinical depression should not be mistaken to imply that grief and depression are one and the same syndrome' (p 23). Features distinguishing grief from depression in general include what Parkes (1985) describes as the 'pangs of grief', episodes of restlessness, angry pining and anxiety occasioned by any reminders of the loss and including the autonomic accompaniments of anxiety and fear. Further differentiating factors include the initial numbness and the experiences of yearning for the lost person, brief hallucinations (including hearing or seeing the lost person), preoccupation with memories of the deceased and identification-related behaviours, e.g. adopting mannerisms or interests of the lost person, or wearing their clothes.

While depression figures prominently in descriptions of complicated grief, it is by no means the only avenue of complication. Although widows may experience depression, males may be susceptible in addition to alcohol-related problems (Mor et al 1986).

Loss may create a vulnerability for the subsequent development of depression. Brown & Harris (1978) found in women in Camberwell that past loss influenced the severity of depression. Past loss by death predisposed those where the loss was early (before 11) to psychotic depression, whereas those whose past loss was by separation were at risk of developing neurotic depression. While vulnerability factors provided the background predisposition, it needed the presence of a provoking agent to lead to depression, the form of which was influenced by symptom formation factors. Congruent with Bowlby's work, Brown & Harris suggested that loss by death led to a sense of abandonment and retarded hopelessness, while loss through separation was less irredeemable but resulted in a sense of rejection and protesting despair.

UNCOMPLICATED GRIEF

Brown & Stoudemire (1983) synthesized the observations of Lindemann (1944), Bowlby (1961, 1963), Parkes (1970) and Greenblatt (1978) to arrive at a three-stage model of the bereavement process.

The first stage, shock, begins with the loss and is particularly marked where the loss is sudden and unanticipated. It encompasses the initial defences used by the individual confronted with an overwhelming painful reality, e.g. denial, disbelief and numbing as well as a range of somatic symptoms such as crying, throat tightness, dysphagia, sighing respirations, chest tightness, nausea and a sensation of abdominal emptiness.

So profound may be the shock that in trying to deal with it the bereaved may be concerned that they are going insane or that the situation seems unreal or unbelievable. They may become dazed or immobilized.

The second stage, commencing 1–14 days after the loss, is characterized by a preoccupation with the deceased in which the bereaved person becomes socially withdrawn, at the same time thinking about and dreaming about the lost person. Past conflicts are re-examined and guilt and anger are frequent.

Parkes (1970) and Bowlby (1962, 1963) emphasize yearning and searching for the lost object. Parkes (1985) points out that restlessness, anger, anxiety and pining (which Parkes considers pathogonomic for the grief reaction), brought on by reminders of the loss and accompanied by the affect of anxiety and fear, have close parallels to the 'separation anxiety' of young children separated from their mothers. In Bowlby's (1961) view the searching phase reaches peak intensity during the period 2–4 weeks following the death. So intense is the preoccupation with the deceased that transient hallucinatory episodes may be experienced in which the deceased's voice is heard or, alternatively, strangers may be mistaken for the deceased.

The bereaved, through processes of identification, may transiently adopt the mannerisms, the habits and even the somatic symptoms of the deceased (Zisook & De Vaul 1985).

Symptoms experienced during this phase include sadness, insomnia, fatigue, anhedonia and anorexia. While symptoms may ameliorate after 6 months, they can be activated at later times by anniversary reactions.

The third phase is described by the term 'resolution', a word widely used in bereavement literature and yet poorly defined. At its simplest level it refers to a subjective self-assessment on the part of the bereaved of having got over the loss. Objectively it might be viewed, for example, as having got to the point where the past, which includes the lost person, can be thought about pleasurably or where new relationships can be formed and interest renewed in work or other activities.

Clearly 'resolution' has many parameters, which range from psychoanalytical concepts of having 'worked through' the loss, to the completion of a social/cultural mourning period; to the diminution of particular symptoms, thoughts or behaviours associated with the loss, to more objective measures of a return to pre-bereavement functioning. The concept of resolution of bereavement is currently being systematically investigated to clarify some of these issues (Middleton 1990). Where the emphasis is placed influences estimates of the time course of uncomplicated grief. While Lindemann (1944) felt that uncomplicated grief averaged 4 months in duration, the subsequent trend has been for bereavement researchers to conceptualize grief as a longer process that may extend beyond the 1–2 years traditionally assumed to encompass it.

While not usually pathogenic, some grief phenomena appear enduring. Zisook & De Vaul (1985) report bereaved 10 years after their loss as still being preoccupied with the lost person, dreaming about them, missing and idealizing them, as well as being prone to respond to reminders by distress or crying.

TYPES OF LOSS

Loss of spouse

The most frequently studied grief has been that of bereaved spouses, with subjects being more usually widows than widowers, a result of men tending to marry women younger than themselves and also on average dying at a younger age.

For bereaved spouses issues may include not only the

loss of the loved or ambivalently loved partner but also the loss of a breadwinner, the loss of a sexual partner, the need to take on responsibilities not previously envisaged and having limited opportunities to develop alternative relationships.

Lopata (1979) characterized younger widows (between 30 and 54) as having to face the difficult challenges of having dependent children and feeling abandoned by their married friends as well as suffering a markedly reduced income. Older women faced the prospect of social isolation.

For some the issue of sexual relationships is conflictual. Sexual feelings may be quite strong, despite the loss or imminent loss. Where there has been a prolonged illness, the survivor may have suppressed his/her sexual feelings and their re-emergence may occasion surprise and perhaps some guilt (Shuchter & Zisook 1987).

Loss of child

In a study of 14 bereaved parents, Sanders (1979–1980) found that the loss of a child (age range 6–49), compared with the loss of a parent or spouse, 'occasioned more intense grief reactions of somatic types, and greater depression. As well parents experienced anger and guilt with accompanying feelings of despair' (p 309). This finding supported Gorer's conclusion that the death of a grown child was the most difficult and longest lasting grief to bear (Gorer 1965).

The untimely death of a child known to the parent for perhaps a few years is seemingly more difficult to cope with than the timely death of an elderly parent who has been known a lifetime. Children often die as a result of accident or chronic illness. The former is likely to be associated with guilt and the latter with feelings of powerlessness and marital stress. The issues are poignantly condensed in Eliot Luby's observation (Osterweis et al 1984). 'When your parent dies, you have lost your past. When your child dies, you have lost your future' (p 4).

Following the loss of a child it is common for parents to be overprotective of remaining children, while the lost child is idealized, a process that can also apply in the replacement-child syndrome (Cain & Cain 1964). Here the lost child is replaced by a baby whom the parents then attempt to shape into a very idealized and often unrealistic image of the child they have lost. While overprotected, this child is also compared unfavourably with the dead sibling.

Miscarriage, stillbirth and perinatal death

Stillbirths illustrate that grief may be marked even when the lost object has not had the opportunity to form a conventional identity. For example, Cullberg (1972) reported that 19 of 56 women who had experienced a stillbirth suffered a variety of major psychological symptoms 1–2 years after their baby's death, including anxiety attacks, phobias and severe depressive states, with those who had initially suppressed their feelings being particularly prone to ongoing symptoms.

Women who experience miscarriage, stillbirth or perinatal death, as Lovell (1983) points out, lose the role of mother and parent simultaneously. Such women may feel anger (Raphael 1983), or be ashamed at their inability to produce a healthy child and are left to mourn a loss which is invisible to others.

As Condon (1986) points out, a repeated finding in the literature is that approximately one-third of parents bereaved by stillbirth perceive the obstetric team as failing to provide adequate support or information in both the short and longer terms.

A number of researchers (e.g. Stringham et al 1982) agree that holding the dead infant is helpful to the grief-resolution process.

Infants who die in the perinatal period do attain a living identify, though some of the same responses elicited in the case of stillbirth may apply (Benfield et al 1978). Mothers blame themselves for the deaths far more than do fathers. Clearly the bonds of parents to the unborn or newborn child may be intense and the loss of the child may induce profound grief.

Loss of parent

The response of adults to the loss of a parent has been little studied, despite it being an almost universal event. It appears that the loss of a parent in adult life, particularly when the death is timely and anticipated, is generally coped with relatively well. It is not infrequently the focus for constructive internalizations and creative outcomes. Nevertheless, those who have not negotiated their own independent adult development may be particularly prone to complicated bereavement.

Childhood grief

There has been considerable debate about whether young children have the developmental prerequisite for mourning. Studies such as Weller's (1989) have indicated that young children do grieve. Grief may be demonstrated in those as young as 2 (Raphael 1982). They may show behavioural disturbance, regression and withdrawal, but also demonstrate features found in bereaved adults such as yearning and pining for the lost person, preoccupation and searching behaviour. The relationship between childhood loss and childhood depression or subsequent depression in adult life remains to be fully clarified particularly as most bereaved children appear to go on to successful adult adaptation.

Anticipatory grief

Anticipatory grief (Lindemann 1944) is a concept applied to grief symptomatology expressed in advance of a loss that is considered inevitable. While anticipatory grief may increase in intensity as the expected loss becomes imminent, when the loss does occur the individual may demonstrate fewer manifestations of acute grief than would have been the case had the death been unexpected.

Extending the model to verification by research, however, has proved difficult in that the ameliorative effect of prior warning may be cancelled out by the difficulties in, for instance, looking after someone with terminal illness. The available evidence indicates that sudden, unexpected deaths lead to greater intensities of grief and health risks than expected deaths. Rando (1988) states that the term is a misnomer, arguing that grieving for a future loss may not necessarily imply detachment, and he goes on to make the point that premature detachment may signify anticipatory grief gone awry.

Jacobs et al (1987) have demonstrated some anticipatory bereavement processes for those facing imminent threatened loss such as pangs of grief, while a bereaved comparison group showed greater levels of searching behaviours and perceptual set for the partner.

COMPLICATED GRIEF

The bereavement literature has failed to achieve consensus on how best to conceptualize and delineate the various ways in which the grieving process can differ significantly from the expected patterns of 'normal' grieving. It is generally agreed that earlier descriptions of grief such as Lindemann's differentiated excessively between normal and pathological. Given the multiple variables that can affect its outcome, it is not surprising that variations in the bereavement experience have proved difficult to classify.

Modifying variables

The sorts of variable suggested or identified as affecting grief can be summarized under the following headings:

1. Type of loss

Evidence suggests that grief is particularly long-lasting where the loss is untimely (such as that of a child) or unexpected. Parkes & Weiss (1983) reported a comparison of bereaved spouses: of a group who had 'brief or no' forewarning, 2–4 years after the loss only one of 18 respondents was rated as doing well or very well whereas, of those with more than 2 weeks forewarning, 63% of 41 respondents were doing well.

Losses which are difficult to acknowledge publicly or which are in some way socially stigmatized, such as death from AIDS or suicide, may prove particularly problematical. Likewise, losses through abortion, miscarriage or adoption may not be easily acknowledged (Lazare 1979). Survivors of suicide deaths have been described as more prone to guilt (Sheskin & Wallace 1976) and search more for explanation than non-suicide survivors.

Death from AIDS occurs in relatively young, recently healthy people and is frequently the result of infection acquired via homosexual contact or intravenous drug use. Close family members may not have had the opportunity to accept the lifestyle associated with AIDS prior to having to deal with the loss. Spouses may have to confront the irrefutable proof that assumptions about the exclusivity of their relationship were false and they may be further outraged at the risk to which they themselves have been put (Houseman & Pheifer 1988).

2. Circumstances of the loss

Where loss occurs in circumstances where there could be cause for blaming the survivor, e.g. a parent failing to supervise a child who drowns (Nixon & Pearn 1977); where the loss occurs in the context of some traumatic event such as a disaster (Raphael 1986); where the circumstances suggest mismanagement, e.g. failure of hospital staff to make a life-saving diagnosis (Raphael 1977); or where there are multiple simultaneous losses (Kastenbaum 1969), grief may not readily resolve.

In a particularly traumatized group of survivors, those who lived through the devastation of Hiroshima, Lifton (1967) described 'death guilt' among survivors who felt that they had been saved at the cost of other's lives. Further, they experienced what Lifton called the 'imprint of death' and in addition to grieving for family members, grieved for all who had died in the bombing. The 'survivor syndrome', consisting of chronic depressive states, anxiety, psychosomatic complaints and psychological numbness, is common to groups such as Holocaust survivors (Krystal 1968) or others exposed to trauma and death in such a way that dissociation becomes a primary defence.

If the trauma or threat is of sufficient magnitude it can produce a post-traumatic syndrome in anyone, the features of which can be very long-lasting and in themselves incapacitating (Raphael 1986) and which may complicate the clinical picture of the bereavement.

The nature of loss may induce post-traumatic symptomatology even in those not actually present at the time. In a retrospective study of 15 relatives who has lost a close family member through homicide over 3 years previously, Rynearson (1984) reported that all subjects perceived their reactions as differing from those experienced in previous bereavements. Despite not witnessing the death all subjects noted the presence of instrusive repetitive images of the homicide.

3. Relationship to the lost person

Lindemann (1944) supported Freud's theoretical position in finding that most severe grief reactions occurred where the preexisting relationship had been ambivalent. Overdependence on the lost person (Lopata 1973, Raphael 1977, Parkes & Weiss 1983) frequently denotes insecurity and greater problems in grieving. Vaillant (1988) suggests that loss in the context of a loving, happy relationship, despite the close attachment, is likely to result in a healthier bereavement.

4. Personality

Given that the personality of the survivor may influence the type of relationship (ambivalent or otherwise) experienced with the lost person and may very much influence such variables as the degree of available social support or choice of marital partner, it is surprising that the contribution of disorders of personality to complicated grief has never been systematically explored.

Bowlby (1981) singled out anxious, insecure, compulsive care-giving and ambivalent persons as being most prone to pathological grief reactions.

Personalities associated with complicated grief and identified as such by other workers have included those troubled by inadequacy, inferiority and insecurity (Sanders 1980) or those who are apprehensive, worried or highly anxious (Vachon et al 1982). Parkes & Weiss, in 1983, described individuals who were insecure, anxious or fearful as being at a high risk of poor outcome. Parkes went on to describe the 'grief-prone personality' (1985) as one characterized by excessive grief and depression, intense clinging behaviour or inordinate pining for the deceased spouse.

It was not until 1984 that a case report specifically described personality disorder as a pathogenic factor in bereavement (Alarcon 1984). Alarcon, noting that the impact of personality on the experience of grief is surprisingly neglected, went so far as to hypothesise that in the absence of major affective disorder, 'complicated' bereavement was primarily a reflection of a personality disorder. If Alarcan's contention is sustained, then the term 'pathological grief' is something of a misnomer, in that the pathology is not specific for the grief, rather the grief accentuates preexisting pathology.

Many clinical descriptions of pathological grief while containing no specific reference to personality disorder, nevertheless contain material which suggests that personality disorder may be a factor influencing outcome. An example is Volkan's paper on pathological grief (1970) where the vignettes used as illustrations frequently make reference to disturbed family relationships and family psychiatric illness, and violent or potentially violent behaviour.

5. Previous History

Volcan (1972) found individuals less likely to have a good outcome if they had coped poorly with a previous loss, while Clayton (1982) hypothesized that the best predictor of poor outcome in bereavement was poor prior physical or mental health. Bunch (1972), in a study of suicide among bereaved persons, reported that 60% of the suicides had a history of psychiatric treatment predating their bereavement.

6. Sociodemographic factors

Age differences have largely been approached in the context of conjugal bereavement. Parkes & Weiss (1983) reported younger widows as suffering more psychological problems, with older widows having more physical problems. It is more likely for younger widows to have experienced an unanticipated and sudden loss (Ball 1977).

Clear-cut trends with respect to gender and health consequences have been difficult to characterize, although in spousal bereavement the trend has been to find that widowers have more health consequences than widows (Sanders 1988). Perhaps more clear-cut is the tendency of mothers, in the event of the death of a young child, to grieve more than fathers (Fish 1986).

Paralleling the general trends of psychiatric epidemiology Stroebe & Stroebe (1987) conclude that the widowed of low socioeconomic status (SES) are less healthy than bereaved of high SES.

Harvey & Bahr (1974), in considering the economic effects of widowhood, went so far as to state that 'the negative impact sometimes attributed to widowhood derives not from widowhood status, but rather from socioeconomic status' (p 106).

The issue of lack of social support contributing to poor outcome has been prominent, at least since Maddison & Walker (1967) found that widows at greater risk perceived themselves to have more unmet needs in interpersonal relationships than did those with good outcome. In what has been termed the buffering hypothesis (e.g. Cohen & Willis 1985), the availability of social support is seen as protecting individuals to some extent from the deleterious effect of stressful life events.

However, social support indices must be assumed to be markedly influenced by personality, SES and the likelihood of those who are depressed or angry to alienate sources of such support.

Evidence is lacking in regard to the impact of race, culture or religion on outcome.

Conceptualizing forms of 'pathological grief'

The above risk factors, viewed from often markedly differing theoretical viewpoints, superimposed on a literature unable to agree on what constitutes 'normal' grief, have led to a situation where a plethora of terms is used to denote pathological forms. A small sample of terms used to describe such forms of grief include: absent (Deutsch 1937), abnormal (Pasnau et al 1987), complicated (Sanders 1989), distorted (Brown & Stoudemire 1983), neurotic (Wahl 1970), morbid (Sireling et al 1988), atypical (Jacobs & Douglas 1979), intensified (Lieberman & Jacobs 1987), prolonged (Lieberman & Jacobs 1987) or unresolved (Zisook & De Vaul 1985).

The general implication from the literature is that 'pathological' grief is maladaptive and differs from normal grief with respect to such features as its inten-sity, symptomatology, time course, interference with social and work function and likelihood of being complicated by physical or psychiatric illness.

Illustrating the problems associated with the diversity of lack of operational criteria for pathological grief would be situations in which a woman loses her spouse and breadwinner in a sudden and violent manner, at a time when they were experiencing financial strain and family illness, and an alternative situation in which a woman with a dependent personality disorder loses her mother, with whom she had had an ambivalent relationship. Although poles apart, both women may attract the 'diagnosis' of prolonged or pathological grief (Middleton & Raphael 1987).

It has proved to be difficult to separate the causes of unresolved grief from the manifestations of it. Lazare (1979) includes in its causes 'guilt', something that many might see as a manifestation of 'unresolved' grief.

Given the limitations of classification it is difficult to be precise but Clayton (1982) estimated that 4–6% of grief cases were 'pathological'. Parkes (1965) identified three forms of pathological grief, derived from observations on the course of grief: *chronic grief*, denoting an indefinite prolongation of grief with symptoms being exaggerated; *inhibited* grief, in which most symptoms of normal grief were absent; and *delayed grief* in which the painful emotions were avoided for a time at least.

Delayed grief may occur in situations where the loss has not been definitively confirmed, e.g. where a body has never been recovered, or alternatively the processes of denial may be utilized for a time by someone who has suffered overwhelming loss (Raphael 1986). Delayed grief reactions are liable to be precipitated by anniversaries or subsequent minor losses. Whilst some denial may be beneficial (e.g. Horowitz 1982), if the delay is so prolonged that the term 'absent grief' is more usefully applied, the longer term result may be depression, often masked by multiple physical symptoms (Brown & Stoudemire 1983).

POSITIVE ASPECTS

Not often emphasized in the literature, where the focus is on pathology, are the positive or productive sequelae of loss. Vaillant (1988) persuasively puts forward his contention that 'loss by itself does not cause psychopathology. Grief hurts, but does not make us ill'. He continues: 'We forget that it is the inconstant people who stay in our lives who drive us mad, not the constant ones who die. We forget that it is failure to internalize those whom we have loved, and not their loss, that impedes adult development' (p 148–149).

Vaillant, while giving examples of individuals who internalized lost loved ones and who matured, acknowledged that it is not known what causes some individuals to internalize more readily than others.

Pollock (1978), whose involvement in the area dates from his own first major bereavement, has made a major theme in work with biographies of his belief that the successful completion of the mourning process results in a creative outcome. For those with the preexisting talent this could be 'a great work of art, music, sculpture, literature, poetry, philosophy or science', while for those less gifted a creative outcome may be a new real relationship, the ability to feel joy, satisfaction and a sense of accomplishment.

Pollock regards some cases of creativity not as the outcome of successful mourning, but rather as an attempt at completing the work of mourning. He reminds us how Sigmund Freud's self analysis began in earnest following his father's death and how this led to the writing of *The Interpretation of Dreams* (Freud 1990).

Freud was later to write of the book: 'It revealed itself to me as a piece of my self-analysis, as my reaction to my father's death; that is, to the most important event, the most poignant loss, in a man's life' (Jones 1953, p 324).

These themes have been systematically investigated by Calhoun and Tedeschi (1990), who found, in a study of 52 adults who had adjusted well to a variety of losses, that most perceived themselves as stronger, more mature and independent as a result.

INTERVENTIONS

Most bereaved persons rely on their personal and social resources to deal with their loss. The issue of treatment then becomes largely focused on complications arising in the bereaved or directed towards assisting the resolution of pathological grief. Given the difficulties in defining pathological grief and given that normal grief may be associated with long-term symptomatology, it has proved difficult to establish what the effect of therapy is. Generally, however, workers have shown beneficial outcomes in controlled studies (Raphael 1977, Parkes 1980).

The concept of 'grief work' dates from Freud (1917) and has been expanded upon by later workers (Lindemann 1944, Parkes 1972, Raphael 1977, Bowlby 1981). The goals have remained similar, i.e. to share the grief work in uncomplicated grief and in more complicated reactions, to facilitate the transformation into 'normal' grief, with the goal being resolution. Expression of the various affects involved in grief is emphasized, as is review of the lost relationship. A psychotherapeutic orientation over 6–10 sessions during the crisis period, or longer (e.g. 15 sessions) at a later stage has been shown to be helpful, with positive outcomes. More complicated or pathological patterns of grief may require special techniques such as 'regrief work' (Raphael & Nunn 1988).

Prominent amongst those approaching grief work from a behavioural standpoint has been Ramsay (1977). He draws on Seligman's learned helplessness (1972) and diminished reinforcement in attributing pathological grief to avoidance caused by depression, producing reduced exposure to grief-provoking stimuli. While for mild cases Ramsay favours supportive psychotherapy, for those unresponsive to this he uses a behaviouralist flooding model which includes use of fantasy play acting, in which the survivor may be asked to force the lost person into a coffin and nail him in.

Illustrative of the difficulties with 'therapy' has been the work of Polak and his colleagues (1975) in using crisis intervention with families immediately following a loss. The experimental group and controls were asessed at 6 and 18 months after bereavement with no demonstrated benefit in those given therapy; indeed it was concluded that such immediate intervention might have delayed or interfered with normal grief.

Not uncommonly the acutely bereaved person's experience is that friends and relatives may be unintentionally thoughtless or relatives may be perceived as not very helpful, with subtle and unsubtle communications that inhibit the free expression of feelings (Maddison & Walker 1967). Arising from such experiences, self-help groups of bereaved people have been formed with the general aims of offering social and emotional support, e.g. CRUSE, the National Association for Loss and Grief, or Compassionate Friends (for parents who have lost a child).

RESEARCH

Systematic research on bereavement has been relatively late in coming. A consistent difficulty has been the very nature of bereavement, particularly in the acute stage, which means that the researcher may represent an intrusive presence at a time of particular emotional pain. Thus many prominent studies have overall participation ratios of less than 50%. Clearly, ethical issues prevent a perfect solution. A feature of much research has been an emphasis on pathology, yet this research has yet to lead to broad agreement about the operational criteria for pathological grief, or to explore in detail the role that personality disorder may have in its aetiology.

The possible protective influence that certain cultures grant to their bereaved members has yet to be clearly delineated. Research into the basic biology of loss, while intriguing, is also in its infancy.

In recent years, the need for more uniformity in defining bereavement phenomenology and its course and complications has led to the development of a number of measuring instruments. These include the Checklist of Grief Feelings, Experiences and Behaviour (Glick et al 1974), the Texas Inventory of Grief (Fashingbauer et al 1977), the Grief Experience Inventory (Sanders et al 1979), the Expanded Texas Inventory of Grief (Zisook et al 1984), the Widowhood Questionnaire (Zisook & Shuchter 1985) the scale devised by Jacobs and his colleagues (1987) and the grief reaction measure of Vargas and his colleagues (1989). Examples of recent scales tailored for use with specific populations include the Perinatal Grief Scale (Toedter et al 1988) and the Grief Experience Questionnaire (Barret & Scott 1989) used in bereavement following suicide. Many of these fail to separate bereavement-specific phenomena and distress from depression.

Despite the emerging trend towards the use of validated instruments designed for measuring the longitudinal responses of various bereaved groups, much of the bereavement literature is fairly subjective and even cornerstones of bereavement theory attract harsh criticism based on the limitations of the research support for them.

REFERENCES

Alarcon R D 1984 Personality disorder as a pathogenic factor in bereavement. Journal of Nervous and Mental Disease 172: 45–47

Averill J 1968 Grief: Its nature and significance. Psychological Bulletin 70: 721–728

Averill J 1979 The functions of grief. In: Izard C E (ed) Emotions in personality and psychopathology. Plenum Press, New York

Ball J F 1977 Widow's grief: the impact of age and mode of death Omega 7: 307–333

Barret T W, Scott T B 1989 Development of the grief experience questionnaire. Suicide and Life-Threatening Behaviour 19(2): 201–215

Bartrop R W, Lazarus L, Luckhurst E, Kiloh L G, Penny R 1977 Depressed lymphocyte function after bereavement. Lancet 2: 834–836

Benfield G, Leib S, Volman J 1978 Grief response of parents to neonatal death and parent participation in deciding care. Pediatrics 62: 171–177

Bowlby J 1960 Grief and mourning in infancy and early childhood. Psychoanalytic Study of the Child 15: 9–52

Bowlby J 1961 Process of mourning. International Journal of Psychoanalysis 42: 317–340

Bowlby J 1963 Pathological mourning and childhood mourning. Journal of the American Psychoanalytic Association 11: 500–541

Bowlby J 1971 Attachment and loss: 1. Attachment. Pelican, Harmondsworth

Bowlby J 1975 Attachment and loss: 2. Loss. Pelican, Harmondsworth

Bowlby J 1979 The making and breaking of affectional bonds. Tavistock Press, London

Bowlby J 1981 Attachment and loss: 3. Sadness and depression. Pelican, Harmondsworth

Bowlby J 1982 Attachment and loss: retrospect and prospect. American Journal of Orthopsychiatry 52(4): 664–678

Brown G W, Harris T 1978 Social origins of depression: a study of psychiatric disorder in women. Free Press, New York

Brown J T, Stoudemire G A 1983 Normal and pathological grief. Journal of the American Medical Association 250: 378–382

Bunch J 1972 Recent bereavement in relation to suicide. Journal of Psychosomatic Research 16: 361–366

Cain A, Cain B 1964 On replacing a child. Journal of the American Academy of Child Psychiatry 3: 443–456

Calhoun L G, Tedeschi R G 1990 Positive aspects of life problems: Recollections of grief. Omega 20: 265–272

Clayton P J 1982 Bereavement. In: Paykel E S (ed) Handbook of affective disorders. Churchill Livingstone, Edinburgh, p 403–415

Clayton P J, Darvish H S 1979 Course of depressive symptoms following the stress of bereavement. In: Barret J, Rose R M, Klerman G L (eds) Stress and mental disorder. Raven Press, New York

Cohen S, Wills T A 1985 Stress, social support, and the buffering hypothesis. Psychological Bulletin 98: 310–357

Condon J T 1986 Management of established pathological grief reaction after stillbirth. American Journal of Psychiatry 14: 987–992

Cullberg J 1972 Mental reactions of women in perinatal death. Psychosomatic medicine in obstetrics and gynaecology, 3rd International Congress. S Karger, Basel

Darwin C 1965 The expression of the emotions in man and animals. University of Chicago Press, Chicago

Deutsch H 1937 Absence of grief. Psycho-Analytic Quarterly 6: 12–22

Eisenbruch M 1984 Cross-cultural aspects of bereavement: II. Ethnic and cultural variations in the development of bereavement practices. Culture, Medicine and Psychiatry 8: 315–347

Engel G 1961 Is grief a disease? Psychosomatic Medicine 23: 18–23

Engel G 1971 Sudden and rapid death during psychological stress. Annals of Internal Medicine 74: 771–798

Fashingbauer T R, DeVaul R A, Zisook S 1977 Development of the Texas Inventory of Grief. American Journal of Psychiatry 134: 696–698

Fish W C 1986 Differences of grief intensity in bereaved parents. In: T A Rando (ed) Parental loss of a child. Research Press, Champaign, IL

Freud A 1958 Adolescence. Psychoanalytic Study of the Child 13: 255–278

Freud S 1900 The interpretation of dreams. Standard Edition, vol 4–5. Hogarth Press, London

Freud S 1917 Mourning and melancholia. In: Sigmund Freud: Collected Papers, vol 4. Hogarth Press, London

Freud S 1923 The ego and the id. Standard Edition, vol 19. Hogarth Press, London

Glick I, Weiss R S, Parkes C M 1974 The first year of bereavement. John Wiley, New York

Goldberg H S 1982 Funeral and bereavement rituals of Kota Indians and Orthodox Jews. Omega 12(2): 117–128

Gorer G D 1965 Death, grief and mourning. Doubleday, New York

Greenblatt M 1978 The grieving spouse. American Journal of Psychiatry 135: 43–47

Harlow H F, Mears L 1979 The human model: Primalo perspectives. John Wiley, New York

Harvey C D, Bahr H M 1974 Widowhood, morale, and affliction. Journal of Marriage and the Family 36: 97–106

Hirsch J, Hofer M, Holland J, Solomon F 1984 Toward a biology of Grieving. In: Osterweis M, Solomon F, Green M (eds) Bereavement: reactions, consequences, and care. National Academy Press, Washington, DC

Hofer M A 1984 Relationships as regulators: a psychobiological perspective on bereavement. Psychosomatic Medicine 46: 183–197

Horowitz M 1982 Psychological processes induced by illness, injury and loss. In: Milton T, Green C, Meagher R (eds) Handbook of clinical health psychology. Plenum Press, New York

Houseman C, Pheifer W G 1988 Potential for unresolved grief in survivors of persons with AIDS. Archives of Psychiatric Nursing 2: 296–301

Izard C 1977 Human emotions. Plenum Press, New York

Jacobs S C 1987 Psychoendocrine aspects of bereavement. In: Zisook S (ed) Biopsychosocial aspects of bereavement. American Psychiatric Press, Washington, DC

Jacobs S C, Douglas L 1979 Grief: a mediating process between a loss and illness. Comprehensive Psychiatry 20: 165–175

Jacobs S C, Kasl S V, Ostfeld A M, Berkman L, Kosten T R, Charpenter P 1987 The measurement of grief: bereaved versus non-bereaved. Hospice Journal 2(4): 21–36

Jones E 1953 The life and work of Sigmund Freud, vol 1. Basic Books, New York

Kastenbaum R 1969 Death and bereavement in later life. In: Kutscher A H (ed) Death and bereavement. C J Thomas, Springfield, IL

Kiecolt-Glaser J K, Glaser R 1986 Psychological influences on immunity. Psychosomatics 27: 621–624

Klein M 1940 Mourning and its relation to manic-depressive states. In: Jones E (ed) Contributions to psychoanalysis. Hogarth Press, London, p 125–153

Kleinman A, Kaplan B, Weiss R 1984 Sociocultural Influences. In: Osterweiss M, Solomon F, Green M (eds) Bereavement: reactions, consequences and care. National Academy Press, Washington, DC, p 199–212

Klerman G L, Izen I 1977 The effects of bereavement and grief on physical health and general well-being. Advances in Psychosomatic Medicine 9: 63–104

Krystal H 1968 Massive psychic trauma. International Universities Press, New York

Laudenslager M L 1988 The psychobiology of loss: lessons from humans and nonhuman primates. Journal of Social Issues 44: 19–36

Lazare A 1979 Unresolved grief. In: Lazare A (ed) Outpatient psychiatry: diagnoses and treatment. Williams & Wilkins, Baltimore, p 498–512

Lieberman P B, Jacobs S C 1987 Bereavement and its complication in medical patients: a guide for consultation-liaison psychiatrists. International Journal of Psychiatry in Medicine 17: 23–39

Lifton R J 1967 Death in life: survivors of Hiroshima. Random House, New York

Lindemann E 1944 Symptomatology and management of acute grief. American Journal of Psychiatry 101: 141–148

Lindemann E 1979 Beyond grief: studies in crisis intervention. Aronson, New York

Lopata H Z 1973 Living through widowhood. Psychology Today 7: 87–92

Lopata H Z 1979 Women as widows: support system. Elsevier-North Holland, New York

Lovell A 1983 Some questions of identity: late miscarriage, stillbirth and parental loss. Social Science in Medicine 17: 755–761

Maddison D C, Walker W L 1967 Factors affecting the outcome of conjugal bereavement. British Journal of Psychiatry 113: 1057–1067

Middleton W 1990 Bereavement phenomenology and the processes of resolution. Current research project (unpublished)

Middleton W, Raphael B 1987 Bereavement: state of the art and state of the science. Psychiatric Clinics of North America 10: 329–343

Miller S I, Schoenfeld L 1973 Grief in the Navajo: psychodynamics and culture. International Journal of Social Psychiatry 19: 187–191

Mor V, McHorney C, Sherwood S 1986 Secondary morbidity among the recently bereaved. American Journal of Psychiatry 143: 158–163

Nixon J, Pearn J 1977 Emotional sequelae of parents and siblings following the drowning or near-drowning of a child. Australian and New Zealand Journal of Psychiatry 11: 265–268

Osterweis M, Solomon F, Green M, quoting Eliot Luby 1984 In: Osterweiss M, Solomon F, Green M (eds) Bereavement: reactions, consequences and care. National Academy Press, Washington, DC

Parkes C M 1965 Bereavement and mental illness. British Medical Journal 38: 1–26

Parkes C M 1970 The first year of bereavement. Psychiatry 33: 444–467

Parkes C M 1972 Bereavement: studies of grief in adult life. International Universities Press, New York

Parkes C M 1980 Bereavement counselling: does it work? British Medical Journal 281: 3–10

Parkes C M 1985 Bereavement. British Journal of Psychiatry 146: 11–17

Parkes C M, Weiss R S 1983 Recovery from bereavement. Basic Books, New York

Parkes C M, Benjamin B, Fitzgerald R G 1969 Broken heart: a statistical study of increased mortality among widowers. British Medical Journal 1: 740–743

Pasnau R O, Fawny F I, Fawny N 1987 Role of the physician in bereavement. Psychiatric Clinics of North America 10: 109–120

Polak P R, Egan D, Vandebergh R, Williams W V 1975 Prevention in mental health: a controlled study. American Journal of Psychiatry 132: 146–149

Pollock G H 1961 Mourning and adaptation. International Journal of Psychoanalysis 42: 341–361

Pollock G H 1978 Process and affect: mourning and grief. International Journal of Psychoanalysis 59: 255–276

Ramsay R W 1977 Behavioural approaches to bereavement. Behavioural Research Therapy 15: 131–135

Rando T A 1988 Anticipatory grief: the term is a misnomer but the phenomenon exists. Journal of Palliative Care 4: 70–73

Raphael B 1977 Preventive intervention with the recently bereaved. Archives of General Psychiatry 34: 1450–1454

Raphael B 1978 Mourning and the presentation of melancholia. British Journal of Medical Psychology 51: 303–310

Raphael B 1982 The young child and the death of a parent. In: Parkes C M, Stevenson-Hinde J (eds) The place of attachment in human behaviour. Basic Books, New York

Raphael B 1983 The anatomy of bereavement. Basic Books, New York

Raphael B 1986 When disaster strikes. Basic Books, New York

Raphael B, Middleton W 1987 Current state of research in the field of bereavement. Israel Journal of Psychiatry and Related Sciences 24: 5–32

Raphael B, Middleton W 1989 Phenomenology of adult bereavement. Proceedings of the American Psychiatric Association 142nd Annual Meeting, May 6–11, San Francisco, CA

Raphael B, Nunn K 1988 Counselling the bereaved. Journal of Social Issues 44: 191–206

Reich P, De Silva P A, Lown B, Murawski B J 1981 Acute psychological disturbance preceding life-threatening ventricular arrhythmias. Journal of the American Medical Association 246: 233–235

Robertson J, Bowlby J 1952 Responses of young children to separation from their mothers. Courrier de la Centre Internationale de l'Enfance 2: 131–142

Rosenblatt P C, Walsh R P, Jackson D A 1976 Grief and mourning in cross cultural perspective. Yale: HRAF, New Haven

Rynearson E K 1984 Bereavement after homocide: a descriptive study. American Journal of Psychiatry 14: 1452–1454

Sanders C M 1980 A comparison of adult bereavement in the death of a spouse, child and parent. Omega 10: 303–322

Sanders C M 1988 Risk factors in bereavement outcome. Journal of Social Issues 44: 97–111

Sanders C M 1989 Grief: the mourning after. John Wiley, New York

Sanders C M, Mauger P A, Strong P N 1979 A manual for the grief experience inventory. Loss and Bereavement Resource Center, University of South Florida

Schleifer S J, Keller S E, Comenno M, Thornton C, Stein M 1983 Suppression of lymphocyte stimulation following bereavement. Journal of the American Medical Association 250: 374–377

Schuchter S R, Zisook S, Kirkorowiez C, Risch C 1986 The dexamethasone test in acute grief. American Journal of Psychiatry 143: 879–881

Shuchter S R, Zisook S 1987 A multidimensional model of spousal bereavement. In: Zisook S (ed) Biopsychosocial aspects of bereavement. American Psychiatric Press, Washington, DC

Seligman M E P 1972 Learned helplessness. Annual Review of Medicine 23: 407–412

Sheskin A, Wallace S E 1976 Differing bereavements: suicide, natural and accidental death. Omega 7: 229–242

Sireling L, Cohen D, Marks I 1988 Guided mourning for morbid grief: a controlled replication. Behaviour Therapy 19: 121–132

Stringham J, Riley J H, Ross A 1982 Silent birth: mourning a stillborn baby. Social Work 27: 322–327

Stroebe W, Stroebe M S 1987 Bereavement and health. Cambridge University Press, Cambridge

Stroebe W, Stroebe M S, Domittner G 1985 The impact of recent bereavement on the mental and physical health of young widows and widowers. Reports from the Psychological Institute of Tübingen University, Tübingen

Toedter L J, Lasker J N, Alhadeff J M 1988 The perinatal grief scale: Development and initial validation. American Journal of Orthopsychiatry 58(3): 435–449

Vachon M, Sheldon A R, Lancee W J, Lyall W J, Rogers W A L, Freeman S J J 1982 Correlates of enduring stress patterns following bereavement: social network, life situation, and personality. Psychological Medicine 12: 783–788

Vaillant G E 1988 Attachment, loss and rediscovery. Hillside Journal of Clinical Psychiatry 10(2): 148–164

Vargas L A, Loya F, Hodde-Vargas J 1989 Exploring the multidimensional aspects of grief reactions. American Journal of Psychiatry 146: 1484–1488

Volkan V 1970 Typical findings in pathological grief. Psychiatric Quarterly 44: 231–250

Volkan V 1972 The linking objects of pathological mourners. Archives of General Psychiatry 27: 215–221

Wahl C W 1970 The differential diagnosis of normal and neurotic grief following bereavement. Archives of the Foundation of Thanatology 1: 137–141

Weller E B 1989 Symptoms of bereavement in normal children. Proceedings of the American Psychiatric Association 142nd Annual Meeting, May 6–11, San Francisco, CA

Wolfenstien M 1966 How is mourning possible? Psychoanalytic Study of the Child 21: 93–123

Zisook S, Shuchter S R 1985 Time course of spousal bereavement. General Hospital Psychiatry 7: 95–100

Zisook S, DeVaul R A 1985 Unresolved grief. American Journal of Psychoanalysis 45: 370–379

Zisook S, DeVaul R A, Click M A 1984 Measuring symptoms of grief and bereavement. American Journal of Psychiatry 139: 1590–1593

Zisook S, Shuchter S R, Lyons L E 1987 Adjustment to widowhood. In: Zisook S (ed) Biopsychosocial aspects of bereavement. American Psychiatric Press, Washington, DC, p 49–74

40. Suicide and attempted suicide

Keith Hawton

Suicidal phenomena can be placed on a continuum ranging from suicidal ideation through attempted suicide to completed suicide. However, this description is too simple to convey a full picture of the spectrum of suicidal cognitions and behaviours. Suicidal ideation can vary in type and degree, from brief fleeting thoughts of wishing oneself dead, which are perhaps experienced by most people at some time, to active planning of a serious suicidal act. Attempted suicide, by which we mean any non-fatal suicidal act, is likewise a complex phenomenon. Thus some 'suicidal' acts are clearly not intended to result in death, but appear to have other conscious or unconscious purposes, while other such acts appear to be failed suicides. Even this distinction is too sharp, many suicidal acts appearing to have multiple purposes (Bancroft et al 1979), of which some degree of suicidal intent may be one. This is why the term 'attempted suicide' has rightly been criticized, and others such as 'parasuicide' (Kreitman et al 1969) or 'deliberate self-harm' (Morgan 1979) proposed. However, since most clinicians understand the meaning of the term 'attempted suicide' it is retained here. Even suicide should not be regarded as an 'all-or-none' phenomenon, as some suicides appear to have involved greater ambivalence than others and some clearly were acts not intended to result in death but went wrong. The first half of this chapter focuses on suicide and the second on attempted suicide.

SUICIDE STATISTICS

The problem of detection of suicide

The accuracy of suicide statistics has long been questioned because of the methods by which they are obtained. First, it has been suggested that because those who decide whether or not deaths are due to suicide, such as English coroners, have to abide by strict rules in making their judgments, figures based on their verdicts are bound to be an underestimate. Misclassified deaths are most likely to be found in the categories of 'death due to undetermined cause' (i.e. open verdicts) and accidental deaths, especially those due to poisoning. Holding & Barraclough (1978) demonstrated some differences but also considerable overlap between the characteristics of individuals whose deaths were recorded as suicides and those assigned to the open verdict category. They found less overlap between suicides and accidental deaths.

Second, it has been suggested that individuals vary in the criteria they use for suicide verdicts. However, while Barraclough (1970) found large changes in rates of suicide in a few English boroughs following a change of coroner, in most boroughs the rates remained fairly stable following such a change.

Third, because the criteria for, and means of reaching verdicts of, suicide differ considerably between countries, international comparisons of suicide cannot be made. Thus differences between the official suicide statistics for England and Wales and for Scotland (which have different judicial systems) are probably due to differences in the extent of use of the 'open verdict' category, especially for poisoning deaths (Barraclough 1972a). Differences have also been demonstrated between English and Danish coroners in their verdicts on identical case material (Atkinson et al 1975). However, in spite of clear evidence of variations in policy for identifying suicides the gross differences between suicide rates for different countries appear to have some validity, since the rank order of suicide rates for people within their own countries is remarkably similar to that of emigrants from those countries living abroad (Sainsbury & Barraclough 1968), irrespective of whether the rates include or exclude open verdicts (Barraclough 1973).

One can therefore conclude that, while considerable unreliability is associated with suicide verdicts, variations in suicide rates at a national level or between countries have sufficient validity to be useful for comparative purposes.

International suicide rates

There are marked differences in suicide rates between countries, with Hungary and Austria having extremely high rates and some Mediterranean countries, especially Greece and Spain, relatively low rates. The rates in the UK are relatively low, those in the USA somewhat higher.

There have also been marked variations in changes in suicide rates between different countries in recent years. Comparing the periods 1961–1963 and 1972–1974 Sainsbury and colleagues (see Sainsbury 1986, p 31–34) were able to identify five social factors whose initial values predicted the change in rates in European countries to a remarkable degree. Thus increasing rates were found where there were higher initial rates of divorce, unemployment, homicide and, interestingly, the proportion of women in employment, but reduction in rates was associated with a larger proportion of the population being aged under 15 years. They also identified four social factors whose *change* during the study period similarly predicted the changes in rates of suicide. Thus increasing rates were associated with higher room occupancy, percentage of women in tertiary education and percentage of the population aged over 65 years, whereas an increase in the proportion of the population aged under 15 was associated with decreasing rates.

Major social changes or events clearly have an impact on suicide rates. Thus most countries showed a considerable increase in suicide rates during the economic depression of the late 1920s and early 1930s and countries involved in the two World Wars had marked reductions in suicide rates (Sainsbury 1986).

Recent trends in suicide rates in England and Wales have been of particular interest since there was a 34% reduction in rates between 1963 and 1974 whereas rates in all but two other European countries increased during that period. The trend was largely attributed to the change in domestic gas supplies from coal gas to non-toxic North Sea Gas (Kreitman 1976), although the view has been questioned (Sainsbury 1986, p 35). Other possible contributory factors include the reduction in prescribing of barbiturates, improved detection and treatment of psychiatric disorders, especially depression, more effective resuscitation of attempters who reached hospital and changes in social factors.

Sociodemographic characteristics of suicides

In virtually every country suicide rates are higher in males and in older people, although peak rates in females are often some years earlier than those in males. Several countries have experienced changes in suicide rates in younger people in recent years (Hawton, 1986), with a substantial increase in rates among young males. The reasons for this are unclear, although increased rates of substance abuse, divorce and unemployment have been suggested as possibilities.

Suicide rates are generally lowest in married individuals, with the widowed, divorced and separated having the highest rates. Rates tend to be highest, at least for males, among those of lower socioeconomic status. High-risk occupation groups include doctors, lawyers, people in the hotel and bar trade, nurses and writers. There is a clear statistical association between suicide and unemployment, which is discussed further below.

FACTORS CONTRIBUTING TO SUICIDE

Psychiatric disorder

The prevalence of psychiatric disorder found in three major studies of suicides, based largely on retrospective diagnoses, is summarized in Table 40.1. The figures, which are only for the principal diagnosis in each case, may overestimate the prevalence of psychiatric disorder among suicides, since the studies included only individuals whose deaths attracted a definite suicide verdict: such a verdict may be more likely in someone with a known psychiatric disorder. Furthermore, much of the information used to assign diagnoses was based on informants' retrospective reports, and these may have overemphasized psychiatric symptoms in an effort to explain or justify the acts. However, they provide a broad picture of the extent and nature of psychiatric disorder in suicides.

Virtually all of the individuals in the studies were judged to have been suffering from psychiatric disorder, with affective illnesses being the most prevalent. In many cases there was more than one diagnosis, with a combination of affective disorder and alcoholism being especially common.

Table 40.1 Psychiatric disorders in completed suicides (%)

	Affective disorders	Alcoholism	Schizophrenia	Other psychiatric disorders	Any psychiatric disorder
Robins et al 1959 St Louis ($n = 134$)	47	25	2	20	94
Dorpat and Ripley 1960 Seattle ($n = 108$)	30	27	12	31	100
Barraclough et al 1974 Southern England ($n = 100$)	70	15	3	5	93

Affective disorders

On the basis of 17 studies of suicide in patients with affective disorders Guze & Robins (1970) calculated that 15% end their lives by suicide, a similar figure to that obtained in a recent more extensive review by Jamison (1986). This amounts to approximately a thirtyfold excess risk compared with that of the general population. Guze & Robins also noted that the risk of suicide appeared to be greatest relatively early in the development of the illness career. The risk in neurotic depression appears to be as great as that in endogenous depression (Miles 1977).

Various attempts have been made to identify specific risk factors for suicide in patients with depression (Table 40.2). In a study by Barraclough & Pallis (1975), which compared 64 suicides retrospectively diagnosed as suffering from depression with 124 living depressed individuals, six times as many of the suicides were living alone compared with the controls, and a history of suicide attempts was found in 41% of the suicides but only 4% of the controls. In a similar comparative study Roy (1983) confirmed the importance of social isolation and previous suicide attempts as specific risk factors.

Table 40.2 Risk factors for suicide in patients with depression (based on Barraclough & Pallis 1975, Roy 1983, Beck et al 1985, 1990)

Male sex	**Symptoms** – insomnia
Older age (females)	impaired memory
Single	self-neglect
Living alone	severity of depression
History of suicide attempts	hopelessness

In terms of specific symptoms distinguishing depres-

sives who killed themselves from surviving depressives, Barraclough & Pallis found insomnia in nearly all their suicides, although almost two-thirds of the controls also had sleep disturbance. Self-neglect and impaired memory were the only other distinguishing symptoms, but were nevertheless relatively uncommon, each being found in only 17% of the suicides. Although in an earlier study Farberow & McEvoy (1966) noted that depressive suicides were more agitated than controls, Barraclough & Pallis commented that almost half of their suicides were retarded, a finding which goes against the dictum that psychomotor retardation makes suicide less likely.

Suicide is more likely at the start as well as towards the end of a depressive episode (Copas et al 1971), and the duration of the illness in those who kill themselves tends to be longer than in surviving depressives (Barraclough et al 1974).

Several recent studies have drawn attention to the importance of hopelessness as a risk factor for suicide. Suicidal intent is more closely related to hopelessness than to degree of depression among suicide attempters (Minkoff et al 1973, Wetzel 1976, Dyer & Kreitman 1984). In follow-up studies of depressed psychiatric inpatients (Beck et al 1985) and outpatients (Beck et al 1990), degree of hopelessness, as measured by the Beck Hopelessness Scale (Beck et al 1974b) at the time of entry to the studies, was significantly related to eventual suicide. In the inpatient sample (but not in the outpatients) the initial level of depression, as measured by the Beck Depression Inventory (Beck et al 1961), also distinguished the eventual suicides from the surviving patients, but the hopelessness measure had greater predictive value. Beck has postulated that a sense of hopelessness in depression arises from the activation of specific underlying cognitive tendencies ('schemata'), which are probably shaped by early experiences, and that individuals differ in the extent to which they are vulnerable to developing pessimistic attitudes, even when suffering from similar levels of depression (Beck et al 1985). Thus a high degree of hopelessness may not only increase the current risk of suicide but may also predict greater hopelessness and therefore greater risk of suicide in subsequent episodes of depression. This suggestion, which is in keeping with clinical impression, clearly has implications for long-term management of patients who suffer from recurrent episodes of depression.

Alcoholism

From the findings of several follow-up studies Miles (1977) estimated that approximately 15% of alcoholics eventually commit suicide. Alcoholic suicides tend to occur relatively late in the development of the disorder and the majority of alcoholics who kill themselves are also suffering from depression (Robins et al 1959, Pitts & Winokur 1966, Barraclough et al 1974). Alcoholic suicides have been distinguished from surviving alcoholics in terms of poor physical health, poor work record and a history of suicide attempts, especially attempts involving serious suicidal intent (Motto 1980). Alcoholic suicides occur particularly frequently shortly after the loss of a close relationship through separation or death (Murphy & Robins 1967, Barraclough et al 1974, Murphy et al 1979).

Schizophrenia

Miles (1977) estimated from a series of follow-up studies that 10% of schizophrenics die by suicide, the risk being especially high during the early years of a chronic illness. On the basis of a comparison of 30 chronic schizophrenics who had killed themselves and 30 surviving chronic schizophrenics Roy (1982a) identified the following distinguishing characteristics of the suicides: male sex, relatively young age, chronic illness characterized by relapses and remissions, depression at the last clinical contact, expression of suicidal ideas, unemployment and recent discharge from psychiatric inpatient care. Some further risk factors have been identified by Drake and co-workers (1984). First, they noted that all of the suicides in their series occurred during a relatively non-psychotic phase of the illness. Second, most of the suicides had attained a relatively high level of educational status prior to their illness, were living alone and had previously indicated suicidal intent. Third, they tended to have high, non-delusional but unrealistic expectations of

themselves, and were largely aware of the effects of their illness and its implications for their future functioning. Finally, they tended to be depressed, with psychological rather than physical symptoms, especially feelings of inadequacy, hopelessness and suicidal ideas. Fears of mental disintegration, suicidal threats and hopelessness were especially strong distinguishing characteristics.

Other psychiatric disorders

Patients with severe neurotic disorders appear to be at increased risk of suicide (Sims & Prior 1978), even when those with depressive neurosis are omitted (Sims 1984). A relatively high risk of suicide has also been demonstrated in patients with panic disorder (Coryell et al 1982) and this is supported by recent data indicating that suicidal ideation and a history of suicide attempts were more common in individuals identified in a community study as having panic disorder than in individuals with other psychiatric disorders (Weissman et al 1989).

A sizeable proportion of people who kill themselves have personality disorders (Barraclough et al 1974). As many as 10% of suicides may have sociopathic disorders (Ovenstone & Kreitman 1974). Relatively little is known about the specific risk factors in such individuals, but those who show marked lability of mood, aggressiveness and impulsivity may be at special risk, particularly if they also misuse alcohol or drugs.

Physical illness

Chronic physical disorders are relatively common among suicides, and were found in half of Dorpat & Ripley's (1960) series of suicides in Seattle. They were particularly common in elderly male suicides and were thought to have contributed directly to the suicide in several cases. Conditions specifically linked to suicide include cancer, diseases of the central nervous system, peptic ulcer and male genitourinary disorders (Whitlock 1986). Suicide risk appears to be especially high in epilepsy. On the basis of several follow-up studies Barraclough (1981) calculated that the risk may be increased fivefold compared with that for the general population and that people with temporal lobe epilepsy may be at even greater risk. The link between suicide and physical illness may be due to several factors, including depression and alcohol abuse as well as rational decisions that suicide is preferable to tolerating the handicaps of debilitating illness.

Serotoninergic abnormalities

There is currently considerable interest in the possibility that suicide risk may be associated with abnormalities of brain serotoninergic systems (Mann et al 1989). Thus suicidal behaviour in depressives has been linked with low CSF 5-HIAA levels (Asberg et al 1976). The occurrence of suicide was found to be greater in attempted suicide patients with low CSF 5-HIAA levels than in those with higher levels (Asberg et al 1986). There is some evidence, although not consistent across all studies, of increased imipramine-binding sites (probably reflecting reduced serotonin release) in the brain tissues of suicides (Asberg et al 1986).

It has been postulated, with some supporting evidence (e.g. Brown et al 1982), that reduced serotonin turnover may be associated with aggression and impulsivity and that this association may underlie the link with suicidal behaviour. This area of research is important in view of its possible therapeutic implications, particularly with the recent advent of antidepressant drugs with specific actions on 5-HT systems.

Family history of suicide

Suicidal behaviour appears to cluster in families (Roy 1986), although one recent study of patients with affective disorder failed to support this view (Scheftner et al 1988). However, the nature of the association, assuming it exists, is less clear. While common environmental influences may be relevant, the risk of suicide appears to be increased in the biological relatives of adoptees who have committed suicide and in the biological relatives of adoptees who have had depressive disorders (Kety 1986). This raises the possibility of a genetic predisposition to suicide in some individuals. The predisposition could possibly be based on genetically-determined abnormalities in brain serotonergic function.

Bereavement

Parental death during childhood may increase the risk of suicide in adulthood (Dorpat et al 1965), although there is a much stronger association between attempted suicide and parental loss, usually through parental separation rather than death (Adam 1986). A likely mechanism is the increased vulnerability to depression associated with early parental loss (Brown & Harris 1978).

Recent bereavement, particularly death of a spouse (McMahon & Pugh 1965) or parent, is also a risk factor. Bunch (1972) found that the risk was increased for at least 4 or 5 years following bereavement, and was particularly high during the first 2 years. The bereaved individuals at most risk appeared to be those who had a history of psychiatric disorder and/or suicidal behaviour before the bereavement and who lacked family support following the loss.

Unemployment

There is an undoubted statistical association between unemployment and suicide, especially in men (Platt 1984). However, the nature of this link is less clear. Thus it is not known whether it is due to the adverse effects unemployment can have on mental health, or whether it is due to the increased risk people with psychiatric disorders have of becoming unemployed (Smith 1985). When commenting on their finding of a markedly larger proportion of unemployed men in a series of suicides compared with matched surviving controls, Shepherd & Barraclough (1980) argued that the association was most likely to be due primarily to psychiatric disorder because this seemed to be responsible for unemployment and suicide in most cases. In some cases unemployment may have exacerbated a pre-existing psychiatric condition and thereby increased the risk of suicide. Whatever the nature of this association, unemployment is nevertheless a risk factor for suicide among patients with psychiatric disorders (Roy 1982a, b) and should be considered when assessing suicide risk.

THE PREVENTION OF SUICIDE

Problems in identifying those at risk

1. A fundamental problem in attempting to identify individuals at special risk of suicide is that we have to use criteria which are relatively crude to predict what is, fortunately, even among higher risk groups such as suicide attempters, a relatively rare event. For example, the risk of suicide during the year following a suicide attempt is approximately 1% (p. 644). Since our ability to predict those who kill themselves is at best 80% efficient, out of 1000 attempters we should be able to identify eight out of the ten who might be expected to die by suicide within a year. However, in doing so we would also incorrectly identify a further 192 individuals as positive for suicide risk. This false-positive rate may

be too high for predictions to be useful in targeting preventive efforts.

2. Although suicide risk factors may be useful in identifying high-risk groups of people, these factors are of less use when the clinician is faced with the problem of prediction in a specific individual.

3. Our knowledge of risk factors is based to a large extent on the characteristics of people who have died in spite of the provision of treatment. Since it is likely that treatment will also have prevented some suicides, what we really have are risk factors for suicide *in spite of* treatment (although treatment in some cases may have been inadequate – see below).

4. Most of the known risk factors concern long-term risk; these may not be identical to short-term risk factors, especially in relation to a time span as short as days or weeks. However, there is evidence that at least some of these factors are also predictive in the relatively short-term (Hawton & Fagg 1988).

5. People are not static in terms of risk factors and risk in an individual may therefore change with time. For example, due to separation and unemployment a relatively low-risk man may move from a low-risk to a high-risk group. The potential instability of risk factors over time may limit their usefulness in long-term prediction.

6. Risk factors are not universal across all populations and circumstances. There are, for example, several differences in risk factors between psychiatric hospital inpatients and suicide attempters.

Methods and results of prevention of suicide

Suicide prevention organizations

In the UK the Samaritans is the principal organization with a specific goal of suicide prevention. Its work is based on confidential counselling, known as 'befriending'. The Samaritans undoubtedly attracts suicidal clients (Barraclough & Shea 1970). An initial study by Bagley (1968) suggested that the Samaritans was effective in preventing suicide. However, a subsequent and better-designed study found no evidence of a significant impact of the Samaritans on suicide rates (Jennings et al 1978).

In the USA during the 1960s and 1970s there was considerable enthusiasm for crisis and suicide prevention centres. Unfortunately, assessment of the effects of these centres has not shown much impact on suicide rates (Weiner 1969, Lester 1974), except for a promising report of a significant effect on suicide rates

in young females, the principal users of crisis centres (Miller et al 1984).

Improved detection and treatment of psychiatric disorder

Since the majority of people who kill themselves have visited doctors during the month before their death (Barraclough et al 1974) it is natural to focus on these contacts to see whether patients at risk can be better identified and managed. The statistical problems associated with the detection of those at risk of suicide have already been discussed. In the study by Barraclough and colleagues of 100 suicides, only a minority of the patients with depressive disorders were receiving antidepressant drugs at the time of their death, in spite of being in contact with medical agencies. In several cases the drugs were thought to be inappropriate or had been prescribed in subtherapeutic doses (Barraclough et al 1974). This emphasizes the need for appropriate treatment when a diagnosis of depression is made. One of the problems of antidepressant treatment is that many of the drugs are dangerous if taken in an overdose, with significant risk of cardiac arrythmia. This applies especially to the older antidepressants (Cassidy & Henry 1987), although many clinicians believe these are the most effective. Limiting the amount of medication available to a patient at any one time and involving relatives in handling it may help reduce the risk of a serious overdose.

At the time of the study by Barraclough and colleagues lithium had not come into common use for the prophylactic management of manic-depressive disorder. Barraclough (1972b) suggested that as many as one-fifth of the suicides in their study might have been prevented if lithium had been used more widely. While this is likely to be an over-estimate, lithium and other prophylactic treatment of patients with recurrent affective disorders may nevertheless have an important role in suicide prevention, although no supportive data are yet available.

Reduced availability of the means for suicide

While undoubtedly some determined suicidal individuals will find a way to kill themselves whatever their circumstances, there is a considerable body of opinion that some suicides will be prevented if obvious methods of suicide cease to be available. The effect of the introduction of non-toxic North Sea Gas in the UK is a possible example of this. Clarke & Lester (1989) have argued that there is evidence that a similar effect might be achieved by a reduction in gun ownership in the USA, although a recent study has suggested that the effect might be minimal and would probably be restricted to persons aged 15–24 years (Sloan et al 1990). However, it would be unwise to generalize from national data to the individual case, where restricting the availability of dangerous medication or other means of suicide might be life-saving by allowing the patient time for therapeutic measures to take effect, possibly in a safe environment.

Positive efforts have been made in relation to some of the major bridges which have become notorious as sites for suicide by erecting barriers or safety nets. The Golden Gate Bridge in San Francisco is a good example of a bridge commonly used for suicide; however in this case aesthetic factors have apparently prevented anti-suicide structures being erected (Clarke & Lester 1989, p 105) in spite of the fact that survivors of jumping from this bridge were unanimous in saying that barriers would have prevented their attempts and that they supported the idea of their being erected (Rosen 1975).

There has been extensive discussion of ways of reducing the availability and toxicity of medicine, including the use of blister packs, combining small doses of emetics with drugs popular for self-poisoning and encouraging the keeping of minimum supplies of medication available in the home. None of these strategies has been tested.

AFTERMATH OF SUICIDE

The effects of suicide on relatives and friends can be devastating, especially in the case of teenage suicides (Hawton 1986, p 49–52). Reactions of family members to suicide are similar to those following other deaths but complicated by the stigma associated with suicide and the considerable guilt that relatives and friends may experience. However, in some cases where the dead individual has long suffered a debilitating psychiatric disorder or one, such as alcoholism, which has severely disrupted family life, relief may be the principal emotion of relatives (Sheskin & Wallace 1976).

Worden (1983) has identified the following common responses of family members to a suicide: 1) *denial*, including refusal to accept the fact of the death, or that it was due to suicide; 2) *anger*, which may be directed towards the deceased, as well as towards medical agencies, friends of the deceased, the coroner, and others; 3) *shame*, because of the stigma associated with suicide; 4) *guilt*, about what the survivor might or

should have done to prevent the suicide, as well as about how he or she may have contributed; 5) *fear*, about the individual's own self-destructive impulses. Physical reactions are also common, including somatization (Rudestam 1977) and, possibly, increased risk of death (Shepherd & Barraclough 1976). Family interactions may also be badly affected by suicide, especially the relationships between parents of adolescents who die by suicide (Herzog & Resnik 1967). Children of parents who have committed suicide can develop learning problems and insecurity, especially if the parental death is concealed or the fact that it was suicide is denied by other family members (Shepherd & Barraclough 1976).

The provision of help for the relatives of suicide is often neglected, partly because potential helpers find this work extremely difficult. Worden (1983) has highlighted strategies which ought to be part of such help, including: 1) establishing accurate communication between family members; 2) helping individuals cope with their feelings of guilt, including getting these responses into perspective; 3) correcting distorted attitudes towards the deceased; 4) helping individuals contemplate the future, including the likely long-term effects of the death; 5) encouraging ventilation of feelings of anger; 6) exploring the sense of abandonment that the relatives are likely to feel.

Special attention needs to be paid to helping relatives of young suicides (Herzog & Resnik 1967). A group counselling approach, involving ten sessions over 12 weeks has been described by Hatton & Valente (1981).

TRENDS IN ATTEMPTED SUICIDE

Attempted suicide statistics are usually obtained on the basis of general hospital referrals for deliberate self-poisoning and self-injury. However, it is known that many more attempts do not come to hospital attention, some being managed by general practitioners (Kennedy & Kreitman 1973) and others not coming to medical notice at all.

During the 1960s and early 1970s there was a massive increase in attempted suicide, mostly self-poisoning, in much of the Western world (Alderson 1974, Weissman 1974, Wexler et al 1978). Rates of general hospital referral for attempted suicide in the UK appeared to peak in the late 1970s (Holding et al 1977, Gibbons et al 1978b, Hawton et al 1982a). Since that time there has been a decline in the problem, especially among females (Platt et al 1988), but deliberate self-poisoning remains the most common reason for emergency medical admission of women to general hospitals and the second most common reason, after acute heart disease, for such admission of men (Hawton & Catalan 1987).

The reasons for the vast changes in the extent of attempted suicide during the past three decades are unclear. While various factors have been proposed, including increasing marital problems, unemployment, rising alcohol problems and changing 'fashion', the pattern of prescribing of psychotropic medication has attracted a lot of attention. There was evidence of a clear correlation between rates of self-poisoning with medication and rates of prescribing of psychotropic drugs (Forster & Frost 1985) for the period when self-poisoning was rapidly becoming more common. The recent decline in self-poisoning has paralleled a reduction in prescribing of psychotropic drugs (Brewer & Farmer 1985). While correlational data of this kind cannot demonstrate a causal association, the very high rates of psychotropic drug prescribing to self-poisoners (Hawton & Blackstock 1976, Prescott & Highley 1985) add further weight to this line of reasoning. However this cannot be the sole explanation, especially since a very large number of overdoses involve non-prescribed drugs, particularly analgesics (Platt et al 1988).

The trends in attempted suicide in the USA are less well-documented. However, a similar pattern to the UK is found in much of the rest of Europe, especially in Northern European countries (Diekstra 1985).

Methods used in attempted suicide

As already noted, attempted suicide is most commonly by self-poisoning, principally with psychotropics, especially minor tranquillizers, or analgesics (Platt et al 1988). Self-poisoning constitutes 80–90% of general hospital attempted suicide referrals, the rest being self-injuries, especially self-cutting (Hawton & Catalan 1987, p 150-160). While many self-injuries are relatively minor in terms of threat to life, some are extremely dangerous, such as those involving deep cutting, jumping and shooting, and these are often 'failed suicides'.

CHARACTERISTICS OF ATTEMPTED SUICIDE PATIENTS

Sociodemographic

In contrast with completed suicide, in nearly all countries attempted suicide is more common in females, the sex ratio of rates being of the order of 1.3–2.0:1.0. Attempted suicide is primarily a behaviour of young people, with at least two-thirds of cases being under 35 years of age. It is rare under the age of 12 years, but is especially common in 15–24-year-old females. Peak rates in males occur in the mid twenties to early thirties (Platt et al 1988). Rates of attempted suicide in older people, while much lower than in the young, show a changed sex pattern, with the sex ratio approximating to unity (Hawton & Fagg 1991).

Attempted suicide rates have a very skewed social class pattern with rates being several times higher in those of lower socio-economic status (Platt et al 1988). Rates tend to be especially high in areas of social deprivation and overcrowding (Morgan et al 1975, Skrimshire 1976, Holding et al 1977).

Clear associations have been demonstrated between unemployment and attempted suicide both for men and women. Unemployed men have been shown to have a risk of attempted suicide some 10–15 times that of employed men, with the risk increasing to approximately 25–35-fold in those unemployed more than a year (Platt & Kreitman 1984, Hawton & Rose 1986). Similar findings have been reported for women (Hawton et al 1988). There has been much debate about the statistical association between unemployment and attempted suicide, a direct cause being unlikely in most cases. Possible factors include the secondary effects of unemployment, such as poverty, domestic upheaval and emotional problems; and the drift of people with longstanding mental health problems, and hence greater risk of attempted suicide, into the ranks of the unemployed, especially the long-term unemployed.

Clinical characteristics

Psychiatric disorder

Although psychiatric symptoms and disorders are common in attempted suicide patients at the time of their attempts, they are by no means universal. Using the Present State Examination (Wing et al 1974) Newson-Smith & Hirsch (1979a) demonstrated that the psychiatric symptoms most often present during the 4 weeks before self-poisoning were feelings of nervous tension (75%), depressed mood (75%), hopelessness (61%), irritability (55%), tension pains (49%), worrying (45%) and poor concentration (43%). However, the proportion of patients with definite psychiatric disorder was only 31%, with a further 29%

reaching criteria for possible disorder. All but one of the patients in these two categories had depressive disorders. A similar picture emerged from a comparable study of self-poisoners conducted by Urwin & Gibbons (1979), although they also identified patients suffering from alcoholism, anxiety disorders and schizophrenia. One-quarter of the men and just over one in ten of the women in this study had personality disorders.

Attempters with high suicidal intent have been distinguished from low-intent attempters in terms of depressive symptoms, with insomnia, pessimism, impaired concentration, loss of interest, social withdrawal, feeling useless or worthless and weight loss being more common in the former (Sainsbury 1986, p 79). Two behaviours observed at interview, namely slow speech and discouraged posture, were also more common among the high-intent attempters.

Other studies have found high rates of alcohol problems, especially in males. Thus Hawton et al (1989) identified alcoholism in 14.6% of male attempters, the prevalence being especially high in the middle and older age groups, and in 4.2% of female attempters.

An association has recently been suggested between attempted suicide and panic disorder (Weissman et al 1989) and also the newly described entity of 'recurrent brief depression' (Angst et al 1990), although the latter may be a feature that occurs in the broader category of borderline personality disorder, suicidal behaviour being one of the criteria for this condition.

Psychological characteristics

Some psychological features have been identified in suicide attempters, although these probably overlap with those of people generally at risk of suicide. The tendency to develop a sense of hopelessness has already been discussed (p 637). The other main psychological characteristics are rigid and constricted thinking (Levenson 1974) and deficient problem-solving skills (Linehan et al 1986), especially with regard to interpersonal problems (McLeavey et al 1987).

Physical disorders

Physical health problems are also common in attempted suicide patients (Bancroft et al 1977), including adolescents (Hawton et al 1982b). As with suicide, patients with epilepsy have an increased risk of attempted suicide (Mackay 1979, Hawton et al 1980).

Considerable attention has been paid to the possible increased risk of attempted suicide in females during the pre- or perimenstrual phase of the menstrual cycle, with some studies showing a positive association (e.g. Tonks et al 1968) and others failing to do so (e.g. Birtchnell & Floyd 1974).

Problems and precipitants associated with attempted suicide

Attempted suicide commonly follows life events. Paykel et al (1975) found that suicide attempters had experienced a mean of 3.3 events during the 6 months before their attempts, compared with a mean of 2.1 events in matched depressed patients during the 6 months before the onset of their symptoms and a mean of 0.8 events in matched general population control subjects during the 6 months before interview. Life events were especially common in the month before attempts and peaked in the week beforehand. The most common event was a serious argument with a partner, a similar finding to that of Bancroft et al (1977).

Relationship difficulties are also the most common persistent problems of attempters, both adults (Bancroft et al 1977) and adolescents (Hawton et al 1982b). Disturbed family relationships are found in many cases, and there is an important association between attempted suicide by parents and risk of child abuse or neglect in young children in the family (Roberts & Hawton 1980, Hawton et al 1985).

Motives for attempted suicide

As has already been noted, the intended outcome of non-fatal suicidal behaviour may not be death. Disentangling the motives for this behaviour is a complex task, reliance having to be placed on the explanations of various people, including the attempter, and on examining the circumstances of the act. Of clinical importance are the differences in explanations of attempts provided by patients themselves and by clinicians and relatives. Thus while the most common reasons chosen by attempters include lack of alternatives, to obtain relief from a distressed state of mind, to escape from a situation and to die, psychiatrists more often attribute hostile and manipulative motives (Bancroft et al 1979), as do relatives (James & Hawton 1985), with both the clinicians and relatives rarely attributing the act to suicidal intent. However, within the population of suicide attempters there is a very important group of patients who have been fairly intent on suicide and who, as discussed below, are at significant risk of eventual suicide.

Repetition of attempted suicide

Repetition of this behaviour is common, with between 12 and 25% of attempters being re-referred to the same hospital for further attempts within a year of a previous one (Bancroft & Marsack 1977, Kreitman 1977, Platt et al 1988). Repeats are especially common during the first 3–6 months following an attempt (Bancroft & Marsack 1977, Sellar et al 1990).

A Risk of Repetition Scale was developed by Bluglass & Horton (1974) to predict further attempts. This includes six items : 1) problems in the use of alcohol; 2) sociopathy; 3) previous inpatient psychiatric treatment; 4) previous outpatient psychiatric treatment; 5) previous attempts resulting in hospital admission; and 6) not living with relatives. One point is allocated for each item positive and the higher the total score the greater the risk of repetition. Buglass & Horton found that of patients with a score of zero only 5% repeated within a year whereas those scoring 5 or 6 had a repetition rate of 48%.

A subgroup of attempters repeats the behaviour on several, even many occasions. Such 'chronic repeaters' are typically from social class V, unmarried, show features of personality disorder, have a history of violence and suffer from alcoholism (Kreitman & Casey 1988). They have a sex ratio close to unity, whereas females considerably outnumber males among people making their first attempt and among 'minor' repeaters. Chronic repeaters have a considerable risk of eventual

suicide (Ovenstone & Kreitman 1974), the risk possibly being especially high following a non-fatal attempt with greater suicidal intent than in previous episodes (Pierce 1981).

Suicide following attempted suicide

Several studies have shown that approximately one out of every 100 suicide attempters will die by suicide within a year of an attempt, a suicide risk approximately 100 times that of the general population. The risk of

Table 40.4 Risk factors for suicide following attempted suicide

Socio-demographic
  Older age (especially females)
  Male sex
  Unemployment; retirement
  Separated, widowed or divorced
  Absence of break-up of a relationship in previous year
  Living alone

Clinical
  Psychiatric disorder, including alcoholism
  Poor physical health

The attempt
  Violent method used
  Suicide note
  High suicide intent
  Did not follow a major argument
  Previous attempts

Table 40.3 Suicide following attempted suicide

	Number of attempted suicide patients	Length of follow-up (years)	Suicides %
Kessel & McCulloch 1966	511	1	1.6
Tuckman & Youngman 1968	1112	1	1.4
Buglass & Horton 1974	2809	1	0.8
Hawton & Fagg 1988	1626	1	1.0
Greer & Bagley 1971	204	$1\frac{1}{2}$	2.0
Stengel & Cook 1958	210	2–5	1.4
Buglass & McCulloch 1970	511	3	3.3
Pokorny 1966	250	4	4.4
Hawton & Fagg 1988	1335	8	2.8

suicide continues to be relatively high during the succeeding years (Table 40.3). Of people who kill themselves approximately half have a history of previous attempts (Ovenstone & Kreitman 1974).

The factors which have been shown to distinguish between suicide attempters who subsequently kill themselves and surviving attempters are summarized in Table 40.4, which is based on the findings of several investigations (Tuckman & Youngman 1968, Pierce 1981, Pallis et al 1982, 1984, Hawton and Fagg 1988). However, despite considerable knowledge of risk factors our ability specifically to identify those at risk is limited (p 639).

MANAGEMENT OF ATTEMPTED SUICIDE PATIENTS

Provision of services for attempted suicide patients in general hospitals is often haphazard. Since psychiatric disorder is by no means universal and social problems are so common in these patients, the necessity of involving psychiatrists in the assessment and aftercare in every case has been questioned. In the UK it is now accepted policy for non-psychiatrists, such as psychiatric nurses, social workers and physicians, to play a major role in the management of attempted suicide patients, provided they receive appropriate training and supervision and have the back-up of psychiatrists (Department of Health and Social Security 1984). Such developments are firmly based on clinical investigations in which well-trained psychiatric nurses and social workers have proved as efficient as junior psychiatrists in assessing attempted suicide patients (Newson-Smith & Hirsch 1979b, Catalan et al 1980), and in providing aftercare (Gibbons et al 1978a, Hawton et al 1981). However, senior psychiatrists need to be an integral part of such services, both to provide training and also to be available to assess patients with significant psychiatric disorder, especially those likely to require psychiatric inpatient admission.

Assessment

The assessment of attempted suicide patients requires care and time, especially since some attempters initially may not be receptive to detailed questioning. The key areas that should be covered during the assessment are listed in Table 40.5.

A thorough assessment should include at least one interview with the patient, enquiry of relatives and friends and discussion with other professionals involved in the patient's care, including general hospital staff, the patient's general practitioner and anyone the patient may recently have seen for psychosocial treatment.

Assessment of the nature of the attempt and probable reasons can best be made by detailed enquiry concerning the 48 hours or so leading up to the attempt. The Beck Suicidal Intent Scale (Beck et al 1974a) is a useful adjunct in the assessment of suicidal intent. Assessment of psychiatric disorder should be based on the usual clinical enquiry and examination. The Risk of Repetition Scale (Buglass & Horton 1974) can assist in assessing whether a repeat is likely, although in predicting immediate risk attention should be paid to factors such as the likelihood that the patient's circumstances will change, the degree of support available from clinical staff, relatives and friends and the potential effectiveness of any planned treatment. The difficulties of assessing risk of suicide in this population have already been discussed (p 639). The best approach is to consider as many factors as possible, including those in Table 40.4 as well as the individual's current circumstances, support, problem-solving ability and attitudes towards the future.

Table 40.5 Assessment of attempted suicide patients: essential items that require attention

1. The nature of the attempt
   Method used
   Circumstances

2. Reason for the attempt
   Problems
   Precipitants
   Motives, including suicidal intent

3. Psychiatric disorder

4. Risk of repetition

5. Risk of suicide

6. Treatment indicated

Treatment

The wide diversity of problems faced by attempted suicide patients demands a broad range of treatment strategies (Hawton & Catalan 1987). Inpatient psychiatric admission, sometimes compulsory, will be necessary in a minority of patients, although there is marked variation in the proportions of cases offered such care in different centres (e.g. Platt et al 1988), possibly reflecting the availability of other treatment resources.

The usual indications are severe psychiatric disorder and/or suicide risk.

The most frequent form of aftercare is outpatient follow-up (Platt et al 1988), usually involving brief problem-orientated counselling. In some areas in the UK the majority of patients are returned to the care of their general practitioners without any specific aftercare arrangements.

In the UK there have been several controlled evaluative studies of aftercare (Hawton 1989). An experimental aftercare service for repeat suicide attempters in Edinburgh, which included regular and frequent outpatient appointments, non-attenders being followed-up at home and an emergency telephone service, was compared with routine care. By the 6-month follow-up the proportions of patients in each group who had made further attempts were virtually identical. However, the patients' social circumstances improved more in the experimental group than in the control group, although this effect was largely confined to women (Chowdhury et al 1973).

In a subsequent study, Gibbons et al (1978a) in Southampton compared a home-based social work aftercare service with routine care. Again no effects on repetition rates were found, but some evidence of improved social adjustment of the attempters in the experimental group was apparent. This effect was again largely confined to women (Gibbons 1979).

Attendance by suicide attempters at outpatient appointments is often poor, and so Hawton et al (1981) in Oxford compared a domiciliary treatment programme, including flexible appointments, with weekly outpatient treatment; problem-orientated counselling was provided in both modalities. In spite of far better compliance with the domiciliary treatment there were no major differences in outcome, including repetition of attempts, between the two groups except that patients with problems in their relationship with their partners showed some evidence of greater improvement in the relationships if treated in the domiciliary group.

The Oxford group then went on to compare outpatient counselling with general practitioner care for patients thought suitable for outpatient care (Hawton et al 1987). Again no major differences in outcome were found, except women and individuals with dyadic problems had a better outcome in the outpatient-treated group. To summarise these studies it appears that: 1) psychosocial intervention has not been shown to have a preventive effect against repetition of attempts; 2) home-based treatment improves compliance but not overall outcome; 3) treatment may have special benefits for women and patients with problems in their relationships with their partners.

Drug therapies for suicide attempters have received less attention. The antidepressant mianserin was found to be ineffective in preventing repeats (Hirsch et al 1982) but depot flupenthixol appeared to reduce the repetition rate of chronic repeaters (Montgomery and Montgomery 1982). This latter interesting result requires replication.

Prevention of attempted suicide

Many attempted suicide patients, like completed suicides, have had contact with helping agencies before their attempts. Thus in one study 82% of self-poisoners had been in contact with such an agency within the month before an overdose and 54% within a week (Bancroft et al 1977). The general practitioner was the person most commonly contacted; this applied to 63% within a month and 36% within a week of their overdoses (Hawton & Blackstock 1976). Many of these patients were experiencing anxiety or depression associated with their social and interpersonal difficulties and often received psychotropic medication as a result of their visits. This raises the question of whether these potential attempters could have been identified at the time and some other treatment tried. For example, counselling might be considered a more appropriate treatment for patients who are distressed as a result of relationship problems, especially those who are known to show poor impulse control and who may be drinking heavily. A major problem in detection of those at risk is that the characteristics of attempters are similar to those of many more patients who do not make attempts.

The Samaritans do not appear to have a significant impact on attempted suicide. Thus Samaritan clients and attempted suicide patients differ considerably (Kreitman & Chowdhury 1973), the Samaritan clients including a greater proportion of men and more socially-isolated individuals. Furthermore, an extensive weekly television series portraying the work of the Samaritans was associated with a very marked increase in the numbers of people seeking help from the Samaritans in Edinburgh but no effect on attempted suicide rates (Holding 1974).

Strategies likely to have the greatest effect on attempted suicide rates include increased availability of psychosocial help, rather than pharmacological treatment, for patients who have relationship difficulties and similar problems but who are not suffering from significant psychiatric illness; changes in attitudes towards this behaviour with encouragement to use other means of seeking help, perhaps through educa-tion in schools and the media; and lastly, and even more ambitiously, major social change leading to reduced levels of unemployment and alcohol abuse.

REFERENCES

Adam K S 1986 Early family influences on suicidal behaviour. In: Psychobiology of suicidal behavior. Annals of the New York Academy of Sciences 487: 63–76

Alderson M R 1974 Self-poisoning: what is the future? Lancet 1: 1040–1043

Angst J, Merikangas K, Scheidegger P, Wicki W 1990 Recurrent brief depression: a new subtype of affective disorder. Journal of Affective Disorders 19: 87–98

Asberg M, Traskman L, Thoren P 1976 5-HIAA in the cerebrospinal fluid – a biochemical suicide predictor? Archives of General Psychiatry 33: 1193–1197

Asberg M, Nordstrom P, Traskman-Bendz L 1986 Biological factors in suicide. In: Roy A (ed) Suicide. Williams & Wilkins, Baltimore, p 47–71

Atkinson M W, Kessel W I N, Dalgaard J B 1975 The comparability of suicide rates. British Journal of Psychiatry 127: 247–256

Bagley C R 1968 The evaluation of a suicide prevention scheme by an ecological method. Social Science and Medicine 2: 1–14

Bancroft J, Marsack P 1977 The repetitiveness of self-poisoning and self-injury. British Journal of Psychiatry 131: 394–399

Bancroft J, Skrimshire A, Casson J, Harvard-Watts O, Reynolds F 1977 People who deliberately poison or injure themselves: their problems and their contacts with helping agencies. Psychological Medicine 7: 289–303

Bancroft J, Hawton K, Simkin S, Kingston B, Cumming C, Whitwell D 1979 The reasons people give for taking overdoses: a further enquiry. British Journal of Medical Psychology 52: 353–365

Barraclough B M 1970 The effect that coroners have on the suicide rate and the open verdict rate. In: Hare E, Wing J (eds) Psychiatric epidemiology. Oxford University Press, Oxford, p 361–365

Barraclough B M 1972a Are the Scottish and English suicide rates really different? British Journal of Psychiatry 120: 267–273

Barraclough B M 1972b Suicide prevention, recurrent affective disorder and lithium. British Journal of Psychiatry 121: 391–392

Barraclough B M 1973 Differences between national suicide rates. British Journal of Psychiatry 122: 95–6

Barraclough B 1981 Suicide and epilepsy. In: Reynolds E H, Trimble M R (eds) Epilepsy and psychiatry. Churchill Livingstone, Edinburgh, p 72–76

Barraclough B M, Pallis D J 1975 Depression followed by suicide: a comparison of depressed suicides with living depressives. Psychological Medicine 5: 55–61

Barraclough B M, Shea M 1970 Suicide and Samaritan clients. Lancet 2: 868–870

Barraclough B, Bunch J, Nelson B, Sainsbury P 1974 A hundred cases of suicide: clinical aspects. British Journal of Psychiatry 125: 355–373

Beck A T, Ward C H, Mendelson M 1961 An inventory for measuring depression. Archives of General Psychiatry 4:561–571

Beck A T, Schuyler D, Herman J 1974a Development of suicidal intent scales. In: Beck A T, Resnik H L P, Lettieri D J (eds) The prediction of suicide. Charles Press, Maryland, p 45–56

Beck A T, Weissman A, Lester D, Trexler L 1974b The measurement of pessimism: the Hopelessness Scale. Journal of Consulting and Clinical Psychology 42: 861–865

Beck A T, Steer O R A, Kovacs M, Garrison B 1985 Hopelessness and eventual suicide: a ten year prospective study of patients hospitalized with suicidal ideation. American Journal of Psychiatry 145: 559–563

Beck A T, Brown G, Berchick R J, Stewart B L, Steer R A 1990 Relationship between hopelessness and ultimate suicide: a replication with psychiatric outpatients. American Journal of Psychiatry 147: 190–195

Birtchnell J, Floyd S 1974 Attempted suicide and the menstrual cycle – a negative conclusion. Journal of Psychosomatic Research 18: 361–369

Brewer C, Farmer R 1985 Self-poisoning in 1984: a prediction that didn't come true. British Medical Journal 290: 391

Brown G W, Harris T 1978 Social origins of depression. Tavistock Press, London

Brown G L, Ebert M H, Goyer P F, Jimerson D C, Klein W J, Bunney W E, Goodwin F K 1982 Aggression, suicide, and a serotonin: relationships to CSF amine metabolites. American Journal of Psychiatry 139: 741–746

Buglass D, Horton J 1974 A scale for predicting subsequent suicidal behaviour. British Journal of Psychiatry 124: 573–578

Buglass D, McCulloch J W 1970 Further suicidal behaviour: the development and validation of predictive scales. British Journal of Psychiatry 116: 483–491

Bunch J 1972 Recent bereavement in relation to suicide. Journal of Psychosomatic Research 16: 361–366

Cassidy S, Henry J 1987 Fatal toxicity of antidepressant drugs in overdose. British Medical Journal 295: 1021–1024

Catalan J, Marsack P, Hawton K E, Whitwell D, Fagg J, Bancroft J H J 1980 Comparison of doctors and nurses in the assessment of deliberate self-poisoning patients. Psychological Medicine 10: 483–491

Chowdhury N, Hicks R C, Kreitman N 1973 Evaluation of an after-care service for parasuicide (attempted suicide) patients. Social Psychiatry 8: 67–81

Clarke R V, Lester D 1989 Suicide: closing the exits. Springer-Verlag, New York

Copas J B, Freeman-Browne D L, Robin A A 1971 Danger periods for suicide in patients under treatment. Psychological Medicine 1: 400–404

Coryell W, Noyes R, Clancy J 1982 Excess mortality in panic disorder: a comparison with primary unipolar depression. Archives of General Psychiatry 39: 701–703

Department of Health and Social Security 1984 The

management of deliberate self-harm HN (84) 25. Department of Health and Social Security, London

Diekstra R F W 1985 Suicide and suicide attempts in the European Economic Community: an analysis of trends, with special emphasis upon trends among the young. Suicide and Life Threatening Behavior 15: 27–42

Dorpat T L, Ripley H S 1960 A study of suicide in the Seattle area. Comprehensive Psychiatry 1: 349–359

Dorpat T L, Jackson J K, Ripley H S 1965 Broken homes and attempted and completed suicide. Archives of General Psychiatry 12: 213–216

Drake R E, Gates C, Cotton P G, Whitaker A 1984 Suicide among schizophrenics: who is at risk? Journal of Nervous and Mental Disease 172: 613–617

Dyer J A T, Kreitman N 1984 Hopelessness, depression and suicidal intent in parasuicide. British Journal of Psychiatry 144: 127–133

Farberow N L, McEvoy T C 1986 Suicide among patients with diagnosis of anxiety reaction or depressive reaction in general medicinal and surgical hospitals. Journal of Abnormal Psychology 71: 287–299

Forster D P, Frost C E B 1985 Medicinal self-poisoning and prescription frequency. Acta Psychiatrica Scandinavica 71: 657–674

Gibbons J L 1979 The Southampton suicide project. Report to the DHSS, Department of Psychiatry, Southampton

Gibbons J S, Butler P, Urwin P, Gibbons J L 1978a Evaluation of social work service for self-poisoning patients. British Journal of Psychiatry 133: 111–118

Gibbons J S, Elliot J, Urwin P, Gibbons J L 1978b The urban environment and deliberate self-poisoning: trends in Southampton 1972–1977. Social Psychiatry 13: 159–166

Greer S, Bagley C 1971 Effect of psychiatric intervention in attempted suicide: a controlled study. British Medical Journal 1: 310–312

Guze S B, Robins E 1970 Suicide among primary affective disorders. British Journal of Psychiatry 117: 437–438

Hatton C L, Valente S M 1981 Bereavement group for parents who suffered suicidal loss of a child. Suicide and Life-threatening Behavior 11: 141–150

Hawton K 1986 Suicide and attempted suicide among children and adolescents. Sage, Beverly Hills

Hawton K 1989 Controlled studies of psychosocial intervention following attempted suicide. In: Platt S D, Kreitman N (eds) Current research on suicide and parasuicide. Edinburgh University Press, Edinburgh, p 180–195

Hawton K, Blackstock E 1976 General practice aspects of self-poisoning and self-injury. Psychological Medicine 6: 571–575

Hawton K, Catalan J 1987 Attempted suicide: a practical guide to its nature and management, 2nd edn. Oxford University Press, Oxford

Hawton K, Fagg J 1988 Suicide and other causes of death following attempted suicide. British Journal of Psychiatry 152: 359–366

Hawton K, Fagg J 1991 Deliberate self-poisoning and self-injury in older people. International Journal of Geriatric Psychiatry 5: 367–373

Hawton K, Rose N 1986 Unemployment and attempted suicide among men in Oxford. Health Trends 18: 29–32

Hawton K, Fagg J, Marsack P 1980 Association between epilepsy and attempted suicide. Journal of Neurology, Neurosurgery and Psychiatry 43: 168–170

Hawton K, Bancroft J, Catalan J, Kingston B, Stedeford A, Welch N 1981 Domiciliary and outpatient treatment of self-poisoning patients by medical and non-medical staff. Psychological Medicine 11: 169–177

Hawton K, Fagg J, Marsack P, Wells P 1982a Deliberate self-poisoning and self-injury in the Oxford area: 1972–80. Social Psychiatry 17: 175–179

Hawton K, O'Grady J, Osborn M, Cole D 1982b Adolescents who take overdoses: their characteristics, problems and contacts with helping agencies. British Journal of Psychiatry 140: 118–123

Hawton K, Roberts J, Goodwin G 1985 The risk of child abuse among attempted suicide mothers with young children. British Journal of Psychiatry 146: 486–469

Hawton K, McKeown S, Day A, Martin P, O'Connor M, Yule J 1987 Evaluation of outpatient counselling compared with general practitioner care following overdoses. Psychological Medicine 17: 756–761

Hawton K, Fagg J, Simkin S 1988 Unemployment and attempted suicide among women in Oxford. British Journal of Psychiatry 152: 632–637

Hawton K, Fagg J, McKeown S P 1989 Alcoholism, alcohol and attempted suicide. Alcohol and Alcoholism 24: 3–9

Hirsch S R, Walsh C, Draper R 1982 Parasuicide: a review of treatment interventions. Journal of Affective Disorders 4: 299–311

Holding T 1974 The BBC 'Befrienders' series and its effects. British Journal of Psychiatry 124: 470–472

Holding T A, Barraclough B M 1978 Undetermined deaths – suicide or accident? British Journal of Psychiatry 13: 542–549

Holding T, Buglass D, Duffy J C, Kreitman N 1977 Parasuicide in Edinburgh – a seven year review 1968–74. British Journal of Psychiatry 130: 534–543

Herzog A, Resnik H L P 1967 A clinical study of parental response to adolescent death by suicide with recommendations for approaching the survivors. In: Proceedings of the 4th International Conference of Suicide Prevention. Delmar, Los Angeles

James D, Hawton K 1985 Overdoses: explanations and attitudes in self-poisoners and significant others. British Journal of Psychiatry 146: 481–485

Jamison K R 1986 Suicide and bipolar disorders. In: Mann J J, Stanley M (eds) Psychobiology of suicidal behaviour. Annals of the New York Academy of Sciences 487: 301–315

Jennings C, Barraclough B M, Moss J R 1978 Have the Samaritans lowered the suicide rate? A controlled study. Psychological Medicine 8: 413–422

Kety S S 1986 Genetic factors in suicide. In: Roy A (ed) Suicide. Williams & Wilkins, Baltimore, p 41–45

Kennedy P, Kreitman N 1973 An epidemiological survey of parasuicide (attempted suicide) in general practice. British Journal of Psychiatry 123: 23–34

Kessel N, McCulloch W 1966 Repeated acts of self-poisoning and self-injury. Proceedings of the Royal Society of Medicine 59: 89–92

Kreitman N 1976 The coal gas story: UK suicide rates

1960–1971. British Journal of Preventive and Social Medicine 30: 86–93

Kreitman N (ed) 1977 Parasuicide. John Wiley, London

Kreitman N, Casey P 1988 Repetition of parasuicide: an epidemiological and clinical study. British Journal of Psychiatry 153: 792–800

Kreitman N, Chowdhury N 1973 Distressed behaviour: a study of selected Samaritan clients and parasuicides ('attempted suicide' patients). British Journal of Psychiatry 123: 1–8

Kreitman N, Philip A E, Greer S, Bagley C R 1969 Parasuicide. British Journal of Psychiatry 115: 746–747

Lester D 1974 The effect of suicide prevention centres on suicide rates in the United States. Health Services Report 89: 37–39

Levenson M 1974 Cognitive correlates of suicide risk. In Neuringer C (ed) Psychological assessment of suicide risk. Charles C Thomas, Springfield, IL, p 150–163

Linehan M M, Chiles J, Egan K J, Devine R H, Laffaw J A 1986 Presenting problems of parasuicides versus suicide ideators and non-suicidal psychiatric patients. Journal of Consulting and Clinical Psychology 54: 880–881

Mackay A 1979 Self-poisoning – a complication of epilepsy. British Journal of Psychiatry 134: 277–282

McLeavey B C, Daly R J, Murray C M, O'Riordan J, Taylor M 1987 Interpersonal problem-solving deficits in self-poisoning patients. Suicide and Life-threatening Behavior 17: 33–49

McMahon B, Pugh T F 1965 Suicide in the widowed. American Journal of Epidemiology 81: 23–31

Mann J J, Arango V, Marzuk P M, Theccanat S, Reis D J 1989 Evidence for the 5-HT hypothesis of suicide: a review of post-mortem studies. British Journal of Psychiatry 155 (supplement 8): 7–14

Miles C P 1977 Conditions predisposing to suicide: a review. Journal of Nervous and Mental Disease 164: 231–246

Miller H L, Coombs D W, Leeper J D, Barton S N 1984 An analysis of the effects of suicide prevention facilities on suicide rates in the United States. American Journal of Public Health 74: 340–343

Minkoff K, Bergman E, Beck A T, Beck R 1973 Hopelessness, depression and attempted suicide. American Journal of Psychiatry 130: 455–459

Montgomery S A, Montgomery D 1982 Pharmacological prevention of suicidal behaviour. Journal of Affective Disorders 4: 291–298

Morgan H G 1979 Death wishes? The understanding and management of deliberate self-harm. John Wiley, Chichester

Morgan H G, Pocock H, Pottle S 1975 The urban distribution of non-fatal deliberate self-harm. British Journal of Psychiatry 126: 319–328

Motto J A 1980 Suicide risk factors in alcohol abuse. Suicide and Life-threatening Behavior 10: 230–238

Murphy G E, Robins E 1967 Social factors in suicide. Journal of the American Medical Association 199: 303–308

Murphy G E, Armstrong J W, Hermele S L, Fischer J R, Clenendin W W 1979 Suicide and alcoholism: interpersonal loss confirmed as a predictor. Archives of General Psychiatry 36: 65–69

Newson-Smith J G B, Hirsch S R 1979a Psychiatric symptoms in self-poisoning patients. Psychological Medicine 9: 493–500

Newson-Smith J G B, Hirsch S R 1979b A comparison of social workers and psychiatrists in evaluating parasuicide. British Journal of Psychiatry 134: 335–342

Ovenstone I M K, Kreitman N 1974 Two syndromes of suicide. British Journal of Psychiatry 124: 336–345

Pallis D J, Barraclough B M, Levey A B, Jenkins J S, Sainsbury P 1982 Estimating suicide risk among attempted suicides: I. The development of new clinical scales. British Journal of Psychiatry 141: 37–44

Pallis D J, Gibbons J S, Pierce D W 1984 Estimating suicide risk among attempted suicides: II. Efficiency of predictive scales after the attempt. British Journal of Psychiatry 144: 139–148

Paykel E S, Prusoff B A, Myers J K (1975) Suicide attempts and recent life events: a controlled comparison. Archives of General Psychiatry 32: 327–333

Pierce D W 1981 Predictive validation of a suicide intent scale: a 5 year follow up. British Journal of Psychiatry 139: 391–396

Pitts F N, Winokur G 1966 Affective disorder - VII: alcoholism and affective disorder. Journal of Psychiatric Research 4: 37–50

Platt S 1984 Unemployment and suicidal behaviour - a review of the literature. Social Science and Medicine 19: 93–115

Platt S, Kreitman N (1984) Trends in parasuicide and unemployment among men in Edinburgh 1968-82. British Medical Journal 289: 1029–1032

Platt S, Hawton K, Kreitman N, Fagg J, Foster J 1988 Recent clinical and epidemiological trends in parasuicide in Edinburgh and Oxford: a tale of two cities. Psychological Medicine 18: 405–418

Pokorny A 1966 A follow-up study of 618 suicidal patients. American Journal of Psychiatry 122: 1109–1116

Prescott L F, Highley M S 1985 Drugs prescribed for self-poisoners. British Medical Journal 290: 1633–1636

Roberts J, Hawton K 1980 Child abuse and attempted suicide. British Journal of Psychiatry 137: 319–323

Robins E, Murphy G E, Wilkinson R H, Gassner S, Kayes J 1959 Some clinical considerations in the prevention of suicide based on a study of 134 successful suicides. American Journal of Public Health 49: 888–899

Rosen D H 1975 Suicide survivors: a follow-up study of persons who survived jumping from the Golden Gate and San Francisco/Oakland Bay Bridges. Western Journal of Medicine 122: 289–294

Roy A 1982a Suicide in chronic schizophrenia. British Journal of Psychiatry 141: 171–177

Roy A 1982b Risk factors for suicide in psychiatric patients. Archives of General Psychiatry 39: 1089–1095

Roy A 1983 Suicide in depressives. Comprehensive Psychiatry 24: 487–491

Roy A 1989 Genetics of suicide. In: Mann J J, Stanley M (eds) Psychobiology of suicidal behaviour. Annals of the New York Academy of Sciences 487: 97–105

Rudestam K E 1977 The impact of suicide among the young. Essence 1: 221–224

Sainsbury P 1986 The epidemiology of suicide. In: Roy A (ed) Suicide. Williams & Wilkins, Baltimore, p 17–40

Sainsbury P, Barraclough B M 1968 Differences between suicide rates. Nature 220: 1252

Sellar C, Hawton K, Goldacre M J 1990 Self-poisoning in adolescents. Hospital admissions and deaths in the Oxford region 1980–85. British Journal of Psychiatry 156: 866–870

Scheftner W A, Young M A, Endicott J, Coryell W, Fogg L, Clark D C, Fawcett J 1988 Family history and five year suicide risk. British Journal of Psychiatry 153: 805–809

Shepherd D M, Barraclough B M 1976 The aftermath of parental suicide for children. British Journal of Psychiatry 129: 267–276

Shepherd D M, Barraclough B M 1980 Work and suicide: an empirical investigation. British Journal of Psychiatry 136: 469–478

Sheskin A, Wallace S E 1976 Differing bereavements: suicide, natural and accidental death. Omega 7: 229–242

Sims A 1984 Neurosis and mortality: investigating an association. Journal of Psychosomatic Research 28: 353–362

Sims A, Prior P 1978 The pattern of mortality in severe neuroses. British Journal of Psychiatry 133: 299–305

Skrimshire A M 1976 A small area analysis of self-poisoning and self-injury in the region of Oxford. Journal of Biosocial Science 8: 85–112

Sloan J H, Rivara F P, Reay D T, Ferris J A J, Kellermann A L 1990 Firearm regulations and rates of suicide. A comparison of two metropolitan areas. New England Journal of Medicine 322: 369–373

Smith R 1985 Occupationless health. 'I couldn't stand it any more': suicide and unemployment. British Medical Journal 291: 1563–1566

Stengel E, Cook N G 1958 Attempted suicide: its social significance and effects. Maudsley Monograph 4. Oxford University Press, Oxford

Tonks C M, Rack P H, Rose M J 1968 Attempted suicide and the menstrual cycle. Journal of Psychosomatic Research 11: 319–323

Tuckman J, Youngman W F 1968 A scale for assessing suicide risk of attempted suicides. Journal of Clinical Psychology 24: 17–19

Urwin P, Gibbons J L 1979 Psychiatric diagnosis in self-poisoning patients. Psychological Medicine 9: 501–507

Weiner I W 1969 The effectiveness of a suicide prevention program. Mental Hygiene 53: 357–363

Weissman M M 1974 The epidemiology of suicide attempts, 1960–71. Archives of General Psychiatry 30: 737–746

Weissman M M, Klerman G L, Markowitz J S, Ouellette R 1989 Suicidal ideation and suicide attempts in panic disorder and attacks. New England Journal of Medicine 321: 1209–1214

Wetzel R D 1976 Hopelessness, depression and suicide intent. Archives of General Psychiatry 33: 1069–1073

Wexler L, Weissman M M, Kasl S V 1978 Suicide attempts 1970–75: updating a United States study and comparisons with international trends. British Journal of Psychiatry 132: 180–185

Whitlock F A 1986 Suicide and physical illness. In: Roy A (ed) Suicide. Williams & Wilkins, Baltimore, p 151–170

Wing J K, Cooper J E, Sartorius N 1974 The measurement and classification of psychiatric symptoms. Cambridge University Press, Cambridge

Worden W 1983 Grief counselling and grief therapy. Tavistock Press, London

41. Depression in general practice

Paul R. Freeling   André Tylee

The chapter on depression in general practice for the first edition of this handbook was written by Dr Arthur Watts, who was among the first to describe systematically the frequency and nature of depressive illness seen in general practice. It seems therefore appropriate to start with a description of his pioneering work.

With the introduction of the National Health Service in 1947, British GPs acquired a defined practice population and the possibility of knowing its distribution by age and sex. Dr Watts, a GP in rural Leicestershire, was immediately aware of the opportunities offered and kept uniquely rigorous records of his depressed patients from 1947 onwards. At the outset (Watts 1947) he was concerned, like many GPs today, that he might be overdiagnosing depression but his psychiatric colleagues largely confirmed his findings. This sense of disbelief about frequency and prevalence and associated concerns about validity and caseness continue to dog consideration of depressive illness in general practice.

Dr Watts continued to treat and observe his depressed patients, mainly in the community, for at least 20 years (Watts 1966) and found a lifetime risk in his practice over 20 years for clinically significant depression of approximately 10 cases per thousand.

Watts was also the first to highlight the extent to which depression went unrecognized by GPs. He described the filtering process which produced a five-tier pyramid. The top layer was the tiny proportion who died by suicide in a single year (0.12 per 1000); the next layer comprised the admissions to mental hospital in a year (0.13 per 1000 compulsory admissions, 0.77 per 1000 informal admissions); and the third layer consisted of people who reached psychiatric outpatients or were seen by the psychiatrist at home or in the courts (1.90 per 1000). The fourth layer (12–15 per 1000) were those depressed patients who consulted GPs, of whom Watts believed about one-half were not recog-

nised. The fifth tier, estimated by Watts at some 150 per 1000, comprised those depressed patients who did not seek medical advice of any kind.

EPIDEMIOLOGICAL ASPECTS

Caseness and workload

That depressive disorder is indeed frequent in general practice was confirmed by Shepherd and colleagues (1966) who demonstrated that 20–25% of a GP's workload concerned psychiatric morbidity, the largest proportion of which involved depressive symptoms. Meanwhile other GPs had pioneered the use of case-report discussion in groups to study the psychological disorders seen by general practitioners (Balint 1957), and some of those discussed also appear to have been suffering from depressive illness (Sowerby 1977).

Much of the early work in general practice dealt with the symptoms of depression, rather than operationally defined syndromes, and the absence of an instrument with an agreed threshold for 'caseness' probably contributed to widely differing rates for depression being reported (Blacker & Clare 1987). Dunn & Skuse (1981) examined an eminent British GP's case-notes over the 20 years up to 1976 and found that one in every six women and one in every 20 men registered in his practice received a diagnosis of depression. A similar retrospective study of one GP's notes in Indiana, in this instance over 15 years, found that 23.5% of those seen continuously had been suffering from depression and 40% of these had presented with 'depression, nervousness or fatigue' (Justin 1976).

The word 'depression' can, of course, mean different things: it can describe a normal variant of mood which is in no way pathological and commonly experienced; it can describe a mood variant of pathological severity symptomatic of a variety of psychiatric disorders; and lastly it can be a syndrome. A diagnosis of pathological disorder requires elucidation of the 'quality' of mood disorder and 'quantity' of associated features and symptoms. In general practice there is a particular risk of overestimating disorder by failing to distinguish between the three meanings and this may well be why there has been so much debate about psychiatric caseness in general-practice populations.

The difficulty of establishing uniformity in the level of severity used to decide 'caseness' of psychiatric disorder is well-rehearsed (Bebbington et al 1981, Wing et al 1978, Goldberg 1982). It is widely exemplified in the literature concerning psychological disorder in general practice. By the late 1960s rating scales were being utilized in general practice to try to resolve problems of caseness and diagnostic accuracy. Salkind (1969) applied the cognitively-oriented Beck Depression Inventory (BDI) (Beck et al 1961) to a sample of 80 consecutive GP attenders. He used a cut-off score of 11, which led to 48% of his sample being classified as being in a 'depressed state'. Salkind considered this 'startling' but possibly related to the social class of his patients and his own consulting style. A later study in the USA (Nielsen & Williams 1980) found that 19.8% of 562 ambulatory primary care medical patients scored 10 and over on the BDI, while 12.2% scored at least 13, which the authors recommended as the caseness threshold. Williamson (1987), also in the USA, found 15.3% of 131 males and 15.7% of 223 females at or over this threshold (Table 41.1).

Table 41.1   Studies of depression in primary care – Beck's Depression Inventory

Study	Sample	Results
Salkind 1969	80	BDI > 11 = 48%
Nielsen & Williams 1980	526	BDI > 9 = 19.8%
Parker et al 1986	564	BDI > 9 = 25% female = 17% male
Williamson 1987	131 (m) 223 (f)	BDI > 9 = 15.3% (m) = 15.7% (f)
Rosenthal et al 1987	123	BDI > 12 = 28%

The Zung Self Rating Depression Scale (SDS) (Zung 1965) identified 13.2% of 1086 attenders in US primary care as 'symptomatically depressed' by scoring over 55 (Zung et al 1983), and 12% in a smaller sample of 499 using the same threshold (Zung & King 1983). However, a cut-off score of 50 on the instrument identified 45% of 212 attenders in a North Carolina

practice as depressed (Moore et al 1978), similar to the 51% (of 95) obtained in Los Angeles (Linn & Yager 1984) and 41% (of 377) in Louisiana (Davis et al 1987) and the rate reported by Salkind using the Beck Inventory. Consecutive attenders in six practices in Sydney, Australia, screened with the SDS, produced 21% considered to be significantly depressed, using a cut-off score of 40 (Bradshaw & Parker 1983) (Table 41.2).

Hankin & Locke (1983) applied another instrument developed for epidemiological studies (the Center for Epidemiological Studies Depression Scale – CES-D; Radloff 1977) and found that 21% of 1921 attenders were rated as cases. Using the same cut-off, two later studies in the USA (Schulberg et al 1985, Duer et al 1988) found that 12% of 1554 attenders and 27% of 262 attenders were depressed respectively. A Canadian study (Barnes & Prosen 1984) identified 33.2% of 1250 attenders as over this threshold for depression (Table 41.3).

Table 41.2   Studies of depression in primary care – Zung Self-rating Depression Scale

Study	Sample	Results
Moore et al 1978	212	SDS > 50 = 45%
Wright et al 1980	199	SDS > 50 = 41%
Zung et al 1983	1086	SDS > 55 = 13.2%
Zung & King 1983	499	SDS > 55 = 12%
Bradshaw & Parker 1983	251	SDS > 40 = 21%
Linn & Yager 1984	95	SDS > 50 = 51%
Davis et al 1987	377	SDS > 50 = 41%
Rosenthal et al 1987	123	SDS > 55 = 21%

Table 41.3   Studies of depression in primary care – Center for Epidemiological Studies Depression Scale (CES-D)

Study	Sample	Results
Hankin & Locke 1983	1921	CES-D > 16 = 21%
Barnes & Prosen 1984	1250	CES-D > 16 = 33.2%
Schulberg et al 1985	1554	CES-D > 16 = 12%
Duer et al 1988	262	CES-D > 16 = 27%

Porter (1970) conducted a treatment study of depression in 1970 in his single-handed English practice and, using rather idiosyncratic criteria, obtained a rate of 1.7% in men and 7.8% in women consulting him, thus producing calculated annual incidences per 1000 patients at risk of 6.5% for men and 29.3 for women. Johnson & Mellor (1977) found GP-diagnosed 'depressive illness' in 3.7% of consecutive attenders at five Manchester practices.

In the Third National Morbidity Study (RCGP/OPCS/DHSS 1986), GPs from England and Wales in 1981–1982 reported 28 patients per year per 1000 at risk to be suffering from depression. The problems caused by relying on non-standardized diagnoses are well illustrated by the fact that the National Morbidity Study 10 years earlier (RCGP/OPCS/DHSS 1979) had obtained an annual case rate for neurotic depression of 31 per 1000 and that this itself had reflected a twentyfold increase over a similar study in the 1950s (Crombie 1974). The increase may have reflected increased recognition and acceptance of depression by GPs and by patients but in some studies GPs have tended to report only patients for whom they have prescribed drugs (Watson & Barber 1981, Burton & Freeling 1982) while choosing to manage similar numbers of depressives in other ways. To this source of inaccuracy must be added false positives: only half of the patients given antidepressants by their GP received diagnoses of major depression (Sireling et al 1985a), although 96% were categorized as having some kind of psychiatric diagnosis by a formal standardized psychiatric interview external to the GP consultation.

Operationally defined criteria and standardized interviews

The use of the rigorously standardized psychiatric interviews with well-defined thresholds for disorder, developed in the UK (Wing et al 1974) and in the USA (American Psychiatric Association 1980), has dramatically affected studies in general practice. Such research interviews, applied externally to the GP's own interview after screening consecutive attenders in a two-stage design, have led to more accurate estimates of the incidence and prevalence of disorder (Table 41.4).

Wright and colleagues (1980) used such a two-stage design. Compliance with the second stage was poor, but they estimated from their data that 17% of their sample of 199 consulting patients in a Kentucky family

Table 41.4 Two-stage studies of depression in primary care

Study	Instruments and rates	
	1st stage	2nd stage
Hoeper et al 1979	(n = 1327) GHQ30 > 4 = 32%	(n = 247) SADS 5.8% major depression
Wright et al 1980	(n = 199) SDS > 50 = 41%	(n = 26) RDC depressive disorder 17%
Nielsen & Williams 1980	(n = 526) BDI > 10 = 19.8%	(n = 88) DSM-II 10% depressive neurosis
Schulberg et al 1985	(n = 1554) CES-D > 16 = 12%	(n = 294) DIS 9.2% current depression
Parker et al 1986	(n = 564) BDI > 9 = 25% f = 17% m	(n = 35) PSE case 83%
Von Korf et al 1987	(n = 1242) GHQ28 > 5 = 39%	(n = 809) DIS 5% major depression
Bridges & Goldberg 1987	(n = 590) GHQ28 > 5 = 45%	(n = 283) DSM-III 13% major depression
Coulehan et al 1988	none	(n = 294) DIS 7.1% major depression
Blacker & Clare 1988	(n = 2308) GHQ30 > 5 = 47%	(n = 1219) SADS/RDC 4.3% major depression
Dhadphale et al 1989	(n = 881) SRQ = 25%	(n = 881) DSM-IIIR 1.2% major depression

practice has depressive disorder as defined by the Research Diagnostic Criteria (RDC) (Spitzer et al 1978).

A brief psychiatric interview applied as a second stage with 41 (47%) of 88 people who had scored more than 10 on the BDI rated just over half as depressed by the Feighner et al (1972) criteria (Nielsen & Williams 1980). Bridges & Goldberg (1987), using the revised third version of the *Diagnostic and Statistical Manual of Mental Disorders* (DSM-IIIR; American Psychiatric Association 1980), found that nearly 13% of 590 consecutive attenders aged 15 and over consulting a GP for a new episode of illness had a diagnosable major depression disorder. Hoeper and colleagues (1979) used the Schedule for Affective Disorders and Schizophrenia (SADS) (Endicott & Spitzer 1978) as the second stage with 1327 patients over 3 months in one primary care setting. They found point prevalence rates of 5.8% for major depressive disorder, 5% for intermittent depression and 3.4% for minor depressive disorder.

Coulehan and colleagues (1968) found that 7.1% of 294 primary case attenders in three practices in Pittsburgh had DSM-III major depressive disorder on the third version of the Diagnostic Interview Schedule (DIS; Robins et al 1981). In the Sydney practices of 12 GPs (Parker et al 1986), only 29% of screen-positive potential depressives accepted further study: 83% were considered cases on subsequent interview, using the Present State Examination (PSE; Wing et al 1974): the effect was that 29 out of 564 attenders (64% female) who were screened were found to be depressed. Block and colleagues (1988) in Pittsburgh found that 9.2% of 294 new attenders to three primary care clinics met DSM-III criteria for depressive disorder. Von Korf and colleagues (1987), in a Baltimore group practice, found a 5% prevalence for DSM-III major depression using the DIS as second stage with 809 patients. In Kenya, 9.2% of 881 patients randomly selected from outpatient queues were depressed (Dhadphale et al 1989).

When a self-completed instrument based on DSM-III was used by attenders to a practice in Nebraska, much higher rates were obtained for depression: 18.5% of 54 males and 19.2% of 146 females (Yates et al 1985).

A well-conducted study of depression in a single Inner London health-centre practice (Blacker & Clare 1988) obtained a prevalence of 4.3% for RDC major depressive disorder among 2308 consecutive attenders. With between 70% and 90% of people with depressive disorder consulting their GP for help (Wing et al 1974, Brown & Harris 1978, Weissman & Myers 1978) this would produce a prevalence rate for depression similar to the common estimate of 5% in the community (Paykel 1989a).

Demography

An excess rate for depression among women of 3:1 or 4:1 has frequently been reported from general practice (Porter 1970, Dunn & Skuse 1981, Sireling et al 1985a, Blacker & Clare 1988). This may not simply represent sex differences in consultation rates or help-seeking behaviour, because differences are seen also in community studies and probably reflect psychosocial, hormonal and genetic factors (Paykel 1989a).

Casey and colleagues (1984) found an excess of depression among women in primary care and of alcoholism and personality disorder among men, although the total of psychiatric disorder did not differ between the sexes, suggesting that men and women express their psychiatric morbidity in different ways. A feature unique to men has been described as interpersonal behaviour change, characterized by social withdrawal, indecisiveness and irritability, and these features can signal depression in males despite the absence of dysphoria (Williamson 1987).

Another factor producing the apparent excess of depression in females may be biased behaviour by GPs: women are more likely to receive prescriptions for psychotropic drugs while men are more likely to receive antibiotics, even for problems which are psychosocial (Raynes 1979). Marks and his colleagues (1979) found that characteristics such as unemployment, female sex and marriages that had ended by separation, divorce or death were associated with an increased likelihood of the doctor detecting a psychiatric illness. That GPs tend to use demographic factors as supporting evidence rather than as cues is suggested in an another study (Freeling et al 1985), which found no differences between the demographic characteristics of patients whose depression was recognized when they consulted their GP and those whose depression went unrecognized.

Jenkins & Shepherd (1983) suggest that environment contributes mainly to the sex difference in psychiatric morbidity. Jenkins & Clare (1985) concluded that there is substantial evidence that the excess of depression in women is environmental rather than genetic and that there is not enough endocrinological evidence to support the notion that their reproductive biology is to blame. A Canadian study (Barnes & Prosen 1984) found depression scores highest in females, patients who were unemployed and patients who were divorced and separated.

The age of people suffering from depression and seen by GPs is generally lower than was traditionally taught (Porter 1970, Sireling et al 1985a). This may reflect the relative preponderance of neurotic rather than psychotic depression in general practice: Grad de Alarcon (1975) reported that the peak age for psychotic depression was in the 50s and for neurotic depression in the 30s. Blacker & Clare (1988) found that 41% of patients with major depression, 48% of patients with minor depression and 49% of people with other psychiatric disorders were aged under 35 years. However, 54% of their sample of 2308 attenders to the inner-city practice were aged under 35, with a median of 34 years old.

There is debate about any relationship between race and depression. Zung and colleagues (1988) found similar depressive symptoms reported by blacks and by whites in two primary care settings in Durham, North Carolina.

When considering seasonal factors, Harris (1986a, b) has described how diagnoses of depression were very significantly more common in April and May, with a much less impressive peak 6 months later, exactly as in studies based on suicide statistics and hospital admissions data. Blacker & Clare's (1988) study confirmed the winter finding in their major depressives.

Socioeconomic status is inversely related to the likelihood that a person in primary care will report depression, (Hesbacher et al 1975, Wright et al 1980, Nielsen & Williams 1980) which does not, of course, imply that respondents of a higher social class are not depressed. In general the social-class distribution of individual general-practice populations in the UK is not well described and findings related to class cannot always be generalized. It is likely, however, that results related to class which are derived from population studies can be extrapolated to general practice.

The importance of provoking agents, such as severe events and major difficulties, and vulnerability factors, such as a lack of social support in a crisis, in the aetiology of depression is well established (Brown & Harris 1978, Brown et al 1986), with 68% of depressed women having seen their GP in the previous year. Other social factors are also likely to apply within individual practices. These would include a reduction in ongoing difficulties and the occurrence of a 'fresh start' event often preceding recovery (Brown et al 1988) and even a threatening life change predicting recovery if

it promised some hope of a better future. It would be important for GPs to be aware that working-class mothers in full-time employment are at risk of depression either because of prior work strain or because of deviant behaviour by a husband, boyfriend or child causing stress (Brown & Bifulco 1990).

Poor physical environment, in objective terms, both of the interior and exterior of the dwellings of a group of women registered with a practice on a South London housing estate was associated with higher depression, as were their personal perceptions about the unpleasantness of their milieu (Birtchnell et al 1988).

DIAGNOSTIC CONSIDERATIONS

The debate over definition and caseness and the variations in some of the findings indicate the difficulties encountered in recognizing depressive disorder, accurately assessing its severity and selecting its management. This makes the diagnosis of depressive disorder in primary care a major challenge to the attitudes, skills and knowledge of the professionals concerned.

A general practitioner needs to pick up and identify any available 'cue' to depression which may appear anywhere in a consultation. Once a cue has been identified, assessment is necessary to establish as soon as is feasible the probability of the patient suffering from a depressive illness. This entails not only exploring the sufferer's experience but also excluding, or identifying and treating, any of a range of physical conditions which may be linked to the depression. If a depressive illness is recognized, the GP needs to acknowledge it to the patient in a non-threatening manner which conveys some hope. Acknowledgment needs to be followed by an explanation of depression as a syndrome rather than a single symptom or normal mood which might be treated by the sufferer 'pulling herself together'. Only after this sequence has been implemented should management be decided upon, in collaboration with the patient who should understand the probabilities, problems, benefits and risks of the different methods available. GPs will sometimes decide to postpone some of these steps to a later interview.

Although British GPs average some 10 minutes per interview they have the advantage of being able to arrange frequent, even daily, contact. This is helped by the continuous nature of the care provided by GPs in the UK and family doctors in many other countries so that a consultation comprises not simply a single doctor – patient contact but a process spread over a number of interviews (RCGP 1972). The opportunity for the patient to consider and review matters between doctor-contacts is fundamental to medical care provided by UK GPs (Freeling & Barry 1982). It allows for proper organization of the rather indefinite descriptions of symptoms provided by people making their first professional contact for a particular episode of illness and, conversely, it reduces the risk of misorganizing the illness itself (Freeling & Harris 1984, Grol 1989).

Perhaps because of its difficulty, depressive illness is among the most rewarding diagnoses which a GP can make. Much of general practice consists of conditions which are self-limiting, though acute, or conditions with an inevitable downhill progression towards chronic handicap and disability (Freeling 1985). The successful management of depressive disorder can produce relief which is dramatic and rewarding because the patient's return to reasonable cognitive function and emotional drive allows the taking and implementation of decisions which can improve social performance and family and working life.

Of fundamental importance is the definition of the syndrome of symptoms and their severity, which is used to help distinguish between the amorphous mass of human malaise on the one hand and those conditions for which there is management of proven efficacy.

Doubt as to the predictive value, in the presence of physical disorder in hospitalized patients, of some symptoms which contribute to depressive diagnoses has led to the construction the Hospital Anxiety and Depression Scale (HADS; Zigmond & Snaith 1983), which excludes somatic symptoms of depression. GPs, faced with the need sometimes to make a diagnosis between different causes of symptoms rather than seeking for simultaneous causes, have a difficulty which is less well understood. Correct definition of emotional state may depend nevertheless on the presence or absence of physical symptoms and the individual GP's ability to tolerate ambiguity. Williams & Skuse (1988) have described how depressive thoughts were commonly reported by a sample of attenders in one practice in South London and that their occurrence corresponded more with the psychiatrist's diagnosis of depression than the GP's. The authors concluded that more attention should be paid to content, rather than simply expressing depression as a total score or as being above a threshold score. Blacker & Clare (1988) used discriminant analysis to show that six symptoms are highly significantly associated with depressive disorder and distinguished between depressive disorder, other forms of psychiatric disorder, taken collectively, and

physical illnesses. In order of statistical importance the symptoms were: insomnia, fatigue, loss of interest, morbid self-opinion and finally (with equal importance) impairment of concentration and hopelessness with or without recurrent suicidal thoughts. Four symptoms distinguished depression from anxiety; loss of interest, morbid self-opinion (with or without morbid guilt) and insomnia.

Errors by GPs in recognizing depressive disorder might arise if they do not require the same number of symptoms to be present as do psychiatrists or if they accept as relevant only a more limited repertoire of symptoms. Such differences in criteria would produce both false-positive and false-negative diagnoses when GPs were assessed against research diagnoses by psychiatrists. It may be, also, that one symptom repeatedly reported carries weight with a GP similar to the mention of a number of different symptoms once each. These differences in diagnostic approaches could easily arise from the tendency for GPs to make diagnoses over a series of relatively short patient contacts.

Table 41.5   Research diagnostic criteria (RDC) for major depression

1) One or more distinct periods with dysphoric mood or pervasive loss of interest (i.e. depressed, sad, blue, can't be bothered or irritable)

2) At least five of the following symptoms for definite and four for probable:
   appetite or weight change
   sleep change
   anergia, fatigue or tiredness
   psychomotor agitation or retardation
   loss of interest or pleasure in usual activities (e.g. sex or socializing)
   feelings of self-reproach or excessive or inappropriate guilt
   diminished thinking or concentration
   recurrent thoughts of suicide or death

Duration of dysphoria at least 1 week (definite = more than 2 weeks, probable = 1–2 weeks). The person needs to have sought help or have been sent by someone or to have difficulty in relationships or have taken medication for the dysphoria. There must be no evidence of schizophrenia.

GPs need, therefore, an effective diagnostic schedule to aid in the recognition of depressive disorder. As we describe below, it has been demonstrated that benefits from drug intervention are predicted at a level of severity equal to or greater than RDC probable major depression (Hollyman et al 1988). Even though the RDC were originally derived by research psychiatrists in the USA we have found the definitions described by

Spitzer and colleagues (1978) (see Table 41.5) easy to memorize and apply in everyday British general practice. The use of such an instrument, which relies upon the presence or absence of a selection from a constellation of symptoms, reduces the problems of 'caseness' and supplies the GP with a response set of suitable questions to be triggered by a depression 'cue' in exactly the same manner as the cue word 'pain' triggers a response set in all medically-trained people. Perhaps in time general practice will generate its own response set and diminish some of the problems encountered by GPs. After all, even the RDC definition of major depression includes key symptoms such as changes in appetite and sleep and easy fatiguability which can just as well be produced by organic disease as by affective disorder.

Structure of general practice

Organizational

The structure of British general practice has changed with increasing rapidity over the past 20 years (Freeling & Fitton 1983), culminating in the changes following the implementation in April 1990 of the 'New GP Contract' within the National Health Service. Large group practices now have several partners sharing lists with each other, and offer clinical experience to vocational and other trainees as well as to medical students, preclinical as well as clinical. The work of these practices is no longer simply reactive to the needs of patients presenting with malaise but proactive, seeking to provide preventive care and to modify lifestyles. This work may in many practices result in patients making their first contact for an episode of care with a member of the primary care team who is not medically trained. Practices with such complex structures may find it difficult to match some of their patients' expectations of a 'family doctor' who knows them well. Balint's (1957) notion of a 'collusion of anonymity' can now occur without the patient ever being referred to a outpatient department but simply moving around within the arrangements of a group practice. The structure described seems to appeal to some patients, who can hide in its interstices and play on the lack of intimacy. A GP covering an absent partner may be less likely to be 'cued' in to underlying depression by recognizing an inconsistency in the patient's behaviour (Freeling 1983) or to have the pre-existing relationship necessary for a patient to open with a statement about mood. It must be said, however,

that, just as with hypothyroidism, depression can be missed by the doctor who regularly sees that patient while a new doctor may recognize it by the incongruity of affect which is produced (Freeling 1983). With the decreased likelihood of patient and doctor acquiring familiarity automatically comes the need for more detailed training in skills to supplement those which, for some doctors and their patients, used to suffice for an encounter which had a major social component of mutual familiarity.

Geographical

It has long been stated that the geography of a consulting room, such as the position of the desk, the doctor and the patient, has a major effect on the development of intimacy within a consultation (Pietroni 1976), and most GPs today routinely avoid having a physical barrier between them and the patient. Patients prefer friendly, less formal consulting rooms without any desk at all (Bevan et al 1979). The absence of a physical barrier, however, does not automatically mean that other non-physical barriers to communication are removed.

It can be seen that changes in the structure of general practice can have unexpected effects upon its process.

The process of care

The medical model of process comprising the sequence of history taking, physical examination, investigation, diagnosis and treatment continues to be taught at medical school but is not always manifest in the consultations of experienced clinicians, especially those of GPs. GPs often seem to make management decisions first and then formulate a diagnosis to justify implementation of those decisions (Howie 1972). This style may have developed because the structure of primary medical care leads to an undifferentiated mixture of physical, psychological and social symptoms being presented in patient-initiated consultations, or perhaps because the early symptoms of serious disease may be impossible to distinguish immediately from those of self-limiting ones. GPs, then, adopt a pragmatic, problem-solving approach, based often on probabilities (Crombie 1963, RCGP 1972) and linked to notions of the threat of a condition together with the effectiveness of available interventions. These processes can be explored in groups and improvements can be produced in the approach which it is intended should be adopted towards the care of specific conditions such as depression, hypertension, diabetes and others (Freeling & Burton 1982). On the other hand, studies of decision-making in psychiatric conditions by GPs (Jenkins et al 1985) and by GP trainees compared with psychiatric trainees (Wilkinson 1988) have shown low agreement within and between groups. This could be related to the ability or the willingness of individual doctors to elicit the symptoms of conditions such as depressive illness. Certainly, when studying associations between scores on a psychiatric screening questionnaire and the number of cues to psychological disturbance given in the consultation, Davenport and his colleagues (1987) concluded that the reason why some doctors are better able than others to detect psychiatric illness is that they are more likely to allow patients to express verbal cues about lowered mood as well as somehow permitting 'vocal' (paraverbal) cues such as sighing. This giving of permission is probably related to, and may account in part for, the wide variation among GPs in their ability to detect psychiatric disorders (Shepherd et al 1966) which has been attributed to the personal bias of individual doctors towards or away from such problems (Marks et al 1979).

This notion of personal idiosyncrasy lying at the root of GP variability has led to a series of efforts to improve GPs' performance with patients who have emotional disorders or psychiatric illnesses. In the 1950s and 1960s these efforts lay largely in the field of what has come to be called Balint training. The training consisted of the discussion, in small groups comprising peers, of case reports made by the responsible doctor. The emphasis was on acquiring an understanding of the patient rather than agreeing a nosological diagnosis, and relied especially on the nature of the relationship and transaction between doctor and patient. Successful training was reported to produce a small but significant change in the doctor's personality (Balint et al 1965). For many doctors such a successful outcome might take 5 years of meeting once weekly for 2 hours for three 13-week terms a year. Originally, all groups were led by psychoanalysts; later, leadership spread to GPs who had themselves experienced the training and for whom a 'group of groups' was often provided. The fact of continuing responsibility of the doctor for the patient was seen originally as very important; nevertheless the technique has been adopted for trainees with considerable success.

Improving the process performance of all GPs, like changing the structure of their practices, might produce some unexpected effects. A patient who wants to avoid the stigmatizing effect of a diagnosis of depression may avoid a doctor known to have a high bias towards the identification of depression, preferring a doctor with a low bias who limits himself to dealing with the presenting physical complaint. What is necessary is a GP who has not only polished the social and interpersonal skills of interviewing but also extended his or her self-knowledge and understanding. These categories of learning are most likely to be achieved within an interactive small group with a skilled leader able to use a range of methods aimed at achieving specific tasks. The most suitable forum for achieving the quality of being open to the emotions of others, unafraid of involvement, yet professionally responsible and able to tolerate one's own uncertainty and helplessness seems to be case discussion and a series of relatively long learning interviews with people needing help. It seems likely that the models used to explain these interviews are much less important than the experience of undertaking them: of sharing a room and a conversation with another human being who has come for help. The learning process may bear a similarity to that of psychotherapy, in which time spent with the patient seems as good a predictor of benefit as the school of origin of the therapist.

A model of the process that GPs thought they used to identify depressed patients and decide upon their management was derived by two groups of GPs (Burton & Freeling 1982). GPs were first 'cued' to consider depressive illness and then applied a check list of symptoms. If depressive illness seemed likely, they assessed recent life events and 'depressive tendencies', which included past or family history of depressive illness or an adverse upbringing. Management decisions were reported to be based on this information.

When the GPs applied their model to an audit of their care of depressive illness their most commonly used cue proved to be the volunteering by the patient of a single symptom of depression (82%), second was the patient saying 'I feel depressed' (52%), third was the ill-defined cue that the doctor 'felt' the patient was depressed (53%), and fourth was the recurrent presentation of symptoms without identifiable organic cause (44%). Only rarely did a single cue trigger the process of seeking supporting evidence.

The doctors had said during their discussions that if a depressed patient had few recent life events and no obvious depressive tendency they would not prescribe but reconsider the diagnosis, and if a patient had a low depressive tendency but many life events they would rely on counselling instead of drugs. When they recorded and audited what they actually did, every patient whom they reported had been prescribed an antidepressant drug, although 36% of them were in one of these 'won't prescribe' groups. This group of GPs conformed to those reported in most other studies by showing great variability in their rates of diagnosis: one of them reported nearly a half of all the cases audited.

The need for GPs to pursue a hypothetico-deductive approach is widely accepted and it would be impossible for a GP to take an extensive formal psychiatric history from every patient.

Attempts have been made to replace the need for GPs to have a high degree of sensitivity to cues of emotional disturbance by providing them with the results of screening questionnaires applied in the waiting room. Providing American family doctors with scores from the 28-item General Health Questionnaire (GHQ; Goldberg & Hillier 1979) produced no increase in the recognition of mental disorder (Hoeper et al 1984) although in a study of one British GP with a known interest in psychiatry the results of the 60-item GHQ proved helpful (Johnstone & Goldberg 1976). It has been suggested that, rather than replacing the emotional antennae of the GP with a print-out of a screening test, it would be sensible to replace the GP with a specially trained worker for some groups known to be at high risk, such as women with postnatal depression. Health visitors trained in Rogerian counselling, seeing such women for eight weekly visits, obtained significant improvements in psychiatric morbidity at 3 months when compared with a control group receiving routine help (Holden et al 1989).

Interviewing behaviours have been taught to, and shown to increase the accuracy of, American family-practice trainees in recognizing psychiatric disorders, although those who performed poorly at onset seemed also to need teaching about approaches to management (Goldberg et al 1980a, b). The technique of problem-based interviewing developed at McMaster University in Canada (Lesser 1985) has successfully been taught to GP trainees (Gask et al 1988) and to a self-selected group of established GPs (Gask et al 1987). The latter improved their skills in psychiatry, which were already good (Gask et al 1987). There must be a suspicion that, as hypothesized above, the improvement in performance is related in part to the group work and not only to the technique learnt. However, it has been demonstrated that communication-skills training of GPs has increased patient satisfaction (Evans et al 1987) and also that interviewing skills taught to medical students persist into professional life (Maguire et al 1986) so that the acquisition of appropriate techniques is in itself likely to be of lasting value. It remains important to identify skills which are associated with accurate identification of depression by GPs.

Recognition of depression

A review of studies (Goldberg & Huxley 1980) estimated that only half of cases of psychiatric disorder are recognized as such by GPs.

Similarly, just over half of those with major depression identified by independent screening in GP waiting rooms are not recognized as depressed by their doctor during the interviews which follow. This remains true whether screening is restricted to patients consulting for a new episode (Bridges & Goldberg 1987) or for any reason, including old episodes and parents bringing children (Skuse & Williams 1984, Freeling et al 1985). Recognition of depression has been reported to be more accurate in the elderly, with acknowledgement being the major problem (MacDonald 1986). The method used in this study included a recording sheet on the GP's desk which could have acted as an aide-memoire, a recurrent cue to the recognition of depression. GPs may recognize depression in the elderly yet decide not to acknowledge it because of a reluctance to prescribe a tricyclic or because it may be felt that depression is characteristic of declining years.

American family physicians also seem to have problems about recognizing depressive illness, whether they are established practitioners (Nielsen & Williams 1980, Hoeper et al 1980, Hankin & Locke 1983, Zung et al 1983, 1985, Zung & King 1983) or doctors in training during family-medicine residencies (Moore et al 1978, Goldberg et al 1980a, b).

Given the frequency with which depressive illness goes unrecognized it seems important to determine whether such failure is disadvantageous. One signal of disadvantageous outcome is flagged by Weissmann and colleagues (1981) in the USA, who suggest that there are some patients who, once missed, stay that way for a long time, although another study has described how depressives are eventually recognized (Widmer & Cadoret 1978). It is clear that a diagnostic method which relies on the a series of short interviews over a period of time (RCGP 1972) will produce cases which appear not to be recognized at first contact.

However, in the UK unrecognized depressives were more likely than recognized ones to have had their illness for more than a year (Freeling et al 1985) and this seems an unacceptably long process of diagnosis.

That GPs fail to make accurate psychiatric diagnoses or to implement appropriate management cannot be solely attributed to the nature of their training or their lack of it. In fact, depressives who go unrecognized are, as a group, significantly less depressed than those whose depression is recognized (Freeling et al 1985); nevertheless, in the study by Freeling et al there was considerable overlap between the two groups in terms of symptoms experienced, such as pessimism, guilt, impaired activity, loss of energy and insomnia, such that there were depressive illnesses unrecognized by some doctors which proved to be of greater severity than those recognized by others. Not only were unrecognized depressives as a group less markedly ill, they were indeed harder to recognize: they were less likely to admit to or complain of the symptom depression, and they looked less miserable and behaved as less depressed (Freeling et al 1985). They were, however, more likely to show a 'distinct quality of mood' (Paykel 1985), a category of symptom representing a change in internal feelings, including descriptions such as 'coldness', 'deadness' or 'emptiness' inside.

We have studied videotaped interviews of depressed people by their GPs to determine any differences in content or interviewing style between consultations which result in major depression being correctly acknowledged and those in which major depression remains' unacknowledged, also using control consultations with patients without depression. Acknowledgment was defined at the minimum as a GP reporting to a researcher at the end of a consulting session that a particular patient might have been depressed *and* arranging for that patient to reattend within 14 days. The two groups of depressed patients had an external psychiatric interview (Sireling et al 1985b) and the videotapes were analysed using the Consultation Analysis by Triggers and Symptoms (CATS; Tylee & Freeling 1987) and the Consultation Analysis by Behaviour and Style (CABS). CATS codes content and GP microbehaviours. CABS covers doctor interviewing behaviours globally, including: interviewing skills; problem definition; the selection, naming, solving or management of key problems; the emotional tone of the consultation; the degree of empathy manifested; and the appropriate use of authority. Preliminary findings using CATS have been reported (Tylee & Freeling 1989) from comparisons of the first approximately 20 trios of consultations. It was found that, in the group in which major depression was correctly acknowledged, a depression cue was presented as the opening utterance in more than a third of the consultations. Three-quarters of these consultations contained the first depression cue within the first four patient utterances. Opening cues included items such as 'depressed', 'so nervous', 'nerves gone', 'can't cope', 'problems sleeping'. Very occasionally, a patient was newly acknowledged by the GP as depressed without a verbal depression cue, suggesting that the communication of emotional disorder occurred at a non-verbal level.

In the group whose major depression went unacknowledged by the GP a fifth of the consultations opened with a possible depression cue including 'at point zero' and 'not eating'. Only a third of these consultations contained a depression cue, including 'bad temper; among the first four patient utterances. One-third contained no utterance which matched our fairly broad definition of a depression cue.

For whatever reason, some patients appear able to volunteer their depressive cue immediately. It is as if those patients see their doctor as having emotionally open arms; just as a trusting child will run to outstretched arms so these patients immediately volunteered intimate and distressing information about themselves.

It remains important to determine the contribution made to correct acknowledgement by doctor interviewing styles and by component behaviours such as listening skills and empathy. Any findings from a global scale need careful interpretation in terms of cause and effect. Global ratings do not allow for the stage in the consultation at which recognition may have occurred: overt empathy, for example, may result in information leading to the diagnosis or be consequent upon a diagnosis having been formulated. A patient who knows that the GP has an open style may feel able to open the consultation with a psychological symptom.

There remain those problems which arise from the responsibility to provide whole-person care in general practice to people who have, simultaneously, physical symptoms and affective disorder. Concern about physical illness is not only reasonable but desirable. On the other hand, it is not appropriate for all patients to be fully investigated for organic disorder before the psychosocial aspects of their problems are tackled. This is reported as happening frequently in the USA (Katon 1984, Rodin & Voshart 1986). There are, of course, patients, who seem to prefer to somatize their complaints and such individuals are reported as comprising the majority of the patients whose major depression goes unrecognized when they present to GPs with a new episode of illness (Bridges & Goldberg 1987). The complexity of the problems faced by GPs is highlighted by the fact that many of these missed and somatizing depressives had not only physical complaints but a physical disorder also. On the other hand, the coexistence of different disorders in a single patient is the very fabric of a generalist discipline and GPs are familiar with the problems of treating for acute and new illness patients with the care of whose chronic disorders they are already involved (Stott & Davis 1979).

TREATMENT

Essential to any consideration of the management of depressive disorder in UK general practice is the fact that virtually all psychiatric disorder presents initially to GPs and that only one in 20 patients with mental illness is referred to a psychiatrist (Fahy 1974, Grad de Alarcon et al 1975). Probably in most other countries psychiatric disorder also presents in this way.

We have touched already upon the possibility that the act of recognition itself may improve outcome: patients with unrecognized major depressive disorder were found in one study (Freeling et al 1985) to do slightly worse over 3 months than the recognized patients, although the latter were prescribed inadequate dosages of antidepressant drugs and rarely had a second contact within the 3 months with anyone in the practice. This finding of little treatment confirmed those of previous studies (Johnson 1973). As well as reducing the likelihood of compliance with drug therapy, such lack of organized follow-up precludes the use of simple support, let alone specific psychotherapeutic techniques.

Antidepressants

Whatever the attitude of GPs may be to following up patients acknowledged as having major depression, there is frequent prescription of drugs specific for the condition. In 1985 alone more than 6.7 million prescriptions for antidepressants were dispensed by the NHS pharmaceutical services in England and Wales.

Sireling and colleagues (1985b) found that patients prescribed antidepressants were more likely to be categorized as having case depression on the Index of Definition (Wing 1976) and had higher scores on the Hamilton Rating Scale for Depression (HRSD; Hamilton 1967) and higher Raskin Three Area Scale for Depression (Raskin et al 1970) than those whose depression was treated in some way other than the prescription of antidepressant drugs. Equally, the

patients for whom those GPs prescribed antidepressants were less depressed than a psychiatric outpatient sample from the same locality.

That very few patients complete a minimal therapeutic course of antidepressant drugs in general practice (Johnson 1973, Parish 1971, Tyrer 1973) has been a matter of concern and may still be true despite the proven value of amitriptyline in Major Depression treated in general practice (Paykel et al 1988, Hollyman et al 1988). In this study general practice depressives were treated for 6 weeks with amitriptyline (reaching mean doses of 119 mg) or placebo. Drug effect was markedly superior to placebo and response was independent of demographic characteristics, history of illness, endogenous symptomatology and precipitating stress. Drug effect was related only to the severity of the depression. In particular, the drug was found to be superior to placebo in patients with initial scores on the 17-item HRSD of 13 or more but not in those with scores below that level, and similarly it was superior to placebo in subjects who at entry satisfied criteria for probable or definite major depression (RDC) but not in those with criteria for minor depression. These findings have confirmed our view that the RDC criteria for probable Major Depression represent a condition which should be acknowledged by GPs as a specific illness whatever decision they take about people with less severe disturbance. Admittedly, people who accept entry into a drug trial and comply with the strict protocols required do not represent, and may respond differently to, patients who do not want drug treatment or who subsequently drop out of it. Optimal management for these patients, therefore, remains to be determined, as it does for unacknowledged depressives. We simply do not know for sure that unacknowledged patients will benefit from the same treatments as acknowledged ones. On the other hand, since severity was the only predictor for outcome for patients within the trial, and since we know that unacknowledged depression often reaches the necessary level of severity, the indications are suggestive. Not only have we yet to prove the outcome of treating previously unacknowledged depression with drugs, we have yet to determine what benefits these patients may receive simply from being acknowledged. In one study, depressed patients about whose outcome their doctors were optimistic and who were therefore not prescribed antidepressants fared significantly worse than those who were treated (Zung et al 1985).

Whether or not GPs will be more willing both to acknowledge depressive illness and to treat it with antidepressant drugs remains to be determined. It remains true that tricyclic antidepressant drugs have unpleasant unwanted effects on cholinergic activity, they have a 2-week delay in producing benefit and they can be lethal in overdose.

Suicide

The ultimate and most distressing outcome of depression is suicide, and in an average GP's practice this may occur once every 3 years or so. Nevertheless, most GPs will remember who these patients were relatively easily because of the impact the news has, whether or not there had been a recent contact with that patient. Most suicide attempters report depressed mood and many are suffering from depression, anxiety, alcohol abuse, personality disorder or schizophrenia (Hawton 1989). Most of them have seen their GPs, two-thirds in the previous month and one-third in the previous week before death (Hawton & Blackstock 1976, Barraclough & Hughes 1987). It is clear why GPs might feel ambivalent towards the prescription of antidepressant drugs, which are dangerous in overdose. However, many GPs seem to act as if drug therapy were not needed for depression related to real problems of living, in spite of the evidence that once a depression is sufficiently severe it will benefit from an antidepressant irrespective of cause.

Supportive sympathy or psychotherapy?

It is important to elicit stresses and life events, even if their presence does not predict the effectiveness of drugs. A depressed patient often needs a certain degree of improvement in function to be able to make decisions and achieve necessary life changes. That this initial 'kick-start' can be achieved by taking drug treatment is helpful, but so may be introducing the patient to improved coping strategies or adopting counselling techniques. Indeed, benefit is likely from simple, sympathetic social support supplied while the effect of the drug is being monitored.

There is a wide range of possible specific psychotherapies which might be chosen to supplement or replace treatment with antidepressant drugs. None is as inexpensive of money or time as drugs, nor are they likely to produce perceptible benefit within the 2 weeks demonstrated for amitriptyline.

Cognitive therapy

Since Beck (1976) described it, cognitive therapy has been used increasingly in primary care, mainly by clinical psychologists. Paykel, in his Maudsley lecture (1989b), has called it the 'Yuppie of the antidepressant therapies: a child of the 1970s, verbal, exciting, a little pushy, perhaps riding for a fall'. One outcome study has shown that either cognitive therapy or a combination of cognitive therapy and drug therapy gave better results than drugs alone (Blackburn et al 1981) in a small general-practice sample. The number of sessions in general practice ranged from 7.5–17.5. There was a disappointing drug response in this group, possibly because of poor compliance, although drug levels were not monitored. Another study in general practice has shown that cognitive therapy combined with routine therapy by the GP was more effective than routine treatment alone (Teasdale et al 1984). Further studies of cognitive therapy are summarized in chapter 31.

An important factor when comparing drug and individual cognitive therapy is the time needed to provide the latter. Often at least 12 weekly sessions of an hour each are involved, although shorter, more focused approaches are being tried. When compared with a control group given simple supportive psychotherapy with relaxation, benefit from the cognitive therapy was still shown (McLean & Hakstian 1979). A cogent argument for possible use of such a time-consuming therapy is suggestive evidence of a reduced relapse rate over a 2-year span when cognitive therapy was added to tricyclic antidepressant medication in the acute phase (Blackburn et al 1986).

It remains to be ascertained what may predict selective benefit from cognitive therapy among general practice depressives. So far a practical procedure has been to reserve it for people unable or unwilling to take drugs. Work published recently (Elkin et al 1989) throws doubt on that practice. A multicentre study compared four treatments, two of them brief psychotherapies (interpersonal psychotherapy and cognitive therapy), imipramine plus clinical management and placebo plus clinical management. Significant differences among the treatments did not occur in patients whose initial score on the 21-item HRSD was less than 20. If these findings are confirmed, then severity will again be the only valuable characteristic on which GPs can base management decisions.

REFERENCES

American Psychiatric Association 1980 Diagnostic and statistical manual of mental disorders, 3rd edn. American Psychiatric Association, Washington, DC

Balint M 1957 The doctor, the patient, and the illness. Pitman Medical, London

Balint M, Balint E, Gosling R, Hildebrand P A 1965 A study of doctors. Pitman Medical, London

Barnes G E, Prosen H 1984 Depression in Canadian general practice attenders. Canadian Journal of Psychiatry 29: 2–10

Barraclough B, Hughes J 1987 Suicide: clinical and epidemiological studies. Croom Helm, London

Bebbington P E, Tennant C, Hurry J 1981 Adversity and the nature of psychiatric disorder in the community. Journal of Affective Disorders 3: 345–366

Beck A T 1976 Cognitive therapy and the emotional disorders. International Universities Press, New York

Beck A T, Ward C H, Mendelson M, Mock J, Erbaugh J 1961 An inventory for measuring depression. Archives of General Psychiatry 4: 561–571

Bevan J, Cunningham D, Floyd C 1979 Doctors on the move. Royal College of General Practitioners, Exeter

Birtchnell J, Masters N, Deahl M 1988 Depression and the physical environment. A study of young married women on a London housing estate. British Journal of Psychiatry 153: 56–64

Blackburn I M, Bishop S, Glen I M, Whalley L J, Christie J E 1981 The efficacy of cognitive therapy in depression: a treatment trial using cognitive therapy and pharmacotherapy, each alone and in combination. British Journal of Psychiatry 139: 181–189

Blackburn I M, Eunson K M, Bishop S 1986 A two year naturalistic follow-up of depressed patients treated with cognitive therapy, pharmacotherapy and a combination of both. Journal of Affective Disorders 10: 67–75

Blacker C V R, Clare A W 1987 Depressive disorder in primary care. British Journal of Psychiatry 150: 737–751

Blacker C V R, Clare A W 1988 The prevalence and treatment of depression in general practice. Psychopharmacology 95: S14–S17

Block M, Schulberg H C, Coulehan J C, McClelland M, Gooding W 1988 Diagnosing depression among new patients in ambulatory trainee settings. Journal of the American Board of Family Practice 1: 91–97

Bradshaw G, Parker G 1983 Depression in general practice attenders. Australian and New Zealand Journal of Psychiatry 17: 361–365

Bridges K, Goldberg D 1987 Somatic presentation of depressive illness in primary care. In: Freeling P, Downey L J, Malkin J C (eds) The presentation of depression: current approaches. Royal College of General Practitioners, London

Brown G W, Bifulco A 1990 Motherhood, employment and the development of depression. A replication of a finding? British Journal of Psychiatry 156: 169–179

Brown G, Harris T 1978 Social origins of depression. Tavistock Press, London

Brown G W, Andrews B, Harris T O, Adler Z, Bridge L 1986 Social support, self-esteem and depression. Psychological Medicine 16: 813–831

Brown G W, Adler Z, Bifulco A 1988 Life events, difficulties and recovery from chronic depression. British Journal of Psychiatry 152: 487–498

Burton R H, Freeling P 1982 How general practitioners manage depressive illness: developing a method of audit. Journal of the Royal College of General Practitioners 32: 558–561

Casey P R, Dillon S, Tyrer P J 1984 The diagnostic status of patients with conspicuous psychiatric morbidity in primary care. Psychological Medicine 14: 673–683

Coulehan J L, Schulberg H C, Block M R, Zettler-Segal M 1988 Symptom patterns of depression in ambulatory medical and psychiatric patients. Journal of Nervous and Mental Disease 176: 284–288

Crombie D L 1963 Diagnostic methods. Journal of the Royal College of General Practitioners 6: 579–589

Crombie E 1974 Changes in patterns of recorded morbidity. In: Taylor D (ed) Benefits and risks in medical care. Office of Health Economics, London

Davenport S, Goldberg D, Millar T 1987 How psychiatric disorders are missed during medical consultations. Lancet ii 439–440

Davis T C, Nathan R G, Crouch M A, Bairnsfather L E 1987 Screening depression in primary care: back to the basics with a new tool. Family Medicine 19: 200–220

Dhadphale M, Cooper G, Cartwright-Taylor 1989 Prevalence and presentation of depressive illness in a primary health care setting in Kenya. American Journal of Psychiatry 146: 659–661

Duer S, Schwenk T L, Coyne J C 1988 Medical and psycho-social correlates of self-reported depressive symptoms in family practice. Journal of Family Practice 27: 609–614

Dunn G, Skuse D 1981 The natural history of depression in general practice: stochastic models. Psychological Medicine 11: 755–764

Elkin I, Shea T, Watkins J T et al 1989 National Institute of Mental Health treatment of depression collaborative research program. Archives of General Psychiatry 46: 971–982

Endicott J, Spitzer R L 1978 A diagnostic interview; the Schedule for affective Disorders and Schizophrenia. Archives of General Psychiatry 35: 837–844

Evans J, Kiellerup F D, Stanley R O, Burrows G D, Sweet B 1987 A communication skills programme for increasing patients' satisfaction with general practice consultations. British Journal of Medical Psychology 60: 373–378

Fahy T J 1974 Pathways of specialist referral of depressed patients from general practice. British Journal of Psychiatry 124: 231–239

Feighner J P, Robins E, Guze S B, Woodruff R A, Winokur G, Munoz R 1972 Diagnostic criteria for use in psychiatric research. Archives of General Psychiatry 26: 57–63

Freeling P 1983 A workbook for trainees in general practice. John Wright, Bristol

Freeling P 1985 Health outcomes in primary care: an approach to the problem Family Practice 2: 177–181

Freeling P, Barry S 1982 In-service training. A study of the Nuffield Courses of the Royal College of General Practitioners. NFER-Nelson, Windsor

Freeling P, Burton R H 1982 General practitioners and learning by audit. Journal of the Royal College of General Practitioners 32: 231–237

Freeling P, Fitton P 1983 Teaching practices revisited. British Medical Journal 287: 535–537

Freeling P, Harris C M 1984 The doctor—patient relationship. Churchill Livingstone, Edinburgh

Freeling P, Rao B M, Paykel E S, Sireling L I, Burton R H 1985 Unrecognized depression in general practice. British Medical Journal 290: 1880–1883

Gask L, McGrath G, Goldberg D P, Millar T 1987 Improving the psychiatric skills of established general practitioners: evaluation of group teaching. Medical Education 21: 362–368

Gask L, Goldberg D, Lesser A L, Millar T 1988 Improving the psychiatric skills of the general practice trainee: an evaluation of a group training course. Medical Education 22: 362–368

Goldberg D 1982 The concept of a psychiatric 'case' in general practice. Social Psychiatry 17: 61–65

Goldberg D P, Hillier V F 1979 A scaled version of the General Health Questionnaire. Psychological Medicine 9: 139–145

Goldberg D, Huxley P 1980 Mental illness in the community. The pathway to psychiatric care. Tavistock Press, London

Goldberg D P, Steele J J, Smith C 1980a Teaching psychiatric interviewing skills to family doctors. Acta Psychiatrica Scandinavica 62: 41–47

Goldberg D P, Steele J J, Smith C, Spivey L 1980b Training family doctors to recognise psychiatric illness with increased accuracy. Lancet 2: 521–523

Grad de Alarcon J, Sainsbury P, Costain W R 1975 Incidence of referred mental illness in Chichester and Salisbury. Psychological Medicine 5: 32–54

Grol R 1989 To heal or to harm. The prevention of somatic fixation in general practice, 3rd edn. Royal College of General Practitioners, London

Hamilton M 1967 Development of a raising scale for primary depressive illness. British Journal of Social and Clinical Psychology 6: 278–296

Hankin J R, Locke B Z 1983 Extent of depressive symptomatology among patients seeking care in a prepaid group practice. Psychological Medicine 13: 121–129

Harris C M 1986a Association between consultations for depression and for other conditions in patients aged 45 or over. Family Practice 3: 97–101

Harris C M 1986b Further observations on seasonal variation: 2. Depression. Journal of the Royal College of General Practitioners 36: 319–321

Hawton K 1989 Suicide and the management of suicide attempts. In: Herbst K, Paykel E S (eds) Depression. An integrative approach. Heinemann, Oxford

Hawton K, Blackstock E 1976 General practice aspects of self-poisoning and self-injury. Psychological Medicine 6: 571–575

Henley C E, Coussens W 1988 The ability of family practice residents to diagnose depression in outpatients. Journal of the American Osteopathic Association 88: 118–122

Hesbacher P T, Rickels K, Goldberg D 1975 Social factors and neurotic symptoms in family practice. American Journal of Public Health 65: 148–155

Hoeper E W, Nycz P D, Cleary P D, Regier D A, Goldberg I D 1979 Estimated prevalence of RDC mental disorder in primary medical care. International Journal of Mental Health 8: 6–15

Hoeper E W, Nycz G R, Regier D A, Goldberg I D, Jacobson A, Hankin J 1980 Diagnosis of mental disorder in adults and increased use of health services in four out-patient settings. American Journal of Psychiatry 137: 207–210

Hoeper E W, Kessler L G, Burke J D, Pierce W 1984 The usefulness of screening for mental illness. Lancet 1: 33–35

Holden J M, Sagovsky R, Cox J L 1989 Counselling in a general practice setting: a controlled study of health visitor intervention in treatment of post-natal depression. British Medical Journal 298: 223–226

Hollyman J A, Freeling P, Paykel E S, Bhat A, Sedgwick P 1988 Double-blind placebo-controlled trial of amitriptyline among depressed patients in general practice. Journal of the Royal College of General Practitioners 38: 393–397

Howie J G R 1972 Diagnosis – the Achilles heel. Journal of the Royal College of General Practitioners 22: 310–315

Jenkins R, Clare A 1985 Women and mental illness. British Medical Journal 291: 1521–1522

Jenkins R, Shepherd M 1983 Mental illness and general practice. In: Bean P (ed) Mental illness: changes and trends. John Wiley, Chichester

Jenkins R, Smeeton N, Marinker M, Shepherd M 1985 A study of the classification of mental ill health in general practice. Psychological Medicine 15: 403–409

Johnson D A W 1973 Treatment of depression in general practice. British Medical Journal 2: 1061–1064

Johnson D A W, Mellor V 1977 The severity of depression in patients treated in general practice. Journal of the Royal College of General Practitioners 27: 419–422

Johnstone A, Goldberg D 1976 Psychiatric screening in general practice: a controlled trial. Lancet 1: 605–608

Justin R G 1976 Incidence of depression in one family physician's practice. Journal of Family Practice 3: 438–439

Katon W 1984 Depression: relationship to somatisation and chronic illness. Journal of Clinical Psychiatry 45: 4–11

Lesser A L 1985 Problem-based interviewing in general practice: a model. Medical Education 19: 209–304

Linn L S, Yager J 1984 Recognition of depression and anxiety by primary physicians. Psychosomatics 25: 8, 593–600

MacDonald A J D 1986 Do general practitioners 'miss' depression in elderly patients? British Medical Journal 292: 1365–1367

McLean P D, Hakstian A R 1979 Clinical depression: comparative efficacy of out-patient treatments. Journal of Consulting and Clinical Psychology 47: 818–836

Maguire G, Fairbairn S, Fletcher C 1986 Benefit of feedback training in interviewing as students persist. British Medical Journal 1: 268–270

Marks J N, Goldberg D, Hillier V F 1979 Determinants of the ability of general practitioners to detect psychiatric illness. Psychological Medicine 9: 337–353

Moore J T, Silimperi D R, Bobula J A 1978 Recognition of depression by family medicine residents: the impact of screening. Journal of Family Practice 7: 509–513

Nielsen A C, Williams T A 1980 Depression in ambulatory medical patients, prevalence by self-report questionnaire and recognition by non-psychiatric physicians. Archives of General Psychiatry 37: 999–1004

Parish P A 1971 The prescription of psychotropic drugs in general practice. Journal of the Royal College of General Practitioners 21 (supplement 4): 1–77

Parker G, Homes S, Manicavasagar V 1986 Depression in general practice attenders. Journal of Affective Disorders 10: 27–35

Paykel E S 1985 The clinical interview for depression: development and validity. Journal of Affective Disorders 9: 85–96

Paykel E S 1989a The background: extent and nature of the disorder. In: Herbst K, Paykel E (eds) Depression. An integrative approach. Heinemann, Oxford

Paykel E S 1989b Treatment of depression. The relevance of research for clinical practice. British Journal of Psychiatry 155: 754–763

Paykel E S, Hollyman J A, Freeling P, Sedgwick P 1988 Predictors of therapeutic benefit from amitriptyline in mild depression: a general practice placebo controlled trial. Journal of Affective Disorders 14: 83–95

Pietroni P 1976 Non-verbal communication in the general practice surgery. In: Tanner B (ed) Language and communication in general practice. Hodder & Stoughton, London

Porter A M W 1970 Depressive illness in a general practice: a demographic study and a controlled trial of imipramine. British Medical Journal 1: 770–778

Radloff L S 1977 The CES-D scale. A self-report depression scale for research in the general population. Applied Psychology Measurements 1: 385–401

Raskin A, Schulterbrandt J, Reatig N, McKeon J J 1970 Differential response to chlorpromazine, imipramine and placebo. A study of sub-groups of hospitalised depressed patients. Archives of General Psychiatry 23: 164–173

Raynes N V 1979 Factors affective the prescribing of psychotropic drugs in general practice consultations. Psychological Medicine 9: 671–679

Robins L, Helzer J, Croughan J et al 1981 National Institute of Mental Health Diagnostic Interview Schedule: its history, characteristics and validity. Archives of General Psychiatry 38: 381–389

Rodin G, Voshart K 1986 Depression in the medically ill: an overview. American Journal of Psychiatry 143: 696–705

Rosenthal M P, Goldfarb N I, Carlson B L, Sagi P C, Balaban D J 1987 Assessment of depression in a family practice center. Journal of Family Practice 25: 143–149

Royal College of General Practitioners 1972 The future general practitioner. Learning and teaching. British Medical Journal, London

Royal College of General Practitioners/Office of Population Censuses and Surveys/Department of Health and Social Security 1979 Morbidity statistics from general practice. Second National Study 1971–1972 HMSO, London

Royal College of General Practitioners/Office of Population Censuses and Surveys/Department of Health and Social Security 1986 Morbidity statistics from general practice. Third National Study 1981–1982 HMSO, London

Salkind M R 1969 Beck Depression Inventory in general practice. Journal of the Royal College of General Practitioners 18: 267–271

Schulberg H C, Saul M, McClelland M, Ganguli M, Christy W, Frank R 1985 Assessing depression in primary medical and psychiatric practices. Archives of General Psychiatry 42: 1164–1170

Shepherd M, Cooper M, Brown A C, Kalton G 1966 Psychiatric illness in general practice. Oxford University Press, Oxford

Sireling L I, Paykel E S, Freeling P, Rao B M, Patel S P 1985a Depression in general practice: case thresholds and diagnosis. British Journal of Psychiatry 147: 113–119

Sireling L I, Freeling P, Paykel E S, Rao B M 1985b Depression in general practice: clinical features and comparison with out-patients. British Journal of Psychiatry 147: 119–125

Skuse D, Williams P 1984 Screening for psychiatric disorder in general practice. Psychological Medicine 14: 365–377

Sowerby P 1977 The doctor, his patient and the illness: a reappraisal. Journal of the Royal College of General Practitioners 27: 583–589

Spitzer R L, Endicott J, Robins E, 1978 Research Diagnostic Criteria: rationale and reliability. Archives of General Psychiatry 35: 773–782

Stott N C H, Davis R H 1979 The exceptional potential of each primary care consultation. Journal of the Royal College of General Practitioners 29: 201–205

Teasdale J D, Fennell M J V, Hibbert G A, Amies P L 1984 Cognitive therapy for major depressive disorders in primary care. British Journal of Psychiatry 144: 400–460

Tylee A T, Freeling P 1987 The Consultation Analysis by Triggers and Symptoms (CATS). A new objective technique for studying consultations. Family Practice 4: 260–265

Tylee A T, Freeling P 1989 The recognition, diagnosis and acknowledgement of depressive disorder by general practitioners. In: Herbst K, Paykel E (eds) Depression. An integrative approach. Heinemann, Oxford

Tyrer P 1973 Drug treatments of depression in general practice. British Medical Journal 2: 18–20

Von Korf M, Shapiro S, Burke J D, Teitelbaum M, Skinner E A, German P, Turner R W, Klein L, Burns B 1987 Anxiety and depression in a primary care clinic. Comparison of Diagnostic Interview Schedule, General Health Questionnaire and practitioner assessments. Archives of General Psychiatry 44: 152–156

Watson J M, Barber J H 1981 Depressive illness in general practice: a pilot study. Health Bulletin 39: 112–116

Watts C A H 1947 Endogenous depression in general practice. British Medical Journal 1: 11

Watts C A H 1966 Depressive disorders in the community. John Wright, Bristol

Weissman M M, Myers J K 1978 Rates and risks of depressive symptoms in a US urban community. Acta Psychiatrica Scandinavica 57: 219–231

Weissman M M, Myers J K, Thompson W D 1981 Depression and its treatment in a US urban community 1975–76. Archives of General Psychiatry 38: 417–421

Widmer R B, Cadoret R J 1978 Depression in primary care: changes in pattern of patient visits and complaints during a developing depression. Journal of Family Practice 7: 293–302

Wilkinson G 1988 A comparison of psychiatric decision-making by trainee general practitioners and trainee psychiatrists using a simulated consultation model. Psychological Medicine 18: 167–177

Williams P, Skuse D 1988 Depressive thoughts in general practice attenders. Psychological Medicine 18: 469–475

Williamson M T 1987 Sex differences in depression

symptoms among adult family medicine patients. Journal of Family Practice 25: 591–594

Wing J K 1976 A technique for studying psychiatric morbidity in inpatient and outpatient series and in general population samples. Psychological Medicine 6: 665–671

Wing J K, Cooper J E, Sartorius N 1974 The measurement and classification of psychiatric symptoms. Cambridge University Press, Cambridge

Wing J K, Mann S A, Leff J P, Nixon J M 1978 The concept of a case in psychiatric population surveys. Psychological Medicine 8: 203–217

Wright J H, Bell R A, Kuhn C C, Rush E A, Patel N, Redmond J E 1980 Depression in family practice patients. Southern Medical Journal 73: 1031–1034

Yates W R, Hill J W, Petty F, Filipi M 1985 Presenting problem and depression in a rural family practice. Nebraska Medical Journal 367–369

Zigmond A S, Snaith R P 1983 The hospital anxiety and depression scales. Acta Psychiatrica Scandinavica 67: 361–370

Zung W W K 1965 A self-rating depression scale. Archives of General Psychiatry 12: 63–70

Zung W W K, King R E 1983 Identification and treatment of masked depression in a general medical practice. Journal of Clinical Psychiatry 44: 365–368

Zung W W K, Magill M, Moore J T, George D T 1983 Recognition and treatment of depression in a family medicine practice. Journal of Clinical Psychiatry 44: 3–6

Zung W W K, Zung E M, Moore J, Scott J 1985 Decision making in the treatment of depression by family medicine physicians. Comprehensive Therapy 11: 19–23

Zung W W K, MacDonald J, Zung E M 1988 Prevalence of clinically significant depressive symptoms in black and white patients in family practice settings. American Journal of Psychiatry 145: 882–883

42. Depression in medical settings

Giovanni A. Fava

Sadness is a common emotional response in a medical setting. An acute serious illness suddenly interrupts a person's way of life and readily arouses feelings of discouragement and loss (Lipowski 1975). Chronic illness, which implies a significant degree of irreversibility of the pathological process and related disability, and terminal illness which connotes impending death, induce highly individualized affective responses based on each patient's psychological assets and liabilities. Convalescence, a transitional period of reintegration after illness, requires a working-through process which is typical of grief in general (Schmale 1979). A number of studies have documented a high prevalence of depressive symptoms in the medically ill (Katon & Roy-Byrne 1988). As judged by self-rating scales scores, at least 20% of general medical inpatients show some evidence of depression (Fava et al 1988).

A depressed mood may influence how a person experiences the pathological process and interaction with others, including medical staff. Some studies have suggested that it may also increase illness susceptibility. An excess mortality was found among persons with depressive symptoms compared to persons without, and this excess particularly involved cardiovascular and neoplastic diseases (Enzell 1984, Rabins et al 1985, Murphy et al 1987, Bruce & Leaf 1989). One study, however, failed to detect such an association (Zonderman et al 1989). Other investigators have found non-suicidal deaths and myocardial infarction to be significantly more frequent in untreated depressed patients compared to an adequately treated group, even though the study did not take into account concomitant medical illness (Avery & Winokur 1976).

Further, the presence of depressive symptoms in association with chronic medical illness is likely to decrease social functioning and to lead to increased health care utilization (Wells et al 1989). Murphy &

Brown (1980) found that the link between severe life events and the onset of physical illness, for women of 50 years or younger, was not a direct causal association, but was mediated by a depressive disorder. For example, almost half of the patients showing a depressive disorder after their first myocardial infarction had suffered from depression prior to the infarct (Lloyd & Cawley 1978). There is much evidence that depression in the medically ill is frequently unrecognized and untreated (Rodin & Voshart 1986, Cassem 1987, Hengeveld et al 1987, Magruder-Habib et al 1990). Such a trend is the result of several converging factors. First, the discrimination of depression worthy of clinical attention is hindered by the widespread occurrence of depressive symptoms in the setting of medical disease. Second, when a mood disorder is associated with a serious medical illness (e.g. cancer), there is a tendency to regard it as a psychological reaction secondary to the distress of illness or to the patient's appreciation of the implications of his condition. Further, in the medical system expression of emotional distress is often discouraged and suppressed and such distress is communicated in a somatic rather than a psychological mode (Lipowski 1990). Finally, the use of antidepressant drugs is limited by fear that side-effects will worsen the existing medical symptomatology or induce serious complications. A survey at Oxford, in fact, showed that only 43% of hospital doctors use antidepressant drugs and the dosages are much lower than those used in psychiatric practice (Mayou & Smith 1986).

DIAGNOSIS OF DEPRESSION

The evaluation of depression in the setting of medical disease is a difficult task that requires considerable clinical skills.

Assessment of severity

The development of diagnostic criteria, such as those in the DSM-IIIR (American Psychiatric Association 1987), provides operational tools whereby mood disorders may be identified and differentiated. In clinical psychiatry, the diagnosis of major depressive disorder generally sets a clinical threshold for the forms of depression requiring specific treatment. In a study concerned with depressions in general practice, amitriptyline was superior to placebo in major, but not in minor depression (Paykel et al 1988). Further, in a follow-up study on the course of depression following myocardial infarction (Schleifer et al 1989), the majority of patients who on initial evaluations met the criteria for major depression still showed evidence of depression at 3 months, unlike those who suffered from minor depression. It has been emphasized that, if the criteria are used in a mere checklist fashion, a heterogenous group of patients is identified (Feinberg et al 1979). This is particularly true in medical patients, where several of the symptoms required for the diagnosis of major depressive disorder may be present regardless of depression. Alternative criteria, where the somatic symptoms were excluded, have been suggested (Endicott 1984). Such criteria have undergone a preliminary validation (Rapp & Vrana 1989). Actually, diagnostic criteria cannot replace clinical judgment and skills in discriminating depressive symptoms and an informed use of standard DSM-IIIR criteria is therefore recommended (Fava et al 1988).

1) Mood

Sadness, complaints of depression, gloom, dejection, crying characterize the depressed mood. Moffic & Paykel (1975) followed on a weekly basis 43 medical patients (found to be depressed on admission) until discharge. For 11 of the 43 patients (28%) the depression completely resolved by the time of discharge. Most were patients in whom the mood showed a dramatic improvement concomitant with recovery from a life-threatening illness. This finding suggests the importance of monitoring the persistence of depressed mood throughout hospitalization in the medically ill. One may observe dramatic changes in a matter of just a few days. In doubtful case, a further assessment after discharge may shed some light.

Depressed mood tends to persist in a substantial proportion of medical inpatients (Hawton 1981,

Mayou et al 1988, Lustman et al 1988, Schleifer et al 1989) and outpatients (Schulberg et al 1987). On a 4–18 month follow-up after initial assessment, such patients made greater demands on medical, social and psychiatric services than matched controls (Mayou et al 1988). Yet mood was found to improve in the majority of patients.

2) Loss of interest or pleasure

Loss of interest or pleasure in usual activities (including sex) frequently accompanies medical disorders (Cavanaugh et al 1983, Fava & Molnar 1987). Limitations on usual activities imposed by physical constraints and/or psychological fears, however, cannot explain the diminished participation in normal activities, with a sense of difficulty and incompetence, which is found in major depressive disorders. Further, in a comparison between depressed and non-depressed medical patients, it was found that loss of interest in usual activities largely involved interpersonal issues in depression, whereas the two groups did not differ in frequencies of pleasant solitary events (Cole & Zarit 1984).

3) Appetite changes

Significant weight loss or weight gain when not dieting occur with greater frequency in a medical population. With both observer rated and self-rated methods, appetite disturbances do not satisfactorily discriminate depressives from general medical patients (Cavanaugh et al 1983, Fava & Molnar 1987).

4) Sleep changes

A number of medical, toxic or environmental (hospitalization) conditions may be associated with insomnias (disorders of initiating and maintaining sleep) or hypersomnias (disorders of excessive somnolence) (Johns et al 1979). As with appetite changes, the discrimination between depressed and non-depressed medical patients is rather poor (Cavanaugh et al 1983, Fava & Molnar 1987). In diagnosing depression, it is very important to differentiate between initial insomnia (difficulty falling asleep) and delayed insomnia (early awakening). The latter symptom, even though it may occur with organic problems such as recurrent pain, abdominal discomfort, sleep apnoea, is certainly more specific to depression, particularly if the patient is unable to sleep during the day. Depressed patients may also display hypersomnia, although less frequently. Excessive somnolence is a feature of many endocrine (e.g. hypothyroidism), metabolic (e.g. uraemia) and central nervous system (e.g. viral encephalitis) disorders. As a result, caution is needed in attributing hypersomnia to depression in a medical patient. The association of hypersomnia with increased appetite and weight gain (Garvey et al 1984) is, however, more specific to depression and should alert the physician to enquire about other depressive symptoms.

5) *Psychomotor agitation or retardation*

In depressed patients, all bodily movements, including gestures, may be diminished (psychomotor retardation); or the patient is restless, apprehensive and unable to finish anything (psychomotor agitation). Psychomotor functioning provides a good index of discrimination between depressed and non-depressed medical patients (Fava & Molnar 1987).

6) *Fatigue*

Engel (1970) remarks that fatigue should be considered a symptom 'when it becomes the occasion for complaint, as when one becomes fatigued with less effort or at unusual times of the day; or when rest is no longer recuperative or diversion as distracting' (p 641). It is probably the most prevalent symptom of illness, whether physical or mental (Engel 1970). Generally, depressed patients feel most fatigued when they get up in the morning and gradually improve as the day goes on, whereas the reverse sequence is the rule when physical factors are responsible. When chronic fatigue is the chief, unexplained, medical complaint, it may be a residual symptom of a previous episode of depression (Manu et al 1989).

7) *Worthlessness and guilt*

Care is necessary in differentiating feelings of self-reproach in the medically ill. Depressed patients frequently report worthlessness and guilt which have a generalized inappropriate and excessive quality. Medical patients may perceive their physical illnesses as a punishment for something wrong done in the past or something for which they are to be blamed (Pilowsky et al 1984). This tendency to attribute one's physical condition to psychological determinants or one's behaviour is weakly correlated with depressed affect (Fava et al 1982).

8) *Poor concentration*

Depressed patients may complain of diminished ability to think or concentrate, such as slowed thinking, or indecisiveness not associated with marked loosening of association and incoherence. Illness and hospitalization are likely to induce mild degrees of cognitive dysfunction, especially in the elderly (Cavanaugh 1983, Cole & Zarit 1984, Feldman et al 1987). Yet reported diminished ability to think and indecisiveness were found to discriminate highly between depressed and non-depressed medical patients (Clark et al 1983, Fava & Molnar 1987). Sometimes, in the elderly, cognitive dysfunction is the prominent feature of depression, with apparent failure of memory and intellectual functions (depressive pseudodementia) (see chapter 38).

9) *Suicidal thoughts*

Cavanaugh et al (1983) used a self-rating scale for depression in 309 medically ill patients, 101 psychiatric depressives and 101 normal subjects. Somatic symptoms were present almost as frequently in the medical population, whereas cognitive-affective symptoms were reported more frequently for the psychiatric than in the medical patients. A study of 40 depressives, 40 medical inpatients matched for sociodemographic variables and 40 healthy controls, using an observer-rated scale, confirmed these findings (Fava & Molnar 1987). Suicidal impulses appeared to be among the most discriminatory symptoms. Their presence in the medically ill and in the terminally ill is less frequent than is generally believed (Brown et al 1986), and should alert the physician to suspect an affective disorder worthy of clinical attention. Many cases of 'suicide by default' (Lipowski 1974) in the medical population (the deliberate omission of therapeutic, dietary and other measures necessary to sustain life or prevent progress of pathology) may mask a major depressive disorder. Examples are provided by diabetic patients who stop taking insulin, those who resume strenuous work after myocardial infarction and those who withdraw from chronic haemodialysis (Lipowski 1974).

Melancholia

The DSM-IIIR concept of melancholia (see chapter 3) entails a more severe spectrum of depressive symptomatology than the diagnosis of major depressive disorder alone. Nelson et al (1981) found that the criteria for melancholia could distinguish those patients having an autonomous syndrome during the first week of hospitalization from those observed to improve upon psychosocial intervention without drug treatment. Further, major depressed episodes secondary to another psychiatric disturbance were found to respond less favourably to desipramine than primary depressions (Coryell & Turner 1985), whereas there were no differences when melancholia was present (Fava et al 1985a). The DSM-IIIR criteria for melancholia may therefore predict stability in the course of depression and a compelling need for drug treatment in the medically ill, although this indication is purely inferential.

Determining aetiological priorities

When depression is found to be associated with a physical disorder, the potential relationships range from a purely coincidental occurrence to a direct causal role of organic factors in the development of the mood disturbance. The latter is often subsumed under the rubric of symptomatic depression (Whitlock 1982) or organic mood syndrome (American Psychiatric Association 1987). Drugs, endocrine disorders, neurological and infectious diseases are common causes of this syndrome. Roth (1977), commenting on the frequency of depression following viral infections, as part of an endocrinopathy or as a side-effect of certain drugs such as reserpine, notes that the remission that follows treatment may be complete and depressive symptoms in such cases may not recur until a further attack of the physical condition.

According to DSM-IIIR, a prominent, persistent depressed mood, not occurring exclusively during the course of delirium, in association with a specific organic factor judged to be aetiologically related to the disturbance, is defined as an organic mood syndrome. Such definition has been criticized, since it perpetuates a false dichotomy (organic versus non-organic depressions) and its retention in DSM-IV is doubtful at present (Popkin et al 1989). This definition reflects the views of Eilenberg (1960) who proposed the following criteria: 1) no past history of psychiatric illness or disturbed premorbid personality; 2) absence of psychologically or socially disturbing events preceding the illness; 3) resolution of the psychiatric disturbance with specific treatment for the organic disease and relapse when treatment is withheld. Unfortunately, these assumptions may be misleading. There are several mechanisms whereby a physical illness may result in a

depressive disorder: by uncovering a latent, inherited or acquired predisposition to depression; by precipitating the recurrence of a disorder that the patient has experienced in the past; or by bringing about a disorder for which both past history and demonstrable predisposition are lacking (Lipowski 1985). Physical illness may play its causative role through structural brain damage (e.g. stroke); by altering neurotransmitter mechanisms (e.g. Cushing's syndrome); as a stressful life event triggering a psychological failure to adapt; or through jointly interlocking processes at neurophysiological, biochemical and experiential levels.

By and large, except in case of structural brain damage, symptomatic or organic depressions are more likely to occur in those individuals who are genetically predisposed to depression or who have had previous depressive illnesses (Whitlock 1982). The model is thus complex and multifactorial. It has been repeatedly shown that clinically significant depression is not an inevitable concomitant of severe medical disability (Rodin & Voshart 1987) and that it is related not to the severity of physical illness but to previous psychiatric history and social problems (Feldman et al 1987). An alternative conceptualization involves the primary/secondary differentiation (Popkin et al 1989). In 1972, Robins & Guze proposed the distinction between primary depression (the affective illness is not a part of another psychiatric or physical disorder) and secondary depression (a mood disorder chronologically superimposed on a non-affective disturbance). In the medically ill, the concept of secondary depression is more in keeping with a multifactorial frame of reference. However, it is probably too vague and its reliance on chronology may be misleading.

Depression may be one of the earliest manifestations of endocrine disease (Fava et al 1987) and the 'early harbinger of serious physical illness which declares itself at a later stage' (Roth 1977). Would it be in these cases primary depression contributing to the occurrence of physical illness? The likelihood of recovery after successful treatment of the underlying disorder (for instance, correction of hypercortisolism in Cushing's syndrome) makes this classification questionable. In Cushing's disease, depression and hypercortisolism may be two distinct yet apparently related manifestations of suprapituitary disease (Sonino et al 1990).

Even though the complex spectrum of relationships of depression to medical illness is acknowledged, there is clinical justification for differentiating one end of the spectrum from an aetiological viewpoint, using criteria that are more specified than those in DSM-IIIR (Table

42.1). Reference to drug-related depressions may be helpful in this respect. Edwards (1989) remarks that much of the depression allegedly caused by drugs appears to be 'a mixture of lethargy, apathy, tiredness, drowsiness and feeling "sluggish" or slowed down', often accompanied by other features of drug-induced toxic reactions such as confusion. One should thus differentiate these depression-like symptoms from the intensity of a major depressive illness. Further, even though a great number of drugs have been associated with depression (Whitlock 1982), only a relatively small number are so associated with any frequency (Whitlock 1982, Edwards 1989). Table 42.2 lists the drugs most clearly associated with depression.

Table 42.1 Diagnostic criteria for differentiating 'symptomatic depressions' (organic mood syndromes) from other affective disorders in the setting of medical disease

---

1) Patient should meet DSM-IIIR criteria for a major depressed episode. Mood disorder should not occur exclusively during the course of delirium.

2) A specific organic factor, on the basis of brain pathology or neurotransmitter balance, is judged to be aetiologically related to the mood disturbance.

3) The organic factor is part of an illness for which there is evidence in the literature for resolution of the psychiatric disturbance with specific treatment for the organic disease and relapse when treatment is withheld (see Table 42.2). It may also be a drug for which depression is included among complications.

4) Patients with family history or personal history of depression are at risk.

Zelnik (1987) appropriately emphasizes the issue of base rate in establishing a specific relationship between drugs and depression. It is easier to detect an adverse drug reaction when the drug commonly induces a rare illness or syndrome than when it induces the common and widespread symptoms of depression. These remarks apply also to the tentative and, at times, controversial nature of the relationships listed in Table 42.2. The issue of generally spontaneous recovery from depression after discontinuation of drug or treatment of underlying disorder is of paramount importance. Except when noted otherwise (Table 42.2), poor response to antidepressant drugs is frequently reported.

Biological markers

In the last decade, biological markers, such as the dexamethasone suppression test (DST) and the REM

latency test in the sleep EEG, have supplemented traditional phenomenological tools in assessing mood disorders. The DST has attracted particular attention (see chapter 17). Its diagnostic use in the medically ill is, however, hindered by three considerations. Firstly, the endocrine literature reports a high percentage (23%) of false-positive results with the DST in hospitalized or chronically ill control patients (Crapo 1979). Secondly, the diagnostic specificity of the DST has also been questioned in psychiatric illness devoid of medical disorders or complications (Fava & Sonino 1986). Finally, there are many factors that may affect the response to DST, such as weight loss, infection, cardiac failure, recent trauma or surgery, fever, dehydration, certain drugs (Carroll 1983a).

Not surprisingly, the specificity of the DST has been shown to be poor or questionable in the setting of depression and gastrointestinal illness (Fava et al 1985b), diabetes mellitus (Cameron et al 1984), secondary amenorrhoea (Fava et al 1984a), cancer (Grandi et al 1987) and following stroke (Lipsey et al 1985). Whether the combination of depression and hypercortisolism may differentiate a subgroup of patients within a specific illness on predictive or other clinical grounds is still open to question. For instance, an abnormal dexamethasone suppression test result has been found to be correlated with a positive response to trazodone in patients participating in a stroke rehabilitation programme (Reding et al 1986).

Depressed patients display a shortened REM latency in the sleep EEG (chapter 19). Discriminatory power of REM density sleep studies has been reported in 61 outpatients with medical-neurological and psychiatric disorders (King et al 1981). The test, replicating previous findings (Foster et al 1976), was able to differentiate depression occurring in somatic disease from depression alone. Therefore, sleep studies may have applicability in evaluating and monitoring depression in the medically ill. However, their clinical potential is at present very limited.

TREATMENT

Treatment of depression in the medical patient is a complex task that requires considerable skill and knowledge. A basic issue is to determine whether specific antidepressant therapy is required, that is, whether the depressive illness 1) reaches the severity threshold of a major depressive disorder and 2) is likely to persist, irrespective of treatment of the associated

Table 42.2 Illnesses and drugs clearly associated with symptomatic depressions (organic mood syndromes)

Physical disorder or drug	Clinical characteristics of depression
1) Endocrine diseases	
Cushing's syndrome	Depression may be severe with suicidal risk; antidepressants are often ineffective while steroid inhibitors, such as metyrapone, are effective (Fava et al 1987)
Addison's disease	Generally responsive to steroid replacement (Cleghorn & Pattee 1954)
Hypothyroidism, thyrotoxicosis, hyperparathyroidism	Often responsive to adequate endocrine treatment; antidepressant drugs are sometimes required (Fava et al 1987)
Hyperprolactinaemia	Depression associated with hostility and largely limited to women (Fava et al 1987); bromocriptine was found to be superior to placebo (Buckman & Kellner 1985) while amitriptyline was ineffective (Fava et al 1987)
2) Neurological disease	
Parkinson's disease	Depression may be severe with suicidal risk (Whitlock 1986) and is more associated with early onset of Parkinson's disease (Starkstein et al 1989); if untreated, it may last more than 1 year (Brown et al 1988). Levodopa is ineffective and may aggravate symptoms (Whitlock 1986), while bromocriptine has yielded improvement (Jouvent et al 1983). Nortriptyline was superior to placebo (Andersen et al 1980)
Cerebrovascular disorders	Major depression is often strongly associated with left frontal or left basal ganglia lesions and pre-existing subcortical atrophy; cortical lesions are associated with anxiety (Starkstein et al 1990); mood disorders may last more than 1 year without treatment (Starkstein & Robinson 1989); nortriptyline was superior to placebo (Lipsey et al 1985) while trazodone was not (Reding et al 1986); ECT has been used with good results (Murray et al 1987)
Huntington's chorea	Depressive symptoms may be associated with delusions and may respond to antidepressant treatment (Folstein et al 1983), including MAO inhibitors (Ford 1986)
Cerebral tumors	Depression may precede other symptoms; it is frequently accompanied by other mental manifestations (Lishman 1987)
Multiple sclerosis	Depression may precede other symptoms; response to antidepressants is very variable (Berrios & Quemada 1990); cognitive therapy was found to be effective (Larcombe & Wilson 1984); amitriptyline was superior to placebo in controlling pathological laughing and weeping (Schiffer et al 1985)
Epilepsy	Patients receiving phenobarbitone were found to be more depressed than those taking carbamazepine (Robertson et al 1987); amitriptyline was superior to placebo (Robertson & Trimble 1985)
Head injury	Depression is more often associated with right-hemisphere damage, particularly to the frontal lobe (Whitlock 1982); amitriptyline and phenelzine were ineffective in minor closed head injury (Saran 1985)
Normal pressure hydrocephalus	Depression often precedes other symptoms (Tucker & Price 1987)
Alzheimer's disease	Imipramine was not superior to placebo (Reifler et al 1989)
3) Infectious diseases	Depression is more common following virus diseases (hepatitis, mononucleosis, influenza, encephalitis) than bacterial infections and has a slow pace of spontaneous remission (Whitlock 1982)
4) Miscellaneous disorders	
Systemic lupus erythematosus	Steroids are often successful in controlling depressive symptoms (Whitlock 1982)
Folate deficiency, pernicious anaemia	Generally responsive to replacement therapy (Eilenberg 1960)
Carcinoma of pancreas, lung cancer	Depression often precedes other symptoms (Holland et al 1986, Hughes 1985)

AIDS	Depression is characterized by lethargy and withdrawal and may respond to zidovudine (AZT) and stimulants (Perry 1990); it is frequently precipitated by CNS opportunistic infections (Cassem 1987); increases in intracellular calcium have been associated with neurotoxicity (Dreyer et al 1990) and calcium channel antagonists may prove useful in future trials

5) Drugs

Reserpine, methyldopa, propranolol, levodopa, steroid hormones, oral contraceptives, sulphonamides, cimetidine, cycloserine, baclofen, ranitidine, fenfluramine, flunarizine	Depressive symptoms tend to be mild and to subside upon drug discontinuation, with the exception of fenfluramine, which induces depression upon cessation (Whitlock 1982, Paykel et al 1982, Pollack et al 1984, Zelnik 1987, Edwards 1989); current low-dose oestrogens of oral contraceptives are less likely to cause depression than was formerly assumed; the use of pyridoxine to prevent depression by compensating oestrogen-derived deficiency is not supported by controlled trials (Edwards 1989)

medical disorder. The latter issue involves discrimination of symptomatic depressions (organic mood syndromes) from other types of depression. Treatment of symptomatic depressions follows treatment (whenever it is feasible) of the underlying medical condition, and includes specific antidepressant therapy only at a subsequent point. While in most cases discontinuation of the drug causing the organic affective syndrome induces remission of depression, treatment of the physical disorder may not always involve disappearance of depression (Fava et al 1988). Replacement therapy may be all that is needed in case of folate deficiency or hypothyroidism. Metyrapone and bromocriptine may be sufficient to treat depression associated with Cushing's disease and hyperprolactinaemia, respectively, and can be used while awaiting a more definitive treatment. However, in many cases, antidepressant drugs or ECT treatment are required and should be tried, even though their outcome is unpredictable. For instance, there are some patients with Cushing's syndrome who have been treated with antidepressant drugs unsuccessfully before correct diagnosis of their condition and display a striking improvement with correction of hypercortisolism (Sonino et al 1990). There are other patients for whom correction of hypercortisolism alone is not sufficient to abate depression and for whom antidepressant drugs are required in addition. This example underscores the great yet insufficiently explored research potential of symptomatic depressions. It is of considerable research interest that some drugs used to treat Cushing's disease or Nelson's syndrome (cyproheptadine, bromocriptine, sodium valproate) have been reported to display antidepressant and/or mood-stabilizing properties in patients with treatment-resistant depressions not suffering from endocrine disease and that, conversely, normalization of the hypothalamic pituitary adrenal axis appears to be

a requirement for successful treatment of depression (Fava et al 1987).

Another issue of clinical importance is the speed of recovery in symptomatic depressions when the organic factor is removed. This may range from a few days to several weeks (Whitlock 1982). The presence of a well-described residual phase in the underlying syndrome (e.g. post-hepatitis syndrome) often connotes a slow pattern of improvement also from the associated depression. In these cases, unless life-threatening depressions are present, a moderate use of benzodiazepines to relieve some depressive symptoms may be of short-term value. In clinical psychiatry, the roll-back phenomenon (as the illness remits, it recapitulates, even though in a reverse order the progression of symptoms leading to the acute illness and the speed of recovery is related to the duration of illness) may have some predictive value as to the pattern of improvement (Detre & Jarecki 1971), but in symptomatic depressions this issue is largely unexplored.

When, despite correction of the underlying organic factors, symptomatic depressions fail to improve, or in the far more common case of non-symptomatic major depressive disorders in the setting of medical disease, specific therapy is required. It may include use of antidepressant drugs, psychotherapy and electroconvulsive treatment.

The use of antidepressant drugs

Several double-blind placebo-controlled studies support the efficacy of antidepressant drugs for major depressive disorders in the medically ill (Andersen et al 1980, Lipsey et al 1984, Rifkin et al 1985, Costa et al 1985, Robertson & Trimble 1985, Lakshmanan et al 1986), although the differences from placebo were far from striking. Schwartz et al (1989), in a retrospective study of 50 patients, found that half of the patients with a previous history of depression improved upon antidepressant treatment, whereas this took place in only 22% of patients without a previous history of depression. The issue of compliance is also important. Popkin et al (1985) found that 32% of antidepressant treatments initiated after psychiatric consultation in patients with major physical illnesses were terminated because of side effects.

The initial choice almost inevitably falls upon one of the tricyclic antidepressants or related compounds. The use of MAO inhibitors in the medically ill is considerably restricted by their potential for serious side-effects and interactions (Ciraulo et al 1988). Although the risks associated with MAO inhibitors have been overstated, tricyclics are generally safer, more effective and thus more versatile in medical patients (Fava et al 1988). The use of stimulants in medical depressives has also been proposed (Kaufman et al 1982, Fisch 1986, Woods et al 1986, Fernandez et al 1987). Their utilization, however, raises serious questions that have not been answered by clinical studies and should be limited to cases where tricyclic antidepressant treatment has failed or is not feasible. The different tricyclics are considered to be roughly equally effective in the average case of depression (Hollister 1978a, b). The effectiveness of the 'second generation' antidepressants (bupropion, fluoxetine, fluvoxamine, maprotiline, mianserin, trazodone, viloxazine) has not been as firmly established, particularly in severe depression (Blackwell 1987). As Carroll (1983b) pointed out, 'one has to wonder how many of the "second generation" antidepressants will survive the test of time in the treatment of classical endogenous depression'. The use of a benzodiazepine, alprazolam, in the treatment of major depression does not seem to have survived the test of time (Fava et al 1988, Rudorfer & Potter 1989). As with any other benzodiazepine, it also has a potential for physical dependence with long-term treatment.

Greater safety has been claimed for the 'second generation' antidepressants. Thus, clinicians may be inclined to select them for the medically ill patient who suffers from a major depressive episode. They have not been used, however, as extensively as the more traditional antidepressants. As Lasagna (1978) notes, the history of toxicology reminds us vividly of the lag that often occurs between the first introduction of a drug into use and the recognition of certain side-effects from that drug. Reviews of the adverse effects of antidepressant drugs (Blackwell 1987, Blackwell & Simon 1988, 1989) provide several examples of this phenomenon.

An increased incidence of seizures has been documented for maprotiline and bupropion; viloxazine may cause nausea, vomiting and migraine; trazodone, despite early claims, has been associated with increased ventricular irritability and irreversible priapism; the neuroleptic properties of amoxapine (potentially including tardive diskinesia) have emerged; a high incidence of gastrointestinal disturbances (nausea and vomiting) has been documented for fluvoxamine. Mianserin has kept its promise as an antidepressant drug with fewer anticholinergic and cardiovascular effects (Blackwell 1987, Jefferson 1989), but a controversy about its haematological effects (potentially including agranulocytosis) has arisen (Blackwell & Simon 1989). The cardiac safety of fluoxetine has not been conclusively demonstrated (Jefferson 1989), but akathisia has emerged as a side-effect (Lipinski et al 1989).

As a result, the use of 'second generation' antidepressants in the medically ill is at present not warranted, with the possible exception of mianserin. At any rate, it requires careful monitoring.

Even though all tricyclics may be considered equally effective, side-effects and pharmacokinetic properties provide clinical rationales for using one antidepressant rather than another when a physical disturbance is present or in the setting of a specific drug treatment. Several reviews on the use of psychotropic drugs in medical patients are available (Siris & Rifkin 1981, Muskin & Glassman 1983, Wheatley 1988, Amdisen & Hildebrant 1988, Silver & Simpson 1988, Ciraulo et al 1988). The clinically relevant interactions of antidepressant drugs and disease states (Table 42.3) or drugs primarily directed to physical disturbances (Table 42.4) should be emphasized. The interactions do not always take place or have clinical significance, and there may be some unpredictable individual susceptibilies to a certain drug or drug—disease combination.

Several studies have shown that antidepressant drugs may be used in the seriously medically ill with the precautions listed in Table 42.3. The last decade has witnessed a considerable modification in the appraisal of cardiovascular side-effects of antidepressant drugs (Jefferson 1989). For instance, antidepressants are not always contraindicated in treatment of depression following ischaemic heart disease, provided that there are no important conduction defects, heart failure or arrhythmias, and after the immediate recovery phase (Raskind et al 1982). What should always be taken into account is the clinical need for such treatment, the severity of symptoms and the likelihood of improve-

Table 42.3 Clinically significant interactions between tricyclic and heterocyclic antidepressants and medical disorders

Disturbance	Interaction	Comments
Cardiac arrhythmias	Increase	Extreme caution; contraindicated when conduction abnormalities are present (Risch et al 1982); consider mianserin or desipramine at low doses
Recovery phase of myocardial infarction	Heart failure, arrhythmias	Contraindicated
Congestive heart failure	Worsening	Caution; monitor blood levels (Muskin & Glassman 1983)
Epilepsy	lowering of seizure threshold	Use antiepileptic drugs; avoid maprotiline, amoxapine and bupropion; consider amitriptyline (Robertson & Trimble 1985)
Oesophageal reflux, hiatus hernia, pyloric stenosis	worsening (anticholinergic effect)	Caution (Tyber 1975); consider desipramine or mianserin
Advanced liver disease	Decreased metabolism of antidepressants	Small doses monitored through blood levels (Morgan & Read 1972)
Angle-closure glaucoma	Precipitation of glaucoma (anticholinergic effect)	Extreme caution; consider mianserin or desipramine
Prostatic hypertrophy	Hesitancy and urinary retention (anticholinergic effect)	Extreme caution; bethanecoline may be used, but cholinergic stimulation of detrusor may lead to rupture (Siris & Rifkin 1981)
Renal failure	Urinary retention compromising renal function and worsening of orthostatic hypotension	Extreme caution (Lieberman et al 1985); small doses monitored through blood levels (Levy 1985)
Hyperthyroidism	Antidepressants may exacerbate tachycardia and cardiac arrhythmias	Caution (Wilson & Jefferson 1985); adjust dosage
Hypothyroidism	Anticholinergic effects and sedating properties of antidepressants may be exaggerated	Caution (Wilson & Jefferson 1985); low doses
Addison's disease	Worsening of hypotension	Extreme caution (Fava et al 1987)
Phaeochromocytoma	Hypertensive crisis	Contraindication (Achong & Keane 1981)

ment following amelioration of physical conditions.

The clinical use of antidepressant drugs in the medically ill does not differ from general use in psychiatry. There is no evidence that lower dosages are required. In a study in general-practice depressives, Blashki et al (1971) found amitriptyline 150 mg daily, but not 75 mg daily, superior to placebo. In a trial on the treatment of depression in patients with epilepsy (Robertson & Trimble 1985), amitriptyline and nomifensine were not superior to placebo when used at low doses.

It should be noted, however, that several illnesses and drugs may alter the metabolism of tricyclic antidepressants (Tables 42.3 and 42.4). These alterations may depend on the metabolic action of the liver, hepatic blood flow and the specific plasma binding of antidepressant drugs (Muskin & Glassman 1983). For drugs like imipramine, unless specific enzymatic induction has taken place (e.g. barbiturates), hepatic clearance may reflect hepatic blood flow more than hepatic metabolic activity (Wilkinson & Shand 1975). As a result, conditions like congestive heart failure or advanced liver disease may increase antidepressants blood levels. Further, the concentration of alpha$_1$ glycoprotein (an acute phase reactant protein that increases with inflammation, stress, malignancy and haematological conditions and decreases with severe hepatic disease, nephrotic syndrome and malnutrition) is negatively correlated with the free fraction of drugs like imipramine (Piafsky & Borga 1977). In the elderly,

Table 42.4   Clinically significant interactions between tricyclic and heterocyclic antidepressants and drugs directed to physical disturbances

Drug	Interaction	Comments
Sympathomimetic agents (noradrenaline, adrenaline, ephedrine, etc.)	Potentiation of hypertensive effect	Contraindicated for parenteral administration (Risch et al 1982); caution for inhalation (Thompson & Thompson 1984)
Quinidine	Synergism	Caution (Muskin & Glassman 1983)
Propranolol	Antidepressants may diminish its cardiovascular effects	Monitor ECG (Risch et al 1982)
Oral anticoagulants (warfarin, dicoumarol)	Antidepressants impair their hepatic metabolism	Monitor prothrombin levels; adjust dosage (Risch et al 1982)
Antihypertensive agents (guanethidine, alphamethyldopa, clonidine, reserpine, verapamil, captopril)	Decrease in hypotensive action	Diuretics or hydralazine preferred (Blackwell 1981); mianserin does not appear to interact with clonidine and alphamethyldopa (Rudorfer & Potter 1989)
Thyroid hormone	Increased cardiac irregularities	Adjust dosage (Wilson & Jefferson 1985)
Methyltestosterone	Paranoid ideation	Reported in men only (Blackwell 1981)
Sulphonylureas	Hypoglycaemic reactions	Monitor glycaemia closely (True et al 1987)
Antacids, levodopa	Impaired gastrointestinal absorption of antidepressants	Adjust dosage (Blackwell 1981); prescribe the two drugs at different times
Anticholinergic agents	Additive effect	Caution, use mianserin or desipramine
Cimetidine	Increased blood levels of antidepressants	Adjust dosage; doxepin or trimipramine can be considered as an alternative to cimetidine or ranitidine in selected cases (Haggerty & Drossman 1985)
Oral contraceptives, barbiturates	Decreased plasma levels of antidepressants	Adjust dosage (Rubinstein et al 1983)
Fenfluramine, allopurinol metronidazole, phenytoin	Increased plasma levels of antidepressants	Adjust dosage (Rubinstein et al 1983)
Chloramphenicol, isoniazid, sulphonamides	Increased plasma levels of antidepressants	Adjust dosage (Bint & Burtt 1980)
Phenylbutazone	Antidepressants delay its absorption	Monitor phenylbutazone blood levels (Ciraulo et al 1988)
Halothane and pancuronium in general anaesthesia	Tachycardia and arrhythmias; additive anticholinergic effects	Discontinue antidepressants 3 days prior to surgery (Kosanin 1981)
Procarbazine	Hypertensive crisis	Contraindication (Massie & Holland 1984)

medical and aging factors may combine to determine a decreased rate of elimination of antidepressants compared to younger subjects (Rubinstein et al 1983). A clear-cut correlation between plasma antidepressant levels and toxicity has not been established (Boyer & Friedel 1984), but it has been shown to be important in several cases, and especially as to cardiovascular effects (Molnar & Gupta 1980). As a result, it appears to be reasonable routinely to monitor antidepressant drug levels when a physical disturbance or an array of different drugs is involved. As Muskin & Glassman (1983) remark, however, blood levels in medical conditions such as renal failure may be misleading, since not all metabolites of antidepressants are routinely assayed (and they may have untoward effects upon organ systems such as the heart) and illnesses or other drugs may affect the unbound portion of the antidepressants in the plasma.

Use of antidepressant drugs in the medically ill should begin therefore with low dosages (such as

25–50 mg of desipramine or its equivalents) with cautious increments (associated with ECG), to a dosage of 100–150 mg after a couple of weeks. A major fault in treatment of depression by non-psychiatrists lies in using doses which are too low (Paykel 1979). Doses below the equivalent of 100 mg of desipramine daily are usually inadequate, except in the elderly, in cancer patients, in renal failure and in advanced liver disease. Both physical and psychiatric conditions should be reevaluated frequently. Treatment may be tapered gradually and eventually discontinued according to clinical judgment. Maintenance doses should be lower than full therapeutic doses. It is widely believed that the agitated insomniac depressive should be treated with a sedating tricyclic (amitriptyline, trimipramine or doxepin), the retarded insomniac patient with a less-sedating drug (imipramine or nortriptyline) and the retarded-hypersomniac case with a non-sedating drug (desipramine or protriptyline). Yet cautious scepticism seems to be appropriate regarding specific antidepressant profiles of tricyclics (Paykel 1979). In the medically ill, consideration of side effects may be far more important (see Tables 42.3 and 42.4).

One should keep in mind that there are significant differences in the anticholinergic activity of antidepressants; among tricyclics, amitriptyline and doxepin are the most potent and desipramine the least active, with imipramine and nortriptyline intermediate; second generation antidepressants such as mianserin and fluoxetine have low anticholinergic activity (Blackwell 1987). Caution is required in attributing less anticholinergic effect to a certain antidepressant (e.g. trazodone) on the basis of receptor-binding studies only, because laboratory findings may not be entirely consistent with clinical observations. Susceptibility to a central anticholinergic syndrome (anxiety, delirium, agitation, hallucinations, hyperpyrexia, myoclonus and convulsions, stupor) appears to increase with age (Van der Kolk et al 1978). There is some evidence that nortriptyline induces less orthostatic hypotension (Muskin & Glassman 1983).

Psychotherapy

Several psychotherapeutic approaches have been proposed to alleviate psychological distress in medical patients (Steinmuller 1978). From controlled studies, however, there is no clear-cut indication that psychotherapy is effective in treating depression in patients with physical illness (Kellner 1975).

Cognitive therapy has emerged as a specific psychotherapeutic treatment of depression and its effectiveness is based on research evidence. Larcombe and Wilson (1984) showed in a controlled study that cognitive therapy improves depression in patients with multiple sclerosis. It is conceivable, even though it has yet to be tested, that cognitive therapy may be of value for those depressed patients in whom physical illness has a personal meaning of punishment or weakness, who develop unrealistic and distorted fears and expectations, or who exhibit an exaggerated pathological response to losses (Steinmuller 1978).

A randomized controlled trial of in-hospital nursing support for first-episode myocardial infarction patients and their partners has shown that a simple programme of counselling may significantly decrease depressive symptoms (Thompson 1989). The scarcity of research in psychotherapy of depression in the medically ill should not lead to underestimation of its potentially powerful effects, particularly in minor depressions.

Electroconvulsive therapy

This modality remains a very effective treatment for depression (see chapter 22), including secondary depression with melancholic features (Rich et al 1984). Its usefulness increases when the patient has been refractory to antidepressant drug treatment, as found in many cases of symptomatic depressions (Whitlock 1982). It can often be used safely in the medically ill, provided that certain precautions concerned with pre-ECT work-up, anticholinergic premedication and ECT administration, are observed (Bidder 1981).

SPECIAL CLINICAL ISSUES

The relationship of depression to somatization, abnormal illness behaviour and pain, and its characteristics in the elderly medical patient, in oncology and in chronic disease merit special attention. The most significant clinical aspects of symptomatic depressions are summarized in Table 42.2. Depression associated with pregnancy and childbirth is described in chapter 36.

Relationship with functional somatic symptoms and abnormal illness behaviour

Functional somatic symptoms are extremely common in medical practice and appear to be caused by physiological function aggravated by emotion (Kellner 1990). Also common are syndromes of abnormal illness behaviour, the persistence of an inappropriate or maladaptive mode of perceiving, evaluating and acting in relation to one's state of health, despite the fact that a doctor has offered a reasonably lucid explanation on the nature of the illness and the appropriate management to be followed (Pilowsky 1986). Hypochondriasis and conversion reactions are the best known manifestations of abnormal illness behaviour. The association between depression and somatization or abnormal illness behaviour has frequently been emphasized (Lipowski 1990). Kellner (1990) remarks that the research evidence for this association has been consistent, regardless of the design of the study: depressed patients tend to have more somatic symptoms than non-depressed individuals and this phenomenon is particularly impressive in general practice (see chapter 41): somatizers tend to be more depressed than patients with physical disease, and within groups there is a consistent positive correlation between depressive and somatic symptoms. In a study on depression and gastrointestinal illness (Fava et al 1985b), about one-quarter of patients with functional gastrointestinal complaints were found to suffer from a major depressive disorder according to DSM-III.

The relationship of depressed mood to abnormal illness behaviour needs to be emphasized. In the general hospital setting, depression was found to be highly correlated with hypochondriasis and irritability (Fava et al 1982). Further, it was found to be related to the patient's perception of physician supportiveness and of illness-related life disruption (Rosenberg et al 1988). A depressed mood may alter the perception of hospitalization. The behaviour of a querulous, self-preoccupied, demanding and irritable patient, with marked bodily preoccupation and many physical complaints, may mask a depressive state (Fava et al 1982). A factor analysis in general hospital patients revealed a common factor underlying depression and abnormal illness behaviour: this factor was characterized by depressed affect, somatic symptoms, psychomotor retardation, hypochondriasis and disease conviction (Fava et al 1984b). A second factor suggested that, in contrast to younger patients, older patients had a tendency to focus on somatic problems and not psychological determinants, were likely to attribute difficulties to physical illness and lacked readiness to report interpersonal friction (Fava et al 1984b). These results were recently replicated (Karanci 1988). Interestingly, however, another study based on patients seen in psychiatric consultation failed to detect a relationship between depression and abnormal illness behaviour (Wise & Rosenthal 1982).

Treatment of a major depressive disorder in the setting of functional somatic symptoms or abnormal illness behaviour may sometimes lead to amelioration of somatization and hypochondriasis (Kellner 1990). In one study (Kellner et al 1986), characteristic hypochondriacal responses occurred in 40% of melancholic patients and in 5% of normals. After 4 weeks of treatment with amitriptyline, the number of patients displaying hypochondriacal fears and beliefs decreased and was the same as in the group of normals (Kellner et al 1986).

Relationship with pain

There is little doubt that chronic pain and depression are closely linked. The majority of published reports suggests that the rate of depressive symptoms is higher in chronic pain patients than in general and medical populations (Romano & Turner 1985). Blumer & Heilbronn (1982) have suggested that chronic pain of uncertain origin is a variant of depressive disease. As Pilowsky & Bassett (1982) remark, this assumption is likely to be an oversimplification of the issue. The research evidence indicates that: 1) because of lack of adequate controlled studies, it cannot be concluded that major depressive disorders are more common among chronic pain patients than among other medical patients; 2) about 50% of patients with chronic pain have developed depression simultaneously, while about 40% became depressed after pain onset (Romano & Turner 1985). In the latter group of patients, pain may be the source of depression (Hendler 1984). The same controversy extends over the use of tricyclic antidepressants to control pain whether of organic or psychogenic origin. The controlled studies show that, if antidepressants relieve pain when used alone, this is likely to be a consequence of relief of depression (Walsh 1983). This suggests that when a major depressive episode is present in the setting of chronic pain, tricyclic antidepressants may be helpful (Fava et al 1988). Caution is needed when an organic cause for pain cannot be established. In some instances, in fact, the pain is clearly protecting the patient from more intense depression and even suicide (Engel 1959) and—by neutralizing guilt and allowing the discharge of aggression through complaint behaviour — possibly ameliorates the depression (Pilowsky 1978).

The concept of masked depression

The relationship of depression to chronic pain, functional somatic symptoms and abnormal illness behaviour has led to the development of the concept of 'masked depression'. The patient denies feeling depressed, volunteers no affective-cognitive symptoms, but merely complains of one or more somatic disturbances, such as fatigue, general malaise and pain. A positive response to antidepressant is frequently regarded as evidence for 'masked depression' (Lesse 1983).

Such therapeutic response has also been related to abnormal DST results (Rihmer et al 1983). There is little room, however, for this diagnostic entity. In most cases of possible masked depression, full assessment either brings to light a major depressive disorder or makes it clear that the patient is not depressed (Paykel & Norton 1982). When depression is clear-cut, treatment follows conventional lines, irrespective of the 'masked' picture (Paykel & Norton 1982). A positive response to antidepressants may only indicate that depression coexists with a physical illness that may declare itself at a later stage (Kerr et al 1969).

Depression in the elderly medical patient

Late in life, depressive syndromes or symptoms are frequently associated with medical (including cerebral) disease, creating difficulties in diagnosis and management. There is no evidence to suggest that elderly medical patients suffer from major depression more frequently than other medical patients (Koenig et al 1988). However, patients with late onset of affective disorders have higher rates of physical illness and lower genetic loadings than those who experienced depression earlier in life (Pollitt 1972, Roth & Kay 1956). Regardless of time of onset, depression in the elderly may be the forerunner of fatal illness (Evans & Whitlock 1983). Depression in elderly medical patients is associated with higher in-patient mortality and higher health-care utilization (Koenig et al 1989). Severe physical illness (associated with recent placement in a nursing home, prior history of depression, the presence of other associated medical illnesses and other stressful life events) was found to increase the development of depressive symptoms in the elderly (Cadoret & Widmer 1988). The clinical differentiation from grief is important. In the medically ill, a grief reaction follows not only the death of a loved one, but also the loss of a body part or bodily function (Schmale 1979). Sight, hearing, speech, reproduction and locomotion are the most valued bodily functions; breast, hair, facial appearance are parts of the body most important in maintaining an integrated sense of self. Apparently, acute or sudden changes are more threatening than gradual changes that take place with chronic progressive diseases (Schmale 1979). Grief has a natural course to run; its symptoms may mimic depression and the speed with which it fades depends on personal and situational determinants (see chapter 39).

Treatment of depression in the elderly medical patient entails the same precautions as for physically healthy geriatric patients (see chapter 38). Use of antidepressant drugs requires a skilful consideration of interactions and side-effects (Koenig & Breitner 1990). There is a general consensus over the use of lower dosages of antidepressants (Koenig & Breitner 1990). The elderly, in fact, may have a decreased rate of elimination of antidepressants compared to younger patients; further, their reduction in acetylcholine-associated enzymes requires caution in using drugs with anticholinergic properties, such as antidepressants (Rubinstein et al 1983); finally, the older patient is more likely to suffer from antidepressant-induced orthostatic hypotension, since several medical factors combine to determine this symptom in the elderly (Davie et al 1981). Use of lower dosages is not always effective. Recently, Slotkin et al (1989) have reported on a reduced inhibition of serotonin uptake into platelets by imipramine in elderly depressed patients. When an increase in dosage is problematic, alternative therapies such as ECT may be contemplated (Koenig & Breitner 1990).

Depression in cancer patients

Silberfarb & Oxman (1988) observe that, if patients are psychologically healthy before the onset of cancer, it is unusual for severe psychiatric consequences to follow the diagnosis or the treatment of cancer.

In research studies, the prevalence of major depressive disorders in cancer patients has been found to be quite low (5–6%) (Derogatis et al 1983, Lansky et al 1985) and similar to that in other general medical populations (Buckberg et al 1984, Hardman et al 1989). Nonetheless, depression in patients with cancer is underdiagnosed (Hardman et al 1989) and undertreated (Derogatis et al 1979) because many physicians believe that all cancer patients are depressed and should be so, given the seriousness of the diagnosis. Antidepressant drugs account for only 1%

of psychotropic prescriptions in an oncology population (Derogatis et al 1979). Yet a double-blind placebo-controlled study (Costa et al 1985) showed that antidepressant drugs are effective in treating depression in cancer patients. Side-effects were not bothersome with the drug used (mianserin). A preliminary open study (Evans et al 1988) suggested that treatment of depression in cancer patients may produce improvement in psychosocial adjustment to illness. Other studies (Noyes & Kathol 1986) have reported the value of psychotherapy or counselling in improving quality of life and depressed mood in cancer patients.

In open studies, tricyclic drugs have been used for treating pain in cancer patients and their prominent feature has been an opiate sparing effect: following relief of pain by antidepressants, subsequent antidepressant withdrawal precipitates pain again (Walsh 1983). As discussed previously, a direct analgesic effect of antidepressants has not been conclusively demonstrated. Clinically, in cancer patients any effect is of limited significance, because the fear of opiate addiction in cancer patients is largely misplaced (Walsh 1983). On the other hand, it may be important to treat the affective component of pain when depressive symptoms are present. A study in 57 patients receiving treatment for cancer suggested that part of the somatic symptoms in cancer patients who are depressed may be caused or aggravated by depression rather than by cancer (Robinson et al 1985).

In several types of cancer, notably in carcinoma of the pancreas (Holland et al 1986) and lung cancer (Hughes 1985), depression may antedate other symptoms. Kerr et al (1969) reported that depression as an early manifestation of occult malignancy has a good although transient response to antidepressant drugs and electro-convulsive therapy. At times, antidepressant treatment may produce an aggravation of signs and symptoms, unmasking diseases such as phaeochromocytoma (Achong & Keane 1981) and cerebellar tumours (Rabej & Avrahami 1985).

Depression and chronic disease

In the past decade there has been an upsurge of interest in the daily functioning and well-being of patients with chronic medical conditions such as arthritis, diabetes and hypertension (Stewart et al 1989). Such psychosocial dimensions have been often subsumed under the rubric of quality of life (Fava & Magnani 1988). Depression has been found to affect quality of life to a considerable degree (Wells et al 1989), whereas the majority of variance in functioning and well-being was not explained by the presence of chronic medical conditions (Stewart et al 1989).

As with cancer patients, even though depressed mood may be a frequent accompaniment of chronic medical disorders, only a small percentage of patients suffer from a major depressive disorder. In haemodialysis patients, such a disorder could be identified in 5–8% of patients (Smith et al 1985, Rodin & Voshart 1987, Hinrichsen et al 1989). Depression was more strongly related to perception of illness than renal disease variables (Sacks et al 1990). Frank et al (1988) reported a 17% prevalence rate for depression in rheumatoid arthritis. Development of depression was more associated with socioeconomic than clinical factors (Hawley & Wolfe 1988, Newman et al 1989). Similar considerations may apply also to other medical disorders, such as diabetes (Rodin 1990) and heart disease (Mayou 1990), and underscore how depression may affect the entire disease process.

ACKNOWLEDGMENT

This work was supported in part by grants from the Ministero della Pubblica Istruzione (Rome, Italy) and the Associazione Italiana per le Ricerche sul Cancro (Milan, Italy). Ms Adele Gentile and Luisella Pezzoli provided expert secretarial assistance.

REFERENCES

Achong M R, Keane PM 1981 Pheochromocytoma unmasked by desipramine therapy. Annals of Internal Medicine 94: 358–359

Amdisen A, Hildebrant J 1988 Use of lithium in the medically ill. Psychotherapy and Psychosomatics 49: 103–119

American Psychiatric Association 1987 Diagnostic and statistical manual of mental disorders, 3rd edn – revised (DSM-IIIR). American Psychiatric Association, Washington, DC

Andersen J, Aabro E, Gulman N, Hjelmsted A, Pedersen H E 1980 Antidepressive treatment in Parkinson's disease. Acta Neurologica Scandinavica 62: 210–219

Avery D, Winokur G 1976 Mortality in depressed patients treated with electroconvulsive therapy and antidepressants. Archives of General Psychiatry 33: 1029–1037

Berrios G E, Quemada J I 1990 Depressive illness in multiple sclerosis. British Journal of Psychiatry 156: 10–16

Bidder T G 1981 Electroconvulsive therapy in the medically ill patient. Psychiatric Clinics of North America 4: 391–405

Bint A, Burtt I 1980 Adverse antibiotic drug interactions Drugs 20: 57–68

Blackwell B 1981 Adverse effects of antidepressant drugs. Drugs 21: 201–209

Blackwell B 1987 Newer antidepressant drugs. In: Meltzer H Y (ed) Psychopharmacology. Raven Press, New York, p 1041–1049

Blackwell B, Simon J S 1988 Antidepressant drugs. In: Dukes M N G, Beeley (eds) Side effects of drugs. Annual 12. Elsevier, Amsterdam, p 8–25

Blackwell B, Simon J S 1989 Antidepressant drugs. In: Dukes M N G, Beeley (eds) Side effects of drugs. Annual 13. Elsevier, Amsterdam, p 6–16

Blashki T G, Mowbray R, Davies B 1971 Controlled trial of amitriptyline in general practice. British Medical Journal 1: 133–138

Blumer D, Heilbronn M 1982 Chronic pain as a variant of depressive disease. Journal of Nervous and Mental Disease 170: 381–394

Boyer W F, Friedel R O 1984 Antidepressant and antipsychotic plasma levels. Psychiatric Clinics of North America 7: 601–610

Brown J H, Henteleff P, Barakat S, Rowe C J 1986 Is it normal for terminally ill patients to desire death? American Journal of Psychiatry 143: 208–211

Brown R G, MacCarthy B, Gotham A M, Der G J, Marsden C D 1988 Depression and disability in Parkinson's disease. Psychological Medicine 18: 49–55

Bruce M L, Leaf P J 1989 Psychiatric disorders and 15-month mortality in a community sample of older adults. American Journal of Public Health 79: 727–730

Buckberg J, Penman D, Holland J C 1984 Depression in hospitalized cancer patients. Psychosomatic Medicine 46: 199–212

Buckman M T, Kellner R 1985 Reduction of distress in hyperprolactinemia with bromocriptine. American Journal of Psychiatry 142: 242–244

Cadoret R J, Widmer R B 1988 The development of depressive symptoms in the elderly following onset of severe physical illness. Journal of Family Practice 27: 71–76

Cameron O G, Kronfol Z, Greden J F, Carroll B J 1984 Hypothalamic—pituitary—adrenocortical activity in patients with diabetes mellitus. Archives of General Psychiatry 41: 1090–1095

Carroll B J 1983a Biologic markers and treatment response. Journal of Clinical Psychiatry 44: 30–40

Carroll B J 1983b Neurobiologic dimensions of depression and mania. In: Angst J (ed) The origins of depression. Springer-Verlag, Berlin, p 163–186

Cassem N H 1987 Depression. In: Hackett T P, Cassem N H (eds) Massachusetts General Hospital handbook of general hospital psychiatry. PSG Publishing, Littleton, MA, p 227–260

Cavanaugh S 1983 The prevalence of emotional and cognitive dysfunction in a general medical population. General Hospital Psychiatry 5: 15–24

Cavanaugh S, Clark D, Gibbons R D 1983 Diagnosing depression in the hospitalized medically ill. Psychosomatics 24: 809–815

Ciraulo D A, Creelman W, Shader R I 1988 Antidepressant drug-drug interactions. In: Ciraulo D A, Shader R I, Greenblatt D J, Creelman W (eds) Drug interactions in psychiatry. Williams & Wilkins, Baltimore, MD, p 21–87

Clark D C, Cavanaugh S, Gibbons R D 1983 The core symptoms of depression in medical and psychiatric patients. Journal of Nervous and Mental Disease 171: 705–713

Cleghorn R A, Pattee C J 1954 Psychologic changes in 3 cases of Addison's disease during treatment with cortisone. Journal of Clinical Endocrinology and Metabolism 14: 344–352

Cole K D, Zarit S H 1984 Psychological deficits in depressed medical patients. Journal of Nervous and Mental Disease 172: 150–155

Coryell W, Turner R 1985 Outcome of desipramine therapy in subtypes of non-psychotic major depression. Journal of Affective Disorders 9: 149–154

Costa D, Mogos I, Toma T 1985 Efficacy and safety of mianserin in the treatment of depression of women with cancer. Acta Psychiatrica Scandinavica 72 (suppl 320): 85–92

Crapo L 1979 Cushing's syndrome. Metabolism 28: 955–977

Davie J W, Blumenthal M D, Robinson-Hawkins S 1981 A model of risk of falling for psychogeriatric patients. Archives of General Psychiatry 38: 463–467

Derogatis L R, Feldstein M, Morrow G, Schmale A H, Schmitt M, Gates C, Murawski B, Holland J, Penman D, Melisaratos N, Enelow A J, McKinney-Adler L 1979 A survey of psychotropic drugs prescriptions in an oncology population. Cancer 44: 1919–1929

Derogatis L R, Morrow G R, Fetting J, Penman D, Piasetsky S, Schmale A H, Henrichs M, Carnicke C L M 1983 The prevalence of psychiatric disorders among cancer patients. Journal of the American Medical Association 249: 751–757

Detre T P, Jarecki H J 1971 Modern psychiatric treatment. J.B. Lippincott, Philadelphia, PA

Dreyer E B, Kaiser P K, Offermann J T, Lipton S A 1990 HIV-1 coat protein neurotoxicity prevented by calcium channel antagonists. Science 248: 364–367

Edwards G J 1989 Drug-related depression. In: Herbst K R, Paykel E S (eds) Depression. Heinemann, Oxford, p 81–108

Eilenberg M D 1960 Psychiatric illness and pernicious anemia. Journal of Mental Science 106: 1539–1548

Endicott J 1984 Measurement of depression in patients with cancer. Cancer 53: 2243–2248

Engel G L 1959 Psychogenic pain and the pain-prone patient. American Journal of Medicine 26: 899–918

Engel G L 1970 Nervousness and fatigue. In: MacBryde C M, Blacklow R S (eds) Signs and symptoms. J.B. Lippincott, Philadelphia, PA, p 632–649

Enzell K 1984 Mortality among persons with depressive symptoms and among responders and non-responders in a health check-up. Acta Psychiatrica Scandinavica 69: 89–102

Evans N J R, Whitlock F A 1983 Mortality and late-onset affective disorders. Journal of Affective Disorders 5: 297–304

Evans D L, McCartney C F, Haggerty J J, Nemeroff C B, Golden R N, Simon J B, Quade D, Holmes V, Droba M, Mason G A, Fowler W C, Raft D 1988 Treatment of depression in cancer patients is associated with better life adaptation. Psychosomatic Medicine 50: 72–76

Fava G A, Magnani B 1988 Quality of life. Medical Science Research 20: 1051–1054

Fava G A, Molnar G 1987 Criteria for diagnosing depression in the setting of medical disease. Psychotherapy and Psychosomatics 48: 21–25

Fava G A, Sonino N 1986 Hypothalamic-pituitary-adrenal axis disturbances in depression. IRCS Medical Science 14: 1058–1061

Fava G A, Pilowsky I, Pierfederici A, Bernardi M, Pathak D 1982 Depressive symptoms and abnormal illness behaviour in general hospital patients. General Hospital Psychiatry 4: 171–178

Fava G A, Trombini G, Grandi S, Bernardi M, Evangelisti L P, Santarsiero G, Orlandi C 1984a Depression and anxiety in secondary amenorrhea. Psychosomatics 25: 905–908

Fava G A, Zielezny M, Pilowsky I, Trombini G 1984b Patterns of depression and illness behaviour in general hospital patients. Psychopathology 17: 105–109

Fava G A, Lisanski J, Kellner R, Zielezny M 1985a Treatment responses in primary and secondary melancholia. Journal of Clinical Psychiatry 46: 332–334

Fava G A, Trombini G, Barbara L, Bernardi M, Grandi S, Callegari C, Miglioli M 1985b Depression and gastrointestinal illness. American Journal of Gastroenterology 80: 195–199

Fava G A, Sonino N, Morphy M A 1987 Major depression associated with endocrine disease. Psychiatric Developments 4: 321–348

Fava G A, Sonino N, Wise T N 1988 Management of depression in medical patients. Psychotherapy and Psychosomatics 49: 81–102

Feinberg M, Carroll B J, Steiner M, Commorato A J 1979 Misdiagnoses of endogenous depression with research diagnostic criteria. Lancet 1: 267

Feldman E, Mayou R, Hawton K, Ardern M, Smith E O B 1987 Psychiatric disorder in medical in-patients. Quarterly Journal of Medicine 63: 405–412

Fernandez F, Adams F, Holmes V F, Levy J K, Neidhart M 1987 Methylphenidate for depressive disorders in cancer patients. Psychosomatics 28: 455–461

Fisch R Z 1986 Methylphenidate for medical in-patients. International Journal of Psychiatry in Medicine 15: 75–79

Folstein S E, Abbott M H, Chase G A, Jensen B A, Folstein M F 1983 The association of affective disorder with Huntington's disease in a case series and in families. Psychological Medicine 13: 537–542

Ford M F 1986 Treatment of depression in Huntington's disease with monoamine oxidase inhibitors. British Journal of Psychiatry 149: 654–656

Foster F G Kupfer D G, Coble P A, McPartland R J 1976 REM density sleep: an objective indicator in severe medical-depressive syndromes. Archives of General Psychiatry 33: 1119–1123

Frank R G, Beck N C, Parker J C, Kashaini J H, Elliott T R, Hant A E, Smith E, Atwood C, Brownlee-Duffeck M, Kay D R 1988 Depression in rheumatoid arthritis. Journal of Rheumatology 15: 920–925

Garvey M J, Mungas D, Tollefson G D 1984 Hypersomnia in major depressive disorders. Journal of Affective Disorders 6: 283–286

Grandi S, Fava G A, Cunsolo A, Ranieri M, Gozzetti G, Trombini G 1987 Major depression associated with mastectomy. Medical Science Research 15: 283–284

Haggerty J J, Drossman D A 1985 Use of psychotropic drugs in patients with peptic ulcer. Psychosomatics 26: 277–284

Hardman A, Maguire P, Crowther D 1989 The recognition of psychiatric morbidity on a medical oncology ward. Journal of Psychosomatic Research 33: 235–239

Hawley D J, Wolfe F 1988 Anxiety and depression in patients with rheumatoid arthritis. Journal of Rheumatology 15: 932–941

Hawton K 1981 The long-term outcome of psychiatric morbidity detected in general medical patients. Journal of Psychosomatic Research 25: 237–243

Hendler N 1984 Depression caused by chronic pain. Journal of Clinical Psychiatry 45: 30–36

Hengeveld M W, Ancion F A J M, Rooijmans H G M 1987 Prevalence and recognition of depressive disorders in general medical inpatients. International Journal of Psychiatry in Medicine 17: 341–349

Hinrichsen G A, Lieberman J A, Pollack S, Steinbeg H 1989 Depression in hemodialysis patients. Psychosomatics 30: 284–289

Holland J C, Korzym A H, Tross S, Silberfarb P, Perry M, Cormis R, Oster M 1986 Comparative psychological disturbance in patients with pancreatic and gastric cancer. American Journal of Psychiatry 143: 982–986

Hollister L E 1978a Tricyclic antidepressants. New England Journal of Medicine 299: 1106–1109

Hollister L E 1978b Tricyclic antidepressants. New England Journal of Medicine 299: 1168–1172

Hughes J E 1985 Depressive illness and lung cancer. European Journal of Surgical Oncology 11: 15–20

Jefferson J W 1989 Cardiovascular effects and toxicity of anxiolytics and antidepressants. Journal of Clinical Psychiatry 50: 368–378

Johns M W, Egan P, Gay T J A, Masterton J P 1970 Sleep habits and symptoms in male medical and surgical patients. British Medical Journal 2: 509–512

Jouvent R, Abensour P, Bonnet A M, Widlocher D, Agid Y, Lhermitte F 1983 Antiparkinsonian and antidepressant effects of high doses of bromocriptine. Journal of Affective Disorders 5: 141–145

Karanci N A 1988 Patterns of depression in medical patients and their relationship with causal attributions for illness. Psychotherapy and Psychosomatics 50: 207–215

Katon W, Roy-Byrne P 1988 Antidepressants in the medically ill. Clinical Chemistry 34: 829–836

Kaufman M A, Murray G B, Cassem N H 1982 Use of psychostimulants in medically ill depressed patients. Psychosomatics 23: 817–819

Kellner R 1975 Psychotherapy in psychosomatic disorders. Archives of General Psychiatry 32: 1021–1028

Kellner R 1990 Somatization. Journal of Nervous and Mental Disease 178: 150–160

Kellner R, Fava G A, Lisansky J, Perini G I, Zielezny M 1986 Hypochondriacal fears and beliefs in DSM-III melancholia. Journal of Affective Disorders 10: 21–26

Kerr T A, Schapira K, Roth M 1969 The relationship between premature death and affective disorders. British Journal of Psychiatry 115: 1277–1282

King D, Akiskal H S, Lemmi H, Wilson W, Belluomini J,

Yerevanian B I 1981 REM density in the differential diagnosis of psychiatric from medical-neurologic disorders. Psychiatry Research 5: 267–276

Koenig H G, Breitner J C S 1990 Use of antidepressants in medically ill older patients. Psychosomatics 31: 22–32

Koenig H G, Meador K G, Cohen H J, Blazer D G 1988 Depression in elderly hospitalized patients with medical illness. Archives of Internal Medicine 148: 1929–1936

Koenig H G, Shelp F, Goli V, Cohen H J, Blazer D G 1989 Survival and health care utilization in elderly medical inpatients with major depression. Journal of the American Geriatrics Society 37: 599–606

Kosanin R 1981 Anesthetic considerations in patients on chronic tricyclic antidepressant therapy. Anesthesiology Reviews 8: 38–41

Lakshmanan M, Mion L C, Frenglej J D 1986 Effective low-dose tricyclic antidepressant treatment for depressed geriatric rehabilitation patients. Journal of the American Geriatrics Society 34: 421–426

Lansky S B, List M A, Herrmann C A, Ets-Hokin E G, Das Gupta T K, Wilbanks G D, Hendrickson F R 1985 Absence of major depressive disorder in female cancer patients. Journal of Clinical Oncology 3: 1533–1540

Larcombe N A, Wilson P H 1984 An evaluation of cognitive behaviour therapy for depression in patients with multiple sclerosis. British Journal of Psychiatry 145: 366–371

Lasagna L 1978 Some adverse interactions with other drugs. In: Lipton M A, Di Mascio A, Killam K F (eds) Psychopharmacology. Raven Press, New York, p 1005–1008

Lesse S 1983 The masked depression syndrome. American Journal of Psychotherapy 37: 456–475

Levy N B 1985 Use of psychotropics in patients with kidney failure. Psychosomatics 26: 699–709

Lieberman J A, Cooper T B, Suckow R F, Steinberg H, Borenstein M, Brenner R, Kane J M 1985 Tricyclic antidepressant and metabolite levels in chronic renal failure. Clinical Pharmacology and Therapeutics 37: 301–307

Lipinski J F, Mallya G, Simmerman P, Pope H G 1989 Fluoxetine-induced akathisia. Journal of Clinical Psychiatry 50: 339–343

Lipowski Z J 1974 Physical illness and psychopathology. International Journal of Psychiatry in Medicine 5: 483–497

Lipowski Z J 1975 Physical illness, the patient and his environment. In: Reiser M (ed) American handbook of psychiatry, vol 4. Basic Books, New York, p 3–42

Lipowski Z J 1985 Psychosomatic medicine and liaison psychiatry. Plenum Press, New York, p 211–225

Lipowski Z J 1990 Somatization and depression. Psychosomatics 31: 13–21

Lipsey J R, Robinson R G, Pearlson G D, Rao K, Price T R 1984 Nortriptyline treatment of post-stroke depression. Lancet 1: 297–300

Lipsey J R, Robinson R G, Pearlson G D, Rao K, Price T R 1985 The dexamethasone suppression test and mood following stroke. American Journal of Psychiatry 142: 318–323

Lishman W A 1987 Organic psychiatry. Blackwell, Oxford

Lloyd G G, Cawley R H 1978 Psychiatric morbidity in men one week after first acute myocardial infarction. British Medical Journal 2: 1453–1454

Lustman P J, Griffith L S, Clouse R E 1988 Depression in adults with diabetes. Diabetes Care 11: 605–612

Magruder-Habib K, Zung W W K, Fenssner J R 1990 Improving physicians' recognition and treatment of depression in general medical care. Medical Care 28: 239–250

Manu P, Matthews D A, Lane T J, Tennen H, Hesselbrock V, Mendola R, Affleck G 1989 Depression among patients with a chief complaint of chronic fatigue. Journal of Affective Disorders 17: 165–172

Massie M J, Holland J C 1984 Diagnosis and treatment of depression in the cancer patient. Journal of Clinical Psychiatry 45: 25–28

Mayou R 1990 Quality of life in cardiovascular disease. Psychotherapy and Psychosomatics 54: 99–109

Mayou R, Smith E O B 1986 Hospital doctors' management of psychological problems. British Journal of Psychiatry 148: 194–197

Mayou R, Hawton K, Feldman E 1988 What happens to medical patients with psychiatric disorder? Journal of Psychosomatic Research 32: 541–549

Moffic H S, Paykel E S 1975 Depression in medical inpatients. British Journal of Psychiatry 126: 346–353

Molnar G, Gupta R N 1980 Plasma levels and tricyclic antidepressant therapy. Part 2. Biopharmaceutics and Drug Disposition 1: 283–305

Morgan M H, Read A E 1972 Antidepressants and liver disease. Gut 13: 697–701

Murphy E, Brown G W 1980 Life events, psychiatric disturbance and physical illness. British Journal of Psychiatry 136: 326–338

Murphy J M, Monson R R, Olivier D C, Sobol A M, Leighton A H 1987 Affective disorders and mortality. Archives of General Psychiatry 44: 473–480

Murray G B, Shea V, Conn D K 1987 Electroconvulsive therapy for post-stroke depression. Journal of Clinical Psychiatry 47: 258–260

Muskin P R, Glassman A H 1983 The use of tricyclic antidepressants in a medical setting. In: Finkel J B (ed) Consultation-liaison psychiatry. Grune & Stratton, New York, p 137–158

Nelson J C, Charney D S, Quinlan D M 1981 Evaluation of the DSM-III criteria for melancholia. Archives of General Psychiatry 38: 555–559

Newman S P, Fitzpatrick R, Lamb R, Shipley M 1989 The origins of depressed mood in rheumatoid arthritis. Journal of Rheumatology 16: 740–744

Noyes R, Kathol R G 1986 Depression and cancer. Psychiatric Developments 2: 77–100

Paykel E S 1979 Management of acute depression. In: Paykel E S, Coppen A (eds) Psychopharmacology of affective disorders. Oxford University Press, Oxford, p 235–247

Paykel E S, Norton K R W 1982 Diagnoses not to be missed. Masked depression. British Journal of Hospital Medicine 28: 151–157

Paykel E S, Fleminger R, Watson J P 1982 Psychiatric side effects of antihypertensive drugs other than reserpine. Journal of Clinical Psychopharmacology 2: 14–39

Paykel E S, Hollyman J A, Freeling P, Sedgwick P 1988 Predictors of therapeutic benefit from amitriptyline in mild depression. Journal of Affective Disorders 14: 83–95

Perry S W 1990 Organic mental disorders caused by HIV. American Journal of Psychiatry 147: 696–710

Piafsky K M, Borga O 1977 Plasma protein binding of basic drugs. Clinical Pharmacology and Therapeutics 22: 545–549

Pilowsky I 1978 Psychodynamic aspects of the pain experience. In: Sternbach R A (ed) The psychology of pain. Raven Press, New York, p 203–217

Pilowsky I 1986 Abnormal illness behaviour. Psychotherapy and Psychosomatics 46: 76–84

Pilowsky I, Bassett D L 1982 Pain and depression. British Journal of Psychiatry 141: 30–36

Pilowsky I, Spence N, Cobb J, Katsikitis M 1984 The Illness Behaviour Questionnaire as an aid to clinical assessment. General Hospital Psychiatry 6: 123–130

Pollack M H, Rosenbaum J F, Cassem N H 1984 Propranolol and depression revisited. Journal of Nervous and Mental Disease 173: 118–119

Pollitt J H 1972 The relationship between genetic and precipitating factors in depressive illness. British Journal of Psychiatry 121: 67–70

Popkin M K, Callies A L, MacKenzie T B 1985 The outcome of antidepressant use in the medically ill. Archives of General Psychiatry 42: 1160–1163

Popkin M K, Tucker G, Caine E, Folstein M, Grant I 1989 The fate of organic mental disorders in DSM-IV. Psychosomatics 30: 439–441

Rabej J M, Avrahami E 1985 Unmasking of cerebellar tumors by amitriptyline in depressive patients. Journal of Neurology Neurosurgery and Psychiatry 48: 291

Rabins P V, Harvis K, Koven S 1985 High fatality rates of late-life depression associated with cardiovascular disease. Journal of Affective Disorders 9: 165–167

Rapp S R, Vrana S 1989 Substituting non-somatic for somatic symptoms in the diagnosis of depression in elderly male medical patients. American Journal of Psychiatry 146: 1197–1200

Raskind M, Veith R, Barnes R, Germbrecht G 1982 Cardiovascular and antidepressant effects of imipramine in the treatment of secondary depression in patients with ischemic heart disease. American Journal of Psychiatry 139: 1114–1117

Reding M J, Orto L A, Winter S W, Fortuna I M, Di Ponte P, McDowell F H 1986 Antidepressant therapy after stroke. Archives of Neurology 43: 763–765

Reifler B V, Teri L, Raskind M, Veith R, Barnes R, White E, McLean P 1989 Double-blind trial with imipramine in Alzheimer's disease patients with and without depression. American Journal of Psychiatry 146: 45–49

Rich C L, Spiker D G, Jewell S W, Neil J F 1984 DSM-III, RDC and ECT. Journal of Clinical Psychiatry 45: 14–18

Rifkin A, Reardon G, Siris S, Karagji B, Kim Y S, Hackstaff L, Endicott N 1985 Trimipramine in physical illness with depression. Journal of Clinical Psychiatry 46: 4–8

Rihmer Z, Szadoczky Z, Arato M 1983 Dexamethasone suppression test in masked depression. Journal of Affective Disorders 5: 293–296

Risch S C, Groom G P, Janowsky D S 1982 The effects of psychotropic drugs on the cardiovascular system. Journal of Clinical Psychiatry 43: 16–31

Robertson M M, Trimble M R, 1985 The treatment of depression in patients with epilepsy. Journal of Affective Disorders 9: 127–136

Robertson M M, Trimble M R, Townsend H R A 1987 Phenomenology of depression in epilepsy. Epilepsia 28: 364–372

Robins E, Guze S B 1972 Classification of affective disorders. In: Williams T A, Katz M M, Shield J A (eds) Recent advances in the psychobiology of the depressive illness. US Government Printing Office, Washington, DC

Robinson J K, Boshier M L, Dansak D A, Peterson K J 1985 Depression and anxiety in cancer patients. Journal of Psychosomatic Research 29: 133–138

Rodin G 1990 Quality of life in adults with insulin dependent diabetes mellitus. Psychotherapy and Psychosomatics 54: 132–139

Rodin G, Voshart K 1986 Depression in the medically ill. American Journal of Psychiatry 143: 696–705

Rodin G, Voshart K 1987 Depressive symptoms and functional impairment in the medically ill. General Hospital Psychiatry 9: 251–258

Romano J M, Turner J A 1985 Chronic pain and depression. Psychological Bulletin 97: 18–34

Rosenberg S J, Peterson R A, Hayes J R, Hatcher J, Headen S 1988 Depression in medical inpatients. British Journal of Medical Psychology 61: 245–254

Roth M 1977 The association of affective disorders and physical somatic disease and its bearing on certain problems of psychosomatic medicine. In: Antonelli F (ed) Therapy in psychosomatic medicine. Pozzi, Roma, p 189–197

Roth M, Kay D W K 1956 Affective disorder arising in the senium. Journal of Mental Science 102: 141–150

Rubinstein G, McIntyre I, Burrows G D, Norman T R, Maguire K P 1983 Metabolism of tricyclic antidepressant drugs. In: Burrows G D, Norman T R, Davies B (eds) Antidepressants. Elsevier, New York, p 57–74

Rudorfer M V, Potter W Z 1989 Antidepressants. Drugs 37: 713–738

Sacks C R, Peterson R A, Kimmel P L 1990 Perception of illness and depression in chronic renal disease. American Journal of Kidney Diseases 15: 31–39

Saran A S 1985 Depression after minor closed head injury. Journal of Clinical Psychiatry 46: 335–338

Schiffer R B, Herndon R M, Rudick R A 1985 Treatment of pathological laughing and weeping with amitriptyline. New England Journal of Medicine 312: 1480–1482

Schleifer S J, Macari-Hinson M M, Coyle D A, Slater W R, Kahn M, Gorlin R, Zucker H D 1989 The nature and course of depression following myocardial infarction. Archives of Internal Medicine 149: 1785–1789

Schmale A H 1979 Reactions to illness. Psychiatric Clinics of North America 2: 321–330

Schulberg H C, McClelland M, Gooding W 1987 Six-month outcomes for medical patients with major depressive disorders. Journal of General Internal Medicine 2: 312–317

Schwartz J A, Speed M, Beresford T P 1989 Antidepressants in the medically ill. International Journal of Psychiatry in Medicine 19: 363–369

Silberfarb P M, Oxman T E 1988 The effects of cancer therapies on the central nervous system. Advances in Psychosomatic Medicine 18: 13–25

Silver P A, Simpson G M 1988 Antipsychotic use in the medically ill. Psychotherapy and Psychosomatics 49: 120–136

Siris S G, Rifkin A 1981 The problem of psychopharmacotherapy in the medically ill patients. Psychiatric Clinics of North America 4: 379–390

Slotkin T A, Whitmore W L, Barnes G A, Krishnan K R R, Blazer D G, Knight D L, Nemeroff C B 1989 Reduced inhibitory effect of imipramine on radiolabeled serotonin uptake into platelets in geriatric depression. Biological Psychiatry 25: 687–691

Smith M D, Hong B A, Robson A M 1985 Diagnosis of depression in patients with end-stage renal disease. American Journal of Medicine 79: 160–166

Sonino N, Fava G A, Fallo F, Boscaro M 1990 Psychological distress and quality of life in endocrine disease. Psychotherapy and Psychosomatics 54: 140–144

Starkstein S E, Robinson R G 1989 Affective disorders and cerebral vascular disease. British Journal of Psychiatry 154: 170–182

Starkstein S E, Berthier M L, Bolduc P L, Preziosi T J, Robinson R G 1989 Depression in patients with early versus late onset of Parkinson's disease. Neurology 39: 1441–1445

Starkstein S E, Cohen B S, Fedoroff P, Parikh R M, Price T R, Robinson R G 1990 Relationship between anxiety disorders and depressive disorders in patients with cerebrovascular injury. Archives of General Psychiatry 47: 246–251

Steinmuller RI 1978 Psychotherapeutic treatment planning in the medically ill. In: Karasu T B, Steinmuller, R I (eds) Psychotherapeutics in medicine. Grune & Stratton, New York, p 35–62

Stewart A L, Greenfield S, Hays R D, Wells K, Rogers W H, Berry S D, McGlynn E A, Ware J E 1989 Functional status and well-being of patients with chronic conditions. Journal of the American Medical Association 262: 907–913

Thompson D R 1989 A randomized controlled trial of in-hospital nursing support for first time myocardial infarction patients and their partners. Journal of Advanced Nursing 14: 291–297

Thompson W L, Thompson T L 1984 Treating depression in asthmatic patients. Psychosomatics 25: 809–812

True B L, Perry B J, Burns E A 1987 Profound hypoglycemia with addition of tricyclic antidepressants to maintenance sulfonylurea therapy. American Journal of Psychiatry 144: 1220–1221

Tucker G J, Price T R P 1987 Depression and neurologic disease. In: Cameron O G (ed) Presentations of depression. John Wiley, New York, p 237–250

Tyber M A 1975 The relationship between hiatus hernia and tricyclic antidepressants. American Journal of Psychiatry 132: 652–653

Van der Kolk B, Shader R I, Greenblatt D J 1978 Autonomic side effects of psychotropic drugs. In: Lipton M A, Di Mascio A, Killam K F (eds) Psychopharmacology. Raven Press, New York, p 1009–1020

Walsh T D 1983 Antidepressants in chronic pain. Clinical Neuropharmacology 6: 271–295

Wells K B, Stewart A, Hays R D, Burnam A, Rogers W, Daniels M, Berry S, Greenfield S, Ware J 1989 The functioning and well-being of depressed patients. Journal of the American Medical Association 262: 914–919

Wheatley D 1988 The use of anti-anxiety drugs in the medically ill. Psychotherapy and Psychosomatics 49: 63–80

Whitlock F A 1982 Symptomatic affective disorders. Academic Press, Sydney

Whitlock F A 1986 The psychiatric complications of Parkinson's disease. Australia and New Zealand Journal of Psychiatry 26: 114–121

Wilkinson G R, Shand D G 1975 A physiological approach to hepatic drug clearance. Clinical Pharmacology and Therapeutics 18: 377–390

Wilson W H, Jefferson J W 1985 Thyroid disease, behaviour, and psychopharmacology. Psychosomatics 26: 481–492

Wise T N, Rosenthal J B 1982 Depression, illness beliefs and severity of illness. Journal of Psychosomatic Research 26: 247–253

Woods S W, Tesar G E, Murray G B, Cassem N H 1986 Psychostimulant treatment of depressive disorders secondary to medical illness. Journal of Clinical Psychiatry 47: 12–15

Zelnik T 1987 Depressive effects of drugs. In: Cameron OG (ed) Presentations of depression. John Wiley, New York, p 355–399

Zonderman A B, Costa P T, McCrae R R 1989 Depression as a risk for cancer morbidity and mortality in a nationally representative sample. Journal of the American Medical Association 262: 1191–1195

Index